PRIMER ON
KIDNEY DISEASES

PRIMER ON KIDNEY DISEASES
Third Edition

EDITOR

ARTHUR GREENBERG

Division of Nephrology
Department of Medicine
Duke University
Durham, North Carolina

ASSOCIATE EDITORS

Alfred K. Cheung
Division of Nephrology and Hypertension
School of Medicine and
Veterans Affairs Salt Lake City Healthcare System
University of Utah
Salt Lake City, Utah

Thomas M. Coffman
Division of Nephrology
Department of Medicine
Duke University Medical Center
Durham, North Carolina

Ronald J. Falk
Division of Nephrology
Department of Medicine
University of North Carolina
Chapel Hill, North Carolina

J. Charles Jennette
Department of Pathology and Laboratory Medicine
University of North Carolina
Chapel Hill, North Carolina

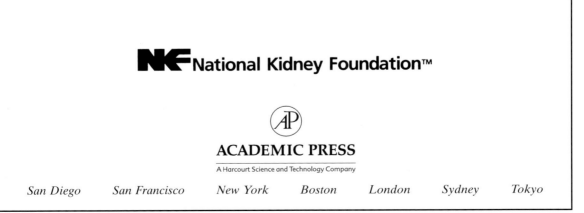

NKF National Kidney Foundation™

ACADEMIC PRESS
A Harcourt Science and Technology Company

San Diego   San Francisco   New York   Boston   London   Sydney   Tokyo

The opinions expressed and approaches recommended are those of the authors and not those of the National Kidney Foundation or Academic Press. Great care has been taken by the authors and editors to maintain the accuracy of the information contained herein. However, neither Academic Press not the National Kidney Foundation nor the editors and authors can be held responsible for errors or for any consequences arising from the use of this information.

This book is printed on acid-free paper. ∞

Academic Press
An imprint of Elsevier Science
525 B Street, Suite 1900, San Diego, California 92101-4495, USA
http://www.academicpress.com

Academic Press
84 Theobalds Road, London WC1X 8RR, UK
http://www.academicpress.com

Library of Congress Catalog Card Number: 00-111101

International Standard Book Number: 0-12-299100-1

PRINTED IN CHINA
02   03   04   05   06   07   CTPS   9   8   7   6   5   4   3   2

CONTENTS

SECTION 9
THE KIDNEY IN SPECIAL CIRCUMSTANCES

SECTION 10
CHRONIC RENAL FAILURE AND ITS THERAPY

SECTION 11
HYPERTENSION

CONTRIBUTORS

Numbers in parentheses indicate the pages on which the authors' contributions begin.

Mahendra Agraharkar, MD (239), Division of Nephrology, Department of Medicine, University of Texas Medical Branch, Galveston, Texas 77555

Michael Allon, MD (98), Division of Nephrology, University of Alabama at Birmingham, Birmingham, Alabama 35233

Gerald B. Appel, MD (154), Division of Nephrology, Columbia-Presbyterian Medical Center, New York, New York 10032

Richard G. Appel, MD (283), Wake Forest University School of Medicine, Winston-Salem, North Carolina 27157

Billy S. Arant, Jr., MD (345), Department of Pediatrics, University of Tennessee College of Medicine—Chattanooga Unit, Chattanooga, Tennessee 37403

Vicente Arroyo, MD (184), Department of Medicine, University of Barcelona Medical School, and Institute of Digestive Diseases, Hospital Clinic, 08036 Barcelona, Spain

Phyllis August, MD (368), Hypertension Center, Weill Medical College of Cornell University, New York, New York 10021

Ellis D. Avner, MD (313), Department of Pediatrics, Case Western Reserve University, Rainbow Babies and Children's Hospital, Cleveland, Ohio 44106

Daniel C. Batlle, MD (71), Division of Nephrology/Hypertension, Department of Medicine, Northwestern University Medical School, Chicago, Illinois 60611

William M. Bennett, MD (290), Department of Solid Organ and Cellular Transplantation, Legacy/Good Samaritan Hospital, Portland, Oregon 97210

Wendy E. Bloembergen, MD (414), Division of Nephrology, Department of Medicine, University of Michigan, Ann Arbor, Michigan 48103

Gregory L. Braden, MD (322), Renal Division, Baystate Medical Center, Springfield, Massachusetts 01199; and Department of Medicine, Tufts University School of Medicine, Boston, Massachusetts 02111

Josephine P. Briggs, MD (3), NIDDK, National Institutes of Health, Bethesda, Maryland 20892

Vardaman M. Buckalew, Jr., MD (283), Section of Nephrology, Department of Medicine, Bowman Gray School of Medicine, Winston-Salem, North Carolina 27157

David A. Bushinsky, MD (107), Department of Medicine and Department of Pharmacology and Physiology, Nephrology Unit, Strong Memorial Hospital, University of Rochester Medical Center, Rochester, New York 14642

Maria Luiza Caramori, MD (212), Department of Pediatrics, University of Minnesota, Minneapolis, Minnesota 55455

Daniel C. Cattran, MD (158), The Toronto Hospital, Toronto, Ontario, Canada M5G 1L7

Dinesh K. Chatoth, MD (264), Division of Nephrology, University of Arkansas for Medical Sciences, and Central Arkansas Veterans Healthcare System, Little Rock, Arkansas 72205

Alfred K. Cheung, MD (396), Division of Nephrology and Hypertension, University of Utah School of Medicine, and Veterans Affairs Salt Lake City Healthcare System, Salt Lake City, Utah 84112

Thomas M. Coffman, MD (251), Division of Nephrology, Department of Medicine, Duke University Medical Center, Durham, North Carolina 27710

Giuseppe D'Amico, MD, FRCP (147), Professor Emeritus of Nephrology, San Carlo Hospital, 20153 Milan, Italy

James A. Delmez, MD (426), Renal Division, Chromalloy American Kidney Center, Washington University School of Medicine, St. Louis, Missouri 63110

Garabed Eknoyan, MD (333), Department of Medicine, Baylor College of Medicine, Houston, Texas 77030

David H. Ellison, MD (116), Division of Nephrology, Oregon Health Sciences University, Portland, Oregon 97201

Jonathan T. Fairbank, MD, FACR (46), Division of Nuclear Medicine, Department of Radiology, Fletcher Allen Health Care and Department of Radiology, University of Vermont College of Medicine, Burlington, Vermont 05401

Ronald J. Falk, MD (129, 196), Division of Nephrology, University of North Carolina, Chapel Hill, North Carolina 27599

Godela M. Fick-Brosnahan, MD (303), University of Colorado Health Sciences Center and Denver Health Medical Center, Denver, Colorado 80262

William F. Finn, MD (319), Division of Nephrology and Hypertension, University of North Carolina, Chapel Hill, North Carolina 27599

John M. Flack, MD, MPH (486), Cardiovascular Epidemiology and Clinical Application Program, Division of Endocrinology, Metabolism, and Hypertension, Department of Internal Medicine, University Health Center, Wayne State University, Detroit, Michigan 48201

Robert N. Foley, MD (434), Department of Renal Medicine, Hope Hospital, Salford Royal Hospitals NHS Trust, Salford M6 8WH, United Kingdom

Alessandro Fornasieri, MD (147), Department of Nephrology, San Carlo Hospital, 20153 Milan, Italy

Richard J. Glassock, MD, MACP (38), Professor Emeritus, UCLA School of Medicine, Los Angeles, California 90095

R. Gokal, MD (405), Department of Renal Medicine, Manchester Royal Infirmary, Manchester M13 9WL, United Kingdom

Martin Goldberg, MD (93), Temple University School of Medicine, Philadelphia, Pennsylvania 19140

R. Ariel Gomez, MD (363), Department of Pediatrics, University of Virginia, Charlottesville, Virginia 22908

Harvey C. Gonick, MD (325), Nephrology Training and Hypertension Research, Nephrology Division, Cedars-Sinai Medical Center, and Department of Medicine, University of California, Los Angeles, California 90048

Arthur Greenberg, MD (28, 261), Division of Nephrology, Department of Medicine, Duke University Medical Center, Durham, North Carolina 27710

Martin C. Gregory, BM. B. Ch., D. Phil. (308), Department of Medicine, University of Utah, Salt Lake City, Utah 84132

Antonio Guasch, MD (299), Renal Division, Department of Medicine, Emory University, Atlanta, Georgia 30322

C. Haller, MD (179), Division of Cardiology, Department of Internal Medicine, University of Heidelberg, D-69115 Heidelberg, Germany

Philip F. Halloran, MD, PhD (377), Division of Nephrology and Immunology, University of Alberta, Edmonton, Alberta, Canada T6G 2S2

Lee A. Hebert, MD (204), Division of Nephrology, The Ohio State University College of Medicine and Public Health, Columbus, Ohio 43210

Jonathan Himmelfarb, MD (438), Division of Nephrology and Renal Transplantation, Maine Medical Center, Portland, Maine 04102

Jean L. Holley, MD (245), Nephrology Unit, University of Rochester Medical Center, Rochester, New York 14642

Florence N. Hutchison, MD (275), Medical Specialty Service, Ralph H. Johnson VA Medical Center, Charleston, South Carolina 29401

T. Alp Ikizler, MD (420), Division of Nephrology, Vanderbilt University Medical Center, Nashville, Tennessee 37232

J. Charles Jennette, MD (129, 196), Department of Pathology and Laboratory Medicine, University of North Carolina, Chapel Hill, North Carolina 27599

Wladimiro Jiménez, PhD (184), Hormonal Laboratory, Hospital Clinic, 08036 Barcelona, Spain

Edward R. Jones, MD (81), Albert Einstein Medical Center, Philadelphia, Pennsylvania 19141

Bruce A. Julian, MD (165), Division of Nephrology, Department of Medicine, University of Alabama at Birmingham, Birmingham, Alabama 35294

Bertram L. Kasiske, MD (455), Division of Nephrology, Department of Medicine, University of Minnesota School of Medicine, Hennepin County Medical Center, Minneapolis, Minnesota 55415

William F. Keane, MD (25), Department of Medicine, Hennepin County Medical Center, Minneapolis, Minnesota 55415

Preston Klassen, MD (480), Department of Nephrology, Duke University Medical Center, Durham, North Carolina 27705

Paul E. Klotman, MD (230), Division of Nephrology, Mount Sinai Medical Center, New York, New York 10029

Stephen M. Korbet, MD, FACP (336), Section of Nephrology, Department of Medicine, Rush Presbyterian-St. Luke's Medical Center, Chicago, Illinois 60612

Eugene C. Kovalik, MD, FRCP, FACP (446), Division of Nephrology, Department of Medicine, Duke University Medical Center, Durham, North Carolina 27710

Wilhelm Kriz, MD (3) Institute for Anatomy and Cell Biology, University of Heidelberg, D-69115 Heidelberg, Germany

Nicolaos E. Madias, MD (87), Department of Medicine, Tufts University School of Medicine, and Division of Nephrology, New England Medical Center, Boston, Massachusetts 02111

Michael Mauer, MD (212), Department of Pediatrics, University of Minnesota School of Medicine, Minneapolis, Minnesota 55455

Catherine M. Meyers, MD (269), Office of Device Evaluation, Center for Devices and Radiological Health, United States Food and Drug Administration, Rockville, Maryland 20850

Alain Meyrier, MD (190), Service de Néphrologie and INSERM U430, Hopital Broussais-HEGP, 75014 Paris, France

Dawn S. Milliner, MD (327), Division of Nephrology, Mayo Clinic, Rochester, Minnesota 55905

Howard J. Mindell, MD, FACR (46), Division of Genitourinary Radiology, Fletcher Allen Health Care and Department of Radiology, University of Vermont College of Medicine, Burlington, Vermont 05401

Marianne Monahan, MD (230), Division of Nephrology, Mount Sinai Medical Center, New York, New York 10029

Carla G. Monico, MD (327), Division of Nephrology, Mayo Clinic, Rochester, Minnesota 55905

Joseph V. Nally, Jr., MD (475), Department of Nephrology and Hypertension, The Cleveland Clinic Foundation, Cleveland, Ohio 44195

Lindsay E. Nicolle, MD (354), Department of Internal Medicine, University of Manitoba, Winnipeg, Manitoba, Canada R3A 1R9

Douglas J. Norman, MD (460), Oregon Health Sciences University, Portland, Oregon 97201

Paul M. Palevsky, MD (64), Renal Section, VA Pittsburgh Healthcare System, and Department of Medicine, University of Pittsburgh School of Medicine, Pittsburgh, Pennsylvania 15240

Neesh Pannu, MD (377), Division of Nephrology and Immunology, University of Alberta, Edmonton, Alberta, Canada T6G 2S2

Patrick S. Parfrey, MD (434), Division of Nephrology, The Health Sciences Center, Saint John's, Newfoundland, Canada A1B 3V6

Roberto Pisoni, MD (385), Mario Negri Institute for Pharmacological Research, Negri Bergamo Laboratories, and Unit of Nephrology and Dialysis, Ospedali Riuniti di Bergamo, 24125 Bergamo, Italy

Charles D. Pusey, M.Sc., FRCP (172), Department of Renal Medicine, Imperial College School of Medicine, London W12 0NN, United Kingdom

Giuseppe Remuzzi, MD, FRCP (385), Mario Negri Institute for Pharmacological Research, Negri Bergamo Laboratories, and Unit of Nephrology and Dialysis, Ospedali Riuniti di Bergamo, 24125 Bergamo, Italy

E. Ritz, MD (179), Division of Nephrology, Department of Medicine, University of Heidelberg, D-69115 Heidelberg, Germany

Robert L. Safirstein, MD (239), John L. McClellan Memorial Veterans' Hospital, Little Rock, Arkansas 72205

Paul W. Sanders, MD (218), Division of Nephrology, University of Alabama at Birmingham, Birmingham, Alabama 35294

Steven J. Scheinman, MD (20) Nephrology Division, Department of Medicine, SUNY Upstate Medical University, Syracuse, New York 13210

Jurgen B. Schnermann, MD (3) NIDDK, National Institutes of Health, Bethesda, Maryland 20892

Sudhir V. Shah, MD (264), Division of Nephrology, University of Arkansas for Medical Sciences, and Central Arkansas Veterans Healthcare System, Little Rock, Arkansas 72205

Norman J. Siegel, MD (143), Department of Pediatrics, Yale University School of Medicine, and Yale–New Haven Children's Hospital, New Haven, Connecticut 06510

Richard L. Siegler, MD (225), Division of Pediatric Nephrology, University of Utah School of Medicine, Salt Lake City, Utah 84132

F. Bruder Stapleton, MD (258), Department of Pediatrics, University of Washington, Seattle, Washington 98105

Laura P. Svetkey, MD (480), Department of Medicine, Duke University Medical Center, and Duke Hypertension Center, Durham, North Carolina 27705

Suzanne K. Swan, MD, FACP (25), Division of Nephrology, Department of Medicine, Hennepin County Medical Center, Minneapolis, Minnesota 55415

Anthony Valeri, MD (154), Division of Nephrology, Columbia-Presbyterian Medical Center, New York, New York 10032

Joseph G. Verbalis, MD (57), Division of Endocrinology and Metabolism, Georgetown University, Washington, DC 20007

Alan G. Wasserstein, MD (348), Renal Division, Hospital of the University of Pennsylvania, Philadelphia, Pennsylvania 19104

Christopher S. Wilcox, MD, PhD (471), Division of Nephrology and Hypertension, Georgetown University Medical Center, Washington, DC 20007

Julian R. Wright, MD (434), Department of Renal Medicine, Hope Hospital, Salford Royal Hospitals NHS Trust, Salford M6 8WH, United Kingdom

FOREWORD

I am pleased to introduce the third edition of the National Kidney Foundation's *Primer on Kidney Diseases*. By all accounts, the *Primer* appears to serve a very useful role. It is designed to provide a succinct yet comprehensive text for practicing physicians, house staff, and students. It is fair to say that consulting nephrologists as well may obtain pearls of wisdom from its pages. House staff and students have enthusiastically embraced the *Primer* as an efficient and relatively easy way to understand many of the complex issues of nephrology, including acid base and fluid disorders and hypertension.

The book continues to maintain its freshness, in part because more than one-third of the chapters are written by new authors. In keeping with the global nature of nephrology advances and expertise, many of the authors are from outside the United States. Many people have worked assiduously to develop this *Primer*. It is clear, however, that Arthur Greenberg, the editor, has contributed the vision and guiding spirit for this book. It is he more than any other individual who is responsible for the comprehensiveness, accuracy, and usefulness of this text. Dr. Greenberg has utilized a rigorous review process wherein each chapter was read by himself, an associate or consulting editor, and a member of the National Kidney Foundation Scientific Advisory Board. The support received from Kerry Willis, Director of Medical Activities of the National Kidney Foundation, as well as the publishers has been invaluable. Finally, the important contribution of the health care industry should be acknowledged. The fact that several corporations have purchased large numbers of the *Primer* for distribution to house staff and students has played no small role in making the *Primer* readily available and increasing its impact on the nephrological skills of future medical practitioners and the medical care of patients everywhere with kidney disease.

Joel D. Kopple

PREFACE

The intent of this third edition of the *Primer* is again to be a comprehensive but accessible source of information on the pathophysiology and treatment of kidney diseases and electrolyte disorders. Each chapter has been written by a nationally or internationally recognized expert in the field who was charged with presenting the essential elements of the topic in a clear and succinct form. Like any rapidly evolving field, the treatment of renal disease is not without controversy. Each author was asked to critically review new developments and put them in perspective for the general audience of students, house staff, and practicing physicians that comprise our anticipated readership.

A number of changes from the previous edition warrant emphasis. As was the case with the last edition, more than a third of the chapters are by new authors. This is not an adverse reflection on the previous contributors, but a deliberate attempt to keep the *Primer* fresh. In a number of cases, several chapters were consolidated into one to streamline the approach to the topic covered. For instance, in one chapter a discussion of the mechanism of progression of renal diseases and the pathogenesis of uremic symptoms now introduces a very practical management strategy for slowing the progression of renal failure and easing the transition to renal replacement therapy. Since the last edition of the *Primer*, the molecular defects responsible for a number of electrolyte disorders have been elucidated. These highly instructive experiments of nature are now outlined in a separate chapter. Coverage of many other areas has been expanded commensurate with the increase in knowledge about pathogenesis or treatment. Nonetheless, the present volume is shorter than the last and contains seven fewer chapters. Many excellent encyclopedic texts are available, but the essence of a primer is brevity.

As an official publication of the National Kidney Foundation, the *Primer* again relied upon peer review to ensure balance and accuracy. Each chapter was read by the editor, a section editor, and a member of the Foundation's Scientific Advisory Board serving as a consulting editor. Our comments were transmitted to the authors, who revised their contributions accordingly. Invariably, these busy experts graciously accepted our suggestions for revision. I also acknowledge the key role of the new consulting editors, Sharon Adler, William F. Keane, and Joel D. Kopple, as well as Shaul G. Massry and William E. Mitch, who reprised their previous roles. Yet again, I am indebted to Alfred Cheung, Tom Coffman, Ron Falk, and Charles Jennette for their insights, extraordinary effort, and devotion to this project.

Arthur Greenberg

SECTION I

STRUCTURE AND FUNCTION OF THE KIDNEY AND THEIR CLINICAL ASSESSMENT

OVERVIEW OF RENAL FUNCTION
AND STRUCTURE

JOSEPHINE P. BRIGGS, WILHELM KRIZ, AND JURGEN B. SCHNERMANN

BASIC CONCEPTS

Functions of the Kidney

The main functions of the kidneys can be categorized as follows:

1. Maintenance of body composition. The volume of fluid in the body, its osmolarity, electrolyte content, and concentration, and its acidity are all regulated by the kidney by variation in urine excretion of water and ions. Electrolytes regulated by changes in urinary excretion include sodium, potassium, chloride, calcium, magnesium, and phosphate.
2. Excretion of metabolic end products and foreign substances. The kidney excretes a number of products of metabolism, most notably urea, and a number of toxins and drugs.
3. Production and secretion of enzymes and hormones.
    a. Renin is an enzyme produced by the granular cells of the juxtaglomerular apparatus and catalyzes the formation of angiotensin from a plasma globulin, angiotensinogen. Angiotensin is a potent vasoconstrictor peptide and contributes importantly to salt balance and blood pressure regulation.
    b. Erythropoietin, a glycosylated, 165-amino acid protein produced by renal cortical interstitial cells, stimulates the maturation of erythrocytes in the bone marrow.
    c. 1,25-Dihydroxyvitamin D_3, the most active form of vitamin D_3, is formed by proximal tubule cells. This steroid hormone plays an important role in the regulation of body calcium and phosphate balance.

In later chapters of this primer, the pathophysiological mechanisms and consequences of derangements in kidney function are discussed in detail. This chapter reviews the basic anatomy of the kidney and the normal mechanisms for urine formation—glomerular filtration and tubular transport.

The Kidney and Homeostasis

Numerous functions of the body proceed optimally only when body fluid composition and volume are maintained within an appropriate range. For example,

- Cardiac output and blood pressure are dependent on optimum plasma volume.

- Most enzymes function best over rather narrow ranges of pH or ion concentration.
- Cell membrane potentials depend on K^+ concentration.
- Membrane excitability depends on Ca^{2+} concentration.

The principal job of the kidneys is the correction of perturbations in the composition and volume of body fluids that occur as a consequence of food intake, metabolism, environmental factors, and exercise. Typically, in healthy people, such perturbations are corrected within a matter of hours so that, in the long term, body fluid volume and the concentration of most ions do not deviate much from normal set points. In many disease states, however, these regulatory processes are disturbed, resulting in persistent deviations in body fluid volumes or ionic concentrations. Understanding these disorders requires an understanding of the normal regulatory processes.

The Balance Concept

The maintenance of stable body fluid composition requires that appearance and disappearance rates of any substance in the body balance each other. Balance is achieved when

$$\text{Ingested amount} + \text{produced amount}$$
$$= \text{excreted amount} + \text{consumed amount.}$$

For a large number of organic compounds, balance is the result of metabolic production and consumption. However, electrolytes are not produced or consumed by the body, balance is achieved by adjusting excretion to match intake. Therefore, when a person is in balance for sodium, potassium, and other ions, the amount excreted must equal the amount ingested. Since the kidneys are the principal organs where *regulated* excretion takes place, urinary excretion of such solutes closely follows the dietary intake. A central theme of physiology of the kidneys is understanding the mechanisms by which urine composition is altered to maintain the body in balance.

Body Fluid Composition

To a large extent, humans are composed of water. Adipose tissue is low in water content; thus, in obese people,

TABLE I
Bedside Estimates of Body Fluid Compartment Volumes

Remember	Example for 60-kg patient
Total body water = 60% × body wt	60% × 60 kg = 36 L
Intracellular water = 2/3 total body water	2/3 × 36 L = 24 L
Extracellular water = 1/3 total body water	1/3 × 36 L = 12 L
Plasma water = 1/4 extracellular water	1/4 × 12 L = 3 L
Blood volume = $\dfrac{\text{Plasma water}}{1 - \text{Hct}}$	3 L ÷ (1 − 0.40) = 6.6 L

the fraction of body weight that is water is lower than that in lean individuals. As a consequence of slightly greater fat content, women, on the average, contain less water than men, about 55% instead of 60%. Useful round numbers to remember for bedside estimates of body fluid volumes are given in Table 1. Typical ionic compositions of the intracellular and extracellular fluid compartments are given in Table 2.

KIDNEY STRUCTURE

The kidneys are two bean-shaped organs lying in the retroperitoneal space, each weighing about 150 g. The kidney is an anatomically complex organ, consisting of many different types of highly specialized cells, arranged in a highly organized three-dimensional pattern. The functional unit of the kidney is called a *nephron* (there are approximately 1 million nephrons in one human kidney); each nephron consists of a *glomerulus* and a long tubule which is made of a single layer of epithelial cells (the nephron is depicted schematically in Fig. 1). The nephron is segmented into

TABLE 2
Typical Ionic Composition of Plasma and Intracellular Fluid

	Plasma (mEq/L)	Intracellular fluid (mEq/L)
Cations		
K+	4	150
Na+	143	12
Ca2+ (ionized)	2	0.001
Mg2+	1	28
Total cations	150 mEq/L	190 mEq/L
Anions		
Cl−	104	4
HCO3−	24	10
Phosphates	2	40
Protein	14	50
Other	6	86
Total anions	150 mEq/L	190 mEq/L

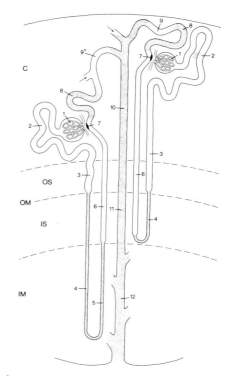

FIGURE I Organization of the nephron. The human kidney is made up of a million nephrons, two of which are shown schematically here. Each nephron consists of the following parts: glomerulus (1), proximal convoluted tubule (2), proximal straight tubule (3), thin descending limb of the loop of Henle (4), thin ascending limb (5), thick ascending limb (6), macula densa (7), distal convoluted tubule (8), and connecting tubule (9). Several nephrons coalesce to empty into a collecting duct, which has three distinct regions: the cortical collecting duct (10), the outer medullary collecting duct (11), and the inner medullary collecting duct (12). As shown, the deeper glomeruli give rise to nephrons with loops of Henle which descend all the way to the papillary tips, while the more superficial glomeruli have loops of Henle that bend at the junction between the inner and outer medulla.

distinct parts—proximal tubule, loop of Henle, distal tubule, collecting duct—each with a typical cellular appearance and special functional characteristics.

The nephrons are packed tightly together to make up the kidney parenchyma, which can be divided into regions. The outer layer of the kidney is called the *cortex:* it contains all the glomeruli, much of the proximal tubule, and some of the more distal portions as well. The inner section, called the *medulla*, consists largely of the parallel arrays of the loops of Henle and collecting ducts. The medulla is formed into cone-shaped regions, called *pyramids* (the human kidney typically has seven to nine), which extend into the renal pelvis. The tips of the medullary pyramids are called *papillae*. The medulla is important for concentration of the urine; the extracellular fluid in this region of the kidney has much higher solute concentration than plasma—as much as four times higher, with highest solute concentrations reached at the papillary tips.

The process of urine formation begins in the *glomerular capillary tuft,* where an ultrafiltrate of plasma is formed. The filtered fluid is collected in *Bowman's capsule* and enters the renal tubule to be carried over a circuitous course, successively modified by exposure to the sequence of specialized tubular epithelial segments with different transport functions. The *proximal convoluted tubule,* which is located entirely in the renal cortex, absorbs approximately two-thirds of the glomerular filtrate. Fluid remaining at the end of the proximal convoluted tubule enters the *loop of Henle,* which dips down in a hairpin configuration into the medulla. Returning to the cortex, the tubular fluid passes close by its parent glomerulus at the *juxtaglomerular apparatus,* then enters the *distal convoluted tubule* and finally the *collecting duct,* which courses back through the medulla, to empty into the renal pelvis at the tip of the renal papilla. Along the tubule, most of the glomerular filtrate is absorbed, but some additional substances are secreted. The final product, the urine, enters the renal pelvis and then the ureter, collects in the bladder, and is finally excreted from the body.

RENAL CIRCULATION

Anatomy of the Circulation

The renal artery, which enters the kidney at the renal hilum, carries about one-fifth of the cardiac output; this represents the highest tissue-specific blood flow of all larger organs in the body (about 350 ml/min per 100 g tissue). As a consequence of this generous perfusion, the renal arteriovenous O_2 difference is much lower than that of most other tissues (and blood in the renal vein is noticeably redder in color than that in other veins). The renal artery bifurcates several times after it enters the kidney and then breaks into the *arcuate arteries,* which run, in an arch-like fashion, along the border between the cortex and the outer medulla. As shown in Fig. 2, the arcuate vessels give rise, typically at right angles, to *interlobular arteries,* which run to the surface of the kidney. The *afferent arterioles* supplying the glomeruli come off the interiobular vessels.

Two Capillary Beds

The renal circulation is unusual in that it breaks into two separate capillary beds: the glomerular bed and the peritubular capillary bed. These two capillary networks are arranged in series so that all the renal blood flow passes through both. As blood leaves the glomerulus, the capillaries coalesce into the *efferent arteriole,* but almost immediately the vessels bifurcate again to form the peritubular capillary network. This second network of capillaries is the site where tubular reabsorbate is returned to the circulation. Pressure in the first capillary bed, that of the glomerulus, is rather high (about 40 to 50 mm Hg), while pressure in the peritubular capillaries is similar to that in capillary beds elsewhere in the body (about 5 to 10 mm Hg).

About 25% of the plasma that arrives at the glomerulus passes through the filtration barrier to become the filtrate.

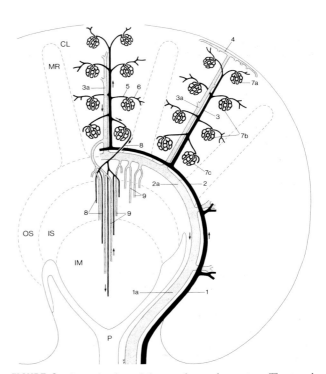

FIGURE 2 Organization of the renal vascular system. The renal artery bifurcates soon after entering the kidney parenchyma and gives rise to a system of arched-shaped vessels that run along the border between the cortex and the medulla. In this diagram, the vascular elements surrounding a single renal pyramid are shown. The human kidney typically has seven to nine renal pyramids. Here the arterial supply and glomeruli are shown in black, and the venous system is shown in gray. The peritubular capillary network which arises from the efferent arterioles is omitted, for simplicity. The vascular elements are named as follows: interlobar artery and vein (1 and 1a), arcuate artery and vein (2 and 2a), interlobular artery and vein (3 and 3a), stellate vein (4), afferent arteriole (5), efferent arteriole (6), glomerular capillaries (7) (from superficial, 7a; mid-cortex, 7b; and juxtamedullary; 7c, regions), juxtamedullary efferent arteriole, supplying descending vasa recti (8), and ascending vasa recti (9).

Blood cells, most of the proteins, and about 75% of the fluid and small solutes stay in the capillary and leave the glomerulus via the efferent arteriole. This postglomerular blood, which has a relatively high concentration of protein and red cells, enters the peritubular capillaries, where the high osmotic pressure from the high protein concentration facilitates the reabsorption of fluid. The peritubular capillaries coalesce to form venules and eventually the renal vein.

Medullary Blood Supply

The blood supplying the medulla is also postglomerular: specialized peritubular vessels, called vasa recta, arise from the efferent arterioles of the glomeruli nearest the medulla (the juxtamedullary glomeruli). Like medullary renal tubules, these vasa recta form hairpin loops dipping into the medulla.

GLOMERULUS

Structure

The structure of the glomerulus is shown schematically in Fig. 3 and photomicrographically in Fig. 4. The glomerulus is a ball of capillaries, consisting of endothelial cells and surrounded by specialized epithelial cells. Directly adherent to the basement membrane that surrounds the capillary loops is an inner layer of epithelial cells called the glomerular podocytes. These are large, highly differentiated cells that form an array of lacelike foot processes over the outer layer of these capillaries. An outer epithelial capsule, called Bowman's capsule, acts as a pouch to capture the filtrate and direct it into the beginning of the proximal tubule. As shown in the accompanying figures, the capillaries are held together by a stalk of cells, called the glomerular mesangium.

Glomerular Filtration Barrier

Urine formation begins at the glomerular filtration barrier. The glomerular filter through which the ultrafiltrate

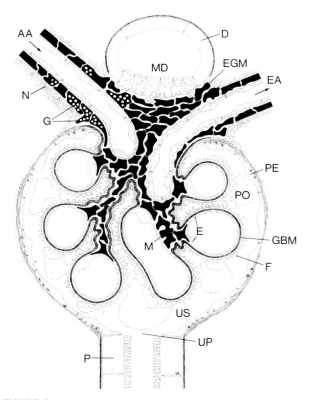

FIGURE 3 Schematic diagram of a section of a glomerulus and its juxtaglomerular apparatus. Structures shown are as follows: afferent arteriole (AA), efferent arteriole (EA), macula densa (MD), distal tubule (D), juxtaglomerular granular cell (G), sympathetic nerve endings (N), mesangial cell (M), extraglomerular mesangial cell (EGM), endothelial cell (E), epithelial podocyte (PO), with foot process (F), parietal epithelial cell (PE), glomerular basement membrane (GBM), urinary space (US), urinary pole (UP), and proximal tubule (P).

has to pass consists of three layers: the fenestrated endothelium, the intervening glomerular basement membrane, and the podocyte layer (Fig. 5). This complex "membrane" is freely permeable to water and small dissolved solutes, but retains most of the proteins and other larger molecules, as well as all blood particles. The main determinant of passage through the glomerular filter is molecular size. A molecule such as inulin (5 kDa) passes freely through the filter, and even a small protein such as myoglobin (16.9 kDa) is filtered to a large extent. Substances of increasing size are retained with increasing efficiency until at a size about 60 to 70 kDa the amount filtered becomes very small. Filtration also depends on ionic charge, and negatively charged proteins, such as albumin, are retained to a greater extent than would be predicted by size alone. In certain glomerular diseases, proteinuria develops because of loss of this charge selectivity.

Ultrafiltration in the Glomerulus

Filtrate formation in the glomerulus is governed by the same forces, often called Starling forces, that determine fluid transport across blood capillaries in general. The glomerular filtration rate (GFR) is equal to the product of the net filtration pressure, the hydraulic permeability, and the filtration area,

$$\text{GFR} = L_p \times \text{area} \times P_{net},$$

where L_p is the hydraulic permeability, and P_{net} is the net ultrafiltration pressure. Net ultrafiltration pressure or effective filtration pressure is the difference between the hydrostatic and osmotic pressure difference across the capillary loop,

$$P_{net} = \Delta P - \Delta \Pi = (P_{GC} - P_B) - (\Pi_{GC} - \Pi_B),$$

where P is hydrostatic pressure, Π is osmotic pressure, and the subscripts GC and B refer to the glomerular capillaries and Bowman's space.

Changes in GFR can result from changes in the permeability/surface area product ($L_p \times$ area) or from changes in net ultrafiltration pressure. One factor influencing P_{net} is the resistance in the afferent and efferent arterioles. An increase in resistance in the afferent arteriolar (before blood gets to the glomerulus) will *decrease* P_{GC} and GFR. However an increase in resistance as blood exits through the efferent arteriole will tend to *increase* P_{GC} and GFR. Changes in P_{net} can also occur as a result of an increase in renal arterial pressure, which will tend to increase P_{GC} and GFR. Obstruction of the tubule will increase P_B and decrease GFR, and a decrease in plasma protein concentration will tend to increase GFR.

Determination of GFR

Glomerular filtration rate is measured by determining the urinary excretion of a marker substance that must fulfill the key requirement that the amount filtered per minute is equal to the amount excreted in the urine per minute. This requirement is met if this substance (1) is neither

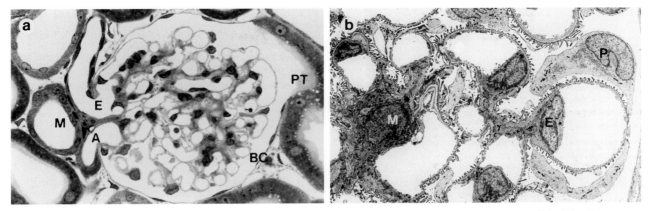

FIGURE 4 Structure of the glomerulus. (a) A light micrograph of a glomerulus, showing the afferent arteriole (A), efferent arteriole (E), macula densa (M), Bowman's capsule (BC), and beginning of the proximal tubule (PT). The typical diameter of a glomerulus is about 100 to 150 μm, which is just barely visible to the naked eye. (b) Higher power view of glomerular capillary loops, showing the epithelial podocyte (P), endothelial cells (E), and mesangial cells (M).

absorbed nor secreted by the renal tubules, (2) is freely filterable across the glomerular membranes, and (3) is not metabolized or produced by the kidneys. These critical properties are ideally met by *inulin,* a large sugar molecule with a molecular weight of about 5000. Inulin is often infused in experimental studies to measure GFR. An endogenous substance that has similar properties and is used in the clinical setting is creatinine. As shown in Table 3, the formula for GFR derives from a simple rearrangement of the statement indicating that the amount filtered per minute

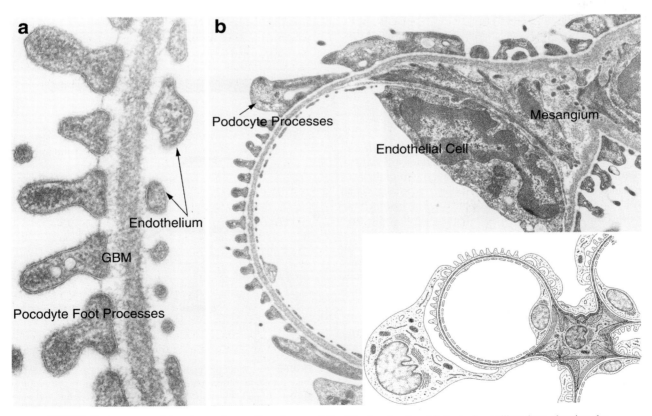

FIGURE 5 Structure of the glomerular capillary loop and the filtration barrier. (a) A single capillary loop showing the endothelial and foot process layers and the attachments of the basement membrane to the mesangium. Pressure in the glomerular capillary bed is substantially higher than in other capillaries. As shown in the diagrammatic insert, the mesangium provides the structural supports which permit these cells to withstand these high pressures. (b) The glomerular filtration barrier.

TABLE 3
Derivation of the Formula for GFR

Step 1. Filtered amount of inulin = excreted amount of inulin

$$GFR \times GF_{in} = U_{in} \times V,$$

where GFR is the glomerular filtration rate, GF_{in} is the concentration of inulin in the filtrate, U_{in} is the concentration of inulin in urine, and V is the urine flow rate.

Step 2. Inulin is freely filterable, so its concentrations in plasma and filtrate are identical. Hence,

$$\text{Filtered amount of inulin} = GFR \times P_{in},$$

where P_{in} is the concentration of inulin in plasma.

Step 3. Substituting produces

$$GFR \times P_{in} = U_{in} \times V$$

and hence

$$GFR = \frac{U_{in} \times V}{P_{in}}.$$

equals the amount excreted per minute. A formula of this general form, called the clearance formula, denotes the volume of plasma (mL/min) cleared of a particular substance by excretion into the urine—its clearance rate. In the case of inulin, the clearance of inulin is equal to GFR. The clearance of creatinine is slightly greater than GFR (15 to 20%) because the excreted amount exceeds the amount filtered as a result of some tubular secretion of creatinine. GFR is typically about 100 mL/min for women and 120 mL/min for men.

Juxtaglomerular Apparatus

Tightly adherent to every glomerulus, in between the entry and the exit of the arterioles, is a plaque of distal tubular cells called the *macula densa,* which is part of the juxtaglomerular apparatus. This cell plaque is in the distal tubule, at the very terminal end of the thick ascending limb of the loop of Henle, right before the transition to the distal convoluted tubule. This is a special position along the nephron, because at this site NaCl concentration is quite variable. Low rates of flow result in a very low salt concentration at this site, 15 mEq/L or less, while at higher flow rates salt concentration rises to 40 to 60 mEq/L. NaCl concentration at this site regulates glomerular blood flow, through a mechanism called tubuloglomerular feedback; increases in salt concentration cause a decrease in glomerular blood flow.

The other unique cells that make up the juxtaglomerular apparatus are the renin-containing juxtaglomerular granular cells. Renin secretion is also regulated locally by salt concentration in the tubule at the macula densa. In addition, the granular cells have extensive sympathetic innervation, and renin secretion is controlled by the sympathetic nervous system.

TUBULAR FUNCTION: BASIC PRINCIPLES

Absorption and Secretion in the Renal Tubules

The glomerular filtrate undergoes a series of modifications before becoming the final urine. These changes consist of removal or absorption and addition or secretion of solutes and fluid. Absorption and secretion indicate directions of transport, not mechanisms.

1. *Absorption.* Absorption, the movement of solute or water from tubular lumen to blood, is the predominant process in the renal handling of Na^+, Cl^-, H_2O, HCO_3^-, glucose, amino acids, protein, phosphates, Ca^{2+}, Mg^{2+}, urea, uric acid, and others.
2. *Secretion.* Secretion, the movement of solute from blood or cell interior to tubular lumen, is important in the renal handling of H^+, K^+, NH_4^+, and a number of organic acids and bases.

Substances can move into or out of the tubule either by the transcellular pathway, which requires traversing the luminal and the basolateral cell membranes, or by the paracellular pathway between cells (Fig. 6). Many specialized

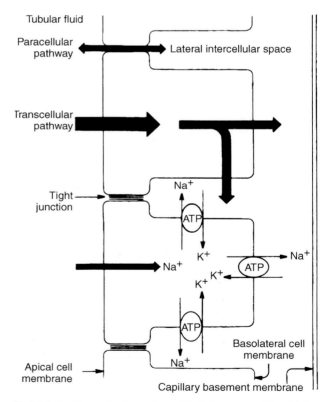

FIGURE 6 General scheme for epithelial transport. The driving force for solute movement is primarily generated by the action of the Na^+, K^+-ATPase in the basolateral membrane. Solute and water can move through either a paracellular pathway between cells or a transcellular transport pathway, which requires movement across both luminal and basolateral membranes. From BM Koeppen, BA Stanton, *Renal Physiology,* Mosby, St. Louis, 1992. With permission.

TABLE 4
Types of Membrane Transport Mechanisms Used in the Kidney

Mechanism	Examples of substances	Examples of transport protein
Facilitated or carrier mediated	Glucose, urea	GLUT1 carrier, urea carrier
Active transport (pumps)	Na^+, K^+, H^+, Ca^{2+}	Na^+, K^+-ATPase, H^+-ATPase, Ca^{2+}-ATPase
Coupled transport		
Cotransport	Cl^-, glucose, amino acids, formate, phosphates	Na^+–K^+–$2Cl^-$ cotransporter
Countertransport	Bicarbonate, H^+	Cl^-/HCO_3^- exchanger, Na^+/H^+ antiporter
Osmosis	H_2O	Water channels (aquaporins)

membrane proteins participate in the movement of substances across cell membranes along the renal tubule. Some of the important membrane transport mechanisms, together with examples of substances that use these mechanisms, and proteins that are important for these processes are given in Table 4.

Segmentation of the Nephron

One of the more striking characteristics of the renal tubule is dramatic cellular heterogeneity. Early renal anatomists recognized that there are marked differences in the appearance of the cells of the proximal tubule, loops of Henle, and distal tubule. These different nephron segments also differ markedly in function, distribution of important transport proteins, and responsiveness to drugs such as diuretics that inhibit transport.

Proximal Tubule

The proximal tubules absorb the bulk of filtered small solutes. These solutes are present in proximal tubular fluid at the same concentration as in plasma. Approximately 60% of the filtered Na^+, Cl^-, K^+, Ca^{2+}, and H_2O and more than 90% of the filtered HCO_3^- are absorbed along the proximal tubule. This is also the segment that normally reabsorbs virtually all the filtered glucose and amino acids by Na^+-dependent cotransport. An additional function of the proximal tubule is phosphate transport, which is regulated by parathyroid hormone. In addition to these reabsorption functions, secretion of solutes also occurs along the proximal tubule. The terminal portion of the proximal tubule, the S3 or pars recta, is the site of secretion of numerous organic anions and cations, a mechanism used by the body for eliminating a number of drugs and toxins. The proximal tubule, as shown in Fig. 7, has a prominent brush border, extensive interdigitated foot basolateral infoldings, and large prominent mitochondria, which supply the energy for Na^+, K^+-ATPase.

Loop of Henle

The loop of Henle consists of the terminal or straight portion of the proximal tubule, thin descending and ascending limbs, and the thick ascending limb and is important for generation of a concentrated medulla and for dilution of the urine. The thick ascending limb is often called the diluting segment, since transport along this water impermeant segment results in development of a dilute tubular fluid. The thick ascending limb is also a major site of Mg^{2+} reabsorption along the nephron. The principal luminal transporter expressed in this segment is the Na^+–K^+–$2Cl^-$ cotransporter, which is the target of diuretics such as furosemide. The morphology of loop of Henle epithelia is illustrated in Fig. 8.

Distal Nephron

The distal nephron, which includes the distal convoluted tubule, the connecting tubule, and the cortical and medullary collecting duct, is the portion of the nephron where final adjustments in urine composition, tonicity, and volume are made. Distal segments are the sites where the most critical regulatory hormones, such as aldosterone and vasopressin, regulate acid and potassium excretion and determine final urinary concentrations of potassium, sodium, and chloride.

Both the distal convoluted tubule and connecting tubule have well-developed basolateral infoldings with abundant mitochondria, like the proximal tubule, although they are easily distinguished from proximal tubule by the lack of brush border (Fig. 9). The distal convoluted tubule is the principal site of action of thiazide diuretics.

The collecting duct cells are cuboidal, and their basolateral folds do not interdigitate extensively. When there is a sizable osmotic gradient, and water moves across this epithelium, the spaces between cells become wide. The collecting duct changes in its appearance as it travels from the cortex to the papillary tip (Fig. 10). In the cortex there are two different cell types in the collecting duct: principal cells and intercalated cells. Principal cells are the main site of salt and water transport, and intercalated cells are the key sites for acid–base regulation. The medullary collecting duct in its most terminal portions comes increasingly to resemble the tall cells typical of transitional epithelium.

SALT AND VOLUME REGULATION

Absorption of Sodium

Because of its high extracellular concentration, large amounts of Na^+ and its accompanying anions are present in the glomerular filtrate, and the absorption of this filtered Na^+ is in a quantitative sense the dominant work performed by the renal tubules. The amount of Na^+ absorbed by the

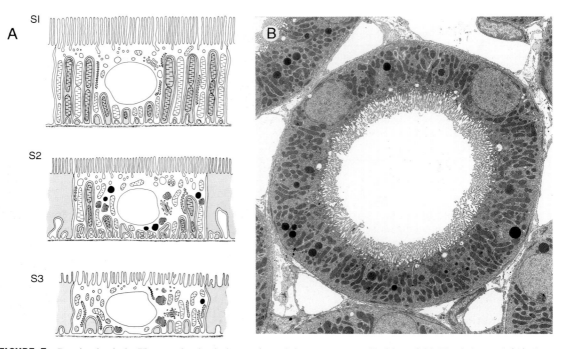

FIGURE 7 Proximal tubule. The proximal tubule consists of three segments: S1, S2, and S3. The left panel (A) shows schematic diagrams of the typical cells from these three segments, the right panel (B) shows a cross section of the S1 segment. The S1 begins at the glomerulus, and extends several millimeters, before the transition to the S2 segment. The S3 segment, which is also called the proximal straight tubule, descends into the renal medulla to the inner medulla. The proximal tubule is characterized by a prominent brush border, which increases the membrane surface area by a factor of about 40-fold. The basolateral infoldings, which are lined with mitochondria, are interdigitated with the basolateral infoldings of adjacent cells (in these diagrams, processes that come from adjacent cells are shaded). These adaptations are most prominent in the first parts of the proximal tubule, and are less well developed later along the proximal tubule.

tubules is the difference between the amount of Na^+ filtered and the amount of Na^+ excreted:

$$Na^+ \text{ absorption} = \text{filtered } Na^+ - Na^+ \text{ excretion}$$

or

$$Na^+ \text{ absorption} = (GFR \times P_{Na}) - (V \times U_{Na}),$$

where U_{Na} is the urinary Na^+ concentration and P_{Na} is the plasma Na^+ concentration. With a GFR of 120 mL/min and a plasma Na^+ concentration of 145 mEq/L, 17.4 mEq of Na^+ is filtered every minute, or about 25,000 mEq or 575 g of Na^+ per day. Since only about 100 to 250 mEq of Na^+ is excreted per day (this reflects the average intake provided by a typical Western diet), or can estimate that the tubule reabsorbs somewhat more than 99% of the filtered Na^+. The fractional excretion of Na^+ (FE_{Na}) is defined as the fraction of filtered Na^+ excreted in the urine. Using creatinine as a GFR estimate, FE_{Na} is calculated from

$$FE_{Na} = \frac{\text{excreted Na}}{\text{filtered Na}} = \frac{U_{Na} \times V}{P_{Na} \times GFR}$$

$$= \frac{U_{Na} \times V}{P_{Na} \times \left(\dfrac{U_{Cr}}{P_{Cr}}\right) \times V} = \frac{U_{Na}/P_{Na}}{U_{Cr}/P_{Cr}}.$$

FE_{Na} is usually less than 1%. However, this value depends on Na^+ intake and can vary physiologically from nearly 0% at extremely low intakes to about 2% at extremely high intakes. FE_{Na} can also exceed 1% in disease states where tubular transport of Na^+ is impaired (e.g., in most cases of acute renal failure).

Mechanisms of Na^+ Absorption

Tubular Na^+ absorption is a primary active transport process driven by the enzyme Na^+, K^+-ATPase. In renal epithelial cells, as in most cells of the body, this pump translocates Na^+ out of cells (and K^+ into cells) and thereby lowers intracellular Na^+ concentration (and elevates intracellular K^+ concentration). A key for the generation of net Na^+ movement from tubular lumen to blood is the asymmetrical distribution of this enzyme: it is present exclusively in the basolateral membrane (the blood side) of all nephron segments, but not in their luminal membranes. Delivery of Na^+ to the pump sites is maintained by Na^+ entry into the luminal side of the cells along a favorable electrochemical gradient. Since Na^+ permeability of the luminal membrane is much higher than that of the basolateral membrane, Na^+ entry is fed from the luminal Na^+ pool. The asymmetric permeability is due to the presence of a variety of

A

tDL

tAL

TAL

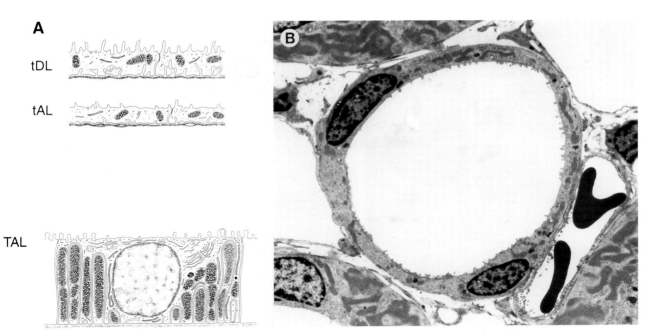

FIGURE 8 Loop of Henle. The loop of Henle makes a hairpin loop into the medulla. Segments included in the loop are terminal portion of the proximal tubule, the thin descending (tDL), and ascending limbs (tAL), as well as the thick ascending limb (TAL). The left panel (A) shows schematic drawings of cell morphology, the right panel (B) shows a cross section through the thin descending limb in the outer medulla. The thin limbs, as their names suggest, are shallow epithelia without the prominent mitochondria of more proximal segments. The thick limb, in contrast, is a taller epithelium with basolateral infoldings and well-developed mitochondria. This segment is water impermeable, and transport along this segment is important for generation of interstitial solute gradients, and a low salt concentration and dilute fluid in the tubular lumen.

A

DCT

CT

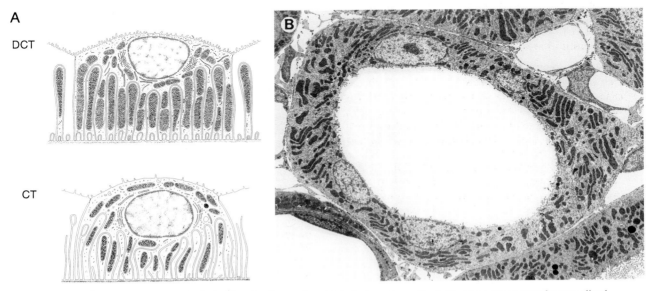

FIGURE 9 Distal convoluted tubule. The distal convoluted tubule is customarily divided into two parts: the true distal convoluted tubule (DCT, shown schematically on the left, and in cross section on the right) and the connecting tubule (CT), where cell morphology is somewhat more similar to collecting duct.

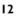

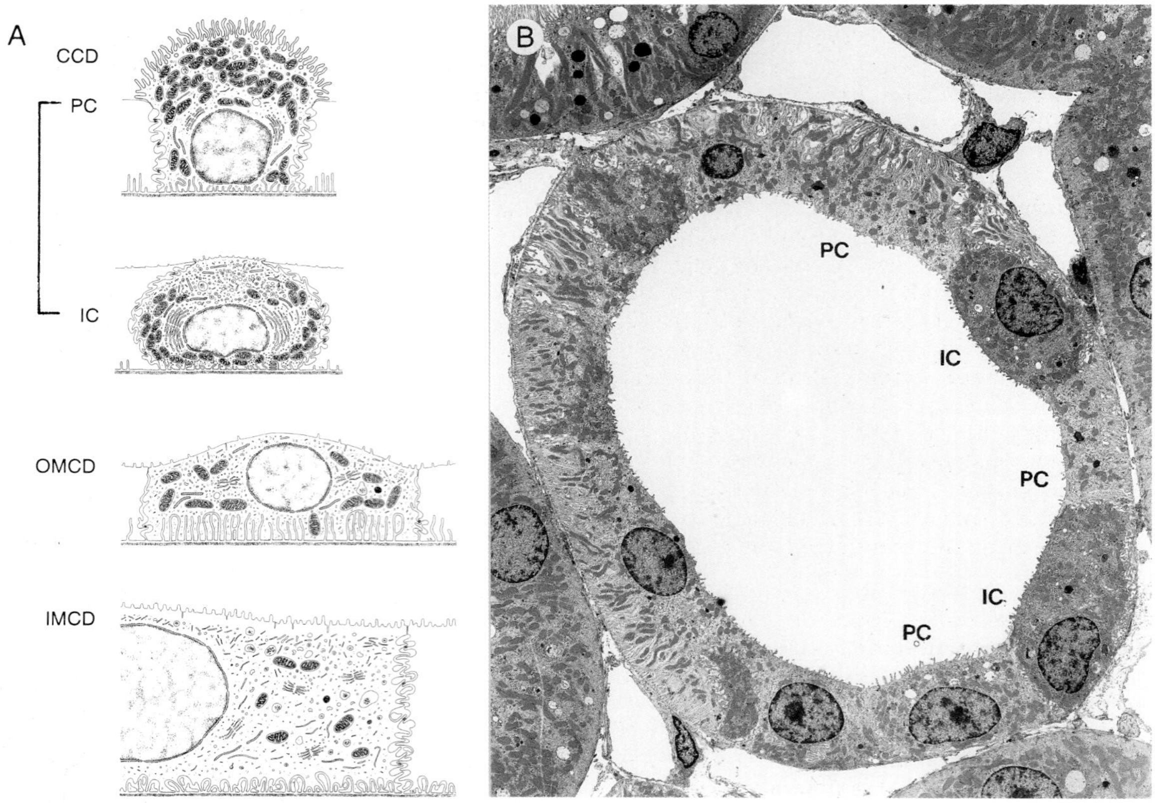

FIGURE 10 Collecting duct. The collecting duct changes its morphology as it travels from cortex to medulla. In the cortex there are two cell types—principal cells (PC) and intercalated cells (IC). Appearance is shown schematically on the left (A) and in cross section on the right (B).

different transport proteins or channels exclusively in the luminal membrane.

A number of these luminal transporters are the target molecules for diuretic action. Principal entry mechanisms for Na^+ and Cl^- in the different nephron segments (and effective diuretics) are

1. Early proximal: Na^+-dependent cotransporter, Na^+/H^+ exchanger
2. Late proximal: Na^+/H^+ exchanger, Cl^-/anion exchanger
3. Thick ascending limb of the loop of Henle: Na^+–K^+– $2Cl^-$ contransporter (furosemide-sensitive carrier)
4. Distal convoluted tubule: Na^+/Cl^- cotransporter (thiazide-sensitive carrier)
5. Collecting duct: Na^+ channel (amiloride-sensitive channel)

Regulation of NaCl Excretion

Because Na^+ salts are the most abundant extracellular solutes, the amount of sodium in the body (the total body sodium) determines extracellular fluid volume. Therefore, excretion or retention of Na^+ salts by the kidneys is critical for the regulation of extracellular fluid volume.[1] A disturbance in volume regulation, particularly enhanced salt retention, is common in disease states. The sympathetic nervous system, the renin–angiotensin–aldosterone system (RAS), atrial natriuretic peptide (ANP), and vasopressin represent the four main regulatory systems that change their activity in response to changes in body fluid volume. These changes in activity mediate the effects of body fluid volume on urinary Na^+ excretion.

Sympathetic Nervous System

A change in extracellular fluid volume is sensed by stretch receptors on blood vessels, principally those located on the low pressure side of the circulation in the thorax, for example, in the vena cava, cardiac atria, and pulmonary vessels. A decreased firing rate in the afferent nerves from these volume receptors enhances sympathetic outflow

---

[1]Plasma Na^+ concentration does not correlate at all with total body sodium or the fullness of the extracellular fluid spaces. In fact, a low serum Na^+ can be observed in states in which there is either excess total body sodium or deficiency of total body sodium. However, plasma Na^+ concentration is the principal determinant of extracellular fluid osmolarity. In general, abnormalities in Na^+ concentration arise from defects in tonicity regulation, not volume regulation.

from cardiovascular medullary centers. Increased renal sympathetic tone enhances renal salt reabsorption and can decrease renal blood flow at higher frequencies. In addition to its direct effects on renal function, increased sympathetic outflow promotes the activation of another salt retaining system: the RAS.

Renin–Angiotensin System

Renin is an enzyme that is formed by and released from granular cells in the wall of renal afferent arterioles near the entrance to the glomerulus. These granular cells are part of the juxtaglomerular apparatus (see Fig. 3). Renin is an enzyme that cleaves angiotensin I from angiotensinogen, a large circulating protein made principally in the liver. Angiotensin I, a decapeptide, is converted by angiotensin-converting enzyme to the biologically active angiotensin II. Renin catalyzes the rate-limiting step in the production of angiotensin II, and it is therefore the plasma level of renin that determines plasma angiotensin II. The three principal mechanisms in control of renin release are as follows:

1. *Macula densa mechanism.* Macula densa refers to a group of distinct epithelial cells in the wall of the thick ascending limb of the loop of Henle, where it makes contact with its own glomerulus. At this location, NaCl concentration is between 30 and 40 mEq/L, and it varies as a direct function of tubular fluid flow rate; that is, it increases when flow rate is high and decreases when flow rate is low. A decrease in NaCl concentration at the macula densa strongly stimulates renin secretion, whereas an increase inhibits it. The connection to the regulation of body fluid volume is the dependence of the flow rate past the macula densa cells on body Na^+ content. The flow rate is high in states of Na^+ excess and low in Na^+ depletion.

2. *Baroreceptor mechanism.* Renin secretion is stimulated by a decrease in arterial pressure, an effect believed to be mediated by a "baroreceptor" in the wall of the afferent arteriole responding to pressure, stretch, or shear stress.

3. *β-Adrenergic stimulation.* An increase in renal sympathetic activity or in circulating catecholamines stimulates renin release through β-adrenergic receptors on the juxtaglomerular granular cells.

Angiotensin II has direct and indirect effects to promote salt retention. It enhances Na^+ reabsorption in the proximal tubule (stimulation of Na^+/H^+ exchange), and, because it is a potent renal vasoconstrictor, it may reduce GFR by reducing glomerular capillary pressure or plasma flow. Angiotensin II affects salt balance indirectly by stimulating the production and release of the steroid hormone aldosterone from the zona glomerulosa of the adrenal gland. Aldosterone acts on the collecting duct to augment salt reabsorption (and K^+ secretion).

Atrial Natriuretic Factor

Atrial natriuretic factor (ANF) is a peptide hormone that is synthesized by atrial myocytes and released in response to increased atrial distension. Thus, ANF secretion is increased in volume expansion and inhibited in volume depletion. The main cause of the ANF-induced natriuresis is an inhibition of Na^+ reabsorption along the collecting duct, but an increase in GFR may sometimes play a contributory role.

Vasopressin or Antidiuretic Hormone

Vasopressin or antidiuretic hormone (ADH) is regulated primarily by body fluid osmolarity. However, in states in which intravascular volume is depleted, the set point for vasopressin release is shifted, so that for any given plasma osmolarity, vasopressin levels are higher than they would be normally. This shift promotes water retention to aid in restoration of body fluid volumes.

WATER AND OSMOREGULATION

Regulation of Body Fluid Osmolarity

When water intake is low or water is lost from the body (in hypotonic fluids such as sweat, for example), the kidneys conserve water by producing a small volume of concentrated urine. In dehydration, urine production is less than a liter per day (less than 0.5 mL/min) and the osmotic concentration may reach 1200 mOsmol/kg H_2O. When water intake is high, urine flow may increase to as much as 14 L/day (10 mL/min) with an osmolality substantially lower than that of plasma (75 to 100 mOsmol/kg). These wide variations in urine volume and osmotic concentration do not obligatorily affect the excretion of the daily solute load. Thus, the daily solute excess of about 1200 mOsmol/day may be excreted in 12 L of urine (with an U_{osm} of 100 mOsmol/L) or in 1 L (with an U_{osm} of 1200 mOsmol/L). The hormone responsible for the regulatory changes in urine volume and tonicity is ADH (synonym: vasopressin).

Role of ADH in Osmolarity Regulation

Antidiuretic hormone is a nonapeptide produced by neurons located in the supraoptic and paraventricular nuclei of the hypothalamus. It is stored in and released from granules in nerve terminals that are located in the posterior pituitary (neurohypophysis). The release of ADH is exquisitely sensitive to changes in plasma osmolality, with increases in P_{osm} above a threshold of about 285 mOsmol/kg leading to increases in ADH secretion and plasma ADH concentrations. As has been pointed out, the actual set point for release depends on body fluid volume as well.

The most important function of ADH is the regulation of water permeability of the distal portions of the nephron, particularly the collecting duct. As shown schematically in Fig. 11, ADH binds to receptors (R) in the basolateral membrane of collecting duct cells. This activates adenylate cyclase (AC) to form cAMP. cAMP activates a protein kinase, which leads to the phosphorylation of undefined proteins. This phosphorylation causes membrane fusion of vesicles that contain preformed water channels. The result is an up to 20-fold increase in water permeability of the apical (luminal) membrane of collecting duct cells. On removal of ADH,

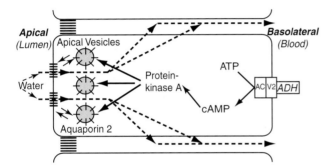

FIGURE 11 Mechanism of action of ADH on the collecting duct. ADH combines with a basolateral receptor (V2) which is coupled with adenylate cyclase (AC). Generation of cyclic AMP (cAMP) leads to activation of protein kinase A which in turn phosphorylates the water channel, aquaporin 2. The vesicles containing aquaporin are then inserted into the luminal membrane, increasing water permeability 10-fold.

water channels are rapidly removed from the apical membrane by endocytosis.

Tubular Water Absorption

At each point along the nephron, the osmotic pressure of the tubular fluid is lower than that in the interstitial space. This transtubular osmotic pressure difference provides the driving force for tubular water reabsorption. The rate of fluid absorption in a given nephron segment is determined by the magnitude of this gradient and the osmotic water permeability of the segment. Even though the osmotic pressure difference across the proximal tubule epithelium is very small (3 to 4 mOsmol/L), the rate of fluid absorption is very high because this segment has a very high water permeability. In contrast, osmotic gradients across the thick ascending limb may be as high as 250 mOsmol/L, and yet virtually no water flows across this segment because it is highly water impermeable. This segment dilutes the urine because it absorbs Na$^+$ and Cl$^-$ without water.

In contrast to the invariability of water conductivity in the proximal tubule and the thick ascending limb, water permeability in the collecting duct can be altered under the influence of ADH. If ADH is absent, water permeability and water absorption are low, and the hypotonicity generated in the thick ascending limb persists along the collecting duct. As a consequence, a dilute urine is excreted. If ADH is present, the collecting duct becomes quite water permeable, and water is reabsorbed until the tubular fluid in the collecting duct equilibrates with the hypertonic interstitium. The final urine in this case is osmotically concentrated and has a low volume.

Medullary Hypertonicity

To allow osmotically driven water absorption, the osmotic concentration in the medullary interstitium must be slightly higher than that in the collecting duct lumen. Thus, when a final urine with an osmolality of 1200 mOsmol/kg is excreted, the medullary interstitium at the tips of the papillae must be a little higher than 1200 mOsmol/kg. The generation of such a unique extracellular environment is achieved by a countercurrent multiplication system that exists in the renal medulla in the form of the countercurrent arrangement of descending and ascending limbs of the loops of Henle.

Countercurrent Multiplication

In two adjacent tubes with flow in opposite directions, the fluid can attain an osmotic concentration difference in the longitudinal axis of the system that can by far exceed that seen at each level along it. This principle of countercurrent multiplication requires energy expenditure and the presence of unique differences in membrane characteristics between the two limbs of the system.

The countercurrent multiplier represented by the loops of Henle is believed to generate an osmotic gradient because

1. Active NaCl transport across the ascending limb (the so-called single effect of the countercurrent system) generates an osmotic difference between tubular fluid and surrounding local interstitium.
2. A low water permeability of the ascending limb prevents dissipation of this gradient.
3. A high water permeability of the descending limb permits equilibration of descending limb contents with the surrounding local interstitium.

How such a system can result in progressive increases in osmotic concentration along the corticopapillary axis is shown in Fig. 12. In Step 1 (time zero), the fluid in the descending and ascending limbs and the interstitium is isoosmotic to plasma. In Step 2, NaCl is absorbed from the ascending limb into the interstitium until a gradient of 200 mOsmol/kg is reached. In Step 3, the fluid in the descending limb equilibrates osmotically with the interstitium by water movement out of the tubule. In Step 4, the hypertonic fluid is presented to the thick ascending limb (TAL) with an increased solute concentration in the region near the tip of the system. Again active NaCl transport along the ascending limb establishes a 200 mOsmol/kg gradient, increasing interstitial concentrations and by water abstraction descending limb contents. Note that concentrations near the tip begin to be higher than those near the base. Continued operation of such a mechanism will gradually result in generation of a gradient of hypertonicity, with the highest osmolarities at the papillary tip.

The tubular fluid leaving the ascending limb of the loop of Henle countercurrent multiplier is hypotonic. However, the medullary interstitium has been osmotically "charged." Since the collecting ducts on their way to the papillary tip return into the hypertonic medullary environment, their content can now be concentrated by water flow along an osmotic gradient.

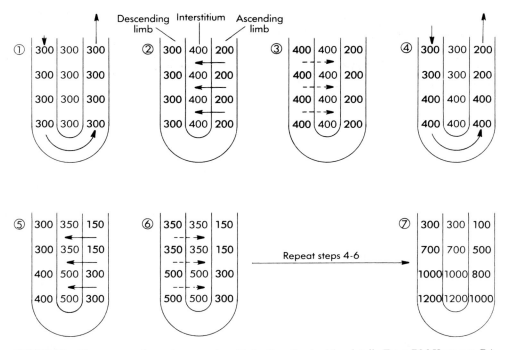

FIGURE 12 The process of countercurrent multiplication. See text for details. From BM Koeppen, BA Stanton, *Renal Physiology,* Mosby, St. Louis, 1992. With permission.

Role of Urea in the Countercurrent Mechanism

In addition to Na^+ and Cl^-, urea is the other major solute present in the renal medulla in an osmotically concentrated form. Urea enters the medulla by reabsorption across the collecting duct. Marked differences in the permeability to urea allow reabsorption to proceed only across the terminal portions of the medullary collecting duct. In the early portions of the collecting duct, urea permeability is low and reabsorption of urea cannot occur. Since water leaves the tubule under the influence of ADH, the urea staying behind is progressively concentrated. As a consequence, a substantial urea gradient develops, providing the driving force for urea reabsorption when the permeability to urea permits it. The contribution of urea accumulation to osmotic water absorption along the inner medullary collecting duct must be sizable since about half of inner medullary tonicity is accounted for by urea. Therefore, a reduction in urea synthesis by reducing protein intake markedly impairs the concentrating ability of the kidneys.

Comparison between Volume Regulation and Osmoregulation

Osmoregulation is under control of a single hormonal system, ADH, whereas volume regulation is under control of a set of redundant and overlapping control mechanisms. Lack or excess of ADH results in defined and rather dramatic clinical syndromes of excess water loss or water retention. In contrast, a defect in a single volume regulatory

mechanism generally results in more subtle abnormalities, because of the redundant regulatory capacity from the other mechanisms. Thus, excess aldosterone results in a mild volume retention followed by "escape" and return to normal Na^+ excretion, due to the action of the other mechanisms. Similarly, excess ANF probably produces only a modest decrement in volume, with no persistent abnormality in Na^+ excretion. Severe salt-retaining states, such as liver cirrhosis and congestive heart failure, are characterized by activation of all the volume regulatory mechanisms. Finally, the symptoms characteristic of disorders of osmoregulation and of volume regulation are different, with hypo- and hypernatremia being the hallmark of deranged osmoregulation, and edema or hypovolemia resulting from deranged volume regulation.

REGULATION OF BODY FLUID POTASSIUM AND ACIDITY

Both potassium and hydrogen ions are present in body fluids at low concentrations, about 4 to 4.5 mEq/L for K^+ and about 40 nEq/L for H^+. Both ions show a number of features:

1. Relatively small deviations in either K^+ or H^+ concentrations can be life threatening, and therefore the regulation of K^+ and H^+ concentration requires control systems with high sensitivity and precision.
2. Constancy of both K^+ and H^+ concentration over the long term is achieved by regulated excretion of these ions in the urine. However, in both cases,

other mechanisms exist that provide immediate protection against excessive deviations of plasma concentrations from normal.

3. Regulation in the renal excretion of both K^+ and H^+ is caused to a large extent by variation in the secretion of these ions by collecting ducts. The principal cell of the collecting duct is the cell type responsible for regulated K^+ secretion; the intercalated cell is the cell type responsible for H^+ secretion (see Fig. 10).

4. The rate of both K^+ and H^+ secretion is increased by aldosterone.

5. A primary derangement of K^+ balance can cause an acidity disturbance and a primary acidity disturbance can derange K^+ homeostasis.

Regulation of Body Fluid Potassium

Distribution of Body K^+

Owing to the presence of Na^+,K^+-ATPase in virtually all cell membranes, K^+ is mostly in the intracellular space. Of the 3500 mEq of body potassium, only about 1 to 2% is present in the extracellular space, where it has a concentration of 4 to 5 mEq/L. The remainder (about 98%) is stored in cells.

The distribution has the potential risk in that the release of even a small amount of K^+ from intracellular stores can elevate plasma K^+ concentration substantially (e.g., in insulin deficiency, cell lysis, severe exercise). On the other hand, the distribution of K^+ between the extracellular and intracellular space is utilized as a means to buffer acute changes in plasma K^+ concentrations. For example, the administration of an acute oral K^+ load induces much smaller changes in plasma K^+ concentration than would occur if all absorbed K^+ were to remain in the extracellular space. Potassium ions are shifted into cells under the stimulatory influence of insulin and epinephrine. The effect of both hormones reflects mainly an activation of the Na^+,K^+-ATPase. Another important factor determining K^+ distribution is plasma H^+ concentration. An increase in H^+ ions causes uptake of H^+ into cells and intracellular buffering and this uptake to some extent occurs in exchange for K^+. Thus, acidosis will tend to increase plasma K^+, and alkalosis will tend to decrease it.

Renal Handling of K^+

Potassium ion nomeostasis in the long term requires the excretion of an amount equivalent to the daily K^+ intake (50 to 150 mEq). This represents a fractional K^+ excretion (FE_{K^+}) of about 10%, much higher than FE_{Na^+}. About 60 to 70% of filtered K^+ is absorbed along the proximal tubule, and further reabsorption of K^+ takes place in the thick ascending limb of the loop of Henle; only about 10% of filtered K^+ enters the distal tubule. Along the collecting duct, K^+ is both secreted and absorbed. Collecting duct K^+ secretion increases when dietary K^+ intake is elevated. On the other hand, when intake is low, collecting duct K^+ secretion virtually ceases and absorption is dominant. Thus,

while K^+ absorption along the proximal tubule and the loop of Henle does not change very much depending on intake, collecting duct K^+ secretion is variable, and this variability accounts almost completely for the variation in urinary K^+ excretion.

Mechanisms of K^+ Secretion

K^+ secretion across the collecting duct epithelium utilizes the transcellular route. K^+ uptake across the basolateral membrane is driven by Na^+,K^+-ATPase, which elevates intracelluar K^+ concentration to a level above electrochemical equilibrium. K^+ can then move along a favorable gradient from cell interior to tubule lumen utilizing potassium channels in the luminal membrane.

Three major variables determine the rate at which K^+ is secreted by collecting duct cells:

1. Changes in the activity of Na^+,K^+-ATPase affect uptake and thereby intracellular K^+ concentration. An increase in pump activity will increase intracellular K^+ levels and will tend to stimulate K^+ secretion.

2. Changes in the electrochemical gradient affect the driving force for K^+ movement across the luminal membrane. Both an increase in intracellular K^+ concentration and in the lumen negative transepithelial potential difference will increase the driving force and will tend to increase K^+ secretion.

3. Changes in the permeability of the luminal membrane determine the amount of K^+ that can be secreted for a given driving force. Thus, an increase in luminal K^+ conductance will increase K^+ secretion.

Regulation of K^+ Excretion

1. *Plasma K^+ concentration.* One important determinant of K^+ excretion is plasma K^+ concentration. For example, the change in K^+ excretion following a change in dietary K^+ intake is mediated by an increase in plasma K^+. The effect of plasma K^+ on secretion is induced partly by a direct effect on intracellular K^+ concentration.

2. *Aldosterone.* At any level of plasma K^+, K^+ secretion will also depend on plasma aldosterone levels. Aldosterone enhances K^+ secretion by activation of Na^+, K^+-ATPase and by an increase in K^+ permeability of the luminal membrane. Aldosterone is partly responsible for the diet-induced increase in K^+ excretion because its production and secretion are directly stimulated by plasma K^+ concentration. This effect is independent of angiotensin.

3. *Tubular flow rate.* An increase in tubular flow rate past the K^+-secreting cells stimulates, and a decrease reduces, K^+ secretion. This effect is the consequence of flow-dependent changes in the K^+ gradient across the apical membrane. K^+ secretion causes an increase in K^+ concentration in the tubular fluid, which eventually decreases the K^+ gradient and the rate of K^+ secretion. An increase in flow diminishes the rate of rise of luminal K^+ concentration so that a more favorable K^+ gradient for K^+ secretion is maintained.

4. *Distal sodium delivery.* When more Na^+ is delivered to the distal nephron, if reabsorption increases, the net electrical charge in the lumen will become more negative. This favorable electrochemical gradient will tend to increase urinary K^+ secretion.

5. *Hydrogen ions.* A decrease in H^+ concentration in alkalotic states causes a stimulation of K^+ secretion. This effect is mediated by the rise in intracellular K^+ concentration that occurs in alkalosis.

Diuretics and K^+ Excretion

Diuretics increase tubular flow rate. Agents such as loop diuretics and thiazides that inhibit NaCl and water absorption in segments prior to the collecting duct (in the loop of Henle and in the distal tubule, respectively) increase the flow of fluid past the collecting duct cells which causes increased K^+ secretion. In addition, the diuretics cause volume depletion, which stimulates aldosterone secretion.

Regulation of Body Fluid Acidity

Basic Considerations

Maintenance of the extracellular pH around 7.4 depends on the operation of buffer systems that accept H^+ when it is produced and liberate H^+ when it is consumed. The state of the demand on total body buffering can be determined by assessing the behavior of the HCO_3^-/CO_2 system, which is the major extracellular buffer. The law of mass action for this buffer system states that

$$pH = 6.1 + \log\frac{[HCO_3^-]}{[CO_2]}.$$

Since $[CO_2]$ equals the solubility coefficient times the P_{CO_2}, this can be rewritten

$$pH = 6.1 + \log\frac{[HCO_3^-]}{0.03 \times P_{CO_2}}.$$

This, the familiar Henderson–Hasselbach equation, tells us that pH constancy depends on a constant ratio in the concentration between the two buffer components. If this ratio increases because either HCO_3^- increases or CO_2 decreases, pH will increase (alkalosis). If the ratio decreases, because either HCO_3^- decreases or CO_2 increases, pH decreases (acidosis). Regulation of HCO_3^- is mainly a function of the kidneys, and regulation of CO_2 is a respiratory function.

The regulation of HCO_3^- concentration by the kidneys consists of two main components:

1. *Absorption of HCO_3^-.* Because of the high GFR and because plasma HCO_3^- concentrations are also relatively high (24 mEq/L), large amounts of HCO_3^- are filtered. Retrieval of this filtered HCO_3^- is absolutely essential for acid–base balance. It is important to note that this process of renal HCO_3^- absorption does not add new HCO_3^- to the blood, but merely prevents a loss of filtered HCO_3^- into the urine. Therefore, renal HCO_3^- absorption cannot correct an existing metabolic acidosis.

2. *Excretion of H^+.* Under normal dietary conditions, approximately 40 to 80 mmol H^+ is generated daily (mostly sulfuric acid from the metabolism of sulfur-containing amino acids). These H^+ are buffered and therefore consume HCO_3^-. The kidneys must excrete these H^+ to regenerate the HCO_3^- pool (this second task can therefore also be labeled as generation of "new" HCO_3^-).

Mechanisms of Bicarbonate Absorption

Filtered HCO_3^- (about 4300 mEq/day) is efficiently absorbed by renal tubules, predominantly the proximal tubules, so that under normal acid–base conditions very little HCO_3^- is found in the urine. As a rule, all tubular HCO_3^- absorption is the consequence of H^+ secretion, and not of direct absorption of HCO_3^- ions. H^+ are continuously generated inside the cells from the dissociation of H_2O (or by CO_2 reacting with H_2O) and transported into the lumen. In the lumen, secreted H^+ combines with filtered HCO_3^- to form carbonic acid, which is broken down to CO_2 and H_2O in a reaction that is catalyzed by a carbonic anhydrase located in the apical brush border membrane. CO_2 and H_2O are then absorbed passively. The OH^- generated in the cell during this process combine with CO_2 to form HCO_3^-, a reaction catalyzed by a cytosolic carbonic anhydrase. HCO_3^- exits across the basolateral side of the cell and returns to the blood in association with Na^+. The net balance of this process can be expressed as

$$H_2O + CO_2 \leftarrow H_2CO_3 \leftarrow HCO_3^- + H^+ \leftarrow H_2O \rightarrow OH^- + CO_2 \rightarrow HCO_3^- + Na^+$$

tubular lumen | cell interior | blood

Specific transport proteins in renal epithelial cells cause the H^+ and HCO_3^- to move in the right directions. Two different mechanisms, both located in the apical membrane, are responsible for the movement of protons into the tubular fluid:

1. The first is a Na^+/H^+ exchanger that is driven by the Na^+ gradient and is found in the proximal tubule. In terms of mEq transported, it contributes most to HCO_3^- absorption.

2. The second is a primary active transport of H^+. An H^+-ATPase has been found in the luminal membrane of one class of intercalated collecting duct cells. There is also some evidence for the presence of an H^+, K^+-ATPase similar to that found in parietal cells of the gastric mucosa. Active H^+ transport is responsible for the secretion of smaller amounts of H^+ than Na^+/H^+ exchange, but it can proceed against a steeper gradient.

There are also at least two mechanisms for the transport of HCO_3^- across the basolateral membrane. The movement of HCO_3^- can be coupled to the movement of Na^+ and this is the major exit mechanism in the proximal tubule. In the collecting duct, HCO_3^- exit occurs predominantly through a basolateral Cl^-/HCO_3^- exchanger (equivalent to the band 3 protein of red cells).

Bicarbonate Secretion

Although net HCO_3^- transport for the whole kidney is always in the reabsorptive direction, certain intercalated cells in the cortical portion of the collecting duct can actually secrete HCO_3^-. The HCO_3^--secreting cells have a polarity that is the reverse of the H^+-secreting cells; that is, they possess a basolateral H^+-ATPase and probably a luminal Cl^-/HCO_3^- exchanger. HCO_3^- secretion may be important during consumption of a diet providing base equivalents and for the correction of metabolic alkalosis.

Excretion of H^+ Ions (Formation of New HCO_3^-)

Urinary acid excretion cannot to any significant extent occur as free H^+. The absolute minimum urinary pH in humans is about 4.5, corresponding to an H^+ concentration of only 0.03 mEq/L. Since about 40 to 80 mEq of H^+ must be excreted per day, it is clear that most H^+ ions must be excreted in a bound or buffered form. Excretion of bound H^+ is achieved (1) by the titration of luminal nonbicarbonate buffers and (2) by the renal synthesis and excretion of ammonium ions.

Titratable Acidity

Binding of secreted H^+ to filtered nonbicarbonate buffer anions leads to the formation and excretion of urinary titratable acidity (titratable acidity is defined as the number of moles of NaOH that has to be added to bring urine back to pH 7.4). The ability to buffer H^+ depends on its dissociation constant (pK) and the quantity of buffer. Under normal conditions only the $HPO_4^{2-}/H_2PO_4^-$ buffer is present in amounts sufficient to act as an intratubular H^+ acceptor. This buffer pair has a pK of 6.8 and is excreted at a daily rate of about 50 mmol. With the Henderson–Hasselbach equation for the phosphate buffer (pH 6.8 + log $[HPO_4^{2-}]/[H_2PO_4^-]$), the following relations can be calculated (considering only that fraction of total phosphate that is actually excreted, about 25 to 30% of the filtered phosphate load):

	pH	HPO_4^{2-} (mmol/day)	$H_2PO_4^-$ (mmol/day)	H^+ buffered (mmol/day)
Filtrate	7.4	40	10	0
End proximal	6.8	25	25	15
Urine	4.8	0.5	49.5	39.5

This tabulation shows that the buffer capacity of HPO_4^{2-} can be fully utilized if the intratubular pH is lowered sufficiently. In some situations other urinary buffers become important. In diabetic ketoacidosis large amounts of β-hydroxybutyrate are excreted (e.g., 300 mmol/L). Even though this buffer component has a pK of 4.8, it will carry up to 150 mmol H^+ per liter.

Ammonium Excretion

The second form of bound H^+ in the urine is ammonium. The excretion of NH_4^+ is equivalent to the generation of HCO_3^- or excretion of H^+. Glutamine, formed in the liver from glutamate and extracted from the blood by uptake mechanisms in the luminal and basolateral membranes of renal proximal tubule cells, is the major source of urinary ammonium. Ammonium is generated in the proximal tubule by a metabolic pathway in which the degradation of glutamine to glutamate and further to α-ketoglutarate yields 2 NH_4^+ and 2 HCO_3^- (rather than NH_3, CO_2, and H_2O. While the NH_4^+ ions are secreted through distinct transport pathways into the lumen of the proximal tubule, the new HCO_3^- ions are added to the blood HCO_3^- pool.

It is essential that the NH_4^+ that is formed by renal proximal tubules is preferentially secreted into the tubular lumen and then excreted in the urine. If the generated NH_4^+ was absorbed by the renal tubular epithelium (or secreted preferentially into the blood), it would be used to form urea (H_2NCONH_2). Ureagenesis forms H^+ that would consume the produced HCO_3^- and thereby negate net base production. This is shown in the following reactions:

$$2NH_4^+ + CO_2 \rightarrow urea + H_2O + 2H^+$$

or

$$2NH_4^+ + 2HCO_3^- \rightarrow urea + CO_2 + 3H_2O.$$

Urinary H^+ excretion in the form of NH_4^+ is of the order of 40 to 50 mmol/day. Renal NH_4^+ formation and excretion are greatly enhanced in metabolic acidosis. Failure of proximal tubules to generate NH_4^+ is the main reason that chronic renal failure leads to metabolic acidosis.

Regulation of H^+ Secretion

1. *Intracellular pH.* Systemic pH changes, whether caused by changes in plasma HCO_3^- (metabolic) or by changes in P_{CO_2} (respiratory), alter H^+ secretion (and therefore HCO_3^- absorption). Intracellular acidification, as occurs in acidosis, stimulates H^+ secretion and intracellular alkalinization (alkalosis) inhibits it.

2. *Aldosterone.* In addition to affecting Na^+ absorption and K^+ secretion, aldosterone stimulates H^+ secretion by collecting ducts.

3. *Potassium.* Changes in plasma K^+ concentration can affect H^+ secretion, in part by changing intracellular pH. Thus, hypokalemia increases intracellular acidity and stimulates H^+ ion secretion. While the effect of hypokalemia alone is relatively small, a marked stimulation of H^+ secretion results when hypokalemia occurs with high plasma aldosterone levels. In this situation, which can occur in primary hyperaldosteronism or with administration of diuretics, metabolic alkalosis may be generated by the kidneys.

RENAL HANDLING OF GLUCOSE AND AMINO ACIDS

An important function of the renal tubule is retrieval of the glucose and amino acids that are present in glomerular filtrate and which would be lost to the body if they were not reabsorbed. To a large extent, this is a proximal tubule function, and disordered glucose and amino acid transport is characteristic of diseases that disturb proximal tubular function.

Glucose transport by the proximal tubule occurs via a transport protein present in the luminal membrane that carries a glucose molecule together with a sodium ion, the

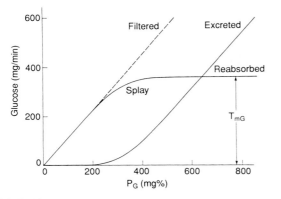

FIGURE 13 Glucose reabsorption. Shown is a typical titration curve for renal glucose reabsorption. At plasma glucose concentrations less than approximately 200 mg%, the filtered glucose is completely reabsorbed, and no glucose is excreted in the urine. When plasma glucose exceeds this level, the filtered load of glucose exceeds the transport capacity of the tubule, and glucose appears in the urine.

glucose–sodium cotransporter. This transporter uses the sodium concentration gradient (sodium concentration is, of course, higher outside the cell than in) to drive the movement of glucose into the cell. Glucose then diffuses out of the cell across the basolateral membrane, a process facilitated by a second carrier protein. The resulting reabsorption process is highly efficient, and in normal circumstances practically all the filtered glucose is removed from the proximal tubule fluid and glucose is virtually absent from urine.

When plasma glucose concentration rises, increasing amounts of glucose are filtered, and at a certain point the filtered load of glucose exceeds the capacity of the proximal transport mechanisms. This maximum reabsorption rate is called the tubular transport maximum for glucose (T_{mG}; Fig. 13). When glucose delivery exceeds the T_{mG}, the excess glucose is excreted in the urine.

Many of the same principles apply to the reabsorption of amino acids. Also a function of the proximal tubule, amino acid absorption is also highly effective. For most amino acids, less than 1% of the amount filtered escapes into the urine. A number of different luminal and basolateral transport proteins are needed to remove the amino acids from the glomerular filtrate. A specific transporter carries the dibasic amino acids, L-arginine and L-lysine, and another carrier is responsible for removal of the acidic amino acids from the tubular fluid. There also are luminal transporters which, like the sodium–glucose cotransporter, exploit the sodium concentration gradient for cotransport of certain amino acids together with sodium. Other carrier molecules in the basement membrane facilitate the exit of the amino acids from the cell.

Bibliography

For a more thorough introduction to normal kidney function:

Berne RM, Levy MN: *Physiology,* 3rd Ed., Chapters 41–43, Mosby-Year Book, St. Louis, 1993.
Guyton AC: *Textbook of Medical Physiology,* 8th Ed., Chapters 25–31, Saunders, New York, 1991.
Koeppen B, Stanton B: *Renal Physiology.* Mosby-Year Book, St. Louis, 1992.
Rose BD: *Clinical Physiology of Acid–Base and Electrolyte Disorders,* 4th Ed. McGraw-Hill, New York, 1994.
Shayman JA: *Renal Physiology,* Lippincott, Philadelphia, 1995.
Vander A: *Renal Physiology,* 4th Ed. McGraw-Hill, New York, 1991.

For more detail on topics covered in this chapter:

Adrogue HJ, Madias NE: Changes in plasma potassium concentration during acute acid–base disturbances. *Am J Med* 71:456–467, 1981.
Baylis C: Glomerular filtration dynamics. In: Lote CJ (ed) *Advances in Renal Physiology.* pp. 33–83, Grune & Stratton, London, 1986.
Beauwkes R, Bonventre JV: Tubular organization and vasculartubular relations in the dog kidney. *Am J Physiol* 229:695–703, 1975.
Debnam ES, Unwin RJ: Hyperglycemia and intestinal and renal glucose transport: Implications for diabetic renal injury. *Kidney Int* 50:1101–1109, 1996.
Kaplan B, Batlle DC: Regulation of potassium balance and metabolism. In: Jacobsen HR, Striker GE, Klahr S (eds) *Principles and Practice of Nephrology.* Mosby, St. Louis, 1995.
Levine SD: Diuretics. *Med Clin North Am* 73:271–282, 1989.
Levey AS: Measurement of renal function in chronic renal disease. *Kidney Int* 38:167–184, 1990.
Lifton RP: Genetic determinants of human hypertension. *Proc Natl Acad Sci USA* 92:8545–8551, 1995.
Robertson GL: Physiology of ADH secretion. *Kidney Int* 32(Suppl 21):S–20, 1987.
Schrier RW: The edematous patient. In: Schrier RW (ed) *Manual of Nephrology.* Little Brown, Boston, 1990.

2

THE GENETIC BASIS OF RENAL TRANSPORT DISORDERS

STEVEN J. SCHEINMAN

The routine measurement of electrolytes and minerals in patient samples produced descriptions of a variety of distinct inherited syndromes of abnormal renal tubular transport. Clinical investigation led to speculation, often quite ingenious, and in some cases controversial, regarding the underlying causes of these syndromes. In the 1990s, the tools of molecular biology made possible the cloning of genes found to be mutated in patients with these monogenic disorders of renal tubular transport. In a sense, these diseases represent experiments of nature that revealed exciting new discoveries. Some of these provided gratifying confirmation of our existing knowledge of transport mechanisms along the nephron. Examples of this include mutations in diuretic-sensitive transporters in Bartter's and Gitelman's syndromes. In other cases, positional cloning led to the discovery of previously unknown proteins, often surprising ones, that appear to play important roles in epithelial transport. The voltage-gated chloride channel ClC-5 and the tight-junction protein paracellin-1, for example, were not known to exist until they were discovered through positional cloning in Dent's disease and inherited hypomagnesemia with hypercalciuria, respectively.

Table 1 summarizes genetic diseases of renal tubular transport for which the molecular basis is known. The diseases listed are each explained by abnormalities of the corresponding protein. Such monogenic conditions tend to be uncommon or rare. Common conditions can often have important genetic components, but they are usually polygenic. In those settings, inheritance is often complex and involves polymorphisms in several genes each of which contributes to the disease phenotype. Some genes responsible for the rare monogenic diseases may also contribute in subtle ways to the common polygenic conditions. Identifying the contribution of these genes, and presumably others yet to be identified, to complex conditions such as hypertension will be the next major challenge of genetics.

DISORDERS OF PROXIMAL TUBULAR TRANSPORT FUNCTION

Selective Proximal Transport Defects

Sodium reabsorption in the proximal tubule occurs through secondary active transport processes in which entry of sodium is coupled to that of glucose, amino acids, or phosphate, or coupled to the exit of protons. Autosomal recessive conditions of impaired transepithelial transport of glucose and dibasic amino acids have been shown to be caused by mutations in these sodium-dependent transporters expressed both in kidney and in the intestine, resulting in urinary losses and intestinal malabsorption of these solutes. Other disorders with renal selective transport defects are also thought, but not yet proven, to result from mutations in transporters expressed specifically in kidney. X-linked (dominant) hypophosphatemic rickets is characterized by impaired Na^+-dependent phosphate reabsorption, in which the maximal transport capacity for phosphate is reduced, as reflected in a reduced number of units of the sodium-dependent phosphate transporter NaPi2 in the apical membrane of proximal tubular cells. In this interesting condition, mutations involve not the gene encoding NaPi2 but rather a neutral endopeptidase expressed in bone that is thought to be involved in processing of a circulating phosphate transport-regulating hormone designated "phosphatonin."

The rare condition of familial proximal renal tubular acidosis was reported in association with mutations that inactivate the basolateral sodium–bicarbonate cotransporter NBC. These patients also suffer ocular abnormalities leading to blindness, probably as a consequence of impaired bicarbonate transport in the eye.

Inherited Fanconi Syndrome

Several inherited forms of the Fanconi syndrome are associated with generalized impairment in reabsorptive function of the proximal tubule. These include the X-linked oculocerebrorenal syndrome of Lowe, in which the gene encoding inositol polyphosphate 5-phosphatase is mutated, and hereditary fructose intolerance, caused by mutations in the gene for aldolase B.

Dent's Disease

In Dent's disease (X-linked recessive nephrolithiasis) the most consistent abnormality is failure to reabsorb low-molecular-weight (LMW) proteins in the proximal tubule. Glycosuria, aminoaciduria, and phosphaturia represent further evidence of proximal tubulopathy. In addition, patients usually are hypercalciuric, often with nephrocalcinosis and kidney stones. The majority of patients progress to renal failure. Some develop rickets. Dent's disease is caused by mutations that inactivate the voltage-gated chloride channel ClC-5. This chloride channel is expressed in the proximal tubule, medullary thick ascending limb (mTAL) of Henle's loop, and the α-intercalated cells of the collecting tubule. In the cells of the proximal tubule, ClC-5 colo-

20

TABLE I

Molecular Bases of Genetic Disorders of Renal Transport

Inherited disorder	Defective protein
Proximal tubule	
Glucose–galactose malabsorption syndrome	Sodium–glucose transporter 1
Dibasic aminoaciduria (lysinuric protein intolerance)	Basolateral dibasic amino acid transporter
X-linked hypophosphatemic rickets	Phosphate regulating gene with homologies to endopeptidases on the X-chromosome (PHEX)
Hereditary hypophosphatemic rickets with hypercalciuria	Unknown
Fanconi's syndrome (hereditary fructose intolerance)	Aldolase B
Oculocerebrorenal syndrome of Lowe	Inositol polyphosphate-5-phosphatase
Cystinuria	Apical cystine–dibasic amino acid transporter
Dent's disease (X-linked nephrolithiasis)[a]	Voltage-gated chloride channel (ClC-5)
Proximal renal tubular acidosis	Basolateral sodium–bicarbonate cotransporter (NBC)
Thick ascending limb of Henle's loop	
Bartter's syndrome	Bumetanide-sensitive Na^+–K^+–$2Cl^-$ cotransporter (NKCC2)
	Apical potassium channel (ROMK)
	Basolateral chloride channel (ClC-Kb)
Familial hypomagnesemia with hypercalciuria	Paracellin-1
Familial benign hypercalcemia[b]	Calcium-sensing receptor (inactivation)
Neonatal severe hyperparathyroidism[b]	Calcium-sensing receptor (inactivation)
Familial hypercalciuric hypocalcemia[b]	Calcium-sensing receptor (activation)
Distal convoluted tubule	
Gitelman's syndrome	Thiazide-sensitive NaCl cotransporter (NCCT)
Pseudohypoparathyroidism Type Ia[c]	Guanine nucleotide-binding protein (G_s)
Collecting duct	
Liddle's syndrome	β and γ subunits of epithelial Na^+ channel (ENaC)
Glucocorticoid-remediable aldosteronism	11β-Hydroxylase and aldosterone synthase (chimeric gene)[d]
Syndrome of apparent mineralocorticoid excess	11β-Hydroxysteroid dehydrogenase type II
Pseudohypoaldosteronism	
Type 1	
Autosomal recessive	α, β, γ subunits of ENaC
Autosomal dominant	Mineralocorticoid (type I) receptor
Type 2 (Gordon syndrome)	Unknown
Distal renal tubular acidosis	
Autosomal recessive	B1 subunit of proton ATPase
Autosomal dominant	Basolateral anion exchanger (AE1)
Carbonic anhydrase II deficiency[e]	Carbonic anhydrase type II
Nephrogenic diabetes insipidus	
X-linked	Arginine vasopressin 2 (V2) receptor
Autosomal	Aquaporin 2 water channel

[a]Gene also expressed in mTAL and collecting duct.
[b]Gene also expressed in collecting duct and elsewhere.
[c]Gene also expressed in proximal tubule where functional abnormalities are clinically apparent.
[d]Gene expressed in adrenal gland.
[e]Clinical phenotype can be of proximal RTA, distal RTA, or combined.

calizes with the H^+-ATPase in subapical endosomes. These endosomes are important in the processing of proteins that are filtered at the glomerulus and taken up by the proximal tubule through adsorptive endocytosis. The activity of the H^+-ATPase acidifies the endosomal space, releasing the proteins from membrane binding sites and making them available for proteolytic degradation. Chloride flow through channels into the endosome appears to be necessary to dissipate the positive charge generated by proton entry. Thus, mutations that inactivate ClC-5 in patients with Dent's disease would interfere with the mechanism for reabsorption of LMW proteins and explain the consistent finding of LMW proteinuria. Glycosuria, aminoaciduria, and phosphaturia are less consistently seen and may be secondary consequences of ClC-5 inactivation through mechanisms that are not yet understood. How inactivation of ClC-5 explains the hypercalciuria and renal failure are other unanswered questions in this disease.

DISORDERS OF TRANSPORT IN THE MEDULLARY THICK ASCENDING LIMB OF HENLE

Bartter's Syndrome

Solute transport in the mTAL involves the coordinated functions of a set of transport proteins depicted in Fig. 1. These are the bumetanide-sensitive Na^+–K^+–2Cl^- cotransporter (NKCC2)

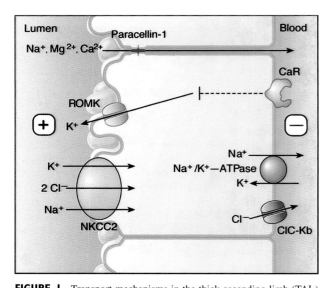

FIGURE I Transport mechanisms in the thick ascending limb (TAL) of Henle's loop indicating transport proteins affected by mutations in genetic diseases. Reabsorption of sodium chloride occurs through the electroneutral activity of the bumetanide-sensitive Na^+–K^+–2Cl^- cotransporter NKCC2. Activity of the basolateral Na^+, K^+-ATPase provides the driving force for this transport, and also generates a high intracellular concentration of potassium which exits through the ATP-regulated apical potassium channel ROMK. This assures an adequate supply of potassium for the activity of the NKCC2 transporter, and also produces a lumen-positive electrical potential which itself is the driving force for paracellular reabsorption of calcium, magnesium, and sodium ions through the tight junctions and involving the protein paracellin-1. Chloride transported into the cell by NKCC2 exits the basolateral side of the cell through the voltage-gated chloride channel ClC-Kb. Activation of the extracellular calcium-sensing receptor CaR inhibits solute transport in the TAL by inhibiting activity of the ROMK potassium channel, and possibly other mechanisms. Mutations that inactivate NKCC2, ROMK, or ClC-Kb occur in patients with Bartter's syndrome, resulting in salt-wasting, hypokalemic metabolic alkalosis, and hypercalciuria. Mutations in paracellin-1 occur in the syndrome of familial hypomagnesemic hypercalciuria. Mutations that inactivate the CaR are associated with enhanced calcium transport and hypocalciuria in familial benign hypercalcemia, and mutations that activate the CaR occur in patients with familial hypercalciuria with hypocalcemia. Adapted from Scheinman *et al.* (1999), with permission. Copyright © 1999, Massachusetts Medical Society. All rights reserved.

and the renal outer medullary potassium channel (ROMK) on the apical surface of cells of the mTAL, and the chloride channel ClC-Kb on the basolateral surface. Mutations in any of the genes encoding these three proteins lead to the phenotype of Bartter's syndrome. The ClC-Kb basolateral chloride channel provides the route for chloride exit to the interstitium. Flow of potassium through the ROMK channel is important in assuring that potassium concentrations in the tubular lumen will not be limiting for the activity of the Na^+–K^+–2Cl^- cotransporter, and also maintains a positive electrical potential in the lumen of this nephron segment. This positive charge is the driving force for paracellular reabsorption of calcium and magnesium.

Bartter's syndrome presents in infancy or childhood, often as a failure to thrive. It is characterized by hypokalemic metabolic alkalosis, typically with hypercalciuria, and these patients thus resemble patients chronically taking loop diuretics that inhibit activity of NKCC2 pharmacologically. Defective function of any of these three proteins leads to impaired salt reabsorption in the mTAL, resulting in volume contraction and activation of the renin–angiotensin–aldosterone axis, which stimulates distal tubular secretion of potassium and protons and produces hypokalemic metabolic alkalosis. Despite impaired reabsorption of magnesium, serum magnesium levels are usually normal in patients with Bartter's syndrome, but occasionally are mildly depressed. The hypercalciuria often leads to nephrocalcinosis, particularly in those patients with mutations in genes encoding NKCC2 and ROMK rather than ClC-Kb. Mutations in these three genes account for most but not all cases of Bartter's syndrome, suggesting that other genes may also be responsible in some patients with Bartter's syndrome.

Familial Hypomagnesemic Hypercalciuria

Reabsorption of calcium and magnesium in the mTAL occurs through the paracellular route driven by the positive electrical potential in the tubular lumen. Selective movement of cations (calcium, magnesium, and sodium) is determined by the tight junctions between the epithelial cells. Disturbance of this selective paracellular barrier would be expected to produce parallel disorders in the reabsorption of calcium and magnesium.

A familial syndrome of hypomagnesemia with substantial renal magnesium losses, and associated with hypercalciuria, has been reported to be inherited in an autosomal recessive fashion. Patients develop nephrocalcinosis, renal failure, and kidney stones. Through investigation of these families by positional cloning, a gene encoding a protein designated paracellin-1 was discovered. Paracellin-1 is homologous to the claudin family of tight-junction proteins. It is expressed at the tight junction between cells of the mTAL (Fig. 1) as well as in the distal convoluted tubule. A range of mutations in this gene have been identified and segregate with disease in families with this syndrome. This is the first instance of a disease shown to result from mutations that alter a tight-junction protein. It is thought that paracellin-1 either itself constitutes the pore in the tight junction that permits selective conductance of cations or is a regulator of the conductance.

Familial Hypocalciuric Hypercalcemia

The extracellular calcium-sensing receptor (CaR) is expressed in many tissues where the ambient calcium concentration triggers a cellular response. In the parathyroid gland, activation of the CaR suppresses synthesis and release of parathyroid hormone. In the kidney, the CaR is expressed on the basolateral surface of cells of the TAL (cortical more than medullary), on the lumenal surface of the cells of the papillary collecting duct, and in other portions of the nephron. Activation of the CaR in the TAL probably mediates the known effects of hypercalcemia to inhibit the transport of calcium, magnesium, and sodium in this nephron segment. For example, CaR activation inhibits activity of the ROMK potassium channel (Fig. 1). This would be expected to reduce the positive electrical potential in the lumen and thereby suppress the driving force for reabsorption of calcium and magnesium. In the papillary collecting duct, activation of the apical CaR could explain the effects of hypercalciuria to impair the hydroosmotic response to vasopressin.

In familial hypocalciuric hypercalcemia (FHH), loss-of-function mutations of the CaR increase the set point for calcium sensing, resulting in hypercalcemia with relative elevation of parathyroid hormone levels. Urinary calcium excretion is low because of enhanced calcium reabsorption in the TAL and PTH-stimulated calcium transport in the distal convoluted tubule. FHH occurs in patients heterozygous for such mutations, and is benign, since tissues are resistant to the high serum calcium levels. A family history is very important in distinguishing FHH from primary hyperparathyroidism, and parathyroidectomy should not be performed. Infants of consanguineous parents with FHH can be homozygous for these mutations, resulting in neonatal severe hyperparathyroidism, which is characterized by severe hypercalcemia with marked hyperparathyroidism, fractures, and failure to thrive.

Other mutations result in constitutive activation of the CaR, and this produces hypocalcemia with hypercalciuria, without elevation in PTH concentrations. It has been speculated but not confirmed that such mutations, if they produce mild gain-of-function of the CaR without frank hypocalcemia, could be responsible for some cases of idiopathic hypercalciuria.

DISORDERS OF TRANSPORT IN THE DISTAL CONVOLUTED TUBULE

Gitelman's Syndrome

Reabsorption of sodium chloride in the distal convoluted tubule occurs through electroneutral transport mediated by the thiazide-sensitive sodium chloride cotransporter (NCCT). Inhibition of NCCT leads to hyperpolarization of distal convoluted tubular cells, and this stimulates the entry of calcium through apical calcium channels. Mutations in the NCCT gene are associated with Gitelman's syndrome, another condition of hypokalemic metabolic alkalosis sometimes considered to be a variant of Bartter's syndrome. An essential distinction between Gitelman's and Bartter's syndrome is the hypocalciuria in Gitelman's syndrome, a consequence of the enhanced calcium transport that results from inactivation of NCCT or its inhibition by thiazide diuretics, in contrast to the hypercalciuria that occurs in Bartter's syndrome or in patients taking loop diuretics. These findings are satisfying in that they connect nicely the clinical physiology with molecular physiology. However, our current understanding of renal transport does not yet allow us to explain the fact that significant hypomagnesemia with renal magnesium wasting is typical of Gitelman's syndrome, whereas in Bartter's syndrome it is much less common and, when it does occur, is milder.

DISORDERS OF TRANSPORT IN THE COLLECTING TUBULE

Liddle's Syndrome

Sodium reabsorption by the principal cells of the cortical collecting duct is under physiological regulation by aldosterone. As in other cells, low intracellular sodium concentrations are maintained by the basolateral Na$^+$, K$^+$-ATPase, and this drives sodium entry through amiloride-sensitive epithelial sodium channels (ENaC) on the apical surface. Mutations that render ENaC persistently open produce, as would be predicted, a syndrome of excessive sodium reabsorption and low-renin hypertension known as Liddle's syndrome. This is an autosomal dominant condition often presenting in children with severe hypertension and hypokalemic alkalosis. It resembles primary hyperaldosteronism; however, serum aldosterone levels are quite low, and for this reason the disease has also been referred to as pseudoaldosteronism. In their original description of the syndrome, Liddle and colleagues demonstrated that aldosterone excess was not responsible for this disease and that while spironolactone had no effect on the hypertension, patients did respond well to triamterene or dietary sodium restriction. They proposed that the primary abnormality was excessive renal salt conservation and potassium secretion independent of mineralocorticoid. This proved to be correct and is explained by the excessive sodium channel activity. Renal transplantation in Liddle's original proband led to resolution of the hypertension, consistent with the defect being intrinsic to the kidneys.

In Liddle's syndrome, gain-of-function mutations in the ENaC produce channels that are resistant to downregulation by physiologic stimuli such as volume expansion. ENaC is formed by three homologous subunits designated αENaC, βENaC, and γENaC. Missense or truncating mutations in patients with Liddle's syndrome alter the carboxyl-terminal cytoplasmic tail of the β or γ subunits in a domain that is important for interactions with the cytoskeletal protein that regulates activity of ENaC. In addition to the severe phenotype of Liddle's syndrome resulting from these mutations, it has been proposed that polymorphisms in the ENaC sequence that have less dramatic effects on sodium channel function could contribute to the much more common low-renin variant of essential hypertension.

Two other hereditary conditions produce hypertension in children with clinical features resembling primary hyperaldosteronism. The syndrome of apparent mineralocorticoid excess (AME) is an autosomal recessive disease in which the renal isoform of the 11β-hydroxysteroid dehydrogenase enzyme is inactivated by mutation. This results in failure to convert cortisol to cortisone locally in the collecting duct, allowing cortisol to activate mineralocorticoid receptors and produce a syndrome resembling primary hyperaldosteronism but, like Liddle's syndrome, with low circulating levels of aldosterone. As in Liddle's syndrome, renal transplantation has been reported to result in resolution of hypertension in AME. Not a renal tubular disorder, the autosomal dominant condition glucocorticoid-remediable aldosteronism (GRA) is caused by a chromosomal rearrangement that produces a chimeric gene in which the regulatory region of the gene encoding the steroid 11β-hydroxylase (which is part of the cortisol biosynthetic pathway and normally is regulated by ACTH) is fused to distal sequences of the aldosterone synthase gene. This results in production of aldosterone that responds to ACTH rather than normal regulatory stimuli. Patients with GRA may have variable elevations in plasma aldosterone levels, and they are often normokalemic. Aldosterone levels suppress with glucocorticoid therapy. Elevated urinary levels of 18-oxacortisol and 18-hydroxycortisol are characteristic of GRA.

Mutations in ENaC that inactivate channel activity also occur, and are responsible for a phenotype of renal salt wasting, hyperkalemia, high plasma renin activity, and high serum aldosterone concentrations. This disease, the mirror image of Liddle's syndrome, is known as pseudohypoaldosteronism and is inherited as an autosomal recessive trait. It presents typically in the neonatal period with vomiting, hyponatremia, and failure to thrive. Respiratory distress and respiratory tract infections also occur. An autosomal dominant form of pseudohypoaldosteronism is associated with mutations that impair function of the mineralocorticoid receptor.

Hereditary Renal Tubular Acidosis

Secretion of acid by the α-intercalated cells of the collecting duct is accomplished by the apical H^+-ATPase. Cytosolic carbonic anhydrase catalyzes the formation of bicarbonate from hydroxyl ions, and this bicarbonate then exits the cell in exchange for chloride through the basolateral anion exchanger AE1. Mutations affecting each of these proteins have been documented in patients with hereditary forms of renal tubular acidosis (RTA). Autosomal recessive distal RTA is associated with mutations in the B1 subunit of the H^+-ATPase. This form of RTA is often severe, presenting in young children, and can be associated with hearing loss, consistent with the fact that this ATPase is expressed in the cochlea and the endolymphatic sac of the inner ear as well as in the kidney. Autosomal dominant RTA, a milder disease often undetected until adulthood, is associated with mutations in the basolateral anion exchanger AE1. Other genetic loci appear to be responsible for additional familial cases of distal RTA. Familial deficiency of carbonic anhydrase II is also characterized by cerebral calcification and osteopetrosis, the latter reflecting the important role of carbonic anhydrase in osteoclast function. The acidification defect in carbonic anhydrase II deficiency affects bicarbonate reabsorption in the proximal tubule as well as in the collecting duct.

Nephrogenic Diabetes Insipidus

Reabsorption of water across the cells of the collecting duct occurs only when arginine vasopressin (AVP) is present. AVP activates V2 receptors on the principal cells and cells of the inner medullary collecting duct, initiating a cascade that results in insertion of aquaporin 2 (AQP-2) water channel pores into the apical membranes of these cells. The V2 receptor is encoded by a gene on the X chromosome, and the most common form of nephrogenic diabetes insipidus is caused by inactivating mutations in the V2 receptor gene. This results in vasopressin-resistant polyuria that is typically more severe in males, and is also associated with impaired responses to the effects of AVP that are mediated by extrarenal V2 receptors, specifically vasodilatation and endothelial release of von Willebrand's factor. Less commonly, families have been described with autosomal recessive inheritance of nephrogenic diabetes insipidus (NDI), and these patients have mutations in the gene encoding AQP-2 that result in either impaired trafficking of water channels to the plasma membrane or defective pore function. Rare autosomal dominant occurrence of NDI with mutation in AQP-2 has also been reported.

Bibliography

Guay-Woodford LM: Bartter syndrome: Unraveling the pathophysiologic enigma. *Am J Med* 105:151–162, 1998.

Hebert S, Brown E, Harris H: Role of the Ca^{2+}-sensing receptor in divalent mineral ion homeostasis. *J Exp Biol* 200:295–302, 1997.

Igarashi T, Inatomi J, Sekine T, *et al.*: Mutations in SLC4A4 cause permanent isolated proximal renal tubular acidosis with ocular abnormalities. *Nat Genet* 23:264–6, 1999.

Karet FE, Finberg KE, Nelson RD, *et al.*: Mutations in the gene encoding B1 subunit of H^+-ATPase cause renal tubular acidosis with sensorineural deafness. *Nat Genet* 21:84–90, 1999.

Knoers NV, Monnens LL: Nephrogenic diabetes insipidus. *Semin Nephrol* 19:344–52, 1999.

Lloyd SE, Pearce SHS, Fisher SE, *et al.*: A common molecular basis for three inherited kidney stone diseases. *Nature* 379:445–449, 1996.

Reilly RF, Ellison DH: Mammalian distal tubule: Physiology, pathophysiology, and molecular anatomy. *Physiol Rev* 80:277–313, 2000.

Scheinman SJ: X-linked hypercalciuric nephrolithiasis: Clinical syndromes and chloride channel mutations. *Kidney Int.* 53:3–17, 1998.

Scheinman SJ, Guay-Woodford LM, Thakker RV, Warnock DG: Genetic disorders of renal electrolyte transport. *N Engl J Med* 340:1177–1187, 1999.

Simon DB, Nelson-Williams C, Bia MJ, *et al.*: Gitelman's variant of Bartter's syndrome, inherited hypokalaemic alkalosis, is caused by mutations in the thiazide-sensitive Na–Cl cotransporter. *Nat Genet* 12:24–30, 1996.

Simon DB, Bindra RS, Mansfield TA, *et al.*: Mutations in the chloride channel gene, CLCNKB, cause Bartter's syndrome type III. *Nat Genet* 17:171–178, 1997.

Simon DB, Lu Y, Choate KA, *et al.*: Paracellin-1, a renal tight junction protein required for paracellular Mg resorption. *Science* 285:103–106, 1999.

Warnock DG: Liddle syndrome: An autosomal dominant form of human hypertension. *Kidney Int* 53:18–24, 1998.

Warnock DG: Hypertension. *Semin Nephrol* 19:374–380, 1999.

CLINICAL EVALUATION OF RENAL FUNCTION

SUZANNE K. SWAN AND WILLIAM F. KEANE

GLOMERULAR FILTRATION RATE

The kidney performs many functions including salt and water balance, excretion of nitrogenous wastes, acid–base regulation, electrolyte homeostasis, bone metabolism, erythropoiesis, and blood pressure control, but the glomerular filtration rate (GFR) is generally considered the best measure of renal function. This consensus is due, in part, to the fact that filtration capacity correlates best with the various functions of the nephron. For example, uremic symptoms generally manifest when the GFR falls below 10 to 15 mL/min. Similarly, alterations in erythropoietic activity as well as calcium and phosphate metabolism can be predicted based on changes in GFR.

Glomerular filtration rate is defined as the renal clearance of a particular substance from plasma, and it is expressed as the volume of plasma that can be completely cleared of that substance in a unit of time. Renal clearance can be mathematically expressed by the following equation:

$$\text{Clearance}_x \,(\text{mL/min}) = \frac{\text{urine}_x \,(\text{mg/dL}) \times \text{volume (mL/min)}}{\text{plasma}_x \,(\text{mg/dL})}$$

where x is the substance being cleared.

The ability of the kidney to filter blood and clear it of nitrogenous wastes while preventing specific solutes, proteins, and blood cells from being excreted from the body constitutes normal glomerular function. An ideal marker for GFR determinations would appear endogenously in the plasma at a constant rate, be freely filtered by the glomerulus, not undergo reabsorption or secretion by the renal tubule, and not be eliminated by extrarenal routes. Although an ideal marker for measuring GFR that could be implemented clinically in an efficient and cost-effective manner has yet to be identified, these characteristics can be helpful for comparing the advantages and disadvantages of the various methods available for GFR estimation or quantification.

Blood Urea Nitrogen

The isolation of urea in 1773 by Rouelle marked the beginning of efforts to quantify renal function. Blood urea nitrogen, or BUN, was first used as a clinical diagnostic test of kidney function in 1903, and urea clearance was introduced in 1929. The BUN concentration remains in wide use today, even though it is well recognized that its many drawbacks make it a poor measure of renal function. It possesses few of the characteristics of an ideal marker. For example, the rate of production of urea is not constant. The urea concentration increases whenever the amount of nitrogenous substrate available for urea production increases. Thus, protein breakdown from increased tissue catabolism, corticosteroids, gastrointestinal bleeding, or hyperalimentation can increase BUN. With cirrhosis and protein malnutrition, the BUN falls because of diminished urea production. Urea is not only filtered at the glomerulus, but also reabsorbed in the tubules. Urea reabsorption parallels proximal and distal nephron fluid reabsorption. Its concentration will rise with volume contraction or prerenal conditions such as congestive heart failure. Conversely, when patients are volume expanded, as with an ongoing saline infusion or with SIADH, urea reabsorption and BUN fall. Table 1 summarizes the nonrenal factors affecting urea levels. Normal BUN concentrations range from 7 to 21 mg/dL. The molecular mass of urea is 60 Da and 28 of the 60 Da are urea nitrogen. To convert from mg/dL to international units (mM/L) divide by 2.8.

Serum Creatinine

Creatinine is a metabolite of the creatine and phosphocreatine found in skeletal muscle. As such, creatinine concentrations reflect muscle mass and vary little from day to day. Nonetheless, significant variability in creatinine production can be seen in a given individual over time as muscle mass changes or acutely with massive myocyte turnover. Similarly, age- and gender-associated differences in creatinine production are proportional to muscle mass. Normal serum creatinine concentrations range from 0.6 to 1.2 mg/dL. The molecular mass of creatinine is 113 Da. To convert from mg/dL to international units (μmol/L), multiply by 88.

Creatinine is a small molecule that is not protein bound and thus freely filtered by the glomerulus. It does, however, undergo tubular secretion into the urinary space; the rate

25

TABLE I

Nonrenal Factors Altering Blood Urea Nitrogen
or Serum Creatinine

	Increased	Decreased
Urea	Prerenal	Cirrhosis
	CHF	Protein malnutrition
	Volume contraction	Water excess
	GI bleeding	(SIADH)
	Catabolic state	
	Corticosteroids	
	Hyperalimentation	
	Tetracyclines	
Creatinine	Overproduction	Decreased muscle mass
	Rhabdomyolysis	Cirrhosis
	Vigorous, sustained	
	exercise	
	Anabolic steroids	
	Dietary supplements	
	(creatine)	
	Blocked tubular secretion	
	Trimethoprim	
	Cimetidine	
	Aspirin	
	Assay interference	
	Cephalosporins	
	Flucytosine	
	Ketosis	
	Methyldopa, levodopa	
	Ascorbic acid	

of which varies within an individual and between individuals as well as with level of renal function. Lastly, like urea, creatinine concentrations can be altered by nonrenal factors as listed in Table 1. Ketones, cephalosporins, glucose, uric acid, and plasma proteins may result in falsely elevated creatinine values when the Jaffe colorimetric method is used. Additionally, cimetidine and trimethoprim block tubular secretion of creatinine. Use of these drugs can lead to a rise in serum creatinine. However, this does not signify a fall in GFR, and an accompanying rise in BUN does not occur. Conversely, low creatinine concentrations independent of any change in GFR may be seen in patients with decreased muscle mass due to malnutrition, cachexia, or cirrhosis.

Finally, the ratio between the BUN and serum creatinine may be helpful when assessing the patient with acute renal failure. Under normal circumstances the BUN:creatinine ratio is 10, but this value will rise to greater than 20 when, for example, the extracellular fluid volume is contracted. Since urea is reabsorbed in the proximal tubule and distal nephron while creatinine is not, any disease process which stimulates reabsorption or promotes a "sodium avid" state will increase BUN relative to creatinine. Thus, prerenal azotemia will have a BUN:creatinine ratio of 20 or greater while acute tubular necrosis ("renal" azotemia) will have a ratio of 10:1 since tubular reabsorption of urea is not preferentially increased. Again, all of the nonrenal factors listed in Table 1 which can increase or decrease BUN and

creatinine must be considered when interpreting the BUN:creatinine ratio.

Serum creatinine has become a standard laboratory measure of renal function due to its convenience and low cost. Unfortunately, it remains a crude marker of GFR. Creatinine concentrations often fail to detect mild to moderate reductions in GFR due to the nonlinear relationship between creatinine concentrations in the blood and GFR as shown in Fig. 1. Stated another way, seemingly small changes in serum creatinine at the low end of the creatinine range, are actually associated with large decrements in GFR. For example, an increase in serum creatinine from 0.6 to 1.2 mg/dL could reflect an approximate 50% reduction in GFR. If no historical creatinine values were available for a patient with a serum creatinine of 1.2 mg/dL, no attention would be paid to this value since it falls within the normal range of creatinine concentrations. When creatinine values rise from 5 to 8 mg/dL, nephrologists are often emergently consulted. This rise is somewhat less critical in that GFR has potentially fallen from 20 to 15 mL/min. Thus, although creatinine can be used to estimate GFR because it varies inversely with the level of renal function, it falls far short of being an ideal marker.

Inulin Clearance

As stated previously, GFR can be quantified as the rate at which a volume of plasma is cleared of a substance per unit time. Inulin, a fructose polymer with molecular mass of 5200 Da, is a substance that is freely filtered, neither reabsorbed nor secreted by the tubules, and eliminated solely

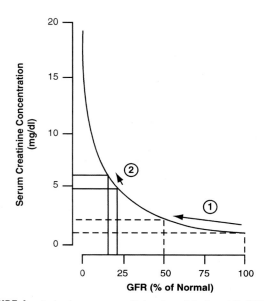

FIGURE 1 A rise in serum creatinine from 1 to 2 mg/dL (①) represents a 50% reduction in GFR. Conversely, a rise in serum creatinine from 4.8 to 6 mg/dL (②) represents a decline in GFR of approximately 20–15%.

by the kidneys. As such, inulin clearance (C_{in}), conventionally considered the gold standard for GFR determination, is one of the most accurate measures of renal function. Inulin clearance can be expressed by the following equation:

$$C_{in} \text{ (mL/min)}$$
$$= \frac{\text{urine inulin (mg/dL)} \times \text{urine volume (mL/min)}}{\text{plasma inulin (mg/dL)}}$$

Inulin, however, is an exogenous compound derived from chicory as well as the Jerusalem artichoke and therefore must be administered as a continuous infusion to achieve steady-state concentrations in the blood. The inconvenience of administration, cost, and limited supply of inulin preclude its routine implementation in clinical practice. In a similar fashion, clearance of radionuclide markers such as ^{125}I-labeled iothalamate, can be used to measure GFR reliably, but such methods are also costly. As they involve radiation exposure, special handling of radioactive samples and skilled staff are needed to perform such testing.

Creatinine Clearance

Unlike inulin, creatinine is produced endogenously by hepatic conversion of skeletal muscle creatine to creatinine thus obviating the need for an intravenous infusion when measuring creatinine clearance (C_{cr}). Further, creatinine is freely filtered and not reabsorbed by the tubule. On average, however, 15 to 25% of urinary creatinine derives from tubular secretion via the organic acid pump in the proximal tubule. Thus, creatinine clearance overestimates GFR. The same formula, discussed earlier with respect to inulin clearance, is used to express C_{cr}:

$$C_{cr} \text{ (mL/min)}$$
$$= \frac{\text{urine creatinine (mg/dL)} \times \text{urine volume (mL/min)}}{\text{plasma creatinine (mg/dL)}}$$

The reproducibility of timed urine collections for C_{cr} determinations is limited by the variability in tubular secretion of creatinine as well as the inability of many patients to accurately collect timed urine samples. For the former, high-dose cimetidine can be prescribed during the urine collection in order to block the tubular secretion of creatinine. For the latter, adequacy of a timed urine collection can be ascertained by estimating the total amount of creatinine that should be excreted in a 24-hr period given the fact that daily excretion of creatinine is 15 to 20 mg/kg lean body weight for women and 20 to 25 mg/kg lean body weight for men. Creatinine excretion significantly less than the normal daily rate is usually indicative of an incomplete urine collection.

Estimated Creatinine Clearance and GFR

Cockcroft and Gault devised a formula to estimate C_{cr} at the bedside using the age of a patient and serum creatinine (S_{cr}) value, since both correlate inversely with GFR, and the ideal body weight (IBW) of the patient as follows:

$$\text{Estimated } C_{cr} = \frac{(140 - \text{age}) \times (\text{IBW in kg})}{S_{cr} \times 72}$$

This equation should be multiplied by 0.85 for women. Although the Cockcroft–Gault approach represents an estimate of C_{cr} and thus an overestimate of GFR, it nonetheless provides a quick and reasonably accurate approximation of GFR as illustrated by the following example:

Do these two patients have the same level of renal function?

1. A 20-year-old MN Viking tackle, weighing 144 kg with a serum creatinine of 1.2 mg/dL.

$$C_{cr} = \frac{(140 - 20)(144)}{(1.2) \times (72)}$$

$$C_{cr} = 200 \text{ mL/min}$$

2. A 93-year-old female nursing home resident, weighing 44 kg with a serum creatinine of 1.2 mg/dL.

$$C_{cr} = \frac{(140 - 93)(44)}{(1.2) \times (72)}$$

$$C_{cr} = 24 \times 0.85 = 20 \text{ mL/min}$$

Thus, the answer to the question is "no" since two very different levels of GFR, estimated by the Cockcroft–Gault equation, are found in these two patients with the same serum creatinine value. This formula can be applied only when the serum creatinine value is at a steady state. It cannot be used when the serum creatinine concentration is rapidly changing, for example, in a patient with acute renal failure.

A new equation to predict renal function has been reported which may provide greater accuracy over the Cockcroft–Gault equation. The so-called MDRD Study prediction equation estimates GFR rather than creatinine clearance. The equation, which also predicts GFR over a wide range of values, has been validated in a cohort of patients that differed from the cohort used to derive the equation, although diabetic patients were not included in the MDRD study. It does not require timed urine collections, and factors in a term for ethnicity as well as the serum albumin concentration as follows:

$$\text{GFR} = 170 \times [Scr]^{-0.999} \times [Age]^{-0.176} \times [0.762 \text{ if female}]$$
$$\times [1.180 \text{ if patient is black}] \times [BUN]^{-0.170}$$
$$\times [\text{albumin}]^{0.318}$$

Whether this equation will be routinely implemented remains to be seen, as it is a good deal more complex than the Cockcroft–Gault formula and requires a separate albumin determination. It does provide a more accurate estimate of GFR than the currently used serum creatinine and BUN values.

Newer Methods for GFR Determination

To avoid all of the aforementioned problems with GFR quantitation, investigators have considered plasma clearance techniques using nonradiolabeled compounds. The plasma "decay" or disappearance of iohexol, a nonionic iodinated contrast agent, represents a newer method for measuring GFR. Like inulin, iohexol is filtered but neither reabsorbed nor secreted, and the rate of fall in plasma iodine levels can be converted to a clearance value. Low concentrations of iodine can be measured with X-ray fluorescence techniques in a single blood sample after a bolus injection of iohexol. Iohexol-derived GFR determinations are generally accurate over a wide range of values and the amount of iohexol used appears to be nonnephrotoxic. In patients with GFR values above 30 mL/min, a blood iodine concentration can be drawn within 4 to 5 hr following iohexol administration; in those with values less than 30, blood samples may be drawn 6 to 12 hr after iohexol injection. The obvious drawback to this technique is that patients must wait or return to the laboratory for phlebotomy. Iodine allergy also precludes its use.

Lastly, cystatin C has been reported to be an accurate marker of GFR. Cystatin C is a small protein linked to the cystatin superfamily of cysteine protease inhibitors which is produced by all nucleated cells at a constant rate. It is eliminated from the body by glomerular filtration but does not appear to undergo tubular secretion. As such, the reciprocal of serum cystatin (1/serum cystatin concentration) has been shown to correlate closely with conventional GFR determinations. Clearly, cystatin C has many of the qualities of an ideal marker of GFR, but further experience with this methodology will be necessary before its role in clinical practice can be validated.

Bibliography

Brown SCW, O'Reilly PH: Iohexol clearance for the determination of glomerular filtration rate in clinical practice: Evidence for a new gold standard. *J Urol* 146:675–679, 1991.

Cockcroft DW, Gault MH: Prediction of creatinine clearance from serum creatinine. *Nephron* 16:31–41, 1976.

Dubb JW, Stote RM, Familiar RG, et al.: Effect of cimetidine on renal function in normal man. *Clin Pharmacol Ther* 24:76, 1978.

Fuller NJ, Elia M: Factors influencing the production of creatinine: Implications for the determination and interpretation of urinary creatinine and creatinine in man. *Clin Chem Acta* 175:199, 1988.

Levey AS, Bosch JP, Breyer Lewis J, Greene T, Rogers N, Roth D for the Modification of Diet in Renal Disease Study Group: A more accurate method to estimate glomerular filtration rate from serum creatinine: A new prediction equation. *Ann Intern Med* 130:461–470, 1999.

Mascioli SR, Bantle JP, Freier EF, et al.: Artifactual elevation of serum creatinine level due to fasting. *Arch Intern Med* 144:1575, 1984.

Newman DJ, Thakkar H, Edwards RG, Wilkie M, White T, Grubb AO, Price CP: Serum cystatin C measured by automated immunoassay: A more sensitive marker of changes in GFR than serum creatinine. *Kidney Int* 47:312–318, 1995.

Saah AJ, Kock TR, Drusano GL: Cefoxitin falsely elevates creatinine levels. *JAMA* 247:205, 1982.

Shemesh O, Golbetz H, Kriss JP, et al.: Limitations of creatinine as a filtration marker in glomerulopathic patients. *Kidney Int* 28:830–838, 1985.

Smith HW, Goldring W, Chasis H: The measurement of tubular excretory mass, effective blood flow, and filtration rate in the normal human kidney. *J Clin Invest* 17:263, 1938.

Swan SK, Halstenson CE, Kasiske BL, Collins AJ: Determination of residual renal function with iohexol clearance in hemodialysis patients. *Kidney Int* 49:232–235, 1996.

4

URINALYSIS

ARTHUR GREENBERG

The microscopic examination of the urine sediment is an indispensable part of the evaluation of patients with renal insufficiency, proteinuria, hematuria, urinary tract infection, or nephrolithiasis. The relatively simple chemical tests performed in the routine urinalysis rapidly provide important information about a number of primary renal and systemic disorders. Examination of the urine sediment provides valuable clues about the renal parenchyma. The dipstick tests can be performed by machine and optical devices, or flow cytometry can identify some cells in the urine. However, automated tests cannot detect unusual cells or distinguish among casts. There is no substitute for careful examination of the urine under the microscope. This task must not be delegated; it should be performed personally. The features of a complete urinalysis are listed in Table 1.

TABLE I
The Routine Urinalysis

Appearance
Specific gravity
Chemical tests (dipstick)
  pH
  Protein
  Glucose
  Ketones
  Blood
  Urobilinogen
  Bilirubin
  Nitrites
  Leukocyte esterase
Microscopic examination (formed elements)
  Crystals: urate; calcium phosphate, oxalate,
    or carbonate, triple phosphate; cystine; drugs
  Cells: leukocytes, erythrocytes, renal tubular
    cells, oval fat bodies, transitional epithelium,
    squamous
  Casts: hyaline, granular, RBC, WBC, Tubular cell,
    degenerating cellular, broad, waxy, lipid-laden
  Infecting organisms: bacteria, yeast,
    Trichomonas, nematodes
  Miscellaneous: spermatozoa, mucous threads,
    fibers, starch, hair, and other contaminants

SPECIMEN COLLECTION AND HANDLING

Urine should be collected with a minimum of contamination. A clean catch midstream collection is preferred. If this is not feasible, bladder catheterization is appropriate in adults; the risk of a urinary tract infection following a single catheterization is negligible. Suprapubic aspiration is employed in infants. In the uncooperative male patient, a clean, freshly applied condom catheter and urinary collection bag may be used. Urine in the collection bag of a patient with an indwelling bladder catheter is subject to stasis, however, a sample suitable for examination may be collected by withdrawing urine from above a clamp placed on the drainage tube.

The chemical composition of the urine changes with standing, and the formed elements degenerate over time. The urine is best examined when fresh; a brief period of refrigeration is acceptable. Since bacteria multiply at room temperature, bacterial counts from unrefrigerated urine are unreliable. High urine osmolality and low pH favor cellular preservation. These two characteristics of the first voided morning urine give it particular value in suspected glomerulonephritis.

PHYSICAL AND CHEMICAL PROPERTIES OF THE URINE

Appearance

Normal urine is clear, with a faint yellow tinge due to the presence of urochromes. As the urine becomes more concentrated, its color deepens. Bilirubin, other pathologic metabolites, and a variety of drugs may discolor the urine or change its smell. Suspended erythrocytes, leukocytes, or crystals may render the urine turbid. Conditions associated with a change in the appearance of the urine are listed in Table 2.

Specific Gravity

The specific gravity of a fluid is the ratio of its weight to the weight of an equal volume of distilled water. The urine specific gravity is a conveniently determined but inaccurate surrogate for osmolality. Specific gravities of 1.001–1.035 correspond to an osmolality range of 50–1000 mOsmol/kg. A specific gravity near 1.010 connotes isosthenuria, with a urine osmolality matching that of plasma. Relative to osmolality, the specific gravity is elevated when dense solutes such as protein, glucose, or radiographic contrast are present.

TABLE 2
Selected Substances That May Alter the Physical Appearance or Odor of the Urine

Change	Substance or condition
Color	
White	Chyle, pus, phosphate crystals
Pink/red/brown	Erythrocytes, hemoglobin, myoglobin, porphyrins, beets, senna, cascara, levodopa, methyldopa, deferoxamine, phenolphthalein and congeners, food colorings, metronidazole, phenacetin
Yellow/orange/brown	Bilirubin, urobilin, phenazopyridine urinary analgesics, senna, cascara, mepacrine, iron compounds, nitrofurantoin, riboflavin, rhubarb, sulfasalazine, rifampin, fluorescein, phenytoin
Brown/black	Methemoglobin, homogentisic acid (alcaptonuria), melanin (melanoma), levodopa, methyldopa
Blue or green or green/brown	Biliverdin, *Pseudomonas* infection, dyes (methylene Blue and indigo carmine), triamterene, vitamin B complex, methocarbamol, indican, phenol, chlorophyll
Odor	
Sweet or fruity	Ketones
Ammoniacal	Urea-splitting bacterial infection
Maple syrup	Maple syrup urine disease
Musty or mousy	Phenylketonuria
Sweaty feet	Isovaleric or glutaric acidemia or excess butyric or hexanoic acid
Rancid	Hypermethioninemia, tyrosinemia

Three methods are available for specific gravity measurement. The hydrometer is the reference standard, but it requires a sufficient volume of urine to float the hydrometer as well as equilibration of the specimen to the hydrometer calibration temperature. The second method is based on the well-characterized relationship between urine specific gravity and refractive index. Refractometers calibrated in specific gravity units are commercially available; they require only a drop of urine. Finally, the specific gravity may also be estimated by dipstick.

The specific gravity is used to determine whether the urine is or can be concentrated. During a solute diuresis accompanying hyperglycemia, diuretic therapy, or relief of obstruction, the urine is isosthenuric. In contrast, with a water diuresis due to overhydration or diabetes insipidus, the specific gravity is typically 1.004 or lower. In the absence of proteinuria, glycosuria, or iodinated contrast administration, a specific gravity more than 1.018 implies preserved concentrating ability. Measurement of specific gravity is useful in differentiating between prerenal azotemia and acute tubular necrosis (ATN) and in assessing the import of proteinuria observed in a randomly voided urine. Since the protein indicator strip responds to concentration of protein, the significance of a borderline reading depends on the overall urine concentration.

Chemical Composition of the Urine—Dipstick Methodology

The urine dipstick is a plastic strip to which paper tabs impregnated with chemical reagents have been glued. The reagents in each tab are chromogenic. After timed development, the color on the paper segment is compared to a chart. Some reactions are highly specific. Others are sensitive to the presence of interfering substances or extremes of pH. Discoloration of the urine with bilirubin or blood may obscure the color changes.

pH

The pH test pads employ indicator dyes that change color with pH. The physiologic urine pH ranges from 4.5 to 8. The determination is most accurate if done promptly, since growth of urea-splitting bacteria and loss of CO_2 raise pH. In addition, bacterial metabolism of glucose may produce organic acids and lower pH. These strips are not sufficiently accurate to be used for the diagnosis of renal tubular acidosis.

Protein

Protein measurement uses the protein-error-of-indicators principle. The pH at which some indicators change color varies with the protein concentration of the bathing solution. Protein indicator strips are buffered at an acid pH near their color change point. Wetting them with a protein containing specimen induces a color change. The protein reaction may be scored from trace to 4+ or by concentration. Their equivalence is as follows: trace, 5–20 mg/dL; 1+, 30 mg/dL; 2+, 100 mg/dL; 3+, 300 mg/dL; 4+, greater than 2000 mg/dL. Highly alkaline urine, especially after

contamination with quaternary ammonium skin cleansers, may produce false positive reactions. Protein strips are highly sensitive to albumin but less so to globulins, hemoglobin, or light chains. When light chain proteinuria is suspected, more sensitive assays should be employed. With acid precipitation tests, an acid that denatures protein is added to the urine specimen and the density of precipitate related to the protein concentration. Urine negative by dipstick but positive with sulfosalicylic acid is highly suspicious for light chains. Tolbutamide, high-dose penicillin, sulfonamides, and radiographic contrast may give false positive turbimetric reactions. More sensitive and specific tests for light chains, including immunoelectrophoresis or immunoprecipitation are preferred, but they require specialized equipment. If the urine is very concentrated, the presence of a modest amount of protein is less likely to correspond to significant proteinuria on a 24-hr basis. The protein indicator used for routine dipstick analysis is not sensitive enough to detect microalbuminuria. Special dipsticks are available fo screening for microalbuminuria in incipient diabetic nephropathy (see Chapters 5 and 28).

Blood

Reagent strips for blood rely on the peroxidase activity of hemoglobin to catalyze an organic peroxide with subsequent oxidation of an indicator dye. Free hemoglobin produces a homogeneous color. Intact red cells cause punctate staining. False positive reactions occur if the urine is contaminated with other oxidants such as povidone-iodine, hypochlorite, or bacterial peroxidase. Ascorbate causes false negatives. Myoglobin is also detected, because it has intrinsic peroxidase activity. A urine that is positive for blood by dipstick but shows no red cells on microscopic examination is suspect for myoglobinuria or hemoglobinuria. Pink discoloration of serum may occur with hemolysis, but free myoglobin is seldom present in a concentration sufficient to change the color of plasma. A specific assay for urine myoglobin will confirm the diagnosis.

Specific Gravity

Specific gravity reagent strips actually measure ionic strength using indicator dyes with ionic strength dependent pK_a's. They do not detect glucose or nonionic radiographic contrast.

Glucose

Modern dipstick reagent strips are specific for glucose. They rely on glucose oxidase to catalyze the formation of hydrogen peroxide which reacts with peroxidase and a chromogen to produce a color change. High concentrations of ascorbate or ketoacids reduce test sensitivity. However, the degree of glycosuria occurring in diabetic ketoacidosis is sufficient to prevent false negatives despite ketonuria.

Ketones

Ketone reagent strips depend on the development of a purple color after acetoacetate reacts with nitroprusside. Some strips can also detect acetone, but none react with

β-hydroxybutyrate. False positives may occur in patients taking levodopa or drugs like captopril or mesna that contain free sulfhydryl groups.

Urobilinogen

Urobilinogen is a colorless pigment produced in the gut from metabolism of bilirubin. Some is excreted in feces and the rest reabsorbed and excreted in the urine. In obstructive jaundice, bilirubin does not reach the bowel and urinary excretion of urobilinogen is diminished. In other forms of jaundice, urobilinogen is increased. The urobilinogen test is based on the Ehrlich reaction in which diethylaminobenzaldehyde reacts with urobilinogen in acid medium to produce a pink color. Sulfonamides may produce false positives and degradation of urobilinogen to urobilin false negatives.

Bilirubin

Bilirubin reagent strips rely on the chromogenic reaction of bilirubin with diazonium salts. Conjugated bilirubin is not normally present in the urine. False positives may be observed in patients receiving chlorpromazine or phenazopyridine. False negatives occur in the presence of ascorbate.

Nitrite

This screening test for bacteriuria relies on the ability of gram-negative bacteria to convert urinary nitrate to nitrite which activates a chromogen. False negative results occur with infection with enterococcus or other organisms that do not produce nitrite, when ascorbate is present, or when urine has not been retained in the bladder long enough (approximately 4 hr) to permit sufficient production of nitrite from nitrate.

Leukocytes

Granulocyte esterases can cleave pyrrole amino acid esters, producing free pyrrole that subsequently reacts with a chromogen. The test threshold is 5–15 white blood cells per high power field (WBC/HPF). False negatives occur with glycosuria, high specific gravity, cephalexin or tetracycline therapy, or excessive oxalate excretion. Contamination with vaginal debris may give a positive test result without true urinary tract infection.

MICROSCOPIC EXAMINATION OF THE SPUN URINARY SEDIMENT

Specimen Preparation and Viewing

The contents of the urine are reported as number of cells or casts per high power (400×) field after resuspension of the centrifuged pellet in a small volume of urine. The accuracy and reproducibility of this semiquantitative method depends on using the correct volume of urine. Twelve milliliters of urine should be spun in a conical centrifuge tube for 5 min at 1500–2000 rpm (450 g). After centrifugation, the tube is inverted and drained. The pellet is resuspended in the few drops of urine that remain in the tube after in-

version by flicking the base of the tube gently with a finger or with the use of a pipette. Care should be taken to fully suspend the pellet without excessive agitation. A drop of urine is poured onto a microscope slide or transferred with the pipette. The drop should be sufficient in size that a standard 22 × 22 mm coverslip just floats on the urine. If too little is used, the specimen rapidly dries out. If an excess of urine is applied, it will spill onto the microscope objective or stream distractingly under the coverslip. Rapid commercial urine stains or the Papanicolaou stain may be used to enhance detail. Most nephrologists prefer the convenience of viewing unstained urine. Subdued light is necessary. The condenser and diaphragm are adjusted to maximize contrast and definition. When the urine is dilute and few formed elements are present, detection of motion of objects suspended in the urine ensures that the focal plane is correct. One should scan the urine at low power (100×) to get a general impression of its contents before moving to high power (400×) to look at individual fields. It is useful to scan large areas at low power and move to high power when a structure of interest is identified. Cellular elements should be quantitated by counting or estimating the number in at least 10 representative high power fields. Casts may be quantitated by counting the number per low power field, although most observers use less specific terms such as rare, occasional, few, frequent, and numerous.

Cellular Elements

The principal formed elements of the urine are listed in Table 1. The figures constitute an atlas of selected formed elements.

Erythrocytes

Red blood cells (Fig. 1A, B) may find their way into the urine from any source between the glomerulus and the urethral meatus. The presence of more than two to three erythrocytes per HPF is usually pathologic. Erythrocytes are biconcave disks 7 μm in diameter. They become crenated in hypertonic urine. In hypotonic urine, they swell or burst, leaving ghosts. Erythrocytes originating in the renal parenchyma are dysmorphic, with spicules, blebs, submembrane cytoplasmic precipitation, membrane folding, and vesicles. Those originating in the collecting system retain their uniform shape. Some experienced observers report success differentiating renal parenchymal from collecting system bleeding by systematic examination of erythrocytes using phase contrast microscopy.

Leukocytes

Polymorphonuclear leukocytes (PMN) (Fig. 1C) are approximately 12 μm in diameter and are most readily recognized in a fresh urine before their multilobed nuclei or granules have degenerated. Swollen PMNs with prominent granules displaying Brownian motion are termed "glitter" cells. PMNs indicate urinary tract inflammation. They may occur with intraparenchymal diseases such as glomerulonephritis or interstitial nephritis. They are a prominent feature of upper or lower urinary tract infection. In addition,

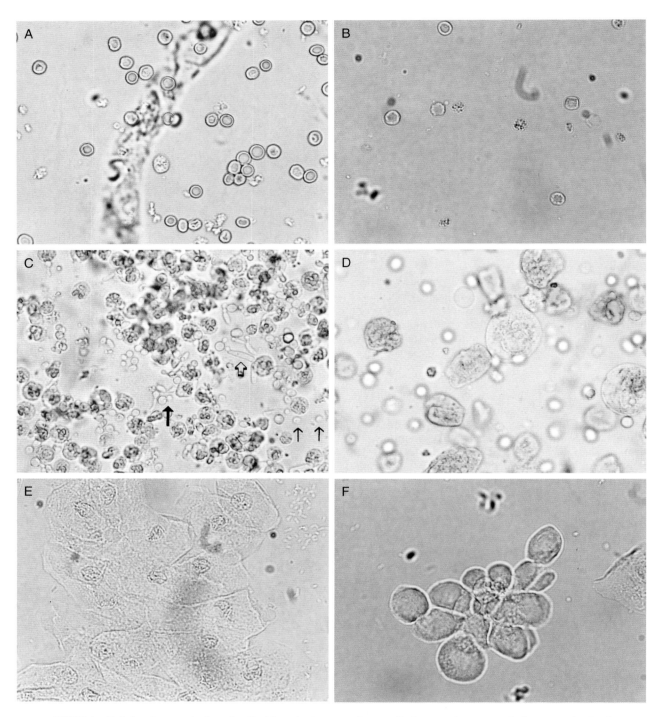

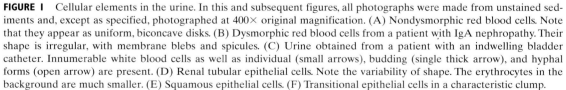

FIGURE 1 Cellular elements in the urine. In this and subsequent figures, all photographs were made from unstained sediments and, except as specified, photographed at 400× original magnification. (A) Nondysmorphic red blood cells. Note that they appear as uniform, biconcave disks. (B) Dysmorphic red blood cells from a patient with IgA nephropathy. Their shape is irregular, with membrane blebs and spicules. (C) Urine obtained from a patient with an indwelling bladder catheter. Innumerable white blood cells as well as individual (small arrows), budding (single thick arrow), and hyphal forms (open arrow) are present. (D) Renal tubular epithelial cells. Note the variability of shape. The erythrocytes in the background are much smaller. (E) Squamous epithelial cells. (F) Transitional epithelial cells in a characteristic clump.

they may appear with periureteral inflammation as in regional ileitis or acute appendicitis.

Renal Tubular Epithelial Cells

Tubular cells (Fig. 1D) are larger than PMNs, ranging from 12 to 20 μm. Proximal tubular cells are oval or egg shaped and tend to be larger than the cuboidal distal tubular cells, but since their size varies with urine osmolality, they cannot be reliably differentiated. In hypotonic urine, it may be difficult to distinguish tubular cells from swollen PMNs. A few tubular cells may be seen in a normal urine. More commonly, they indicate tubular damage or inflammation from ATN or interstitial nephritis.

Other Cells

Squamous cells (Fig. 1E) of urethral, vaginal, or cutaneous origin are large, flat cells with small nuclei. Transitional epithelial cells (Fig. 1F) line the renal pelvis, ureter, bladder, and early urethra. They are rounded cells several times the size of leukocytes and often occur in clumps. In hypotonic urine, they may be confused with swollen tubular epithelial cells.

Casts and Other Formed Elements

Based on their shape and origin, casts are appropriately named. Immunofluorescence studies demonstrate that they consist of a matrix of Tamm–Horsfall urinary mucoprotein in the shape of the distal tubular or collecting duct segment in which they were formed. The matrix has a straight margin helpful in differentiating casts from clumps of cells or debris.

Hyaline Casts

Hyaline casts consist of mucoprotein alone. Because their refractive index is very close to that of urine, they may be difficult to see, requiring subdued light and careful manipulation of the iris diaphragm. Hyaline casts are nonspecific. They occur in concentrated normal urine as well as in numerous pathologic conditions (Fig. 2A).

Granular Casts

Granular casts consist of finely or coarsely granular material. Immunofluorescence studies show that fine granules derive from altered serum proteins. Coarse granules may result from degeneration of embedded cells. Granular casts are nonspecific but usually pathologic. They may be seen after exercise or with simple volume depletion and as a finding in ATN, glomerulonephritis, or tubulointerstitial disease (Fig. 2B).

Waxy Casts

Waxy casts or broad casts are made of hyaline material with a much greater refractive index than hyaline casts, hence their waxy appearance. They behave as though they are more brittle than hyaline casts and frequently have fissures along their edge. Broad casts form in tubules that have become dilated and atrophic due to chronic parenchymal disease Fig. 2C).

Red Blood Cell Casts

Red blood cell casts indicate intraparenchymal bleeding. The hallmark of glomerulonephritis, they are less frequently seen with tubulointerstitial disease. RBC casts have been described along with hematuria in normal individuals after exercise. Fresh RBC casts retain their brown pigment and consist of readily discernable erythrocytes in a tubular shaped cast matrix (Fig. 2D). Over time, the heme color is lost along with the distinct cellular outline. With further degeneration, RBC casts are hard to distinguish from coarsely granular casts. RBC casts may be diagnosed by the company they keep. They appear in a background of hematuria with dysmorphic red cells, granular casts, and proteinuria. Occasionally, the evidence for intraparenchymal bleeding is a hyaline cast with embedded red cells. These have the same pathophysiologic implication as RBC casts.

White Blood Cell Casts

White blood cell casts consist of white cells in a protein matrix. They are characteristic of pyelonephritis and useful in distinguishing this disorder from lower tract infection. They may also be seen with interstitial nephritis and other tubulointerstitial disorders.

Tubular Cell Casts

These casts consist of a dense agglomeration of sloughed tubular cells or just a few tubular cells in a hyaline matrix. They occur in concentrated urine, but are more characteristically seen with the sloughing of tubular cells that occurs with ATN (Fig. 2E).

Bacteria, Yeast, and Other Infectious Agents

Bacillary or coccal forms of bacteria may be discerned even on an unstained urine. Examination of a Gram's stain preparation of unspun urine allows estimation of the bacterial count. One organism per HPF of unspun urine corresponds to 20,000 organisms/mm^3. Individual and budding yeasts and hyphal forms occur with candida infection or colonization. *Candida* organisms are similar in size to erythrocytes, but they are greenish spheres, not biconcave disks. When budding forms or hyphae are present, yeast are obvious (Fig. 1C). *Trichomonas* organisms are identified by their teardrop shape and motile flagellum.

Lipiduria

In the nephrotic syndrome with lipiduria, tubular cells reabsorb luminal fat. Sloughed tubular cells containing fat droplets are called oval fat bodies. Fatty casts contain lipid laden tubular cells or free lipid droplets. By light microscopy, lipid droplets appear round and clear with a green tinge. Cholesterol esters are anisotropic; cholesterol containing droplets rotate polarized light, producing a Maltese cross appearance under polarized light. Triglycerides appear similar by light microscopy, but they are

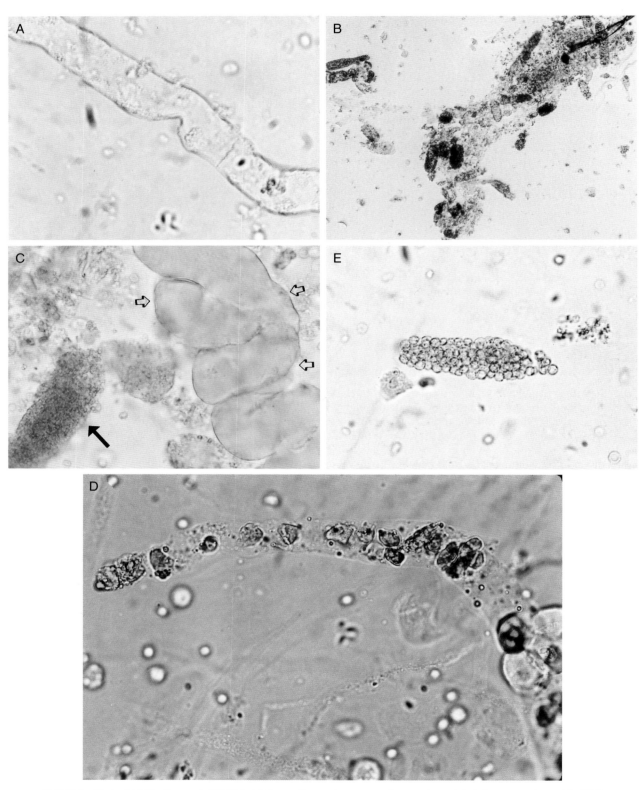

FIGURE 2   Casts. (A) Hyaline cast. (B) "Muddy brown" granular casts and amorphous debris from a patient with ATN (original magnification, 100×). (C) Waxy cast (open arrows) and granular cast (solid arrow) from a patient with lupus nephritis and a telescoped sediment. Note background hematuria. (D) Tubular cell cast. Note the hyaline cast matrix. (E) Red blood cell cast. Background hematuria is also present.

isotropic. Crystals, starch granules, mineral oil, and other urinary contaminants are also anisotropic. Before concluding that anisotropic structures are lipid, the observer must compare polarized and bright field views of the same object (Fig. 3).

Crystals

Crystals may be present spontaneously or precipitate with refrigeration of a specimen. They may be difficult to identify because of similar shapes; the common urinary crystals are described in Table 3. The pH is an important clue to identity, since solubility of a number of urinary constituents is pH dependent. The three most distinctive crystal forms are cystine, calcium oxalate, and magnesium ammonium (triple) phosphate. Cystine crystals are hexagonal plates resembling benzene rings. Calcium oxalate crystals are classically described as "envelope shaped," but when viewed as they rotate in the urine under the microscope, they appear bipyramidal (Fig. 4A). "Coffin-lid" shaped triple phosphates are rectangular with beveled ends

(Fig. 4B). Oxalate may also occur in dumbell shaped crystals (Fig. 4C). Urate may have several forms, including rhomboids (Fig. 4D) and needles (Fig. 4E).

Characteristic Urine Sediments

The urine sediment is a rich source of diagnostic information. Occasionally, a single finding, for example, cystine crystals, is pathognomonic. More often, the sediment must be considered as a whole and interpreted in conjunction with clinical and other laboratory findings. Several patterns bear emphasis.

In the acute nephritic syndrome, the urine may be pink or pale brown and turbid. Blood and moderate proteinuria are present by dipstick. The microscopic examination shows RBCs and RBC casts as well as granular and hyaline casts. WBC casts are rare. In the nephrotic syndrome, the urine is clear or yellow. Increased foaming may be noted because of the elevated protein content. In comparison to the sediment of nephritic patients, the nephrotic sediment is bland. Hyaline casts and lipiduria with oval fat bodies or lipid-laden casts predominate. Granular casts and

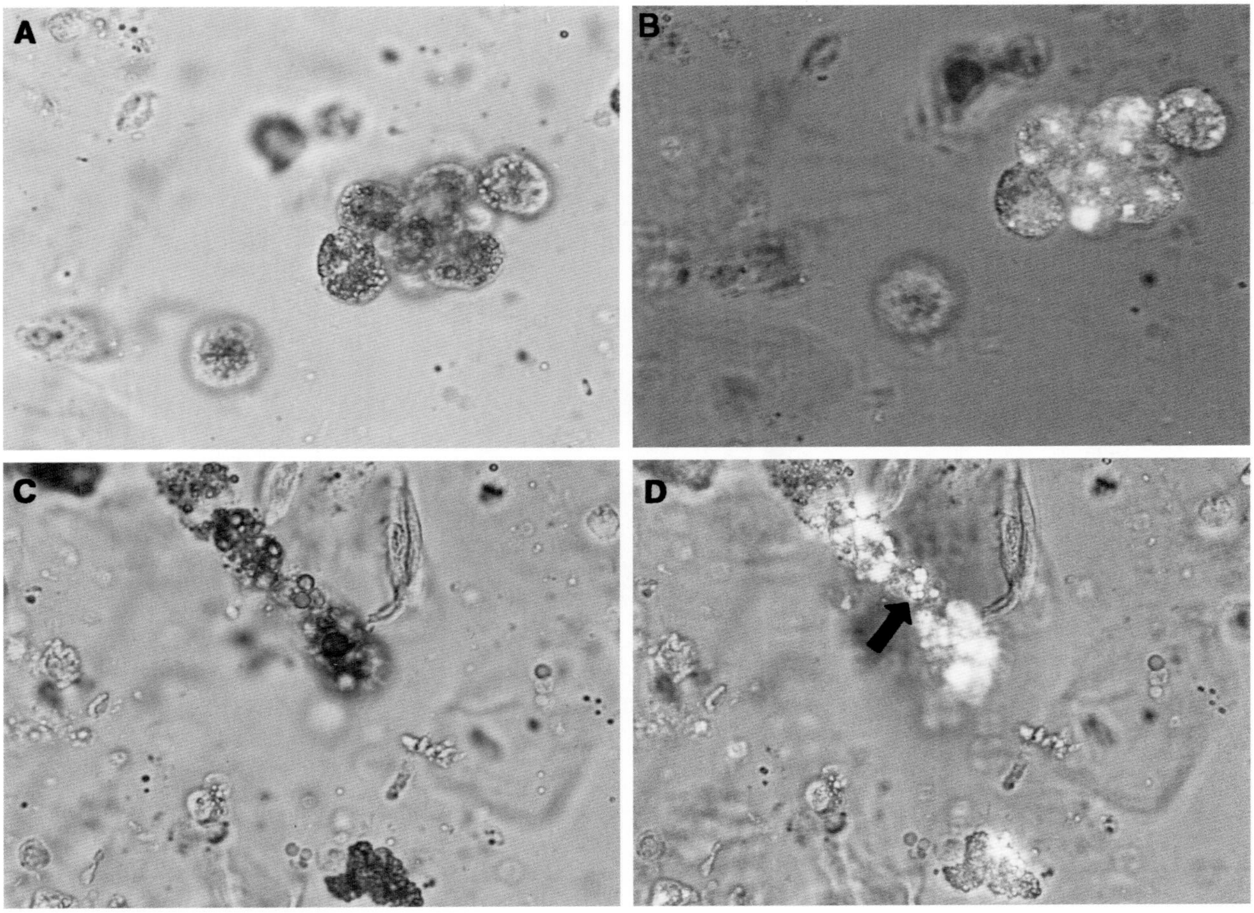

FIGURE 3   Lipid. (A) Oval fat bodies, bright field illumination. (B) Same field under polarized light. (C) Lipid-laden cast, bright field illumination. (D) Same field under polarized light. Characteristic Maltese cross shown at arrow.

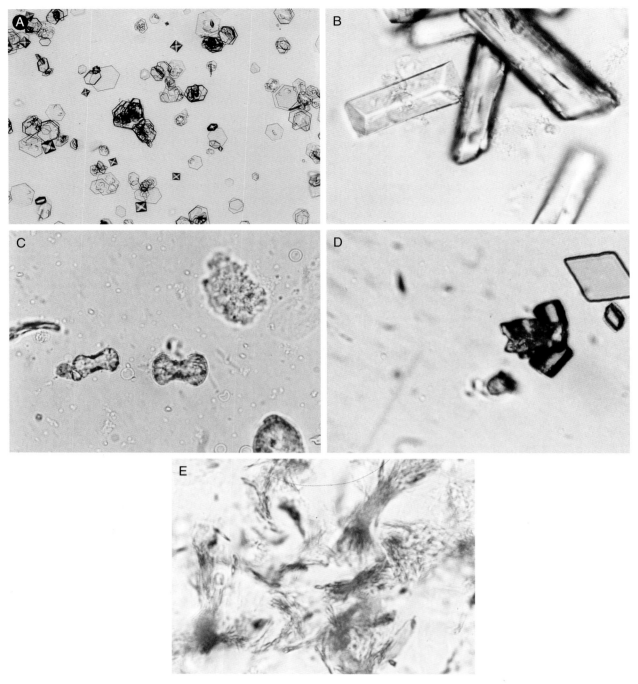

FIGURE 4   Crystals. (A) Hexagonal cystine and bipyramidal or "envelope shaped" oxalate. Photo courtesy of Dr. Thomas O. Pitts. (B) "Coffin-lid shaped" triple phosphate. (C) Dumbell shaped oxalate. (D) Rhomboid urate.(E) Needle shaped urate.

a few tubular cells may also be present along with a few RBCs. With some forms of chronic glomerulonephritis, a telescoped sediment is observed. This term refers to the presence of the elements of a nephritic sediment together with broad or waxy casts indicative of tubular atrophy and dipstick findings of heavy proteinuria (Fig. 2C). In

pyelonephritis, WBC casts and innumerable WBCs are present along with bacteria. In lower tract infection, WBC casts are absent. The sediment in ATN shows tubular cells, tubular cell casts, and muddy brown granular casts (Fig. 2B). The typical urinary findings in individual renal disorders are discussed in their respective chapters.

TABLE 3
Common Urinary Crystals

Description	Composition	Comment
Crystals found in acid urine		
Amorphous	Uric acid Sodium urate	Cannot be distinguished from amorphous phosphates except by urine pH, may be orange tinted by urochromes
Rhomboid prisms	Uric acid	
Rosettes	Uric acid	
Bipyramidal	Calcium oxalate	Also termed "envelope-shaped"
Dumbbell shaped	Calcium oxalate	
Needles	Uric acid Sulfa drugs Radiographic contrast	Clinical history provides useful confirmation Sulfa may resemble sheaves of wheat; urate and contrast crystals are thicker
Hexagonal plates	Cystine	Presence may be confirmed with nitroprusside test
Crystals found in alkaline urine		
Amorphous	Phosphates	Indistinguishable from urates except by pH
Coffin-lid (beveled rectangular prisms)	Triple (magnesium ammonium) phosphate	Seen with urea-splitting infection and bacteriuria
Granular masses or dumbbells	Calcium carbonate	Larger than amorphous phosphates
Yellow brown masses with or without spicules	Ammonium biurate	
Platelike rectangles, fan shaped, starburst	Indinavir	Causes nephrolithiasis or renal colic; *in vitro* solubility increased at very low pH; the lowest urine pH achievable *in vivo* may not actually be acid enough to lessen crystalluria

Bibliography

Birch DF, Fairley KF, Becker GJ, Kincaid-Smith P: *A Color Atlas of Urine Microscopy.* Chapman & Hall, New York, 1994.

Braden GL, Sanchez PG, Fitzgibbons JP, Stupak WJ, Germain MJ: Urinary doubly refractile lipid bodies in nonglomerular renal disease. *Am J Kidney Dis* 16:332–337, 1988.

Fairley KF, Birch DF: Hematuria: A simple method for identifying glomerular bleeding. *Kidney Int* 21:105–108, 1982.

Fassett RG, Owen JE, Fairley J, Birch DF, Fairley KF: Urinary red-cell morphology during exercise. *Br Med J* 285:1455–1457, 1982.

Fogazzi GB, Cameron JS: Urinary microscopy from the seventeenth century to the present day. *Kidney Int* 50:1058–1068, 1996.

Graff L: *A Handbook of Routine Urinalysis.* Lippincott, Philadelphia, 1983.

Henry JB, Lauzon RB, Schumann GB: Basic examination of the urine. In: Henry JB. (eds) *Clinical Diagnosis and Management by Laboratory Methods,* 19th Ed., pp. 411–456. Saunders, Philadelphia, 1991.

Kincaid-Smith P: Haematuria and exercise-related haematuria. *Br Med J* 285:1595–1597, 1982.

Kopp JB, Miller KD, Mican JM, Feuerstein IM, Vaughan E, Baker C, Pannell LK, Falloon J: Crystalluria and urinary tract abnormalities associated with indinavir. *Ann Intern Med* 127:119–125, 1997.

Raymond JR, Yarger WE: Abnormal urine color: Differential diagnosis. *South Med J* 81:837–841, 1988.

Rutecki GJ, Goldsmith C, Schreiner GE: Characterization of proteins in urinary casts. Fluorescent-antibody identification of Tamm–Horsfall mucoprotein in matrix and serum proteins in granules. *N Engl J Med* 284:1049–1052, 1971.

Schumann GB, Harris, S, Henry JB: An improved technic for examining urinary casts and a review of their significance. *Am J Clin Pathol* 69:18–23, 1978.

Stamey TA, Kindrachuk RW: *Urinary Sediment and Urinalysis. A Practical Guide for the Health Professional.* Saunders, Philadelphia, 1985.

Voswinckel P: A marvel of colors and ingredients. The story of urine test strips. *Kidney Int* 46:S3–S7, 1994.

HEMATURIA AND PROTEINURIA

RICHARD J. GLASSOCK

Hematuria and proteinuria are cardinal manifestations of renal disease. Because of their simplicity and ready availability, the tests used to detect these abnormalities are cornerstones of nephrologic diagnosis. All physicians should be cognizant of the analytical methods and significance of the results of these tests as well as their pitfalls, and should be prepared to logically follow-up abnormal results. While hematuria or proteinuria do not always signify an abnormality arising in the kidneys or urinary tract, the investigation of both abnormalities requires a systematic approach.

HEMATURIA

Definition and Normal Values

Hematuria is defined as the excretion of abnormal quantities of erythrocytes (either intact or damaged) in the urine. It must be distinguished from pigmenturia (e.g., hemoglobinuria or myoglobinuria) in which proteins or other substances impart an abnormal coloration to urine, sometimes resembling hematuria. Many of these substances are delivered to the kidney from the circulation and filtered into urine.

Normal individuals excrete small numbers of erythrocytes in the urine. Estimation of the degree of hematuria is most commonly performed by counting the number of erythrocytes present per high power field (hpf) when the resuspended sediment obtained by light centrifugation (3000 rpm for 5 min) of a freshly voided urine specimen is examined under high power magnification (400×). In normal individuals, usually three or fewer erythrocytes are observed per highpower field (hpf). Menstruation or urethral trauma (e.g., urethral catheterization) may increase this value substantially.

Hematuria can be gross or macroscopic, covert or microscopic, and can occur in several patterns: persistent, intermittent, or recurrent. The coexistence or absence of symptoms referable to the urinary tract confer the designation symptomatic or asymptomatic hematuria, respectively. The term isolated hematuria refers to the presence of erythrocytes in the urine in abnormal quantities without any other abnormality in the urine. These patterns of hematuria may have diagnostic significance.

Detection and Quantification

Hematuria can be detected in either of two ways. The first method is the direct microscopic examination of centrifuged or uncentrifuged urine. Microscopic examination is always the preferred method, since it provides information about shape and size of erythrocytes and information regarding the presence of other cells (e.g., leukocytes) and formed elements (e.g., erythrocyte casts) which may have diagnostic value. The detection of erythrocyte dysmorphism is a critical and vital step in the microscopic examination of urine. Small, fragmented, poorly hemoglobinized (dysmorphic) erythrocytes are a sign of glomerular bleeding. These abnormalities in shape and size of erythrocytes can be best determined by phase contrast microscopy or supravital staining of the urinary sediment. They are more difficult to reliably identify when fresh unstained urinary sediments are examined by standard light microscopy. On the other hand, normal sized and shaped, well-hemoglobinized (normomorphic) erythrocytes are a sign of urinary tract bleeding or bleeding from within the kidney parenchyma of a nonglomerular origin (e.g., from a renal tumor). Not all distorted erythrocytes in the urine are suggestive of glomerular bleeding. Acanthocytes, small erythrocytes with multiple spinelike or bubblelike projections, are most specific for glomerular bleeding. Crenated erythrocytes may be seen in very hypertonic urine which is not freshly examined, irrespective of whether the erythrocytes are from a glomerular or nonglomerular source. Very hypotonic urine may cause hemoglobin release leaving erythrocyte ghosts. Candida spherules, air bubbles, and starch granules can all be mistaken for erythrocytes. Dysmorphic erythrocytes accompanied by cellular casts (particularly erythrocyte casts) are almost always indicative of a glomerular source for hematuria. Automated cell sorters may allow determination of the mean corpuscular volume (MCV) of erythrocytes in urine. A MCV less than 70 fL is usually indicative of a glomerular source.

The second method of detecting hematuria is by orthotolidine impregnated paper strips (Hemastix). These test strips will detect as few as five erythrocytes per hpf of centrifuged urine. The test strip will also be positive in hemoglobinuria and myoglobinuria. Thus, all positive dipstick tests must be accompanied by a microscopic examination of the urine in order to differentiate hematuria from pigmenturia. False negative tests may occur in patients taking large amounts of vitamin C.

While any erythrocyte count greater than the upper limit of normal is by definition a sign of potential disease, additional information can be obtained by quantification of erythrocyte excretion rates. In gross (macroscopic) hematuria, a urocrit may be obtained in the same way a hematocrit is obtained. A urocrit greater than 1% often signifies lower urinary tract bleeding. When microscopic hematuria is present, timed overnight or random morning urine specimens (centrifuged or noncentrifuged) may be examined with a hemocytometer chamber and the number of erythrocytes excreted per hour (or per 12 hr) or the number of erythrocytes excreted per milliliter urine readily calculated. The excretion of large numbers of dysmorphic erythrocytes (e.g., greater than 10^6/ml) may be an indication of an underlying crescentic glomerulonephritis.

Pathophysiology

Abnormal numbers of erythrocytes in the urine may arise anywhere from the glomerular capillaries to the tip of the distal urethra. As discussed, dysmorphic erythrocytes tend strongly to be associated with a glomerular source. Presumably, glomerular hematuria arises from small breaks or discontinuities in the integrity of the glomerular capillary wall. As such, other circulating elements, especially plasma proteins (low and high molecular weight) may also escape into Bowman's space and be excreted in the urine (see later). Dysmorphic erythrocyturia accompanied by abnormal proteinuria is a quite reliable sign of glomerular disease. On the other hand, disruption of tubular architecture including the peritubular capillaries, may also lead to the passage of erythrocytes from the peritubular capillaries into tubular lumina leading to hematuria. In this circumstance, proteinuria is less conspicuous and usually is of tubular origin (see later). Urinary tract abnormalities (e.g., in the renal pelvis down to the distal urethra) lead to microscopic or macroscopic but normomorphic hematuria. Because plasma proteins are excreted only in proportion to the degree of bleeding, lower urinary tract hematuria seldom leads to marked proteinuria. For example, urinary tract bleeding sufficient to result in a urocrit of 0.5% would give a semiquantitative estimate of proteinuria (dipstick) of approximately 2+ (or less than 100 mg/dL). Hemolysis of red cells, giving a pinkish hue to the supernatant in urine, will increase protein concentration further. The concentration of hemoglobin to urinary protein can be assessed by urinary electrophoresis (hemoglobin migrates as a β globulin). Thus, macroscopic hematuria accompanied by 3+ or greater qualitative proteinuria, in the absence of erythrocyte hemolysis in the urine, should always be suspected as being due to glomerular disease. The causes of glomerular, tubulointerstitial and urinary tract bleeding are quite diverse as listed in Table 1.

The Approach to Hematuria

All patients with hematuria should have a complete and thorough history and physical examination with particular attention to weight changes, symptoms referable to the urinary tract, drug ingestion, family history, bleeding tendency, corneal and hearing abnormalities, and costovertebral angle or bladder tenderness. One of the first steps in the evaluation of a patient who has been found to have hematuria (assuming pigmenturia has been excluded) is to assign the patient to one of three categories of probable diagnosis (Table 2): glomerular hematuria, indeterminate hematuria, and urinary tract hematuria.

Patients with glomerular hematuria should be further evaluated to detect and diagnose the cause of glomerular disease (see Table 3). In many patients, the cause will be quite evident (e.g., systemic lupus erythematosus, Henoch-Schönlein purpura) while in others, a systematic clinical and laboratory evaluation will be required. A history of systemic features, such as fever or weight loss, may suggest a multisystem disease such as vasculitis. A family history of hematuria may suggest Alport syndrome, Fabry's disease, or thin basement membrane nephropathy.

The laboratory evaluation of patients with glomerular hematuria will depend largely on the history and physical examination, but most patients will require a hemogram, tests of renal function, (serum creatinine and blood urea nitrogen), and a renal-metabolic panel (electrolytes, calcium, phosphorus, total protein, albumin, globulin, cholesterol, alkaline phosphatase, alanine aminotransferase (ALT), aspartate aminotransferase (AST), lactate dehydrogenase, uric acid, and blood glucose) (see also Table 3). Urinary excretion of protein should be quantitated by a 24-hr collection or a protein to creatinine ratio in a random, untimed morning urine sample (see later). Renal size and contour should be evaluated by renal ultrasound. A chest X-ray and stool for occult blood would be a prudent step in many situations, particularly in older patients and those with weight loss or abdominal or pulmonary symptoms. Serologic studies, again critically depending on the clinical findings and history and physical examination, might include C3, C4, C^1H50, antineutrophil cytoplasmic antibodies (antimyeloperoxidase and antiproteinase 3), antiglomerular basement membrane antibody, fluorescent antinuclear antibody, anti-double stranded DNA antibody, antistreptolysin O titer, and/or cryoglobulins. An audiogram should be performed when Alport syndrome is suggested and a slit lamp examination of the cornea might be performed in Fabry's disease. Obviously, the selection of noninvasive diagnostic tests will be greatly influenced by the a priori probability of the presence of specific diseases. In many patients, a renal biopsy will be required for definitive diagnosis but the decision to carry out this procedure will be determined by the likelihood of finding a treatable lesion or the necessity to acquire information of either diagnostic or prognostic value. Patients with isolated hematuria with normal blood pressure and normal renal function have a low probability of finding information which will lead to a specific therapeutic intervention.

Patients with indeterminate hematuria can have either glomerular or nonglomerular disease as a cause for the hematuria, and further evaluation will depend heavily on clues obtained in the history and physical examination. The greater the degree of erythrocyte dysmorphism, the greater the likelihood that a glomerular disease will be present. At a minimum, all patients should undergo testing of kidney function, quantification of urine protein, a renal-metabolic panel, and renal ultrasound. Many patients will also require further

TABLE I
Causes of Hematuria

Renal parenchymal diseases	Urinary tract diseases

Glomerular disease
  Primary
    Mesangial IgA nephropathy (Berger's disease)
    Thin basement membrane nephropathy
    Mesangial proliferative glomerulonephritis with IgM and/or
      C3 deposits
    Membranoproliferative glomerulonephritis
    Crescentic glomerulonephritis
    Focal glomerulosclerosis
    Membranous glomerulopathy (<20%)
    Minimal change disease (<20%)
    Fibrillary glomerulonephritis
  Multisystem
    Systemic lupus crythematosus nephritis
    Microscopic polyangiitis
    Wegener's granulomatosis
    Henoch-Schönlein purpura
    Goodpasture's disease
    Thrombotic microangiopathies (e.g., hemolytic-uremic
      syndrome)
  Infection
    Poststreptococcal glomerulonephritis
    Infective endocarditis
    Shunt nephritis
    Other postinfectious glomerulonephritis
  Hereditary disease
    Alport syndrome
    Nail-patella syndrome
    Fabry's disease
  Other
    Primary idiopathic renal hematuria with or without
      hypercalciuria
Vascular and tubulointerstitial diseases
  Hypersensitivity
    Acute hypersensitivity interstitial nephritis
    Tubulointerstitial nephritis with uveitis
  Neoplastic
    Tumors (renal cell carcinoma, Wilms tumor, leukemic
      infiltrates, angiomyolipoma)
    Metastatic tumors (uncommon)
  Hereditary
    Polycystic kidney disease (autosomal dominant variety)
    Medullary sponge kidney
  Vascular
    Malignant hypertension
    Renal arterial emboli or thrombosis
    Loin pain-hematuria syndrome
    Arteriovenous malformations
  Papillary necrosis
    Analgesic abuse nephropathy
    Sickle cell trait
    Diabetes mellitus
    Alcoholism
    Ankylosing spondylitis
    Obstructive uropathy
	Renal pelvis
	  Transitional cell carcinoma
	  Varices
	  Calculi
	  Trauma
	  Severe hydronephrosis
	  Nevi
	Ureter
	  Calculi (uric acid, calcium oxalate, calcium phosphate,
	    struvite, cystine, adenine, xanthine)
	  Transitional cell carcinoma
	  Periureteritis (appendicitis, ileocolitis, abscess)
	  Retroperitoneal fibrosis
	  Ureterocele
	  Varices
	  Endometriosis
	  Tuberculosis
	Bladder
	  Carcinoma of the bladder
	  Cystitis (bacterial, viral, parasitic, fungal)
	  Chronic interstitial cystitis (Hunner's ulcers)
	  Schistosoma haematobium
	  Radiation cystitis
	  Nitrogen mustard or cyclophosphamide cystitis
	  Hypersensitivity (allergic) cystitis
	  Bladder calculi
	  Sudden decompression of severe overdistention
	  Foreign bodies
	  Vascular anomalies
	  Amyloidosis
	  Trauma
	  Jogger's or marathon runner's hematuria (?)
	  Tuberculosis
	Prostate
	  Benign prostatic hypertrophy
	  Carcinoma of the prostate
	  Acute or chronic prostatitis
	Urethra
	  Meatal ulcers
	  Urethral prolapse
	  Urethral caruncle
	  Acute or chronic urethritis
	  Carcinoma of the urethra or penis
	  Vascular anomalies
	  Trauma
	  Foreign body
	  Condyloma acuminatum
	  Other (endometrosis)
	In association with a systemic coagulation disturbance
	  (with or without diseases previously listed)
	Platelet defect
	  Idiopathic or drug-induced
	  Thrombocytopenic purpura
	  Thrombasthenia
	  Bone marrow diseases

(continues)

TABLE 1 *(continued)*

Renal parenchymal diseases	Urinary tract diseases
Trauma	Coagulation protein deficiency
Acute bacterial pyelonephritis	Hemophilia A or B
Acquired cystic disease of renal failure and dialysis	Heparin therapy
	Warfarin therapy
	Other congenital and acquired defect in coagulation
	Other
	Scurvy
	Hereditary telangiectasia
	Surreptitious (malingering)

From Glassock, R. *Hematuria and Pigmenturia Textbook of Nephrology*. 3rd ed. Williams & Wilkins, Philadelphia, 1995.

imaging studies such as intravenous urograms and computerized tomography (CT) scans of the abdomen and kidney. Invasive procedures such as cystoscopy can usually be deferred unless features strongly suggest a malignancy (e.g., positive urine cytology, history of weight loss, and a history of heavy smoking in older males). Further evaluation, according to the glomerular or urinary tract hematuria based approach, may be necessary if findings lead to a suspicion of renal parenchymal or urinary tract abnormalities, respectively.

In patients with urinary tract hematuria, in addition to routine tests of renal function, hemogram and serum biochemistry will nearly always require a thorough and meticulous investigation of the urinary tract, which may include cystoscopy, intravenous urogram, and abdominal CT or magnetic resonance imaging (MRI) (see Table 4). The sequence of these examinations may vary, but cystoscopy will often be the first step, unless the preliminary ultrasound reveals a renal mass. CT scans are usually done with administration of contrast media. Patients with urinary tract hematuria and a renal mass should undergo an abdominal CT scan as the next test. Intravenous urograms are useful for detection of lesions on the upper urinary tract (ureter or pelvis), such as stones or tumors. Urine cytology for the detection of transitional cell carcinoma of the bladder, should be performed in smokers, those who abuse

analgesics, or those who have been exposed to other potential carcinogens (e.g., cyclophosphamide, plant or fungal toxins). If macroscopic hematuria is present, cystoscopy should be performed on a semiurgent basis to detect the source of active bleeding. If cystoscopy, urine cytology, intravenous urograms, CT scans, MRI, and ultrasound are all unrevealing, an angiogram may be necessary to detect an occult arteriovenous malformation.

Coagulation tests (prothrombin time, partial thromboplastin time, bleeding time, and platelet count) will be required if a bleeding tendency is elicited in the history or if anticoagulants have been administered. African-Americans should be tested for sickle cell hemoglobin. A tuberculin

TABLE 2
Clinical Categories of Hematuria

Glomerular hematuria
  Microscopic or gross hematuria
  >70% of erythrocytes are dysmorphic and/or
  Proteinuria >1000 mg/day or ≥2+ present
  Cellular casts (including erythrocyte casts) present

Indeterminate hematuria
  Microscopic or gross hematuria
  >30 and <70% of erythrocytes are dysmorphic and/or
  Proteinuria <1000 mg/day or ≥2+ present
  Cellular casts (except erythrocyte casts) are variably present

Non-glomerular (urinary tract) hematuria
  Microscopic or gross hematuria
  >70% of erythrocytes are normomorphic and/or
  Protein excretion rate normal or slightly increased (≤2+)
  Cellular casts absent

TABLE 3
Glomerular Hematuria: Laboratory Testing Based on Suspected Disease Causation

Suspected cause	Laboratory tests[a]
Vasculitis	ANCA, Cryo-Ig, CRP, blood cultures, Anti-GBM, FANA
Systemic lupus erythematosus	FANA, anti-DNA, C3, C4
Goodpasture's disease	anti-GBM, ANCA, Cryo-Ig
Crescentic GN	ANCA, anti-GBM, C3, C4, Cryo-Ig
Henoch–Schönlein purpura	IgA-fibronectin, serum IgA
Poststreptococcal GN	ASLOT, anti-DNAase, C3, C4
Membranoproliferative GN	C3, C4, Cryo-Ig, anti-hepatitis C, C3 NeF
Alport syndrome	Audiogram, Slit lamp exam
Infective endocarditis	Blood cultures, rheumatoid factor, C3, C4
Acute interstitial nephritis	Hansel's stain for urine eosinophils, CRP
Fibrillary glomerulonephritis	Serum and urinary electrophoreses, C3, C4

[a]ANCA, antineutrophil cytoplasmic antibody; Cryo-Ig, cryo-immunoglobulins; CRP, C-reactive protein; Anti-GBM, anti-glomerular basement membrane antibody; FANA, fluorescent antinuclear antibody; Anti-DNA, anti double-stranded (native) DNA antibody; ASLOT, antistreptolysin O titer; Anti-DNAase, anti-desoxyribonuclease; C3 NeF, C3 nephritic factor.

TABLE 4
Nonglomerular (Urinary Tract) Hematuria: Evaluation
Based on Suspected Cause

Suspected cause	Test[a]
Parenchymal renal mass; cystic or solid	Abdominal CT, IVU, puncture for cytology (if cystic)
Bilateral enlarged kidneys, cystic	Abdominal CT
Pelvic mass or filling defect	IVU, cystoscopy, urine cytology
Papillary necrosis	Urine cytology, cystoscopy, hemoglobin electrophoresis, review analgesic exposure
Medullary sponge kidney	Urine calcium, urine culture
Ureteral stricture	Urine for *M. tuberculosis,* ANCA
Urinary calculus	Urine calcium, oxalate, cystine, urine culture, serum calcium, phosphorus, PTH
Retroperitoneal mass	Abdominal CT
Bladder/prostatic neoplasm	Cystoscopy, IVU, urine cytology

[a]IVU, intravenous urogram; PTH, parathyroid hormone; ANCA, antineutrophil cytoplasmic antibody.

skin test is indicated when patients are suspected of having mycobacterium tuberculosis. Urine should be tested for ova and parasites in patients who have traveled in areas endemic for *Schistosoma hematobium.*

The pattern of urinary bleeding in patients with macroscopic hematuria can be helpful in estimating the site of bleeding. Urinary tract bleeding confined to the first 10–15 mL of urine suggest a urethral site, bleeding in the final 10–30 mL of urine suggest bladder bleeding, and bleeding through-out all phases of urination suggest upper urinary tract bleeding. Significant bleeding at the very end of voiding should suggest *Schistosoma hematobium* or a urinary bladder source. Twenty-four-hour urine calcium or uric acid may detect hypercalcuria or hyperuricosuria in patients with unexplained hematuria, particularly in children.

Using this approach, 85% or more of patients discovered to have hematuria can be correctly diagnosed. In the 15% of patients remaining with "idiopathic hematuria," the diagnosis may become evident with follow-up and the emergence of new symptoms or signs. Follow-up of patients with idiopathic hematuria should be strongly encouraged as some may have a treatable disease (e.g., occult small bladder or renal tumors, vascular malformations, or low-grade infections). Malingering is a rare cause of hematuria.

PROTEINURIA
Definition and Abnormal Values

The normal rate of excretion of protein in urine is 80 ± 24 mg/24 hr (1 SD) in healthy individuals. Thus, over 95% of normal adults excrete less than 130 mg/day of protein. Protein excretion rates are somewhat higher in children and adolescents, and a value for the upper limit of normal

may be set as high as 200 mg/day in these individuals. Urinary protein excretion rates rise modestly in normal pregnancy. Over 75% of the total 24-hr urine protein excretion occurs during quiet, upright ambulation. Fever, severe exercise, and the acute infusion of hyperoncotic solutions or certain pressor agents (e.g., angiotensin II, norepinephrine) may transiently cause abnormal protein excretion in otherwise normal individuals.

Abnormal proteinuria can be intermittent or constant and can occur predominantly in the upright position (orthostatic proteinuria). It may be isolated, when it occurs in the absence of hematuria or other signs of renal disease. On quantification, it can be nephrotic (greater than 3.5 g/day in adults or 40 mg/hr/m^2 in children) or subnephrotic (less than 3.5 g/day). Overt proteinuria is usually defined as that level which is easily detectable using routine screening methods (greater than 500 mg/day) (see later).

Detection and Quantification

Abnormal proteinuria may be detected in a variety of ways. The simplest and least expensive is the use of a dye impregnated strip (Multistix, Albustix, Ames) which depend on a color change of a pH sensitive dye (tetrabromophenol blue) buffered to pH 3. These tests detect protein, principally albumin, down to concentrations of approximately 20 mg/dL and provide semiquantitative estimates of protein concentration up to 300 mg/dL. These strips are relatively insensitive to globulins (including Bence Jones proteins) and false positives may occur in highly buffered alkaline urine. The semiquantitative estimates of proteinuria are greatly influenced by urinary concentration (as assessed by urine osmolality or specific gravity). Although a highly concentrated urine (e.g., 1200 mOsmol/kg H$_2$O or specific gravity of 1.030) may show "abnormal" concentration results (e.g., 1+, 30 mg/dL) the total daily excretion rate may still be normal (e.g., 130 mg/day) because daily urine volume is low (less than 500 ml/day). Contrariwise, highly dilute urine (50 mOsmol/kg H$_2$O, specific gravity 1.004) may show "normal" protein results (negative to trace, less than 30 mg/dL) even when abnormal amounts of protein (e.g., 1000 mg/day) are excreted because in the presence of a water diuresis, the urine flow rate is very high (5000 ml/day). Dye impregnated strips that can detect albumin excretion rates below the usual detection limits (microalbuminuria, between 15 and 200 μg/min, or 20–300 mg/day) have been developed and are commercially available. Colorimetric (e.g., biuret) or turbidometric (heat and acetic acid or 3% sulfosalicylic acid) methods can detect lower levels of proteinuria (down to about 5–10 mg/dL), close to the upper limit of normal. These tests also detect a broader class of proteins (both albumin and globulins react equally). Thus a negative or borderline test result with dye impregnated strips and a strongly positive test by a colorimetric or turbidometric assay usually indicates the presence of globulins (often light chains) in the urine. False positive turbidometric tests may occur after the administration of certain agents (e.g., tolmetin, radiocontrast agents, cephalosporins).

Quantitation of urine protein excretion rates can be determined by subjecting timed urine samples, (e.g., 12–24 hr) to chemical or immunochemical assay. Alternatively, quantitation of protein excretion rate can be approximated by comparison of a urine protein concentration (mg/dL) to a reference substance (in mg/dL) excreted predominantly by glomerular filtration and whose concentration in urine is principally determined by the extraction of water from urine. Creatinine is conventionally chosen as this substance even though, in certain states, it may undergo substantial tubular secretion. The protein/creatinine ratio in random urine samples correlates highly with 24-hr urine protein. A protein to creatinine ratio of greater than 3.0 corresponds to a protein excretion rate exceeding 3.0 to 3.5 g/day. Other tests may be useful in evaluating proteinuria, including cellulose acetate electrophoresis, immunoelectrophoresis, immunofixation, and spectrophotometry. These are particularly well suited for examining the chemical nature of the excreted protein (e.g., hemoglobin, myoglobin, globulins, monoclonal light chains).

Composition of Urine Proteins

The protein in normal and abnormal urine is derived from three sources: (1) plasma proteins normally or abnormally filtered at the glomerular capillaries and escaping reabsorption by the proximal tubule; (2) proteins normally secreted by renal tubules or leaking into tubular lumina as a result of cellular injury; and (3) proteins derived from the lower urinary tract, secreted by lining cells or associated glands or leaking into the urine as a result of tissue injury or inflammation.

The composition of normal urine is shown in Table 5. It is noteworthy that albumin makes up 15% of the total urinary protein excreted with values for excretion rate ranging from 4 to 15 μg/min (5.8 to 21.6 mg/day) in normal urine. Values above the upper limit of normal (greater than 15 μg/min) to values which are usually detected by semiquantitating screening methods (about 200 μg/min) are commonly termed microalbuminuria. This corresponds to an albumin/creatinine ratio of 30 μg protein/mg creatinine. Approximately one-half of the protein in normal urine is derived from the kidney and about one-half represents filtered proteins escaping reabsorption by the proximal tubules or arising from the lower urinary tract (e.g., secretory immunoglobulin A).

The Pathophysiology of Abnormal Proteinuria

Four pathophysiologic varieties of abnormal proteinuria are recognized: (1) glomerular; (2) tubular; (3) overflow; and (4) tissue proteinuria. Each has diagnostic significance and requires a different approach to evaluation.

Glomerular proteinuria is the result of a disturbance in the permeoselectivity of the glomerular capillary wall leading to the abnormal filtration of plasma proteins (chiefly albumin), which quickly saturate maximal tubular reabsorption capacity and thus are excreted into the urine. Two

TABLE 5

Protein Composition of Normal Urine

	Urinary protein		
		Excretion rate	Percentage of total
	μg/min	mg/day	%
Plasma proteins			
Albumin	8	12	15
	(4–5)	(5–25)	
IgG	2	3	
	(1–3)	(2–7)	
IgA (secretory)	0.7	1	5.4
	(0.2–2.0)	(0.4–3.0)	
IgM	0.2	0.3	
Light chains	2.6	3.7	4.6
κ		2.3	
λ		1.4	
β_2-Microglobulin	0.8	0.12	<0.2
Other plasma proteins and enzymes (total)	13.8	≈20	25
Subtotal of all plasma proteins	27.5 μg/min	40 mg/day	50%
Nonplasma proteins			
Tamm–Horsfall protein	28	40	50
Other renal-derived proteins	<0.7	<1	<1
Subtotal of nonplasma proteins	28 μg/min	40 mg/day	50%
Total protein	55 ± 17 μg/min (1 SD)	80 ± 24 mg/day (1 SD)	100%

From Glassock, R: Proteinuria. In: *Textbook of Nephrology*, 3rd Ed. Williams & Wilkins, Baltimore, 1995.

subvarieties are described. Selective proteinuria, in which albumin and other relatively low molecular weight plasma proteins (e.g., transferrin) are excreted results from a disturbance in the charge-sensitive barrier of the glomerular capillary. It is principally seen in diseases associated with minimal structural glomerular abnormalities (e.g., minimal change disease). Nonselective proteinuria, in which globulins and other higher molecular weight proteins are excreted in addition to albumin, is another subvariety and is a reflection of a disturbance in the size selective barrier of the glomerular capillary wall, and is seen particularly in diseases associated with significant glomerular structural abnormalities (e.g., focal and segmental glomerulosclerosis).

The quantity of protein excreted in these various pathophysiologic states varies from slightly above normal (e.g., 200 mg/day) to over 20 g/day. Protein excretion rates greater than 3.5 g/day in the adult (corresponding to a protein/creatinine ratio of greater than 3.0) or greater than 40 mg/m^2/hr in children are usually termed nephrotic range proteinuria while lower values are termed non-nephrotic or subnephrotic proteinuria. Nephrotic range proteinuria is very frequently, but not exclusively, associated with underlying glomerular disease. The nephrotic syndrome comprise nephrotic range proteinuria with hypoalbuminemia, edema, and hyperlipidemia; an underlying glomerular disease will almost invariably be present.

Tubular proteinuria results from inadequate reabsorption of normal or abnormal filtered proteins. Glomerular and tubular proteinuria can coexist, especially when tubulointerstitial injury complicates the picture of glomerular disease. Isolated tubular proteinuria chiefly consists of the excretion of α and β migrating proteins on electrophoresis. An increase in β_2-microglobulin excretion relative to albumin excretion is characteristic of tubular proteinuria. The total amount of protein excretion in tubular proteinuria is usually modest, generally in the range of 200 to 2000 mg/day, corresponding to a urine protein to creatinine ratio of less than 3.0. The detection of tubular proteinuria requires analytical methods that separate proteins based on size or charge such as electrophoresis or gel filtration.

Overflow proteinuria is due to the filtration of low molecular weight proteins across a normal glomerular capillary bed accompanied by incomplete tubular reabsorption. The abnormal filtration is due to an increase in the plasma concentration of the protein in a form which can be readily filtered. Examples include free hemoglobin (e.g., not bound to haptoglobin), myoglobin, and the excretion of fragments of monoclonal immunoglobulins (e.g., monoclonal light chains). The amount of protein excreted in overflow proteinuria may range widely from trace amounts to massive quantities, even exceeding the lower limits of the nephrotic range. Detection and identification of overflow proteinuria depends on electrophoretic, immunochemical, or spectrophotometric analysis of urine protein composition. Monoclonal light chains are best detected by immunochemical techniques.

Tissue proteinuria is generally associated with inflammatory or neoplastic abnormalities within the urinary tract. It seldom exceeds 500 mg/day and is best detected by electrophoretic or immunochemical assays.

These four pathophysiologic categories of abnormal proteinuria can be caused by a wide variety of underlying disorders or outlined in Table 6. The approach to diagnosing these conditions in a patient with abnormal proteinuria depends on appropriate initial classification.

Approach to Evaluation

The approach to a patient in whom abnormal protein excretion has been detected on random urine samples using semiquantitative methods involves three phases: (1) initial confirmation of abnormal proteinuria; (2) preliminary investigation designed to determine the pathophysiologic category; and (3) definitive evaluation leading to precise diagnosis.

Initial Confirmation

The first step is to assess whether the abnormal result of a test using dye impregnated strips for proteinuria is likely to be a true or a false positive. False positive tests occur more frequently in highly concentrated, highly buffered alkaline urine. The clinical significance of the test

TABLE 6

Differential Diagnosis of Proteinuria Based on Pathophysiologic Mechanism[a]

Glomerular proteinuria
  Primary glomerular disease
    Minimal change lesion
    Mesangial proliferative GN (including IgA and IgM nephropathy)
    Focal and segmental glomerulosclerosis
    Membranous GN
    Mesangiocapillary GN
    Fibrillary glomerulonephritis
    Crescentic glomerulonephritis
  Secondary glomerular disease
    Medications (mercurials, gold compounds, heroin, penicillamine, probenecid, captopril, lithium, NSAID)[b]
    Allergens (bee sting, pollen, milk)
    Infectious (bacterial, viral, protozoal, fungal, belminthic)
    Neoplastic (solid tumors, leukemia)
    Multisystem (SLE,[c] Henoch-Schönlein purpura, amyloidosis)
    Heredofamilial (diabetes mellitus, congenital nephrotic syndrome, Fabry's disease, Alport syndrome)
    Other (transplant rejection, reflux nephropathy, toxemia of pregnancy)
    Other glomerular proteinuria
      Postexercise proteinuria
      Benign orthostatic proteinuria
      Febrile proteinuria

Tubular proteinuria
  Toxins and drugs
    Endogenous
      Light chain damage to proximal tubule
      Lysozyme (myclomonocytic leukemia)
    Exogenous
      Mercury
      Lead
      Cadmium
      Outdated tetracycline
      Arginine or lysine infusions
  Tubulointerstitial disease (chiefly and predominantly involving proximal nephron)
    Lupus erythematosus
    Acute hypersensitivity interstitial nephritis
    Acute bacterial pyelonephritis
    Obstructive uropathy
    Chronic interstitial nephritis (e.g., Sjögren's syndrome, Balkan endemic nephropathy, tubulointerstitial nephritis with uveitis)
    Fanconi syndrome

Overflow proteinuria
  Multiple myeloma
  Light chain disease
  Amyloidosis (see also Glomerular proteinuria)
  Hemoglobinuria
  Myoglobinuria
  Certain pancreatic or colon carcinomas (rare)

Tissue proteinuria
  Acute inflammation of urinary tract
  Uroepithelial tumors

[a]From Glassock, RJ: Proteinuria. In: *Textbook of Nephrology*, 3rd Ed. Williams & Wilkins, Baltimore, 1995.
[b]NSAID, nonsteroidal antiinflammatory drugs.
[c]SLE, systemic lupus erythematosus.

is decreased if the specimen has been collected during a high fever, following vigorous exercise, or during the infusion of vasopressor agents. A confirmatory qualitative test using a colorimetric or turbidimetric assay on a first morning urine (after overnight recumbency) is quite useful and often indicated, particularly if the initial test reveals only modest proteinuria (trace to 2+). A negative test suggests an initial laboratory error or possibly orthostatic proteinuria (see later). A positive test confirms proteinuria. If the confirmatory test is strongly positive associated with a weakly positive result on the dye impregnated paper strip, excretion of globulins (e.g., light chains) rather than albumin is suggested, and further evaluation of urinary protein composition is indicated. A fresh urinary sediment should always be examined. If hematuria or other formed elements, especially red cell casts, are present, glomerular or tubulointerstitial renal parenchymal disease should be suspected, and additional testing undertaken as indicated later. The confirmatory steps previously mentioned can be omitted if the initial tests demonstrated heavy proteinuria (e.g., 3–4+ on dipstick) or if the urinary sediment is distinctly abnormal (e.g., dysmorphic hematuria).

Preliminary Investigation

In patients with confirmed abnormal qualitative proteinuria, the urine protein excretion rate should next be quantitated (24-hr collection or urine protein to creatinine ratio). If the protein excretion rate is greater than 3.5 g/day, or the protein/creatinine ratio greater than 3.0, then a glomerular or overflow cause should be suspected. A test of kidney function [serum creatinine, blood urea nitrogen (BUN)] should also be performed and a hemogram and biochemical studies of serum undertaken (this should include albumin, globulin, cholesterol, calcium, phosphorus, uric acid, alkaline phosphatase, bilirubin, ALT, and AST). An ultrasound of the kidney should also be performed. The history and physical examination should be thoroughly reevaluated for possible signs and symptoms of diseases listed in Table 6 with particular attention to systemic diseases and concomitant use of therapeutic agents. Clues present in the history and physical examination and initial screening studies should be used to direct further preliminary investigations and definitive evaluation. For example, a disparity between the dipstick and turbidometric urine tests of protein accompanied by a normocytic, normochromic anemia, a reduced anion gap, impaired renal function, and elevated serum globulins would lead to a test for overflow proteinuria (cellulose acetate electrophoresis of serum and urine and immunofixation of urine protein) and later to a bone marrow biopsy for diagnosis of multiple myeloma. Heavy proteinuria and dysmorphic hematuria, accompanied by abnormal renal function would lead to preliminary investigation of glomerular disease (e.g., serology, complement components) and later to a renal biopsy for definitive diagnosis. Modest proteinuria less than 2 g/day, accompanied by signs of tubular dysfunction including renal tubular acidosis, hypophosphatemia, hypouricemia, or renal glycosuria would lead to an evaluation of tubular proteinuria (including a β_2-microglobulin/albumin excretion ratio). Patients with features consistent with a systemic disease, a drug related disorder, or a heredofamilial disorder will require additional directed studies. As previously stated, abnormalities in the urinary sediment, especially dysmorphic hematuria, will direct the investigation to glomerular diseases. Nephrotic range proteinuria accompanied by hypoalbuminemia and hypercholesterolemia strongly indicate a further evaluation for glomerular disease.

In the absence of urinary sediment abnormalities, including hematuria, an evaluation for tubular or overflow proteinuria, which includes cellulose acetate electrophoresis, immunoelectrophoresis, or a β_2-microglobulin/albumin excretion ratio, may be in order.

An evaluation of the anatomy of the urinary tract is usually not needed unless there is a history of recurrent urinary tract infections or unless renal masses, hydronephrosis, or renal cysts are noted in the preliminary investigations. A voiding cystourethrogram may be indicated if vesicoureteral reflux nephropathy is suspected.

Definitive Evaluation

Precise diagnosis of patients with abnormal proteinuria will be guided by the results of preliminary investigations (Table 7). Nephrotic range proteinuria, accompanied by hypoalbuminemia, regardless of findings in the urinary sediment, will lead to a renal biopsy unless a systemic, heredofamilial, or drug-associated cause is apparent. In some circumstances, even when the diagnosis is evident, a renal biopsy may be indicated for prognostic purposes or therapeutic decision making. In patients with the nephrotic syndrome without underlying disease (e.g., idiopathic nephrotic syndrome) serologic investigations including C3,

TABLE 7
Proteinuria: Initial Evaluation Based on Pathophysiologic Category

Pathophysiologic category	Test
Glomerular	24-hr protein or $U_{protein}/U_{creatinine}$ ratio
	Urine sediment
	C3, C4
	Serum albumin
	Serum cholesterol
	Serum and urine immunoelectrophoresis (if amyloid suspected)
	Renal biopsy
Tubular	β_2-Microglobulin/albumin excretion ratio
	Heavy metal screen
	Urinary electrophoresis
Overflow	Urinary electrophoresis
	Serum electrophoresis
	Urinary light chains
	Urinary spectrophotometry

C4, C^{1}H50, ANCA, anti-GBM, and antistreptolysin O titer may be indicated. Older patients with nephrotic syndrome should be suspected of having covert primary amyloidosis and should undergo urine and serum electrophoresis for paraproteinuria.

Non-nephrotic glomerular proteinuria, especially if accompanied by changes in the urinary sediment may be another indication for renal biopsy. Patients with non-nephrotic proteinuria, less than 1g/day, without changes in the urinary sediment, and with normal renal function and blood pressure can often be observed without renal biopsy, providing overflow and tubular proteinuria have been excluded. Patients with overflow proteinuria due to abnormal light chain excretion will require investigation for multiple myeloma, including bone survey and bone marrow biopsy. Patients with myoglobinuria may require an evaluation for an inherited muscle enzyme deficiency. Patients with hemoglobinuria should be evaluated for causes of intravascular hemolysis. Patients with tubular proteinuria, confirmed by a cellulose acetate electrophoresis showing α- and β-globulins and by high β_2-microglobulin/albumin excretion ratio, should undergo evaluation for heavy metal intoxication (cadmium, lead), systemic diseases such as Sjögren's syndrome, leukemia, exposure to other biological toxins such as mycotoxins, and endemic (Balkan) nephropathy. Occasionally, a renal biopsy is indicated for definitive diagnosis. Patients with fixed and reproducible orthostatic proteinuria, normal renal function, normal blood pressure, and normal urine sediment do not need further evaluation but should be followed at yearly intervals to be sure that evolution to constant proteinuria has not occurred.

Bibliography

Fairley K, Birch DF: Hematuria: A simple method for identifying glomerular bleeding. *Kidney Int* 21:105–108, 1982.

Fogazzi GB, Passerini P, Ponticelli C, Ritz E: *The Urinary Sediment,* 2nd Ed. Masson, Milan, 2000.

Glassock R: Proteinuria. In: Massry S, Glassock R (eds) *Textbook of Nephrology,* 3rd Ed., pp. 600–604. Williams & Wilkins, Baltimore, 1995.

Glassock R: Hematuria and pigmenturia. In: Massry S, Glassock R (eds) *Textbook of Nephrology,* 3rd Ed., pp. 557–566. Williams & Wilkins, Baltimore, 1995.

Mallick N, Short CP: The clinical approach to hematuria and proteinuria. In: Davison A, Cameron JS, Grunfeld J-P, Kerr DS, Ritz E, Winearls C (eds) *Oxford Textbook of Clinical Nephrology,* 2nd Ed., pp. 227–236. Oxford Medical Publ., Oxford, 1998.

6

RENAL IMAGING TECHNIQUES

HOWARD J. MINDELL AND JONATHAN T. FAIRBANK

GENERAL CONSIDERATIONS

Investigation of patients with renal disorders often requires obtaining images of the kidneys and urinary tract. Although more helpful in evaluating renal masses or disorders of the urinary outflow tract than intrinsic renal parenchymal disease, imaging studies can either establish the general pathway for further investigation or lead to a specific diagnosis. In general, the choice of studies proceeds from less to more invasive or expensive studies, unless the expensive or invasive study is much more likely to be definitive. The current medical–economic environment favors the use of the simplest, safest, and cheapest approach that can answer the question at hand.

ULTRASONOGRAPHY

Ultrasonography (US) is entirely safe, independent of renal function, capable of multiplanar display, and does not require contrast agents or prior patient preparation. However, it lacks specificity in many instances (e.g., in differentiating among renal parenchymal diseases), and technical problems may arise in large patients in whom tissue degrades the interrogating sound waves or when intestinal gas reflects sound, and prevents delineation of the underlying structure. Although US can exquisitely demonstrate vascular occlusive disease, in many patients it is inapplicable because of the technical reasons previously cited. Doppler US, even with the use of color to show flow direction, has

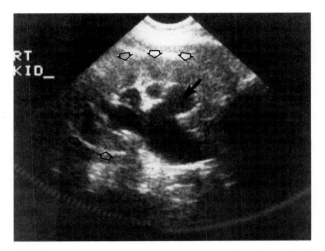

FIGURE 1 Ultrasound showing a sagittal section through the right kidney. The single black arrow indicates a dilated calyx in the lower pole. Note how the calyx connects to the dilated renal pelvis (black, fluid filled). Multiple open arrows indicate the margin of the renal cortex.

not enjoyed wide or universal success in screening for renovascular hypertension. In addition to the limitations noted, multiple renal arteries may be impossible to sort out by US alone. Nevertheless, US is a mainstay of renal imaging and is frequently the first study chosen. US can easily differentiate hydronephrosis (Fig. 1) from intrinsic renal parenchymal disease and renal cysts from solid tumors. Color Doppler US has unique potential, such as easily showing the presence of moving blood, as in a renal artery

aneurysm (Fig. 2). US is also a useful method for delineating perinephric collections, pyelonephritic scars, and nephrocalcinosis. US can assist in evaluating renal transplants and guide a variety of interventional approaches to the kidney, including biopsy, aspiration, and percutaneous nephrostomy.

EXCRETORY (INTRAVENOUS) UROGRAPHY

Intravenous urography (IVU) depends on glomerular filtration and subsequent tubular excretion of iodinated water-soluble contrast media by the kidneys, permitting noninvasive visualization of the entire urinary tract, the kidneys, the ureters, and the bladder. Although other imaging modalities, such as US, may provide more detail regarding the renal parenchyma, the IVU remains an inexpensive, widely available test that gives excellent detail of the entire urinary tract, and remains indispensable for evaluation of the urothelium, and lesions such as transitional cell carcinoma of the renal pelvis, ureters, and bladder. The IVU remains the first choice in most patients with hematuria or pyuria. Other indications for the IVU include tuberculosis, evaluation for scarring in chronic pyelonephritis, papillary necrosis, and a variety of congenital anomalies. In a recent innovation, limited currently to a few centers and depending on local logistics, computerized tomography (CT) sections have been added to the IVU, the result being a new hybrid, the "CTU." The CTU can offer increased parenchymal resolution over the linear tomographic sections ordinarily available with the IVU. Unenhanced helical CT is largely replacing the IVU for the diagnosis of renal colic (see Urolithiasis, later). When the

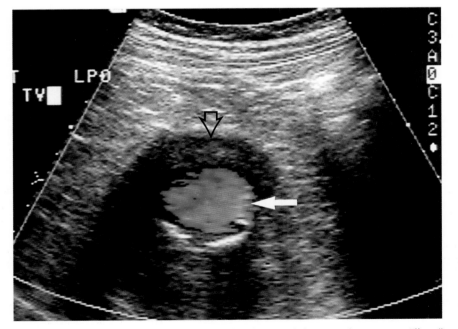

FIGURE 2 Renal artery aneurysm, color Doppler ultrasound. Arrow to the aneurysm "lit up" in red by turbulent arterial flow.

collecting systems must be examined, but the IVU is inadequate because renal failure limits excretion of radiographic contrast and urinary tract visualization, retrograde urography or percutaneous antegrade urography may be needed. The former requires cystoscopy and ureteral catheter placement; the latter is performed after imaging guided puncture of the calyceal system. The IVU is used to evaluate renal donors and in the pre- and postoperative assessment of patients with nephrolithiasis and other lesions that can be treated with endoscopic manipulation of the ureter.

The contrast media used for intravenous urography and other studies may result in acute reactions as an untoward side effect, so-called "idiosyncratic" reactions, or, alternatively may cause contrast media induced nephropathy, that is, acute renal failure. The former category, idiosyncratic reactions, involves some 0.1 to 0.2% of patients, and such events may result in "allergiclike" symptoms of urticaria, wheezing, and dyspnea, and may also result in hypotension or chest pain, and in rare instances anaphylaxis and cardiovascular collapse. The fatality rate, difficult to estimate because of its rarity, may approach 1 in 100,000. Pretreatment with steroids or the use of newer nonionic or low osmolality contrast may reduce the frequency of mild or severe reactions, but there is no conclusive evidence of a lower fatality rate with the nonionic contrast agents. Although the cost of the low osmolality contrast agents has come down in recent years, the cost differential between the long established conventional high osmolar agents and the newer LOM (low osmolar media) remains significant, and although wide differences can be found between institutions, many centers still use the LOM selectively rather than universally. If used selectively, standard indications for the LOM would include, at least, a prior history of significant reaction, a general allergic history—especially asthma, and procedures where a large bolus of contrast is injected rapidly or where extravasation of the contrast into the soft tissues is likely. The role of LOM in preventing acute renal failure (ARF) remains uncertain, and any contrast agent should be avoided if possible in diabetic patients who also have underlying renal failure, as they are at highest risk.

The risk of contrast nephropathy is highest in patients with diabetic nephropathy, intermediate in patients with renal insufficiency due to other causes, and low or normal for diabetics without renal disease. There are no absolute contraindications to the use of IV contrast, but it should be used with circumspection in such settings as advanced age, debility, congestive heart failure, and multiple myeloma. Patients with volume depletion are at much higher risk. Intravascular volume should be restored by fluid administration before contrast is given. Overnight expansion with 0.5% saline affords protection in patients who are not volume depleted (see Chapter 34).

It also bears emphasis that these comments about side effects of administration of radiographic contrast apply no matter what the procedure for which contrast is employed. They are not specific to IVU, and concern about contrast administration must be taken into account when CT with contrast or angiography is requested. Finally, the

visualization of the urinary tract is diminished when the serum creatinine exceeds 2 to 3 mg/dL; the IVU is unlikely to successfully visualize the collecting system when the serum creatinine exceeds 4 mg/dL. Therefore, the risk of increased contrast administration should be weighed against its diminished potential benefit in these patients. In patients with end stage renal disease who are maintained on dialysis, the issue of contrast induced nephropathy is not relevant. The sole risks of contrast administration are the idiosyncratic reactions previously described and volume overload due to the small amount intravascular expansion produced by administration of approximately 100 mL of contrast agent. It is not necessary to follow contrast administration with dialysis unless clinical evidence of volume overload develops after the radiographic procedure.

PLAIN ABDOMINAL RADIOGRAPH

The plain abdominal radiograph (KUB), while a standard prelude (scout film) for the IVU, may be requested alone or in conjunction with US. Renal or ureteric calculi usually contain calcium and are visible on the KUB, although the former may require oblique views to confirm an intrarenal location (as opposed to the more anterior gallbladder, etc.), and the latter may require IVU to differentiate from pelvic phleboliths.

COMPUTED TOMOGRAPHY

Computed tomography (CT) offers far greater contrast resolution than conventional radiography, with detailed anatomic cross-sectional anatomic imaging unaffected by overlying structures such as bone or gas. Virtually the entire urinary system and retroperitoneum are well visualized on CT. This modality has the main role in staging renal neoplasms, and has superseded IVU in trauma. CT is useful in the diagnosis of pyelonephritis and its complications and in renal cystic disorders. With arterial occlusive disease, CT can show perfusion defects, where contrast fails to opacify segments of the renal parenchyma, and recent work has shown that three-dimensional reconstruction with helical CT may show the renal arteries directly. With venous occlusive disease, CT can show flow abnormalities and stasis in the affected kidney and can directly show thrombus in the renal vein. Unenhanced helical CT is now replacing the IVU in renal colic, as it may show tiny calculi precisely, even urate stones that were invisible on conventional radiography, and also demonstrate hydronephrosis, hydroureter, and other pertinent findings (Fig. 3). Very recently, CT sections through the kidneys have been added at a few centers to the IVU, for a new combined procedure, the "CTU."

MAGNETIC RESONANCE IMAGING

Magnetic resonance imaging (MRI) depends on first aligning the hydrogen nuclei (protons) of body tissues with a powerful magnetic field and then applying radiofrequency

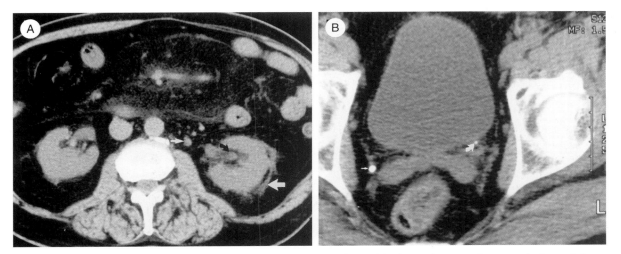

FIGURE 3 (A) Unenhanced CT at the level of the kidneys. Patient with obstruction secondary to calculus at left ureterovesical junction. Black arrow to dilated renal pelvis; small white arrow to proximal hydroureter. Large white arrow to extravasation of urine secondary to ruptured calyx due to acute obstruction. (B) Same patient, unenhanced CT at the level of the bladder. Curved arrow to 3-mm calculus in the left ureterovesical junction. Note flattening of the ipsilateral bladder wall, left ureter coursing to the calculus. Straight arrow to an incidental phlebolith; note the pelvic vein containing the phlebolith.

(RF) pulses. Energy released in these circumstances can be measured and used to create anatomic images dependent on characteristics of the tissues and the introduced magnetic and RF energy sources. MRI offers superb tissue contrast, with multiplanar imaging capabilities, although calcification is not well shown. MRI is safe, and uses no ionizing radiation, although MR contrast agents such as gadolinium may rarely cause side effects or reactions. MR may not be suitable for use in claustrophobic patients or those with implanted ferromagnetic devices, such as pacemakers. MRI has a limited role in defining specific parenchymal lesions at present, although its sensitivity to iron in hemoglobin permits its use to image the kidneys in patients with paroxysmal nocturnal hemoglobinuria, myoglobinuria, and epidemic Korean fever. MRI can beautifully show the renal vasculature, and magnetic resonance angiography (MRA) has replaced conventional angiography or is a rival to CTA at many centers in assessing various arterial lesions such as renal artery stenosis. MRI has the following roles in renal imaging:

1. Delineating complex masses, where CT is not definitive.
2. Staging renal neoplasm, particularly in evaluating for renal vein or inferior vena caval extension of tumor, usually after CT is not definitive or where the patient is reactive to iodinated contrast agents.
3. Diagnosing renovascular lesions.
4. Where renal failure or contrast media reactivity precludes the use of other modalities. Magnetic resonance urography (MRU), the MR equivalent of a KUB, after the use of IV gadolinium, offers imaging roughly comparable to an IVU. This technique is used at some centers, mainly to show hydronephrosis or hydroureter.

RADIONUCLIDE IMAGING

For nuclear medicine studies, radiopharmaceutical agents with specific renal handling characteristics are employed (see Table 1). These agents are administered and then the patient is imaged with a γ camera that can record the number of counts emitted and the location of their source. This permits quantification of function in a region as well as anatomic delineation. Nuclear medicine techniques are particularly useful in assessing the adequacy of renal perfusion and in determining whether the outflow tract is intact. Renal parenchymal integrity may also be assessed.

The scanning method is varied according to the nature of the information sought. When anatomic information is desired, the scanning interval for each image typically encompasses several minutes. Late views may be obtained after a delay of hours. In contrast, when flow is being studied, images are typically of only a few seconds in duration. Although the spatial resolution of nuclear medicine studies cannot match the other imaging modalities, it is superior in assessing renal physiology. Modern γ cameras are equipped with SPECT (single photon emission computed tomography), which renders three-dimensional images that greatly enhance anatomic detail. The most common uses of nuclear medicine studies are listed next.

1. Measurement of renal function. Radionuclide studies permit calculation of glomerular filtration rate (GFR) and effective renal plasma flow (ERPF), even in cases of renal impairment. Appropriate radionuclides are injected intravenously and images obtained. The most accurate calculations of GFR and EPFR are obtained by withdrawing blood samples at predetermined intervals and using standard clearance calculations, but strictly count-based computer imaging methods now closely rival this method, without requiring blood samples.

TABLE I
Most Commonly Used Radiopharmaceuticals in Renal Imaging

Radionuclide	Mechanism of renal action	Major clinical usefulness
^{99m}Tc DTPA	Glomerular filtration	Perfusion Parenchymal imaging Estimate GFR Excretion
^{99m}Tc DMSA	Tubular binding and tubular secretion	Pyelonephritis Estimation of tubular mass (i.e., cortical scar)
^{99m}Tc GHP	Glomerular filtration and tubular secretion and tubular binding	Perfusion Excretion Estimation of tubular mass
^{99m}Tc MAG 3	Tubular secretion and glomerular filtration	High renal extraction and useful images even with moderate renal dysfunction Estimate ERPF
^{67}Ga citrate	N/A	Pyelonephritis Interstitial nephritis Renal abscess
^{99m}Tc-, ^{111}In-labeled WBCs	N/A	Renal abscess

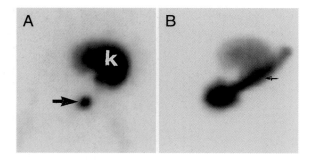

FIGURE 4 (A) Renal transplant scan (5 min after injection) with ^{99m}Tc MAG3 showing tracer in kidney and bladder. K = kidney; arrow to urinary bladder. (B) Scan at 30 min showing leak of tracer due to ureteric necrosis at anastomosis site. Arrow to extravasation of radioactive urine. Note fading activity in kidney, increased size of bladder overlapping inferior margin of extravasation.

2. Measurement of "split" renal function. To determine whether nephrectomy is warranted or safe, it is often important for the surgeon to know the relative contribution to total renal function of each kidney. Computer-enhanced scan techniques can determine the contribution of each kidney to ERPF or GFR. Split renal function measurements are also helpful in follow up of surgical procedures that relieve unilateral obstruction.

3. Renovascular hypertension. Differential renal blood flow studies using ^{99m}Tc mercaptoacetyltriglycine (MAG3) before and after administration of an angiotensin converting enzyme (ACE) inhibitor such as captopril in an appropriately screened hypertensive patient with intact renal function will detect renovascular disease with a sensitivity and specificity exceeding 90%.

4. Contraindication to contrast media. While radionuclide methods do not provide the anatomic detail of other imaging methods, they may be particularly suitable for patients with renal failure or severe contrast media sensitivity. Allergic reactions to radiotracers are extremely rare. Aside from pregnancy, there are no contraindications to the use of radionuclides for diagnostic purposes.

5. Evaluation of renal transplants. Radionuclide imaging may detect impaired blood flow at the renal arterial anastomotic site, urinary tract obstruction, and extravasation of urine due to disruption at the ureteric anastomosis (Figs. 4A, B). This modality complements US for these purposes.

6. Obstructive uropathy. The diuretic renogram is very helpful, particularly in children, who demonstrate an enlarged renal pelvis by US or IVU. This test distinguishes between true obstruction at the ureteropelvic junction and nonobstructive hydronephrosis. Furosemide is injected before or after administration of ^{99m}Tc diethylenetreaminepenta-acetic acid (DTPA) or MAG 3, renal images are obtained, and a renogram curve of activity in each kidney is constructed. Dilatation without significant obstruction is suggested when radionuclide accumulation in the dilated area is reduced at high urine flow rates.

7. Renal infection or scar. The IVU may appear normal in patients with pyelonephritis and the differentiation between this and cystitis may be difficult. 99m-dimercaptosuccinic acid (DSMA) and glucoheptonate (GHP) are renal cortical scanning agents. Areas of inflammation or scar will demonstrate no uptake. The agents are also helpful in determining the amount of remaining renal cortex in children with chronic urinary tract infections and vesicoureteric reflux. ^{99m}Tc- or ^{111}Indium (^{111}In)-labeled WBCs may be used to identify renal abscesses. In patients with low WBC counts, gallium-67 may be used.

ANGIOGRAPHY

Intravenous administration of contrast medium has not proved suitable for renal angiography, and direct intra-arterial injections, either into the main renal arteries or selectively into smaller branches, are generally necessary in this modality. Renal angiography can be used for diagnostic and/or therapeutic purposes.

Diagnostic Angiography

1. Suspected renal artery lesions. Renal angiography is the definitive imaging procedure where renovascular hypertension is suspected, although catheter angiography is increasingly challenged at many centers, as previously indicated, by computed tomographic angiography (CTA) (Fig. 5A, B) and MRA. Such angiography is indicated if

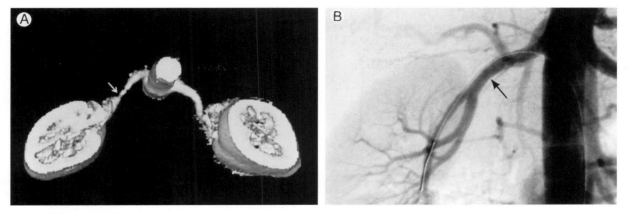

FIGURE 5 (A) Computed tomographic angiography (CTA) showing the computer-generated three-dimensional reconstruction of the aorta and the main renal arteries, possible after a simple IV injection of contrast media. The arrow indicates a significant stenosis in the main right renal artery. (B) Selective right renal angiogram after successful angioplasty, in the same patient as in Fig. 4A, with an arrow showing the now patent right main renal artery. Figures courtesy of Dr. Ken Najarian, FAHC, Burlington, Vermont.

medical therapy for hypertension is ineffective, or in young patients with significant hypertension where medication may be needed for many decades. The patient also should be a suitable candidate for surgical or angioplastic therapy. Renal vein sampling for renin levels may assist selecting patients for treatment. Patients with acute occlusion or thrombosis of the renal arteries, embolic processes, or post-traumatic renal vascular injury may be candidates for renal angiography. In patients with polyarteritis nodosa, renal angiography is the only method with sufficient resolution to detect the characteristic tiny peripheral aneurysms.

2. Unexplained hematuria. Because of the availability of helical CT, angiography is now less likely to be required to investigate the cause of unexplained hematuria, but occasionally angiography is still indispensable. Vascular malformations may be suspected on US or CT but generally require angiography for definitive delineation, especially if the use of catheter injected coils, Gelfoam, or other therapeutic agents is contemplated.

3. Renal transplantation. Angiography is frequently required to map the arterial system in prospective renal donors, where multiple renal arteries or vascular anomalies may complicate transplant surgery. Angiography is required to diagnose post-transplant renal artery stenoses or occlusions. CTA or MRA are increasingly assuming this role, depending on local circumstances and preferences.

4. Renal vein disorders. Although renal vein thrombosis or occlusion may be shown by US, CT, or MRI, rarely direct angiographic renal venography may be required, if there are problems or uncertainties with the other methods.

5. Miscellaneous. Complex or highly unusual renal masses, complications of polycystic disease such as superimposed neoplasm, or trauma, may require angiography.

Interventional Angiography

Angiography has become increasingly important as a therapeutic maneuver rather than only a diagnostic test, and in many angio-interventional radiology sections, therapy far overshadows straight diagnostic imaging in terms of daily workload. Balloon angioplasty treatment is now widely accepted, and may be used to dilate renal artery stenosis, both in native and transplanted kidney (Fig. 5B). Ostial lesions previously thought to be refractory to this method may be amenable to endovascular stenting. Angiography may also be used to embolize bleeding sites within the kidney that may have resulted from trauma or as a complication of interventional procedures such as percutaneous biopsy. Angiography may also be used for selective infusion of thrombolytic agents for treatment of renal artery or vein thrombosis.

Voiding Cystourethrography

This study is useful in demonstrating vesicoureteric reflux. Voiding cystourethrography (VCUG) is mostly commonly performed with fluoroscopic techniques, but radio-nuclide methods have similar sensitivities in the detection of vesico–ureteric reflux.

CHOICE OF IMAGING PROCEDURE FOR SPECIFIC CLINICAL SITUATIONS

Arterial Disease

Ultrasonography can readily diagnose aortic aneurysm, but CT is more accurate where aneurysmal bleeding is suspect, and CT or CTA are better for surgical planning, especially to show the exact levels of the renal arteries. CT can diagnose acute renal infarction by showing parenchymal perfusion defects with a peripheral "rim sign" of collateral flow. As previously suggested, although color Doppler US may demonstrate renal artery stenosis in an individual patient, it is insufficiently reliable to be recommended as a screening tool for renovascular hypertension. In selected patients where significant hypertension is not amenable to medical control, and where surgical or angioplastic therapy is contemplated, some combination of captopril radionuclide renography or MRA and angiography is required.

Congenital Disorders

The most common congenital renal anomalies for which imaging is used are the various forms of renal ectopia, fusion anomalies such as horseshoe kidney, and obstructive processes of the ureteropelvic junction (UPJ) or distal ureter. US and IVU are the primary imaging tools in evaluating these lesions, although occasionally horseshoe kidney (Fig. 6) or other anomaly presents as an incidental finding or CT, MRI, or nuclear medicine study such as a bone scan, where the radiopharmaceutical is excreted by the kidneys. UPJ obstruction may be further evaluated by diuretic urography or radionuclide renography.

Inflammatory Diseases

In acute pyelonephritis, the IVU is usually not indicated and in any case ordinarily not diagnostic. In selected patients, CT can diagnose acute pyelonephritis by showing peripheral perfusion defects in the renal parenchyma, frequently with edema in the perinephric fat. When urinary tract infections follow an atypical or protracted course, US, and with better specificity CT, can delineate infected renal cysts, abscesses, or infected perirenal collections. Either US or CT can guide interventional procedures for diagnosis and treatment, that is, drainage of these lesions. Tuberculosis causes strictures of the renal collecting systems or ureters, and the diagnosis may be suggested by the IVU. Chronic pyelonephritis, frequently associated with reflux nephropathy, produces scarred, and in advanced disease shrunken kidneys readily shown on IVU or cross-sectional imaging.

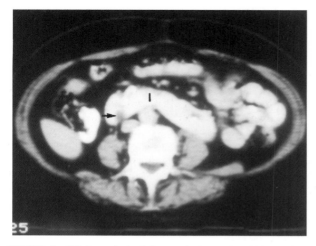

FIGURE 6 CT through the isthmus of a horseshoe kidney. I is on the isthmus, and the arrow points to an incidental cyst in the attached lower pole of the right kidney.

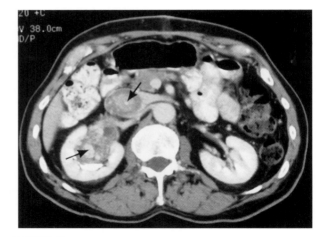

FIGURE 7 CT showing renal carcinoma. This cross section through the level of the kidneys was obtained using oral and IV contrast media. The lower black arrow points to the irregularly radiolucent, necrotic tumor mass. The second black arrow, higher in position as the reader views the illustration, points to a filling defect in the inferior vena cava, representing tumor thrombus. A normal cava would be homogeneously bright with enhancing blood, like the aorta.

Neoplasia

The main grouping of renal tumors divides renal parenchymal masses from urothelial lesions. Although cystic or solid renal parenchymal masses may be first detected by IVU, they require US and/or CT for further differentiation and staging (Fig. 7). MRI is available in some instances where the patient is sensitive to iodinated intravascular contrast media, or where a question about the renal vasculature is unresolved. Urothelial tumors, nearly always transitional cell carcinoma (TCC), are best shown on IVU or retrograde pyelography—the latter serving as a guide for brush biopsy. The detection of small TCCs of the ureter or bladder is one reason CT has not supplanted the IVU as a screening tool in hematuria, although in selected patients cross-sectional imaging may be required to confirm or further delineate such lesions. In some centers geometric reconstruction with three-dimensional CT or even more recently three-dimensional MRI of renal tumors may be used to stage renal neoplasm, especially where partial nephrectomy is considered. Three-dimensional reconstruction of the urinary bladder can depict the geometry of TCC down to the millimeter range, so called "virtual cystoscopy."

Cystic Disorders

Benign renal cysts occur in up to 30% of normal adults and can nearly always be readily differentiated from solid neoplasm by US. Complex cysts may require CT for definitive evaluation. Both infantile autosomal recessive and adult autosomal dominant polycystic renal disease are readily diagnosed by US; the former may be detected *in utero,* and the latter lends itself to US where indicated (see Chapter 43). Medullary sponge kidney (renal tubular ectasia) is diagnosed by IVU.

Trauma

Helical CT, where very rapid CT of the entire upper abdomen can be done in a single breath hold, has supplanted the IVU for evaluating renal trauma, because of its speed and accuracy, and its multiorgan sweep. CT also may assess the renal vascular supply, although conventional angiography is required in selected cases or major renovascular trauma, where diagnosis and/or therapy are required. For suspected bladder rupture, CT cystography, where CT sections through the bladder are done after retrograde injection of contrast media is becoming the method of choice. For suspected urethral rupture, in males, retrograde urethrography remains the procedure of choice.

Parenchymal Disorders

Renal parenchymal disease consists of a broad range of processes, from inflammatory or immunologic disorders to toxic or ischemic lesions. Imaging can show small kidneys, and US may demonstrate echogenic, abnormal parenchyma, but rarely pinpoints the diagnosis, which may require renal biopsy, the latter amenable to US guidance. The main goal of imaging is to rule out obstruction, polycystic kidney disease, renal papillary necrosis, vascular disease, or reflux nephropathy. For patients presenting in renal failure, US is an excellent noninvasive method to differentiate intrinsic parenchymal disease from obstructive uropathy.

Urolithiasis

Most urinary calculi are calcified and therefore are readily detectable by KUB. Radiolucent stones on plain radiography, primarily composed of uric acid, appear as filling defects within the opacified urinary tract on the IVU. The IVU also shows obstruction by virtue of demonstrating hydronephrosis or hydroureter related to the obstructing calculus. Retrograde pyelography may be required to plan therapy where stent placement is needed, and KUBs may assist in follow up of calculus material treated by ESWL (extracorporeal shock wave therapy). US has a limited role in patients with urinary calculi: it can show nephrocalcinosis or nephrolithiasis, and occasionally urinary bladder calculi, but is insensitive for ureteric stones. The major innovation in the diagnosis of renal colic has been the conversion of the use of IVU to unenhanced helical abdominal CT, the so-called renal colic CT protocol. Helical CT (Fig. 3A, B) has completely replaced the IVU in many centers, where renal colic is suspect. CT is quick (5 min on the CT table), requires no patient preparation, is without any side effects since no IV contrast is used, is highly accurate and sensitive, and can precisely locate and measure the size of ureteric stones. CT will show calculi not visible on the KUB, the urate stones; virtually all calculi, regardless of their chemical composition, will be visible. CT can show obstruction and extravasation of urine and help plan therapy. In addition, CT has the virtue of showing many nonurinary causes of acute abdominal pain, such as appendicitis, ovarian cysts, pancreatitis, etc., conditions which typically are not diagnosable by the IVU.

Renal Transplantation

Renal transplantation donors need at least an IVU preoperatively, and as previously indicated, depending on institutional preferences, angiography, CTA, or MRA, to assess vascular anatomy. In recipients post-transplantation, color flow Doppler US documents the status of vascular perfusion to the transplanted kidney, and US can document hydronephrosis, renal volumes, and extrarenal collections such as lymphocele, but cannot reliably differentiate rejection from acute tubular necrosis. Radionuclide studies can also assess perfusion or obstruction, and rarely retrograde or even percutaneous antegrade pyelography is required to assess ureteral patency. Angiography may be needed to show renal artery stenoses to the transplant.

Ureteral Obstruction

Bilateral ureteric obstruction causing renal failure is rare in adults in the absence of malignancy. Although specific lesions such as retroperitoneal fibrosis must be considered, US can show hydronephrosis, and is generally used as the first imaging procedure in patients with acute renal failure. US is a noninvasive, inexpensive study that can readily differentiate obstructive hydronephrosis with ureterectasis from other causes of renal failure where the calyces may be normal, but the renal parenchyma may be diminished or scarred, such as chronic pyelonephritis. Acute unilateral ureteric obstruction, commonly due to renal colic with passage of a ureteric calculus, is readily diagnosed by IVU. As previously indicated, however, helical CT is rapidly completely supplanting the IVU as the method of choice in the diagnosis of renal colic, for the reasons noted.

Renal Vein Lesions

Diagnostic imaging of the renal vein is now nearly always done during the course of cross-sectional imaging—US, CT, or MRI. Conventional renal venography via angiographic methods is rarely done. Contrast injections into the renal vein via catheter might be done during the course of renal vein renin sampling, which itself is institution specific, and not universally used. During the course of US or CT evaluation of a renal neoplasm, for instance, either method may show tumor thrombus in the renal vein. MRI can nicely show the renal vein if thrombosis is suspected, if other methods are problematic.

Bibliography

Bude RO, Rubin JA: Detection of renal artery stenosis with Doppler sonography: It is more complicated than originally thought. *Radiology* 96:612–613, 1995.

Dodd GD, Tublin ME, Shah A, Zajko AB: Review. Imaging of vascular complications associated with renal transplants. *AJR* 157:449–459, 1991.

Dunnick NR, Cohan RH: Commentary. Cost, corticosteroids, and contrast media. *AJR* 162:527–529, 1994.

Fielding JR, Silverman SG, Rubin GD: Helical CT of the urinary tract. Review. *AJR* 172:1199–1206, 1999.

Gilfeather M, Yoon HC, Siegelman ES, *et al.:* Renal artery stenosis: Evaluation with conventional angiography versus gadolinium-enhanced MR angiography. *Radiology* 210:367–372, 1999.

Lanoue MZ, Mindell HJ: Pictorial essay. The use of unenhanced helical CT to evaluate suspected renal colic. *AJR* 169:1579–1584, 1997.

Mindell HJ, Cochran ST: Commentary. Current perspectives in the diagnosis and treatment of urinary stone disease. *AJR* 163:1314–1315, 1994.

Solomon R, Warner C, Mann D, *et al.:* Effects of saline, mannitol and furosemide on acute decreases in renal function produced by radiocontrast agents. *N Engl J Med* 331:1416–1420, 1994.

Taylor A: Radionuclide renography: A personal approach. *Semin Nucl Med* 29(2):102–127, April 1999.

Tublin ME, Murphy ME, Tessler FN, Review. Current concepts in contrast media-induced nephropathy. *AJR* 171:933–939, 1998.

Zagoria RJ, Berchtold RE, Dyer RB: Staging of renal adenocarcinoma: Role of various imaging procedures. *AJR* 164:363–370, 1995.

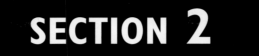

SECTION 2

ACID–BASE, FLUID, AND ELECTROLYTE DISORDERS

HYPONATREMIA AND HYPOOSMOLAR DISORDERS

JOSEPH G. VERBALIS

The incidence of hyponatremia depends on the nature of the patient population and also the criteria used to establish the diagnosis. Hospital incidences of 15–22% are common if hyponatremia is defined as a serum $[Na^+] < 135$ mEq/L, but in most studies only 1–4% of patients have a serum $[Na^+] \leq 130$. Although most cases are mild, hyponatremia is important clinically because: (1) acute severe hyponatremia can cause substantial morbidity and mortality; (2) mild hyponatremia can progress to more dangerous levels during management of other disorders; (3) general mortality appears to be higher in patients with even asymptomatic hyponatremia; and (4) overly rapid correction of chronic hyponatremia can produce severe neurological deficits and death.

DEFINITIONS

Hyponatremia is of clinical significance only when it reflects corresponding hypoosmolality of the plasma. Plasma osmolality can be measured directly by osmometry, or calculated as:

$$P_{osm} \text{ (mOsmol/kg } H_2O) = 2 \times \text{serum } [Na^+] \text{ (mEq/L)} + \text{glucose (mg/dL)}/18 + \text{BUN (mg/dL)}/2.8$$

Both methods produce comparable results under most conditions, as does simply doubling the serum $[Na^+]$. However, total osmolality is not always equivalent to *effective osmolality*, sometimes referred to as the *tonicity* of the plasma. Solutes compartmentalized to the extracellular fluid (ECF) are effective solutes, since they create osmotic gradients across cell membranes leading to osmotic movement of water from the intracellular fluid (ICF) to ECF compartments. In contrast, solutes that freely permeate cell membranes (urea, ethanol, methanol) are not effective solutes, since they do not create osmotic gradients across cell membranes and therefore are not associated with secondary water shifts. Only the concentration of effective solutes in plasma should be used to determine whether clinically significant hypoosmolality is present.

Hyponatremia and hypoosmolality are usually synonymous, but with two important exceptions. First, *pseudohy-ponatremia* can be produced by marked elevation of serum lipids and/or proteins. In such cases the concentration of Na^+ per liter of serum water is unchanged, but the concentration of Na^+ per liter of serum is artifactually decreased because of the increased relative proportion occupied by lipid or protein. Fortunately, measurement of serum or plasma $[Na^+]$ by ion-specific electrodes, which is now commonly employed by most clinical laboratories, is much less influenced by high concentrations of lipids or proteins than is measurement of serum $[Na^+]$ by flame photometry, although such errors can nonetheless still occur. However, because direct measurement of plasma osmolality is based on the colligative properties of solute particles in solution, the measured plasma osmolality will *not* be affected by the increased lipids or proteins. Second, high concentrations of effective solutes other than Na^+ can cause relative decreases in serum $[Na^+]$ despite an unchanged plasma osmolality; this commonly occurs with hyperglycemia. Misdiagnosis can be avoided again by direct measurement of plasma osmolality, or by correcting the serum $[Na^+]$ by 1.6 mEq/L for each 100 mg/dL increase in blood glucose concentration above 100 mg/dL.

PATHOGENESIS

The presence of significant hypoosmolality always indicates excess water relative to solute in the ECF. Because water moves freely between the ICF and ECF, this also indicates an excess of total body water relative to total body solute. Imbalances between water and solute can be generated initially either by *depletion* of body solute more than body water, or by *dilution* of body solute from increases in body water more than body solute (Table 1). It should be recognized, however, that this distinction represents an oversimplification, because most hypoosmolar states include variable components of both solute depletion and water retention (e.g., isotonic solute losses, as occurs during an acute hemorrhage, do not produce hypoosmolality until the subsequent retention of water from ingested or infused hypotonic fluids causes a secondary dilution of the remaining ECF solute). Nonetheless, this concept has proven to be useful because it provides a simple framework for understanding the diagnosis and therapy of hypoosmolar disorders.

TABLE I
Pathogenesis of Hypoosmolar Disorders[a]

Depletion (primary decreases in total body solute + secondary water retention)[b]

1. Renal solute loss
   Diuretic use
   Solute diuresis (glucose, mannitol)
   Salt wasting nephropathy
   Mineralocorticoid deficiency

2. Nonrenal solute loss
   Gastrointestinal (diarrhea, vomiting, pancreatitis, bowel obstruction)
   Cutaneous (sweating, burns)
   Blood loss

Dilution (primary increases in total body water ± secondary solute depletion)[c]

1. Impaired renal free water excretion

   A. Increased proximal reabsorption
      Hypothyroidism

   B. Impaired distal dilution
      Syndrome of inappropriate antidiuresis (SIAD)
      Glucocorticoid deficiency

   C. Combined increased proximal reabsorption and impaired distal dilution
      Congestive heart failure
      Cirrhosis
      Nephrotic syndrome

   D. Decreased urinary solute excretion
      Beer potomania

2. Excess water intake
   Primary polydipsia
   Dilute infant formula

[a]Modified from Verbalis (1995).

[b]Virtually all disorders of solute depletion are accompanied by some degree of secondary retention of water by the kidneys in response to the resulting intravascular hypovolemia; this mechanism can lead to hypoosmolality even when the solute depletion occurs via hypotonic or isotonic body fluid losses.

[c]Disorders of water retention primarily cause hypoosmolality in the absence of any solute losses, but in some cases of SIAD secondary solute losses occur in response to the resulting intravascular hypervolemia, and this can then further aggravate the dilutional hypoosmolality in the plasma (however, this pathophysiology does not likely contribute to the hyponatremia of edema-forming states such as congestive heart failure and cirrhosis, since in these cases multiple factors favoring sodium retention will result in an increased total body sodium).

DIFFERENTIAL DIAGNOSIS

The diagnostic approach to hypoosmolar patients should include a careful history (especially concerning medications); clinical assessment of the ECF volume status; a thorough neurological evaluation; serum or plasma electrolytes, glucose, blood urea nitrogen (BUN), creatinine, and uric acid; calculated and/or directly measured plasma osmolality; and simultaneous urine electrolytes and osmolality. Although incidences will vary according to the population being studied, sequential analysis of hyponatremic patients admitted to a large university teaching hospital have revealed that approximately 20% were hypovolemic, 20% had edema-forming states, 33% were euvolemic, 15% had hyperglycemia-induced hyponatremia, and 10% had renal failure. Consequently, euvolemic hyponatremia generally constitutes the largest single group of hyponatremic patients found in this setting. A definitive diagnosis is not always possible at the time of presentation, but an initial categorization according to the clinical ECF volume status of the patient will allow a determination of the appropriate initial therapy in the majority of cases (Fig. 1).

Decreased ECF Volume (Hypovolemia)

Clinically detectable hypovolemia, generally determined most sensitively by careful measurement of orthostatic changes in blood pressure and pulse rate, always indicates some degree of solute depletion. Elevation of BUN is a useful laboratory correlate of decreased ECF volume. Even isotonic or hypotonic volume losses can lead to hypoosmolality if water or hypotonic fluids are ingested or infused as replacement. A low urine Na$^+$ concentration (U_{Na}) in such cases suggests a nonrenal cause of the solute depletion, whereas a high U_{Na} suggests renal causes of solute depletion (Table 1). Diuretic use is the most common cause of hypovolemic hypoosmolality, and thiazides are more commonly associated with severe hyponatremia than are loop diuretics such as furosemide. Although this represents a prime example of solute depletion, the pathophysiological mechanisms underlying the hypoosmolality are complex and are composed of multiple potential components, including free water retention. Furthermore, many such patients do not present with clinical evidence of marked hypovolemia, in part because ingested water has been retained in response to nonosmotically stimulated vasopressin (AVP) secretion, as is often true for all disorders of solute depletion. To further complicate diagnosis, the U_{Na} may be high or low depending on when the last diuretic dose was taken. Consequently, almost any suspicion of diuretic use mandates careful consideration of this diagnosis. A low serum [K$^+$] is an important clue to diuretic use, since few other disorders that cause hyponatremia and hypoosmolality also produce appreciable hypokalemia. Whenever the possibility of diuretic use is suspected in the absence of a positive history, a urine screen for diuretics should be performed. Most other etiologies of renal or nonrenal solute losses causing hypovolemic hypoosmolality will be clinically apparent, although some cases of salt wasting nephropathies (chronic interstitial nephropathy, polycystic kidney disease, obstructive uropathy, or Bartter's syndrome), or mineralocorticoid deficiency (Addison's disease), can be challenging to diagnose during early phases of these diseases.

Normal ECF Volume (Euvolemia)

Virtually any disorder associated with hypoosmolality can potentially present with a volume status that appears normal by standard methods of clinical evaluation. Because

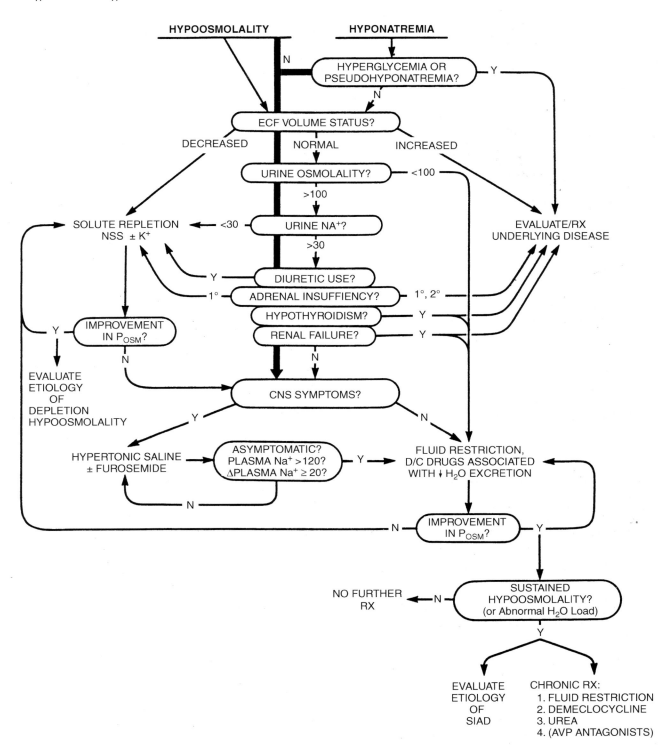

FIGURE I   Algorithm for evaluation and therapy of hypoosmolar patients. The dark arrow in the center emphasizes that the presence of central nervous system dysfunction due to hyponatremia should always be assessed immediately, so that appropriate therapy can be started as soon as possible in symptomatic patients even while the outlined diagnostic evaluation is proceeding. Abbreviations: N = no; Y = yes; ECF = extracellular fluid volume; NSS = normal (isotonic) saline; Rx = treat; 1° = primary; 2° = secondary; P_{osm} = plasma osmolality; d/c = discontinue; SIAD = syndrome of inappropriate antidiuresis; numbers referring to osmolality are in mOsmol/kg H_2O, numbers referring to serum Na^+ concentration are in mEq/L (modified from Verbalis, 1995).

clinical assessment of volume status is not very sensitive, the presence of normal or low levels of serum BUN and uric acid are very helpful laboratory correlates of relatively normal, or even slightly expanded, ECF volume. In these cases, a low U_{Na} suggests a depletional hypoosmolality secondary to ECF losses with subsequent volume replacement by water or other hypotonic fluids; as discussed earlier, such patients may appear euvolemic by all the usual clinical parameters used to assess hydrational status. Primary dilutional disorders are less likely in the presence of a low U_{Na} (≤ 30 mEq/L), although this pattern can occur in hypothyroidism. A high U_{Na} (>30 mEq/L) generally indicates a dilutional hypoosmolality such as SIAD (Table 1). Although originally described as the syndrome of inappropriate antidiuretic hormone secretion (SIADH), approximately 10 to 20% of patients who meet all established criteria for SIADH do not have measurably elevated plasma AVP levels, so it is actually more accurate to use the term syndrome of inappropriate antidiuresis (SIAD) rather than SIADH to describe this entire group of disorders. SIAD is the most common cause of euvolemic hypoosmolality in clinical practice. The clinical criteria necessary for a diagnosis of SIAD remain essentially as defined by Bartter and Schwartz in 1967 (Table 2), but several points deserve emphasis. First, true ECF hypoosmolality must be present and hyponatremia secondary to pseudohyponatremia or hyperglycemia excluded. Second, urinary osmolality must be inappropriate for plasma hypoosmolality. This does *not* require a $U_{osm} > P_{osm}$, but simply that the urine osmolality is

TABLE 2
Criteria for the Diagnosis of SIAD[a]

Essential

1. Decreased effective osmolality of the extracellular fluid ($P_{osm} < 275$ mOsmol/kg H_2O).

2. Inappropriate urinary concentration ($U_{osm} > 100$ mOsmol/kg H_2O with normal renal function) at some level of hypoosmolality.

3. Clinical euvolemia, as defined by the absence of signs of hypovolemia (orthostasis, tachycardia, decreased skin turgor, dry mucous membranes) or hypervolemia (subcutaneous edema, ascites).

4. Elevated urinary sodium excretion while on a normal salt and water intake.

5. Absence of other potential causes of euvolemic hypoosmolality: hypothyroidism, hypocortisolism (Addison's disease or pituitary ACTH insufficiency) and diuretic use.

Supplemental

6. Abnormal water load test (inability to excrete at least 80% of a 20 ml/kg water load in 4 hr and/or failure to dilute U_{osm} to <100 mOsmol/kg H_2O).

7. Plasma AVP level inappropriately elevated relative to plasma osmolality.

8. No significant correction of serum $[Na^+]$ with volume expansion but improvement after fluid restriction.

---

[a]Modified from Verbalis (1995).

greater than maximally dilute (i.e., $U_{osm} > 100$ mOsmol/kg H_2O in adults). Furthermore, urine osmolality need not be inappropriately elevated at all levels of P_{osm} but simply at some level under 275 mOsmol/kg H_2O, since in patients with a *reset osmostat*, AVP secretion can be suppressed at some level of osmolality resulting in maximal urinary dilution and free water excretion at plasma osmolalities below this level. Although some consider a reset osmostat to be a separate disorder rather than a variant of SIAD, such cases nonetheless illustrate that some hypoosmolar patients can exhibit an appropriately dilute urine at some, though not all, plasma osmolalities. Third, clinical euvolemia must be present to diagnose SIAD, and this diagnosis *cannot* be made in a hypovolemic or edematous patient. This does not mean that patients with SIAD cannot become hypovolemic for other reasons, but in such cases it is impossible to diagnose the underlying SIAD until the patient is rendered euvolemic. The fourth criterion, renal salt wasting, has probably caused the most confusion regarding SIAD. The importance of this criterion lies in its usefulness in differentiating hypoosmolality caused by a decreased relative intravascular volume in which case renal Na^+ conservation occurs, from dilutional disorders in which urinary Na^+ excretion is normal or increased due to ECF volume expansion. However, U_{Na} can also be high in renal causes of solute depletion such as diuretic use or Addison's disease, and conversely patients with SIAD can have a low urinary Na^+ excretion if they subsequently become hypovolemic or solute depleted, conditions sometimes produced by imposed salt and water restriction. Consequently, although high urinary Na^+ excretion is the rule in most patients with SIAD, its presence does not confirm this diagnosis nor does it absence rule out the diagnosis. The final criterion emphasizes that SIAD remains a diagnosis of exclusion, and the absence of other potential causes of hypoosmolality must always be verified. Glucocorticoid deficiency and SIAD can be especially difficult to distinguish, since hypocortisolism can cause elevated plasma AVP levels and in addition has direct renal effects to prevent maximal urinary dilution. Therefore, no patient with chronic hyponatremia should be diagnosed as having SIAD without a thorough evaluation of adrenal function, preferably via a rapid ACTH stimulation test (acute hyponatremia of obvious etiology, such as postoperatively or in association with pneumonitis, may be treated without adrenal testing as long as there are no other clinical signs or symptoms suggestive of adrenal dynfunction). Many different disorders have been associated with SIAD, and these can be divided into several major etiologic groups (Table 3).

Some cases of euvolemic hyponatremia do not fit particularly well into either a dilutional or depletional category. Chief among these is the hyponatremia that sometimes occurs in patients who ingest large volumes of beer with little food intake for prolonged periods, often called *beer potomania*. Even though the volume of fluid ingested may not seem sufficiently excessive to overwhelm renal diluting mechanisms, in these cases free water excretion is limited by very low urinary solute excretion thereby causing water retention and dilutional hyponatremia. However,

TABLE 3
Common Etiologies of SIAD

1. **Tumors**

Pulmonary/mediastinal (bronchogenic carcinoma; mesothelioma; thymoma)

Nonchest (duodenal carcinoma; pancreatic carcinoma; ureteral/prostate carcinoma; uterine carcinoma; nasopharyngeal carcinoma; leukemia)

2. **Central nervous system disorders**

Mass lesions (tumors; brain abscesses; subdural hematoma)

Inflammatory diseases (encephalitis; meningitis; systemic lupus)

Degenerative/demyelinative diseases (Guillian-Barré; spinal cord lesions)

Miscellaneous (subarachnoid hemorrhage; head trauma; acute psychosis; delirium tremens; pituitary stalk section)

3. **Drug induced**

Stimulated AVP release (nicotine; phenothiazines; tricyclics; serotonin reuptake inhibitors)

Direct renal effects and/or potentiation of AVP effects (desmopressin; oxytocin; prostaglandin synthesis inhibitors)

Mixed or uncertain actions [angiotensin converting enzyme inhibitors; chlorpropamide; clofibrate; carbamazepine; cyclophosphamide; 3,4-methylenedioxymeth-amphetamine ("ecstasy"); vincristine]

4. **Pulmonary diseases**

Infections (tuberculosis; aspergillosis; pneumonia; empyema)

Mechanical/ventilatory (acute respiratory failure; COPD; positive pressure ventilation)

because such patients have very low sodium intakes as well, it is likely that relative depletion of body Na^+ stores also is a contributing factor to the hypoosmolality in some cases.

Increased ECF Volume (Hypervolemia)

The presence of hypervolemia, as detected clinically by the presence of edema and/or ascites, indicates whole body sodium excess, and hypoosmolality in these patients suggests a relatively decreased intravascular volume and/or pressure leading to water retention as a result of both elevated plasma AVP levels and decreased distal delivery of glomerular filtrate. Such patients usually have a low U_{Na} because of secondary hyperaldosteronism, but under certain conditions the U_{Na} may be elevated (e.g., glucosuria in diabetics, diuretic therapy). Hyponatremia generally does not occur until fairly advanced stages of diseases such as congestive heart failure, cirrhosis, and nephrotic syndrome, so diagnosis is usually not difficult. Renal failure can also cause retention of both sodium and water, but in this case the factor limiting excretion of excess body fluid is not decreased effective circulating volume but rather decreased glomerular filtration. It should be remembered that even though many edema-forming states have *secondary* increases in plasma AVP levels as a result of decreased effective arterial blood volume, nonetheless they are not classified as cases of SIAD, since they fail to meet the criterion of clinical euvolemia

(Table 2, point 3). Although it can be argued that this represents a semantic distinction, nonetheless it is important because it allows segregation of identifiable etiologies of hyponatremia that are associated with different methods of evaluation and therapy. Primary polydipsia also can cause hypoosmolality in a small subset of patients with some degree of underlying SIAD, particularly psychiatric patients with long-standing schizophrenia on neuroleptic drugs, or even more rarely in patients with normal kidney function if the volumes ingested exceed the maximum renal free water excretory rate of approximately 500–1000 ml/hr. However, these patients rarely manifest overt signs of volume excess since water retention alone without sodium excess does not cause clinically apparent hypervolemia.

CLINICAL MANIFESTATIONS OF HYPONATREMIA

Hypoosmolality is associated with a broad spectrum of neurological manifestations, ranging from mild nonspecific symptoms (e.g., headache, nausea) to more significant disorders (e.g., disorientation, confusion, obtundation, focal neurological deficits, and seizures). In the most severe cases death can result from respiratory arrest after tentorial cerebral herniation with subsequent brain stem compression. This neurological symptom complex has been termed *hyponatremic encephalopathy,* and primarily reflects brain edema resulting from osmotic water shifts into the brain because of the decreased effective plasma osmolality. Significant symptoms generally do not occur until the serum $[Na^+]$ falls below 125 mEq/L, and the severity of symptoms can be roughly correlated with the degree of hypoosmolality. However, individual variability is marked, and for any single patient the level of serum $[Na^+]$ at which symptoms will appear cannot be predicted. Furthermore, several factors other than the severity of the hypoosmolality also affect the degree of neurological dysfunction. Most important is the period over which hypoosmolality develops. Rapid development of severe hypoosmolality is frequently associated with marked neurological symptoms, whereas gradual development over several days or weeks is often associated with relatively mild symptomatology despite profound degrees of hypoosmolality. This is because the brain can counteract osmotic swelling by excreting intracellular solutes (including both electrolytes and organic osmolytes), a process called *volume regulation.* Since this is a time-dependent process, rapid development of hypoosmolality can result in brain edema before this adaptation occurs, but with slower development of the same degree of hypoosmolality brain cells can lose solute sufficiently rapidly to prevent brain edema and neurological dysfunction.

Underlying neurological disease also can significantly affect the level of hypoosmolality at which CNS symptoms appear (e.g., moderate hypoosmolality is generally of little concern in an otherwise healthy patient, but can cause substantial morbidity in a patient with an underlying seizure disorder). Non-neurological metabolic disorders (hypoxia, hypercapnia, acidosis, hypercalcemia, etc.) similarly can affect the level of plasma osmolality at which CNS symptoms occur. Studies have suggested that some patients may be susceptible to a vicious cycle in which hypoosmolality-induced brain edema causes noncardiogenic pulmonary edema, and the resulting hypoxia and hypercapnia then further impair the ability of the brain to volume regulate, thus leading to more brain edema with neurological deterioration and death in some cases. Other clinical studies have suggested that menstruating females and young children may be particularly susceptible to the development of neurological morbidity and mortality during hyponatremia, especially in the acute postoperative setting. The true clinical incidence as well as the underlying pathophysiological mechanisms responsible for these sometimes catastrophic cases remains to be determined.

TREATMENT

Despite some continuing controversy regarding the optimal speed of correction of osmolality in hyponatremic patients, there is now a relatively uniform consensus about appropriate therapy in most cases (Fig. 1). If any degree of clinical hypovolemia is present, the patient should be considered to have a solute depletion-induced hypoosmolality and should be treated with isotonic (0.9%) NaCl at a rate appropriate for the estimated volume depletion. If diuretic use is known or suspected, the replacement fluids should be supplemented with potassium (30–40 mEq/L) even if the serum [K$^+$] is not low because of the propensity of such patients to have total body potassium depletion. Most often the hypoosmolar patient will be clinically euvolemic, but several situations will dictate a reconsideration of potential solute depletion even in the patient without clinically apparent hypovolemia: a decreased U_{Na}, any history of recent diuretic use, and any suggestion of primary adrenal insufficiency. Whenever a reasonable likelihood of depletional rather than dilutional hypoosmolality exists it is appropriate to treat initially with a trial of isotonic NaCl. If the patient has SIAD no harm will have been done with a limited (1–2 L) saline infusion, since such patients will simply excrete excess NaCl without significantly changing their P_{osm}. However, this therapy should be abandoned if the serum [Na$^+$] does not improve, since longer periods of continued isotonic NaCl infusion can worsen the hyponatremia by virtue of gradual water retention. The treatment of euvolemic hypoosmolar patients will vary depending on their presentation. A patient meeting all criteria for SIAD except that U_{osm} is low should simply be observed since this may represent spontaneous reversal of a transient form of SIAD. If there is any suspicion of either primary or secondary adrenal insufficiency, glucocorticoid replacement should be started immediately after completion of a rapid ACTH stimulation test. Prompt water diuresis following initiation of glucocorticoid treatment strongly supports glucocorticoid deficiency, but the absence of a quick response does not negate this diagnosis since several days of glucocorticoids are sometimes required for normalization of P_{osm}. Hypervolemic hypoosmolar patients are generally treated initially by diuresis and other measures directed at their underlying disorder. Such patients rarely require any therapy to increase plasma osmolality acutely, but often

benefit from varying degrees of sodium and water restriction to reduce body fluid retention.

In any significantly hyponatremic patient one is faced with the question of how quickly the plasma osmolality should be corrected. Although hyponatremia is associated with a broad spectrum of neurological symptoms, sometimes leading to death in severe cases, too rapid correction of severe hyponatremia can produce *pontine and extrapontine myelinolysis,* a brain demyelinating disease that also can cause substantial neurological morbidity and mortality. Clinical and experimental results suggest that optimal treatment of hyponatremic patients must entail balancing the risks of hyponatremia against the risks of correction for each patient. Several factors should therefore be considered when making a treatment decision in hyponatremic patients: the severity of the hyponatremia, the duration of the hyponatremia, and the symptomatology of the patient. Neither sequelae from hyponatremia itself nor myelinolysis after therapy are very likely in patients whose serum [Na$^+$] remains $\geq$120 mEq/L, although significant symptoms can develop even at higher serum [Na$^+$] levels if the rate of fall of plasma osmolality has been very rapid. The importance of duration and symptomatology relate to how well the brain has volume-adapted to the hyponatremia, and consequently its degree of risk for subsequent demyelination with rapid correction. Cases of acute hyponatremia ($\leq$48 hr duration) are usually symptomatic if the hyponatremia is severe (i.e., $\leq$120 mEq/L). These patients are at greatest risk from neurological complications from the hyponatremia itself and should be corrected to higher serum [Na$^+$] levels promptly. Conversely, patients with more chronic hyponatremia (>48 hr in duration) who have minimal neurological symptomatology are at little risk from complications of hyponatremia itself, but can develop demyelination following rapid correction. There is no indication to correct these patients rapidly, and they should be treated using slower-acting therapies such as fluid restriction.

Although the previously mentioned extremes have clear treatment indications, most hyponatremic episodes will be of indeterminate duration and the patients will have varying degrees of milder neurological symptomatology. This group represents the most challenging treatment decision, since the hyponatremia will have been present sufficiently long enough to allow some degree of brain volume regulation, but not long enough to prevent some brain edema and neurological symptomatology. Most authorities recommend prompt treatment of such patients because of their symptoms, but using methods that allow a *controlled and limited correction* of their hyponatremia. Reasonable correction parameters consist of a maximal rate of correction of serum [Na$^+$] in the range of 1–2 mEq/L/hr as long as the total magnitude of correction does not exceed 25 mEq/L over the first 48 hr. Some argue that these parameters should be even more conservative with magnitudes of correction that do not exceed 12 mEq/L over the first 24 hr and 18 mEq/L over the first 48 hr of correction. Treatments for individual patients should be chosen within these limits depending on their symptomatology. In patients who are only moderately symptomatic one should proceed at the lower recommended limits of ≤0.5 mEq/L/hr, while in those who manifest more severe neurological symptoms an initial correction at a rate of 1–2 mEq/L/hr would be more appropriate. Controlled corrections are generally best accomplished with hypertonic (3%) NaCl solution given via continuous infusion, since patients with euvolemic hypoosmolality such as SIAD generally will not respond to isotonic NaCl. An initial infusion rate can be estimated by multiplying the body weight of the patient, in kilograms by the desired rate of increase in serum [Na$^+$], in mEq/L/hr (e.g., in a 70 kg patient an infusion of 3% NaCl at 70 ml/hr will increase serum [Na$^+$] by approximately 1 mEq/L/hr, while infusing 35 ml/hr will increase serum [Na$^+$] by approximately 0.5 mEq/L/hr). Furosemide (20–40 mg iv) should be used to treat volume overload; in patients with known cardiovascular disease preemptive use is appropriate. Patients with diuretic-induced hyponatremia usually respond well to isotonic NaCl and do not require 3% NaCl. Regardless of the initial rate of correction chosen, acute treatment should be interrupted once any of three endpoints is reached: (1) the symptoms of the patient are abolished, (2) a safe serum [Na$^+$] (generally ≥120 mEq/L) is achieved, or (3) a total magnitude of correction of 20 mEq/L is achieved. It follows from these recommendations that serum [Na$^+$] levels must be carefully monitored at frequent intervals (at least every 4 hr) during the active phases of treatment in order to adjust therapy so that the correction stays within these guidelines. Regardless of the therapy or rate initially chosen, it cannot be emphasized too strongly that it is only necessary to correct the plasma osmolality acutely to a safe range rather than completely to normonatremia. In some situations patients may spontaneously correct their hyponatremia via a water diuresis. If the hyponatremia is acute (e.g., psychogenic polydipsia with water intoxication) such patients do not appear to be at risk for subsequent demyelination; however, in cases where the hyponatremia has been chronic (e.g., hypocortisolism) intervention should be considered to limit the rate and magnitude of correction of serum [Na$^+$] (e.g., administration of desmopressin 1–2 μg iv or infusion of hypotonic fluids) using the same endpoints as for active corrections.

Treatment of chronic hyponatremia entails choosing among several suboptimal therapies. One important exception are those patients with the reset osmostat syndrome; because the hyponatremia of such patients is not progressive but rather fluctuates around their reset level of serum [Na$^+$], no therapy is generally required. For most other cases of mild to moderate SIAD, fluid restriction represents the least toxic therapy by far, and is the treatment of choice. This should always be tried as the initial therapy, with pharmacological intervention reserved for refractory cases where the degree of fluid restriction required to avoid hypoosmolality is so severe that the patient is unable, or unwilling, to maintain it. If pharmacological treatment is necessary the preferred drug at present is the tetracycline derivative demeclocycline, which causes nephrogenic diabetes insipidus thereby decreasing urine concentration. The effective dose of demeclocycline ranges from 600 to 1200 mg/day; several days of therapy are necessary to achieve maximum effects, so one should wait 3–4 days before increasing the dose. Demeclocycline can cause reversible nephrotoxicity, especially in patients with cirrhosis; renal function should be monitored and the medication stopped if increasing azotemia occurs. Several other drugs can decrease AVP hypersecretion in selected cases (diphenylhydantoin, opiates, ethanol), but responses are unpredictable. Despite current unavailability of an ideal therapeutic agent for chronic SIAD, this will likely change in the near future with development of specific *vasopressin receptor antagonists*. Such agents will likely become the treatments of choice for SIAD in the future. However, their use to correct established hyponatremia will require judicious adherence to the same guidelines already established for other therapies to prevent complications from brain demyelination.

Bibliography

Anderson RJ, Chung H-M, Kluge R, et al.: Hyponatremia: A prospective analysis of its epidemiology and the pathogenetic role of vasopressin. Ann Intern Med 102:164–168, 1985.

Arieff AI, Llach F, Massry SG: Neurological manifestations and morbidity of hyponatremia: Correlation with brain water and electrolytes. Medicine 55:121–129, 1976.

Ayus JC, Arieff AI: Pulmonary complications of hyponatremic encephalopathy. Noncardiogenic pulmonary edema and hypercapnic respiratory failure. Chest 107:517–521, 1995.

Ayus JC, Arieff AI: Chronic hyponatremic encephalopathy in postmenopausal women. JAMA 281:2299–2304, 1995.

Ayus JC, Wheeler JM, Arieff AI: Postoperative hyponatremic encephalopathy in menstruant women. Ann Intern Med 117:891–897, 1992.

Bartter FC, Schwartz WB: The syndrome of inappropriate secretion of antidiuretic hormone. Am J Med 42:790–806, 1967.

Berl T: Treating hyponatremia: Damned if we do and damned if we don't. Kidney Int 37:1006–1018, 1990.

Saito T, Ishikawa S, Abe K, et al.: Acute aquaresis by the nonpeptide arginine vasopressin (AVP) antagonist OPC-31260 improves hyponatremia in patients with syndrome of inappropriate secretion of antidiuretic hormone (SIADH). J Clin Endocrinol Metab 82:1054–1057, 1997.

Schrier RW: Pathogenesis of sodium and water retention in high-output and low-output cardiac failure, nephrotic syndrome, cirrhosis and pregnancy. N Engl J Med 319:1065–1072 and 1127–1134, 1988.

Sterns RH: Severe symptomatic hyponatremia: Treatment and outcome. A study of 64 cases. Ann Intern Med 107:656–664, 1987.

Sterns RH, Cappuccio JD, Silver SM, Cohen EP: Neurologic sequelae after treatment of severe hyponatremia: A multicenter perspective. J Am Soc Nephrol 4:1522–1530, 1994.

Verbalis JG: Inappropriate antidiuresis and other hypoosmolar states. In: Becker KG (ed) Principles and Practice of Endocrinology and Metabolism, pp. 265–276, Lippincott, Philadelphia, 1995.

Verbalis JG: The syndrome of inappropriate antidiuretic hormone secretion and other hypoosmolar disorders. In: Schrier RW, Gottschalk CW (eds) Diseases of the Kidney, pp. 2393–2427. Little, Brown, Boston, 1996.

Verbalis JG: Adaptation to acute and chronic hyponatremia: Implications for symptomatology, diagnosis, and therapy. Semin Nephrol 18:3–19, 1998.

Zerbe R, Stropes L, Robertson G: Vasopressin function in the syndrome of inappropriate antidiuresis. Annu Rev Med 31:315–327, 1980.

HYPERNATREMIA

PAUL M. PALEVSKY

Hypernatremia is one of the two cardinal disturbances of water homeostasis. Decreases in total body water relative to total body electrolyte are characterized by an increase in the electrolyte concentration in all body fluids. In the intracellular compartment this is manifested by a decrease in cell volume and an increase in the intracellular potassium concentration. In the extracellular space, the primary manifestation is an increase in the sodium concentration, resulting in the laboratory finding of hypernatremia.

The development of hypernatremia does not imply an abnormality in sodium homeostasis. Total body sodium content is the primary determinant of extracellular volume. In the setting of intact water homeostasis, alterations in sodium balance result in isotonic volume expansion or volume depletion but do not alter the extracellular fluid sodium concentration. Hypernatremia may, however, be accompanied by either volume depletion or hypervolemia, when impaired water homeostasis is accompanied by a disturbance in sodium balance.

Hypernatremia is a common clinical problem, with a prevalence in hospitalized patients of 0.5 to 2%. In adults, two distinct groups of hypernatremic patients may be identified. Patients developing hypernatremia outside of the hospital setting are generally elderly and debilitated, and often have an intercurrent acute infection. In contrast, patients developing hypernatremia during the course of hospitalization have an age distribution similar to that of the general hospital population. In these patients, hypernatremia is an iatrogenic complication that is usually associated with impaired thirst or restricted access to water, combined with an inadequate prescription for water administration.

REGULATION OF WATER HOMEOSTASIS

The physiologic response to hypertonicity includes both renal water conservation and stimulation of thirst. Hypertonicity is sensed by osmoreceptors located adjacent to the anterior wall of the third ventricle in the hypothalamus. Activation of these osmoreceptors stimulates the secretion of arginine vasopressin by neurons whose cell bodies are in the supraoptic and paraventricular nuclei in the hypothalamus and whose axons terminate in the posterior pituitary gland. In the kidney, arginine vasopressin modulates the hydraulic permeability of the collecting duct. In the absence of vasopressin, the collecting duct is relatively impermeant to water. Vasopressin exerts its effect on the collecting duct through the activation of V_2-vasopressin receptors located on the basolateral aspect of the tubular epithelium. The V_2-receptor is coupled to adenylate cyclase by GTP-binding proteins; receptor binding activates adenylate cyclase, which catalyzes the conversion of ATP to the second messenger, cyclic-AMP (cAMP). Through incompletely elucidated mechanisms, cAMP stimulates the insertion of aquaporin 2 water channels into the apical cell membrane. The resulting increase in the hydraulic permeability of the apical cell membrane permits the passive reabsorption of water from the collecting duct into the isotonic cortical and hypertonic medullary interstitium. The excretion of a concentrated urine is therefore dependent on the generation and maintenance of the corticomedullary osmotic gradient as well as the utilization of the gradient through a normal tubular response to vasopressin secretion.

The osmotic regulation of vasopressin secretion is extremely sensitive. Below a body fluid osmolality of 280 to 285 mmol/kg, vasopressin secretion is inhibited and plasma vasopressin levels are virtually undetectable. As body fluid osmolality increases above this threshold, vasopressin secretion increases linearly, with increases in body fluid osmolality of as little as 1–2% resulting in detectable increases in plasma vasopressin levels. The renal response to changes in vasopressin secretion is also extremely sensitive. Urine is maximally dilute when vasopressin secretion is suppressed; urinary concentration increases linearly as plasma vasopressin levels rise in response to rising plasma tonicity, with maximal urinary concentration achieved at vasopressin levels that correspond to a plasma osmolality of approximately 295 mmol/kg.

Although renal water conservation is important in preventing further renal losses, water conservation is not sufficient for either the prevention of progressive hypertonicity or the restoration of normal plasma tonicity. The ultimate defense against the development of hypertonicity and hypernatremia is the osmotic stimulation of thirst and its resultant increase in water ingestion. Thirst is also mediated by hypothalamic osmoreceptors located in the anterior wall of the third ventricle. These thirst-osmoreceptors, although in proximity to the osmoreceptors modulating vasopressin secretion, are anatomically distinct. Impulses from these osmoreceptors are projected to higher levels in the cerebral cortex where they result in the perception of thirst and water-seeking behavior. The osmotic threshold for thirst is approximately 5 mmol/kg greater than the osmotic threshold for vasopressin secretion; once this threshold is exceeded, thirst increases in proportion to increases in body fluid osmolality.

PATHOPHYSIOLOGY

Hypernatremia results when there is net water loss or hypertonic sodium gain. In the normal individual, thirst is stimulated by any rise in body fluid tonicity. Water ingestion increases and the hypernatremic state is rapidly corrected. Therefore, sustained hypernatremia can occur only when the thirst mechanism is impaired and water intake does not increase in response to hypertonicity. Although increased water losses or hypertonic sodium gain usually contribute to the development of hypernatremia, abnormalities in the osmoregulation of thirst or in thirst perception, or the inability to gain access to water are required for sustained hypernatremia.

The importance of thirst in the pathogenesis of hypernatremia is illustrated by patients with severe diabetes insipidus. These patients are unable to concentrate their urine and excrete large volumes of dilute urine, occasionally in excess of 10 to 15 L/day. Under normal circumstances they do not develop hypernatremia—in response to their renal water losses, thirst is stimulated and they maintain body fluid tonicity at the expense of profound secondary polydipsia. If, however, they are unable to drink in response to thirst, as may occur during an intercurrent illness, hypernatremia rapidly develops.

Isolated defects in thirst (primary hypodipsia) are uncommon but may result from any process involving the hypothalamus in proximity to the anterior wall of the third ventricle (Table 1). Lesions may include a wide range of intracranial pathology, including primary and metastatic tumors, granulomatous diseases, vascular abnormalities (most commonly involving the anterior communicating artery), trauma, and hydrocephalus. Hypodipsia has also been described in elderly patients (geriatric hypodipsia) in

whom overt hypothalamic pathology is absent. Essential hypernatremia is a rare disorder in which there is an upward resetting of the thresholds for both thirst and vasopressin secretion. Patients with this condition are able to concentrate and dilute their urine, albeit around an elevated body fluid osmolality, and have an elevated set point for thirst perception. More commonly, impaired thirst results from diffuse neurologic disease which interferes with the less well defined cerebral cortical pathways subserving thirst perception and water ingestion (secondary hypodipsia). Thus, defects in thirst are commonly associated with cerebrovascular disease, dementia, and acute illnesses that result in delirium or obtundation.

CLINICAL CLASSIFICATION

Although impaired thirst and restricted water intake underlie the development of sustained hypernatremia, the hypernatremic states are most commonly classified on the basis of the associated water loss or electrolyte gain and corresponding changes in extracellular fluid volume (Table 2). Pure water deficits are associated with minimal change in total body sodium and relative preservation of extracellular fluid volume. When hypotonic fluid deficits are present, hypernatremia coexists with total body sodium depletion and extracellular fluid volume contraction. Hypertonic sodium gain results in hypernatremia and extracellular fluid volume expansion.

TABLE 1
Defects in Thirst

Primary hypodipsia
  Hypothalamic lesions affecting the osmostat
    Trauma
    Craniopharyngioma or other primary suprasellar tumor
    Metastatic tumor
    Granulomatous disease
    Vascular lesions
  Essential hypernatremia
  Geriatric hypodipsia
Secondary hypodipsia
  Cerebrovascular disease
  Dementia
  Delirium
  Mental status changes

TABLE 2
Classification of Hypernatremia on the Basis of Associated Changes in Extracellular Volume

Pure water deficit (normal extracellular volume)
  Diabetes insipidus
    Hypothalamic
    Nephrogenic
  Increased insensible losses
Hypotonic fluid deficit (decreased extracellular volume)
  Renal losses
    Diuretic administration
    Osmotic diuresis
    Postobstructive diuresis
    Polyuric phase of ATN[a]
  Gastrointestinal losses
    Vomiting
    Nasogastric drainage
    Enterocutaneous fistulae
    Diarrhea
  Cutaneous losses
    Burn injuries
    Excessive perspiration
Hypertonic sodium gain (increased extracellular volume)
  Salt ingestion
  Hypertonic NaCl
  Hypertonic $NaHCO_3$
  Total parenteral nutrition

[a]ATN, acute tubular necrosis.

Pure Water Deficits

Isolated water deficits are generally not associated with clinical evidence of intravascular volume depletion. Only one-third of a pure water deficit is derived from the extracellular compartment, and only one-twelfth from the intravascular compartment. In a 70 kg individual, a 5% decrease in total body water, which would result in an increase in the plasma sodium concentration by approximately 7 mmol/L, results in a reduction in ECF volume by less than 700 mL and intravascular volume by less than 200 mL. This modest degree of volume depletion is generally not detectable on physical examination and may be manifest only by mild prerenal azotemia. With more severe water deficits, hemodynamically significant intravascular volume depletion may develop.

Pure water deficits may occur when thirst is impaired, even in the absence of increased water losses. In patients with significant hypodipsia, voluntary water ingestion may not be sufficient to replace obligate gastrointestinal and insensible water losses. Despite maximal renal water conservation, progressive hypernatremia will result if supplemental water intake is not provided. More commonly, pure water deficits develop when thirst is impaired or water intake is restricted despite increased insensible or renal water losses. Insensible water losses are approximately 0.6 mL/kg/hr, or about 1 L per day in the average adult. These losses are not subject to osmotic regulation but may be increased by a wide variety of factors, including fever, exercise, increased ambient temperature and hyperventilation. Increased renal electrolyte-free water losses result from diabetes insipidus. Patients with increased insensible losses manifest oliguria with a maximally concentrated urine (urine osmolality >700 mmol/kg). In contrast, patients with diabetes insipidus have polyuria and a less than maximally concentrated urine.

Diabetes Insipidus

Diabetes insipidus results either from failure of the hypothalamic–pituitary axis to synthesize or release adequate amounts of vasopressin (hypothalamic diabetes insipidus) or from failure of the kidney to produce a concentrated urine despite appropriate circulating vasopressin levels (nephrogenic diabetes insipidus). In both forms of the disorder, the inability of the kidney to concentrate the urine leads to polyuria and secondary polydipsia. If water intake is adequate to replace urinary electrolyte-free water losses, hypertonicity and hypernatremia will not develop. Thus, hypernatremia is not a hallmark of diabetes insipidus.

Diabetes insipidus may occur in either complete or partial forms. In complete hypothalamic diabetes insipidus, vasopressin secretion is absent, resulting in the production of large volumes of dilute urine (urine osmolality <150 mmol/L). In partial hypothalamic diabetes insipidus, vasopressin secretion is detectable but subnormal, and a less severe defect in renal water conservation is present. Similarly, in complete nephrogenic diabetes insipidus, renal responsiveness to the hydro-osmotic effect of vasopressin is absent, whereas an impaired response occurs in partial nephrogenic diabetes insipidus.

Any pathologic process involving the hypothalamic–pituitary axis may lead to vasopressin deficiency and hypothalamic diabetes insipidus (Table 3). Common etiologies include pituitary surgery, head trauma, primary and metastatic tumors, leukemia, hemorrhage, thrombosis, and granulomatous diseases. Diabetes insipidus following head trauma or surgery may be transient, permanent, or may follow a triphasic course. The transient form is most common, with an abrupt onset followed by resolution over a period of days to weeks. In the triphasic pattern, there is an initial period of vasopressin deficiency lasting 2 to 4 days as the result of axonal injury, a 5 to 7 day period of inappropriate vasopressin release thought to result from release of hormone by degenerating neurons, and finally permanent diabetes insipidus following neuronal death. In 30% of patients, hypothalamic diabetes insipidus is idiopathic, most probably occurring on an autoimmune basis. A rare, hereditary form is due to mutations in the vasopressin–neurophysin gene, which result in an abnormal structure and processing of the vasopressin prohormone and ultimately cell death of the vasopressin-secreting neurons.

The term nephrogenic diabetes insipidus should be restricted to those situations in which there is an intrinsic abnormality of the collecting duct that leads to vasopressin-insensitivity or hyporesponsiveness. Patients with chronic tubulointerstitial renal disease may be unable to generate or maintain a normal corticomedullary osmotic gradient and are therefore unable to concentrate their urine normally. However, they rarely have significant polyuria and should not be considered to have nephrogenic diabetes insipidus.

TABLE 3
Hypothalamic Diabetes Insipidus

Pituitary surgery

Head trauma

Neoplasia
  Primary: dysgerminoma, craniopharyngioma, suprasellar pituitary tumors
  Metastatic: carcinoma of the breast, carcinoma of the lung, lymphoma
  Leukemia

Vascular lesions
  Aneurysms
  Cerebrovascular accidents
  Sheehan's syndrome (postpartum pituitary hemorrhage)

Infections
  Encephalitis
  Meningitis
  Tuberculosis
  Syphilis

Granulomatous disease
  Sarcoidosis
  Histiocytosis

Autoimmune

Vasopressin–neurophysin gene mutations

TABLE 4

Nephrogenic Diabetes Insipidus

Drug induced
  Lithium
  Demeclocycline
  Methoxyflurane
  Amphotericin B

Electrolyte disorders
  Hypercalcemia
  Hypokalemia

Obstructive uropathy

Congenital
  Vasopressin V_2-receptor mutations
  Aquaporin 2 mutations

Nephrogenic diabetes insipidus may be either acquired or congenital (Table 4). The acquired form is far more common, and is most often associated with pharmacologic therapy with lithium or demeclocycline. Both agents have been demonstrated to inhibit intracellular generation of cAMP in response to vasopressin. In addition, demeclocycline also inhibits the intracellular action of cAMP. Acquired nephrogenic diabetes insipidus may also result from obstructive uropathy, hypercalcemia, or severe hypokalemia.

A congenital form of nephrogenic diabetes insipidus has been identified in multiple kindreds and is usually inherited in a sex-linked pattern with variable penetrance in hemizygous females. The genetic defect has been localized in the majority of kindreds to the vasopressin V_2-receptor gene; however, mutations in the aquaporin 2 gene have been identified in rare patients with an autosomal recessive form of nephrogenic diabetes insipidus.

The polyuria of diabetes insipidus needs to be differentiated from other forms of polyuria, including primary polydipsia, solute diuresis secondary to glycosuria, mannitol, urea or diuretics, or resolving acute renal failure. Polyuria due to solute diuresis can usually be excluded by demonstrating that the urine osmolality is less than 150 mmol/kg. In patients with severe polyuria, formal dehydration testing is usually unnecessary and may result in severe hypernatremia and hypotension. Dehydration testing may be required, however, to diagnose partial forms of diabetes insipidus.

During a dehydration test, the patient is placed on a strict fast with special care taken to ensure that the patient consumes no fluids. During the test, urine osmolality is measured hourly and plasma osmolality every 4 to 6 hr. Water deprivation is continued until body weight has declined by 3%, plasma osmolality has reached 295 mmol/kg, or urine osmolality has reached a plateau (variation of less than 5% over 3 hr). In patients with severe diabetes insipidus, urine osmolality will remain less than plasma osmolality, while in partial diabetes insipidus urine osmolality will be greater than plasma osmolality, although submaximally concentrated (Table 5). The urinary response to exogenous vasopressin usually differentiates between the hypothalamic and nephrogenic forms. Measurement of plasma vasopressin levels at maximal dehydration (prior to exogenous vaso-

pressin), although not routinely available, may be extremely useful in equivocal cases.

Hypotonic Fluid Deficits

Patients with inadequately replaced hypotonic fluid losses will develop both hypernatremia and extracellular volume depletion. Unlike patients with pure water losses, these individuals manifest the classic findings of intravascular volume depletion, that is, tachycardia, hypotension, and decreased central venous pressure. Hypotonic fluid may be lost from the skin, gastrointestinal tract, or kidney. Cutaneous losses of electrolyte-containing hypotonic fluids may be significant in patients with severe burn injuries and patients with increased sensible perspiration (as opposed to insensible transpirational skin loss). The majority of gastrointestinal fluids, with the exception of pancreatic and biliary secretions, are also hypotonic. Protracted vomiting, nasogastric drainage, and diarrhea commonly contribute to the development of hypovolemic hypernatremia. Excessive hypotonic renal fluid losses most commonly result from diuretic therapy, but may also be associated with osmotic diureses due to glucose, mannitol, or urea. Postobstructive diuresis, the polyuric phase of acute tubular necrosis, adrenal insufficiency, and a variety of chronic renal diseases, especially medullary cystic disease and renal tubular acidosis (types I and II) are also associated with renal-salt wasting and hypotonic urinary losses. Hypovolemic hypernatremia may also develop in patients with "third-space" fluid losses (e.g., bowel obstruction, pancreatitis, or peritonitis) if the sequestration of isotonic fluid is combined with inadequate replacement of ongoing electrolyte-free water losses.

Urinary indices are helpful in ascertaining the source of hypotonic fluid losses. When the losses have a renal origin, the urine sodium concentration is usually elevated (>20 mmol/L) and the urine is less than maximally concentrated. In contrast, nonrenal losses are associated with renal sodium avidity (urine sodium <10 mmol/L) and a maximally concentrated urine (urine osmolality >700 mmol/kg).

Hypertonic Sodium Gain

Hypertonic sodium gain produces hypernatremia and extracellular volume overload. When both thirst and renal function are intact, the volume and tonicity disturbances are transient. The increase in tonicity stimulates thirst, with a resultant increase in water intake that corrects the hypertonicity. In addition, the volume expansion stimulates a natruresis. Persistent hypernatremia implies impaired thirst or restricted water intake. Hypertonic sodium gain may result from the accidental ingestion of large quantities of sodium salts but is more commonly iatrogenic, resulting from the administration of hypertonic sodium chloride or sodium bicarbonate solutions, inappropriate electrolyte prescription for parenteral hyperalimentation solutions, or inappropriate sodium supplementation of enteral nutrition. Errors in formula preparation may result in hypernatremia in infants.

TABLE 5

Diagnosis of Diabetes Insipidus

	Urine osmolality		
Diagnosis	**After dehydration**	**After exogenous vasopressin**	**Plasma vasopressin level**
Normal individuals	>700 mmol/kg	<10% increase	>2.0 pg/mL
Hypothalamic DI			
Complete	<300 mmol/kg	>50% increase	<1.0 pg/mL
Partial	>300 mmol/kg	>10% increase	<1.5 pg/mL
Nephrogenic DI			
Complete	<300 mmol/kg	<50% increase	>5.0 pg/mL
Partial	>300 mmol/kg	<10% increase	>2.0 pg/mL

Hypertonicity Due to Nonelectrolyte Solutes

Although all hypernatremic patients are hypertonic, hypertonicity can also occur in the absence of hypernatremia. When osmotically active nonelectrolyte solutes accumulate in the extracellular compartment, hypertonicity may be accompanied by a normal, or even depressed, serum sodium concentration. The accumulation of a nonelectrolyte solute increases the osmolality of the extracellular fluids. If the solute is impermeable to cell membranes, water will exit the intracellular compartment to maintain osmotic equilibrium. The net result is intracellular dehydration, cell shrinkage, expansion of the extracellular compartment, and dilution of the extracellular fluid sodium concentration. It is important to recognize nonhypernatremic hypertonicity so as to avoid institution of inappropriate therapy for the resultant dilutional hyponatremia.

The most common nonelectrolyte solute associated causing hypertonicity is glucose. In patients with hyperglycemia, the serum sodium concentration usually declines by 1.6–2.0 mmol/L for each 100 mg/dL increase in plasma glucose. Isonatremic and hyponatremic hypertonicity have also been described following administration of mannitol, maltose, sorbitol, glycerol, and radiocontrast agents. The presence of an unmeasured solute may be identified by comparison of the measured plasma osmolality with the estimate of plasma osmolality derived from measurement of serum sodium, glucose, and urea nitrogen concentrations:

$$(P_{Osm} = 2 \times [Na^+] + glucose \ (mg/dL)/18 + BUN \ (mg/dL)/2.8).$$

The presence of an "osmolar gap" between these two values for plasma osmolality suggests the presence of an unmeasured solute. The specific solute responsible is usually ascertainable from a review of medications administered and may be confirmed by specific biochemical testing.

DIAGNOSTIC APPROACH

The algorithm in Fig. 1 provides a diagnostic approach to the patient with hypernatremia. The initial step is evaluation of intravascular volume. If intravascular volume is preserved,

the hypernatremia is due to pure water loss. Measurement of urine osmolality permits differentiation between nonrenal etiologies (isolated hypodipsia, increased insensible losses) and renal water loss (diabetes insipidus). Intravascular volume contraction implies combined water and sodium deficits due to gastrointestinal, cutaneous, or renal losses. Intravascular volume expansion suggests hypertonic sodium gain, but may also be seen when hypernatremia is superimposed on a preexisting edematous disorder.

CLINICAL MANIFESTATIONS

The major clinical manifestations of hypernatremia result from alterations in brain water content. In response to hypertonicity, fluid shifts from the intracellular compartment into the extracellular compartment, maintaining osmotic equilibrium and resulting in a decrease in intracellular volume. In the central nervous system, acute hypernatremia is associated with a rapid decrease in water content and brain volume (Fig. 2). Within 24 hr, however, adaptive processes result in the uptake of electrolyte into brain cells with a partial restoration of brain volume. Subsequently, there is an increase in intracellular organic solute content, primarily through the accumulation of amino acids, polyols, and methylamines, which restores brain volume to normal. The accumulation of these intracellular solutes ("idiogenic osmoles") has important therapeutic implications. Although they minimize cerebral dehydration during hypertonicity, their accumulation increases the risk of cerebral edema during rehydration.

The clinical manifestations of hypernatremia reflect its rapidity of onset, its duration, and its magnitude. In severe acute hypernatremia brain shrinkage may be substantial, placing traction on the venous sinuses and intracerebral veins and causing their rupture. The resulting intracerebral and subarachnoid hemorrhage may produce irreversible neurologic defects or death. The manifestations of less profound hypernatremia are nonspecific and include nausea, muscle weakness and fasciculations, and alterations in mental status ranging from lethargy to coma. Seizures, while uncommon in chronic hypernatremia, may develop after initiation of therapy in as many as 40% of patients.

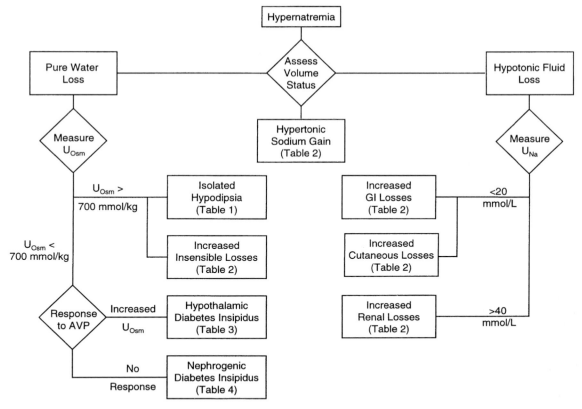

FIGURE I Algorithm for the evaluation of hypernatremia.

The mortality rate associated with hypernatremia has been reported to range between 40 to greater than 70%, depending on its magnitude and the rapidity of its onset. The majority of deaths, however, are not a direct consequence of the hypernatremia but result from underlying illnesses. In a recent study, the mortality in 103 consecutive hypernatremic patients was 41%; however, in only 16% of the patients did the hypernatremia contribute to the cause of death. When mortality was analyzed on the basis of adequacy of therapy, hypernatremia contributed to mortality in 25% of patients in whom it persisted for more than 72 hr as compared to only 8% of patients in whom the hypernatremia was promptly treated and resolved within 72 hr.

TREATMENT

The treatment of hypernatremia is water. The existing water deficit should be repleted and any ongoing electrolyte-free water losses replaced. The water deficit may be estimated based on the current serum sodium concentration ($[Na^+]$) and a normal serum sodium concentration of 140 mmol/L. Assuming that the hypernatremia is due to pure water loss and that total body solute has remained constant:

$$[Na^+] \times TBW_{current} = 140 \times TBW_{usual}$$

where TBW_{usual} and $TBW_{current}$ are the normal and current body water contents of the patient, respectively. Since the water deficit is the difference between the usual and current total body water, the equation can be arranged as:

$$Water\ Deficit = TBW_{current} \times [([Na^+]/140) - 1]$$

If we assume that total body water is 60% of body weight,

$$Water\ Deficit = 0.6 \times [Body\ Weight\ (kg)] \times [([Na^+]/140) - 1]$$

Despite inaccuracies inherent in this formula, the calculation provides a useful first approximation for initiating water replacement.

In acute hypernatremia, repletion of the water deficit may be rapid. The electrolytes that accumulate in the brain during acute hypernatremia are rapidly extruded into the extracellular compartment during treatment, minimizing the risk of cerebral edema. In contrast, overly rapid therapy of chronic hypernatremia may produce cerebral edema if the water replacement occurs more rapidly than the brain can dissipate the accumulated organic solutes, a process requiring approximately 24 to 48 hr. Well-controlled studies to ascertain the optimal treatment of chronic hypernatremia do not exist. However, based on knowledge of the rate of solute loss by the brain following chronic hypernatremia, an approach of prompt but gradual correction is

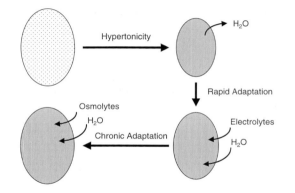

FIGURE 2 Brain adaptation to hypernatremia. Brain cell volume is indicated by the size of the oval, intracellular osmolality by the density of shading. Following the acute onset of hypernatremia, there is a rapid loss of water from the intracellular compartment, resulting in a decrease in brain cell volume and an increase in brain cell osmolality. Adaptive processes are then activated which restore brain cell volume to normal. An initial phase of rapid adaptation, occurring over the first 24 hr, consists of electrolyte uptake into brain cells, partially restoring brain volume. In chronic adaptation, which is complete by day 7, organic solutes accumulate within brain cells leading to restoration of brain volume to normal although intracellular osmolality remains elevated.

most prudent. In symptomatic patients, initial rapid water replacement should be provided; however, the serum sodium concentration should be reduced by no more than 1–2 mmol/L/hr. Once symptoms have resolved, replacement of the remainder of the water deficit should occur over 24 to 48 hr. Throughout treatment, the neurologic status of the patient should be closely monitored; deterioration after an initial improvement in neurologic symptoms suggests the development of cerebral edema and mandates temporary discontinuation of water replacement.

No individual regimen of water replacement is of documented superiority. Water may be administered enterally, either orally or by nasogastric tube, or intravenously. Intravenous repletion can consist of either hypotonic saline or 5% dextrose in water; pure water cannot be administered intravenously as the local hypotonicity at the site of administration can produce severe intravascular hemolysis. When using glucose containing solutions, the blood glucose concentration should be monitored carefully and insulin therapy initiated, if necessary, to forestall hyperglycemia.

In addition to replacing the calculated water deficit, ongoing fluid losses must also be replaced. Urinary, gastrointestinal, and other losses should be quantified and should be replaced on the basis of their volume and electrolyte content. Insensible losses must also be replaced, recognizing that they increase by approximately 20% for each 1° C increase in body temperature.

Prompt attention to reducing excessive water losses is also important. Insensible losses may be reduced by normalizing body temperature with cooling blankets and antipyretics. Hyperglycemia should be controlled and protein loading decreased in order to limit osmotic diuresis. Nasogastric drainage can be reduced by therapy with H$_2$-receptor antagonists or proton pump inhibitors. Altering enteral feeding, treating infectious causes, discontinuing cathartic agents, or administering antidiarrheal agents can reduce diarrhea. Specific therapy for diabetes insipidus should be initiated, when appropriate.

Hypothalamic diabetes insipidus is readily treated with hormone replacement. Although the native hormone, aqueous arginine vasopressin, is available, treatment is most often with desamino-8-D-arginine vasopressin (dDAVP), a synthetic analog of vasopressin with a longer half-life and less vasoconstrictive effects. Hormone replacement therapy is generally ineffective in nephrogenic diabetes insipidus. Restriction of dietary protein and sodium intake may attenuate the polyuria by reducing obligate urinary solute excretion. Thiazide diuretics may also be of benefit in mitigating the renal water losses. Thiazides directly inhibit urinary diluting capacity, reducing free-water generation. In addition, they decrease distal tubular fluid delivery by inducing mild intravascular volume contraction. The net effect is decreased delivery of free-water to the collecting duct and enhanced vasopressin-independent water reabsorption, thereby moderating the polyuria. Nonsteroidal antiinflammatory drugs are also useful as adjunctive therapy. Amiloride is useful in the treatment of lithium-induced nephrogenic diabetes insipidus. It is postulated that in addition to its diuretic effects, amiloride blocks lithium entry into collecting duct cells, thereby reducing cellular toxicity.

Initial treatment of the patient with coexistent hypernatremia and extracellular volume depletion should be directed at restoring intravascular volume. Frank circulatory compromise should be promptly treated with isotonic saline or colloid solutions. Once adequate volume replacement has been achieved, treatment should then be directed toward replacing the water deficit.

Treatment of hypernatremia in patients with volume overload generally requires both water repletion and solute removal. Because hypernatremia often develops rapidly in these patients, the compensatory mechanisms defending brain volume are ineffective and neurologic symptoms may be accentuated. In addition, the concomitant intravascular volume expansion may result in pulmonary edema and exacerbate respiratory failure. Treatment must therefore be promptly instituted in order to prevent neurologic and cardiopulmonary complications. Since water repletion will further exacerbate intravascular volume overload, a loop diuretic should be simultaneously administered to facilitate solute excretion. In patients with massive volume overload or renal failure, initiation of hemodialysis or hemofiltration may be necessary.

Bibliography

Ayus JC, Armstrong DL, Arieff AI: Effects of hypernatremia in the central nervous system and its therapy in rats and rabbits. *J Physiol* 492:243–255, 1996.

DeRubertis FR, Michelis MF, Beck N, Field JB, Davis BB: "Essential" hypernatremia due to ineffective osmotic and intact volume regulation of vasopressin secretion. *J Clin Invest* 50:97–110, 1971.

Fitzsimons JT: Physiology and pathophysiology of thirst and sodium appetite. In: Seldin DW, Giebisch G (eds) *The Kidney: Physiology and Pathophysiology,* 2nd Ed., pp. 1615–1648. Raven, New York, 1992.

Gullans SR, Verbalis JG: Control of brain volume during hyperosmolar and hypoosmolar conditions. *Annu Rev Med* 44:289–301, 1993.

Holtzman EJ, Ausiello DA: Nephrogenic diabetes insipidus: Causes revealed. *Hospital Practice* 29:67–82, 1994.

Lien YH, Shapiro JI, Chan L: Effects of hypernatremia on organic brain osmoles. *J Clin Invest* 85:1427–1435, 1990.

Miller M, Dalakos T, Moses AM, Fellerman H, Streeten DHP: Recognition of partial defects in antidiuretic hormone secretion. *Ann Intern Med* 73:721–729, 1970.

Palevsky PM: Hypernatremia. *Semin Nephrol* 18:20–30, 1998.

Palevsky PM, Bhagrath R, Greenberg A: Hypernatremia in hospitalized patients. *Ann Intern Med* 124:197–203, 1996.

Phillips PA, Rolls BJ, Ledingham JGG, Forsling ML, Morton JJ, Crowe MJ, Wollner L: Reduced thirst after water deprivation in healthy elderly men. *N Engl J Med* 311:753–759, 1984.

Robertson GL: Regulation of vasopressin secretion. In: Seldin DW, Giebisch G (eds) *The Kidney: Physiology and Pathophysiology,* 2nd Ed., pp. 1595–1613. Raven, New York, 1992.

Ross EJ, Christie SBM: Hypernatremia. *Medicine* 48:441–473, 1969.

Seckl JR, Dunger DB: Diabetes insipidus: Current treatment recommendations. *Drugs* 44:216–224, 1992.

Snyder NA, Feigal DW, Arieff AI: Hypernatremia in elderly patients. *Ann Intern Med* 107:309–319, 1987.

Zerbe RL, Robertson GL: A comparison of plasma vasopressin measurements with a standard indirect test in the differential diagnosis of polyuria. *N Engl J Med* 305:1539–1546, 1981.

9

METABOLIC ACIDOSIS

DANIEL BATLLE

METABOLIC ACIDOSIS

Metabolic acidosis is an acid–base disorder characterized by a fall in blood bicarbonate concentration and a fall in blood pH (i.e., a rise in the hydrogen ion concentration [H^+]). Respiratory compensation provides for a predictable decrease of the blood CO_2 tension (pCO_2). For each 1 mEq decrease in bicarbonate concentration the pCO_2 falls by 1.0 to 1.5 mm Hg. The importance of respiratory compensation, or its lack, on blood pH is illustrated in Fig. 1. The presence of an inappropriate response suggests the existence of a mixed acid–base disturbance. Severe metabolic acidosis, unlike respiratory alkalosis, cannot be fully compensated despite maximal hyperventilation. Accordingly, if the blood pH is not reduced when bicarbonate is very low, a respiratory alkalosis must be present.

Metabolic acidosis occurs when bicarbonate is lost from the body (via the gastrointestinal tract or the kidney), when the kidneys fail to regenerate bicarbonate via adequate acid excretion, or when bicarbonate is consumed in the titration of excessive acid produced endogenously or from the ingestion of acid-producing compounds.

THE PLASMA ANION GAP IN THE INITIAL EVALUATION OF METABOLIC ACIDOSIS

The plasma anion gap (AG) is useful in the evaluation of the type of metabolic acidosis and the initial classification of its various causes. The AG is simply a calculation that allows the clinician to infer whether there has been a change in unmeasured anions or cations in plasma.

The use of the anion gap takes advantage of the principle of electroneutrality which dictates that the number of positively charged particles in any solution must be equal to the number of negatively charged particles. The major unmeasured anions in plasma include albumin, phosphate, sulfate, and other organic anions. The major unmeasured cations in plasma include calcium, magnesium, and other less-abundant cations. That the anion gap actually reflects the difference between unmeasured anions (UA) and the unmeasured cations (UC) can be easily appreciated by examining the following basic equations:

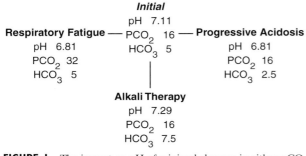

Initial
pH 7.11
Respiratory Fatigue — PCO_2 16 — Progressive Acidosis
pH 6.81 HCO_3 5   pH 6.81
PCO_2 32 PCO_2 16
HCO_3 5 HCO_3 2.5

Alkali Therapy
pH 7.29
PCO_2 16
HCO_3 7.5

FIGURE I The impact on pH of minimal changes in either pCO_2 or HCO_3^- when plasma bicarbonate is very low is illustrated.

Since the sum of all cations = the sum of all anions,

$$(Na^+ + K^+) + UC = (Cl^- + HCO_3^-) + UA$$
$$(Na^+ + K^+) - (Cl^- + HCO_3^-) = UA - UC.$$

Accordingly, the anion gap (AG) reduces to

$$AG = UA - UC$$
$$AG = (Na^+ + K^+) - (Cl^- + HCO_3^-)$$

(normally the AG is 16 ± 4 mEq/L, assuming a "normal range" of plasma Cl^- between 100 and 108 mEq/L).

Due to the small magnitude of changes in potassium concentration in the plasma, potassium is often omitted from the calculation of the AG. Thus,

$$AG = [Na^+ - (Cl^- + HCO_3^-)] \text{ (normally } 12 \pm 4 \text{ mEq/L).}$$

The AG provides a convenient tool to estimate whether there has been a change in either UA or UC faster than such changes can be documented by direct measurements. For instance, in metabolic acidosis due to the addition of nonchloride-containing acid (e.g., lactic acid) the added protons will buffer the bicarbonate while the retained anion (lactate) will add to the unmeasured anions. The anion gap therefore will increase as a result of an increase in an unmeasured anion (lactate) such that the increase in the anion gap will match the fall in plasma bicarbonate. In contrast, when a chloride-containing acid is added to the blood, the hydrogen ion titrates bicarbonate while exogenous chloride ion is largely retained by the kidneys. This results in a rise in the chloride concentration that is equivalent to the fall in bicarbonate; the anion gap will not change. This is described as hyperchloremic or normal anion gap metabolic acidosis. When the decrement in plasma bicarbonate is not matched by either an equivalent increment in plasma chloride or in the plasma anion gap, a mixed hyperchloremic and high anion gap metabolic acidosis is present. For instance, a mixed hyperchloremic/high anion gap metabolic acidosis can develop in a setting where the metabolic acidosis originates from two different mechanisms (e.g., diarrhea in someone with preexisting renal failure or shock).

Because the AG reflects changes in UA or UC, there are certain situations other than metabolic acidosis where the plasma anion gap can be altered. The level of plasma albumin influences the plasma anion gap and should be taken into consideration. For every fall of albumin of 10g/L, the anion gap drops by about 4 mEq/L. An abnormally high concentration of unmeasured cations, as seen with the accumulation of abnormal cationic paraproteins in patients with IgG myeloma, can depress the anion gap. These interpretative pitfalls in the use of the plasma anion gap stress the need to pay careful attention to all the laboratory variables and to look for appropriate clinical correlates.

HYPERCHLOREMIC METABOLIC ACIDOSIS (NORMAL ANION GAP TYPE METABOLIC ACIDOSIS)

Hyperchloremic metabolic acidosis should be distinguished from chronic respiratory alkalosis. In either acid–base disorder plasma chloride is elevated and plasma bicarbonate is reduced. An arterial blood gas is needed to properly diagnose each acid–base disorder.

With the administration of HCl or other HCl-generating compounds, a hyperchloremic metabolic acidosis develops as blood bicarbonate is titrated while plasma chloride increases proportionally due to retention of exogenous chloride. One basic alteration underlying the generation of hyperchloremic metabolic acidosis is the loss of bicarbonate, usually in the urine or in the stools (Table 1). In individuals with metabolic acidosis associated with chronic diarrhea due to protracted laxative abuse, a chronic volume deficit ensues despite avid renal sodium retention. The virtual absence of urine sodium in some of these patients may impede a normal distal acidification response to the prevailing acidemia. This is because distal sodium delivery is necessary for optimal distal hydrogen ion secretion. When sodium excretion is increased to normal by salt replacement, urine pH falls and acid excretion increases, resulting in amelioration of the metabolic acidosis.

Diversion of urine through intestinal segments can result in hyperchloremic metabolic acidosis, hypokalemia, and other electrolyte abnormalities, for example, hypomagnesemia and hypocalcemia. Various intestinal segments

TABLE I
Causes of Hyperchloremic (or Normal Anion Gap) Metabolic Acidosis

Administration of chloride containing acid
  NH_4Cl, HCl
  Hyperalimentation
  Cholestyramine

Bicarbonate wastage
  GI tract (diarrhea, ileus, fistula, villous adenoma)
  Urinary tract diversions to intestine
    (ureterosigmoidostomy, ileal conduit)

Impaired renal H^+ secretion and reduced NH_4^+ excretion
  Distal RTA (hypokalemic and some hyperkalemic types)
  Posthypocapnia (transient)

Impaired NH_3 formation and reduced NH_4^+ excretion
  Advanced renal insufficiency (GFR < 20 mL/min)
  Hyperkalemia
  Aldosterone deficiency

have been used as conduits to substitute for the bladder. The anastomosis of a ureter into the sigmoid colon (ureterosigmoidostomy) almost always results in hyperchloremic metabolic acidosis. Consequently this technique was supplanted by the ileal conduit. Hyperchloremic metabolic acidosis, however, is still a problem in about 10% of patients with an ileal conduit, particularly those where the ileal conduit is obstructed.

RENAL CAUSES OF HYPERCHLOREMIC METABOLIC ACIDOSIS

Ingestion of an average protein-containing diet generates a net fixed acid excess of approximately 1 mEq/kg body weight daily during the course of metabolism. Addition of acid (HA) to the blood compartment results in the titration of the bicarbonate anion according to the equation:

$$HA + NaHCO_3 = H_2O + CO_2 + NaA.$$

In addition to reclaiming all filtered bicarbonate, the kidney must excrete the acid anion and regenerate the bicarbonate that was consumed in the initial titration by the acid. Regeneration of bicarbonate is largely accomplished by hydrogen ion secretion in the distal nephron. Hydrogen ions secreted by the renal tubules are titrated by urinary buffers, primarily ammonia. Phosphate due to its favorable pK (6.8) and relatively high concentration in the urine is also a major urinary buffer and contributes greatly to titratable acid excretion. Increased ammonium excretion is, by far, the major mechanism by which the kidneys can regenerate bicarbonate. Net renal acid excretion (NAE) is calculated as urinary ammonium excretion (NH_4^+) plus urinary titratable acid (TA) minus bicarbonate (HCO_3^-) or other potential bases (PB) that are excreted in the urine:

$$NAE = (NH_4^+ + TA) - (HCO_3^- + PB).$$

The kidneys may fail to provide for an adequate excretion of acid because of either decreased acid excretion (NH_4^+, TA, or both) or increased alkali excretion (i.e., HCO_3^- wastage). The former mechanism underlies an array of syndromes collectively termed distal renal tubular acidosis. The latter mechanism accounts for proximal renal tubular acidosis. With advanced renal failure NH_4^1 excretion is also reduced, resulting in metabolic acidosis which is usually mixed (i.e., hyperchloremic and high anion gap).

PROXIMAL RENAL TUBULAR ACIDOSIS

In normal individuals, the urine bicarbonate concentration is usually very low (less than 1 mEq/24 hr). In patients with proximal renal tubular acidosis (RTA) (type II RTA), a large fraction of the filtered load of bicarbonate is excreted when the concentration of bicarbonate in plasma is normal or even only moderately reduced. In contrast, the urine of such patients is virtually bicarbonate-free when the concentration of bicarbonate in plasma falls below a critical level referred to as the renal threshold. The renal bicarbonate threshold in patients with proximal RTA

varies between 15 and 20 mEq/L (normal about 24 mEq/L). When plasma bicarbonate is below the renal bicarbonate threshold, urine pH falls to levels almost as low as those seen in normal subjects (less than 5.5). This feature is helpful to distinguish proximal RTA from some types of distal RTA (dRTA) where urine pH is higher than 5.5 despite severe acidemia (type I RTA and some cases of hyperkalemic RTA, see later).

In both children and adults, bicarbonate wastage may occur as a part of the Fanconi syndrome, a generalized defect in proximal tubular transport that results in inhibition of reabsorption of glucose, phosphate, uric acid, and amino acids. In this setting, glycosuria develops at normal plasma glucose concentrations, and reduced plasma phosphate and plasma uric acid levels as well as aminoaciduria may be observed.

OVERVIEW OF DEFECTS IN COLLECTING TUBULE ACIDIFICATION CAUSING THE VARIOUS DISTAL RTA SUBTYPES

The collecting tubule is the major site of urinary acidification within the distal nephron. This nephron segment displays axial heterogeneity both anatomically and functionally. In cortical collecting tubules active sodium reabsorption generates an electrical potential (lumen-negative) that favors the secretion of H^+ and potassium. In contrast, in outer medullary collecting tubules, H^+ secretion is neither under the influence of sodium transport nor accompanied by potassium secretion. The collecting tubule contains a proton pump at its luminal surface. This pump, a proton-translocating ATPase, secretes H^+ in an electrogenic manner and can operate independently of sodium transport and despite an unfavorable transtubular electrical gradient. Alterations causing an impairment of collecting tubule acidification by primarily interfering with active H^+ secretion are secretory types of distal RTA (Table 2). Alterations in transepithelial voltage caused by either inhibition of sodium transport or enhancement of lumen to cell chloride transport can also reduce the rate of H^+ secretion, albeit indirectly, and are voltage-dependent types of distal RTA. A primary H^+ secretory defect, by definition, is limited to a defect in either the H^+-ATPase pump or the H^+, K^+-ATPase pump (Table 2).

Most patients with distal RTA appear to have a secretory defect due to H^+-ATPase failure, including patients with different diseases causing acquired as well as hereditary distal RTA. Hypokalemia can develop in such patients as a consequence of secondary hyperaldosteronism and accelerated potassium secretion in the distal nephron. Theoretically, a defect in the H^+, K^+-ATPase pump could better explain the development of severe hypokalemia in some of these cases, but evidence that such a defect causes distal RTA in humans is so far lacking. It is nevertheless attractive to consider that a defect in this pump could be involved in the causation of both potassium wastage and impaired H^+ secretion which is characteristic of hypokalemic distal RTA.

In a typical patient with distal RTA (type I or classic RTA), urine pH during spontaneous acidosis or after acid loading cannot be lowered below 5.5, and ammonium

TABLE 2
Classification of dRTA

Type	Examples
Secretory defects[a]	
Diffuse collecting tubule H$^+$-ATPase defect	Sjögren's syndrome
Medullary collecting tubule H$^+$-ATPase defect	Nephrocalcinosis (some cases)
Diffuse H$^+$-ATPase secretory defect	Chronic kidney transplant rejection
Rate-dependent defects	
Impaired Na$^+$ transport Na$^+$ channel (Ec Na$^+$) mutations	Amiloride, trimethoprin Pseudohypoaldosteronism type I
Enhanced Cl$^-$ transport	Pseudohypoaldosteronism type II
Aldosterone deficiency	Selective aldosterone deficiency
Aldosterone resistance	Pseudohypoaldosteronism type I[b]
Reduced urinary buffers	Hyperkalemia of any cause
Increased intracellular pH	Cystosolic CA II deficiency
Permeability defects	
H$^+$ and K$^+$ backleak	Amphotericin B
Enhanced HCO$_3^-$ secretion	AE-1 gene mistargeting (?)

[a]A defect in H$^+$K$^+$-ATPase has been postulated to be a cause of dRTA (for instance the endemic hypokalemic dRTA of Thailand), but so far there is no convincing evidence to support it.

[b]Pseudohypoaldosteronism type I has been associated with mutations in both the Na$^+$ channel and the mineralocorticoid receptor.

excretion is reduced. The latter can be inferred at the bedside from the finding of a positive urine anion gap (see later). In such patients, the urine pCO$_2$ measured after bicarbonate loading does not increase normally (i.e., above 70 mmHg), reflecting the reduced rate of collecting tubule H$^+$ secretion. The latter feature is useful in distinguishing a secretory from a permeability defect. It is not useful, however, in differentiating a secretory from a voltage-dependent defect, which also decreases the rate of H$^+$ secretion (albeit indirectly). Except for permeability defects (i.e., amphotericin B-induced RTA) any other perturbation leading to a decrease in the rate of collecting tubule H$^+$ secretion impairs the generation of a normally high urine pCO$_2$.

Recent studies have provided new insights into our understanding of the molecular basis of hereditary (primary) distal RTA. Primary DRTA can be inherited in an autosomal dominant or autosomal recessive manner. Autosomal dominant DRTA has been associated with mutations that involve the gene that encodes the Cl$^-$/HCO$_3^-$ exchanger (AE-1). These patients often present in their adulthood, and the severity of their disease is mild to moderate. The recessive form, by contrast, may result either from mutations in the carbonic anhydrase II gene (CA II) or a defect in the gene that encodes the β1-subunit of H$^+$-ATPase. Patients with CA II gene defects present very early in life, with severe disease and often with profound hypokalemia. In addition, these patients may be physically and mentally

retarded and develop nephrocalcinosis and cerebral calcifications. Deafness (conductive type) has been reported in the patients with CA II gene defect, whereas a sensorineural type of deafness is seen in some of the patients with a H$^+$-ATPase defect. Patients with a CA II gene defect appear to have a mixed form of distal and proximal RTA.

Hyperkalemic RTA

Two pathogenic subtypes of hyperkalemic distal RTA that are frequently encountered in adults with underlying renal disease have been well described (Table 3). One subtype, which corresponds to the animal model of selective aldosterone deficiency (SAD), is characterized by hyperkalemic hyperchloremic metabolic acidosis associated with low plasma and urinary aldosterone levels, reduced ammonium excretion, and preserved ability to lower urine pH below 5.5. This constellation of findings is also termed type IV distal RTA. The findings associated with selective aldosterone deficiency or type IV RTA are typified by the syndrome of hyporeninemic hypoaldosteronism. Although hyperkalemia is the usual manifestation of this syndrome, the development of hyperchloremic metabolic acidosis is also very common (more than 75% of cases). In these subjects, acidosis develops because of impaired acid excretion secondary to reduced urinary buffer (ammonia) availability. Ammonia formation in these patients is suppressed as a result of both hyperkalemia and aldosterone deficiency.

TABLE 3
Causes of Hyperkalemic Metabolic Acidosis

Selective aldosterone deficiency
  Low renin
    Hyporeninemic hypoaldosteronism (e.g., diabetic nephropathy)
    Prostaglandin synthesis inhibitors
  Normal or high renin
    Normoreninemic hypoaldosteronism
    Hyperreninemic hypoaldosteronism in critically ill patients
    Converting enzyme inhibitors
    Corticosterone methyloxidase deficiency
    Heparin therapy
    Cyclosporine A
Hyperkalemic distal renal tubular acidosis
  Obstructive uropathy
  Sickle cell hemoglobinopathies
  Renal amyloidosis
  Acute hypersensitivity interstitial nephritis
  Amiloride administration
  Trimethoprim[a]
  Cyclosporine A
  Pentamidine
Aldosterone resistance
  Pseudohypoaldosteronism type I (infants)
  Pseudohypoaldosteronism type II (Gordon's syndrome)
  Adult aldosterone hyporesponsiveness and renal insufficiency
  Spironolactone administration

[a]Denotes that metabolic acidosis is usually not a feature of trimethoprim-induced hyperkalemia.

TABLE 4
Causes of Metabolic Acidosis with Increased Plasma Anion Gap

Etiology	Major circulating anion	Characteristic features and other comments
Ketoacidosis	β-Hydroxybutyrate, acetoacetate	Diabetes, alcohol, starvation
Lactic acidosis	Lactate	Shock, tissue hypoxia, liver failure
Renal failure	Sulfate, phosphate, variety of organic acids	Increased BUN
Methanol	Formate	Increased osmolal gap, hyperemic optic disk
Ethylene glycol	Glycolate, lactate	Increased osmolal gap; ARF, urinary oxalate crystals
Salicylates	Variety of organic acids, salicylate	Concomitant respiratory alkalosis; tinnitus; fever
Toluene	Hippurate	It also causes distal RTA and hypokalemia
Paraldehyde	Acetate?	Very rare nowadays

In the other subtype of hyperkalemic RTA, ammonium excretion is also reduced but, characteristically, urine pH cannot be lowered below 5.5. This is true not only during acidemia, but also after stimulation of sodium-dependent distal acidification by the administration of sodium sulfate or loop diuretics. In this type, referred to as hyperkalemic distal RTA, plasma aldosterone levels may be normal or elevated but are more often reduced. The finding of low aldosterone levels suggests the existence of a combined defect, that is, SAD combined with a tubular defect that interferes with the ability to maximally lower urine pH despite the presence of acidosis. The mechanism underlying this subtype of hyperkalemic distal RTA, which was first described in patients with obstructive uropathy, was originally attributed to a failure to generate a favorable transtubular voltage gradient (lumen negative) in the collecting tubule that interferes with both H^+ and K^+ secretion. A study in patients with this subtype of hyperkalemic distal RTA suggests, however, that the defect in H^+ secretion is related to H^+-ATPase dysfunction and is independent of the associated defect in K^+ secretion.

RTA: CLINICAL FEATURES AND TREATMENT

A common feature of children with proximal and distal RTA is failure to thrive. Acidemia, by mechanisms not yet fully delineated, interferes with normal growth. Distal RTA may also lead to nephrolithiasis or nephrocalcinosis.

The treatment of distal RTA is alkali therapy. When alkali is started early in the course of the disease, growth is normalized. The alkali requirements of these patients are usually small compared with those of patients with proximal RTA. A dose of 1 to 2 mEq/kg body weight of sodium bicarbonate daily is sufficient in most cases. Many patients with hereditary distal RTA have a bicarbonate wastage tendency during the first years of life that gradually abates with advancing age. Hence, the dose of alkali needed to correct the acidosis decreases beyond 6 years of age. Alkali can be provided in the form of a sodium citrate solution, which is well tolerated because it causes less abdominal distention than bicarbonate. Each milliliter of citrate solution provides 1 mEq of bicarbonate after hepatic con-

version of citrate into bicarbonate. Potassium supplements are indicated in patients with hypokalemia.

The hyperkalemic types of distal RTA usually develop in patients with an underlying tubulointerstitial renal disease and/or moderate renal insufficiency who have aldosterone deficiency. The syndrome of selective aldosterone deficiency is particularly common in patients with either type I or type II diabetes and especially so in those who have developed nephropathy. Other common causes are listed in Table 4. Patients with hyperkalemic distal RTA should be differentiated from those with pure selective aldosterone deficiency because some of the patients with the latter condition are more likely to respond to treatment with mineralocorticoids. Tubular hyporesponsiveness to the action of exogenous mineralocorticoid, however, is common in some patients with the syndrome of selective aldosterone deficiency. High doses of mineralocorticoid may be needed to correct the hyperkalemia.

Hyperkalemia can also be treated using exchange resins such as sodium polystyrene sulfonate, which increase gastrointestinal potassium excretion. Correction of hyperkalemia has an additional salutory effect in that it improves the acidosis by increasing ammonium excretion. Loop diuretics are effective in increasing potassium excretion, and they also ameliorate the metabolic acidosis associated with selective aldosterone deficiency.

DIAGNOSTIC APPROACH TO HYPERCHLOREMIC METABOLIC ACIDOSIS

After history and physical examination, the next step in the diagnostic approach to hyperchloremic metabolic acidosis is to determine whether urinary acidification is normal (Fig. 2). Ideally, this should involve measurement of urine pH, titratable acidity, and ammonium excretion. Whether ammonium is appropriately increased or inappropriately low for the prevailing acidosis can be inferred at bedside by a simple calculation of the urine anion gap (UAG):

$$UAG = (Na^+ + K^+) - (Cl^- + HCO_3^-).$$

In a relatively acid urine (pH <6.5), urine bicarbonate concentration is very low, and its contribution to the urine

I. HYPERCHLOREMIC ACIDOSIS WITH NORMAL OR LOW PLASMA POTASSIUM

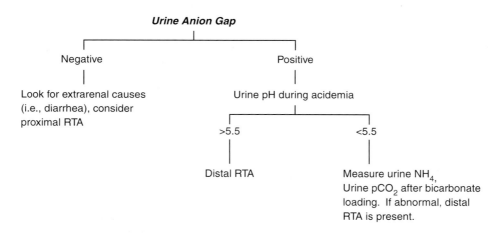

II. HYPERCHLOREMIC ACIDOSIS WITH HYPERKALEMIA

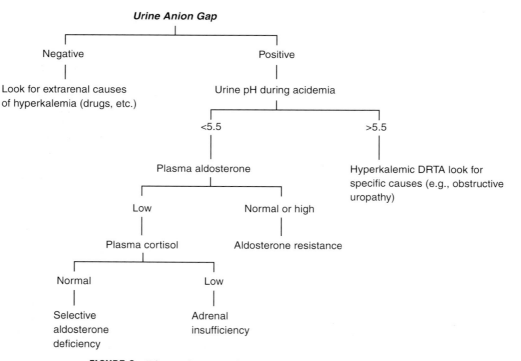

FIGURE 2   Diagnostic approach to hyperchloremic acidosis.

anion gap can be considered negligible. Under usual circumstances, provided that a stimulus for ammonium excretion (i.e., acidosis) is present, the UAG will have a negative value (0 to −50) since ammonium's accompanying anion is chloride. The UAG, by contrast, is positive in the patients with various types of defects in distal urinary acidification. This reflects the inability of patients with distal RTA to excrete ammonium appropriately in the face of spontaneous acidosis.

Accordingly, the UAG is useful in the separation of patients with reduced ammonium excretion because of impaired distal acidification from those with hyperchloremic metabolic acidosis from other causes, namely, gastrointestinal bicarbonate losses (Fig. 2). Normal subjects with diarrhea or those given an acid load to produce metabolic acidosis display a negative anion gap. The negative urine anion gap in patients with diarrhea reflects an abundance of ammonium in the urine because the response of the kidney to acidosis is appropriate (i.e., to excrete acid). In patients with diarrhea, renal acidification is greatly stimulated by acidemia, and the urine pH should be low. In some patients, however, urine pH rises because of the addition of large amounts of ammonia buffer into the collecting tubule. In addition, many of these patients are volume-depleted from protracted diarrhea, so that the delivery of sodium to the collecting tubule is impaired. In this situation, urine pH may not be lowered below 5.5 despite acidemia, until distal sodium delivery is restored by the administration of salt or diuretics. The findings of hypokalemia, hyperchloremic metabolic acidosis, and a high urine pH could erroneously suggest the diagnosis of distal RTA in these patients. The key differential finding is the UAG, which is positive if the patient has distal RTA but negative if the patient has hypokalemic hyperchloremic metabolic acidosis associated with diarrhea. Patients with proximal RTA display a negative UAG insofar as they are capable of excreting substantial amounts of ammonium. Chronic respiratory alkalosis increases the urine anion gap, because in this condition urinary ammonium excretion is reduced as part of a normal adaptation to hypocapnia.

Provided that respiratory alkalosis is excluded, patients with hypobicarbonatemia who have a positive UAG should be suspected to have distal RTA, which can be separated into hyperkalemic and hypokalemic (classic) distal RTA on the basis of the plasma potassium (Fig. 2). The diagnosis of distal RTA can be confirmed by the finding of a urinary pH above 5.5 in the face of spontaneous or ammonium chloride-induced metabolic acidosis. In general, if the patient is spontaneously acidotic (pH < 7.35), there is no need to induce severe acidosis in order to evaluate urinary acidification. If the patient is suspected of having distal RTA and acidosis is mild or not present, ammonium chloride can be given (0.1 g/kg body weight daily for 3 consecutive days). Measurements of urine pH, urinary ammonium, and titratable acidity should be performed at the end of day 3 to confirm or exclude the diagnosis of distal RTA. Some patients with a defect in distal acidification can lower urine pH below 5.5 in the face of metabolic acidosis. This typically occurs in patients with hyperkalemic RTA associated with selective aldosterone deficiency (see Fig. 2). In some patients without hyperkalemia, the ability to lower urine pH below 5.5 may also be preserved, even when distal acidification assessed by the urine pCO_2 after bicarbonate loading is defective (i.e., urine pCO_2 does not increase above 50–60 mm Hg (normal >70 mm Hg) (Table 2). This has been well documented in individuals receiving chronic lithium therapy, subjects with medullary sponge kidney, and some patients with idiopathic hypercalciuria. These patients can be considered to have incomplete distal RTA since metabolic acidosis is often absent.

HIGH ANION GAP TYPES OF METABOLIC ACIDOSIS
Renal Failure

Renal failure, both acute and chronic, is a common cause of metabolic acidosis that is usually classified as a high an-

ion gap type (Table 4). It should be appreciated, however, that the fall in plasma HCO_3^- associated with renal failure is largely due to an absolute decrease in ammonium excretion as a result of reduced renal mass and that a reciprocal increase in the anion gap does not need to occur. Variable degrees of anion retention (sulfate, phosphate, and organic anions) occurring as renal insufficiency progresses determine whether a high anion gap metabolic acidosis will develop or not. The predominant pattern among patients with end stage renal disease on maintenance hemodialysis is a mixed one, that is, a combined high anion gap and hyperchloremic metabolic acidosis.

In patients with chronic renal disease an increase in ammonia production by remaining nephrons is capable of maintaining normal acid–base balance until the glomerular filtration rate has dropped below 20–25 mL/min. Some of the metabolic abnormalities with chronic renal insufficiency, however, may interfere with urinary acidification. In particular, chronic hyperkalemia worsens the acidosis by suppressing ammoniagenesis. An absolute decrease in overall renal ammonia production ensues when glomerular filtration rate (GFR) is less than 20 mL/min and acidosis develops. Even with advanced renal insufficiency the urine is acid (pH less than 5.5), suggesting that the collecting tubules of residual nephrons are capable of adequate H^+ secretion. In fact, when acidosis is seen in patients with moderate degrees of renal failure, a distal acidification defect should be suspected.

The acidosis is usually nonprogressive and relatively asymptomatic. The goal of alkali therapy in this group is mainly to avert the consequences of protracted acidosis on bone tissue which may be through a direct demineralization effect of acidemia or through its effects on the hormones that regulate calcium metabolism, namely, parathyroid hormone and vitamin D.

Lactic Acidosis

Lactate is formed in the cell cytosol from pyruvate. The enzyme catalyzing this reaction is lactate dehydrogenase (LDH). Under normal conditions, the rates of lactic acid regeneration and utilization are matched (about 15 to 20 mEq/day). The liver and, to a lesser extent, the kidneys are the major sites of lactic acid uptake and metabolism. Lactic acidosis, resulting from the accumulation of excess lactate, is usually seen in severely ill patients, many of whom have tissue hypoxia due to tissue hypoperfusion from hypotension with or without hypoxemia. When the tissue oxygen supply does not meet the cellular oxygen demand lactic acidosis occurs and is referred to as type A lactic acidosis.

Some patients with lactic acidosis, however, lack any evidence of tissue hypoxia. This condition is known as type B lactic acidosis and almost always results from liver insufficiency causing impaired lactate clearance. In type A lactic acidosis, the diagnosis is usually made on the basis of the clinical setting (shock, hypoxemia, severe anemia). Type B lactic acidosis should be suspected when there is evidence of liver impairment or ingestion of substances known to produce this condition. Type B lactic acidosis can also occur with large tumors producing a large cell turnover and a marked increase in pyruvate production.

A distinctive type of lactic acidosis can occur in patients with bacterial overgrowth due, for example, to jejunoileal bypass or small-bowel resection. In this situation, intestinal bacteria can metabolize glucose into D-lactic acid (the usual form is L-lactate) which then accumulates in the blood.

Treatment of lactic acidosis must be directed to the correction of the underlying cause. Levels of plasma lactate higher than 20 mEq/L reflect very severe acidosis and are associated with a high mortality. In monitoring the patient one should not rely on an isolated lactate level because of the rapidly changing nature of the underlying condition. Monitoring the plasma anion gap provides an estimate of serum lactate changes over time and obviates the need for serial lactate levels.

The administration of bicarbonate is usually indicated when blood pH is very low (i.e., less than 7.10) despite adequate respiratory compensation. In lactic acidosis, to counteract the excessive lactic acid production, large amounts of bicarbonate are usually needed and this may lead to increased systemic CO_2 generation, a rise in cell CO_2, and thus a fall in intracellular pH. Despite this theoretical problem I favor the use of bicarbonate therapy in cases of severe acidemia provided that blood pCO_2 is reduced. A more specific approach to correct lactic acidosis entails the use of dichloroacetate. This agent, now available in some hospital pharmacies, is effective in lowering lactate levels by stimulating pyruvate dehydrogenase and stimulating mitochondrial pyruvate oxidation. Despite clear-cut improvement of the acidosis, however, controlled studies have failed to demonstrate an improvement in survival in patients with lactic acidosis treated with this agent.

Diabetic Ketoacidosis

This condition is characterized by hyperglycemia of variable degree and metabolic acidosis secondary to overproduction of ketoacids. The hormonal profile of patients with diabetic ketoacidosis is characterized by low insulin levels, hyperglucagonemia, high cortisol levels, high level of circulating catecholamines, and elevated growth hormone levels. These hormonal alterations trigger and maintain the ketogenesis. The accumulation of acetoacetic and β-hydroxybutyric acids results in metabolic acidosis. Some of the acetoacetic acid is nonenzymatically converted to acetone. Acetone is a volatile ketone that is excreted via the lungs producing the characteristic acetone odor of the breath.

The acidosis is usually of the high anion gap type, but a striking hyperchloremic type of acidosis may be seen when ketones are rapidly lost in the urine. If volume contraction is severe, ketoacids are retained and the AG is elevated. In this situation, the retained ketoacids provide a source of potential bicarbonate. This may contribute to a fast recovery from acidosis owing to the equimolar conversion of retained ketone salts to bicarbonate.

Metabolic acidosis in diabetic ketoacidosis is often severe. The diagnosis of ketoacidosis is established by demonstrating ketonemia or ketonuria, metabolic acidosis, and hyperglycemia (Fig. 3). Ketonuria may be undetectable if most of the offending acetoacetic acid has been converted to β-hydroxybutyric acid which is not detected on the routine urine dipstick. Lack of a marked elevation in blood sugar may result in delayed diagnosis. Uncontrolled hyperglycemia usually has caused an osmotic diuresis which has resulted in substantial loss of sodium, chloride, and potassium. Many of such patients therefore develop various degrees of prerenal failure. A significant total body potassium deficit is usually present even in the presence of a normal serum potassium concentration. Some patients may have hyperkalemia which is mainly due to impaired potassium transport into cells caused by the insulin deficiency. Significant phosphate depletion is usually present as a result of poor food intake and urinary phosphate wasting.

The goal of therapy is to reverse and halt the ketogenesis and to replace the electrolyte and water deficits. Insulin is needed to inhibit ketogenesis and break the cycle of lipolysis and ketogenesis. Insulin should be preferably administered as a low-dose constant intravenous infusion. Insulin should not be stopped as glucose concentrations

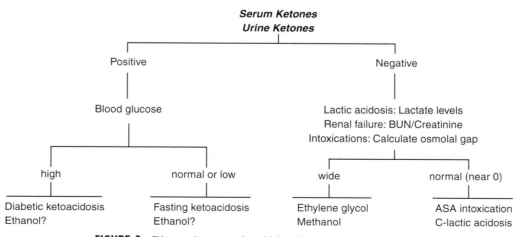

FIGURE 3 Diagnostic approach to high anion gap metabolic acidosis.

approach the normal range. Rather, glucose should be infused and insulin continued until the ketosis has cleared. Although these patients often have more of a water than sodium deficit, isotonic saline is usually needed initially to achieve a rapid correction of the volume deficit. Correction of the potassium deficit should be initiated early, even when plasma potassium concentration is normal, provided that insulin has been given and an adequate urine output is present.

The role of bicarbonate therapy in patients with diabetic ketoacidosis has been debated. In general, the use of bicarbonate is warranted when the acidosis is severe, because its potential benefits seem to outweigh the risks. Bicarbonate should be administered to patients whose arterial blood pH is less than 7.20 despite adequate hyperventilation and to those with a bicarbonate concentration below 10. During recovery, a high anion gap metabolic acidosis is sometimes replaced by a hyperchloremic type of acidosis. The excretion of ketoanions, which represent potential bicarbonate, coupled with the administration of intravenous saline infusion and avid renal retention of chloride leads to hyperchloremia. The development of hyperchloremic acidosis is an indication for continuation of HCO_3^- therapy.

Starvation Ketoacidosis

During starvation, lipolysis and gluconeogenesis provide the body with the needed calories for survival. The low insulin levels induced by hypoglycemia and the associated increase in glucagon, epinephrine, cortisol, and growth hormone levels stimulate lipolysis with release of fatty acids. The accumulation of ketone bodies may result in metabolic acidosis which is often of mild severity. Increased net acid excretion by the kidneys may correct the acidosis over the next few days, obviating the need for bicarbonate therapy. Previously malnourished individuals, however, may have inadequate ammoniagenesis and thus develop a more severe acidosis. Patients may develop metabolic alkalosis with refeeding, which may be related to the abrupt cessation of ketogenesis while urinary acidification remains stimulated.

Alcoholic Ketoacidosis

This condition is characterized by acidosis secondary to increased ketogenesis and variable blood glucose levels in the absence of clinical diabetes. Typically, the condition develops following an alcoholic binge and an episode of vomiting and starvation. Unlike starvation ketoacidosis, the acidosis in alcoholic ketoacidosis may be severe. The combination of low insulin levels (related to low food intake), high levels of epinephrine (which may be related, in part, to withdrawal of alcohol), and elevation of cortisol levels result in the stimulation of glycogenolysis, gluconeogenesis, and lipolysis. The net result is acidosis of variable severity, hyperglycemia or hypoglycemia, and a clinical picture easily confused with diabetic ketoacidosis.

There is usually a prompt improvement in response to hydration and glucose administration without need for exogenous insulin. Bicarbonate should be given if the acidosis is severe (blood pH less than 7.20). Therapy also includes correction of other concomitant electrolyte disturbances such as hypophosphatemia, hypomagnesemia, and hypokalemia.

Salicylate Intoxication

Two distinct forms of intoxication may result from salicylate ingestion, (1) an acute form which usually follows an acute overdose ingested accidentally or intentionally and (2) a chronic form which results from gradual accumulation of the drug during long-term administration. Acid–base disturbances are predominant in the acute form. Typical manifestations of acute salicylate intoxication include intense hyperventilation, fever, stupor, coma, and convulsions. Tinnitus, deafness, and vertigo are common complaints particularly in patients with chronic salicylism. Hypouricemia due to inhibition of renal tubule urate reabsorption by high salicylate levels may be observed.

The diagnosis of salicylate intoxication is usually obvious from the history, but may be difficult. It can be rapidly confirmed by checking the blood salicylate level. Severe toxicity occurs when blood salicylate levels reach 100 mg/dL. In chronic salicylism, however, dose nomograms are not useful and death can occur at low blood salicylate levels.

Combined metabolic acidosis and respiratory alkalosis is a frequent finding in adult patients with acute salicylate intoxication. In children, metabolic acidosis is predominant, often overshadowing the attendant respiratory alkalosis. In adults, the respiratory alkalosis usually predominates. Respiratory alkalosis is the result of direct stimulation of the respiratory center by salicylate. The amount of salicylate required to produce this effect is much less than that required to produce metabolic acidosis. The mechanism of metabolic acidosis in patients with salicylate intoxication is not totally clear. Only a small fraction of the decrement in plasma bicarbonate and the increment in unmeasured anions may be directly attributed to salicyclic acid accumulation. Ketoacidosis as well as lactic acidosis may contribute to the metabolic acidosis in patients with salicylate intoxication.

Removal of the salicylate from the body starts with gastric lavage if the patient presents within 6 hr of drug administration. Repetitive administration of oral-activated charcoal, which possesses a large surface area for drug adsorption, enhances whole-body drug elimination and interferes with drug absorption. Sodium bicarbonate not only corrects the acidosis but it also augments the renal clearance of salicylates by producing an alkaline diuresis (urine pH > 7.0) and may limit the amount of the drug that enters the cerebrospinal fluid and brain cells. Hemodialysis is a very efficient way of removing salicylate from the body and also helps correct the acidosis and other electrolyte abnormalities.

Ethylene Glycol

Ethylene glycol is commonly found as a component of antifreeze and as a solvent in a number of industrial applications. It can cause damage to the central nervous system, the kidneys, and the cardiopulmonary system. Ethylene glycol is metabolized by alcohol dehydrogenase to glycoaldehyde, which is further metabolized to glycolic, glyoxilic, and oxalic acids, all potentially toxic compounds. Suppression of the citric acid cycle and altered intracellular redox state may lead to lactic acid overproduction. A high concentration of ethylene glycol in plasma will result in a disparity between measured and calculated plasma osmolality, such that there is a high plasma osmolar gap (Normally 6 ± 4 mOsmol). The plasma osmolality may be estimated according to the formula:

$$P_{osm} = (Na^+ \times 2) + \frac{glucose}{18} + \frac{BUN}{28}$$

A high plasma "osmolal gap," may also be seen in ethanol and methanol intoxications as well as in some cases of diabetic ketoacidosis (Fig. 2). Calcium oxalate crystalluria is a hallmark of oxalate intoxication and may cause obstructive renal failure when crystals precipitate in the renal tubules. The urine should be examined for the presence of the crystals which may be needle-shaped (monohydrate) or envelope-shaped (dihydrate).

Treatment includes supportive measures, diuresis, bicarbonate, and the provision of thiamine and pyridoxine supplements. Hemodialysis is usually indicated to quickly lower ethylene glycol plasma levels; it can also remove other potentially toxic metabolites and correct the acidosis. Ethanol administration is also useful as ethanol competes with ethylene glycol metabolism by alcohol dehydrogenase and thus it slows its metabolism. A serum ethanol level of 100 mg/dL can be achieved by either nasogastric or intravenous administration of ethanol. 4-Methylpyrazole (fomepizole) can also be used as an effective antidote in treatment of ethylene glycol poisoning. It is an alcohol dehydrogenase inhibitor and acts by preventing the formation of the toxic metabolites of ethylene glycol. Though treatment with fomepizole may be more costly than ethanol, it may yield cost savings by eliminating the need for frequent measurements of blood ethanol, decreasing the time in the intensive care unit, and potentially lessening the need for hemodialysis.

Methanol

Methanol, also known as wood alcohol, is a common solvent and fuel component. It may be ingested as a substitute for ethanol or in suicide attempts. Methanol is metabolized via alcohol dehydrogenase to formaldehyde which is rapidly converted to formate, the anion responsible for the anion gap and most of the toxicity. It can cause severe optic nerve as well as central nervous system injury. Symptoms may include blurred vision which suggest serious toxicity, respiratory depression, cyanosis, altered mental status, and cardiovascular collapse. There is a latent period before the onset of symptoms that averages 12 to 24 hr but that may be delayed up to 3 to 4 days if there is concomitant consumption of ethanol. Acidosis, often severe, is related to the accumulation of formate as well as lactate,

ketoacids, and other organic acids. An osmolal gap is usually present. The finding of optic nerve swelling coupled with the absence of crystalluria strongly suggest the diagnosis of methanol as opposed to ethylene glycol intoxication. Therapy includes osmotic diuresis, administration of ethanol, bicarbonate infusion, and hemodialysis.

Alcohol dehydrogenase inhibitors such as 4-methylpyrazole (fomepizole) can also be used either orally or intravenously in the treatment of methanol poisoning. They act by preventing the degradation of methanol to formic acid, thereby making the level of formic acid undetectable in the serum and thus preventing the toxic effects of methanol.

Bibliography

Adrogue HJ, Wilson H, Boyd AE, Suki WN, Eknoyan G: Plasma acid–base patterns in diabetic ketoacidosis. *N Engl J Med* 307:1603–1610, 1982.

Batlle D: Segmental characterization of defects in collecting tubule acidification. *Kidney Int* 30:546–553, 1986.

Batlle D: Hyperchloremic acidosis. In: Giebisch G, Seldin D (eds) *The Regulation of Acid–Base Balance,* pp. 107–121. Raven, New York, 1989.

Batlle D, Flores G: Underlying defects in distal renal tubular acidosis. New understandings. *Am J Kidney Dis* 27(6):896–915, 1996.

Batlle D, Arruda JAL, Kurtzman NA: Hyperkalemic distal renal tubular acidosis associated with obstructive uropathy. *N Engl J Med* 304:373–380, 1981.

Batlle D, Grupp M, Gaviria M, Kurtzman NA: Distal renal tubular acidosis with intact ability to lower urine pH. *Am J Med* 72:751–758, 1982.

Batlle D, vonRiotte A, Schlueter W: Urinary sodium in the evaluation of hyperchloremic metabolic acidosis. *N Engl J Med* 316:140–144, 1987.

Batlle D, Hizon M, Cohen E, Gutterman C, Gupta R: The use of the urinary anion gap in the diagnosis of hyperchloremic metabolic acidosis. *N Engl J Med* 318:594–599, 1988.

Batlle D, Sabatini S, Kurtzman NA: On the mechanism of toluene-induced renal tubular acidosis. *Nephron* 49:210–218, 1988.

Bruce LJ, Cope DL, Jones GK, Schofield AE, Burly M, Povey s, Unwin RJ, Wrong O, Tanner MJA: Familial dRTA is associated with mutations in red cell anion exchanger (Band 3 AE1) gene. *J Clin Invest* 100:1693–1707, 1997.

Burns MJ, Graudins A, Aaron CK, McMartin K, Brent J: Treatment of methanol poisoning with intravenous 4-methyl pyrazole Report of clinical and toxicogenic data. *Ann Emergency Med* 30(6):829–832, 1997.

Emmett M, Seldin D: Overproduction acidosis. In: Giebisch G, Seldin D (eds) *The Regulation of Acid–Base Balance,* 3rd Ed., pp. 391–429. Raven, New York, 1989.

Fernandez PC, Cohen RM, Feldman GM: The concept of bicarbonate distribution space: The crucial role of body buffers. *Kidney Int* 36:747–752, 1989.

Green J, Kleeman CR: Role of bone in regulation of systemic acid–base balance. *Kidney Int* 39:9–26, 1991.

Jacobsen D: New treatment for ethylene glycol poisoning. *N Engl J Med* 340:879–881, 1999.

Karet FE, Lifton RP, *et al.*: Mutations in the gene encoding B subunit of H+- ATPase cause RTA with sensory neural deafness. *Nat Genet* 21:84–89, 1999.

Oh MS, Phelps KR, Traube M, Barbosa-Saldiar JL, Boxhill C, Carroll HJ: D-Lactic acidosis in a man with the short-bowel syndrome. *N Engl J Med* 301:249–252, 1979.

Schlueter W, Batlle D: Electrolyte abnormalities in obstructive
nephropathy and diversions of the urinary tract. In: Kokko JP,
Jannen RK (eds) *Fluids and Electrolytes,* 3rd Ed., pp. 561–579.
Saunders, Philadelphia, 1996.
Schlueter W, Keilani T, Hizon M, Kaplan B, Batlle D: On the mech-
anism of impaired distal acidification in hyperkalemic renal

tubular acidosis: Evaluation with amiloride and bumetanide.
J Am Soc Nephrol 3:953–964, 1992.
Stacpoole PW, Wright EC, Baumgartner TG, *et al.*: Dichloroacetate
for lactic acidosis in adults: A controlled clinical trial of
dichloroacetate for treatment of lactic acidosis in adults. *N Engl
J Med* 327:1564–1569, 1992.

10

METABOLIC ALKALOSIS

EDWARD R. JONES

Metabolic alkalosis is characterized by a primary increase in the plasma bicarbonate concentration. The resultant alkalemia suppresses ventilation yielding a secondary increase in $p\,CO_2$. Hyperbicarbonatemia may also
be observed as compensation for hypercapnia (respiratory acidosis) attempting to normalize plasma pH. Distinguishing between these disturbances, each associated
with hyperbicarbonatemia and hypercapnia, requires a
blood gas determination to define pH. The history and
physical examination are critical in distinguishing between these two disorders and in identifying patients who
have both metabolic alkalosis and respiratory acidosis.
The distinctive physical characteristics of patients with
chronic lung disease are helpful clues. Formulae and confidence bands to predict metabolic adaptation to hypercapnia and define the presence of simple metabolic
alkalosis, respiratory alkalosis, or mixed disturbances are
discussed in Chapter 12.

In a study of 13,000 arterial blood gases in 3300 hospitalized patients, metabolic alkalosis was the most frequent
acid–base disturbance. Although its direct cause is poorly
defined, morbidity and mortality are increased in surgical
patients with multisystem organ failure and metabolic alkalosis (blood pH > 7.55). Therefore, the recognition and
correction of metabolic alkalosis is important.

CLINICAL MANIFESTATION OF METABOLIC ALKALOSIS

Patients with metabolic alkalosis manifest symptoms related to the cause of the alkalosis, that is, postural symptoms, weakness, and thirst are associated with volume
depletion; neuromuscular symptoms and arrhythmias are
associated with hypokalemia. The clinical presentation is
generally a consequence of the alkalemia, which exerts significant effects on the central nervous and neuromuscular
systems, cardiovascular system, and pulmonary vasculature
as well as contributing to various metabolic derangements.
These signs and symptoms occur with both metabolic and
respiratory alkalosis. It is difficult to differentiate most of
the side effects of alkalemia from the numerous other concomitant metabolic derangements in patients with metabolic alkalosis such as hypocalcemia and hypomagnesemia.

Alkalemia may contribute to the changes in mental status seen in patients with metabolic alkalosis and to a lowering of the seizure threshold. Tetany and neuromuscular irritability including carpopedal spasm, and positive
Chovstek and Trousseau signs may be seen.

Ventricular and supraventricular irritability as well as increased sensitivity to digoxin appears to be more frequent.
Antiarrhythmics may be ineffective until the alkalemia is
corrected. Decrements in cardiac output and cardiovascular instability are common.

Alkalemia decreases ionized calcium by shifting ionized
calcium onto plasma proteins. Therefore, despite normocalcemia, the alkalemic patient may present with seizures
or carpopedal spasms. The clinical significant of the anti-
calciuresis seen in metabolic alkalosis is not well defined.

Alkalemia shifts potassium intracellularly, resulting in
hypokalemia. In addition, metabolic alkalosis causes potassium depletion, which is generally correlated with the magnitude of the alkalosis. The consequences of potassium depletion are discussed in Chapter 13.

Metabolic alkalosis causes an elevated plasma anion
gap. Alkalosis stimulates glycolysis, more specifically

phosphofructokinase, increasing lactate production. The plasma lactate level may increase as much as 5 mEq/L, thereby raising the anion gap by an equivalent amount. Volume contraction concentrates plasma proteins, which increases the unmeasured anion. Finally, alkalemia is associated with the loss of protons from plasma proteins, uncovering negative charges and contributing to the rise in unmeasured anion.

Alkalemia also alters the oxyhemoglobin curve, shifting the curve leftward and potentially limiting oxygen availability. The clinical significant of this is unknown.

PATHOPHYSIOLOGY

Recognition and appropriate intervention to correct the many processes that result in a metabolic alkalosis demands a basic understanding of the pathogenesis of metabolic alkalosis. Under normal conditions, the kidney can effectively excrete an excess of bicarbonate from any source by suppressing renal acid excretion and bicarbonate reabsorption. A sustained rise in serum bicarbonate concentration can only occur if two factors are present. First there must be a source of the alkali (the generation of alkalosis). Second, there must be factors in place that retain the alkali or limit the ability of the kidney to excrete bicarbonate (maintenance of the alkalosis). In those clinical settings where metabolic alkalosis occurs, bicarbonate excretion is impaired as a result of factors which both generate and maintain the alkalosis.

Generation of Metabolic Alkalosis

The generation of bicarbonate (Table 1) results from either the renal or extrarenal loss of acid or gain of base to the extracellular fluid (ECF). Net negative hydrogen ion balance (acid excretion exceeding production) results in a rise in ECF bicarbonate concentration. The loss of acid translates into an equimolar gain of bicarbonate.

Secretion of hydrogen ion from the gastric mucosa is associated with the addition of bicarbonate to blood. Vomiting or gastric drainage are common causes of metabolic alkalosis. Intestinal acid loss can also occur with chloride-losing diarrhea (congenital or acquired chloridorrhea).

A minor rise in serum bicarbonate concentration can occur due to a translocation of protons across cells in exchange for potassium during hypokalemia. This mechanism has little or no clinical significance.

Renal loss of acid is probably the most common cause of metabolic alkalosis. Loop diuretics like furosemide as well as the thiazides stimulate acid excretion by increasing distal nephron sodium delivery and by causing secondary hyperaldosteronism. Hypokalemia enhances proton secretion and ammoniagenesis thus increasing net acid excretion.

Excessive alkali gains can be seen during the administration of bicarbonate or its equivalents during cardiopulmonary resuscitation with massive blood transfusions (sodium citrate is used as an anticoagulant) or the administration of total parenteral nutrition formula (acetate). The

TABLE I
Pathophysiologic Approach to Metabolic Alkalosis

Generation of metabolic alkalosis
　Loss of acid from extracellular fluid
　　Nonrenal acid loss
　　Gastrointestinal fluid losses
　　　Gastric losses
　　　Chloride losing diarrhea
　　Cellular shifts: potassium–hydrogen exchange
　　Renal acid losses
　　　Acid secretion due to diuretics
　　　Nonreabsorbable anions: enhanced distal sodium–
　　　　hydrogen exchange
　　　Severe potassium depletion
　Gain of bicarbonate to the extracellular fluid
　　Conversion of bicarbonate equivalents (citrate, acetate,
　　　lactate)
　　Bicarbonate administration: parenteral or oral
　　Resin exchanges plus antacids
　Unchanged bicarbonate content
　　Contraction of ECF bicarbonate
　　Posthypercapnic state

Maintenance of metabolic alkalosis
　Decreased glomerular filtration rate (GFR)
　　(decreased filtered load of bicarbonate)
　Enhanced proximal bicarbonate reabsorption
　　Reduced arterial blood volume
　　absolute or effective
　　Potassium depletion (also decreased GFR)
　　Hypercapnia
　　Decreased parathyroid hormone
　　Hypercalcemia

　Increased distal tubular bicarbonate reabsorption
　　Mineralocorticoid excess
　　Hypokalemia
　　Nonreabsorbable anion
　　Chloride depletion

addition of alkali from the gastrointestinal tract occurs during the concomitant use of exchange resins (Kayexalate) and poorly absorbable antacids.

Contraction alkalosis results from the loss of chloride-rich, bicarbonate-free fluid which increases serum bicarbonate concentration by 3–5mEq/L. The metabolic alkalosis commonly seen with loop diuretics results predomi- nately from enhanced renal acid excretion and the concomitant hypovolemia, and not contraction of the ECF bicarbonate alone.

Maintenance of Metabolic Alkalosis

A sustained rise in bicarbonate concentration implies a decreased renal bicarbonate excretion. Under normal circumstances, the addition of alkali to the extracellular fluid volume is associated with volume expansion and hypochloremia. The normal kidney senses the volume expansion, the alkali is excreted along with sodium, and the hypochloremia is corrected. Sustained hyperbicarbonatemia requires either a decreased glomerular filtration rate (GFR), enhanced proximal tubular bicarbonate reabsorption (both of the latter are volume dependent stimuli) or increased distal tubular bicarbonate reabsorption (a volume independent mechanism).

Decrements in GFR translate into diminished filtered bicarbonate loads limiting bicarbonate excretion. Enhanced proximal tubular bicarbonate reabsorption will sustain the ECF bicarbonate and maintain the alkalosis. Reduced effective arterial blood volume (EABV) is associated with a decreased bicarbonate excretion. Hypokalemia and hypercapnia stimulate proton secretion and thus bicarbonate addition to blood. Hypokalemia may also decrease GFR, further limiting bicarbonate excretion.

Enhanced distal nephron bicarbonate reabsorption is an important factor in maintaining metabolic alkalosis. Persistent hypermineralocorticoidism, hypokalemia, and the presence of a poorly reabsorbable anion stimulates acid excretion and subsequent addition of alkali to blood.

The importance of hypochloremia in the maintenance of metabolic alkalosis is not established. Some suggest that chloride depletion itself may maintain the metabolic alkalosis and that this effect is independent of plasma volume. Indeed, chloride depletion appears to enhance bicarbonate reabsorption while distal bicarbonate secretion decreases. Differences in location of the chloride/bicarbonate (Cl^-/HCO_3^-) exchanger within intercalated cells of the cortical collecting tubule play a role in maintenance of metabolic alkalosis. Type A intercalated cells have the transporter on the basolateral membrane. In type B cells, these transporters are on the luminal side. Hydrogen ion secretion via the H^+-ATPase pump and passive chloride cosecretion are enhanced on the luminal side during decreased chloride delivery. A concomitant enhancement of chloride entry into, and subsequent HCO_3^- addition to blood, occurs in type A cells. Recent studies have further elucidated the role of transporters in the intercalated cells (IC) of the cortical collecting tubule. Metabolic alkalosis is associated with increased activity of type B IC cells. There is good evidence that augmented distal tubular acidification in alkalotic animals is due to enhanced H^+, $K+$-ATPase along with N^+/H^+ exchange. The H^+-ATPase in type A IC cells redistributes to the basolateral surface and plays little role in the enhanced acidification seen in metabolic alkalosis. The Cl^-/HCO_3^- exchange is reversed in type B cells; thus enhanced chloride secretion into the lumen results in decreased bicarbonate secretion. Consequently both cell types play important roles in maintaining metabolic alkalosis in chloride depleted states. Interestingly endogenous endothelins appear to stimulate Na^+/H^+ exchangers in metabolic alkalosis, suggesting a potential role in the pathophysiology of metabolic alkalosis.

In essence, the recognition of metabolic alkalosis and intervention for this disorder depend on the understanding that metabolic alkalosis is a result of the dependent processes of generation of alkali and maintenance of the alkalosis. Correction of either component alone does not resolve the alkalosis. Cessation of vomiting alone will not lower serum bicarbonate, but correction of the accompanying

TABLE 2
Differential Diagnosis of Metabolic Alkalosis

Urine chloride <15 mEg/L (chloride-responsive)
　Gastric fluid losses
　Stool losses: Chloride losing diarrhea
　Diuretic therapy[a] (diuretic screen negative)
　Posthypercapnic state
　Refeeding
Urine chloride >20 mEg/L (chloride-resistant)
　Primary hyperaldosteronism
　Exogenous steroids
　Bartter's syndrome
　Cushing's syndrome
　Severe hypokalemia
　Alkali loading
　Hypercalcemia

[a] Urinary chloride will vary depending on proximity to ingestion of diuretics. Generally, a negative diuretic screen is associated with remote diuretic use and a low urine chloride.

hypovolemia along with cessation of vomiting will permit normalization of the ECF bicarbonate concentration.

Clinical Conditions Resulting in Metabolic Alkalosis

In keeping with the pathophysiology previously presented, metabolic alkalosis is best categorized according to the volume status of the patient (Table 2). Hypovolemic, chloride-deficient patients excrete less than 15 mEq/L of chloride in a spot urine specimen. These patients have been classified as saline-responsive alkalosis and when their plasma volumes are restored with sodium chloride, bicarbonaturia and renal chloride retention ensue.

On the other hand, the ECF volume expanded (chloride-rich) patient excretes greater than 20 mEg/L of chloride. These patients do not respond to sodium chloride administration and they are thus said to have saline-resistant alkalosis.

Metabolic Alkalosis Associated with ECF Volume Contraction

Hyperbicarbonatemia can be generated either from renal or extrarenal sources. The maintenance of the hyperbicarbonatemia results from the hypovolemia and hypokalemia which enhance proximal bicarbonate reabsorption as well as a decreased GFR which limits bicarbonate excretion. In addition, the hypokalemia and excess mineralocorticoid state enhance distal acid excretion and bicarbonate addition to blood.

Renal Alkalosis

Thiazide and loop diuretics cause hypokalemic metabolic alkalosis. They lead to hypokalemia, hypovolemia, and, as expected, hyperaldosteronism. The incidence of metabolic alkalosis associated with diuretic use ranges from 3 to 50% of diuretic users. Thiazide diuretics increase bicarbonate concentration by only 2 to 7 mEq/L. The use of loop diuretics either alone or in combination with metalazone, particularly in patients with anasarca, can increase bicarbonate concentration by 15–20 mEq/L.

Laboratory findings vary depending on whether the patient is still taking the diuretic. Continued diuretic consumption results in a sustained natriuresis into a high urinary chloride despite hypovolemia. Once the diuretic is stopped, the urinary sodium and chloride fall below 15 mEq/L. This electrolyte pattern may occur with the surreptitious use of diuretics for weight loss, and may be confirmed with a urinary diuretic screen.

The administration of poorly reabsorbable anions in the form of ampicillin, carbenicillin, and other penicillin result in an obligatory natriuresis with enhanced distal tubular potassium and proton losses. The resultant hypokalemia, hypovolemia, and metabolic alkalosis can be blunted or aborted with adequate potassium supplementation and volume repletion.

Bartter's Syndrome, a rare disorder, is not a single entity but comprises several related tubular transport abnormalities that differ somewhat in their presenting symptoms, age of onset, magnitude of urinary prostaglandin excretion, and urinary calcium excretion. At least three phenotypic expressions have been described: the antenatal hypercalciuric variant; the hypocalciuric-hypomagnesemic variant known as Gitelman's syndrome, and classic Bartter's syndrome.

The clinical presentation of Bartter's syndrome consists of hypokalemia, metabolic alkalosis, hypomagnesemia, hyperuricemia, hyperreninism, and hyperaldosteronism without hypertension. Prostaglandin production is increased. Patients are hyperchloruresis and have urinary potassium wasting. The majority of patients are less than 25 years old, with common presenting symptoms of polyuria, paresthesias, muscle weakness, cramping, and failure to thrive. The antenatal variant is characterized by hydramnios, prematurity, and dehydration at birth. Gitelman's syndrome is associated with hypokalemia, hypomagnesemia, and hypocalciuria. Urinary chloride levels are low, and there is juxtaglomerular apparatus hyperplasia. There is impaired transport in the cortical thick limb of Henle and reduced sodium reabsorption in the distal tubule. The former defect probably accounts for magnesium wasting and the later hypocalciuria. The major differences in Bartter's syndrome and Gitelman's syndrome is divalent ion metabolism. Bartter's syndrome is generally associated hypercalciuria, nephrocalcinosis and a normal serum magnesium.

Bartter's syndrome and its variant have an autosomal recessive mode of inheritance. Cloning of genes encoding renal transporters explain the Bartter variants. Bartter's syndrome results from defective transepithelial transport of sodium chloride in the thick ascending limb of the loop of Henle. The genes encoding several proteins in the thick ascending limb have been identified: the bumetanide-sensitive sodium–potassium–chloride cotransporter, the luminal ATPase regulated K^+ channel, and the kidney specific basolateral chloride channel. Gene mutations for each of the transport proteins have been identified. Gitelman's syndrome results from a defect in the gene for the thiazide-sensitive distal tubular sodium-chloride cotransporter. (See Chapter 2.)

Nonrenal Alkalosis

Vomiting is associated with the loss of water, electrolytes, and protons from the ECF. The loss of hydrogen ion into the gastric lumen is associated with delivery of equimolar quantities of bicarbonate into gastric venous blood. The loss of 3 or 4 L of gastric content will result in marked electrolyte and fluid losses. The hypovolemia and concomitant hyperaldosteronism induce a marked kaliuresis, resulting in profound potassium depletion and subsequent hypokalemia (the gastric potassium losses are trivial in this setting), hypochloremia, and severe metabolic alkalosis. The clinical setting of vomiting is approached best by evaluating the various phases of development of the alkalosis. The early developmental phase is associated with a rapid rise in bicarbonate, mild hypovolemia, and hypochloremia. The filtered load of bicarbonate exceeds the reabsorptive capacity of the proximal tubule. Therefore, bicarbonaturia with an alkaline urine are present. Despite hypovolemia, there is a natriuresis due to the obligatory bicarbonate diuresis. It should be noted that the combination of an ongoing natriuresis with hypovolemia is also seen with diuretic use. Kaliuresis is marked while the urine is chloride deplete. There is a positive urinary anion gap (defined as the urinary sodium plus potassium minus chloride). A positive urinary anion gap with alkaline urine implies that bicarbonate is the unmeasured anion; with an acid urine, nonreabsorbable anions, including, ketones, lactate, and penicillin account for the gap. See Chapter 9 for a more extensive discussion of the urine anion gap. When vomiting ceases, the gastric losses end, but the patient remain profoundly hypovolemic. During this maintenance phase, proximal sodium reabsorption is maximized, GFR is depressed, bicarbonaturia is absent, and sodium is reabsorbed. The kaliuresis is lessened but persists and approximates the low urine chloride plus an undefined quantity of anion. A paradoxical aciduria exists, and the urinary anion gap is no longer significantly positive. During the correction of the alkalosis (reparative phase), as plasma volume is restored and GFR improves, bicarbonaturia resumes as does the natriuresis, with an alkaline urine and a positive urinary anion gap. The urine remains low in chloride until volume repletion is complete. The commonality in these phases is the low urinary chloride with persistent kaliuresis.

The provision of chloride as sodium and potassium salts to avoid volume depletion can prevent significant metabolic alkalosis. The use of parenteral H_2-receptor blockers or proton pump inhibition will limit gastric acid losses. Once alkalosis is present both the generative and maintenance phase of the alkalosis must be resolved. Stopping the gastric losses is critical as is replenishment of plasma volume in these saline-responsive patients with sodium chloride and appropriate KCl supplementation.

Metabolic Alkalosis Associated with ECF Volume Expansion

The kidneys are responsible for both the generation and maintenance of this setting of metabolic alkalosis but the alkalosis is not responsive to saline. These patients have urinary chloride excretion greater than 20 mEq/L.

The saline unresponsive alkaloses are generally divided into those associated with or without hypertension. Further categorization according to renin/aldosterone profiles may also be helpful. The later are generally not measured in clinical practice; this characterization is most helpful as a conceptual tool.

Hypertension with Mineralocorticoid Excess

The mineralocorticoid excess, be it endogenous or exogenous, is associated with enhanced salt reabsorption with volume expansion, hypokalemia, kaliuresis, chloruresis, increased net acid excretion (enhanced ammoniagenesis), and decreased GFR. The severity of the metabolic alkalosis is related to the severity of the potassium depletion.

High renin, mineralocorticoid excess states are seen most commonly with renal vascular hypertension. Approximately 20% of patients with renal artery stenosis (RAS) present with severe hypokalemia and metabolic alkalosis. Malignant hypertension is generally associated with hyperreninemia due to renal ischemia. Hypokalemic metabolic alkalosis is seen in 10–20% of these cases. Renin-secreting tumors of juxtaglomerular apparatus origin are associated with hypertension and metabolic alkalosis.

Low renin, mineralocorticoid excess states are most commonly seen with primary hyperaldosteronism (Conn's syndrome). Hypokalemic, metabolic alkalosis, hypernatremia, and hypertension are hallmarks of this low renin state. It accounts for less than 1–2% of all cases of hypertension. Marked potassium depletion (as much as 1000 mEq have been reported) along with the hyperaldosteronism is responsible for the alkalosis in that aldosterone administration alone or hypokalemia alone only marginally increase serum bicarbonate concentration. Serum bicarbonate concentrations above 30 mEq/L in 85% of cases and above 35 mEq/L in 40% of cases have been reported.

Hypertension with Low Renin and Aldosterone

Nonaldosterone mineralocorticoids will exert the same identical physiologic effects as aldosterone. In this setting measurements of serum aldosterone will be negative. The clinical syndromes include Cushing's syndrome, exogenous steroids, and adrenal enzyme deficiencies (11β- and 17β-hydroxylase). Licorice use has also been associated with metabolic alkalosis due to glycyrrhizic acid in licorice. Glycyrrhizic acid ingestion is associated with a mineralocorticoid excess state. This component had been thought to exert a direct mineralocorticoid activity, but it appears that it inhibits 11β-hydroxysteroid dehydrogenase which is responsible for the conversion between the active steroid cortisol and inactive cortisone.

Volume Expanded States with Low Renin and Mineralocorticoid

Exogenous consumption of sodium bicarbonate, calcium carbonate, baking soda, Tums (10 mEq of alkali/tablet), or Rolaids (4.6 mEq/tablet) in the face of decreased renal excretion of bicarbonate can cause metabolic alkalosis.

In patients with renal failure, the consumption of poorly absorbable antacids, particularly aluminum hydroxide gets used to control hyperphosphatemia, sucralfate, or sodium polystyrene sulfonate resin used to treat hyperkalemia, will generate bicarbonate from the gastrointestinal tract. The later resin binds cations leaving a more soluble form of bicarbonate which is absorbed by the intestinal cell from the lumen. Renal failure perpetuates the alkalosis because of the concomitant inability to excrete the excess bicarbonate added from the gastrointestinal tract.

The administration of multiple blood transfusions can be associated with metabolic alkalosis. Each unit of whole blood contains 17 mEq of sodium citrate while packed cells contain 5 mEq. Citrate is converted to bicarbonate and therefore a large volume transfusion can result in metabolic alkalosis.

Milk-alkali syndrome is a rare but frequently mentioned cause of metabolic alkalosis. The consumption of calcium carbonate containing absorbable antacids along with large quantities of milk (2–3 quarts/day) can result in the milk-alkali syndrome. Hypercalcemia, hypoparathyroidism, hypercalciuria, and alkalinuria favor renal calcium phosphorous deposition and can result in nephrocalcinosis and renal failure.

DIAGNOSIS OF METABOLIC ALKALOSIS

To recognize and appropriates intervene in metabolic alkaline require a full appreciation of the underlying pathophysiology. A thorough history and physical is necessary, focusing on potential sources of alkali. Particular attention to the volume status of the patient is also required. Comparison of the change (delta) in bicarbonate to the change in anion gap, the so-called delta–delta gaps can disclose the presence of an otherwise unsuspected metabolic alkalosis. Acid added to the extracellular fluid dissociates to form a proton and the related anion. The former is buffered by bicarbonate and the rise in anion concentration is accompanied by an equimolor fall in bicarbonate. This results in a delta anion to delta bicarbonate ratio (delta–delta) of one. If the delta anion gap exceeds the delta bicarbonate, a potential excess of alkali is implied. This indication tract a metabolic alkalosis is present along with the metabolic acidosis. For example, if a patient has a bicarbonate level of 20 mEq/L (delta bicarbonate of 5 mEq/L assuming a starting value of 25 m Eq/L) and an anion gap of 22 mEq/L (assuming a normal upper limit of anion gap of 12 mEq/L), the delta–delta ratio is 10:5 or 2:1. Alternatively, to yield an anion gap of 22 mEq/L, 10 mEq/L of bicarbonate must have been titrated. Since the final bicarbonate concentration is 20 mEq, the starting concentration must have been 30 mEq/L (10 + 20). Either means of assessment implies that both a metabolic alkalosis and acidosis are present.

The use of urinary electrolytes to define causes of metabolic alkalosis and make inferences about plasma volume is predicated upon the presence of normal renal and adrenal function and the absence of diuretics. Screening for the latter may be necessary. A urinary chloride less than 15 mEq/L implies decreased effective or absolute arterial blood volume or very low salt intake. In the absence of edema, volume expansion to restore plasma volume results in bicarbonaturia and subsequent correction of the alkalosis as long as the generation of the alkalosis is also uncovered and corrected. In the presence of edema and low urinary chloride, improving EABV rather than saline infusions (which will only worsen the edema) is necessary.

Urinary chloride concentrations greater than 20 mEq/L, in the absence of polyuria, suggest that plasma volumes are normal or increased. Obviously patients with salt wasting states in the face of volume depletion (diuretic use, salt-wasting nephropathies, and the setting where nonreabsorbable anions are present, as is the early and late phases of vomiting, or penicillin use) will have high urinary chlorides and need to be differentiated on clinical grounds. Generally mineralocorticoid excess, Bartter's syndrome, and similar disorders are the likely culprits. Hypokalemic alkalosis from occult vomiting or diuretic use can be differentiated from Bartter's syndrome, but only with difficulty. Indeed, some authorities have referred to these two conditions as pseudo-Bartter's syndrome. Urinary electrolytes are especially helpful in differentiating, between these states.

TREATMENT OF METABOLIC ALKALOSIS

As discussed earlier correcting the processes responsible for the generation of the alkali is necessary. Antiemetics, H_2-blockers, proton pump inhibition, stopping diuretics, and preventing and correcting hypokalemia, are critical. Defining and reestablishing plasma volume is mandatory. Rarely, severe alkalemia can be treated with acetazolamide (250 to 500 mg) with appropriate replacement of saline and potassium.

Severe metabolic alkalosis in the setting of acute or chronic renal failure, where bicarbonaturia (to correct the alkalosis) is not anticipated may require an acidifying agent particularly in the symptomatic patient. The goal is to lower arterial pH below 7.5. Either 0.1 or 0.2 M hydrochloric acid (100–200 mEq/L) is infused into a central vein. The HCl distributes initially in the ECF, and the amount of acid to be infused is 20% of body weight times the fall in bicarbonate (in mEq/L) calculated as necessary to lower pH.

Frequent monitoring of arterial pH is necessary. Finally, in the anuric patient, an alternative is dialysis against a non-bicarbonate containing dialysate.

Bibliography

Bastani B, Purcell H, Henken P, *et al.:* Expression and distribution of renal vacuolar proton-translocating adenosine triphosphatase in response to chronic acid and alkali loads in the rat. *J Clin Invest* 88:126, 1991.

Bettinelli A, Bianchetti MG, Borella P, *et al.:* Genetic heterogeneity in tubular hypomagnesemia–hypokalemia with hypocalciuria (Gitelman's syndrome). *Kidney Int* 47:547, 1995.

Carrneiro AV, Sebastian A, Cogan MG: Reduced glomerular filtration rate can maintain a rise in plasma bicarbonate concentration in humans. *Am J Nephrol* 7:450, 1987.

Cogan MG, Liu FY, Berger BE, Sebastian A, *et al.:* Metabolic alkalosis. *Med Clin North Am* 67:903, 1983.

Gabow PA: Disorders associated with an altered anion gap. *Kidney Int* 27:472, 1985.

Guay-Woodford LM: Bartter syndrome: Unraveling the pathophysiologic enigma. *Am J Med* 105:151, 1998.

Halperin ML, Kamel KS, Narins RG: Use of urine electrolytes and osmolality: Bringing physiology to the bedside. In: Narins RG, Stein JH (eds) *Diagnostic Techniques in Renal Diseases, Volume 52 Contemporary Issues in Nephrology*, p.q. Churchill Livingstone, New York, 1992.

Hodgkin JE, Soepranoff, Chan DM: Incidence of metabolic alkalemia in hospitalized patients. *Crit Care Med* 8:725, 1980.

Kassirer JP, London AM, Goldman DM, *et al.:* On the pathogenesis of metabolic alkalosis in hyperaldosteronism. *Am J Med* 49:306, 1970.

Koch SM, Taylor RW: Chloride ion in intensive care medicine. *Crit Care Med* 20:227, 1992.

Kurtz I: Molecular pathogenesis of Bartter's and Gitelman's syndromes. *Kidney Int* 54:1396, 1998.

Narins RG, Jones ER, Townsend R: *Metabolic Acid Base Disorders: Pathophysiology, Classification, and Treatment, Fluid, Electrolytes and Acid Base Disorders*, pp. 335–385. Churchill Livingstone. New York, 1985.

Norris SH, Kurtzman NA: Does chloride play an independent role in the pathogenesis of metabolic alkalosis. *Semin Nephrol* 8:101, 1988.

Scheinman SJ, Guay-Woodford LM, Thakker RV, Warnock DG: Genetic disorders of renal electrolyte transport. *N Engl J Med* 340:1177, 1999.

Seldin DW, Rector FC, Jr: The generation and maintenance of metabolic alkalosis. *Kidney Int* 1:305, 1972.

Stone DK, Xie XS: Proton translocating ATPases: Issues in structure and function. *Kidney Int* 33:767, 1988.

Tsukamoto T, Kobayashi T, Kawamoto K, *et al.:* Possible discrimination of Gitelman's syndrome from Bartter's syndrome by renal clearance study: Report of two cases. *Am J Kidney Dis* 25:637, 1995.

RESPIRATORY ACIDOSIS AND ALKALOSIS

NICOLAOS E. MADIAS

RESPIRATORY ACIDOSIS

Respiratory acidosis, or primary hypercapnia, is the acid–base disturbance initiated by an increase in carbon dioxide tension of body fluids. Hypercapnia acidifies body fluids and elicits an adaptive increment in plasma bicarbonate that should be viewed as an integral part of the respiratory acidosis. Arterial carbon dioxide tension (pCO_2) measured at rest and at sea level is greater than 45 mm Hg in simple respiratory acidosis. Lower values of pCO_2 might still signify the presence of primary hypercapnia in the setting of mixed acid–base disorders (e.g., eucapnia, rather than the expected hypocapnia, in the presence of metabolic acidosis).

Pathophysiology

Hypercapnia develops whenever carbon dioxide excretion by the lungs is insufficient to match carbon dioxide production, thus leading to positive carbon dioxide balance. Hypercapnia could result from increased carbon dioxide production, decreased alveolar ventilation, or both. Overproduction of carbon dioxide is usually matched by increased excretion such that hypercapnia is prevented. However, patients with marked limitation in pulmonary reserve and those receiving constant mechanical ventilation might experience respiratory acidosis due to increased carbon dioxide production. Established clinical circumstances include increased physical activity, augmented work of breathing by the respiratory muscles, shivering, seizures, fever, and hyperthyroidism. Increments in carbon dioxide production might also be imposed by the administration of large carbohydrate loads (greater than 2000 kcal per day) and parenteral nutrition to semistarved, critically ill patients as well as during the decomposition of bicarbonate infused in the course of treating metabolic acidosis. By far, most cases of respiratory acidosis reflect a decrease in alveolar ventilation. Decreased alveolar ventilation can result from decreased minute ventilation, increased dead space ventilation, or a combination of the two.

The major threat to life from carbon dioxide retention in patients breathing room air is the associated obligatory hypoxemia. Thus, in the absence of supplemental oxygen, patients suffering respiratory arrest develop critical hypoxemia within a few minutes, long before extreme hypercapnia ensues. Because of the constraints of the alveolar gas equation, it is not possible for pCO_2 to reach values much higher than 80 mm Hg while the level of pO_2 is still compatible with life. Extreme hypercapnia can only be seen during oxygen administration and, in fact, is often the result of uncontrolled oxygen therapy.

Secondary Physiological Response

An immediate increment in plasma bicarbonate concentration owing to titration of nonbicarbonate body buffers occurs in response to acute hypercapnia. This adaptation is complete within 5 to 10 min from the rise in pCO_2. On average, plasma bicarbonate increases by about 0.1 mEq/L for each mm Hg acute increment in pCO_2; as a result, plasma hydrogen ion concentration rises by about 0.75 nEq/L for each mm Hg acute rise in pCO_2. Therefore, the overall limit of adaptation of plasma bicarbonate in acute respiratory acidosis is quite small; even when pCO_2 rises to levels of 80 to 90 mm Hg, the increment in plasma bicarbonate does not exceed 3 to 4 mEq/L. Moderate hypoxemia does not alter the adaptive response to acute respiratory acidosis. On the other hand, preexisting hypobicarbonatemia (whether due to metabolic acidosis or chronic respiratory alkalosis) enhances the magnitude of the bicarbonate response to acute hypercapnia, whereas such a response is diminished in hyperbicarbonatemic states (whether due to metabolic alkalosis or chronic respiratory acidosis). Other electrolyte changes observed in acute respiratory acidosis include a mild rise in plasma sodium (1 to 4 mEq/L), potassium (0.1 mEq/L for each 0.1 unit fall in pH), and phosphorus, and a small decrease in plasma chloride and lactate concentrations. A small reduction in the plasma anion gap is also observed, reflecting the fall in plasma lactate and the acidic titration of plasma proteins.

The adaptive increase in plasma bicarbonate concentration observed in the acute phase of hypercapnia is amplified markedly during chronic hypercapnia as a result of generation of new bicarbonate by the kidneys. Both proximal and distal acidification mechanisms contribute to this adaptation, which requires 3 to 5 days for completion. The renal response to chronic hypercapnia includes chloruresis and generation of hypochloremia. On average, plasma bicarbonate increases by about 0.3 mEq/L for each mm Hg chronic increment in pCO_2; as a result, plasma hydrogen ion concentration rises by about 0.3 nEq/L for each mm Hg chronic rise in pCO_2. Empirical observations indicate a limit of adaptation of plasma bicarbonate on the order of 45 mEq/L. The renal response to chronic hypercapnia is not altered appreciably by dietary sodium or chloride restriction, moderate potassium depletion, alkali loading, or moderate hypoxemia. It is currently unknown to what extent renal insufficiency of variable severity limits the renal response to chronic hypercapnia. Obviously, patients with end stage renal disease cannot mount a renal response to chronic hypercapnia and, thus, they are more subject to severe acidemia. The degree of acidemia is more pronounced in patients receiving hemodialysis rather than peritoneal dialysis because the former treatment maintains, on average, a lower plasma bicarbonate concentration. Recovery from chronic hypercapnia is crippled by a chloride-deficient diet. In this circumstance, despite correction of the level of pCO_2, plasma bicarbonate concentration remains elevated as long as the state of chloride deprivation persists, thus creating the entity of "posthypercapnic metabolic alkalosis." Chronic hypercapnia is not associated with appreciable changes in the plasma concentrations of sodium, potassium, phosphorus, or anion gap.

Etiology

Respiratory acidosis can develop in patients with normal or abnormal airways and lungs. Tables 1 and 2 present causes of acute and chronic respiratory acidosis, respectively. This classification takes into consideration the usual mode of onset and duration of the various causes and emphasizes the biphasic time course that characterizes the secondary physiological response to hypercapnia. Primary hypercapnia can result from disease or malfunction within any element of the regulatory system controlling respiration, including the central and peripheral nervous system, the respiratory muscles, the thoracic cage, the pleural space, the airways, and the lung parenchyma. Not infrequently, more than one cause contributes to the development of respiratory acidosis in a given patient. Chronic lower airways obstruction resulting from bronchitis and emphysema is the most common cause of chronic hypercapnia.

Clinical Manifestations

Clinical manifestations of respiratory acidosis arising from the central nervous system are collectively known as "hypercapnic encephalopathy" and include irritability, inability to concentrate, headache, anorexia, mental cloudiness, apathy, confusion, incoherence, combativeness, hallucinations, delirium, and transient psychosis. Progressive narcosis or coma might develop in patients receiving oxygen therapy, especially those with an acute exacerbation of chronic respiratory insufficiency in whom pCO_2 levels up to 100 mm Hg or even higher can occur. In addition, frank papilledema (pseudotumor cerebri) and motor disturbances, including myoclonic jerks, flapping tremor identical to that observed in liver failure, and seizures might develop. The occurrence of neurological symptomatology in patients with respiratory acidosis depends on the magnitude of the hypercapnia, the rapidity with which it

TABLE I
Causes of Acute Respiratory Acidosis[a]

Normal airways and lungs	Abnormal airways and lungs
Central nervous system depression	Upper airways obstruction
General anesthesia	Coma-induced hypopharyngeal obstruction
Sedative overdosage	
Head trauma	Aspiration of foreign body or vomitus
Cerebrovascular accident	
Central sleep apnea	Laryngospasm or angioedema
Cerebral edema	
Brain tumor	Obstructive sleep apnea
Encephalitis	Inadequate laryngeal intubation
Neuromuscular impairment	
High spinal cord injury	Laryngeal obstruction postintubation
Guillain-Barré syndrome	
Status epilepticus	Lower airways obstruction
Botulism, tetanus	Generalized broncho-spasm
Crisis in myasthenia gravis	
Hypokalemic myopathy	Severe asthma (status asthmaticus)
Familial hypokalemic periodic paralysis	
	Bronchiolitis of infancy and adults
Drugs or toxic agents (e.g., curare, succinylcholine, aminoglycosides, organophosphorus)	Disorders involving pulmonary alveoli
	Severe bilateral pneumonia
Ventilatory restriction	
Rib fractures with flail chest	Acute respiratory distress syndrome
Pneumothorax	
Hemothorax	Severe pulmonary edema
Impaired diaphragmatic function (e.g., peritoneal dialysis, ascites)	Pulmonary perfusion defect
	Cardiac arrest
Iatrogenic events	Severe circulatory failure
Misplacement or displacement of airway cannula during anesthesia or mechanical ventilation	Massive pulmonary thromboembolism
	Fat or air embolus
Bronchoscopy-associated hypoventilation or respiratory arrest	
Increased CO_2 production with constant mechanical ventilation (e.g., due to high carbohydrate diet or sorbent-regenerative hemodialysis)	

[a]Adapted from Madias and Adrogué (1991).

develops, the severity of the acidemia, and the degree of the accompanying hypoxemia.

The hemodynamic consequences of respiratory acidosis reflect a variety of mechanisms, including a direct depressing effect on myocardial contractility. An associated sympathetic surge, sometimes intense, leads to increases in plasma catecholamines, but, during severe acidemia (generally blood pH below 7.20), receptor responsiveness to catecholamines is markedly blunted. Hypercapnia results

TABLE 2
Causes of Chronic Respiratory Acidosis[a]

Normal airways and lungs	Abnormal airways and lungs
Central nervous system depression	Upper airways obstruction
Sedative overdosage	Tonsillar and peritonsillar hypertrophy
Methadone/heroin addiction	Paralysis of vocal cords
Primary alveolar hypoventilation (Ondine's curse)	Tumor of the cords or larynx
	Airway stenosis post prolonged intubation
Obesity-hypoventilation syndrome (Pickwickian syndrome)	Thymoma, aortic aneurysm
Brain tumor	Lower airways obstruction
Bulbar poliomyelitis	Chronic obstructive lung disease (bronchitis, bronchiolitis, bronchiectasis, emphysema)
Neuromuscular impairment	
Poliomyelitis	
Multiple sclerosis	Disorders involving pulmonary alveoli
Muscular dystrophy	Severe chronic pneumonitis
Amyotrophic lateral sclerosis	Diffuse infiltrative disease (e.g., alveolar proteinosis)
Diaphragmatic paralysis	Interstitial fibrosis
Myxedema	
Myopathic disease	
Ventilatory restriction	
Kyphoscoliosis, spinal arthritis	
Obesity	
Fibrothorax	
Hydrothorax	
Impaired diaphragmatic function	

[a]Adapted from Madias and Adrogué (1991).

in systemic vasodilation by a direct action on vascular smooth muscle; this effect is most obvious in the cerebral circulation where blood flow increases in direct relation to the level of pCO_2. By contrast, carbon dioxide retention can produce vasoconstriction in the pulmonary circulation as well as in the kidneys; in the latter case, the hemodynamic response might be mediated via an enhanced sympathetic activity. The composite effect of these inputs is such that mild to moderate hypercapnia is usually associated with an increased cardiac output, normal or increased blood pressure, warm skin, a bounding pulse, and diaphoresis. However, when hypercapnia is severe or considerable hypoxemia is present, decreases in both cardiac output and blood pressure might be observed. Concomitant therapy with vasoactive medications or the presence of congestive heart failure might further modify the hemodynamic response. Cardiac arrhythmias, particularly supraventricular tachyarrhythmias not associated with major hemodynamic compromise, are common. They do not result primarily from the hypercapnia, but rather reflect the associated hypoxemia and sympathetic discharge, concomitant medication, electrolyte abnormalities, and underlying cardiac disease. Salt and water retention is commonly observed in sustained hypercapnia, especially in the presence of cor pulmonale. In addition to the effects of heart

failure on the kidney, multiple other factors might be involved, including the prevailing stimulation of the sympathetic nervous system and the renin–angiotensin–aldosterone axis, the increased renal vascular resistance, and the elevated levels of antidiuretic hormone and cortisol.

Diagnosis

In general, one never should rely on clinical evaluation alone to assess the adequacy of alveolar ventilation. Whenever hypoventilation is suspected, arterial blood gases should be obtained. If the acid–base profile of the patient reveals hypercapnia in association with acidemia, at least an element of respiratory acidosis must be present. However, hypercapnia might be associated with a normal or an alkaline pH because of the simultaneous presence of additional acid–base disorders. Information from the patient's history, physical examination, and ancillary laboratory data should be utilized for an accurate assessment of the acid–base status.

Therapeutic Principles

Treatment of acute respiratory acidosis must be directed at prompt removal of the underlying cause whenever possible. Immediate therapeutic efforts should focus on establishing and securing a patent airway, restoring adequate oxygenation by delivering an oxygen-rich inspired mixture, and providing adequate ventilation in order to repair the abnormal gas composition. As noted, acute respiratory acidosis poses its major threat to survival not because of hypercapnia or acidemia, but because of the associated hypoxemia. Mechanical ventilation must be initiated in the presence of apnea, severe hypoxemia unresponsive to conservative measures, or progressive hypercapnia (pCO_2 >80 mm Hg). Despite its overall merit, noninvasive oximetry should not substitute for arterial blood gas measurements in titrating FiO_2. The presence of a component of metabolic acidosis is the primary indication for alkali therapy in patients with acute respiratory acidosis. Administration of sodium bicarbonate to patients with simple respiratory acidosis is not only of questionable efficacy, but also involves considerable risk. Concerns include pH-mediated depression of ventilation, enhanced carbon dioxide production due to bicarbonate decomposition, and volume expansion. Alkali therapy might have a special role in patients with severe bronchospasm by restoring the responsiveness of the bronchial musculature to β-adrenergic agonists. Successful management of intractable asthma in patients with blood pH below 7.00 by administering sufficient sodium bicarbonate to raise blood pH to above 7.20 has been reported.

Recent evidence indicating that large tidal volumes often lead to alveolar overdistention and volutrauma has led to a new strategy for management of disorders requiring mechanical ventilation, such as acute respiratory distress syndrome (ARDS) and severe airway obstruction. The strategy entails prescription of tidal volumes of <7 mL/kg body weight (instead of the conventional level of 10 to 15 mL/kg body weight) to achieve plateau airway pressures of <30 cm H_2O. Because an increase in pCO_2 might develop, this approach is termed permissive hypercapnia or controlled hypoventilation. If the resultant hypercapnia reduces blood pH below 7.15 to 7.20, many physicians prescribe bicarbonate; however, this strategy is controversial and others intervene only for pH values on the order of 7.00. Some observations suggest that permissive hypercapnia affords improved clinical outcomes, but other studies have failed to demonstrate benefit; thus, the available results remain inconclusive. Heavy sedation and neuromuscular blockade are frequently needed with this therapy. Following discontinuation of neuromuscular blockade, some patients develop prolonged weakness or paralysis. Contraindications to permissive hypercapnia include cerebrovascular disease, brain edema, increased intracranial pressure, and convulsions; depressed cardiac function and arrhythmias; and severe pulmonary hypertension. Notably, most of these entities can develop as adverse effects of permissive hypercapnia itself, especially when associated with substantial acidemia.

Patients with chronic respiratory acidosis frequently develop episodes of acute decompensation that can be serious or life-threatening. Common culprits include pulmonary infection, use of narcotics, or uncontrolled oxygen therapy. In contrast to acute hypercapnia, injudicious use of oxygen therapy in patients with chronic respiratory acidosis can produce further reductions in alveolar ventilation. Respiratory decompensation superimposes an acute element of carbon dioxide retention and acidemia on the chronic baseline. Unfortunately, only rarely can one remove the underlying cause of chronic respiratory acidosis. Nonetheless, maximizing alveolar ventilation with relatively simple maneuvers is often rewarding in managing respiratory decompensation. Such maneuvers include treatment with antibiotics, bronchodilators, or diuretics; avoidance of irritant inhalants, tranquilizers, or sedatives; elimination of retained secretions; and gradual reduction of supplemental oxygen aiming at a pO_2 of about 60 mm Hg. Administration of adequate quantities of chloride (usually as the potassium salt) prevents or corrects a complicating element of metabolic alkalosis (commonly diuretic induced) that can further dampen the ventilatory drive. Acetazolamide can be used as an adjunctive measure, but care must be taken to avoid potassium depletion. Potassium and phosphate depletion should be corrected, because they can contribute to the development or the maintenance of respiratory failure by impairing the function of skeletal muscles. The use of pharmacologic stimulants of ventilation has been generally disappointing, but a measure of benefit can been derived by some patients with central sleep apnea, obesity-hypoventilation syndrome, or chronic obstructive lung disease. Whereas an aggressive approach that favors the early use of ventilator assistance is most appropriate for acute respiratory acidosis, a more conservative approach is advisable in decompensated chronic hypercapnia, because of the great difficulty often encountered in weaning such patients from ventilators. As a general rule, if the patient is alert, able to cough, and can cooperate with the treatment program,

mechanical ventilation is usually not necessary. On the other hand, if the patient is obtunded or unable to cough, and if hypercapnia and acidemia are worsening, mechanical ventilation should be instituted. Restoration of the pCO_2 of the patient to near its chronic baseline should proceed gradually over a period of many hours to a few days. Overly rapid reduction in pCO_2 in such patients risks the development of sudden, posthypercapnic alkalemia with potentially serious consequences, including reduction in cardiac output and cerebral blood flow, cardiac arrhythmias (including predisposition to digitalis intoxication), and generalized seizures. Noninvasive mechanical ventilation with a nasal or facial mask is increasingly being used to avoid the potential complications of endotracheal intubation. In the absence of a complicating element of metabolic acidosis and with the possible exception of the severely acidemic patient with intense generalized bronchoconstriction undergoing mechanical ventilation, there is no role for alkali administration in chronic respiratory acidosis.

RESPIRATORY ALKALOSIS

Respiratory alkalosis, or primary hypocapnia, is the acid–base disturbance initiated by a reduction in carbon dioxide tension of body fluids. Hypocapnia alkalinizes body fluids and elicits an adaptive decrement in plasma bicarbonate that should be viewed as an integral part of the respiratory alkalosis. The level of pCO_2 measured at rest and at sea level is lower than 35 mm Hg in simple respiratory alkalosis. Higher values of pCO_2 might still indicate the presence of an element of primary hypocapnia in the setting of mixed acid–base disorders (e.g., eucapnia, rather than the anticipated hypercapnia, in the presence of metabolic alkalosis).

Pathophysiology

Primary hypocapnia most commonly reflects pulmonary hyperventilation owing to increased ventilatory drive. The latter results from signals arising from the lung, the peripheral chemoreceptors (carotid and aortic), the brain stem chemoreceptors, or influences originating in other centers of the brain. Additional mechanisms for the generation of primary hypocapnia include maladjusted mechanical ventilators, the extrapulmonary elimination of carbon dioxide by a dialysis device or extracorporeal circulation (e.g., heart–lung machine), and decreased carbon dioxide production (e.g., due to sedation, skeletal muscle paralysis, hypothermia) in patients receiving constant mechanical ventilation.

A condition termed pseudorespiratory alkalosis occurs in patients with profound depression of cardiac function and pulmonary perfusion but with relative preservation of alveolar ventilation, including patients with advanced circulatory failure and those undergoing cardiopulmonary resuscitation. In these patients, there is venous (and tissue) hypercapnia due to the severely reduced pulmonary blood flow that limits the CO_2 delivered to the lungs for excretion.

On the other hand, arterial blood evidences hypocapnia owing to the increased ventilation-to-perfusion ratio that causes a larger than normal removal of CO_2 per unit of blood traversing the pulmonary circulation. Absolute carbon dioxide excretion is decreased, however, and body carbon dioxide balance is positive. Therefore, respiratory acidosis, rather than respiratory alkalosis, is present. Such patients may have severe venous acidemia (often owing to mixed respiratory and metabolic acidosis) accompanied by an arterial pH that ranges from the mildly acidic to the frankly alkaline. In addition arterial blood might reveal normoxia or hyperoxia despite the presence of severe hypoxemia in venous blood. Thus, both arterial and mixed (or central) venous blood sampling is needed to assess the acid–base status and oxygenation of patients with critical hemodynamic compromise.

Secondary Physiological Response

Adaptation to acute hypocapnia is characterized by an immediate decrement in plasma bicarbonate that is principally due to titration of nonbicarbonate body buffers. This adaptation is completed within 5 to 10 min after the onset of hypocapnia. Plasma bicarbonate falls, on average, by approximately 0.2 mEq/L for each mm Hg acute decrement in pCO_2; consequently, plasma hydrogen ion concentration decreases by about 0.75 nEq/L for each mm Hg acute reduction in pCO_2. The limit of this adaptation of plasma bicarbonate is on the order of 17 to 18 mEq/L. Concomitant small rises in plasma chloride, lactate, and other unmeasured anions balance the fall in plasma bicarbonate; each of these components accounts for about one-third of the bicarbonate decrement. Small decreases in plasma sodium (1–3 mEq/L) and potassium (0.2 mEq/L for each 0.1 unit rise in pH) might be observed. Severe hypophosphatemia can occur in acute hypocapnia due to translocation of phosphorus into the cells.

A larger decrement in plasma bicarbonate occurs in chronic hypocapnia as a result of renal adaptation to the disorder and involves suppression of both proximal and distal acidification mechanisms. Completion of this adaptation requires 2 to 3 days. Plasma bicarbonate decreases, on average, by about 0.4 mEq/L for each mm Hg chronic decrement in pCO_2; as a consequence, plasma hydrogen ion concentration decreases by approximately 0.4 nEq/L for each mm Hg chronic reduction in pCO_2. The limit of this adaptation of plasma bicarbonate is on the order of 12 to 15 mEq/L. About two-thirds of the fall in plasma bicarbonate is balanced by a rise in plasma chloride concentration, the remainder reflecting an increase in plasma unmeasured anions; part of the remainder is due to the alkaline titration of plasma proteins, but most remains undefined. Plasma lactate does not rise in chronic hypocapnia, even in the presence of moderate hypoxemia. Similarly, no appreciable change in the plasma concentration of sodium occurs. In sharp contrast with acute hypocapnia, the plasma concentration of phosphorus remains essentially unchanged in chronic hypocapnia. Although plasma potassium is in the normal range in patients with chronic

hypocapnia at sea level, hypokalemia and renal potassium wasting have been described in subjects in whom sustained hypocapnia was induced by exposure to high altitude. Patients with end stage renal disease are obviously at risk of developing severe alkalemia in response to chronic hypocapnia because they cannot mount a renal response. Such a risk is higher in patients receiving peritoneal dialysis rather than hemodialysis because the former treatment maintains, on average, a higher plasma bicarbonate concentration.

Etiology

Primary hypocapnia is the most frequent acid–base disturbance encountered, occurring in normal pregnancy and high-altitude residence. Table 3 lists the major causes of respiratory alkalosis. Most are associated with the abrupt appearance of hypocapnia but, in many instances, the process might be sufficiently prolonged to permit full chronic adaptation to occur. Consequently, no attempt has been made to separate these conditions into acute and

TABLE 3
Causes of Respiratory Alkalosis[a]

Hypoxemia or tissue hypoxia	Central nervous system stimulation
Decreased inspired O_2 tension	Voluntary
High altitude	Pain
Bacterial or viral pneumonia	Anxiety
Aspiration of food, foreign body, or vomitus	Psychosis
Laryngospasm	Fever
Drowning	Subarachnoid hemorrhage
Cyanotic heart disease	Cerebrovascular accident
Severe anemia	Meningoencephalitis
Left shift deviation of HbO_2 curve	Tumor
Hypotension[b]	Trauma
Severe circulatory failure[b]	Drugs or hormones
Pulmonary edema	Nikethamide, ethamivan
Stimulation of chest receptors	Doxapram
Pneumonia	Xanthines
Asthma	Salicylates
Pneumothorax	Catecholamines
Hemothorax	Angiotensin II
Flail chest	Vasopressor agents
Acute respiratory distress syndrome	Progesterone
Cardiac failure	Medroxyprogesterone
Noncardiogenic pulmonary edema	Dinitrophenol
Pulmonary embolism	Nicotine
Interstitial lung disease	Miscellaneous
	Pregnancy
	Sepsis
	Hepatic failure
	Mechanical hyperventilation
	Heat exposure
	Recovery from metabolic acidosis

[a]Adapted from Madias and Adrogué (1991).
[b]Might produce "pseudorespiratory alkalosis."

chronic categories. Some of the major causes of respiratory alkalosis are benign, whereas others are life threatening. Primary hypocapnia is particularly common among the critically ill, occurring either as the simple disorder or as a component of mixed disturbances. Its presence constitutes an ominous prognostic sign, mortality increasing in direct proportion to the severity of the hypocapnia.

Clinical Manifestations

Rapid decrements in pCO_2 to half the normal values or lower are typically accompanied by paresthesias of the extremities, chest discomfort, circumoral numbness, light-headedness, confusion, and infrequently, tetany or generalized seizures. These manifestations are seldom present in the chronic phase. Acute hypocapnia decreases cerebral blood flow, which, in severe cases, might reach values less than 50% of normal, resulting in cerebral hypoxia. This hypoperfusion has been implicated in the pathogenesis of the neurological manifestations of acute respiratory alkalosis along with other factors, including hypocapnia per se, alkalemia, pH-induced shift of the oxyhemoglobin dissociation curve, and decrements in the level of ionized calcium and potassium. Some evidence indicates that cerebral blood flow returns to normal in chronic respiratory alkalosis.

Actively hyperventilating patients manifest no appreciable changes in cardiac output or systemic blood pressure. By contrast, acute hypocapnia in the course of passive hyperventilation typically observed during mechanical ventilation in patients with a depressed central nervous system or those under general anesthesia, frequently results in a major reduction in cardiac output and systemic blood pressure, increased peripheral resistance, and substantial hyperlactatemia (exceeding 2 mEq/L). Neither cardiac arrhythmias nor clinically evident signs or symptoms of coronary insufficiency develop in actively hyperventilating normal volunteers. However, patients with underlying coronary artery disease might occasionally suffer hypocapnia-induced coronary vasoconstriction, resulting in angina pectoris, ischemic electrocardiographic changes, and arrhythmias. Increased cardiac excitability has been attributed to the same factors that have been held responsible for the enhanced excitability of the central nervous system associated with acute hypocapnia.

Diagnosis

Careful observation can detect abnormal patterns of breathing in some patients, yet marked hypocapnia can be present without a clinically evident increase in respiratory effort. Thus, arterial blood gases should be obtained whenever hyperventilation is suspected. In fact, the diagnosis of respiratory alkalosis, especially the chronic form, is frequently missed; physicians often misinterpret the electrolyte pattern of hyperchloremic hypobicarbonatemia as indicative of normal anion gap metabolic acidosis. If the acid–base profile of the patient reveals hypocapnia in association with alkalemia, at least an element of respiratory alkalosis must be present. Primary hypocapnia, however,

might be associated with a normal or an acidic pH due to the concomitant presence of other acid–base disorders. Notably, mild degrees of chronic hypocapnia commonly leave blood pH within the high-normal range. As always, proper evaluation of the acid–base status of the patient requires careful assessment of the history, physical examination, and ancillary laboratory data. Once the diagnosis of respiratory alkalosis has been made, a search for its cause should be carried out. The diagnosis of respiratory alkalosis can have important clinical implications: It often provides a clue to the presence of an unrecognized, serious disorder (e.g., sepsis) or signals the severity of a known underlying disease.

Therapeutic Principles

Management of respiratory alkalosis must be directed toward correcting the underlying cause, whenever possible. Taking measures to treat the respiratory alkalosis itself is not commonly required, because the disorder, especially in its chronic form, leads to minimal or no symptoms and poses little risk to health. A notable exception is the patient with the anxiety-hyperventilation syndrome; in addition to reassurance or sedation, rebreathing into a closed system (e.g., a paper bag) might prove helpful by interrupting the vicious cycle that can result from the reinforcing effects of the symptoms of hypocapnia. Administration of acetazolamide can be beneficial in the management of signs and symptoms of high-altitude sickness, a syndrome characterized by hypoxemia and respiratory alkalosis. Considering the risks of severe alkalemia, sedation or, in rare cases, skeletal muscle paralysis and mechanical ventilation might be required to temporarily correct marked respiratory alkalosis. Management of pseudorespiratory alkalosis must be directed at optimizing systemic hemodynamics.

Bibliography

Adrogué HJ, Madias NE: Management of life-threatening acid–base disorders. *N Engl J Med* 338:26–34, 107–111, 1998.

Adrogué HJ, Rashad MN, Gorin AB, Yacoub J, Madias NE: Assessing acid–base status in circulatory failure. Differences between arterial and central venous blood. *N Engl J Med* 320:1312–1316, 1989.

Al-Awqati Q: The cellular renal response to respiratory acid–base disorders. *Kidney Int* 28:845–855, 1985.

Amato MB, Barbas CSV, Medeiros DM, *et al.*: Effect of a protective-ventilation strategy on mortality in the acute respiratory distress syndrome. *N Engl J Med* 338:347–354, 1998.

Arbus GS, Hebert LA, Levesque PR, Etsten BE, Schwartz WB: Characterization and clinical application of the "significance band" for acute respiratory alkalosis. *N Engl J Med* 280:117–123, 1969.

Brackett NC Jr, Cohen JJ, Schwartz WB: Carbon dioxide titration curve of normal man. Effect of increasing degrees of acute hypercapnia on acid–base equilibrium. *N Engl J Med* 272:6–12, 1965.

Brackett NC Jr, Wingo CF, Muren O, Solano JT: Acid–base response to chronic hypercapnia in man. *N Engl J Med* 280:124–130, 1969.

Dries DJ: Permissive hypercapnia. *J Trauma* 39:984–989, 1995.

Feihl F, Perret C: Permissive hypercapnia. How permissive should we be? *Am J Respir Crit Care Med* 150:1722–1737, 1994.

Gennari FJ, Kassirer JP: Respiratory alkalosis. In: Cohen JJ, Kassirer JP (eds) *Acid–Base*, pp. 349–376. Little, Brown, Boston, 1982.

Jardin F, Fellahi J, Beauchet A, *et al.*: Improved prognosis of acute respiratory distress syndrome 15 years on. *Intensive Care Med* 25:936–941, 1999.

Krapf R, Beeler I, Hertner D, Hulter HN: Chronic respiratory alkalosis. The effect of sustained hyperventilation on renal regulation of acid–base equilibrium. *N Engl J Med* 324:1394–1401, 1991.

Madias NE, Adrogué HJ: Respiratory acidosis and alkalosis. In: Adrogué HJ (ed) *Contemporary Management in Critical Care:*

Acid–Base and Electrolyte Disorders, pp. 37–53. Churchill Livingstone, New York, 1991.

Madias NE, Adrogué HJ: Acid–base disturbances in pulmonary medicine. In: Arieff AI, DeFronzo RA (eds) *Fluid, Electrolyte, and Acid–Base Disorders*, pp. 223–253. Churchill Livingstone, New York, 1995.

Madias NE, Cohen JJ: Respiratory acidosis. In: Cohen JJ, Kassirer JP (eds) *Acid–Base*. pp. 307–348. Little, Brown, Boston, 1982.

Madias NE, Wolf CJ, Cohen JJ: Regulation of acid–base equilibrium in chronic hypercapnia. *Kidney Int* 27:538–543, 1985.

Stewart TE, Meade MO, Cook DJ, *et al.*: Evaluation of a ventilation strategy to prevent barotrauma in patients at high risk for acute respiratory distress syndrome. *N Engl J Med* 338:355–361, 1998.

Tobin MJ: Mechanical ventilation. *N Engl J Med* 330:1056–1061, 1994.

APPROACH TO ACID–BASE DISORDERS

MARTIN GOLDBERG

Acid–base disorders occur commonly in medical and surgical patients. They are particularly important in severely ill hospitalized patients. They may be present as single (simple) disorders or as a combination of simple disorders (mixed acid–base disturbances). Systematic diagnostic recognition and correction of these simple or mixed disorders is important because they may not only affect the prognosis of the patient, but also may provide clues to the nature of the underlying primary disease(s). Before discussing a systematic approach to the diagnosis of acid–base disorders, several fundamental terms require definition.

ACIDEMIA VERSUS ALKALEMIA

These terms represent abnormal hydrogen ion concentrations of blood: either higher (acidemia) or lower (alkalemia) than the normal range of 35–45 nEq/l (pH = 7.35–7.45).

$$[H^+] = \text{hydrogen ion concentration}$$
$$pH = \log 1/[H^+] = -\log [H^+]$$

The Henderson–Hasselbalch equation is

$$pH = pK + \log ([HCO_3^-]/[0.03 \times pCO_2]).$$

Normally,

$$\text{Blood pH} = 6.10 + \log (24/0.03 \times 40)$$
$$= 6.10 + \log (20/1) = 7.40.$$

The Henderson Equation (modified) is

$$[H^+] = 24 \times pCO_2/[HCO_3^-].$$

Normally,

$$[H^+] = 24 \times (40/24) = 40 \text{ nEq/L}.$$

ACIDOSIS VERSUS ALKALOSIS

These are pathophysiological processes or abnormal states which, if unopposed by therapy or disease, would cause deviations of extracellular fluid $[H^+]$ from normal levels. They are defined independently of the $[H^+]$ or pH since two or more concomitant processes may be present simultaneously. In this instance they may either produce no net change in $[H^+]$ and/or may modify the body's adaptive response to a single disorder.

Alkalosis is a primary process (e.g., loss of H^+ from vomiting) which, if unopposed, would produce alkalemia.

Acidosis is a primary process (e.g., retention of $[H^+]$ due to renal failure) which, if unopposed, would produce acidemia.

RESPIRATORY VERSUS METABOLIC DISTURBANCES

Respiratory disturbances are those caused by abnormal pulmonary elimination of CO_2, producing an excess (acidosis) or deficit (alkalosis) of H_2CO_3 (in equilibrium with pCO_2) in extracellular fluid. These primarily alter the pCO_2 in the denominator of the Henderson–Hasselbalch equation. Compensatory (adaptive) adjustments involve changes in $[HCO_3^-]$ accumulation in body fluids. Adaptation via the kidneys is slow (3–4 days); hence there are operationally four respiratory disorders: acute and chronic respiratory acidosis; acute and chronic respiratory alkalosis.

Metabolic disturbances are those caused by excessive intake, metabolic production, or losses of fixed (nonvolatile) acids or bases in the extracellular fluid. These are reflected by changes in $[HCO_3^-]$ in blood and therefore alter primarily the numerator of the Henderson–Hasselbalch ratio. Adaptation to metabolic disorders is relatively rapid (12–36 hr); hence there are two: Metabolic acidosis (a process which lowers plasma $[HCO_3^-]$) and metabolic alkalosis (a process which raises plasma $[HCO_3^-]$).

COMPENSATORY (ADAPTIVE) RESPONSES

Primary changes in the metabolic component ($[HCO_3^-]$) stimulate adaptive changes in ventilation, producing changes in pCO_2. Additional adaptive changes occur in extracellular and cellular buffers and in the kidney (adjustments in H^+ secretion, HCO_3^- reabsorption and secretion, and generation of HCO_3^-).

Primary changes in the respiratory component (pCO_2) stimulate adaptive changes in $[HCO_3^-]$ via reactions with extra- and intracellular buffers and by slower (renal) adjustments in H^+ secretion, HCO_3^- reabsorption and secretion, and HCO_3^- generation.

As a rule compensation restores $[H^+]$ or pH towards normal, but not to complete normality.

SIMPLE (SINGLE) VERSUS MIXED DISORDERS

A *simple disorder* includes the primary process with the initial changes in $[H^+]$, pCO_2 or $[HCO_3^-]$ and all compensatory processes in reaction to these initial changes.

A *mixed disorder* is the simultaneous occurrence of two or more simple disturbances in a patient. Mixed disorders may be additive or counterbalancing regarding their net effect on $[H^+]$ or pH; they are frequently difficult to diagnose and reflect serious illness. A mixed disorder in which there are three simultaneous primary acid–base disorders present is commonly termed a triple acid–base disturbance.

ACID–BASE MAPS AND FORMULAS IN DIAGNOSIS OF ACID–BASE DISORDERS

The adaptive responses for the six simple disorders (including the acute and chronic respiratory disorders) have been quantified experimentally. The 95% confidence limits can be defined, and several formulas have been developed to reflect the ranges of compensation. The acid–base map provides the graphic representation of these ranges. See Table 1 and Fig. 1.

In a patient with a clinical condition suggesting a simple acid–base disorder, values of pH, pCO_2, and $[HCO_3^-]$ lying within the ranges defined by the formulas or map are compatible with the diagnosis of the specified simple disorder. This does not, however, rule out the possibility of a mixed disorder due to two or more counterbalancing processes, the net effects of which might produce values lying in the normal range, or in an area of a simple disorder. Furthermore, whereas values lying outside the range of a simple disorder suggest the diagnosis of a mixed disorder, a mixed disorder may sometimes be simulated during a transient state in which the adaptive processes to a simple disorder have not yet been completed.

TABLE I

Patterns of Arterial Blood Changes and Adaptation in Simple Acid–Base Disorders[a]

| Primary disorder | Blood acid–base pattern | | | | Adaptive response[b] | Limits of adaptation |
	pH	$[H^+]$	$[HCO_3^-]$	pCO_2		
Metabolic acidosis	↓	↑	↓[c]	↓[d]	$pCO_2 = 1.5 \times [HCO_3^-] + 8 \pm 2$	pCO_2 not <10 mm Hg
Metabolic alkalosis	↑	↓	↑[c]	↑[d]	$\Delta pCO_2 = 0.5 \times \Delta[HCO_3^-]$	pCO_2 not >55 mm Hg
Respiratory acidosis						
Acute	↓	↑	↑[d]	↑[c]	$\Delta[HCO_3^-] = 0.1 \times \Delta pCO_2$	$[HCO_3^-]$ not >30 mEq/L
Chronic	↓	↑	↑↑[d]	↑[c]	$\Delta[HCO_3^-] = 0.4 \times \Delta pCO_2$	$[HCO_3^-]$ not >45 mEq/L
Respiratory alkalosis						
Acute	↑	↓	↓[d]	↓[c]	$\Delta[HCO_3^-] = 0.2 \times \Delta pCO_2$	$[HCO_3^-]$ not <17–18 mEq/L
Chronic	↑	↓	↓↓[d]	↓[c]	$\Delta[HCO_3^-] = 0.5 \times \Delta pCO_2$	$[HCO_3^-]$ not <12–15 mEq/L

[a]Arrows indicate direction of change from normal. A double arrow indicates that the magnitude of the change is considerably greater in the chronic disorder compared to the acute disorder. Units for pCO_2 are mm Hg, and units for $[HCO_3^-]$ mEq/L.

[b]Δ = Change from normal.

[c]Initial event.

[d]Secondary adaptive response.

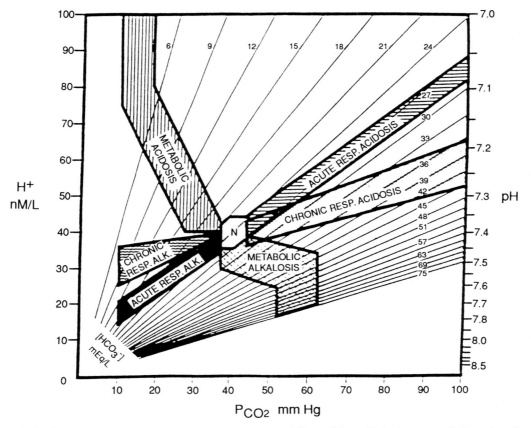

FIGURE I The acid–base map. Shaded areas represent the 95% confidence limits for zones of adaptation of the simple acid–base disorders. Numbered diagonal lines represent isopleths of plasma bicarbonate concentration. This map has been modified and updated from Goldberg M, Green SB, Moss ML, Marbach MS, Garfinkel D: Computer-based instruction and diagnosis of acid–base disorders. *JAMA* 223:269–275, 1973.

ANION GAP

The anion gap (AG) is the concentration of unmeasured anions (proteinate, phosphates, sulfates, organic acid anions) which are typically associated with H^+ as it is initially generated in body fluids. It is commonly calculated as

$$AG = plasma\ [Na^+] - (plasma\ [Cl^-] + plasma\ [HCO_3^-]).$$

Normal values for AG are 6–13 mEq/L. An AG > 15 mEq/L generally indicates one type of metabolic acidosis (i.e., due to accumulation of organic acids as occurs in lactic acidosis or diabetic ketoacidosis, or after ingestion of toxins). An exception is the widening of the anion gap that occurs during infusions of fluids containing salts of organic anions (e.g., lactate, amino acids, high doses of penicillins).

APPROACH TO THE DIAGNOSIS OF ACID–BASE DISORDERS

Appropriate diagnosis of acid–base disorders involves analysis and synthesis of all relevant information based on the patient's history, physical examination, and laboratory data. Use of data from one of these areas alone is insufficient to define the various processes that determine the primary disorder and the adaptational responses of the body. An outline of the important steps in this approach is as follows:

1. Suspect acid–base disturbances from the *history*.
2. Suspect acid–base disturbances from the *physical examination*.
3. *Evaluate the venous total CO_2 (tCO_2), [Cl^-], [K^+], and anion gap to support suspected diagnoses and to suggest possible additional primary disorders.*
4. *Obtain arterial pH, pCO_2, and [HCO_3^-] to establish definitive diagnoses using formulas, acid–base map, and limits of compensation.*

A careful review of the *patient's history* may reveal several commonly encountered clinical conditions which are typically associated with one or more acid–base disturbances (Table 2). The presence of these conditions should cause one to add the potential disorders to the differential diagnosis. One needs to assess the specific disease states, various drugs, the presence of mechanical ventilation, and nasogastric suction, all of which may be either causative of

TABLE 2
Common Clinical Conditions Associated with Acid–Base Disorders

Condition	Metabolic acidosis	Metabolic alkalosis	Respiratory acidosis	Respiratory alkalosis
Cardiovascular disease				
Cardiopulmonary arrest	+[a]	+[b]	+	+[b]
Pulmonary edema				+
CNS disease			+ or	+
Diabetes mellitus	+[a]			
Drugs				
Diuretics		+		
Poisonings	+[a]		+	+
Fever				+
GI disease				
Diarrhea	+			
Vomiting/gastric suction		+		
Hepatic failure	+[a]			+
Hyperkalemia	+			
Hypokalemia		+		
Pulmonary disease				
Acute asthma				+
COPD/respiratory failure			+	
Emboli				+
Pneumonia				+
Renal disease				
Renal failure	+[a]			
Renal tubular acidosis	+			
Sepsis	+[a]			+

[a] High anion gap metabolic acidosis.
[b] During treatment and recovery.

primary acid–base disorders or modifiers of the adaptive response to a disorder. Thus a history of renal failure suggests metabolic acidosis; pneumonia, sepsis, or hepatic failure should raise the suspicion of respiratory alkalosis, and therapy with the common diuretics should alert one to the possibility of metabolic alkalosis. In particular, certain clinical catastrophes such as cardiac arrest, septic shock, various intoxications, and the hepatorenal syndrome typically involve mixed acid–base disorders (see Table 2).

The *physical examination* may provide additional clues to potential acid–base disorders or may provide evidence in support of those suspected from the history. For example, normocalcemic tetany is compatible with severe alkalemia, and cyanosis may indicate severe hypoxia, and the possibility of respiratory acidosis or lactic metabolic acidosis. Rapid and/or deep respirations in the absence of cardiac or pulmonary failure are compatible with the hyperventilation associated with severe metabolic acidosis. Metabolic alkalosis is common in patients with signs of extracellular fluid volume contraction, while high fever typically stimulates respiratory alkalosis.

Careful analysis of the routine laboratory data including the venous electrolytes may provide useful quantitative information enabling the *identification* of the possible predominant acid–base disturbance and clues to additional disorders. The presence of azotemia strengthens support for the diagnosis of renal metabolic acidosis.

Most useful is examination of the venous plasma tCO_2, $[Cl^-]$, $[K^+]$, and the AG. In the clinical laboratory, measurement of venous plasma or serum electrolytes includes an estimation of the tCO_2 (total CO_2). This measurement reflects the sum of the numerator and the denominator of the Henderson or Henderson–Hasselbalch equations, that is, $[HCO_3^-] + H_2CO_3 + $ dissolved CO_2 gas. Since, normally and in pathophysiological states the $[HCO_3^-]$ is >90% of the tCO_2, then the venous tCO_2 is a reasonable approximation of the venous $[HCO_3^-]$. An abnormal plasma $[HCO_3^-]$ indicates an acid–base disorder (Table 1). An increased $[HCO_3^-]$ indicates either a primary metabolic alkalosis or adaptation to respiratory acidosis. A decreased $[HCO_3^-]$ indicates either primary metabolic acidosis or adaptation to respiratory alkalosis. Applying knowledge of the limits of adaptation (Table 1) may enable the elimination of some diagnostic considerations. For example, if the plasma $[HCO_3^-]$ is less than 12 mEq/L, a value which exceeds the limits of adaptation (Table 1) to respiratory alkalosis, then metabolic acidosis is definitely present. Conversely, if plasma $[HCO_3^-]$ is greater than 45 mEq/L, exceeding the adaptive limit for respiratory acidosis, then metabolic alkalosis may be diagnosed. A plasma $[HCO_3^-]$ in the normal range, on the other hand, does not exclude either a mixture of disorders which have opposing effects on $[HCO_3^-]$ (e.g., metabolic acidosis + metabolic alkalosis such as may occur in a patient with renal failure with a high anion gap metabolic acidosis who is also vomiting due to uremia and is losing HCl), or acute respiratory disorders in which the early adaptive changes in $[HCO_3^-]$ are small (Table 1).

Evaluating changes in plasma $[Cl^-]$ may provide additional insights into possible acid–base disorders. Remember, however, that changes in $[Cl^-]$ are important from the standpoint of acid–base disorders only when they are disproportionate to changes in plasma $[Na^+]$. When this occurs the changes in plasma $[Cl^-]$ are typically associated with reciprocal changes in plasma $[HCO_3^-]$. Thus in primary metabolic alkalosis and in the adaptation to chronic respiration acidosis, plasma $[Cl^-]$ falls as $[HCO_3^-]$ rises, whereas in primary metabolic acidosis (with normal AG) and in the adaptation to chronic respiratory alkalosis, plasma $[Cl^-]$ rises as $[HCO_3^-]$ decreases.

Abnormalities in plasma $[K^+]$ are common in patients with acid–base disorders. There is, however, no consistent quantitative relationship between changes in pH or $[HCO_3^-]$ and changes in $[K^+]$. This is because $[K^+]$ is influenced by many metabolic and physiological factors besides acid–base disturbances. Alterations in plasma $[K^+]$ are more pronounced in metabolic than in respiratory disorders. A rise in serum $[K^+]$ is more likely to be associated with an acute metabolic acidosis with normal AG and is least likely to be observed in lactic acidosis. In general a change in $[K^+]$ is useful only as a qualitative indicator in acid–base disorders; a high K^+ plus a low $[HCO_3^-]$ implies metabolic acidosis, and a low $[K^+]$ with high $[HCO_3^-]$ suggests metabolic alkalosis.

Calculation of the AG is essential in the evaluation of acid–base disorders. An elevated AG commonly signifies the presence of a metabolic acidosis regardless of the change in plasma $[HCO_3^-]$. One should be aware, however, that uncommonly the AG may be moderately increased (5–9 mEq/L) by severe volume contraction, metabolic alkalosis, and infusions of sodium salts of unmeasured anions (e.g., sulfates, lactate, carbenicillin). Nevertheless, the AG is a valuable tool in suspecting the presence of metabolic acidosis: an AG > 30 mEq/L almost always signifies a metabolic acidosis, and an AG between 20 and 30 mEq/L usually signifies metabolic acidosis.

Examination of the relationship between the changes in AG (ΔAG) and the change in $[HCO_3^-]$ (ΔHCO_3^-) may be useful in diagnosing mixed acid–base disorders. In simple high AG metabolic acidosis each mEq of H^+ accumulation is associated with 1 mEq of unmeasured anion accumulation; furthermore, each mEq of H^+ has consumed 1 mEq of HCO_3^-. Therefore increases in the AG are associated with corresponding decreases in plasma $[HCO_3^-]$, and ΔAG approximates ΔHCO_3^-. If ΔAG > ΔHCO_3^-, this suggests the presence of an additional process that generates HCO_3^- (either a metabolic alkalosis or chronic respiratory acidosis), whereas ΔAG < ΔHCO_3^- suggests the additional presence of a hyperchloremic metabolic acidosis or a chronic respiratory alkalosis.

Arterial blood gases are used to confirm the predominant acid–base disorder and to identify and confirm mixed disturbances. From information derived from the history, physical examination, and the routine analyses of venous blood, potential acid–base disturbances can be identified, and in many instances a reasonable acid–base diagnosis can be established without obtaining arterial blood gases. On the other hand, it is extremely difficult to diagnose acute respiratory disturbances and most mixed acid–base disorders without knowledge of arterial pH, pCO_2, and $[HCO_3^-]$. Thus if these are distinct possibilities or if the patient is critically ill (a setting in which mixed disorders are common), arterial studies should be obtained.

The data on arterial pH, pCO_2, and $[HCO_3^-]$ should be analyzed and applied to the acid–base formulas, to the acid–base map, and to knowledge of limits of adaptation (see Table 1 and Fig. 1). The results of these analyses should be coordinated with the differential and potential diagnostic inferences derived from the history, physical exam, and routine laboratory data. Before proceeding further, however, one must ensure the internal consistency of the blood values and their compatibility with the Henderson–Hasselbalch or Henderson equations. This can readily be accomplished using the acid–base map (which also serves as a nomogram for these equations) or by converting pH values to $[H^+]$ and applying the Henderson equation. In the pH range 7.20–7.50, each 0.1 unit change in pH from a normal value of 7.40 corresponds to a 10 nEq/L change in $[H^+]$ from a normal value of 40 nEq/L.

If the pH is abnormal then the major acid–base disturbance may be identified. Acidemia denotes a predominant acidosis, and alkalemia indicates a predominant alkalosis. Reference should then be made to the patterns for each acid–base disorder summarized in Table 1. This will enable confirmation of the major disorder. For example, acidemia, a low $[HCO_3^-]$, and a low pCO_2 support the diagnosis of metabolic acidosis. In order to rule out an additional primary disorder as a component of a mixed disturbance, the data must be compared to the expected range of adaptation by either plotting the data on the acid–base map (Fig. 1), or using one of the formulas for adaptive response in Table 1. When the pCO_2 is above or below the predicted range of compensation for a metabolic disturbance or when the $[HCO_3^-]$ is above or below the predicted levels for a respiratory disorder, a mixed disturbance is present.

Although many mixed acid–base disorders can be diagnosed using the arterial blood values in conjunction with the map or formulas, the final diagnostic conclusions require a coordinated synthesis of information derived from the clinical and laboratory data in conjunction with the arterial data. Thus use of the map alone will not identify triple mixed acid–base disorders. Values lying within a specific zone on the map (while suggesting a simple disorder) are also compatible with a mixed disorder with counter-balancing effects on pH, $[HCO_3^-]$, or pCO_2. In order to dissect out the various components of a mixed disorder, we must apply information on changes in AG, plasma $[Cl^-]$, and the plasma $[K^+]$. In fact a normal plasma $[HCO_3^-]$ or a normal pH or a normal pCO_2 by themselves do not rule out mixed disorders; nor are normal levels of all three variables simultaneously incompatible with mixed disorders.

Mixed disorders should be suspected in the following circumstances:

1. pH is normal and:
   a. [HCO$_3^-$] is high (mixed metabolic alkalosis + respiratory acidosis).
   b. [HCO$_3^-$] is low (mixed metabolic acidosis + respiratory alkalosis).
   c. [HCO$_3^-$] is normal and AG is high (mixed metabolic acidosis + metabolic alkalosis).
2. [HCO$_3^-$] is normal and:
   a. pH is in the acidemic range (mixed chronic respiratory acidosis and metabolic acidosis).
   b. pH is in the alkalemic range (mixed metabolic alkalosis and chronic respiratory alkalosis).
3. pCO$_2$ and [HCO$_3^-$] are shifted from normal in opposite directions.
4. AG is elevated, and clinical/laboratory data suggest a diagnosis other than a simple metabolic acidosis (metabolic acidosis is a component of a mixed disorder).
5. When AG is high and the ΔAG $\neq$ ΔHCO$_3^-$ (see previous discussion of AG and ΔAG). Remember that a mixed disorder may include two different types or etiologies of a simple disorder (e.g., a high AG + a normal AG metabolic acidosis or an acute respiratory disorder superimposed on an underlying chronic respiratory disorder).

In conclusion, a successful approach to resolving the sometimes complex dilemmas associated with the diagnosis of acid–base disorders involves the application of a systematic, orderly, and logical series of steps. Building on a knowledge of pathophysiology, these involve a coordinated analysis and resynthesis of information derived from taking a proper history, performing an adequate physical examination, and obtaining relevant laboratory data. Final success is measured not only by the intellectual satisfaction of the physician in making the correct evaluation(s), but also by the well being of the patient who has benefited from the appropriate corrective therapy.

Bibliography

Bia M, Thier SO: Mixed acid–base disturbances: A clinical approach. *Med Clin North Am* 65:347–361, 1981.

DuBose, TD Jr: Acid–base disorders, In: Brenner BM (ed) *The Kidney*, 6th Ed., pp. 925–997. Saunders, Philadelphia, 2000.

Goldberg M, Green SB, Moss ML, Marbach MS, Garfinkel D: Computer-based instruction and diagnosis of acid–base disorders. *JAMA* 223:269–275, 1973.

Gabow PA: Disorders associated with an altered anion gap. *Kidney Int* 27:472–483, 1985.

Hamm L: Mixed acid–base disorders. In: Kokko JP, Tannen RL (eds) *Fluids and Electrolytes*, pp. 490–495. Saunders, Philadelphia, 1990.

Kraut JA, Adrogue HJ, Madias NE: Respiratory and mixed acid–base disorders. In: Brady HR, Wilcox CS (eds) *Therapy in Nephrology and Hypertension*, pp. 292–301. Saunders, Philadelphia, 1999.

McCurdy, DK: Mixed metabolic and respiratory acid–base disturbances: Diagnosis and treatment. *Chest* 62:35S–44S, 1972.

DISORDERS OF POTASSIUM METABOLISM

MICHAEL ALLON

MECHANISMS OF POTASSIUM HOMEOSTASIS

Total body potassium is about 3500 mmol. Approximately 98% of the total is intracellular, primarily in skeletal muscle, and to a lesser extent in liver. The remaining 2% (about 70 mmol) is in the extracellular fluid. Two homeostatic systems help to maintain potassium homeostasis. The first system regulates potassium excretion (kidney and intestine). The second regulates potassium

shifts between the extracellular and intracellular fluid compartments.

External Potassium Balance

The average American diet contains about 100 mmol of potassium per day. Dietary potassium intake may vary widely from day to day. To stay in potassium balance, it is necessary to increase potassium excretion when dietary potassium increases, and decrease potassium excretion when dietary potassium decreases. Normally, the kidneys excrete 90–95% of dietary potassium, with the remaining 5 to 10% excreted by the gut. Potassium excretion by the kidney is a relatively slow process. It takes 6–12 hr to excrete an acute potassium load.

Renal Handling of Potassium

To understand the physiologic factors that determine renal excretion of potassium, it is critical to review the main features of tubular potassium handling. Plasma potassium is freely filtered across the glomerular capillary into the proximal tubule. It is subsequently completely reabsorbed by the proximal tubule and loop of Henle. In the distal tubule and the collecting duct potassium is secreted into the tubular lumen. For practical purposes, urinary excretion of potassium can be viewed as a reflection of potassium secretion into the lumen of the distal tubule and collecting duct. Thus, any factor that stimulates potassium secretion increases urinary potassium excretion; conversely, any factor that inhibits potassium secretion decreases urinary potassium excretion.

Physiologic Regulation of Renal Potassium Excretion

Five major physiologic factors stimulate distal potassium secretion (increase excretion): aldosterone; high distal sodium delivery; high urine flow rate; high $[K^+]$ in tubular cell; and metabolic alkalosis. Aldosterone directly increases the activity of the Na^+, K^+-ATPase in the collecting duct cells, thereby stimulating secretion of potassium into the tubular lumen. Medical conditions that impair aldosterone production or secretion (e.g., diabetic nephropathy, chronic interstitial nephritis) or drugs that inhibit aldosterone production or action [e.g., nonsteroidal antiinflammatory drugs (NSAIDs), angiotensin converting enzyme (ACE) inhibitors, heparin, spironolactone] decrease potassium secretion by the kidney. Conversely, medical conditions associated with increased aldosterone levels (primary aldosteronism, secondary aldosteronism due to diuretics or vomiting) increase potassium excretion by the kidney. Although there is profound secondary hyperaldosteronism in congestive heart failure and cirrhosis, each of these conditions may be associated with hyperkalemia due to decreased delivery of sodium. Many diuretics increase renal potassium excretion by a number of mechanisms, including high distal sodium delivery, high urine flow rate, metabolic alkalosis, and hyperaldosteronism due to volume depletion. Poorly controlled diabetes commonly increases urinary potassium excretion due to osmotic diuresis with high urinary flow rate and high distal delivery of sodium.

Reabsorption of sodium in the collecting duct occurs through selective sodium channels. This creates an electronegative charge within the tubular lumen relative to the tubular epithelial cell, which in turn promotes secretion of cations (K^+ and H^+) into the lumen. Therefore, drugs that block the sodium channel in the collecting duct decrease potassium secretion. Conversely, in Liddle's syndrome, a rare genetic disorder, this sodium channel is constitutively open, resulting in avid sodium reabsorption and excessive potassium secretion.

Adaptation in Renal Failure

In patients with renal failure, the kidney compensates by increasing the efficiency of potassium excretion. Clearly, there is a limit to renal compensation, and a significant loss of kidney function impairs the ability to excrete potassium, thereby predisposing to a positive potassium balance and a tendency to hyperkalemia. In most patients with chronic renal failure overt hyperkalemia does not occur until the creatinine clearance falls below 10 mL/min. Serum aldosterone levels are elevated in many patients with chronic renal failure. Aldosterone stimulates the activity of both Na^+, K^+-ATPase and H^+, K^+-ATPase, thereby promoting secretion of potassium in the collecting duct, and defending against hyperkalemia. These adaptive mechanisms are less effective in patients with acute renal failure, as compared with chronic renal failure. Therefore, severe hyperkalemia occurs more frequently in the former group.

A subset of patients with chronic renal failure fail to increase aldosterone levels appreciably; as a result, they develop hyperkalemia at moderate levels of renal insufficiency (CrCl <50 mL/min), typically in association with hyperchloremic, normal anion gap metabolic acidosis [type IV renal tubular acidosis (RTA) or hyporeninemic hypoaldosteronism]. This condition is most commonly associated with diabetic nephropathy and chronic interstitial nephritis. Moreover, administration of drugs that inhibit aldosterone production or secretion (e.g., ACE inhibitors, angiotensin II antagonists, NSAIDs, heparin) may provoke hyperkalemia in patients with mild to moderate chronic renal failure.

Intestinal Potassium Excretion

Like the renal collecting duct, the small intestine and colon secrete potassium. Aldosterone stimulates potassium excretion by the gut. In normal individuals intestinal potassium excretion plays a minor role in potassium homeostasis. However, in patients with significant renal failure, intestinal potassium secretion is increased three- to four fold, thereby contributing significantly to potassium homeostasis. This adaptation is limited, and is inadequate to compensate for the loss of excretory function in patients with advanced renal failure.

Internal Potassium Balance

Overview

Extracellular fluid $[K^+]$ is ~4 mEq/L, whereas the intracellular $[K^+]$ is ~150 mEq/L. Because of the uneven distribution of potassium between the fluid compartments, a relatively small net shift of potassium from the intracellular to the extracellular fluid compartment produces marked increases in plasma potassium. Conversely, a relatively small net shift from the extracellular to the intracellular fluid compartment produces a marked decrease in plasma potassium. Unlike renal excretion of potassium, which requires several hours, potassium shift between the extracellular and intracellular fluid compartment (also referred to as extrarenal potassium disposal) is extremely rapid, occurring within minutes.

Clearly, in patients with advanced renal failure, whose capacity to excrete potassium is marginal, extrarenal potassium disposal plays a critical role in the prevention of life-threatening hyperkalemia following potassium-rich meals. The following example will illustrate this important principle. Suppose that a 70 kg dialysis patient with a serum potassium of 4.5 mmol/L eats one cup of pinto beans (~35 mmol potassium). Initially, the dietary potassium is absorbed into the extracellular fluid compartment (0.2 × 70 = 14 L). This amount of dietary potassium will increase the serum potassium by 2.5 mmol/L (35 mmol/14 L). In the absence of extrarenal potassium disposal, the serum potassium of the patient would rise acutely to 7.0 mmol/L, a level frequently associated with serious ventricular arrhythmias. In practice, the increase in serum potassium is much smaller, due to efficient physiologic mechanisms that promote potassium shifts into the intracellular fluid compartment.

Effects of Insulin and Catecholamines on Extrarenal Potassium Disposal

The two major physiologic factors that stimulate transfer of potassium from the extracellular to the intracellular fluid compartments are insulin and epinephrine. The stimulation of extrarenal potassium disposal by insulin and β-2 adrenergic agonists are both mediated by stimulation of the Na^+,K^+-ATPase activity, primarily in skeletal muscle cells. Interference with these two physiologic mechanisms (insulin deficiency or β-2 adrenergic blockade, respectively) predisposes to hyperkalemia. On the other hand, excessive insulin or epinephrine levels predispose to hypokalemia.

The potassium-lowering effect of insulin is dose-related within the physiologic range of plasma insulin. The potassium-lowering effect of insulin is independent of its effect on plasma glucose. Even the low physiologic levels of insulin present during fasting promote extrarenal potassium disposal. In nondiabetic individuals hyperglycemia stimulates endogenous insulin secretion, thereby decreasing the serum potassium. In insulin-dependent diabetics, endogenous insulin production is limited, and significant hyperglycemia may occur. Hyperglycemia results in plasma hypertonicity, which promotes potassium shifts out of the cells, and produces paradoxic hyperkalemia.

The potassium-lowering action of epinephrine is mediated by β-2 adrenergic stimulation, and is blocked by nonselective β blockers, but not by selective β-1 adrenergic blockers. Alpha-adrenergic stimulation promotes shifts of potassium out of the cells into the extracellular fluid compartment, tending to increase serum potassium. Epinephrine is a mixed α- and β-adrenergic agonist, such that its net effect on serum potassium reflects the balance between its β-adreneric (potassium-lowering) and α-adrenergic (potassium-raising)

effects. In normal individuals the β-adrenergic effect of epinephrine predominates over the α-adrenergic effect, such that the serum potassium decreases. In contrast, the α-adrenergic effect of epinephrine on potassium shifts is much more prominent in patients with severe renal failure; as a result, dialysis patients are refractory to the potassium-lowering effect of epinephrine.

Effect of Acid–Base Disorders on Extrarenal Potassium Disposal

Acid–base disorders produce internal potassium shifts in a less predictable manner. As a general rule, metabolic alkalosis shifts potassium into the cells, whereas metabolic acidosis shifts potassium out of the cells. However, the nature of the metabolic acidosis determines its effect on serum potassium. Thus, mineral acidosis (i.e., hyperchloremic, normal anion gap metabolic acidosis) typically shifts potassium out of the cells, thereby predisposing to hyperkalemia. In contrast, organic metabolic acidosis (e.g., lactic acidosis) does not affect the serum potassium. Bicarbonate administration to individuals with normal renal function decreases serum potassium, but this effect is largely due to enhanced urinary excretion of potassium. In contrast, bicarbonate administration to dialysis patients (in whom the capacity for urinary potassium excretion is negligible) does not lower plasma potassium acutely. Moreover, bicarbonate administration does not potentiate the potassium-lowering effects of insulin or albuterol in dialysis patients.

LABORATORY TESTS FOR DIFFERENTIAL DIAGNOSIS OF POTASSIUM DISORDERS

Differential Diagnosis of Hypokalemia and Hyperkalemia

The clinical history, review of medications, family history, and physical examination are sufficient in the rapid differential diagnosis of the etiology of most potassium disorders. In selected patients the etiology of hypokalemia or hyperkalemia is not apparent, and additional specialized laboratory tests may be useful. Measurements of the fractional excretion of potassium (FE_K) and transtubular potassium gradient (TTKG) may be useful in distinguishing between renal and nonrenal etiologies of hyperkalemia and hypokalemia. The general principle underlying these tests is that the kidney compensates for hyperkalemia by increasing potassium excretion, and compensates for hypokalemia by decreasing potassium excretion. In contrast, when potassium excretion is inappropriate for the serum potassium, this suggests a renal etiology. The optimal use of FE_K or TTKG in the differential diagnosis requires that these values be obtained before the potassium abnormality (hyperkalemia or hypokalemia) is corrected.

Fractional Excretion of Potassium

FE_K is the percentage of potassium filtered into the proximal tubule that appears in the urine. It represents potassium clearance corrected for glomerular filtration rate (GFR), or Cl_K/Cl_{CR}. Since the clearance of any substance can be calculated from UV/P, this ratio (in bold type) can be algebraically transformed to $[U_K V/P_K)/(U_{CR} V/P_{CR})] \times 100\%$. The V in the numerator and denominator cancel out, giving the simplified formula

$$\frac{[U_K/S_K] \times 100\%}{[U_{CR}/S_{CR}]},$$

where U_K and U_{CR} are the concentrations of potassium and creatinine in the urine, and S_K and S_{CR} are the corresponding serum concentrations. For an individual with normal renal function on an average dietary potassium intake the FE_K is approximately 10%. When hypokalemia is due to extrarenal causes (low potassium diet, GI losses, potassium shifts into cells) the kidney conserves potassium, and the FE_K is low. In contrast, hypokalemia due to renal potassium losses is associated with an increased FE_K. Similarly, in the setting of hyperkalemia, a high FE_K suggests an extrarenal etiology, whereas a low FE_K is consistent with a renal etiology. If a urine creatinine measurement is not available, one can often use U_K alone to differentiate between renal and extrarenal causes of hyperkalemia. Specifically, in a hypokalemic patient, $U_K > 20$ mEq/L suggests a renal etiology, whereas $U_K < 20$ mEq/L suggests an extrarenal etiology.

Transtubular Potassium Gradient

The TTKG is a formula that estimates the potassium gradient between the urine and the blood in the distal nephron. It is calculated from $[U_K/(U_{osm}/P_{osm})]/P_K$, where U_{osm} and P_{osm} are the urine and plasma osmolalities. The numerator is an estimate of the luminal potassium concentration. The U_{osm}/P_{osm} term is included to correct for the rise in U_K that is due purely to water abstraction and concentration of urine overall. TTKG values have been derived from empiric measurements in normal individuals under a variety of physiologic conditions. In a normal individual under normal circumstances the TTKG is about 6–8. Hypokalemia with a high TTKG suggests excessive renal potassium losses, whereas hypokalemia with a low TTKG suggests an extrarenal etiology. Similarly, hyperkalemia with a low TTKG suggests a renal etiology, whereas hyperkalemia with a high TTKG is consistent with an extrarenal etiology.

Several factors limit the utility of the FE_K and TTKG in the differential diagnosis of potassium disorders. The FE_K and TTKG are increased when dietary potassium is increased, and decreased when dietary potassium is decreased. Furthermore, in patients with chronic renal failure there is an adaptive increase in potassium excretion per functioning nephron, such that FE_K and TTKG increase. This means that the "normal" value for a given individual can vary substantially, making it difficult to determine the significance of a high or low FE_K or TTKG.

HYPOKALEMIA

Hypokalemia versus Potassium Deficiency

It is important to distinguish between potassium deficiency and hypokalemia. Potassium deficiency is the state resulting from a persistent negative potassium balance, that is, potassium excretion exceeding potassium intake. Hypokalemia refers to a low plasma potassium concentration. Hypokalemia can be due either to potassium deficiency (inadequate potassium intake or excessive potassium losses) or to net potassium shifts from the extracellular to the intracellular fluid compartment. A patient may have severe potassium depletion without manifesting hypokalemia. An important example is a patient presenting with diabetic ketoacidosis. Such patients have typically had severe hyperglycemia with osmotic diuresis for several days, leading to high levels of renal potassium excretion and potassium deficiency. However, as a result of insulin deficiency, there is a concomitant shift of potassium out of the cells into the extracellular fluid compartment. At presentation to the hospital, such patients are frequently normokalemic or even hyperkalemic. Once they are treated with exogenous insulin, there is a rapid shift of potassium back into the cells, and within a few hours the patients develop significant hypokalemia. Conversely, patients hospitalized with an acute myocardial infarction commonly have hypokalemia due to stress-induced catecholamine release and enhanced extrarenal potassium disposal, even though they have a normal external potassium balance.

Clinical Disorders Associated with Hypokalemia

Table 1 provides a list of the most common causes of hypokalemia. The kidney can avidly conserve potassium, such that hypokalemia due to inadequate potassium intake is a rare event requiring prolonged starvation ("tea and toast diet"). Therefore, hypokalemia is usually due excessive potassium losses from the gut or the urine or is due to potassium shifts from the extracellular to the intracellular fluid compartment. Prolonged vomiting causes potassium losses, in part due to potassium present in the gastric juice (~10 mEq/L), but primarily due to renal losses because of secondary aldosteronism from volume depletion. Severe diarrhea, either due to disease or laxative abuse, results in significant potassium excretion in the stool.

Excessive renal potassium losses as a cause of hypokalemia is seen with a number of clinical syndromes. Conceptually, it is useful to distinguish between hypokalemia associated with hypertension and hypokalemia associated with a normal blood pressure. When hypokalemia is associated with hypertension, measurements of plasma renin and aldosterone may be helpful in the differential diagnosis. Several physiologic observations are relevant in this regard.

1. Aldosterone, a mineralocortocoid, stimulates sodium reabsorption and potassium secretion in the collecting duct.
2. The physiologic stimulus for aldosterone secretion is activation of the renin–angiotensin axis. Moreover,

TABLE I
Causes of Hypokalemia

Inadequate potassium intake (severe malnutrition)

Extrarenal potassium losses
    Vomiting
    Diarrhea

Hypokalemia due to urinary potassium losses
    Diuretics (loop diuretics, thiazides, acetazolamide)
    Osmotic diuresis (e.g., hyperglycemia)
    Hypokalemia with hypertension
        Primary aldosteronism
        Glucocorticoid remediable hypertension (GRA)
        Malignant hypertension
        Renovascular hypertension
        Renin-secreting tumor
        Essential hypertension with excessive duretics
        Liddle's syndrome
        11 β-Hydroxysteroid dehydrogenase deficiency
            Genetic
            Drug induced (chewing tobacco, licorice,
                some French wines)
        Congenital adrenal hyperplasia
    Hypokalemia with a normal blood pressure
        Distal RTA[a] (type I)
        Proximal RTA (type II)
        Bartter's syndrome
        Gitelman's syndrome
        Hypomagnesemia (cisplatinum, alcoholism, diuretics)

Hypokalemia due to potassium shifts
    Insulin administration
    Catecholamine excess (acute stress)
    Familial periodic hypokalemic paralysis
    Thyrotoxic hypokalemic paralysis

[a]RTA, renal tubular acidosis.

aldosterone-induced sodium retention suppresses the renin–angiotensin axis by negative feedback.

3. Glucocorticoids at high concentrations bind to mineralocorticoid receptors and mimic their physiologic actions.

4. Glucocorticoids are stimulated by ACTH, and suppress ACTH production by negative feedback.

Primary aldosteronism is due to autonomous (nonrenin-mediated) secretion of aldosterone by the adrenal cortex. This results in avid sodium retention and potassium secretion by the distal nephron. The patients present with volume-dependent hypertension, hypokalemia, and metabolic alkalosis. Biochemical evaluation reveals a high serum aldosterone level and suppressed plasma renin. Abdominal computerized tomography (CT) scan reveals either a unilateral adrenal adenoma or bilateral adrenal hyperplasia. The former is treated surgically, and the latter with spironolactone. Glucocorticoid-remediable aldosteronism (GRA) is a rare, autosomal dominant condition in which there is fusion of the 11 β-hydroxylase and aldosterone synthase genes. As a result, aldosterone secretion is stimulated by ACTH, and can be suppressed by an exogenous mineralo-

corticoid, dexamethasone. Patients with GRA have a very similar clinical presentation to those with primary aldosteronism (volume dependent hypertension, hypokalemia, high serum aldosterone, and low serum renin), except that they are younger and have a family history of hypertension.

Patients with renovascular hypertension, renin-secreting tumors, and severe malignant hypertension may also present with severe hypertension and hypokalemia. In contrast to patients with primary aldosteronism, these patient have secondary aldosteronism, that is, high serum renin and aldosterone levels. Of course, patients with essential hypertension may also have hypokalemia and high plasma renin and aldosterone levels if they are treated with loop or thiazide diuretics and are volume depleted.

Patients with 11 β-hydroxysteroid dehydrogenase deficiency, a rare genetic disorder, have a defect in the conversion of cortisol to cortisone in the peripheral tissues. This results in high tissue cortisol levels that activate the mineralocorticoid receptors, producing hypokalemia and hypertension. Such patients have low serum renin and aldosterone levels. Chewing tobacco, certain brands of licorice, and some French red wines contain glycyrrhizic acid, which inhibits 11 β-hyroxysteroid dehydrogenase. Ingestion of these foods may produce hypokalemia, volume-dependent hypertension, and low serum renin and aldosterone levels, similar to the clinical presentation of congenital 11 β-hyroxysteroid dehydrogenase deficiency.

Patients with congenital adrenal hyperplasia have a deficiency of 11 β-hydroxylase, an enzyme required in the common pathways for mineralocorticoids and glucocorticoids. These patients have low serum renin and aldosterone levels, high levels of DOCA (a mineralocorticoid), and high levels of androgen. Males have early puberty, and females exhibit virilization, with hirsutism and clitorimegaly. This condition improves with exogenous corticosteroids to suppress ACTH.

Liddle's syndrome is a rare autosomal dominant disorder caused by a defect of the sodium channel, such that there is increased sodium absorption and potassium secretion in the collecting duct. The patients present with hypokalemia, hypertension, and volume overload. Their biochemical profile reveals a low serum renin and aldosterone level. The patients' blood pressure and serum potassium improves dramatically with inhibitors of the sodium channel, such as amiloride.

Hypokalemia due to excessive renal potassium excretion is also seen in a number of clinical conditions in which hypertension is infrequent. Both type I (distal) and type II (proximal) RTA are associated with kaliuresis and hypokalemia; both conditions present with a normal anion gap metabolic acidosis. Type I RTA is frequently associated with hypercalciuria and calcium oxalate kidney stones. Type II RTA is rare in adults, and is often associated with a generalized defect in proximal tubular function, manifesting with glycosuria (with a normal serum glucose), hypophosphatemia with phosphaturia, and a low serum uric acid with uricosuria.

Bartter's syndrome is a rare familial disease characterized by hypokalemia, metabolic alkalosis, hypercalciuria, normal blood pressure, and high plasma renin and aldosterone levels. It has been associated with a number of mutations which inhibit active sodium reabsorption in the thick ascending limb of Henle, including mutations in the Na^+-K^+-$2Cl^-$ transporter, ClC-Kb, and ROMK (see Chapter 2). These patients act as if they are chronically ingesting loop diuretics; for this reason they are difficult to distinguish clinically from patients with surreptious diuretic ingestion. Patients with Gitelman's syndrome, a variant of Bartter's syndrome, differ in that they have hypocalciuria and hypomagnesemia. Recently, Gitelman's syndrome has been linked to a mutation in the renal thiazide-sensitive Na^+-Cl^- transporter. These patients act as if they are chronically ingesting thiazide diuretics.

Familial hypokalemic periodic paralysis is a rare, autosomal dominant disorder in which affected individuals develop periodic episodes of severe muscle weakness in association with profound hypokalemia, due to rapid shifts of potassium from the extracellular to the intracellular fluid compartment. Interestingly, even when the patient has complete paralysis, the diaphragm and bulbar muscles are spared, such that the patient is able to breathe, swallow, talk, and blink. The paralysis resolves within hours of potassium ingestion. The patients are asymptomatic with a normal serum potassium in between the acute episodes. Thyrotoxic hypokalemic paralysis is an unusual manifestation of hyperthyroidism, seen primarily in Asian patients. The clinical presentation is similar to that of hypokalemic periodic paralysis, except that the paralytic episodes cease when the hyperthyroidism is corrected.

Drug-Induced Hypokalemia

A number of drugs have the potential to cause hypokalemia, either by stimulating renal potassium excretion or by blocking extrarenal disposal. Exogenous mineralocorticoids mimic the effects of aldosterone, thereby stimulating distal potassium secretion. High doses of glucocorticoids posses some mineralocorticoid activity and have a similar effect. Most diuretics, including loop diuretics, thiazide diuretics, and acetazolamide increase renal potassium excretion. A number of drugs, including alcohol, diuretics, and cisplatinum, cause renal magnesium-wasting and hypomagnesemia. For reasons that are not well understood, hypomagnesemia impairs renal potassium conservation. Thus, these patients may have associated hypokalemia that is refractory to potassium supplementation until the magnesium deficit is corrected. (Paradoxically, cyclosporine may produce hypomagnesemia in conjunction with hyperkalemia.)

Drugs that promote extrarenal potassium disposal may also result in hypokalemia. This phenomenon can be seen after the administration of an acute dose of insulin. Similarly, administration of β-2 agonists (either intravenous or nebulized), including albuterol and terbutaline, frequently result in acute hypokalemia.

Clinical Manifestations of Hypokalemia

Hypokalemia may produce electrocardiographic abnormalities, including a flattened T wave and a U wave (Fig. 1). Hypokalemia also appears to increase the risk of ventricular arrhythmias in patients with ischemic heart disease or patients taking digoxin. Severe hypokalemia is associated with variable degrees of skeletal muscle weakness, even to the point of paralysis. On rare occasions diaphragmatic paralysis from hypokalemia can lead to respiratory arrest. There may also be decreased motility of smooth muscle, manifestor ileus or urinary retention. Rarely, severe hypokalemia may result in rhabdomyolysis.

Severe hypokalemia also interferes with the urinary concentrating mechanism in the distal nephron, resulting in nephrogenic diabetes insipidus. Such patients have a low urine osmolality in the face of high serum osmolality, and are refractory to vasopressin.

Treatment of Hypokalemia

The acute treatment of hypokalemia requires potassium supplementation. This can be given either intravenously or orally. The correlation between serum potassium and total

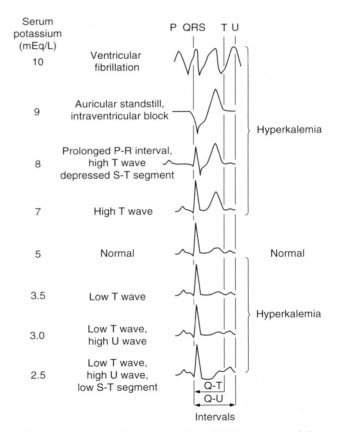

FIGURE I A schematic representation of ECG changes and the serum potassium levels at which such changes are typically seen. From Seldin DW, Giebisch G (eds): *The Regulation of Potassium Balance.* Raven, New York, 1989, by permission of Lippincott.

potassium deficit in hypokalemia patients is quite poor. A given patient's serum potassium is a reflection of both external potassium balance and transcellular potassium shifts. The percentage of administered exogenous potassium that remains in the extracellular fluid compartment is variable. Thus, it is difficult to predict how much potassium replacement a given hypokalemic patient will require. Without adequate monitoring, it is possible to give too much potassium and make the patient hyperkalemic. Therefore, one should give multiple small doses of potassium, with frequent checks of serum potassium values.

Oral potassium administration is safer than the intravenous route, and less likely to produce an overshoot in the serum potassium. Each oral dose should not exceed 20–40 mEq of potassium. Intravenous KCl should be reserved for severe, symptomatic hypokalemia (<3.0 mEq/L) or for patients who cannot ingest oral potassium. Intravenous KCl should not be given any faster than 10 mmol/hr in the absence of continuous EKG monitoring. The serum potassium should be rechecked every 2–3 hr to confirm a clinical response and to avoid an overshoot.

Correction of the underlying medical condition may prevent recurrence of hypokalemia after its correction. If the patient has a chronic condition associated with persistent urinary potassium losses, such that hypokalemia is likely to recur, the patient should be encouraged to increase the intake of foods high in potassium (especially fresh fruits, nuts, and legumes). In some patients, chronic oral potassium supplementation may be necessary.

HYPERKALEMIA

Pseudohyperkalemia is a factitious elevation of the serum potassium due to *in vitro* release of potassium from blood cells. It may be seen with *in vitro* hemolysis, thrombocytosis, or severe leukocytosis. Pseudohyperkalemia due to hemolysis is readily apparent because the serum is pink. Pseudohyperkalemia due to severe thrombocytosis or leukocytosis can be confirmed by drawing simultaneus blood samples in tubes with and without anticoagulant; if serum potassium is higher than plasma potassium, this confirms the diagnosis.

True hyperkalemia is caused by a positive potassium balance (increased potassium intake or decreased potassium excretion) or an increase in net potassium shift from the intracellular to the extracellular fluid compartment. Table 2 provides a list of the most common causes of hyperkalemia. In practice, most patients who develop severe hyperkalemia have more than one contributory factor. For example, a patient with moderate renal failure due to diabetic nephropathy may be medicated with an ACE inhibitor and have mild hyperkalemia. However, when he is started on indomethacin for acute gouty arthritis, the patient rapidly develops severe hyperkalemia.

Drug-Induced Hyperkalemia

A large number of drugs have the potential to cause hyperkalemia, either by inhibiting renal potassium excre-

TABLE 2
Causes of Hyperkalemia

Pseudohyperkalemia
  Hemolysis
  Thrombocytosis
  Severe leukocytosis
  Fist clenching

Decreased renal excretion
  Acute or chronic renal failure
  Aldosterone deficiency (e.g., type IV renal tubular acidosis)
    Frequently associated with diabetic nephropathy, chronic interstitial nephritis, or obstructive nephropathy)
  Adrenal insufficiency (Addison's disease)
  Drugs that inhibit potassium excretion (see Table 3)
  Kidney diseases that impair distal tubule function
    Sickle cell anemia
    Systemic lupus erythematosis

Abnormal potassium distribution
  Insulin deficiency
  β blockers
  Metabolic or respiratory acidosis
  Familial hyperkalemic periodic paralysis

Abnormal potassium release from cells
  Rhabdomyolysis
  Tumor lysis syndrome

tion or by blocking extrarenal disposal (Table 3). Most individuals taking these drugs will not develop hyperkalemia. Patients at risk are those with renal failure, especially if they have a high dietary potassium intake or are on an additional medication that predisposes to hyperkalemia. Most diuretics (loop diuretics, thiazide diuretics, acetazolamide) increase urinary potassium excretion and tend to cause hypokalemia. However, potassium-sparing diuretics inhibit urinary potassium excretion and predispose to hyperkalemia by one of two mechanisms. Spironolacton is a competitive inhibitor of aldosterone; it binds to the aldosterone receptors in the collecting duct, thereby inhibiting Na^+,K^+-ATPase activity, and indirectly limiting potassium secretion. Interestingly, the immunosuppresant drug, cyclosporine, also blocks Na^+,K^+-ATPase activity in the distal nephron. Two other potassium-sparing diuretics, amiloride and triamterene, bind to the sodium channel in the collecting duct. This inhibits sodium reabsorption in the distal nephron, and thereby limits the establishment of an electrochemical gradient required for potassium secretion. Interestingly, two antibiotics, trimethoprim (one of the components of Bactrim) and pentamidine, have also been shown to block the sodium channel in the collecting duct, and therefore predispose patients to hyperkalemia. In addition, trimethoprim has been shown to inhibit the collecting tubule H^+,K^+-ATPase.

Because aldosterone plays an important role in enhancing renal potassium excretion in patients with renal failure, drugs that inhibit aldosterone production (either directly or indirectly) predispose such patients to hyperkalemia. Angiotensin II is a potent stimulator of aldosterone

TABLE 3
Mechanisms for Drug-Induced Hyperkalemia

Decrease renal potassium excretion

Block sodium channel in the distal nephron
  Potassium-sparing diuretics: amiloride, triamterene
  Antibiotics: trimethoprim, pentamidine

Block aldosterone production
  ACE inhibitors
  Angiotensin II antagonists
  NSAIDs
  Heparin
  Tacrolimus

Block aldosterone receptors
  Spironolactone

Block Na$^+$,K$^+$-ATPase activity in the distal nephron
  Cyclosporine

Inhibit extrarenal potassium disposal
  Block β-2 adrenergic mediated extrarenal
    potassium disposal—nonselective β blockers
    (e.g., propranolol, nadolol, timolol)
  Block Na$^+$,K$^+$-ATPase activity in skeletal
    muscles: digoxin overdose (not therapeutic doses).
  Inhibit insulin release (e.g., somatostatin)

Potassium release from injured cells
  Drug-induced rhabdomyolysis (e.g., lovastatin, cocaine)
  Drug-induced tumor lysis syndrome (chemotherapy agents in
    acute leukemias, high-grade lymphomas)

Drug-induced acute renal failure

production in the adrenal cortex. Angiotensin converting enzyme (ACE) inhibitors inhibit the production of angiotensin II, thereby decreasing aldosterone levels. Similarly, angiotensin II receptor blockers also inhibit aldosterone production. Prostaglandin inhibitors (nonsteroidal antiinflammatory drugs) inhibit the production of renin, thereby indirectly decreasing aldosterone production. This effect is seen even with "renal-sparing NSAIDs," such as sulindac. Hyperkalemia may also be caused by selective cyclo-oxygenase-2 (COX-2) inhibitors. Heparin has been shown to directly inhibit the production of aldosterone in the renal cortex, primarily by decreasing the number and affinity of angiotensin II receptors in the zona glomerulosa. This effect occurs even with the low doses of subcutaneous heparin used for prophylaxis of venous thrombosis in hospitalized patients (e.g., 5000 units q 12 hr). The immunosuppressant tacrolimus may also cause hyperkalemia by inhibiting aldosterone synthesis.

Given the stimulation of extrarenal potassium disposal by β-adrenergic agonists, it is not surprising that β-2 antagonists can predispose to hyperkalemia. This effect is seen primarily with nonselective β blockers (e.g., proparnolol and nadolol), rather than β-selective blockers (e.g., atenolol, metoprolol). There is significant systemic absorption of topical β blockers, and severe hyperkalemia may rarely be provoked by timolol eyedrops. Drugs inhibiting endogenous insulin release, such as somatostatin, have been implicated rarely as a cause of hyperkalemia in

patients with renal failure. Presumably, long-acting somatostatin analogs, such as octreotide, would have a similar effect on serum potassium. Digoxin overdose causes inhibition of Na$^+$,K$^+$-ATPase activity in skeletal muscle cells, and may manifest with hyperkalemia. This effect is rarely seen at therapeutic doses of the drug.

Finally, drugs can also cause hyperkalemia indirectly by causing release of intracellular potassium from injured cells (e.g., rhabdomyolysis with lovastatin and cocaine, or tumor lysis syndrome when chemotherapy is administered in patients with acute leukemia or high grade lymphoma). Moreover, drug-induced acute renal failure may be associated with secondary hyperkalemia.

Fasting Hyperkalemia in Dialysis Patients

Prolonged fasting decreases plasma insulin concentrations, thereby promoting potassium shifts from the intracellular to the extracellular fluid compartments. In normal individuals the excess potassium is excreted in the urine, such that the plasma potassium remains constant. In dialysis patients the potassium entering the extracellular fluid compartment during fasting cannot be excreted, thereby resulting in progressive hyperkalemia. The phenomenon of fasting hyperkalemia may be clinically significant in dialysis patients who are fasted longer than 8–12 hr prior to a surgical or radiologic procedure. Occasionally, such patients develop life-threatening hyperkalemia during a prolonged fast. The hyperkalemia can be prevented by the administration of intravenous dextrose (to stimulated endogenous insulin secretion) for the duration of the fast. If the patient is diabetic, insulin must be added to the dextrose infusion, to prevent paradoxic hyperkalemia.

Clinical Manifestations of Hyperkalemia

Hyperkalemia may produce progressive electrocardiographic (EKG) abnormalities, including peaked T waves, flattening or absence of P waves, widened QRS complexes, and sine waves (see Fig. 1). The major risk of severe hyperkalemia is the development of life-threatening ventricular arrhythmias. Severe hyperkalemia with EKG changes is a medical emergency.

Severe hyperkalemia, like severe hypokalemia, can cause skeletal muscle weakness, even to the point of paralysis and respiratory failure. Hyperkalemia impairs urinary acidification by decreasing collecting tubule apical H$^+$,K$^+$-ATPase, which may result in a renal tubular acidosis (type IV RTA). Hyperkalemia stimulates endogenous aldosterone secretion. Hyperkalemia stimulates insulin secretion in dogs, but not in humans.

Treatment of Hyperkalemia

Severe hyperkalemia associated with electrocardiographic changes (see Fig. 1) is a life-threatening state requiring emergent intervention. If the patient's EKG is suspicious for hyperkalemia, one should initiate therapy without waiting for the laboratory confirmation. If the patient has renal failure, urgent dialysis is required for removal of potassium from the body. Because of the inevitable delay in initiating dialysis, the following temporizing measures must be initiated promptly:

1. Stabilize the myocardium. Acute administration of intravenous calcium gluconate does not change plasma potassium, but does transiently improve the EKG. The effect is almost immediate. Give 10 mL of calcium gluconate over 1 min. If there is no improvement in the EKG appearance within 3–5 min, the dose should be repeated.

2. Shift potassium from the extracellular to the intracellular fluid, so as to rapidly decrease the serum potassium. This involves administration of insulin and a β-2 agonist.

a. Intravenous insulin is the fastest way to lower the serum potassium. The plasma potassium starts to decrease within 15 min. Intravenous glucose is given concurrently to prevent hypoglycemia. One should give 10 units of regular insulin and 50 mL of 50% dextrose (1 ampoule of D_{50}) as a bolus, followed by a continuous infusion of 5% dextrose at 100 mL/hr to prevent late hypoglycemia. In diabetic patients the serum glucose should be ascertained with a glucometer; if it is >300 mg/dL, one can administer the intravenous insulin alone (without concomitant 50% dextrose). One should never give dextrose without insulin for the acute treatment of hyperkalemia; in patients with inadequate endogenous insulin production, the resulting hyperglycemia can produce a paradoxical increase in serum potassium.

b. β-Agonists. One should give 20 mg of albuterol (a β_2-agonist) by inhalation over 10 min. The onset of action is 30 min. Make sure they use the concentrated from (5 mg/mL) of the drug to minimize the volume that needs to be inhaled. The dose required to lower plasma potassium is considerably higher than that used to treat asthma, because only a small fraction of nebulized albuterol is absorbed systemically. Thus, 0.5 mg of intravenous albuterol (not available in the United States) produces a comparable change in plasma potassium to that seen after 20 mg of nebulized albuterol. The potassium-lowering effect of albuterol is additive to that of insulin.

c. Sodium bicarbonate. This is NOT useful acutely, because it takes 3–4 hr for the serum potassium to start to decrease. Moreover, bicarbonate administration does not enhance the potassium lowering effects of insulin or albuterol. Bicarbonate administration is still indicated if the patient has severe metabolic acidosis (serum bicarbonate <10 mmol/L).

3. Once the previous temporizing measures have been performed, further interventions are done to remove potassium from the body.

a. Diuretics. These only work if the patient has adequate kidney function.

b. Kayexalate. This resin-exchanger removes potassium from the blood into the gut, in exchange for an equal amount of sodium. It is relatively slow-acting, requiring 1–2 hr before plasma potassium decreases. Each gram of Kayexalate removes 0.5–1.0 mmol of potassium. Give 50 g

in 30 mL sorbitol by mouth, or 50 g in a retention enema. The rectal route is faster and more reliable. A recent study suggested that a single standard oral dose of Kayexalate may not be efficacious in decreasing the serum potassium within 4 hr in normokalemic hemodialysis patients, despite a documented increase in potassium excretion by the gut. Whether this modality is effective in hyperkalemic dialysis patients, or when given in multiple doses, remains to be determined. Given this uncertainty, frequent monitoring of plasma potassium in patients treated with Kayexalate is warranted.

c. Hemodialysis. This is the definitive treatment for patients with advanced renal failure and severe hyperkalemia.

For patients with moderate hyperkalemia, not associated with electrocardiographic changes, it is frequently sufficient to discontinue the drugs predisposing to hyperkalemia.

To prevent a recurrence of hyperkalemia once the acute treatment has been provided, the following measures are useful:

1. Counsel the patient on dietary potassium restriction, 40–60 mEq/day (Table 4).
2. Avoid medications that interfere with renal excretion of potassium, for example, potassium-sparing diuretics, NSAIDs, and converting enzyme inhibitors.
3. Avoid drugs that interfere with potassium shifts from the extracellular to the extracellular compartments, for example, nonselective β blockers.
4. When hemodialysis patients are fasted in preparation for surgery or a radiologic procedure, administer intravenous 10% dextrose at 50 mL/hr to prevent hyperkalemia. If the patient is diabetic add 10 units of regular insulin to each liter of 10% dextrose.
5. In selected patients, chronic medication with loop diuretics can be used to stimulate urinary potassium excretion.
6. Specific therapy may be indicated for the underlying etiology, when available. For example, patients with adrenal insufficiency require replacement with

TABLE 4
Potassium Content of Selected Foods

Food	Potassium (mg)	Potassium (mEq)
Pinto beans (1 cup)	1370	35
Raisins (1 cup)	1106	28
Honeydew (1/2 melon)	939	24
Nuts (1 cup)	688	18
Blackeyed peas (1 cup)	625	16
Collard greens (1 cup)	498	13
Banana (1 medium)	440	11
Tomato (1 medium)	366	9
Orange (1 large)	333	9
Milk (1 cup)	351	9
Potato chips (10)	226	6

exogenous glucocorticoids and mineralocorticoids. In patients with hyperkalemic periodic paralysis (a rare, autosomal dominant disorder in which affected individuals develop periodic episodes of severe muscle weakness in association with profound hyperkalemia), prophylactic aerosolized albuterol can prevent both exercise-induced hyperkalemia and muscle weakness.

Bibliography

Allon M: Treatment and prevention of hyperkalemia in end-stage renal disease. *Kidney Int* 43:1197–1209, 1993.

Allon M: Hyperkalemia in end-stage renal disease: Mechanisms and management. *J Am Soc Nephrol* 6:1134–1142, 1995.

Allon M, Takeshian A, Shanklin N: Effect of insulin-plus-glucose infusion with or without epinephrine on fasting hyperkalemia. *Kidney Int* 43:212–217, 1993.

DuBose TD: Hyperkalemic hyperchloremic metabolic acidosis: Pathophysiologic insights. *Kidney Int* 51:591–602, 1997.

Ethier JH, Kamel KS, Magner PO, Lemann J, Halperin ML: The transtubular potassium concentration in patients with hyperkalemia and hypokalemia. *Am J Kidney Dis* 15:309–315, 1990.

Farese RV, Biglieri EG, Shackleton CHL, Irony, I, Gomez-Fontes R: Licorice-induced hypermineralocorticoidism. *N Engl J Med* 325:1223–1227, 1991.

Field MJ, Giebisch GJ: Hormonal control of renal potassium excretion. *Kidney Int* 27:379–387, 1985.

Gruy-Kapral C, Emmett M, Santa Ana CA, Porter JL, Fordtran JS, Fine KD: Effect of single dose resin-cathartic therapy on serum potassium concentration in patients with end-stage renal disease. *J Am Soc Nephrol* 9:1924–1930, 1998.

Kamel KS, Halperin ML, Faber MD, Steigerwalt SP, Heilig CW, Narins RG: Disorders of potassium balance. In: Brenner BM (ed) *The Kidney,* pp. 999–1037. Saunders, Philadelphia, 1996.

Krishna GG, Steigerwalt SP, Pikus R, Kaul R, Narins RG, Raymond KH, Kunau RT: Hypokalemic states. In: Narins RG (ed) *Clinical Disorders of Fluid and Electrolyte Metabolism,* pp. 659–696. McGraw-Hill, New York, 1994.

Kurtz I: Molecular pathogenesis of Bartter's and Gitelman's syndromes. *Kidney Int* 54:1396–1410, 1998.

Lifton RP, Dluhy RG, Powers M, *et al.*: A chimaeric 11 β-hydroxylase/aldosterone synthase gene causes glucocorticoid-remediable aldosteronism and human hypertension. *Nature* 355:262–265, 1992.

Salem MM, Rosa RM, Batlle DC: Extrarenal potassium tolerance in chronic renal failure: Implications for the treatment of acute hyperkalemia. *Am J Kidney Dis* 18:421–40, 1991.

Shimkets RA, Warnock DG, Bositis CM, *et al.*: Liddle's syndrome: Heritable human hypertension caused by mutations in the beta subunit of the epithelial sodium channel. *Cell* 79:407–414, 1994.

Tannen RL: Approach to the patient with altered potassium concentration. In: Kelley WN (ed) *Textbook of Internal Medicine,* pp. 848–855. Lippincott, Philadelphia, 1992.

14

DISORDERS OF CALCIUM AND PHOSPHORUS HOMEOSTASIS

DAVID A. BUSHINSKY

CALCIUM

Calcium Homeostasis

Distribution

The vast majority (99%) of total body calcium is contained within the bone mineral while only about 0.1% of body calcium is in the extracellular fluid. The mineral phases of bone provide a reservoir of calcium for the smaller extra and intracellular pools.

The concentration of calcium in the cell cytosol is approximately 100 nmol/L or approximately one-thousandth of the extracellular calcium concentration. Within the cell, the mitochondria and the sarcoplasmic and endoplasmic reticula contain the highest concentrations of calcium.

Serum Concentration

In humans the concentration of serum calcium is maintained at a constant level between 9.0 and 10.4 mg/dL or

2.25–2.6 mmol/L. Of the total serum calcium approximately 40% is protein bound, especially to albumin and to a lesser extent globulins and other proteins. Approximately 10% of the calcium is complexed to phosphate, citrate, carbonate, and other anions; the remaining 50% exists in the ionized form. The ionized and complexed calcium together constitute that which is filtered by the kidney, the ultrafiltrable calcium, which has a concentration of approximately 1.5 mmol/L.

The concentration of ionized calcium is of physiological importance and remains remarkably constant even with marked variations in the levels of total calcium. Increases in total calcium concentration lead to an increase in calcium binding to albumin, lessening the increase in ionized calcium concentration. While a fall in serum albumin of 1 g/dL is usually associated with a fall of 0.8 mg/dL in total calcium concentration, the proportional fall in ionized calcium will be less. The fall in albumin will lessen the fraction of bound calcium and result in only a small decrease in the concentration of ionized calcium. Alterations in systemic pH will alter calcium binding by albumin. A fall in pH of 0.1 unit will cause approximately a 0.1 mEq/L rise in the concentration of ionized calcium as the increase in hydrogen ions displaces calcium from albumin. However, the concentration of ionized calcium is difficult to predict using these "rules of thumb," so it should be measured directly.

Intestinal Absorption

The average American diet contains approximately 800 mg (20 mmol) of calcium of which there is generally a net absorption of approximately 160 mg (4 mmol). Calcium absorption varies widely depending on the presence of other dietary components that may bind calcium (oxalate or phosphate) or promote absorption (lactose) and the level of serum $1,25(OH)_2D_3$. $1,25(OH)_2D_3$ is the principal hormonal regulator of intestinal calcium absorption; it stimulates calcium absorption. Calcium is absorbed in the duodenum, jejunum, and ileum. Calcium moves across the brush border down its concentration gradient by a $1,25(OH)_2D_3$ facilitated mechanism, and then through the cell bound to $1,25(OH)_2D_3$ induced calcium binding proteins. It is then transported across the basolateral membrane against a steep gradient utilizing a calcium ATP-ase or through a sodium for calcium exchange mechanism.

Renal Excretion

A 70 kg male with a glomerular filtration rate of 180 L/day filters approximately 270 mmol of calcium/day (180 L/day × 1.5 mmol/L). This quantity of calcium, over 10 g, is far more than the entire extracellular fluid calcium content. The kidney reabsorbs approximately 98% of the ultrafiltered calcium leading to a urine calcium excretion of approximately 4 mmol/day. Approximately 65% of filtered calcium is reabsorbed in the proximal tubule. Proximal reabsorption is linked to sodium reabsorption and does not appear to be under hormonal control. Approximately 25% of filtered calcium is reabsorbed in the loop of Henle. In this segment, the lumen-positive voltage provides a strong driving force for calcium reabsorption. In addition there appears to be active transport of calcium. Loop diuretics, such as furosemide, decrease reabsorption in this segment. The distal convoluted tubule is responsible for approximately 8% of calcium reabsorption and is the major site for the regulation of urine calcium excretion. In this segment, active calcium transport occurs against both electrical and chemical gradients. Distal convoluted tubule calcium reabsorption is stimulated by parathyroid hormone (PTH), phosphorus depletion, and thiazide diuretics and is inhibited by metabolic acidosis and adrenocortical excess. There appears to be some, albeit quite small, calcium reabsorption in the collecting tubule.

In health, daily urine calcium excretion equals intestinal calcium absorption. However during renal insufficiency, urine calcium excretion falls owing not only to the decreased glomerular filtration rate but also owing to enhanced calcium reabsorption secondary to the usual increase in PTH. The increase in PTH is multifactorial. Both the decrease in renal $1,25(OH)_2D_3$ synthesis, that results from a decrease in renal mass and the increase in serum phosphorus that follows the decrease in phosphorus excretion are responsible. The fall in $1,25(OH)_2D_3$ not only decreases calcium absorption resulting in hypocalcemia and subsequent increased PTH secretion, but $1,25(OH)_2D_3$ itself has a significant inhibitory effect on PTH secretion. Increased levels of serum phosphorus will increase serum levels of PTH independent of alterations in calcium or $1,25(OH)_2D_3$. (Renal osteodystrophy is covered in detail in Chapter 63.)

Regulation of Serum Levels

Large amounts of calcium must be transported through the extracellular fluid during periods of rapid skeletal growth and pregnancy, yet the concentration of serum calcium usually varies by less than 10%. This precise regulation of serum calcium concentration is accomplished by a complex interaction of the intestine, bone, and kidney involving the principal calcium regulating hormones PTH and $1,25(OH)_2D_3$. PTH stimulates renal calcium reabsorption and bone mineral turnover and increases the serum level of $1,25(OH)_2D_3$. A principal role of $1,25(OH)_2D_3$ is to stimulate intestinal calcium absorption. Numerous cellular activities are regulated by calcium, or dependent on a stable serum calcium concentration, for normal function. Alterations in serum calcium concentration result in disturbances of cellular, especially neuronal, function.

DISORDERS OF CALCIUM HOMEOSTASIS
Hypocalcemia

Hypocalcemia is defined as a reduction in the ionized component of serum calcium. Patients who have a decrease in total serum calcium concentration may, or may not, have a reduction in ionized calcium as hypoalbuminemia is very prevalent in hospitalized patients and albumin binds the majority of protein bound calcium. If there is doubt about the diagnosis, ionized calcium should be measured directly.

Clinical Presentation

The clinical presentation of patients with hypocalcemia correlates with the rapidity and magnitude of the fall in serum calcium, but symptoms are manifest in many patients with a total serum calcium of 7.0 mg/dL or less. The principal clinical manifestations of hypocalcemia are neurologic. Perioral paresthesias are followed by carpopedal spasm involving the hands and feet. Occasionally patients develop laryngeal stridor. Tetany may be evoked by acute respiratory alkalosis caused by hyperventilation, due to the rapid fall in ionized calcium concentration. As the pH rises (a decrease in hydrogen ion concentration), hydrogen ions are dissociated from albumin, promoting increased calcium binding.

Two clinical signs may indicate hypocalcemia: Chvostek's and Trousseau's. Chvostek's sign is evoked by tapping the facial nerve and observing a grimace. Trousseau's sign is evoked by inflating a blood pressure cuff 3 mm Hg above the systolic pressure for at least 3 min and observing spasm of the outstretched hand. Trousseau's sign is more specific, as Chvostek's sign is present in approximately 10% of normocalcemic individuals.

Patients with hypocalcemia may also present with generalized seizures, which represent whole body tetany. The electrocardiogram (EKG) in hypocalcemic patients has a characteristic prolonged corrected QT and ST interval. There may be peaked T waves, arrhythmias, and heart block.

Causes (Table 1)

Chronic Renal Insufficiency. Decreased glomerular filtration decreases renal phosphorus excretion, resulting in hyperphosphatemia. The increased serum phosphorus not only complexes with serum calcium, producing hypocalcemia but also downregulates the 1α-hydroxylase responsible for the renal conversion of 25(OH)D3 to 1,25(OH)$_2$D$_3$. Chronic renal insufficiency also results in a reduction of functional renal mass and decreased 1,25(OH)$_2$D$_3$ production. Serum levels of 1,25(OH)$_2$D$_3$ are low, resulting in decreased intestinal calcium absorption and hypocalcemia, and levels of PTH and the osteoblastic enzyme alkaline phosphatase tend to be elevated.

TABLE 1

Principal Causes of Hypocalcemia

Chronic renal insufficiency
Following parathyroidectomy
Hypoparathyroidism
Pseudohypoparathyroidism
Malignant disease
Rhabdomyolysis
Hypomagnesemia
Acute pancreatitis
Septic shock
Vitamin D deficiency

Following Parathyroidectomy. Surgical reduction of the parathyroid mass in patients with renal failure and secondary or tertiary hyperparathyroidism usually leads to profound hypocalcemia due to bone remineralization. This "hungry bone syndrome" may require prolonged and vigorous calcium replacement. Simultaneous oral or intravenous 1,25(OH)$_2$D$_3$ supplementation will promote intestinal calcium absorption, providing substrate for bone mineralization.

Hypoparathyroidism. Either idiopathic or postsurgical hypoparathyroidism results in a deficiency of PTH and an increase in renal calcium excretion, a decrease in 1,25(OH)$_2$D$_3$ production, and a decrease in bone turnover. Serum levels of PTH are low for the level of serum calcium or may be undetectable.

Pseudohypoparathyroidism. In this hereditary disorder there is a decrease in the target cell response to PTH. These patients have an elevated PTH level, and in most there is a failure of cyclic AMP to respond to PTH. Patients also commonly have shortened metacarpals and metatarsals in addition to short stature, obesity, and heterotopic calcification.

Malignant Disease. The most frequent cause of a decrease in total calcium concentration in ill patients with malignant disease is a decrease in serum albumin concentration; ionized calcium may be normal. Certain malignancies, such as prostate and breast, may cause enhanced osteoblastic activity and accelerated bone formation resulting in hypocalcemia. In the tumor lysis syndrome, the rapid cell destruction in response to chemotherapy may result in an increase in serum phosphorus which then complexes serum calcium, resulting in hypocalcemia. Certain antineoplastic agents such as cisplatinum induce hypocalcemia, owing in this case to promotion of hypomagnesemia (see later).

Rhabdomyolysis. Cellular injury, especially due to crush injuries, causes a rapid release of cellular phosphorus which complexes with extracellular calcium, resulting in hypocalcemia.

Hypomagnesemia. Hypocalcemia and hypomagnesemia frequently coexist, and they are often due to decreased absorption of dietary divalent cations or poor dietary intake. Hypomagnesemia may impair PTH secretion and interfere with its peripheral action.

Acute Pancreatitis. Acute pancreatitis leads to the release of pancreatic lipase. Pancreatic lipase degrades retroperitoneal and omental fat which then binds calcium in the peritoneum removing it from the extracellular fluid which results in hypocalcemia. Hypomagnesemia and hypoalbuminemia also have been reported to contribute to the hypocalcemia of acute pancreatitis.

Septic Shock. Endotoxic shock is associated with hypocalcemia through mechanisms that are not clear at this time. As myocardial function is correlated directly with ionized calcium concentration, hypocalcemia in this condition may be responsible, in part, for the hypotension.

Vitamin D Deficiency. There are numerous causes of vitamin D deficiency including renal insufficiency as previously noted. Dietary deficiency is uncommon in the United States as vitamin D is added to various foods. This fat-soluble vitamin is subject to malabsorption, and levels may be low in chronic liver disease and primary biliary cirrhosis. Anticonvulsant therapy with any of several agents increases the turnover of vitamin D into inactive compounds and results in a decrease in serum levels of 1,25 $(OH)_2D_3$.

Treatment
Acute. Patients with symptoms attributable to hypocalcemia must be treated promptly. In addition, asymptomatic patients with a serum calcium of approximately 7.0 to 7.5 mg/dL or less also should be treated prophylactically. Intravenous calcium is the mainstay of treatment. Calcium gluconate may be administered as 10 ml of a 10% solution (94 mg of elemental calcium) administered over 5 to 10 min. Patients on digoxin require EKG monitoring because administration of calcium may potentiate digitalis toxicity and cause death. Calcium must not be given in the same intravenous line as bicarbonate or the insoluble salt, calcium carbonate, will rapidly precipitate. If a patient is acidemic and hypocalcemic, in general the hypocalcemia must be treated first, as the acidemia increases the proportion of ionized calcium and thus protects the patient against symptomatic hypocalcemia. If the patient has renal failure, dialysis against a high calcium, high bicarbonate bath will correct both the hypocalcemia and acidemia. More prolonged correction can be accomplished with a constant infusion of calcium gluconate (50 mL of 10% calcium gluconate in 450 mL of 5% glucose), administered over 4 hr, the rate being titrated according to the level of serum calcium. Infusion of 15 mg/kg of elemental calcium over 4–6 hr generally increases the total serum calcium by 2–3 mg/dL.

Chronic. Treatment of chronic hypocalcemia in patients with normal renal function generally involves administration of oral calcium and 1,25$(OH)_2D_3$. The former, often given as calcium carbonate, must provide at least 1 g of elemental calcium each day. 1,25$(OH)_2D_3$ therapy will promote intestinal calcium absorption; however, in the case of hypoparathyroidism it will also increase urine calcium excretion as PTH is not present to stimulate renal calcium reabsorption. Thus the goal of therapy in treating patients with hypoparathyroidism and normal renal function is to keep serum calcium concentration at the lower limit of normal, approximately 8.0 mg/dL, and keep urine calcium excretion below 350 mg/day. Thiazide diuretics may be utilized to help prevent hypercalciuria and promote normocalcemia. 1,25$(OH)_2D_3$ administered without oral calcium may result in resorption of bone mineral and osteopenia.

Hypercalcemia
Hypercalcemia is defined as an increase in the concentration of serum ionized calcium.

Clinical Presentation
The clinical signs and symptoms present in patients with hypercalcemia correlate with the rapidity of the rise and the magnitude of the elevation in serum calcium. As with hypocalcemia, neurologic abnormalities predominate. Patients present with drowsiness and lethargy followed by headache, irritability, confusion, and then stupor and coma. Muscle weakness, emotional problems, and depression may be observed.

Polyuria is frequent in patients with hypercalcemia due to a defect in renal concentration. The excess calcium is thought to impair the renal response to antidiuretic hormone. Hypercalcemia can lead to a decline in renal function due to a variety of mechanisms. The polyuria may lead to volume depletion and prerenal azotemia. Excess calcium excretion may produce nephrocalcinosis, especially in the presence of alkaline urine, which decreases the solubility of calcium phosphate complexes.

Calcium directly increases cardiac contractility, and patients with hypercalcemia are thought to have an increased incidence of hypertension. Hypercalcemia shortens the corrected QT interval, may broaden the T waves, and produce first degree AV block. Anorexia, nausea, and severe vomiting are associated with hypercalcemia, as is constipation.

Causes (Table 2)
Primary Hyperparathyroidism. Accounting for more than 50% of patients with hypercalcemia, primary hyperparathyroidism is the leading cause of hypercalcemia. Typical patients are females 60 years of age or older, and most have a benign adenoma of a single parathyroid gland. Others have hyperplasia of all four glands. Parathyroid carcinoma is extremely rare. The elevated PTH level in these patients increases renal calcium reabsorption and decreases renal phosphorus reabsorption. Proximal tubule bicarbonate reabsorption is impaired and, as expected, urinary cyclic-AMP is elevated. The excess PTH also increases the serum level

TABLE 2
Principal Causes of Hypercalcemia

Primary hyperparathyroidism

Malignancy

Renal failure

Following renal transplant

Thiazide diuretics

Lithium

Immobilization

Milk-alkali syndrome

Granulomatous disease

Familial hypocalciuric hypercalcemia

Thyrotoxicosis

Vitamin intoxication

of $1,25(OH)_2D_3$ enhancing intestinal calcium absorption and bone turnover, with bone resorption predominating over bone formation.

Approximately 6% of patients with calcium containing kidney stones have hyperparathyroidism. In this case, the increased filtered load of calcium exceeds the increased renal calcium reabsorption, leading to hypercalciuria, renal stone formation, and occasionally nephrocalcinosis. Increased urinary bicarbonate alkalinizes the urine promoting precipitation of calcium phosphorus complexes. With current automated blood chemical analysis, hypercalcemia and the causative hyperparathyroidism are generally detected before stone formation or nephrocalcinosis occurs.

Malignancy. Patients with malignancy are the second largest group presenting with hypercalcemia. The hypercalcemia may be related to direct bone destruction by the growing tumor or to secretion of calcemic factor(s) by malignant cells. Patients with squamous cell lung carcinoma and metastatic carcinoma of the breast develop hypercalcemia most frequently. Patients with myeloma, T-cell tumors, renal cell carcinoma, and other squamous cell tumors are also prone to hypercalcemia. Many tumors produce a PTH-related peptide (PTH-rP) in which the first 13 amino acids are very similar to those in PTH and which binds to PTH receptors in the kidney and bone, yet is not detected on standard PTH assays. Commercial assays are now available for PTH-rP. Other tumors produce factors such as transforming growth factor α or interleukin-1, cytokines such as lymphotoxin, or hormones such as $1,25(OH)_2D_3$.

Usually, the malignancy is evident when patients present with hypercalcemia. The finding of a low level of PTH and an elevated level of PTH-rP support the diagnosis. While hypercalcemia due to an occult malignancy is rare, associated symptoms such as weight loss and fatigue should focus the search for tumors that are frequently associated with hypercalcemia such as those in the lung, kidney, breast, and urogenital tract.

Renal Failure. Hypocalcemia, and not hypercalcemia, is generally found in patients with renal failure. In these patients, it is important to determine if the hypercalcemia was responsible for the renal failure. The hypercalcemia caused by diseases such as sarcoidosis, myeloma, immobilization, and milk-alkali syndrome frequently cause renal failure. Hypercalcemia may occur during the recovery phase of rhabdomyolysis induced renal failure as calcium recently deposited in muscle and soft tissues is rapidly mobilized.

Hypercalcemia is frequently observed during excessive $1,25(OH)_2D_3$ replacement therapy of patients on dialysis, especially if they are simultaneously being given large amounts of oral calcium as a phosphorus binder. Some patients may develop severe secondary hyperparathyroidism with marked hyperplasia of the parathyroid glands and subsequent hypercalcemia. In addition, patients may have aluminum intoxication, a disorder characterized by low bone turnover, which predisposes them to hypercalcemia. These aluminum intoxicated patients often have modestly elevated PTH and alkaline phosphatase levels.

Following Renal Transplant. Frequently patients on long-term dialysis develop parathyroid hyperplasia leading to autonomous secretion of PTH. After a successful renal transplant, the PTH secretion will still continue, and hypercalcemia may develop due to enhanced, PTH induced, renal calcium reabsorption. The hypercalcemia is generally mild and tends to decrease over the ensuing 6 to 12 months as the hypertrophied parathyroid glands involute; however, patients with prolonged and marked hypercalcemia may require surgical parathyroidectomy.

Thiazide Diuretics. Many patients with hypertension or renal disease are on thiazide diuretic therapy, with which with mild hypercalcemia may result from increased renal calcium reabsorption. If the hypercalcemia does not resolve when the thiazides are discontinued, then the patient must be investigated for other causes of hypercalcemia.

Lithium. Approximately 5% of patients treated with lithium carbonate develop hypercalcemia. The hypercalcemia is due to a resetting of the parathyroid gland calcium set point such that PTH secretion is inhibited only by higher than normal elevations of serum calcium.

Immobilization. Immobilization leads to a rapid increase in bone resorption and may lead to hypercalcemia especially if there is any decrement in renal calcium excretion. This disorder is most prevalent in younger patients who sustain a traumatic, especially spinal cord, injury.

Milk-Alkali Syndrome. Ingestion of large amounts of calcium-containing antacids may lead to hypercalcemia, alkalemia, nephrocalcinosis, and renal insufficiency. While this disorder has become less common as ulcers are being treated with antibiotics and agents that inhibit gastric acid secretion, the use of calcium and alkali preparations has increased with efforts to prevent and treat osteoporosis.

Granulomatous Disease. Granulomatous diseases, such as sarcoidosis, tuberculosis, and leprosy may produce hypercalciuria and hypercalcemia due to the conversion of $25(OH)D_3$ to $1,25(OH)_2D_3$ by the granulomatous tissue. This has been observed in anephric patients.

Familial Hypocalciuric Hypercalcemia. This autosomal dominant disorder causes mild hypercalcemia, hypophosphatemia, and reduced renal calcium excretion (often less than 100 mg/day). These patients have a mutation in the recently identified calcium receptor that causes a reduction in receptor activity. PTH levels are normal, and parathyroidectomy is not indicated.

Thyrotoxicosis. Excess thyroid hormone can stimulate osteoclastic bone resorption, resulting in hypercalcemia. The hypercalcemia is generally mild, and coexistent hyperparathyroidism must be excluded.

Vitamin Intoxication. Vitamin D intoxication, as previously noted, is often observed in patients with end stage

disease treated with $1,25(OH)_2D_3$. Vitamin D intox-
n can also occur in food or vitamin faddists. Vitamin
:ess also causes hypercalcemia; it may be seen in the
same patients.

Treatment

Rational therapy depends on the severity of the hypercalcemia and its cause and should ideally be directed at the
underlying disorder. However, if the patient is symptomatic
and the serum calcium level is 13.5 mg/dL or higher acute
therapy is indicated. A mainstay of treatment in patients
with reasonable renal and cardiac function is intravenous
saline. Rates as high as 200–250 ml/hr of normal saline may
be used to facilitate renal calcium excretion. Furosemide
is calciuric and is often necessary (40 mg intravenously in
patients with normal renal function) during volume repletion with saline to avoid pulmonary congestion. Thiazide
diuretics must be avoided as they decrease renal calcium
excretion. Patients with renal insufficiency may not be able
to excrete the sodium load, and hemodialysis against a low
calcium bath may be necessary to lower serum calcium concentration. Patients with cardiac or renal insufficiency are
at particular risk for volume overload during saline treatment and may require central various pressure monitoring
and a more modest rate of normal saline infusion.

Patients with hypercalcemia mediated by enhanced osteoclastic bone resorption, and general patients with malignancy or immobililzation, will benefit from the osteoclastic inhibitor calcitonin (4–8 units/kg subcutaneously
or intramuscularly every 6–12 hr). However, the hypocalcemic effect of calcitonin is often transient. The bisphosphonate etidronate (7.5 mg/kg body weight/day infused
intravenously for 3 days) will lower serum calcium in a
few days with a maximal effect in 7 days. Pamidronate
(30–90 mg/day given as a single 24-hr infusion for 3 days)
is a more potent bisphosphonate than etidronate and is
generally the preferred agent. Pamidronate is not metabolized and is exclusively eliminated by renal excretion;
there is a direct correlation between renal excretion and
creatinine clearance. Both bisphosphonates have been
shown to cause renal insufficiency and should be avoided
in patients with renal impairment. Pamidronate has been
used to treat intractable hypercalcemia, with a reduction
in dosage amount and frequency, in patients with renal
failure. Gallium nitrate will effectively lower serum calcium; however, it is contraindicated in patients with
renal insufficiency or those receiving other nephrotoxic
agents.

Patients with hypercalcemia due to enhanced intestinal
calcium absorption may benefit from a reduction of dietary
calcium intake. Normally Americans consume approximately 800 mg of calcium/day, reducing this by one-third
is generally effective. However, this should only be a short-
term remedy as the provision of a low calcium diet in a patient with normal renal function and excess $1,25(OH)_2D_3$
will promote bone demineralization. Glucocorticoids (initial dose 40 mg of prednisone) will inhibit intestinal calcium absorption but may require a week for maximal
effect.

Oral phosphorus can be utilized to treat hypercalcemia
only if the serum phosphorus is at or below the lower limit
of normal in order to prevent soft tissue calcium deposition; however, in general, this form of outdated therapy
should be avoided.

Treatment of hypercalcemia in dialysis patients involves
reduction or elimination of both $1,25(OH)_2D_3$ and calcium,
the latter is often being used as a phosphorus binder.
Patients can be treated exclusively with the noncalcium
containing phosphorus binder sevelamer hydrochloride
until the serum calcium returns to the normal range.
$1,25(OH)_2D_3$ and oral calcium binders can then be cautiously reinstituted at lower doses while continuing with
the sevelamer hydrochloride. Some new analogs of vitamin
D may also be less hypercalcemic than $1,25(OH)_2D_3$ itself.

PHOSPHORUS

Phosphorus Homeostasis

Distribution

The majority (~90%), of total body phosphorus is contained within the bone mineral while ~10% is contained
within the cells and ~1% in the extracellular fluid.

Serum Concentration

The concentration of serum phosphorus in adults ranges
between 2.5 and 4.5 mg/dL or 0.81 to 1.45 mM. Serum phosphorus levels are highest in infants and decrease in childhood reaching adult levels in late adolescence. Approximately 70% of blood phosphorus is termed organic and
contained within phospholipids. The remaining 30% is
termed inorganic. Of the inorganic phosphorus, the majority, 85%, is free and circulates as monohydrogen or dihy-
drogen phosphate or is complexed with sodium, magnesium, or calcium while the minority, 15%, is protein bound.

Intestinal Absorption

Dietary phosphorus intake varies between 800 and 1850
mg of phosphorus/day (26–60 mmol/day), and approximately
25 mmol/day is absorbed. Diets that are adequate in calories and protein generally contain adequate phosphorus.
Phosphorus absorption is regulated by $1,25(OH)_2D_3$ via a
sodium dependent active transport mechanism principally
in the duodenum and by a passive phosphorus concentration dependent mechanism in the jejunum and ileum. The
absorption of phosphorus is hindered by complex formation in the intestine; both aluminum and calcium will form
insoluble complexes with phosphorus and hinder its absorption. During renal failure, phosphorus absorption continues and the complexing of intestinal phosphorus by aluminum or calcium is used to advantage in these patients
who are unable to excrete absorbed phosphorus. Use of
calcium or the newer binding gels to complex intestinal
phosphorus is favored over aluminum as the latter is toxic
to many organs, including brain and bone.

Renal Excretion

A 70 kg male with a glomerular filtration rate of 180 L/day
and a mean serum phosphorus concentration of 1.25 mM

filters approximately 200 mmol of phosphorus/day as approximately 85% of serum phosphorus is ultrafiltrable (180 L/day × 1.25 mmoles/L × 0.85). Urine phosphorus excretion averages about 25 mmol/day so that approximately 12.5% of the glomerular filtrate is excreted in the urine. The bulk of phosphorus reabsorption, approximately 85%, occurs in the proximal tubule. In this nephron segment, transport across the apical membrane occurs by a rate limiting sodium–phosphorus cotransport. Phosphorus resorption occurs in the pars recta but not in the loop of Henle. A small quantity of phosphorus is reabsorbed in the distal convoluted tubule, especially in the absence of PTH. Whether there is phosphorus reabsorption more distally is not well defined.

Parathyroid hormone is the major hormonal regulator of renal phosphorus excretion while variation in dietary phosphorus intake is the major nonhormonal regulator. PTH is phosphaturic as is $1,25(OH)_2D_3$, extracellular fluid volume expansion, and a high phosphorus diet while a low phosphorus diet leads to a decrease in renal excretion. The hypophosphaturia of phosphorus depletion overrides the hyperphosphaturia induced by PTH. During renal insufficiency urine phosphorus excretion remains relatively constant until the glomerular filtration rate falls to about 25% of normal. Phosphorus excretion is maintained in the face of a fall in glomerular filtration rate and the subsequent decline in the filtered load of phosphorus by the phosphaturic effects of elevated PTH levels as previously discussed (See Renal Calcium Excretion).

Regulation of Serum Levels

Serum levels of phosphorus are not as tightly regulated as those of calcium, and they may vary by as much as 50% over the course of a day. Although there is diurnal variation in phosphorus levels, alterations in dietary phosphorus intake are principally responsible for the swings in serum levels. In addition serum levels are controlled by hormones such as PTH and $1,25(OH)_2D_3$ and by the status of extracellular fluid volume and renal function.

DISORDERS OF PHOSPHORUS HOMEOSTASIS

Hypophosphatemia

A decrease in the level of serum phosphorus may or may not reflect total body phosphorus content since only ~1% of body phosphorus is in the extracellular fluid. Moderate hypophosphatemia may be defined as a serum phosphorus between 1 mg/dL and the lower limit of normal and severe hypophosphatemia as a serum level below 1 mg/dL. While moderate hypophosphatemia is generally asymptomatic, severe hypophosphatemia is associated with a variety of clinical disturbances and occasionally, death. Hypophosphatemia may result from a decrease in intake, an increase in excretion, or a shift of phosphorus from the extracellular environment into cells.

Clinical Presentation

Patients with severe hypophosphatemia may have neurologic dysfunction characterized by weakness, paresthe-

sias, confusion, seizures, and coma. The weakness may be associated with muscle edema and rhabdomyolysis. Respiratory muscle paralysis may result in death.

Causes (Table 3)

Alcohol Related. Many chronic ethanol abusers are hypophosphatemic on hospital admission or become hypophosphatemic with treatment. The etiology of their hypophosphatemia is multifactorial but has a large component of poor oral intake.

Refeeding. When patients are fed after prolonged poor intake or starvation the calories provide a stimulus for tissue growth and utilization of phosphorus in phosphorylated intermediates such as ATP. If the diet does not contain adequate phosphorus then severe hypophosphatemia may develop after several days. Analogously, if total parenteral nutrition solutions contain inadequate phosphorus then hypophosphatemia may become evident as the patient regains body mass.

Diabetes Mellitus. In severe diabetic ketoacidosis, especially of prolonged duration, there is excessive urinary phosphorus loss, which accompanied by poor oral phosphorus intake, may lead to hypophosphatemia and also hypokalemia. The severity of the hypophosphatemia may become manifest only during treatment of the diabetic ketoacidosis.

Alkalosis. Both respiratory and metabolic alkalosis may induce hypophosphatemia; however, hypophosphatemia is far more severe in prolonged respiratory alkalosis. The extracellular alkalosis appears to cause intracellular alkalosis, which results in a shift of phosphorus into the intracellular space and hypophosphatemia.

Postrenal Transplant. Hypophosphatemia is commonly observed following renal transplantation. The etiology is multifactorial but related to a persistent elevation in serum PTH levels and an intrinsic renal tubular defect in phosphorus reabsorption both resulting in hyperphosphaturia. In addition, glucocorticoids used in immunosuppression inhibit renal phosphorus transport.

Urinary Loss. Renal tubular acidosis, hypokalemia, hypomagnesemia, and other renal tubular disorders are

TABLE 3
Principal Causes of Hypophosphatemia

Alcohol related
Refeeding
Diabetes mellitus
Alkalosis
Postrenal transplant
Urinary loss
Total parenteral nutrition

associated with an increased urinary excretion of phosphorus. Hyperparathyroidism results in a marked increase in phosphorus excretion and hypophosphatemia.

Treatment

The treatment of hypophosphatemia is best directed at reversing the underlying disease or nutritional process. Moderate hypophosphatemia can often be treated with oral phosphorus supplementation in the form of milk, an excellent source of phosphorus containing about 1 g of phosphorus/L, or Neutra-Phos tablets (250 mg of phosphorus). Oral phosphorus can cause diarrhea which is usually seen at doses of over 1 g/day. Severe hypophosphatemia usually indicates a significant loss of total body phosphorus. In asymptomatic patients, if oral replacement is possible then the patient should receive approximately 3 g/day for a week. Often the patient will be symptomatic and require intravenous therapy. In this case treatment may be initiated with 2 mg/kg of body weight of phosphorus as the sodium salt infused over 6 hr. Serum phosphorus levels must be checked frequently during replacement. Intravenous phosphorus may produce hypocalcemia and metastatic calcification especially if the calcium phosphorus product exceeds 60. Concurrent electrolyte, hypokalemia, and mineral disorders, including hypomagnesemia, are often found in patients with hypophosphatemia.

Hyperphosphatemia

Hyperphosphatemia is defined as an increase in the concentration of serum phosphorus to greater than 5.0 mg/dL in adults. Because cells contain abundant phosphorus, hemolysis of the collected sample should be excluded especially if there is associated hyperkalemia. Hyperphosphatemia may be caused by decreased phosphorus excretion, an increase in phosphorus load, or a shift of phosphorus from cells into the extracellular fluid.

Clinical Presentation

The clinical presentation of patients with hyperphosphatemia is dominated by the associated fall in serum calcium. In general, as serum phosphorus rises there is a reciprocal fall in serum calcium. This fall is multifactorial but includes a decrease in $1,25(OH)_2D_3$ synthesis, leading to a decrease in intestinal calcium absorption, and formation of calcium phosphorus complexes resulting in ectopic calcification especially of previously injured tissues. The symptoms of patients with hyperphosphatemia are those of patients with hypocalcemia, names tetany, seizures, and decreased myocardial contractility. In addition, ectopic calcification may occur in virtually any organ in the body especially when the calcium phosphorus product with both concentration expresses as mg/L exceeds 60. Calcification is especially prominent in proton secreting organs, such as the stomach or kidney, in which basolateral bicarbonate secretion results in an increase in pH promoting calcium hydrogen phosphate (brushite) precipitation. On a chronic basis, the hyperphosphatemia of renal failure

TABLE 4
Principal Causes of Hyperphosphatemia

Renal failure
Hypoparathyroidism
Cell injury
Exogenous administration

can result in secondary hyperparathyroidism and renal osteodystrophy.

Causes (Table 4)

Renal Failure. With a fall in the glomerular filtration rate below approximately 25 ml/min, renal excretion of phosphorus is less than intestinal absorption and hyperphosphatemia ensues. Increased levels of phosphorus directly increase the level of PTH. The increased levels of phosphorus also suppress renal $1,25(OH)_2D_3$ production, resulting in less calcium absorption, and the excess phosphorus may bind serum calcium if the calcium phosphorus product exceeds approximately 60. Additionally, levels of serum $1,25(OH)_2D_3$ fall due to the reduction in the renal tissue responsible for the conversion of $25(OH)D_3$ to $1,25(OH)_2D_3$. The resulting hypocalcemia and low levels of $1,25(OH)_2D_3$ further increase PTH secretion and urine phosphorus excretion lowering the level of serum phosphorus at the cost of hyperparathyroidism. In spite of the additional phosphorus excretion per nephron, with more profound renal insufficiency serum phosphorus increases as the patient is unable to excrete the absorbed phosphorus. During chronic renal failure, the hyperphosphatemia is less severe than during the same decrement in glomerular filtration rate in acute renal insufficiency when there has been insufficient time for adaptation (see Chapter 63).

Hypoparathyroidism. PTH promotes renal phosphorus excretion, and hyperphosphatemia is associated with clinical disorders in which there is a lack of PTH or a resistance to its action.

Cell Injury. During chemotherapy of rapidly lysing cells, such as those of lymphomas, a marked increase in phosphorus release from cells can exceed renal excretory capacity. The hyperphosphatemia is often associated with hyperkalemia and hyperuricemia and leads to hypocalcemia. Phosphorus can also be released from cells during acute rhabdomyolysis, crush injuries, or tissue infarction (see Chapter 37). Hyperphosphatemia is especially severe when the release of cellular phosphorus occurs in the setting of acute renal failure.

Exogenous Administration. Excess phosphorus in TPN solutions, or phosphorus in laxatives may result in hyperphosphatemia. Phosphorus-containing enemas can result in hyperphosphatemia and should be avoided in patients with renal failure. Excess vitamin D not only increases calcium absorption but phosphorus absorption as well and can result in hyperphosphatemia.

Treatment

The treatment of hyperphosphatemia must be directed at the underlying cause. If renal function is intact, then phosphaturia should be promoted. Extracellular fluid volume expansion with saline will lower renal phosphorus reabsorption as will increasing urine pH with sodium bicarbonate or acetazolamide. In patients with hyperphosphatemia and acute renal failure, phosphorus is best removed from the extracellular space with dialysis.

The successful treatment of hyperphosphatemia in chronic renal failure requires a coordinated effort among the patient, dietician, and physician. A diet devoid of phosphorus is unpalatable; however, dietary phosphorus can be reduced substantially with proper dietary supervision. Both hemodialysis and peritoneal dialysis remove phosphorus; however, even with a low phosphorus diet dialysis alone is unable to restore phosphorus balance. Agents which bind dietary phosphorus and prevent its absorption are generally necessary to prevent and treat hyperphosphatemia. Calcium salts given with meals are effective in binding dietary phosphorus. Doses are gradually increased until the serum phosphorus is less than approximately 5 mg/dL. If hypercalcemia occurs before the serum phosphorus is controlled, then the patient may require institution of alternative intestinal phosphorus binders. Aluminum is toxic to the brain, bone, and bone marrow and should be avoided whenever possible. Sevelamer hydrochloride is a new polymer that binds intestinal phosphate. If patients present with severe hyperphosphatemia and serum phosphorus greater than 6.5 mg/dL, the serum phosphorus should be lowered with sevelamer prior to adding calcium salts to avoid soft tissue calcification.

Acknowledgments
This work was supported by Grants DK-36788, AR-46289 and DK-57716 from the National Institutes of Health.

Bibliography
Brown EM, Pollock AS, Hebert SC: The extracellular calcium-sensing receptor: Its role in health and disease. *Annu Rev Med* 49:15–29, 1998.

Bushinsky DA: Calcium, magnesium, and phosphorus: Renal handling and urinary excretion. In: Favus MJ (ed) *Primer on the Metabolic Bone Diseases and Disorders of Mineral Metabolism,* 4th Ed., pp. 67–74. Lippincott Williams & Wilkins, Philadelphia, 67–74, 1999.

Bushinsky DA, Krieger NS: Integration of calcium metabolism in the adult. In: Coe FL, Favus, MJ (eds) *Disorders of Bone and Mineral Metabolism,* pp. 417–432. Raven, New York, 1992.

Bushinsky DA, Krieger NS: Role of the skeleton in calcium homeostasis. In: Seldin DW, Giebisch G (eds) *The Kidney: Physiology and Pathophysiology,* pp. 2395–2430. Raven, New York, 1992.

Bushinsky DA, Monk RD: Calcium. *Lancet* 352:306–311, 1998.

Chertow GM, Burke SK, Lazarus JM, Stenzel KH, Wombolt D, Goldberg D, et al.: Poly[allylamine hydrochloride] (RenaGel): A noncalcemic phosphate binder for the treatment of hyperphosphatemia in chronic renal failure. Am J Kidney Dis 29:66–71, 1997.

Hruska KA, Lederer ED: Hyperphosphatemia and hypophosphatemia. In: Favus MJ, (ed) *Primer on the Metabolic Bone Diseases and Disorders of Mineral Metabolism,* 4th Ed., pp. 245–253. Lippincott-Raven, Philadelphia, 1999.

Kovach KL, Hruska KA: Phosphate balance and metabolism. In: Jacobson HR, Striker, GE, and Klahr, S. (eds) *The Principles and Practice of Nephrology,* pp. 986–992. Mosby, St. Louis, 1995.

Kumar R: Calcium metabolism. In: Jacobson HR, Striker GE, Klahr S (eds) *The Principles and Practice of Nephrology,* pp. 964–971. Mosby, St. Louis, 1995.

Levi M, Cronin RE, Knochel JP: Disorders of phosphate and magnesium metabolism. In: Coe FL, Favus FL (eds) *Disorders of Bone and Mineral Metabolism,* pp. 587–610. Raven, New York, 1992.

Monk RD, Bushinsky D: Treatment of calcium, phosphorus, and magnesium disorders. In: Halperin M (ed) *Therapy in Nephrology and Hypertension: A Companion to Brenner and Rector's The Kidney,* pp. 303–315. Saunders, Philidelphia, 1999.

Monk RD, Bushinsky DA: Pathogenesis of idiopathic hypercalciuria. In: Coe F, Favus M, Pak C, Parks J, Preminger G (eds) *Kidney Stones: Medical and Surgical Management,* pp. 759–772. Raven, New York, 1996.

Pollak MR: Disturbances of calcium metabolism. In: Brenner BM (ed) *Brenner & Rector's the kidney,* 6th Ed., pp. 1037–1054. Saunders, Philadelphia, 2000.

Shane E: Hypocalcemia; Pathogenesis, differential diagnosis, and management. In: Favus MJ (ed) *Primer on the Metabolic Bone Diseases and Disorders of Mineral Metabolism,* 4th Ed., pp. 223–226. Lippincott Williams & Wilkins, Philadelphia, 1999.

Shane E: Hypercalcemia: Pathogenesis, clinical manifestations, differential diagnosis, and management. In: Favus MJ (ed) *Primer on the Metabolic Bone Diseases and Disorders of Mineral Metabolism,* 4th Ed. pp. 183–187. Lippincott Williams & Wilkins, Philadelphia, 1999.

Slatopolsky E, Finch J, Denda M, Ritter C, Zhong M, Dusso A, et al.: Phosphorus restriction prevents parathyroid gland growth. High phosphorus directly stimulates PTH secretion in vitro. *J Clin Invest* 97:2534–2540, 1996.

Suki WN, Lederer ED, Rouse D. Renal transport of calcium, magnesium, and phosphate. In: Brenner BM (ed) *Brenner & Rector's The Kidney,* 6th Ed., pp. 520–574. Saunders, Philadelphia, 2000.

Yu ASL: Disturbances of magnesium metabolism. In: Brenner BM (ed) *Brenner & Rector's The kidney,* 6th Ed. pp. 1055–1070. Saunders, Philadelphia, 2000.

15

EDEMA AND THE CLINICAL
USE OF DIURETICS

DAVID H. ELLISON

Edema is usually a manifestation of expanded extracellular fluid (ECF) volume resulting from congestive heart failure, hepatic cirrhosis, nephrotic syndrome, or renal failure. Extracellular fluid volume expands when the kidneys retain NaCl in excess of dietary NaCl intake. Renal NaCl retention may reflect an adaptive response to inadequate effective arterial blood volume, as in patients with congestive heart failure, or it may reflect a pathological response of kidney tubules to damage, as in patients with acute renal failure. Regardless of its cause, the best treatments for edema are to restrict dietary NaCl intake and to correct the primary disorder. Despite these interventions, or when they are impossible, ECF volume frequently remains expanded unacceptably. For this reason, diuretics are commonly prescribed. All of the diuretics used to treat edema increase both Na^+ and water excretion. They are powerful drugs which, if used carefully, play an important role in treating symptomatic edema. The prompt and dramatic improvement of symptoms when intravenous diuretics are administered to a patient suffering from acute pulmonary edema remains one of the most gratifying responses in clinical medicine. Data suggest that some diuretics may prolong life, as well, under specific circumstances.

In addition to their use for edema, diuretic drugs are indicated for a wide variety of nonedematous disorders. Specific details of diuretic treatment of hypertension, acute renal failure, nephrolithiasis, and hyponatremia are discussed elsewhere in this primer. This chapter will focus on renal mechanisms of diuretic action and diuretic therapy of edema.

THE PHYSIOLOGICAL BASIS OF DIURETIC ACTION

The amount of NaCl excreted by the kidneys is equal to the difference between the filtered amount of Na^+ (plasma Na^+ concentration times glomerular filtration rate) and the quantity reabsorbed by the renal tubules. Assuming a normal glomerular filtration rate ($\sim$150 L/day) and a normal plasma Na^+ concentration ($\sim$150 mM), $\sim$23 mol of Na^+ are filtered each day in normal humans (equivalent to about 3 pounds of table salt). To maintain a normal fractional Na^+ excretion (FE_{Na}) of <1%, more than 99% of the filtered Na^+ is reabsorbed. All of the diuretic drugs in clinical use act primarily on the renal tubules to inhibit Na^+ reabsorption and increase fractional Na^+ excretion.

A simple and clinically useful classification of diuretic drugs is based on the sites and mechanisms of their actions along the nephron (see Table 1). All active NaCl reabsorption by renal epithelial cells is driven by the Na^+, K^+-ATPase pump, which is expressed at the basolateral membrane (the blood side) of epithelial cells along the nephron. This pump uses metabolic energy (derived from hydrolysis of ATP) to extrude Na^+ from the cell into the blood and to move K^+ into the cell. The action of the Na^+, K^+-ATPase keeps the cellular Na^+ concentration low and the cellular K^+ concentration high. It also contributes to making the cell interior electrically negative with respect to the extracellular fluid (the high intracellular K^+ concentration being the other factor). The low cellular Na^+ concentration and the cell-negative voltage drive positively charged Na^+ ions into the cell across the luminal membrane from tubule fluid. Although Na^+, K^+-ATPase pumps are present at the basolateral cell membranes of nearly all epithelial cells, each nephron segment possesses unique apical mechanisms that permit Na^+ to move across the luminal membrane; these specific transport pathways at the luminal membrane form the molecular bases of diuretic action. Together, active Na^+ extrusion from the basolateral membrane and passive Na^+ entry across the luminal membrane permit vectorial Na^+ transport in the absorptive direction.

Proximal Tubule Diuretics

Approximately two-thirds of filtered water and NaCl are reabsorbed along the proximal tubule. Sodium moves down its electrochemical gradient from tubule lumen into proximal tubule cells coupled to the movement of other solutes against their electrochemical gradients; among these solutes are glucose, amino acids, and phosphate. The reabsorption of bicarbonate and chloride is indirectly coupled to Na^+ absorption (see later). Because the epithelium is electrically "leaky" (highly permeable to ions), large transepithelial ion gradients do not develop, and solute absorption along this segment is isosmotic.

An important pathway by which Na^+ crosses the luminal membrane of proximal tubule cells involves electroneutral exchange of Na^+ for H^+ (see Fig. 1). Protons that are

TABLE I

Physiological Classification of Diuretic Drugs

Proximal diuretics	Loop diuretics	DCT[a] Diuretics	CD[b] Diuretics
Carbonic anhydrase inhibitors	Na⁺–K⁺–2Cl⁻ inhibitors	Na⁺–Cl⁻ inhibitors	Na⁺ channel blockers
Acetazolamide	Furosemide	Hydrochlorothiazide	Amiloride
	Bumetanide	Metolazone	Triameterene
	Torsemide	Chlorthalidone	Aldosterone antagonists
	Ethacrynic acid	Indapamide[c]	Spironolactone
		Many others	

[a]DCT, distal convoluted tubule.
[b]CD, collecting duct.
[c]Indapamide may have other actions as well.

extruded across the luminal membrane of proximal cells titrate bicarbonate (HCO_3^-), which has been filtered by the glomeruli. This forms carbonic acid (H_2CO_3), which is dihydrated to CO_2 and H_2O, a reaction catalyzed by the enzyme carbonic anhydrase in the brush border of proximal tubule cells. Via these events, Na^+ and HCO_3^- are functionally reabsorbed across the luminal membrane into the cell. For transepithelial $NaHCO_3$ reabsorption to continue at steady state, Na^+ and HCO_3^- must leave the cell across the basolateral membrane via the Na^+, K^+-ATPase pump and a $NaHCO_3$ transport pathway. Carbonic anhydrase located within proximal tubule cells generates H ions for extrusion across the apical membrane and bicarbonate ions which exit across the basolateral membrane.

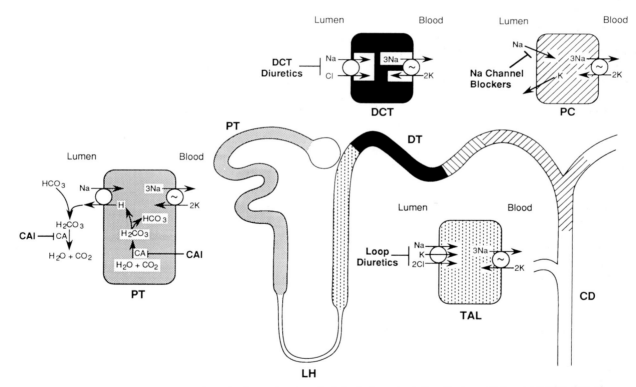

FIGURE I Predominant sites and mechanisms of action of clinically important diuretic drugs. Patterns identify sites of action along the nephron and corresponding cell types. □ PT, proximal tubule; LH, loop of Henle; ▦ TAL, thick ascending limb cell; DT, distal tubule; ■ DCT, distal convoluted tubule cell; CD, collecting duct; ▨ PC, principal cell; CA, carbonic anhydrase; CAI, carbonic anhydrase inhibitors. Both intracellular and luminal actions of carbonic anhydrase inhibitors are important in their ability to reduce Na^+ reabsorption by the renal proximal tubule. Note that Na^+ channel blockers probably act along the connecting tubule ▨ as well as the collecting duct ▨. Spironolactone (not shown) is a competitive aldosterone antagonist and acts primarily in the cortical collecting tubule. Reproduced with permission from Ellison DH: The physiological basis of diuretic synergism: Its role in treating diuretic resistance. *Ann Intern Med* 114:887, 1991.

Carbonic anhydrase inhibitors interfere with enzyme activity both inside the cell and within the brush border. Their action in the brush border inhibits Na^+/H^+ exchange by slowing the rate of carbonic acid dehydration. Thus, carbonic acid accumulates and acidifies the tubule fluid. Carbonic anhydrase inhibition inside the cell inhibits HCO_3^- production, thereby interfering with basolateral base exit. The net result of carbonic anhydrase inhibition is impaired Na^+, HCO_3^-, Cl^-, and H_2O reabsorption by the proximal tubule and increased renal Na^+, Cl^-, HCO_3^- and H_2O excretion. When administered acutely, these drugs provoke a moderate alkaline diuresis. When administered chronically, their natriuretic potency is relatively weak because compensatory processes develop. First, when $NaHCO_3$ reabsorption along the proximal tubule is inhibited, much of the solute and fluid that escapes reabsorption by the proximal tubule can be reabsorbed by more distal nephron segments. Second, inhibition of solute reabsorption along the proximal tubule leads to increased solute delivery to the macula densa. This activates the tubuloglomerular feedback mechanism, which suppresses glomerular filtration rate and decreases the amount of Na^+, Cl^-, and HCO_3^- that is filtered. Finally, alkaline diuresis induces metabolic acidosis; when serum HCO_3^- concentrations decline, less HCO_3^- is filtered and the carbonic anhydrase-dependent component of Na^+ reabsorption declines.

Because carbonic anhydrase inhibitors are relatively weak diuretics in chronic use and because they often result in metabolic acidosis, their use as diuretic drugs is limited. They are commonly employed, however, to treat open angle glaucoma, where they reduce the formation of aqueous humor by as much as 50%. Furthermore, they can be used to prevent acute mountain sickness and to treat metabolic alkalosis at times when Cl^- cannot be administered because of ECF volume expansion. This is especially useful when respiratory drive is compromised by metabolic alkalosis; careful use of carbonic anhydrase inhibitors may correct alkalosis and improve respiratory drive. Carbonic anhydrase inhibitors may also be used in combination with other classes of diuretics to induce diuresis in otherwise resistant patients (see Resistance to Diuretics, later).

Loop Diuretics

Approximately 25% of the filtered NaCl is reabsorbed along the loop of Henle. Transcellular NaCl reabsorption along the medullary and cortical thick ascending limbs is driven by Na^+, K^+-ATPase at the basolateral membrane. An electroneutral pathway at the luminal membrane carries 1 Na^+, 1 K^+, and 2 Cl^- from tubule fluid into the cell, driven by the electrochemical gradient for Na^+ (see Fig. 1). Much of the K^+ that is taken up via this pathway recycles across the luminal membrane through K^+ channels. The Na^+–K^+–$2Cl^-$ pathway, therefore, generates net NaCl reabsorption and (because of the K^+ recycling) a voltage across the wall of the tubule that is oriented with the lumen positive relative to blood.

Loop diuretics such as furosemide, bumetanide, and torsemide inhibit the action of the Na^+–K^+–$2Cl^-$ pathway directly. These diuretics are anions that circulate bound to protein so that very little diuretic reaches tubule fluid via filtration. Instead, they are secreted into the lumen of the proximal tubule by the organic anion transport pathway and travel downstream to the thick ascending limb where they bind to the transport protein and inhibit its action. Although the mechanism by which ethacrynic acid inhibits NaCl reabsorption is not as clear, its net effect on transport along the thick ascending limb is qualitatively similar. Loop diuretics are potent ("high ceiling") drugs that promote the excretion of Na^+ and Cl^-, together with K^+. Although they inhibit K^+ reabsorption along the thick ascending limb, their effects on K^+ excretion reflect predominantly their tendency to increase K^+ secretion along the distal nephron (see Complications of Diuretic Treatment, later). Loop diuretics increase magnesium and calcium excretion. Bumetanide, furosemide, and torsemide reduce the magnitude of the lumen-positive voltage in the thick ascending limb. This tends to impair Ca^{2+} and Mg^{2+} reabsorption because the reabsorption of these cations is driven across the paracellular pathway by the lumen-positive voltage. This accounts for the ability of loop diuretics to increase urinary calcium excretion, a clinically useful phenomenon.

Loop diuretics impair the ability of the kidney to elaborate urine that is either very concentrated or very dilute. The Na^+–K^+–$2Cl^-$ pathway removes Na^+ and Cl^- from the lumen as fluid courses up the thick ascending limb. Because this segment of the nephron is impermeable to water, solute removal dilutes the tubule fluid. By blocking the predominant solute removal pathway, loop diuretics inhibit free water generation. The action of the Na^+–K^+–$2Cl^-$ pathway also provides the "single effect" that is responsible for countercurrent multiplication. Solute removal from the thick ascending limb contributes to generating a high solute concentration in the medullary interstitium, which drives water reabsorption from the medullary collecting tubule. By blocking the Na^+–K^+–$2Cl^-$ pathway, loop diuretics inhibit the ability of the kidney to generate a concentrated urine; this is one reason these diuretics can be useful in treating patients with the syndrome of inappropriate antidiuretic hormone secretion.

Loop diuretics have important hemodynamic effects, both within the kidney and systemically. They increase secretion of vasodilatory prostaglandins and often reduce cardiac preload, when administered acutely. In some situations, however, they elicit a vasoconstrictor response that may impair cardiac performance acutely; this anomalous response is probably due to enhanced renin secretion and may be blocked by angiotensin converting enzyme inhibitors. Loop diuretics tend to maintain or increase the rate of glomerular filtration, even in the face of ECF volume depletion, because they block the tubuloglomerular feedback mechanism and because diuretic-induced prostaglandin secretion dilates the afferent arteriole.

Distal Convoluted Tubule Diuretics

The distal tubule, the nephron segment just beyond the loop of Henle, reabsorbs 5–10% of the filtered NaCl. As in other cells along the nephron, the concentration of Na^+ in distal convoluted tubule (DCT) cells is maintained at a low level by Na^+, K^+-ATPase. Sodium and Cl^- enter the cell across the luminal membrane via a distinct Na^+–Cl^- cotransport pathway (see Fig. 1). DCT diuretics are anions that, like the loop diuretics, circulate in the bloodstream bound to protein and are secreted into the lumen of the proximal tubule by the organic anion transport pathway. They are carried downstream to the distal tubule where they bind to the Na^+–Cl^- transport protein and inhibit its action. Because the distal tubule is relatively water impermeable, NaCl reabsorption along the DCT contributes to urinary dilution. DCT diuretics therefore impair urinary diluting capacity, but they have no effect on urinary concentrating ability. Most DCT diuretics, with the possible exception of metolazone, become less effective when the glomerular filtration rate declines below 40 ml/min.

DCT diuretics increase magnesium excretion but, in contrast to loop diuretics, inhibit urinary calcium excretion. Two mechanisms have been invoked to explain the effects of DCT diuretics on calcium excretion. First, DCT diuretics stimulate calcium reabsorption along the proximal tubule because they contract ECF volume and increase proximal Na^+ reabsorption (Na^+ and Ca^{2+} transport vary in parallel along the proximal tubule). Second, DCT diuretics stimulate calcium reabsorption along the distal tubule through their action on the Na^+–Cl^- cotransporter. When this pathway is blocked intracellular concentrations of Na^+ and Cl^- decline. Low intracellular Cl^- concentrations make the cell interior more electrically negative, with respect to interstitium. This is because more chloride, which is negatively charged, tends to diffuse into the cell from the interstitium. This opens the voltage-sensitive epithelial calcium channel, ECaC, in the luminal membrane. It also stimulates $3Na^+/Ca^{2+}$ exchange at the basolateral cell membrane, which is an electrogenic process. Diuretic-induced reductions in intracellular Na^+ concentrations also stimulate $3Na^+/Ca^{2+}$ exchange because they increase the electrochemical gradient favoring sodium entry. Both processes increase calcium reabsorption. The effects of DCT diuretics on calcium excretion form the basis for their use in prevention of calcium nephrolithiasis.

Collecting Duct Diuretics

Sodium reabsorption by the collecting duct system, which amounts to only 3% of the filtered NaCl load, is primarily electrogenic (current generating) unlike transport along more proximal segments. Current moves because Na^+ enters cells across the luminal membrane through ion channels. As in the other segments, the concentration of Na^+ inside collecting duct (also called principal) cells is maintained below electrochemical equilibrium by the action of the Na^+, K^+-ATPase. As Na^+ moves out of the lumen, it generates a voltage across the tubule wall that is oriented with the lumen negative, relative to blood. This lumen-negative voltage helps to drive K^+ movement in the secretory direction. Although Na^+ and K^+ do not traverse the same channel, their transport is coupled functionally by the transepithelial voltage.

Two major groups of diuretics act predominantly in the collecting duct. Sodium channel blockers, such as triamterene and amiloride, act from the lumen to inhibit Na^+ movement through Na^+ channels in collecting duct cells. Because these drugs impair Na^+ movement, the transepithelial voltage declines, inhibiting K^+ secretion secondarily. This effect accounts for their K^+ sparing action. It should be emphasized that, although amiloride inhibits renal Na^+/H^+ exchange in the proximal tubule, the proximal effect probably does not contribute to its diuretic action in humans because the concentrations of amiloride achieved in the lumen of the proximal tubule during oral administration are insufficient to interfere with Na^+/H^+ exchange. The second class of collecting duct diuretics is represented by spironolactone, a competitive antagonist of aldosterone. Aldosterone, a mineralocorticoid hormone secreted by the adrenal gland in response to renin or high serum potassium concentrations, stimulates Na^+ reabsorption and K^+ secretion along the collecting duct. It also increases the magnitude of the lumen-negative transepithelial voltage. By inhibiting the action of aldosterone, spironolactone causes mild natriuresis and potassium retention.

Because the collecting duct reabsorbs only a small percentage of the filtered Na^+ load, collecting duct diuretics are relatively modest in potency, at least when given acutely. In the past, their use as sole agents has been limited to situations in which excessive aldosterone secretion plays a central pathogenic role; in patients with cirrhotic ascites, for example, spironolactone has been reported to be more effective than loop diuretics, as a single agent. Further, when hypertension is caused by adrenocortical hyperplasia, adequate blood pressure control can often be obtained with oral spironolactone or amiloride. The most common use of the collecting duct diuretics is to prevent excessive potassium wasting when combined with other, more potent, diuretics. Interest in the utility of CD diuretics has been stimulated by suggestions that nonrenal actions of aldosterone may contribute to the pathogenesis of congestive heart failure, and that addition of these drugs may reduce the number of premature ventricular contractions. The results of a large multicenter trial showed that adding a small dose of spironolactone (25 to 50 mg daily) to traditional therapy of congestive heart failure reduced mortality by 30%, at 2 years.

Osmotic Diuretics

Unlike other classes of diuretics, osmotic diuretics do not interfere directly with specific transport proteins but rather act as osmotic particles in tubule fluid. Water reabsorption throughout the nephron is driven by the osmotic gradients that are generated by solute transport. When an agent such as mannitol is administered, it is filtered but very poorly reabsorbed. Because the mannitol is retained in the tubule lumen, the osmolality of tubule fluid remains higher than normal, inhibiting fluid reabsorption. NaCl reabsorption is also inhibited, in this case because solute reabsorption dilutes tubule fluid, predisposing to NaCl backflux. Thus, these drugs tend to increase the excretion not only of fluid but also that of Na^+, K^+, Cl^-, bicarbonate, and other solutes. The urinary osmolality during osmotic diuresis tends to approach that of plasma, regardless of the state of hydration. Osmotic diuretics increase renal blood flow and wash out the medullary solute gradient, effects which contribute to the diuretic induced impairment in urinary concentrating capacity.

Osmotic diuretics have been used to prevent acute renal failure following cardiopulmonary bypass, rhabdomyolysis, and radiocontrast exposure, although controlled studies with mannitol have not shown a benefit. Mannitol is also frequently employed to reduce cerebral edema, first by osmotic fluid removal from the brain and then by promoting diuresis.

ADAPTATION TO DIURETIC DRUGS

When a loop diuretic drug is administered acutely, Na^+ and fluid excretion increase transiently. This natriuresis is followed by a period of positive NaCl balance, termed postdiuretic NaCl retention (see Fig. 2). The net effect of the diuretic on ECF volume during a 24-hr period is equal to the sum of NaCl losses during diuretic action (excretion > intake), and NaCl retention during periods when the drug concentration is low (intake > excretion). Factors that influence the relation between natriuresis and postdiuretic NaCl retention include the dietary NaCl intake, the dose of diuretic, its half-life, and the frequency with which it is administered. When loop diuretics are administered once daily to patients ingesting a high NaCl diet, postdiuretic NaCl retention often compensates entirely for NaCl losses during the period of drug action; net Na^+ balance remains neutral from the first day. When NaCl intake is restricted, Na^+ avidity during the postdiuretic period cannot overcome the initial NaCl losses, Na^+ balance is negative, and ECF volume declines. This relation between dietary NaCl intake and the net effect of diuretics accounts for the central role of dietary NaCl restriction in effective diuretic therapy.

Even when diuretic treatment does induce negative NaCl and fluid balance initially, neutral NaCl balance is achieved after several days to weeks because other adaptive mechanisms come into play, limiting the magnitude of the diuretic response (the "Braking Phenomenon," see Fig. 2). Several mechanisms contribute to adaptation during chronic diuretic treatment. Contraction of the ECF volume, at least relative to pretreatment levels, may stimulate

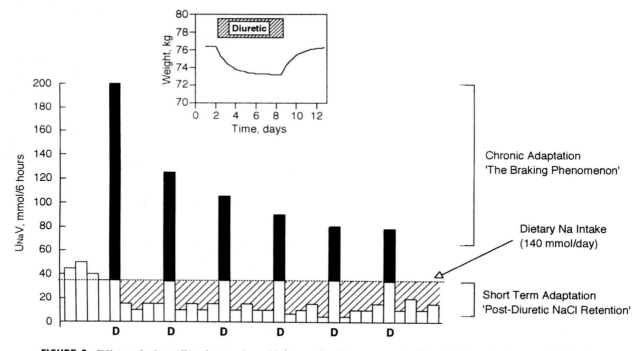

FIGURE 2 Effects of a loop diuretic on urinary Na^+ excretion. Bars represents 6 hr. Black bars indicate periods during which urinary Na^+ excretion exceeds dietary intake. Hatched areas indicate postdiuretic NaCl retention, periods during which dietary Na^+ intake exceeds urinary Na^+ excretion. Changes in the magnitude of natriuretic response during several days are indicative of diuretic "braking." Dashed line indicates dietary Na^+ intake/6-hr period. Inset is effect of diuretics on weight (and extracellular fluid volume) during several days of diuretic administration. Used with permission from Ellison DH: In Seldin DW, Giebisch G (eds) *Diuretic Agents: Physiology and Pharmacology,* Academic Press, San Diego, 1997.

secretion of renin, aldosterone, and antidiuretic hormone which mediate renal NaCl and fluid retention. Contraction of the ECF volume may increase the activity of renal nerves which stimulate renal NaCl retention via direct effects on renal tubules. Contraction of the ECF volume may also reduce renal perfusion pressure and the glomerular filtration rate. In addition to adaptations that depend on changes in ECF volume, however, specific intrarenal effects of diuretics may also contribute to adaptation. Loop diuretics inhibit solute reabsorption along the thick ascending limb of Henle's loop, thereby increasing solute delivery to and solute reabsorption from the distal nephron. When solute delivery to the distal tubule is increased chronically (as during long-term diuretic therapy) distal tubule cells undergo substantial hypertrophy and increases in the expression of transport proteins. These changes are associated with increases in NaCl transport capacity, which participates in returning the patient to neutral NaCl balance. When these adaptive mechanisms occur prior to the achievement of acceptable levels of ECF volume (the therapeutic response to diuretics), they may contribute importantly to diuretic resistance, as discussed later.

The goal of diuretic treatment of edema is not simply to increase urinary NaCl or fluid excretion. Instead, the goal is to reduce ECF volume to a clinically acceptable level and to maintain that volume chronically. To achieve this goal, urinary NaCl excretion must increase initially (Fig. 2), but excretion rates of NaCl and fluid always return to pretreatment levels once steady state occurs. Thus, during successful diuretic treatment of edema, when the weight of the patient has stabilized, urinary NaCl excretion matches dietary intake; it is not increased above normal values.

COMPLICATIONS OF DIURETIC TREATMENT

The most common complications of diuretic treatment result directly from the effects of these drugs on renal fluid and electrolyte excretion. They include ECF volume depletion, hyponatremia, and hypokalemia. Although both DCT and loop diuretics predispose to hypokalemia, disorders of K^+ homeostasis occur more frequently with DCT diuretics. Serum K^+ concentration declines by approximately 0.5 mM, when DCT diuretics are administered without KCl supplementation. Mild hypokalemia (<3.5 mM) occurs in up to 48% of patients during treatment with DCT diuretics (50 mg hydrochlorothiazide); moderate hypokalemia (<3.0 mM) occurs in up to 17%. During furosemide treatment, mild hypokalemia occurs in 5% of patients, moderate hypokalemia in less than 1%. Frank hypokalemia during treatment of hypertension with a DCT diuretic should alert the clinician that increased renin or aldosterone secretion may be responsible for the hypertension (as occurs in Conn's syndrome or renovascular disease).

Several mechanisms contribute to the tendency of loop and DCT diuretics to cause hypokalemia. First, both classes of diuretics increase fluid flow through the distal nephron, the site at which K^+ secretion determines urinary K^+ excretion rates. High fluid flow rates stimulate K^+ secretion

directly. Second, both loop and DCT diuretics stimulate secretion of aldosterone which also increases K^+ secretion along the distal nephron. Finally, both DCT and loop diuretics predispose to hypomagnesemia, which contributes to the development of hypokalemia through unknown mechanisms. Hypokalemia has several adverse consequences. These include ventricular arrhythmias, especially during the administration of digitalis glycosides or when hypomagnesemia is present, and glucose intolerance. Hypokalemia may make control of blood pressure more difficult.

Methods to prevent or treat hypokalemia during diuretic therapy include, (1) using the lowest effective diuretic dose (especially for hypertension), (2) supplementing dietary K^+ (best administered as KCl), (3) preventing hypomagnesemia, and (4) using CD (K^+ sparing) diuretics together with loop or DCT diuretics. Serum concentrations of Na^+ and K^+ should be monitored in every patient who is treated with diuretics, and most patients should be encouraged to consume a diet that is rich in K^+ and low in Na^+. Many physicians treat patients whose serum K^+ concentration falls below 3.5 mM, although some have suggested that K^+ concentrations between 3.0 and 3.5 mM do not require treatment. Certainly, if a patient is at risk for complications of hypokalemia, such as patients receiving digitalis glycosides or patients with hepatic cirrhosis, K^+ concentrations should be maintained above 3.5 mM. Of note, adding a CD diuretic not only corrects hypokalemia in many patients, but may also prevent hypomagnesemia; hypomagnesemia may act synergistically with hypokalemia to predispose to ventricular arrhythmias.

Hyperkalemia is a complication of CD diuretics. Hyperkalemia occurs most commonly in patients with renal failure or in patients taking angiotensin converting enzyme inhibitors. Anecdotal reports suggest that the use of spironolactone in patients treated for heart failure with angiotensin converting enzyme inhibitors may increase the incidence of clinically important hyperkalemia in these patients. Triamterene metabolism is impaired in patients with cirrhosis; this drug can precipitate hyperkalemia in this group of patients.

Mild metabolic alkalosis occurs frequently during treatment with loop and DCT diuretics. These drugs promote urinary losses of NaCl (leaving HCO_3^- behind). Further, they increase aldosterone secretion, which stimulates H^+ secretion directly. Metabolic alkalosis can exacerbate hepatic encephalopathy and can inhibit the respiratory drive. Severe metabolic alkalosis is often a manifestation of overly aggressive therapy. Loop diuretics or combination diuretic therapy (see later) may also lead to excessive ECF volume depletion and vascular collapse.

Hyponatremia may develop during treatment with loop diuretics, but this complication is more common with DCT diuretics (thiazides and their congeners). Some patients treated with thiazide diuretics develop severe and potentially life-threatening hyponatremia, often several days to weeks after initiation of diuretic therapy. The tendency for hyponatremia to recur on rechallenge of these individuals can be assessed by measuring body weight and serum [Na^+]

before and 6–8 hr after a single dose of DCT diuretic. If the serum [Na$^+$] falls below 136 mM following diuretic administration, the patient is at high risk for severe hyponatremia. In these patients, DCT diuretics appear to stimulate fluid intake which contributes to weight gain and hyponatremia. DCT diuretics and, less commonly, loop diuretics also predispose to glucose intolerance, hyperlipidemia, and hyperuricemia, when administered chronically. Although the mechanisms by which these complications develop are not completely clear, hypokalemia and ECF volume contraction may contribute. Serum concentrations of glucose, lipids, and uric acid should be monitored in patients on chronic diuretic treatment, but the clinical significance of these adverse effects was probably overemphasized in the past.

Some complications of diuretic treatment are drug or group specific and reflect toxic side effects; allergic interstitial nephritis is an idiosyncratic reaction to diuretics that may precipitate skin rash and acute renal failure. Ototoxicity is a toxic effect of loop diuretics that occurs most commonly when high doses are administered rapidly (furosemide IV >15 mg/min) to patients with renal insufficiency. Triamterene can cause renal stones and may precipitate acute renal failure when administered with indomethacin. Spironolactone causes gynecomastia, especially in patients with cirrhosis of the liver.

DIURETIC TREATMENT OF EDEMA

Edema is a manifestation of disordered NaCl homeostasis. The NaCl retention often reflects a physiological response to inadequate effective arterial blood volume, as occurs in congestive heart failure. In other situations, NaCl retention may reflect an abnormal renal response, resulting from damage to the kidney, as occurs in renal failure and nephrotic syndrome. In either case, therapeutic maneuvers should be aimed first at correcting the primary disorder. Often, however, such maneuvers are not available or do not contract the ECF volume adequately and, more direct methods of effecting NaCl removal are needed. Before initiating treatment with diuretic drugs, it is important to institute a low NaCl diet. ECF volume varies directly with NaCl intake, both in normal and edematous individuals. For patients with mild ECF volume expansion, a "no added salt" diet may be appropriate (4 g Na$^+$/day); for more severe edema, a low Na$^+$ diet (2 g Na$^+$/day) should be prescribed. Even when dietary restriction alone is unsuccessful and diuretic drugs are administered, the dietary Na$^+$ intake must be restricted below 4 g/day for diuretics to be effective. A second important consideration before initiating diuretic therapy is to improve the general management of the patient by discontinuing, when possible, drugs that predispose to NaCl retention or interfere with diuretic efficacy. Nonsteroidal antiinflammatory drugs (NSAIDs) promote renal NaCl retention directly and interfere with the efficacy of loop and DCT diuretics. Many vasodilators promote edema; minoxidil frequently causes significant ECF volume expansion; nifedipine promotes edema despite intrinsic natriuretic properties, perhaps

through local vasodilation. Other antihypertensive drugs may also predispose to NaCl retention by reducing renal perfusion.

Once the decision to initiate diuretic therapy has been made, the initial choice of drug and dosage depends on the underlying cause of edema and its severity. Hypertension often responds to a very low dose of a DCT diuretic (12.5 mg/day of hydrochlorothiazide, for example), a dose associated with few side effects. Cirrhotic edema and ascites frequently respond to spironolactone (50–300 mg daily); spironolactone appears to be more effective than furosemide in these patients. Moderate edema associated with congestive heart failure may respond to a DCT diuretic such as hydrochlorothiazide, in doses of 25 to 50 mg/day; some studies suggest that a DCT diuretic may reduce extracellular fluid volume more effectively than loop diuretics in patients with very mild congestive heart failure. But when edema from congestive heart failure, cirrhosis, or nephrotic syndrome is more than mild, when renal failure is present, or in the presence of pulmonary congestion or severe symptoms, loop diuretics are the drugs of choice. As previously mentioned, the addition of a small dose of spironolactone (25 to 50 mg/day) to traditional therapy of heart failure was shown to reduce morbidity and mortality in patients with left ventricular dysfunction.

Loop diuretics have the highest natriuretic potency, are active at all levels of renal function, and act rapidly even following oral administration. The drugs have steep dose–response relationships; as the dose is increased, there is little response until a critical threshold is reached, above which diuretic effectiveness increases rapidly to a maximum (see Fig. 3). When a loop diuretic is administered in a dose that exceeds the threshold, most patients experience an increase in urine output that is noticeable during the several hours after diuretic ingestion. To be effective, each dose of loop diuretic must exceed this threshold. When initiating oral diuretic therapy, a target is set for weight loss and a low dose of loop diuretic (20 mg furosemide or its equivalent) is begun once or twice daily. If urine output rises during 4 to 6 hr after diuretic ingestion, the same dose is continued on a daily basis (unless weight loss exceeds the target value). If urine output does not rise, the patient may double the dose the following day (to 40 mg once daily). If there is no response, the dose can be doubled each day until a response is obtained or until the maximum safe dose is achieved (usually ≤240 mg). In normal individuals, 40 mg of furosemide orally produces maximal diuresis, but in patients with edema or renal failure, larger doses are frequently necessary (see Fig. 3). Renal failure shifts the loop diuretic dose–response curve to the right. When the fractional Na$^+$ excretion is plotted, the maximal effectiveness is unchanged. In contrast, when absolute Na$^+$ excretion is plotted, it can be seen that the maximal effectiveness of loop diuretics is dramatically reduced in the setting of chronic renal failure (Fig. 3). Even in renal failure, however, there is little to be gained by increasing intravenous doses beyond 240 mg furosemide or 8 mg bumetanide, because these doses reach the plateau of the dose–response curve. Some clinicians have reported that much higher

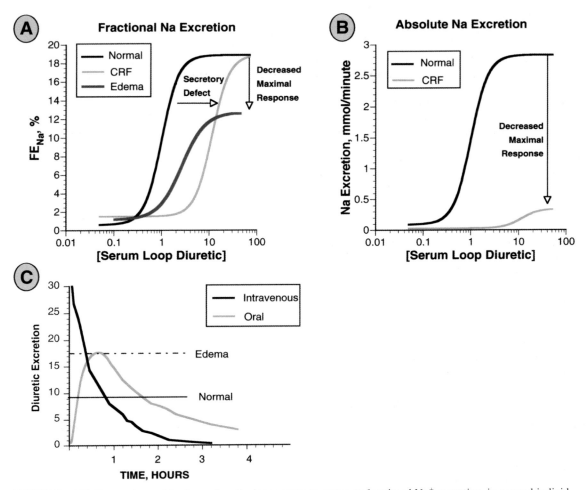

FIGURE 3 (A) Comparison of the loop diuretic dose–response curve, as fractional Na$^+$ excretion, in normal individuals and in patients with chronic renal failure (CRF) and edematous conditions (edema). The diuretic threshold is indicated by the serum concentration at which natriuresis increases. Note that the curve is shifted rightward in CRF owing to impaired diuretic secretion. Note that the maximal effect is reduced in edema. (B) Comparison of the loop diuretic dose–response curve, expressed as absolute Na$^+$ excretion rate, in normal individuals and CRF. Note that the maximal absolute natriuretic response is reduced in CRF even though the fractional response is not. (C) Pharmacokinetics of intravenous and oral loop diuretics. The diuretic thresholds for normal and edematous individuals are shown as horizontal lines. Note that, whereas a normal individual will respond to a given dose of either intravenous or oral diuretic, some edematous individuals will achieve therapeutic drug levels following an intravenous dose but not the same dose given orally.

doses of loop diuretics can be effective. Figure 3C suggests that this increased natriuresis reflects a longer duration at which serum diuretic levels are above the diuretic threshold. This prolonged duration, however, comes at the price of potential for toxicity and most investigators believe that more frequent but more moderate doses are just as effective and better tolerated. Often, the dose that elicits an increase in urine output can be continued indefinitely, because adaptive mechanisms such as those previously discussed, bring the patient back into NaCl balance once ECF volume has been reduced. Sometimes, however, patients may be maintained with lower doses than were necessary to elicit diuresis initially, once control of the ECF volume is achieved.

DIURETIC RESISTANCE: CAUSES AND TREATMENT

Control of ECF volume expansion can be attained in most edematous patients using the approach previously outlined. In some circumstances, however, moderate or high doses of loop diuretics do not reduce ECF volume to the desired level even when used appropriately, and the patient is deemed resistant to diuretic therapy. Determining what ECF volume is acceptable depends on many factors, including the severity of the underlying disease, patient preference, and comorbid illness. When further reductions in ECF volume are necessary, a systematic approach (see Fig. 4) to diuretic resistance usually leads to a treatment regimen that is safe and effective. One of the most com-

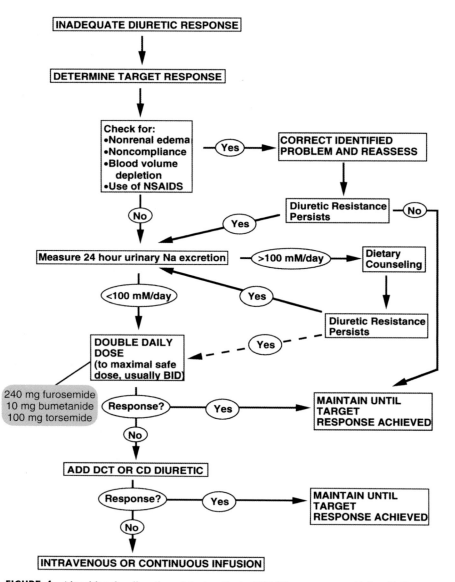

FIGURE 4 Algorithm for diuretic resistant patients. NSAIDs are nonsteroidal antiinflammatory drugs. Regimens for combination therapy are given in the text. Maximal individual doses are provided in the gray box. Note that higher doses have been used to treat patients with acute renal failure. Modified with permission from Wilcox CS: In: Brenner B (ed) *The Kidney,* 5th Ed. Saunders, Philadelphia, 1996.

mon causes of apparent resistance to diuretic drugs is dietary indiscretion because, as previously discussed, dietary NaCl excess abrogates the effect of most diuretic regimens; the influence of dietary NaCl intake is most pronounced for the loop diuretics. If the weight of the patient is stable, dietary compliance can be assessed by measuring the amount of Na^+ excreted during 24 hr. A urinary Na^+ excretion rate greater than 100–120 mmol (equivalent to 2.3–2.8 g Na^+/day) indicates both that the patient is ingesting too much NaCl and that true diuretic resistance is not present; daily Na^+ excretion rates above 120 mmol/day should be sufficient to effect weight loss when patients ingest less than this quantity on a daily basis. Of course, di

etary compliance cannot always be assured, and more intensive regimens (see later) may provide effective diuresis for patients who continue to ingest too much NaCl.

Absorption of many diuretics is variable. The gastrointestinal absorption of furosemide varies by as much as 60% from day to day in a single individual, averaging around 50 to 60% (this effect is true of both Lasix and other brands of furosemide). Gastrointestinal absorption may be slowed further by edema of the gut, such as occurs in some patients with congestive heart failure. In contrast, the bioavailability of torsemide and bumetanide exceeds 80%, and some studies suggest this may provide more reliable diuresis. Alternatively, intravenous therapy may be neces sary until edema is controlled; at this time, diuretic absorption may improve again, and oral therapy may once again become effective.

Once a loop or DCT diuretic drug has been absorbed into the bloodstream, it reaches the lumen of kidney tubule via the organic anion secretory pathway located in the proximal tubule. This pathway also interacts with nonsteroidal antiinflammatory drugs and probenecid, as well as with endogenous anions that accumulate in renal failure. When nonsteroidal antiinflammatory drugs have been administered and in patients with renal failure, diuretic secretion into the lumen of the proximal tubule is inhibited and less diuretic reaches its active site for any given serum concentration. To overcome the inhibition, higher serum levels are needed, this is one reason that high doses of diuretic drugs are required to effect a diuresis in patients with renal failure (up to 400 mg of furosemide in severe renal failure). Of note, although the ratio of equipotent doses of furosemide to bumetanide is 40:1 in patients with normal renal function, it falls to 20:1 in patients with renal failure because the clearance of furosemide is reduced (leading to relatively higher serum levels), whereas the clearance of bumetanide is maintained. Torsemide has both renal and nonrenal clearance so that its clearance rate is relatively stable in the face of either renal or hepatic disease. In general, when switching from intravenous to oral furosemide, twice the oral dose is given. When switching from intravenous to oral torsemide or bumetanide, the conversion is one to one. In each case, however, it is necessary to confirm that an effective oral dose has been selected.

Diuretic resistance is common in patients with the nephrotic syndrome. Hypoalbuminemia reduces the serum concentration of diuretics because it increases their volume of distribution (diuretics are extensively protein bound). Further, hypoalbuminemia may predispose to renal vasoconstriction. Because albumin is filtered by the abnormal glomeruli, renal clearance of diuretics is actually increased, but the diuretic in the tubule lumen may be inactive because it is bound to filtered albumin in tubule fluid and is not free to interact with the transport protein. In these situations, increasing the dose, changing from oral to intravenous therapy, or infusing diuretic mixed together with albumin (ratio of 5 mg furosmide/g of albumin) may improve the therapeutic response. A controlled study showed a modest improvement in natriuresis when 40 g of albumin were infused with furosemide, versus furosemide alone in patients with nephrotic syndrome. Another randomized controlled study examined the efficacy of albumin in promoting diuresis in patients with cirrhotic ascites. In patients with more resistant ascites, albumin infusions were effective in increasing natriuresis and reducing hospitalization; thus they appeared to be cost effective.

Inadequate renal perfusion from any cause compromises diuretic effectiveness. For patients in whom low cardiac output contributes to Na$^+$ retention, low dose dopamine (2–4 μg/kg/min) may increase renal plasma flow and increase urine flow (dopamine may also increase urine flow in patients with acute renal failure), but the effects of "renal dose" dopamine are controversial and poorly docu-

mented. When edema results from cirrhosis of the liver, removal of ascitic fluid by paracentesis or peritoneovenous shunting may improve renal function and Na$^+$ excretion. Arterial hypoxemia causes renal vasoconstriction resulting in antinatriuresis, which reverses promptly when the arterial oxygen tension increases above 60 mm Hg. Renal vasoconstrictors, such as nonsteroidal antiinflammatory drugs and adrenergic agonists may also lead to diuretic resistance, in part by reducing glomerular filtration rate, and should be avoided in the diuretic resistant patient. The effects of drugs used to reduce cardiac afterload on renal NaCl excretion are complex. When angiotensin converting enzyme inhibitors or nitroprusside increase cardiac output effectively, they may stimulate natriuresis and reduce edema. On the other hand, when aggressive therapy reduces blood pressure beyond a critical threshold (which may be surprisingly high in patients with severe vascular disease), they may lead to NaCl retention and even renal failure. This is especially common during concomitant administration of nonsteroidal antiinflammatory drugs, when bilateral renal artery stenosis is present, or during very aggressive diuretic therapy.

Not uncommonly, simple approaches to diuretic resistance fail. Several strategies are available to achieve effective control of ECF volume in such patients. First, loop diuretics often must be administered more frequently than once a day, especially if "postdiuretic Na$^+$ retention" is contributing importantly to NaCl retention. Recall, however, that each dose must be above the diuretic threshold to be effective. Second, a diuretic of another class may be added to a regimen that contains a loop diuretic. This strategy produces true synergism; the combination of agents is more effective than the sum of the responses to each agent alone. DCT diuretics are the class of drug most commonly combined with loop diuretics, although diuretic synergism occurs when loop diuretics are combined with carbonic anhydrase inhibitors and theophylline as well. These drugs may act synergistically for several reasons. First, loop diuretics increase NaCl delivery to the distal tubule, a site at which NaCl transport depends on the luminal NaCl concentration. Loop diuretics, therefore, stimulate NaCl reabsorption in the DCT diuretic-sensitive segment. Adding a DCT diuretic will inhibit NaCl transport along the stimulated segment. Second, when loop diuretics are administered chronically, cells in the distal tubule enlarge, further increasing their ability to transport NaCl. DCT diuretics inhibit the increased NaCl reabsoriion that accompanies hypertrophy of the distal nephron and therefore counteract the effects of hypertrophy. Third, as previously discussed, the efficacy of loop diuretics reflects the balance between natriuresis during diuretic action and Na$^+$ retention when diuretic concentrations decline. DCT diuretics have longer half-lives than loop diuretics. These drugs therefore prevent or attenuate NaCl retention during the periods between doses of loop diuretics, thereby increasing their net effect. Thus, at least three mechanisms contribute to the ability of DCT diuretics to act synergistically with loop acting drugs.

When two diuretics are combined, the DCT diuretic is generally administered sometime before the loop Diuretic

TABLE 2
Continuous Diuretic Infusion[a]

Diuretic	Loading dose (mg)	Creatinine clearance <25 mL/min (mg/hr)	Creatinine clearance 25–75 mL/min (mg/hr)	Creatinine clearance >75 ml/min (mg/hr)
Furosemide	40	20–40	10–20	10
Torsemide	20	10–20	5–10	5
Bumetanide	1	1–2	0.5–1.0	0.5

[a]Data from Brater DC: Diuretic therapy. *N Engl J Med* 339:387–395, 1998.

(1 hr is reasonable) in order to insure that NaCl transport in the distal nephron is blocked when it is flooded with solute. When intravenous therapy is indicated, chlorothiazide (500–1000 mg) may be employed. Metolazone is the DCT diuretic most frequently combined with loop diuretics because its half-life is relatively long (as formulated in Zaroxylin) and because it has been reported to be effective even when renal failure is present. Other thiazide and thiazide-like diuretics, however, may be equally effective. The dramatic effectiveness of combination diuretic therapy, is accompanied by complications in a significant number of patients. Massive fluid and electrolyte losses have led to circulatory collapse during combination therapy, and patients must be followed carefully. The lowest effective dose of DCT diuretic should be added to the loop diuretic regimen; patients can frequently be treated with combination therapy for only a few days and then placed back on a single drug regimen; when continuous combination therapy is needed, low doses of DCT diuretic (2.5 mg metolazone or 25 mg hydrochlorothiazide) administered only two or three times per week may be sufficient.

For hospitalized patients who are resistant to diuretic therapy, a different approach is to infuse loop diuretics continuously (see Table 2 and Fig. 4). Continuous diuretic infusions have several advantages over bolus diuretic administration. First, because they avoid peaks and troughs of diuretic concentration, continuous infusions prevent periods of positive NaCl balance (postdiuretic NaCl retention) from occurring. Second, continuous infusions are more efficient than bolus therapy (the amount of NaCl excreted/mg of drug administered is greater). Third, some patients who are resistant to large doses of diuretics given by bolus have responded to continuous infusion. Fourth, diuretic response can be titrated; in the intensive care unit where obligate fluid administration must be balanced by fluid excretion, excellent control of NaCl and water excretion can be obtained. Finally, complications associated with high doses of loop diuretics, such as ototoxicity, appear to be less common when large doses are administered as continuous infusion. Total daily furosemide doses exceeding 1 g have been tolerated well when administered over 24 hr, but a more cautious dosing regimen is provided in Table 2.

Most patients who are deemed resistant to diuretics respond to these approaches. Rather than lack of efficacy, side effects of diuretic therapy such as increases in serum creatinine concentration often limit the ability to reduce ECF volume further. Obtaining effective control of ECF volume without provoking complications requires a thorough understanding of diuretic physiology and a commitment to use diuretics rationally and carefully. When used in this manner, they remain among the most powerful drugs in clinical medicine.

Bibliography

Brater DC: Diuretic therapy. *N Engl J Med* 339:387–395, 1998.

Denton MD, Chertow GM, Brady HM: "Renal-dose" dopamine for the treatment of acute renal failure: Scientific rationale, experimental studies and clinical trials. *Kidney Int* 49:4–14, 1996.

Ellison DH: Diuretic drugs and the treatment of edema: From clinic to bench and back again. *Am J Kidney Dis* 23:623–643, 1994.

Ellison DH: Diuretic resistance: Physiology and therapeutics. *Semin Nephrol* 19:581–597, 1999.

Fliser D, Schröter M, Neubeck M, Ritz E: Coadministration of thiazides increases the efficacy of loop diuretics even in patients with advanced renal failure. *Kidney Int* 46:482–488, 1994.

Fliser D, Zurbruggen I, Mutschler E, Bischoff I, Nussberger J, Franek E, Ritz E: Coadministration of albumin and furosemide in patients with the nephrotic syndrome. *Kidney Int* 55:629–634, 1999.

Gentilini P, Casini-Raggi V, Di Fiore G, Romanelli RG, Buzzelli G, Pinzani M, La Villa G, Laffi G: Albumin improves the response to diuretics in patients with cirrhosis and ascites: Results of a randomized, controlled trial. *J Hepatol* 30:639–645, 1999.

Martin SJ, Danziger LH: Continuous infusion of loop diuretics in the critically ill: A Review of the literature. *Crit Care Med* 22:1323–1329, 1994.

Pitt B, Zannad F, Remme WJ, Cody R, Castaigne A, Perez A, Palensky J, Wittes J: The effect of spironolactone on morbidity and mortality in patients with severe heart failure. *N Engl J Med* 341:709–717, 1999.

Rudy DW, Voelker JR, Greene PK, Esparza FA, Brater DC: Loop diuretics for chronic renal insufficiency: A continuous infusion is more efficacious than bolus therapy. *Ann Intern Med.* 115:360–366, 1991.

Seldin DW, Giebisch G: *Diuretic Agents: Clinical Physiology and Pharmacology.* Academic Press, San Diego, 1997.

Solomon R, Werner C, Mann D, D'Elia J, Silva P: Effects of saline, mannitol, and furosemide on acute decreases in renal function induced by radiocontrast agents. *N Engl J Med.* 331:1416–1420, 1994.

Stevens MA, McCullough PA, Tobin KJ, Speck JP, Westveer DC, Guido-Allen DA, Timmis GC, and O'Neill WW: A prospective randomized trial of prevention measures in patients at high risk for contrast nephropathy: Results of the P.R.I.N.C.E. Study. Prevention of Radiocontrast Induced Nephropathy Clinical Evaluation. *J Am Coll Cardiol* 33:403–411, 1999.

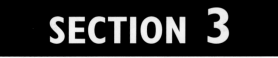

SECTION 3

GLOMERULAR DISEASES

GLOMERULAR CLINICOPATHOLOGIC SYNDROMES

J. CHARLES JENNETTE AND RONALD J. FALK

Injury to glomeruli results in a multiplicity of signs and symptoms of disease, including proteinuria caused by altered permeability of capillary walls, hematuria caused by rupture of capillary walls, azotemia caused by impaired filtration of nitrogenous wastes, oliguria or anuria caused by reduced urine production, edema caused by salt and water retention, and hypertension caused by fluid retention and disturbed renal homeostasis of blood pressure. The nature and severity of disease in a given patient is dictated by the nature and severity of glomerular injury.

Specific glomerular diseases tend to produce characteristic syndromes of renal dysfunction, however, multiple different glomerular diseases can produce the same syndrome (Tables 1 and 2). The diagnosis of a glomerular disease requires recognition of one of these syndromes followed by collection of data to determine which specific glomerular disease is present. Alternatively, if reaching a specific diagnosis is not possible or not necessary the physician should at least narrow down the differential diagnosis to a likely candidate disease.

Evaluation of pathologic features identified in a renal biopsy specimen is often required for a definitive diagnosis. The pathologic features of various glomerular diseases are described in the corresponding chapters of this book. Figure 1 depicts some of the clinical and pathologic features used to resolve the differential diagnosis in patients with antibody-mediated glomerulonephritis, Figs. 2–5 illustrate the distinctive ultrastructural features of some of the major categories of glomerular disease, and Fig. 6 illustrates some of the major patterns of immune deposition identified by immunofluorescence microscopy.

ASYMPTOMATIC HEMATURIA AND RECURRENT GROSS HEMATURIA

Hematuria is usually defined as greater than three red blood cells per high power field observed by microscopic examination of a centrifuged urine sediment (see Chapters 4 and 5 for more details). Hematuria is asymptomatic when a patient is unaware of its presence and it is not accompanied by clinical manifestations of nephritis or nephrotic syndrome, that is, without azotemia, oliguria, edema, or hypertension. Asymptomatic microscopic hematuria occurs in

5 to 10% of the general population. Recurrent gross hematuria may be superimposed on asymptomatic microscopic hematuria, or may occur in isolation. The patient observes urine discoloration, which often is described as tea colored or cola colored.

All hematuria is not of glomerular origin. In fact, most hematuria is not of glomerular origin. Glomerular diseases cause less than 10% of hematuria in patients with no proteinuria, with almost 80% being caused by bladder, prostate, or urethral disease. Hypercalciuria and hyperuricosuria also can cause asymptomatic hematuria, especially in children.

Microscopic examination of the urine can help determine whether hematuria is of glomerular or nonglomerular origin. Chemical (e.g., osmotic) trauma to red blood cells as they pass through the nephron causes structural changes that are not present in red blood cells that have passed directly into the urine from a gross parenchymal injury in the kidney (e.g., a neoplasm) or from a lesion in the urinary tract (e.g., renal pelvis traumatized by stones or an inflamed bladder). Dysmorphic red blood cells that have transited the urinary tract from the glomeruli usually have lost their biconcave configuration and hemoglobin, and often have multiple membrane blebs, sometimes producing acanthocytes and "Mickey Mouse cells." The presence of red blood cell casts and other sediment abnormalities typical of glomerulonephritis also supports a glomerular origin for hematuria.

Published renal biopsy series carried out in patients with asymptomatic hematuria show differences in the frequencies of identified underlying glomerular lesions. Differences in the nature of the population analyzed (e.g., military recruits versus routine physical examination patients), and differences in pathologic analysis (e.g., failure of the earlier studies to recognize thin basement membrane nephropathy) account for the observed disparities. The data presented in Table 3 are derived from patients with hematuria who underwent diagnostic renal biopsy. The data in the first column equate with asymptomatic hematuria, and are similar to other recent series. In these patients with hematuria, less than 1 g/24 hr proteinuria and serum creatinine less than 1.5 mg/dL, the three major findings were no pathologic abnormality (30%), thin basement membrane

TABLE I
Clinical Manifestations of Glomerular Diseases, and Representative
Diseases That Present with these Manifestations[a]

Asymptomatic proteinuria	Acute nephritis
Focal segmental glomerulosclerosis	Acute diffuse proliferative GN
Mesangioproliferative GN	Poststreptococcal GN
	Poststaphylococcal GN
Nephrotic syndrome	Focal or diffuse proliferative GN
Minimal change glomerulopathy	IgA nephropathy
Membranous glomerulopathy	Lupus nephritis
Idiopathic (primary)	Type I membranoproliferative GN
Secondary (e.g., lupus)	Type II membranoproliferative GN
Focal segmental glomerulosclerosis	Fibrillary GN
Mesangioproliferative GN	Rapidly progressive nephritis
Type I membranoproliferative GN	Crescentic GN
Type II membranoproliferative GN	Anti-GBM GN
Fibrillary GN	Immune complex GN
Diabetic glomerulosclerosis	ANCA GN
Amyloidosis	Pulmonary–renal vasculitic syndrome
Light chain deposition disease	Goodpasture's (anti-GBM) syndrome
Asymptomatic microscopic hematuria	Immune complex vasculitis
Thin basement membrane nephropathy	Lupus
IgA nephropathy	ANCA vasculitis
Mesangioproliferative GN	Microscopic polyangiitis
Alport's syndrome	Wegener's granulomatosis
Recurrent gross hematuria	Churg–Strauss syndrome
Thin basement membrane nephropathy	Chronic renal failure
IgA nephropathy	Chronic sclerosing GN
Alport's syndrome	

[a]Note that the same manifestations can be caused by different diseases, and that the same disease can manifest in different ways. GN, glomerulonephritis; GBM, glomerular basement membrane; ANCA, antineutrophil cytoplasmic autoantibodies.

nephropathy (26%), and IgA nephropathy (28%). Whereas thin basement membrane nephropathy virtually always manifests as asymptomatic hematuria or recurrent gross hematuria, IgA nephropathy can manifest any of the syndromes listed in Table 1.

Alport's syndrome (Chapter 44) is an hereditary disease caused by a defect in the genes that code for basement membrane type IV collagen α-3 chain or α-5 chain. Approximately 85% of patients have a mutation in the X-chromosomal α-5 gene and 15% in the autosomal α-3 and α-4 genes. In affected males, Alport's syndrome initially manifests as asymptomatic microscopic hematuria, sometimes with superimposed episodes of gross hematuria. The hematuria usually begins in the first decade of life. Progressively worsening proteinuria and renal insufficiency eventually develop, although the rate of progression is quite variable. Affected females, who are almost always heterozygous, often have intermittent microscopic hematuria but may have no other manifestations of renal disease.

Renal biopsy is not usually performed to evaluate asymptomatic hematuria. Renal biopsy diagnoses rarely affect treatment in patients with asymptomatic hematuria, but occasional patients will be found to have disease that might benefit from treatment (e.g., the one patient with early crescentic glomerulonephritis identified in the cohort

of patients in the first column of Table 3). Renal biopsy can also be of some prognostic value. For example, thin basement membrane nephropathy has a better prognosis and a much greater propensity for familial occurrence than IgA nephropathy. Many patients with asymptomatic hematuria are subjected to repeated invasive urologic evaluations until a definitive diagnosis is be made. In these patients, additional urologic evaluation can be prevented if renal biopsy provides a diagnosis.

In renal biopsy specimens, thin basement membrane nephropathy is diagnosed based on thinning of the glomerular basement membrane lamina densa (Fig. 3), whereas Alport's syndrome is suspected if there is marked lamination of the lamina densa. The kidney and skin also have abnormalities in immunohistologic staining for α chains of type IV collagen. The presence of mesangial immune deposits with a dominance or codominance of immunohistologic staining for IgA is diagnostic for IgA nephropathy (Fig. 6).

ACUTE GLOMERULONEPHRITIS AND RAPIDLY PROGRESSIVE GLOMERULONEPHRITIS

Acute and rapidly progressive glomerulonephritis often present with acute onset of manifestations of nephritis, such as azotemia, oliguria, edema, hypertension, proteinuria, and

TABLE 2
TABLE 2
Tendencies of Glomerular Diseases to Manifest Nephrotic
and Nephritic Features[a,b]

	Nephrotic features	Nephritic features
Minimal change glomerulopathy	++++	−
Membranous glomerulopathy	++++	+
Diabetic glomerulosclerosis	++++	+
Amyloidosis	++++	+
Focal segmental glomerulosclerosis	+++	++
Fibrillary glomerulonephritis	+++	++
Mesangioproliferative glomerulopathy[c]	++	++
Membranoproliferative glomerulonephritis[d]	++	+++
Proliferative glomerulonephritis[c]	++	+++
Acute diffuse proliferative glomerulonephritis[e]	+	++++
Crescentic glomerulonephritis[f]	+	++++

[a]Note that most diseases can manifest both nephrotic and nephritic features, but there usually is a tendency for one to predominate.

[b]Modified with permission from Jennette JC, Mandal AK: The nephrotic syndrome. In: Mandal AK, Jennette JC (eds) *Diagnosis and Management of Renal Disease and Hypertension.* Carolina Academic Press, Durham, North Carolina, 1994.

[c]Mesangioproliferative and proliferative glomerulonephritis (focal or diffuse) are structural manifestations of a number of glomerulonephritides, including IgA nephropathy and lupus nephritis.

[d]Both type I (mesangiocapillary) and type II (dense deposit disease).

[e]Often a structural manifestation of acute poststreptococcal glomerulonephritis.

[f]Can be immune complex mediated, antiglomerular basement membrane antibody mediated or associated with antineutrophil cytoplasmic autoantibodies.

hematuria with an "active" urine sediment that often contains red blood cell casts, pigmented casts, and cellular debris. Rapidly progressive glomerulonephritis leads to a 50% or greater loss of renal function within weeks to months. If renal failure is severe, manifestation of uremia develop, such as nausea and vomiting, hiccups, dyspnea, lethargy, pericarditis, and encephalopathy. Severe volume overload can cause congestive heart failure and pulmonary edema.

The pathologic processes that most often produce the clinical manifestations of acute or rapidly progressive nephritis are inflammatory glomerular lesions. The nature and severity of the glomerular inflammation correlate with the clinical features of the nephritis (Fig. 7). Note in Fig. 7 that the structural stages of glomerular inflammation can change over time, and this is reflected by changes in the clinical manifestations of nephritis.

The structurally least severe injury is mesangial hyper-

plasia alone, which usually is associated with asymptomatic proteinuria or hematuria rather than overt nephritis. Proliferative glomerulonephritis, which may be focal (affecting less than 50% of glomeruli) or diffuse (affecting greater than 50% of glomeruli), is characterized histologically not only by the proliferation of glomerular cells (e.g., mesangial, endothelial, and epithelial cells) but also by the influx of leukocytes, especially neutrophils and mononuclear phagocytes. Necrosis and sclerosis also may be present.

Lupus nephritis (see Chapter 27) provides a paradigm of the interrelationships between pathogenic mechanisms, pathologic consequences, and clinical manifestations of glomerular disease (Fig. 4). The mildest expression of lupus nephritis (mesangioproliferative lupus glomerulonephritis, class II lupus nephritis) is induced by exclusively mesangial localization of immune complexes that usually causes only mild nephritis or asymptomatic hematuria and proteinuria. Localization of substantial amounts of nephritogenic immune complexes in the subendothelial zones of glomerular capillaries where they are adjacent to the inflammatory mediator systems in the blood induces overt glomerular inflammation (focal or diffuse proliferative lupus glomerulonephritis, class III or IV lupus nephritis) and usually causes severe clinical manifestations of nephritis. Qualitative and quantitative characteristics of the pathogenic immune complexes that result in localization predominantly in subepithelial zones where they are not in contact with the cellular inflammatory mediator systems in the blood induces membranous lupus glomerulonephritis (class V lupus nephritis). This variant is usually associated with the nephrotic syndrome rather than nephritis. As the nephritogenic immune response in a given patient changes over time, sometimes modified by treatment, transitions may occur between different lupus nephritis phenotypes.

The structurally most severe form of active glomerulonephritis is crescentic glomerulonephritis, which usually manifests clinically as rapidly progressive glomerulonephritis. In patients with new onset renal disease who have a nephritic sediment and a serum creatinine >3 g/24 hr, glomerulonephritis with crescents is the most common finding in renal biopsy specimens (Table 3). Crescents are proliferations of cells within Bowman's capsule that include both mononuclear phagocytes and glomerular epithelial cells. Crescent formation is a response to glomerular rupture, and therefore is a marker of severe glomerular injury. Crescents do not indicate the cause of glomerular injury, however, because many different pathogenic mechanisms can cause crescent formation. There is no consensus on how many glomeruli should have crescents in order to use the term crescentic glomerulonephritis. Most pathologists use the term when greater than 50% of glomeruli have crescents, but the percentage of glomeruli with crescents should be specified in the diagnosis even if it is less than 50% (e.g., IgA nephropathy with focal proliferative glomerulonephritis and 25% crescents). Within a specific pathogenic category of glomerulonephritis [e.g., anti-glomerular basement disease (GBM) disease, lupus nephritis, IgA nephropathy, poststreptococcal

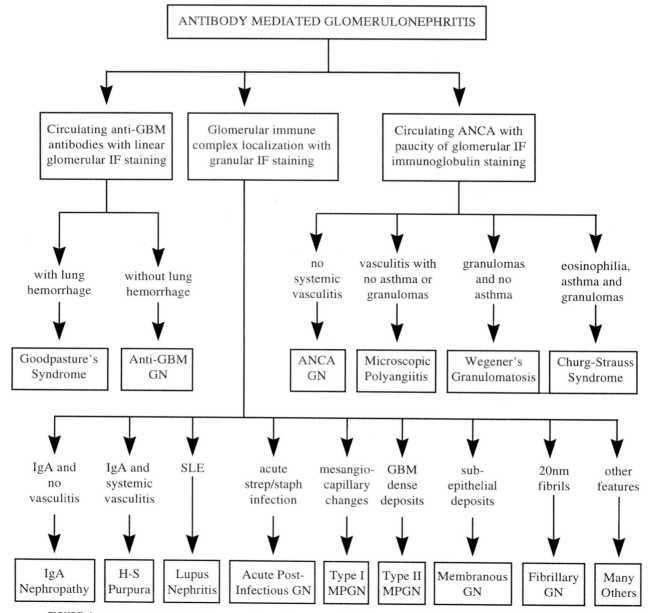

FIGURE I Features that distinguish among different immunopathologic categories of antibody mediated glomerulonephritis. GBM, glomerular basement membrane; IF, immunofluorescence microscopy; ANCA, antineutrophil cytoplasmic autoantibodies; GN, glomerulonephritis; H-S, Henoch–Schönlein; MPGN, membranoproliferative glomerulonephritis; SLE, systemic lupus erythematosus.

glomerulonephritis], the higher the fraction of glomeruli with crescents the worse the prognosis. Among pathogenetically different glomerulonephritides, however, the pathogenic category may be more important in predicting outcome than the presence of crescents. For example, a patient with poststreptococcal glomerulonephritis with 50% crescents has a much better prognosis for renal survival, even without immunosuppressive treatment, than a patient with anti-GBM glomerulonephritis or antineutrophil cytoplasmic autoantibodies (ANCA) glomerulonephritis with 25% crescents.

This importance of pathogenic category in predicting the natural history of glomerulonephritis indicates that the pathologic diagnosis of glomerulonephritis into the light microscopic morphologic categories in Fig. 7 is not adequate for optimum patient management. In addition to determining the morphologic severity of glomerular inflammation, the pathogenic or immuno-pathologic category of disease must be determined. If a renal biopsy is performed, this is usually done by immunohistology and electron microscopy (Figs. 1–6). Immunohistology reveals the presence or absence of immunoglobulins and

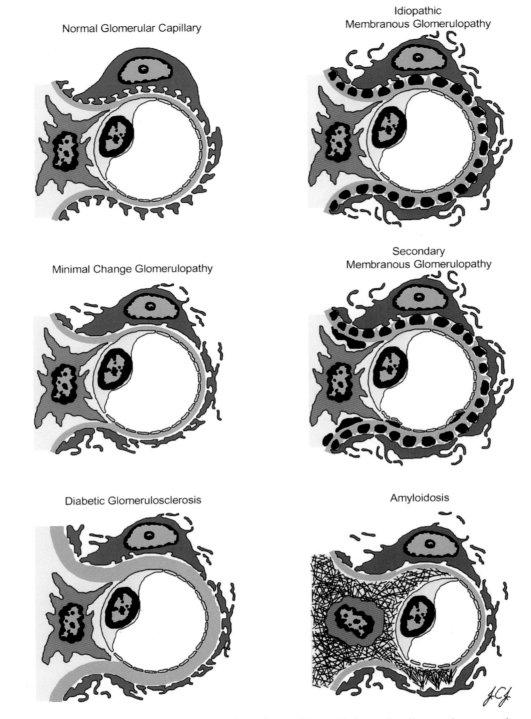

Normal Glomerular Capillary

Idiopathic
Membranous Glomerulopathy

Minimal Change Glomerulopathy

Secondary
Membranous Glomerulopathy

Diabetic Glomerulosclerosis

Amyloidosis

FIGURE 2 Ultrastructural changes in glomerular capillaries of glomerular diseases that cause the nephrotic syndrome. Normal glomerular capillary: note the visceral epithelial cell with intact foot processes (green), endothelial cell with fenestrations (yellow), mesangial cell (red) with adjacent mesangial matrix (light gray), and basement membrane with lamina densa (dark gray) that does not completely surround the capillary lumen but splays out as the paramesangial basement membrane. Minimal change glomerulopathy: note the effacement of foot processes and microvillous transformation. Diabetic glomerulosclerosis: note the thickening of the lamina densa and expansion of mesangial matrix. Idiopathic membranous glomerulopathy: note the subepithelial dense deposits with adjacent projections of basement membrane (see also Fig. 5). Secondary membranous glomerulopathy: note the mesangial and small subendothelial deposits in addition to the requisite subepithelial deposits. Amyloidosis: note the fibrils within the mesangium and capillary wall. From JC Jennette, with permission.

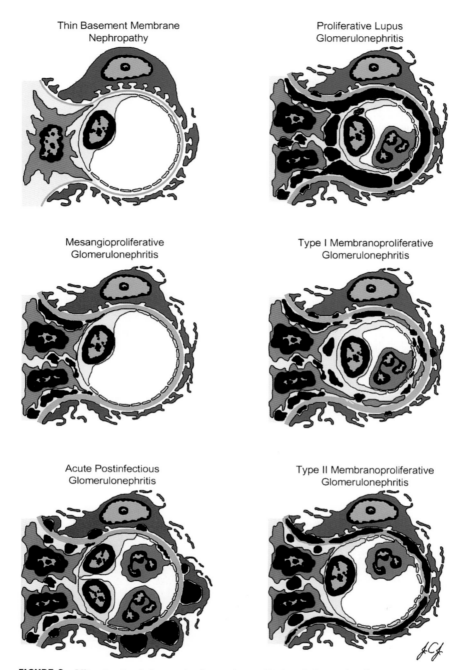

FIGURE 3 Ultrastructural changes in glomerular capillaries of glomerular diseases that cause hematuria and the nephritic syndrome. Thin basement membrane nephropathy: note the thin lamina densa of the basement membrane. Mesangioproliferative glomerulonephritis (e.g., mild lupus nephritis or IgA nephropathy): note the mesangial dense deposits and mesangial hypercellularity. Acute diffuse proliferative glomerulonephritis (e.g., poststreptococcal glomerulonephritis): note the endocapillary hypercellularity contributed to by leukocytes, endothelial cells, and mesangial cells, and the dense deposits, including not only conspicuous subepithelial "humps" but also inconspicuous subendothelial and mesangial deposits. Proliferative lupus glomerulonephritis (see also Fig. 4): note the extensive subendothelial and mesangial dense deposits. Type I membranoproliferative glomerulonephritis (mesangiocapillary glomerulonephritis): note the subendothelial deposits with associated subendothelial interposition of mesangial cytoplasm and deposition of new matrix material resulting in basement membrane replication. Type II membranoproliferative glomerulonephritis (dense deposit disease): note the intramembranous and mesangial dense deposits. From JC Jennette, with permission.

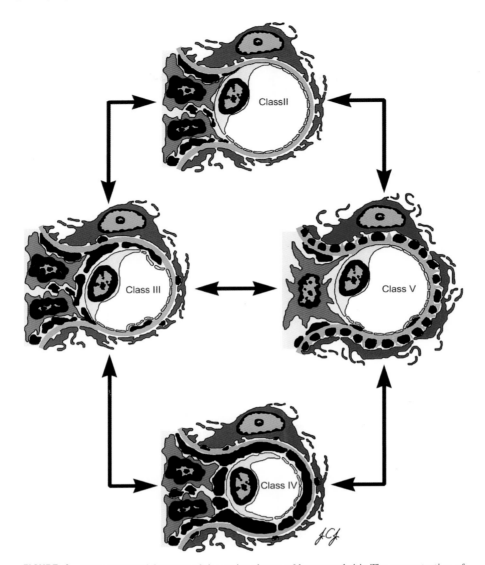

FIGURE 4 Ultrastructural features of the major classes of lupus nephritis. The sequestration of immune deposits within the mesangium in class II (mesangioproliferative) lupus glomerulonephritis causes only mesangial hyperplasia and mild renal dysfunction. Substantial amounts of subendothelial immune deposits, which are adjacent to the inflammatory mediator systems of the blood, cause focal (class III) or diffuse (class IV) proliferative lupus glomerulonephritis with overt nephritic signs and symptoms. Localization of immune deposits predominantly in the subepithelial zone causes membranous (class V) lupus glomerulonephritis, which usually manifests predominantly as the nephrotic syndrome. From JC Jennette, with permission.

complement components. The distribution (e.g., capillary wall, mesangium), pattern (e.g., granular, linear), and composition (e.g., IgA-dominant, IgG-dominant, IgM-dominant) of immunoglobulin is useful for determining specific types of glomerulonephritis, as will be discussed in detail in later chapters in this primer that deal with specific types of glomerular disease.

Table 4 gives the frequencies of the major immunopathologic categories of glomerulonephritis in patients with crescents who have undergone renal biopsy. The immune

complex category contains a variety of diseases, including lupus nephritis, IgA nephropathy, and poststreptococcal glomerulonephritis. Note that most patients with >50% crescents have little or no immunohistologic evidence for immune complex or anti-GBM antibody localization within glomeruli (i.e., pauciimmune glomerulonephritis). Over 80% of these patients with pauciimmune crescentic glomerulonephritis have circulating ANCA.

Because both the structural severity (e.g., morphologic stages in Fig. 7) and immunopathologic category of

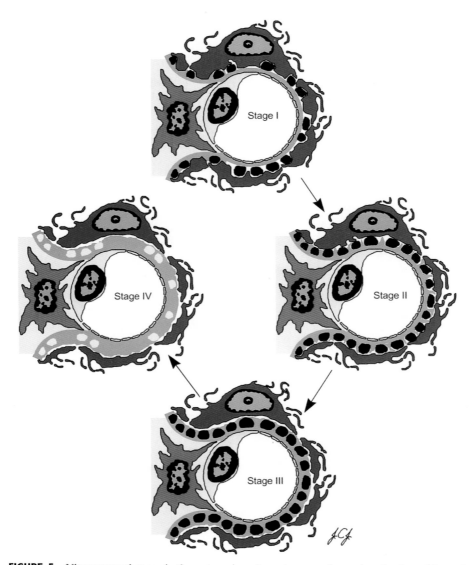

FIGURE 5 Ultrastructural stages in the progression of membranous glomerulopathy. Stage I has subepithelial electron dense immune complex deposits without adjacent projections of basement membrane material. Stage II has adjacent glomerular basement membrane (GBM) projections that eventually surround the electron dense immune deposits in stage III. Stage IV has a markedly thickened GBM with electron lucent zones replacing the electron dense deposits. From JC Jennette, with permission.

disease (e.g., the categories given in Figs. 1–6, such as IgA nephropathy, lupus nephritis, anti-GBM disease) are important in predicting the course of disease in a patient with glomerulonephritis, the most useful diagnostic term should include information about both (e.g., focal proliferative IgA nephropathy, diffuse proliferative lupus glomerulonephritis, crescentic anti-GBM glomerulonephritis).

Because they often are immune-mediated inflammatory diseases, many types of glomerulonephritis are treated with corticosteroids, cytotoxic drugs, or other antiinflammatory and immunosuppressive agents. The aggressiveness of the

treatment, of course, should match the aggressiveness of the disease. For example, active class IV lupus nephritis warrants immunosuppressive treatment whereas class II lupus nephritis does not.

The two most aggressive forms of glomerulonephritis are anti-GBM crescentic glomerulonephritis and ANCA crescentic glomerulonephritis. The most important factor in improving renal outcome is early diagnosis and treatment. Once extensive sclerosis of glomeruli and advanced chronic tubulointerstitial injury have developed, response to treatment is unlikely. Both diseases are treated with immunosuppressive regimens, for example, pulse methylprednisolone and

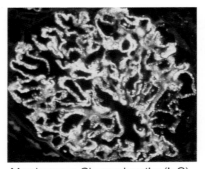

Membranous Glomerulopathy (IgG)

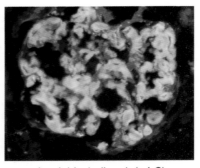

Amyloidosis (Lambda LC)

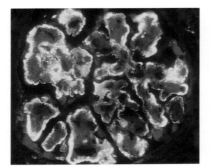

Type I MPGN (C3)

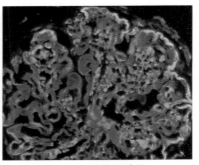

Type II MPGN (C3)

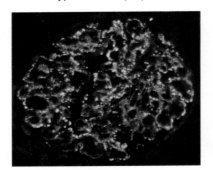

Postinfectious GN (C3)

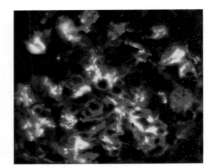

IgA Nephropathy (IgA)

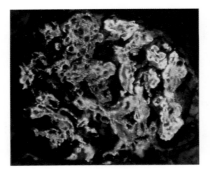

Class IV Lupus GN (IgG)

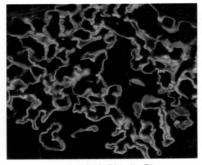

Anti-GBM GN (IgG)

FIGURE 6 Immunofluorescence microscopy staining patterns for membranous glomerulopathy: note the global granular capillary wall staining for IgG. AL amyloidosis: note the irregular fluffy staining for light chains. Type I membranoproliferative glomerulonephritis (MPGN): note the peripheral granular to bandlike staining for C3. Type II MPGN: note the bandlike capillary wall and coarsely granular mesangial staining for C3. Acute postinfectious glomerulonephritis: note the coarsely granular capillary wall staining for C3. IgA nephropathy: note the mesangial staining for IgA. Class IV lupus nephritis: note the segmentally variable capillary wall and mesangial staining for IgG. Anti-GBM glomerulonephritis: note the linear GBM staining for IgG.

TABLE 3
Renal Disease in Patients with Hematuria Undergoing Renal Biopsy[a]

	Prot <1 Cr <1.5	Prot 1–3	Cr 1.5–3.0	Cr >3
No abnormality	30%	2%	1%	0%
Thin BM nephropathy	26%	4%	3%	0%
IgA nephropathy	28%	24%	14%	8%
GN without crescents[c]	9%	26%	37%	23%
GN with crescents[c]	2%	24%	21%	44%
Other renal disease[d]	5%	20%	24%	25%
Total	100%	100%	100%	100%
	n = 43	n = 123	n = 179	n = 255

[a]An analysis of renal biopsy specimens evaluated by the University of North Carolina Nephropathology Laboratory. Patients with systemic lupus erythematosus have been excluded from the analysis. GN, glomerulonephritis; BM, basement membrane; Prot, proteinuria (g/24 hr); Cr, serum creatinine (mg/dL).

[b]Derived from Caldas MLR, Jennette JC, Falk RJ, Wilkman AS: NC Glomerular Disease Collaborative Network: What is found by renal biopsy in patients with hematuria? *Lab Invest* 62:15A, 1990.

[c]Proliferative or necrotizing GN other than IgA nephropathy or lupus nephritis.

[d]Includes causes for the nephrotic syndrome, such as membranous glomerulopathy and focal segmental glomerulosclerosis.

intravenous or oral cyclophosphamide. Plasmapheresis is usually added to the regimen for anti-GBM disease. Immunosuppressive treatment generally can be terminated after 4 to 5 months in patients with anti-GBM glomerulonephritis with very little risk of recurrence (see Chapter 22). The initial induction of remission for ANCA-glomerulonephritis often is carried out for 6 to 12 months, and even then there is an approximately 25% risk for recurrence that will require additional immunosuppression (see Chapter 26).

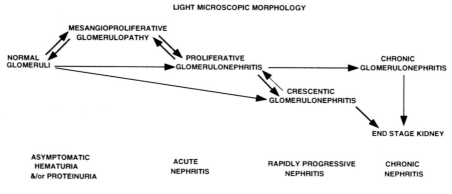

FIGURE 7 Morphologic stages of glomerulonephritis (top of diagram) aligned with the usual clinical manifestations (bottom of diagram). Certain glomerular diseases, such as anti-GBM and ANCA glomerulonephritis, usually have crescentic glomerulonephritis with rapid progression of renal failure if not promptly treated: Others, such as lupus nephritis, have a predilection for causing focal or diffuse proliferative glomerulonephritis with variable rates of progression dependent on the activity of the glomerular lesions. IgA nephropathy tends to begin as mild mesangioproliferative lesions but may progress into more severe proliferative lesions. Poststreptococcal glomerulonephritis typically initially develops a very active acute proliferative glomerulonephritis but then resolves through a mesangioproliferative phase to normal. Still others, such as IgM mesangial nephropathy, rarely progress past the mesangioproliferative phase. Reprinted with permission from Jennette JC, Mandal AK: Syndrome of glomerulonephritis. In: Mandal AK, Jennette JC (eds) *Diagnosis and Management of Renal Disease and Hypertension*, 2nd Ed., Carolina Academic Press, Durham, North Carolina, 1994.

TABLE 4

Frequency of Immunopathologic Categories of Crescentic Glomerulonephritis in More Than 3000 Consecutive Nontransplant Renal Biopsies Evaluated by Immunofluorescence Microscopy in the University of North Carolina Nephropathology Laboratory

	Any crescents (n = 540)	>50% Crescents (n = 195)	Arteritis in biopsy (n = 37)
Immunohistology			
Pauciimmune (<2+ Ig)	51% (277/540)	61% (118/195)[b]	84% (31/37)
Immune complex (≥2+ Ig)	44% (238/540)	29% (56/195)	14% (5/37)[c]
Anti-GBM	5% (25/540)[d]	11% (21/195)	3% (1/37)[e]

[a]Modified with permission from Jennette JC and Falk RJ: The pathology of vasculitis involving the kidney. *Am J Kidney Dis* 24:130–144, 1994.

[b]70 of 77 patients tested for ANCA were positive (91%). (44 P-ANCA and 26 C-ANCA).

[c]Four patients had lupus and one had poststreptococcal glomerulonephritis.

[d]Three of 19 patients tested for ANCA were positive (16%). (2 P-ANCA and 1 C-ANCA).

[e]This patient also had a P-ANCA (MPO-ANCA).

GLOMERULONEPHRITIS ASSOCIATED WITH SYSTEMIC DISEASES

Some patients with acute or rapidly progressive glomerulonephritis have a pathogenetically related systemic disease. Immune complex mediated glomerulonephritides that are induced by infections may have an antecedent or concurrent infection, such as streptococcal pharyngitis or pyoderma preceding acute poststreptococcal glomerulonephritis or hepatitis C infection concurrent with type I membranoproliferative glomerulonephritis. As noted earlier, glomerulonephritis with any of the morphologic expressions shown in Fig. 7, as well as membranous glomerulopathy, can be caused by systemic lupus erythematosus (Fig. 4).

Because glomeruli are vessels, glomerulonephritis is a frequent manifestation of systemic small vessel vasculitides, such as Henoch–Schönlein purpura, cryoglobulinemic vasculitis, microscopic polyangiitis, Wegener's granlomatosis, or Churg–Strauss syndrome. Henoch–Schönlein purpura is caused by vascular localization of IgA-dominant immune complexes, which manifests as IgA nephropathy in the glomeruli. Cryoglobulinemic vasculitis is caused by cryoglobulin deposition in vessels, and often is associated with hepatitis C infection. In glomeruli, cryoglobulinemia usually causes type I membranoproliferative glomerulonephritis, but other phenotypes of proliferative and even membranous glomerulonephritis may develop. Microscopic polyangiitis, Wegener's granulomatosis, or Churg–Strauss syndrome have a paucity of immune deposits in vessel walls and are associated with circulating ANCA. Glomerulonephritis with ANCA is characterized pathologically by fibrinoid necrosis and crescent formation, and often manifests as rapidly progressive renal failure. Patients with vasculitis-associated glomerulonephritis typically have clinical manifestations of vascular inflammation in multiple organs, such as skin purpura caused by dermal angiitis, hemoptysis caused by alveolar capillary hemorrhage, abdominal pain caused by gut infarcts, and mononeuritis multiplex caused by vasculitis in the epineural and perineural vessels of peripheral nerves.

A distinctive and severe clinical presentation for glomerulonephritis is pulmonary–renal vasculitic syndrome, which usually has rapidly progressive glomerulonephritis combined with pulmonary hemorrhage. Table 1 lists the most common causes for pulmonary–renal vasculitic syndrome. Histologic and immunohistologic examination of involved vessels, including glomeruli in renal biopsy specimens, is useful in making a definitive diagnosis (Fig. 1). Serologic analysis for anti-GBM antibodies, ANCA, and markers for immune complex disease (e.g., antinuclear antibodies, cryoglobulins, anti-hepatitis C and B antibodies, complement levels) also may indicate the appropriate diagnosis (Fig. 1). ANCA small vessel vasculitis is the most frequent cause for pulmonary–renal vasculitic syndrome.

ASYMPTOMATIC PROTEINURIA AND NEPHROTIC SYNDROME

When proteinuria is severe, it causes the nephrotic syndrome. Less severe proteinuria, or severe proteinuria of short duration, may be asymptomatic. The nephrotic syndrome is characterized by massive proteinuria (>3 g/24 hr/1.73 m^2), hypoproteinemia (especially hypoalbuminemia), edema, hyperlipidemia, and lipiduria. The most specific microscopic urinalysis finding is the presence of oval fat bodies. These are sloughed tubular epithelial cells that have resorbed some of the excess lipids and lipoproteins in the urine (see Chapter 4, Fig. 3).

Severe nephrotic syndrome predisposes to thrombosis secondary to loss of hemostasis control proteins (e.g., antithrombin III, protein S, and protein C), infection secondary to loss of immunoglobulins, and, possibly, accelerated atherosclerosis because of the hyperlipidemia. Volume depletion and inactivity may increase the risk for venous thrombosis in nephrotic patients. In nephrotic patients with frequent bacterial infections, administration of intravenous γ globulin may be required.

Any type of glomerular disease can cause proteinuria. In fact, proteinuria is a very sensitive indicator of glomerular damage. All proteinuria, however, is not of glomerular origin. For example, tubular damage can cause proteinuria, but rarely more than 2 g/24 hr.

As noted in Table 2, some glomerular diseases are more likely to manifest the nephrotic syndrome than others, although virtually any form of glomerular disease may cause it. The two primary renal diseases that most often manifest as nephrotic syndrome are minimal change glomerulopathy and membranous glomerulopathy, and the two secondary forms of renal disease that most often manifest as nephrotic syndrome are diabetic glomerulosclerosis and amyloidosis.

Age has a major influence of the frequency of causes for the nephrotic syndrome. In children under 10-years-old, about 80% of the nephrotic syndrome is caused by minimal change glomerulopathy. Throughout adulthood, minimal change glomerulopathy accounts for only about 10 to 15% of primary nephrotic syndrome.

Membranous glomerulopathy is the most common cause for primary nephrotic syndrome in adults, but it accounts for less than 50% of cases. As shown in Fig. 8, a variety of glomerular diseases account for the remaining cases of nephrotic syndrome that are identified at the time of renal biopsy. The data in Fig. 8 are derived from patients with nephrotic range proteinuria who have undergone renal biopsy. The frequency of causes for the nephrotic syndrome that are not always examined by renal biopsy, especially diabetic glomerulosclerosis, are not accurately represented in Fig. 8.

Membranous glomerulopathy, (see Chapter 20) is most frequent in the fifth and sixth decades of life. It is characterized pathologically by numerous subepithelial immune complex deposits (Figs. 2, 5, and 6). The glomerular lesion evolves over time, with progressive accumulation of basement membrane material around the capillary wall immune complexes (Fig. 5) and eventual development of chronic tubulointerstitial injury in those patients with progressive disease. If the Heymann nephritis animal model is analogous to human disease, idiopathic (primary) membranous glomerulopathy may be caused by autoantibodies specific for antigens on visceral epithelial cells, which would allow immune complex formation in the subepithelial zone but not in the subendothelial zone or mesangium of glomeruli. In addition to the numerous subepithelial immune deposits, membranous glomerulopathy secondary to immune complexes composed of antigens and antibodies in the systemic circulation often has immune complex deposits in the mesangium, and may have small subendothelial deposits (Fig. 2). Thus, the ultrastructural identification of mesangial or subendothelial deposits should raise the level of suspicion for secondary membranous glomerulopathy, such as membranous glomerulopathy caused by a systemic autoimmune disease (e.g., lupus, mixed connective tissue disease, autoimmune thyroiditis), infection (e.g., hepatitis B or C, syphilis), or

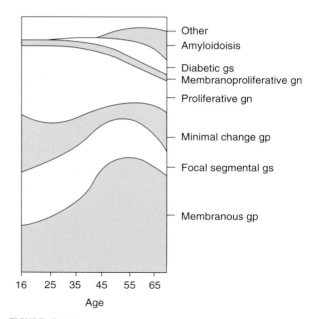

FIGURE 8 Diagram demonstrating the approximate frequency of different renal diseases in patients with the nephrotic range proteinuria who had renal biopsies that were evaluated in the University of North Carolina Nephropathology Laboratory. Note the variation in frequency with age. The proliferative glomerulonephritis category includes all forms of proliferative glomerulonephritis, including lupus nephritis, IgA nephropathy, IgM mesangial nephropathy, and others. gn, Glomerulonephritis; gp, glomerulopathy; gs, glomerulosclerosis. Reprinted with permission from Jennette JC, Mandal AK: The nephrotic syndrome. In: Mandal AK, Jennette JC (eds). *Diagnosis and Management of Renal Disease and Hypertension.* Carolina Academic Press, Durham, North Carolina, 1994.

neoplasm (e.g., lung or gut carcinoma). In very young and very old patients, the likelihood of secondary membranous glomerulopathy is greater, although still uncommon. Membranous glomerulopathy occurring in young patients raises the possibility of systemic lupus erythematosus or hepatitis B infection, and in very old patients raises the possibility of occult carcinoma.

Both type I and II membranoproliferative glomerulonephritis (MPGN), (see Chapter 18) typically manifest mixed nephrotic and nephritic features, sometimes accompanied by hypocomplementemia and C3 nephritic factor, which is an autoantibody against the C3 convertase of the alternative complement activation pathway. Both types often have glomerular capillary wall thickening and hypercellularity by light microscopy. Type I MPGN (mesangiocapillary glomerulonephritis) is characterized ultrastructurally by subendothelial immune complex deposits that stimulate subendothelial mesangial interposition and replication of basement membrane material, whereas type II MPGN (dense deposit disease) has pathognomonic intramembranous dense deposits (Fig. 3). Both types have extensive glomerular staining for C3 (Fig. 6), with type I having more immunoglobulin staining than type II. Type I

MPGN may be secondary to cryoglobulinemia, neoplasms, or chronic infections (e.g., hepatitis C and B, and infected prostheses, such as a ventriculoatrial shunt, chronic bacterial endocarditis, chronic mastoiditis.

When taken as a group, focal and diffuse proliferative glomerulonephritides account for a substantial proportion of patients who have nephrotic range proteinuria. Patients with proliferative glomerulonephritis and marked proteinuria usually also have features of nephritis, especially hematuria. Included in this group would be patients with lupus nephritis and IgA nephropathy who have nephrotic range proteinuria.

Amyloidosis as a cause for the nephrotic syndrome is most frequent in older adults (Fig. 8). Currently in the United States, amyloid causing the nephrotic syndrome is approximately 75% AL amyloid rather than AA. Approximately 75% of AL amyloid is composed of λ rather than κ light chain. Patients with κ light chain paraproteins and the nephrotic syndrome are more likely to have light chain deposition disease (i.e., nodular sclerosis without amyloid fibrils) rather than amyloidosis (see Chapter 29). Amyloid composition can be determined by immunofluorescence microscopy (Fig. 6). In less developed areas of the world, where chronic infections are more prevalent, AA amyloidosis is more frequent than AL amyloidosis.

CHRONIC GLOMERULONEPHRITIS AND END STAGE RENAL DISEASE

Most glomerular disease, with possible exceptions being uncomplicated minimal change glomerulopathy and thin basement membrane nephropathy, can progress to chronic glomerular sclerosis with progressive renal failure and eventually to end stage renal disease (ESRD). Chronic glomerular disease is the third leading cause of ESRD in the United States, following hypertensive and diabetic renal disease in frequency. Clinicopathologic studies of different glomerular diseases have revealed marked differences in their natural histories. Some diseases have high risk for rapid progression to ESRD unless treated, such as anti-GBM and ANCA crescentic glomerulonephritis. Other diseases have more indolent but persistent courses, with renal failure eventually ensuing in a significant number of patients, such as IgA nephropathy and focal segmental glomerulosclerosis. A few glomerulonephritides, for example, poststreptococcal glomerulonephritis, may initially manifest a rather severe nephritis, but usually resolve completely with little risk for progression to ESRD. And some diseases are very unpredictable, for example, membranous glomerulopathy, which may remit spontaneously, have persistent nephrosis for decades without renal failure, or progress over several years to ESRD.

Chronic glomerulonephritis is characterized pathologically by varying degrees of glomerular scarring, which is always accompanied by cortical tubular atrophy, interstitial fibrosis, interstitial infiltration by chronic inflammatory cells, and arteriosclerosis. As the glomerular, interstitial, and vascular sclerosis worsen, they eventually reach a point at which histologic evaluation of the renal tissue cannot reveal the initial cause for the renal injury, and a pathologic diagnosis of ESRD is all that can be concluded.

Clinically, chronic glomerulonephritis that is progressing to ESRD eventually results in uremia that must be managed by dialysis or renal transplantation. As the term implies, patients with uremia have accumulation of nitrogenous wastes (urea, uric acid, creatinine) in the blood. Other clinical manifestations of uremia include nausea and vomiting, hiccups, anorexia, pruritis, lethargy, pericarditis, myopathies, neuropathies, and encephalopathy.

RENAL BIOPSY: INDICATIONS AND METHODS

In a patient with renal disease, a renal biopsy provides tissue that can be used to determine the diagnosis, indicate the cause, predict the prognosis, direct treatment, and collect data for research, although not all potential applications are accomplished by every renal biopsy.

Renal biopsy is indicated in a patient with renal disease when all three of the following conditions are met: (1) the cause cannot be determined or adequately predicted by less invasive diagnostic procedures, (2) the signs and symptoms suggest parenchymal disease that can be diagnosed by pathologic evaluation, and (3) the differential diagnosis includes diseases that have different treatments, different prognoses, or both. Situations in which a renal biopsy serves an important diagnostic function include nephrotic syndrome in adults, steroid-resistant nephrotic syndrome in children, glomerulonephritis in adults other than clear-cut acute poststreptococcal glomerulonephritis or lupus nephritis, and acute renal failure of unknown cause. In some renal diseases for which the diagnosis is relatively definite from clinical data, a renal biopsy may be of value not only for confirming the diagnosis but also for assessing the activity, chronicity, and severity of injury; for example, in patients with suspected lupus nephritis. Although the diagnosis is strongly supported by positive serologic results in patients with anti-GBM and ANCA-glomerulonephritis, the extremely toxic treatment that is used for these diseases warrants the additional level of confirmation that a renal biopsy provides; and a renal biopsy also provides information about the severity and potential reversibility of the glomerular damage. Table 5 demonstrates the types of native renal disease that have prompted renal biopsy among the nephrologists who refer specimens to the University of North Carolina Nephropathology Laboratory. Approximately 80% of these biopsies were performed by nephrologists in community practice. Diseases that typically cause nephrotic syndrome were the most frequent impetus for biopsy, followed by diseases that cause nephritis.

Contraindications to percutaneous renal biopsy include an uncooperative patient, solitary kidney, hemorrhagic diathesis, uncontrolled severe hypertension, severe anemia or dehydration, cystic kidney, hydronephrosis, multiple renal arterial aneurysms, acute pyelonephritis or perinephric abscess, renal neoplasm, and end stage renal disease. Transjugular renal biopsy and wedge renal biopsy are advocated by some as safer procedures in patients with these risk factors.

TABLE 5

Frequency of Various Diagnoses among 7257 Renal Biopsies Evaluated in the University of
North Carolina Nephropathology Laboratory[a]

Diseases that often cause nephrotic syndrome (42%)	3067	Diseases that often cause hematuria and nephritis (29%)	2109
Idiopathic membranous glomerulopathy	847	Lupus nephritis (all classes)	636
Focal segmental glomerulosclerosis (FSGS)	768	IgA nephropathy	538
Minimal change glomerulopathy	398	Other immune complex proliferative GN	375
Diabetic glomerulosclerosis	246	Pauciimmune/ANCA GN	301
Type I membranoproliferative GN	190	Acute diffuse proliferative (postinfectious) GN	86
Mesangioproliferative GN	145	Thin basement membrane nephropathy	82
Amyloidosis	108	Anti-GBM GN	56
Clq nephropathy	99	Alport's syndrome	35
Collapsing variant of FSGS	87	Diseases that often cause chronic renal failure (8%)	583
Glomerular tip lesion variant of FSGS	65	Arterionephrosclerosis	229
Fibrillary GN	59	Chronic sclerosing GN	166
Light chain deposition disease	26	End stage renal disease	114
Type II membranoproliferative GN	14	Chronic tubulointerstitial nephritis	74
Preecalmpsia/eclampsia	6	Miscellaneous other diseases (3%)	199
Immunotactoid glomerulopathy	6	No pathologic lesion identified (2%)	141
Collagenofibrotic glomerulopathy	3	Adequate tissue with nonspecific abnormalities (5%)	370
Diseases that often cause acute renal failure[b] (5%)	371	Inadequate tissue for definitive diagnosis (6%)	417
Thrombotic microangiopathy (all types)	126		
Acute tubulointerstitial nephritis	101		
Acute tubular necrosis	69		
Atheroembolization	34		
Light chain cast nephropathy	31		
Cortical necrosis	10		

[a]Specimens with nonspecific abnormalities (e.g., interstitial fibrosis, tubular atrophy, glomerular scarring, arteriosclerosis), specimens with no identifiable pathologic abnormality (e.g., in a patient with asymptomatic hematuria), and some specimens with inadequate tissue for definitive diagnosis (e.g., a very small specimen with only a few glomeruli but with negative immunofluorescence microscopy) may never the less provide useful clinical information, especially with respect to ruling out diseases that were in the differential diagnosis. GN = glomerulonephritis.

[b]Other than glomerulonephritis.

Clinically significant complications of renal biopsy are relatively infrequent but must be kept in mind when determining the risk/benefit ratio of the procedure. Small perirenal hematomas that can be seen by imaging studies (e.g., ultrasound) are relatively common if looked for carefully. Gross hematuria occurs in <10% of patients, arteriovenous fistula in <1%, hemorrhage that requires surgery in <1%, and mortality in <0.1%.

Current percutaneous needle biopsy procedures usually employ localization of the kidney by real-time ultrasound guidance determination of kidney location and depth by ultrasound immediately prior to biopsy, or computed tomography (CT) guided localization of the kidney. Many varieties of biopsy needles have been used over the years, most of which are effective in experienced hands. Recently, there has been a major shift toward utilization of spring-loaded disposable gun devices.

Light microscopy alone is not adequate for the diagnosis of most native kidney diseases, although it may be adequate for assessing the basis for renal allograft dysfunction during the first few weeks after transplantation. All native kidney biopsies should be processed for at least light microscopy and immunofluorescence microscopy. Most renal pathologists advocate performing electron microscopy on all native kidney biopsies, but some believe that tissue for electron microscopy should be fixed as a contingency and electron microscopy performed only if the other microscopic findings suggest that it will be useful.

The needle biopsy core should be examined with a magnifying glass (e.g., 15×) or a dissecting microscope to confirm that renal tissue is present and to determine whether it is cortex or medulla. When gently prodded and pulled with forceps, adipose tissue is mushy and strings out, skeletal muscle tissue falls apart into little clumps, and renal tissue maintains a cylindrical shape. At 15× magnification, adipose tissue looks like clusters of tiny fat droplets (cells), skeletal muscle is red-brown with irregular fiber bundles, and renal tissue is pale pink-tan. Glomeruli in the renal cortex appear as reddish blushes or hemispheres projecting from the surface of the core. Straight red striations produced by the vasa recta are markers for the medulla. When there is extensive glomerular hematuria, the convoluted tubules in the cortex appear as red corkscrews. Once the tissue landmarks are identified, portions of tissue should be separated for processing for light, immunofluorescence, and electron microscopy.

In our experience with renal biopsy specimens sent to us from over 100 different nephrologists per year, most of whom are in private practice, approximately 6% of renal biopsy specimens are inadequate for a definitive diagnosis (Table 5). The most common inadequacy is renal tissue with too little or no cortex. This can be remedied by beginning the sampling procedure with the biopsy needle just barely into the outer cortex. Obviously, if the biopsy needle is inserted too deeply into or through the cortex, the specimen will contain only medulla. Even specimens that are considered inadequate for a definitive diagnosis may provide useful information. For example, in a patient with the nephrotic syndrome, a renal biopsy specimen that has no glomeruli for light or electron microscopy, but has one glomerulus that stains negative for immunoglobulins and complement by immunofluorescence microscopy, rules out any form of immune complex glomerulonephritis, such as membranous glomerulopathy, and focuses the differential diagnosis on minimal change glomerulopathy versus focal segmental glomerulosclerosis.

Bibliography

Appel GB: Renal biopsy: The clinician's viewpoint. In: Silva FG, D'Agati VD, Nadasdy T (eds) *Renal Biopsy Interpretation,* pp. 21–29. Churchill Livingstone, New York, 1996.

Bolton WK: Goodpasture's syndrome. *Kidney Int* 50:1753–1766, 1996.

Cameron JS: The nephrotic syndrome and its complications. *Am J Kidney Dis* 10:157–171, 1987.

Cameron JS: Nephrotic syndrome in the elderly. *Semin Nephrol* 16:319–329, 1996.

Cohen AH, Nast CC, Adler SG, Kopple JD: Clinical utility of kidney biopsies in the diagnosis and management of renal disease. *Am J Nephrol* 9:309–315, 1989.

Couser WG: Rapidly progressive glomerulonephritis: Classification, pathogenetic mechanisms, and therapy. *Am J Kidney Dis* 11:449–464, 1988.

Dische F, Parsons V, Taube D: Thin-basement-membrane nephropathy. *N Engl J Med* 320:1752–1753, 1989.

Feneberg R, Schaefer F, Zieger B, Waldherr R, Mehls O, Scharer K: Percutaneous renal biopsy in children: A 27-year experience. *Nephron* 79:438–446, 1998.

Galla JH: IgA nephropathy. *Kidney Int* 47:377–387, 1995.

Glassock RJ, Cohen AH: The primary glomerulopathies. *Disease A Month* 42:329–383, 1996.

Haas M, Spargo BH, Coventry S: Increasing incidence of focal-segmental glomerulosclerosis among adult nephropathies: A 20-year renal biopsy study. *Am J Kidney Dis* 26:740–750, 1995.

Jennette JC, Falk RJ: Diagnosis and management of glomerulonephritis and vasculitis presenting as acute renal failure. In: Mandal AK, Hebert LA (eds) *Medical Clinics of North America: Renal Failure and Transplantation,* pp. 893–908. Saunders, Philadelphia, 1990.

Jouet P, Meyrier A, Mal F, Callard P, Guettier C, Stordeur D, Trinchet JC, Beaugrand M: Transjugular renal biopsy in the treatment of patients with cirrhosis and renal abnormalities. *Hepatology* 24:1143–1147, 1996.

Mariani AJ, Mariani MC, Macchioni C, Stams UK, Hariharan A, Moriera A: The significance of adult hematuria: 1,000 hematuria evaluations including a risk–benefit and cost–effectiveness analysis. *J Urol* 141:350–355, 1989.

Niles JL, Bottinger EP, Saurina GR, Kelly KJ, Pan G, Collins AB, McCluskey RT: The syndrome of lung hemorrhage and nephritis is usually an ANCA-associated condition. *Arch Intern Med* 156:440–445, 1996.

Schena FP: Survey of the Italian Registry of Renal Biopsies. Frequency of the renal diseases for 7 consecutive years. The Italian Group of Renal Immunopathology. *Nephrology, Dialysis, Transplantation* 12:418–426, 1997

Tiebosch ATMG, Frederik PM, van Breda Vriesman PJC, Mooy JMV, van Rie H, van de Wiel TWM, Wolters J, Zeppenfeldt E: Thin-basement-membrane nephropathy in adults with persistent hematuria. *N Engl J Med* 320:14–28, 1989.

van der Loop FT, Monnens LA, Schroder CH, Lemmink HH, Breuning MH, Timmer ED, Smeets HJ: Identification of COL4A5 defects in Alports' syndrome by immunohitochemistry of skin. *Kidney Int* 55(4):1217–1224, 1999.

MINIMAL CHANGE DISEASE

NORMAN J. SIEGEL

TERMINOLOGY AND HISTOPATHOLOGY

Minimal change nephropathy or minimal change disease (MCD) is a histopathologic lesion which is almost always associated with the nephrotic syndrome at the onset of disease. Other terms such as lipoid nephrosis, nil disease, and idiopathic nephrotic syndrome have been used, interchangeably, with minimal change nephropathy.

Primer on Kidney Diseases, Third Edition

Minimal change disease is defined on light microscopy by a lack of definitive alteration in glomerular structure from that seen in normal patients. While the degree of alterations which may remove a biopsy from this category has been debated, it is generally agreed that the cellularity of the glomerulus must be minimal and that the tubular and interstitial structures must also be normal. There may be some doubly refractile appearance or lipid droplets in the tubule cells but there should be no evidence of tubular atrophy or interstitial fibrosis. Immunofluorescent staining also shows no change from normal and an absence of immunoglobulin or complement protein deposition. The most obvious and consistent finding in patients with MCD is a characteristic swelling of epithelial foot processes seen on electron microscopy (Fig. 1). Fenestration of the endothelial cells lining the capillary loop is normal. The glomerular basement membrane is uniform in thickness and structure, but the epithelial cells show swelling and a continuous layer of contact with the glomerular basement membrane. Because a biopsy is susceptible to sampling error, it must be remembered that lesions which affect only some glomeruli, such as focal and segmental glomerulosclerosis, may be inadvertently misdiagnosed as MCD.

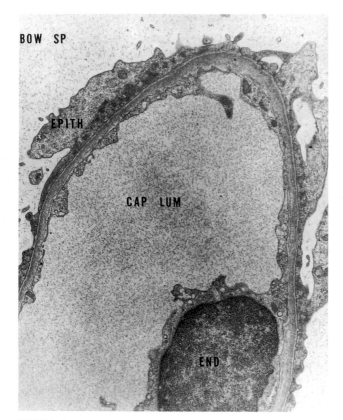

FIGURE 1 Electron micrograph of glomerular capillary loop in patient with MCD. The endothelial cell (End) and basement membrane are normal in content and structure. The epithelial cell (Epith) demonstrates diffuse swelling of the pseudopods, foot-process fusion. There are no electron dense deposits.

The role of a renal biopsy in the initial management of patients who present with nephrotic syndrome is controversial. In most cases, children are treated with a course of steroids, and biopsies are reserved for those who are steroid resistant. Because of their lower prevalence of steroid-responsive lesions, adolescents and adults are usually biopsied prior to treatment. In patients of any age with a complicated clinical presentation or course of disease, an assessment of histopathologic changes is recommended.

CLINICAL PRESENTATION

The pathogenesis of MCD is poorly understood. Although generally thought to be a childhood disease, MCD presents in both children and adults. The insidious onset of nephrotic syndrome, usually manifested by edema formation, is the most common presentation. In children, the onset of disease is after the first year of life, with a peak incidence between 24 and 36 months of age and a strong male predominance. In preadolescent children, 85–95% with idiopathic or primary nephrotic syndrome will have MCD. In adolescents and young adults, the prevalence of MCD declines to approximately 50%, and the male predominance begins to disappear. In patients over the age of 40 years with primary nephrotic syndrome, the incidence of MCD is 20–25%, and there is a nearly equal distribution between males and females.

In patients presenting with the typical features of MCD, a relatively "pure" nephrotic syndrome is usually observed. Nephritic features such as hypertension, hematuria, and reduced renal function are relatively uncommon. Any one of these features may occur in 15–20% of patients with MCD but the presence of two or more is decidedly unusual and should make one consider a different diagnosis. The finding of gross hematuria or red cell casts would generally not be considered to be compatible with the diagnosis of MCD. Thus, the predominant clinical features are those of nephrotic syndrome with heavy proteinuria, low serum albumin, edema formation, and elevated serum cholesterol. Other than the findings of oval fat bodies which appear as maltese crosses on examination of the urine under a polarized lens, the urinalysis is normal (see Chapter 4, Fig. 3). Serum complement levels are normal, and antinuclear antibodies and cryoglobulins are absent. Serum immunoglobulins may be abnormal with a reduction of serum IgG levels to 20% or less of normal values, a less severe reduction in IgA, and a mild increase in IgM and IgE levels.

Although MCD is usually associated with a primary or idiopathic nephrotic syndrome, secondary MCD also occurs (Table 1). In 80–90% of children, MCD is idiopathic although cases associated with the ingestion of heavy metals such as mercury or lead as well as acquired immunodeficiency syndrome have been reported. In adult patients, especially the elderly, the association of this MCD with nonsteroidal antiinflammatory drugs is particularly important because of their very frequent use. Hodgkin's disease and lymphoproliferative disorders must be kept in mind when older patients present with MCD. Although most patients with obesity and nephrotic syndrome have focal segmental

TABLE I

Secondary Causes of Minimal Change Nephropathy

Drugs
    Nonsteroidal antiinflammatory agents
    Ampicillin/penicillin
    Trimethadione

Toxins
    Mercury
    Lead
    Bee stings

Infection
    Mononucleosis
    HIV
    Immunizations

Tumors
    Hodgkin's lymphoma
    Other lymphoproliferative diseases
    Carcinoma

Obesity

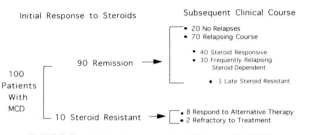

FIGURE 2 Clinical outcome for children with MCD.

glomerulosclerosis, some of these patients have responded to steroids or have been documented to have MCD.

RESPONSE TO THERAPY

The benchmark for therapy in MCD is the use of corticosteroids. No other cause of nephrotic syndrome is as exquisitely sensitive to treatment with steroid therapy as MCD. Because of the high prevalence of this lesion in children, disappearance of proteinuria in response to the oral administration of prednisone is considered diagnostic for MCD. Characteristically, these young children respond to treatment with a diuresis and clearing of proteinuria within about 2 weeks of initiation of prednisone therapy, usually at a dose of 2 mg/kg/day not to exceed 60 mg daily. Some children may have a slower response to initial therapy and not clear their proteinuria for 6 to 8 weeks. A response to therapy in 80–90% of adolescents and adults with MCD has also been documented. However, in these age groups, the response is slower and a prolonged period of therapy, in some cases up to 16 weeks, may be required before complete remission of proteinuria is achieved. In addition, adults more frequently develop a partial remission of proteinuria which is uncommon in children with MCD.

The clinical course of MCD is frequently described in terms of the response of the patient to steroids. Complete remission is defined as complete resolution of proteinuria for at least 3–5 consecutive days; a partial remission is a reduction in the degree of proteinuria without complete clearing, and a relapse is a reoccurrence of proteinuria for at least 3–5 consecutive days. The clinical outcome for children with MCD, as related to steroid therapy, is outlined in Fig. 2. About 10% of children initially treated with steroid therapy will not respond to treatment and will have early steroid resistance. Alternative methods of administration of steroids have been attempted in this group of patients, but have not been particularly successful. These patients frequently respond to

cytotoxic or immunosuppressive therapies. A similar, although not identical, pattern can be expected in adults. In adult patients, consideration for alternative initial therapy should be given in situations in which an underlying condition such as diabetes mellitus, hypertension, or osteoporosis may complicate steroid usage. In those circumstances, initial therapy with an alkylating agent may be preferred.

Of the patients who achieve a remission on initial steroid therapy, the vast majority, 75–85% experience one or more relapses (Fig. 2). Reports have suggested that prolonged treatment of the initial episode can reduce the incidence of subsequent relapses. In those patients who are destined to follow a relapsing course, the first relapse usually occurs within 6 to 12 months of the onset of their disease, although in some patients the first relapse may be delayed as long as 24–30 months. In patients with a relapsing course, 50–65% can be expected to have a steroid-responsive clinical profile with frequent relapses occurring over a 3- to 5-year period. However, for 25–30% of patients with MCD, a more protracted clinical course occurs, and their disease is described as being frequently relapsing or steroid-dependent. A small proportion of these patients may develop late steroid resistance at which point a repeat renal biopsy may show evolution to other histopathologic patterns such as focal segmental glomerular sclerosis. Thus, the majority of patients with MCD have a good response to initial steroid therapy, and a disease course characterized by relapses of their nephrotic syndrome but, overall, an excellent long-term prognosis.

Patients with frequently relapsing/steroid-dependent MCD present the greatest therapeutic challenge. In the long run, the relapsing nature of their disease is likely to disappear but, over the short term, deleterious side effects of continued steroid therapy may occur; particularly in adults and geriatric patients. To decrease the frequency of relapses, these patients may be treated with low doses of prednisone on a daily or alternate day basis without significant side effects. For those patients who require large doses of medication to remain in remission or who develop significant side effects, alternative therapy must be considered.

Cyclophosphamide and chlorambucil have proven to be the most effective alternative therapies for patients with MCD. These drugs have been shown to be effective in both children and adults with frequently relapsing/steroid-dependent nephrotic syndrome. Typically, prednisone will be used to induce remission, then an 8- to 12-week course of cyclophosphamide in a dose of 2 mg/kg/day or chlorambucil in a dose of 0.1–0.2 mg/kg/day will be added. The most pronounced and dramatic effect is the prolonged period of remission of the nephrotic syndrome which is achieved in patients treated with these agents. After cessation of the cytotoxic agent, 30–40% of patients will have no subsequent relapses. Among relapsers, the average period of remission is 18–24 months. Subsequent relapses are usually more steroid responsive than prior to cytotoxic therapy. Thus, steroid related side effects such as a cushingoid appearance, growth retardation in children, or abnormalities in bone metabolism can be markedly diminished and reversed. In patients who are intolerant of steroids, particularly adults, these agents may be used earlier in the clinical course than in children. These agents have a number of serious side effects which include cystitis, alopecia, leukopenia, gonadal toxicity, potential for malignancy formation, and seizures; their use requires caution and careful judgment.

Other medications have also been used for the treatment of patients with either steroid refractory or frequently relapsing/steroid-dependent disease. Cyclosporine has been reported to be effective in some adult and pediatric patients with an initial steroid resistant course. Its primary utility is to achieve a steroid-sparing effect since the relapse rate is high and prolonged remission is not sustained after cyclosporine is discontinued. Levamisole and mycophenolic acid have been used to achieve a steroid-sparing effect.

For patients unresponsive to these therapeutic interventions, symptomatic control of edema with the use of diuretics and a low salt diet are the mainstay of therapy. If complications of anasarca occur such as pleural or pericardial effusions, severe hyponatremia, or cellulitis, the infusion of albumin can be beneficial to mobilize the extracellular fluid and prevent pulmonary or cardiac decompensation. This therapy, however, should be undertaken with caution because the shifts in intravascular volume associated with albumin infusion can result in severe hypertension or congestive heart failure, particularly in children, and because the beneficial effect is short-term since the albumin is rapidly excreted in a patient with heavy proteinuria. Proteinuria can be reduced with nonsteroidal antiinflammatory drugs and angiotension converting enzyme inhibitors. These therapies may be of benefit in patients who are refractory to treatment of their nephrotic syndrome, have severe proteinuria, and are developing malnutrition because of the quantity of protein lost in the urine. However, the reduction in proteinuria in patients treated with either of these medications is, in large part, related to alterations in renal blood flow and glomerular filtration rate rather than a direct effect on the mechanisms of the proteinuria. Consequently, patients with MCD who are treated with either of these agents are particularly prone to the development of acute renal failure. While these drugs are generally well tolerated and may be beneficial in a selected subset of patients, the associated complications must be carefully monitored.

COMPLICATIONS AND LONG-TERM OUTCOME

The primary complications of MCD are related to persistent nephrotic syndrome or to side effects of therapy.

The most common complications of steroid therapy include cushingoid facies, stria, and acne as well as cataracts. However, steroid therapy is also associated with alterations in glucose, lipid, and bone metabolism, cosmetic appearance, and emotional stability. In general, these medications are much better tolerated in children than in adults. The induction of a prolonged remission by a cytotoxic agent permits regression of the majority of the steroid-related side effects. Stria and cataracts usually persist; however, catch-up growth in children frequently occurs and the cushingoid appearance disappears. Complications of cytotoxic agents are substantial but can be avoided with the careful dosing of these drugs, limitations of their use to short courses, and appropriate precautions such as adequate hydration. Indeed, in the majority of studies in children and adults, minimal side effects of either chlorambucil or cyclophosphamide have been reported, and the drugs have been well tolerated. One of the most disturbing side effects of cyclophosphamide therapy, gonadal toxicity, appears to be dose-related and reversible in the majority of young patients treated with this medication. For adult patients oligospermia and cessation of menses may occur during a course of treatment but are frequently reversible.

Peritonitis is an important complication of the nephrotic syndrome for those patients who are unable to achieve a remission of their proteinuria. Peritonitis occurs during periods of severe edema formation particularly when ascites is present. The most common infecting agent is *Streptococcus* pneumonia. However, infections with *Escherichia coli* and *Hemophilus* influenza have also been reported. Prior to antibiotic therapy, peritonitis was the major cause of death in children and adults with MCD.

Reversible acute renal failure has also been reported in patients with MCD. This complication appears to occur much more frequently in adult patients than in children. It usually develops in patients with severe edema formation and those who have been taking nonsteroidal antiinflammatory drugs or angiotensin converting enzyme (ACE) inhibitors. A period of rapid weight accumulation immediately precedes the onset of the renal failure. The pathophysiology of acute renal failure in patients with MCD is poorly understood and cannot be clearly related to intravascular volume depletion, acute tubular necrosis, or vascular obstruction such as renal vein thrombosis. In some cases, the combination of infusions of albumin and diuretics to reduce interstitial edema have been effective.

The development of chronic renal failure in patients with MCD is rare in children or adults with a steroid-responsive clinical course. Patients at highest risk are those who either do not have an initial response to steroid therapy or those who become late steroid nonresponders (Fig. 2). In both of these situations the possibility that the histopathologic lesion may be different or have evolved into a pattern different than MCD must be considered and may be the dominant factor in overall prognosis. For the majority of children the relapsing nature of their disease will begin to dissipate after about 10 years from onset, and the majority will be free of proteinuria after puberty. However, late relapses after long-term remissions of the nephrotic syndrome in patients who have had their initial episode at a very young age have been well documented. Similarly, adult patients with MCD have a very good prognosis with 85–90% survival rate 10 years or more after the onset of disease. The major morbidity is related to complications of therapy.

Bibliography

Berns JS, Gaudio KM, Krassner LS, Anderson FP, Durante D, McDonald BM, Siegel NJ: Steroid-responsive nephrotic syndrome of childhood: A long-term study of clinical course, histopathology, efficacy of cyclophosphamide therapy, and effects on growth. *Am J Kidney Dis* 9:108–114, 1987.

Habib R, Kleinknecht C: The primary nephrotic syndrome of childhood: Classification and clinicopathologic study of 406 cases. In: Sommers SC (ed) *Pathology Annual,* pp. 417–474. Appleton-Century-Crofts, New York, 1971.

International Study of Kidney Disease in Children: Nephrotic syndrome in children: Prediction of histopathology from clinical and laboratory characteristics at time of diagnosis. *Kidney Int* 13:159–165, 1996.

Nolasco F, Cameron JS, Heywood EF, *et al.*: Adult-onset minimal change nephrotic syndrome: A long-term follow-up. *Kidney Int* 29:1215–1223, 1986.

Schnaper HW, Robson AM: Nephrotic syndrome: Minimal change disease, focal glomerulosclerosis and related disorders. In: Schrier RW, Gottschalk CW (eds) *Diseases of the Kidney,* 6th Ed., pp. 1725–1780. Little, Brown, Boston, 1996.

Smith JD, Hayslett JP: Reversible renal failure in the nephrotic syndrome. *Am J Kidney Dis* 21:201–213, 1992.

Korbet SM: Management of Idiopathic nephrosis in adults, including steroid-resistant nephrosis. *Curr Opin Nephrol Hypertens* 4(2): 169–176, 1995.

Bargman JM: Management of minimal lesion glomerulonephritis: Evidence-based recommendations. *Kidney Int* 55:S3–S16, 1999.

18

MEMBRANOPROLIFERATIVE GLOMERULONEPHRITIS AND CRYOGLOBULINEMIA

GIUSEPPE D'AMICO AND ALESSANDRO FORNASIERI

The term membranoproliferative glomerulonephritis (MPGN) is employed to describe a histopathological entity characterized by intense glomerular hypercellularity, capillary loop thickening due to subendothelial or intramembranous deposits, and interposition of mesangial cells and matrix into the capillary loops which produces a double contour appearance to the basement membrane.

This entity includes both forms of unknown cause (idiopathic MPGN) and forms associated with systemic and infectious disorders (Table 1). Its morphologic pattern should be integrated within an etiologic context whenever possible.

IDIOPATHIC MPGN

Epidemiology

In Africa and Asia, "idiopathic" MPGN is a common disease, probably related to uncharacterized infectious or parasitic diseases. In the United States and in Europe, however, it is rare, and its incidence has declined over the past three decades. It occurs equally in males and females, and presents mainly in childhood.

Pathology

Two major and distinct categories of idiopathic MPGN have been identified, termed type I and type II. Type I is characterized by the presence of glomerular subendothelial deposits, associated with proliferation of mesangial cells and mesangial matrix expansion, moderate leukocyte infiltration, and duplication of the peripheral glomerular basement membrane (GBM), with a double contour appearance due to interposition of mesangial cells (and sometimes also monocytes) in the capillary wall. A more marked mesangial expansion, occluding the capillary lumina of

TABLE I
Classification of Membranoproliferative Glomerulonephritis

Primary
  Idiopathic MPGN

Secondary
  Infectious diseases
    Hepatitis C with type II mixed cryoglobulinemia
    Subacute endocarditis
    Infected ventriculoatrial shunt
    Malaria
    Schistosomiasis
  Systemic connective tissue disorders
    Systemic lupus erythematosus (SLE)
  Neoplasms
    Leukemia and lymphoma

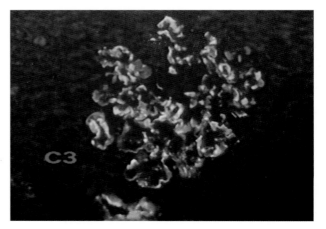

FIGURE 2 Type I MPGN. Immunofluorescence: Diffuse and intense mesangial and capillary loop deposits (C_3, × 250).

some loops, gives some cases a "lobular" pattern (Fig. 1). By immunofluorescence, deposition of IgM, IgG, C3, and sometimes also C1q and C4, in a granular capillary wall distribution, is seen (Fig. 2).

In type II, homogeneous dense deposits in many renal basement membranes (glomerular, tubular, and arteriolar) are the characteristic feature by electron microscopy (Fig. 3), and sometimes also by light microscopy. The immunofluorescence pattern is similar to that seen in type I, but only C3 stains the capillary wall.

A variant of type I MPGN, designated type III MPGN, has also been described. It is characterized by the simultaneous presence of subendothelial and subepithelial deposits associated with lamination and disruption of the lamina densa of GBM.

Pathogenesis

Three interrelated mechanisms contribute to the development of the morphological features of MPGN: (1) accumulation on the subendothelial side of the GBM (type I) or within the GBM (type II) of electron-dense deposits that are probably immune complexes (IC) in the first type and

deposits of undefined origin in the second, (2) mesangial proliferation involving both cells and matrix, with a tendency of the activated mesangium to expand the peripheral capillary walls and to extend into the subendothelial space, causing the specific splitting ("double contour" appearance) of the GBM, and (3) inflow of blood-borne inflammatory cells, mainly monocytes.

The accumulated experience with experimental models of chronic immune complex-induced GN and with humans, in whom IC deposit on the internal aspect of the GBM (chronic infectious diseases, systemic lupus erythematosus, cryoglobulinemia), suggests that deposits come first. The activation of the mesangium such that it expands to the periphery of capillary walls with cytoplasmic extensions that engulf the deposits, and the inflow of leukocytes are both secondary events. However, these two mechanisms of defense are not necessarily activated to the same extent. When the broad spectrum of lesions associated with protracted deposition of IC and complement is considered, sometimes (lupus, cryoglobulinemic GN, exudative variant

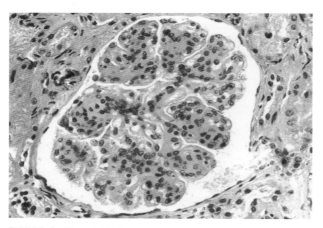

FIGURE 1 Type I MPGN. Marked mesangial proliferation with mesangial matrix expansion and pronounced lobulation of the glomerular tuft (Hematoxylin and eosin × 250).

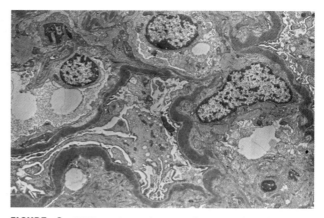

FIGURE 3 Diffuse dense intramembranous deposits within glomerular basement membrane. Some portions of glomerular basement membrane are preserved (original magnification: lead citrate, uranyl acetate, × 2800).

of idiopathic MPGN) the predominant mechanism of defense is the accumulation of monocytes and neutrophils in the subendothelial space. This is also responsible for the thickening and duplication of the GBM, with mesangial interposition being less evident. At the other end of the spectrum, as in the classic type I idiopathic MPGN, little or no cell influx occurs, and mesangial activation with peripheral interposition is the principal mechanism of defense.

It is possible that not only the amount, but also the nature and composition of the subendothelial deposits accounts for the endothelial damage and the prevailing cytokine-mediated activation of mesangium or inflammatory cells, mainly monocytes. It is also possible that the recruitment of monocytes and polymorphonuclear cells is the important mechanism when IC are deposited acutely on the subendothelial aspect of the GBM (see Cryoglobulinemic Glomerulonephritis), whereas mesangial activation and peripheral interposition are later, more chronic phenomena, favored by the cytokine-mediated stimulation of resident glomerular cells induced by the infiltrating monocytes. However, in some circumstances (cryoglobulinemic GN and some cases of idiopathic MPGN), monocyte infiltration can be demonstrated even in less acute stages of the disease, in the absence of evident mesangial interposition.

When IC are deposited on the internal side of the GBM, it can be postulated that mesangial interposition is a consequence of deposition of complement and immunoglobulins. The regression of the mesangial expansion when exogenous bacterial antigens are eliminated from the body, as in shunt nephritis, confirms this hypothesis. However, it is more difficult to explain mesangial interposition when no deposits are present or when such deposits stain only with complement, without accompanying immunoglobulins. It is possible that other mechanisms of injury of the capillary wall, especially if they induce endothelial cell damage and detachment from the basement membrane, may also eventually stimulate the accumulation of plasma proteins and the ingrowth of the mesangium in the resulting subendothelial space, independent of the presence of deposits.

A very characteristic feature, when the sequence of immunopathogenetic events described above (i.e., long-term accumulation of electron-dense deposits on the internal aspect of the GBM, recruitment of monocytes, and chronic mesangial activation with peripheral interposition) takes place, is the frequent coexistence of persistent hypocomplementemia. In idiopathic MPGN, the association with low complement levels is so frequent that this GN has also been called hypocomplementemic GN.

However, the cause of hypocomplementemia in idiopathic and secondary MPGN, its relationship to the pathogenesis, and its possible role in perpetuating the glomerular disease are still obscure. We also do not yet understand why in some cases (type II idiopathic MPGN) the activation of the alternative pathway predominates, whereas in other cases (type I idiopathic MPGN, lupus nephritis, cryoglobulinemic GN, shunt nephritis), there is activation of the classic pathway. Similary, it is unknown whether the hypocomplementemia is always a secondary phenomenon, derived from increased consumption triggered by subendothelial or intramembranous deposits, or whether it may precede such deposition and favor it, as proposed many years ago. To make things more complicated, hypocomplementemia per se does not appear to correlate with the clinical course of MPGN. Complement levels are not of value for monitoring the course or predicting the final outcome of MPGN. When persistently depressed, they can only be considered markers of this group of glomerular diseases.

It is now evident that hypocomplementemia can be ascribed to at least two mechanisms: (1) the activation of the classic pathway produced by circulating IC and (2) the presence in the blood of anticomplement autoantibodies, called nephritic factors (Nef). At least two nephritic factors have been described, one that acts on the amplification loop of the complement cascade (Nef_a) and another that acts on the terminal pathway (Nef_t). Activation of the classic pathway by circulating IC is probably the major mechanism responsible for hypocomplementemia in idiopathic type I MPGN, lupus nephritis, and shunt nephritis. Nef_a is probably the major mechanism responsible for the hypocomplementemia of type II idiopathic MPGN. However, nephritic factors are sometimes found in sera of patients of the former group, and hypocomplementemia may be multifactorial in origin. The classic pathway is activated in some. In others, the presence of the nephritic factors Nef_t or Nef_a better explains the abnormalities of the serum complement profile. In other words, different nephritic factors can be present in the same morphological type of MPGN, and the same nephritic factor can coexist in heterogeneous types of MPGN with quite different abnormalities of glomerular ultrastructure.

Clinical Features and Outcome

Idiopathic MPGN presents with nephrotic syndrome in more than 50% of cases, and with nonnephrotic proteinuria together with microscopic hematuria in another 20% of cases. Less marked urinary abnormalities occur in the remaining patients. An impairment of renal function, usually slowly progressive, is present in 20–25% of cases at presentation, while an acute nephritic syndrome, with rapid deterioration of renal function, usually associated with the presence of crescents at biopsy, characterizes the onset in less than 10% of patients. Arterial hypertension, sometimes very severe, is present in more than half of the patients. Hypocomplementemia is frequently, but not invariably noted at presentation. In type I MPGN, the classic pathway is preferentially activated (normal or low C_3, low C_4, and low CH_{50}). In type II, the alternative pathway is activated (low C_3, normal C_4, and low CH_{50}). With type III, C_3 is generally low, in association with a depression of terminal complement components (C_3–C_9).

The clinical course of idiopathic MPGN is characterized by spontaneous variation in severity of proteinuria and a variable rate of deterioration of renal function, with periods of prolonged remission in many patients (total remission being reported in 7–10% of patients), or episodes of acute deterioration of renal function. The few studies on the final outcome of the disease report renal survivals at 10 years after onset between 60 and 64%. These studies showed that an elevated serum creatinine, severe proteinuria, and arterial hypertension at presentation are the most significant clinical predictors of an unfavorable outcome, while the presence of marked tubulointerstitial lesions is the only significant histological sign of bad prognosis.

Treatment

The role of steroids or cytotoxic drugs in the treatment of idiopathic MPGN, both in children and adults, has remained controversial. In the absence of convincing controlled trials, in our opinion, the use of these drugs is not recommended. Cyclosporine and anticoagulants have been used in some studies, without beneficial results.

Antiplatelet drugs (aspirin and persantine) demonstrated a beneficial effect in a single trial in the United States. They are now commonly used as a long-term therapy, in part because they lack significant adverse effects.

As in all proteinuric diseases, ACE inhibitors should be administered, even in the absence of arterial hypertension, to reduce urinary protein loss. When patients are hypertensive, blood pressure should be treated aggressively.

CRYOGLOBULINEMIC GLOMERULONEPHRITIS

Mixed cryoglobulins (MC) are immunoglobulins that precipitate from cooled serum. They are composed of a polyclonal immunoglobulin G (IgG) bound to another immuno-globulin with rheumatoid factor (RF) activity (usually IgM). According to the classification of Brouet, two types of mixed cryoglobulins can be identified. In type II, the antiglobulin component is monoclonal (usually an IgM κ); in type III MC, it is polyclonal. The majority of MC, defined as "secondary mixed cryoglobulinemias," have been detected in patients with connective tissue disorders, lymphoproliferative disorders, noninfectious hepatobiliary diseases, or immunologically mediated glomerular diseases. Until recently, in 30% of all MC, the etiology was undetermined and cryoglobulinemia was termed essential. With the availability of new serological markers of hepatitis C virus (HCV) infection, it was recognized that nearly all these patients have antibodies against viral antigens and HCV RNA. This finding may explain why the prevalence of MC differs according to geographical area and is greater in countries such as in Italy, France, Spain, and Israel where HCV infection is endemic.

The clinical syndrome of MC is characterized by purpura, weakness, arthralgias and, in some patients, by glomerular involvement. This syndrome can be associated with both type II and type III MC, whereas renal involvement has a higher prevalence in type II MC with monoclonal IgM component (usually IgM κ). Although in the few reported cases of type III MC with renal involvement,

glomerular lesions were variable and nonspecific, in type II MC a specific and well-characterized pattern of glomerular lesions has been described.

Pathology

In most patients with type II MC a peculiar type of exudative membranoproliferative glomerulonephritis (MPGN) is found. Especially in its more acute stage, this "cryoglobulinemic glomerulonephritis" has distinctive features which differentiate it from idiopathic type I MPGN as well as lupus nephritis.

The glomeruli are markedly hypercellular, due to an evident infiltration of leukocytes, which are mainly monocytes (Fig. 4). The average number of infiltrating leukocytes is greater than in diffuse proliferative lupus nephritis. Electron microscopy demonstrates that these leukocytes are in close contact with endocapillary and subendothelial IC deposits, and contain phagolysosomes, indicative of their phagocytic function.

The intraglomerular deposits, which are commonly found in a subendothelial position, as is typical of all glomerulonephritides with the membranoproliferative pattern, may sometimes also fill the capillary lumen, especially in patients with an acute and rapidly progressive deterioration of renal function. Both these intraluminal deposits and the subendothelial deposits are eosinophilic, periodic acid–schiff (PAS)-positive, and usually amorphous. They are electron-dense and resemble IC. However, electron microscopic examination sometimes demonstrates a specific fibrillar or cylindrical structure identical to that seen in the *in vitro* cryoprecipitate of the same patients. These structures are 100 to 1000 μm long and have a hollow axis, appearing in cross sections like annular bodies (Fig. 5).

The peripheral interposition of mesangial matrix and mesangial cells between the GBM and the newly formed

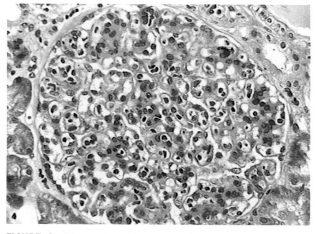

FIGURE 4 Glomerulus with prominent endocapillary hypercellularity, mainly due to massive infiltration of inflammatory mononuclear leukocytes. Mesangial cell proliferation and mesangial matrix expansion are mild (Masson trichrome × 250).

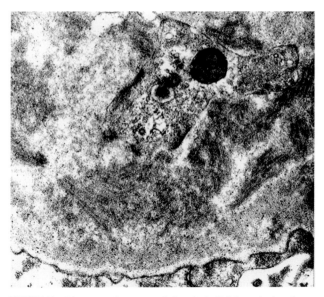

FIGURE 5 Electron microscopy: Subendothelial deposit showing a specific annular and cylindrical structure (original magnification × 22,000-Uranyl acetate and lead citrate. Courtesy of Dr. E. Schiaffino-Pathology Department S. Carlo Borromeo Hospital, Milan).

basement membranelike material, which accounts for the double contour appearance on stains that show basement membrane, is usually less evident than in other primary and secondary type I MPGN. This milder mesangial involvement may explain both why glomerular segmental and global sclerosis is less severe than in other types of idiopathic or secondary MPGN, even many years after the onset of the renal disease and why evolution toward renal failure with sclerosing nephritis is so rarely observed. In about 20% of cases, these distinctive features may be absent, and the histologic and immunohistologic picture at biopsy can be that of a type I lobular MPGN indistinguishable from that of idiopathic MPGN. Lobular MPGN is more likely to be found in patients with marked proteinuria associated with a moderate reduction in renal function without a rapidly progressive course. In these patients, when signs of systemic involvement due to mixed cryoglobulinemia, especially purpura, are mild or absent at the time of biopsy, only serological data, particularly detection of circulating cryoglobulins make a correct diagnosis possible.

The histologic features of MPGN with subendothelial deposits including the lobular type are found in about 80% of patients with HCV-associated type II mixed cryoglobulinemia and glomerular involvement. In the remaining 20% of cases, the biopsy at presentation (the clinical renal syndrome usually being characterized by mild urinary abnormalities) shows the histologic pattern of a mild mesangial proliferative GN, with moderate or no infiltration of leukocytes. A similar pattern may be observed after intensive immunosuppresive therapy.

At least one-third of patients with cryoglobulinemic GN have acute vasculitis of the small and medium sized renal arteries, which is characterized by fibrinoid necrosis of the arteriolar wall and infiltration of monocytes in and around the vessel wall. This renal vasculitis, which is sometimes associated with other signs of systemic vasculitis, including purpura and mesenteric vasculitis, can also be found in the absence of obvious glomerular involvement. Even when the fibrinoid necrosis of the renal arterial walls is severe, segmental necrosis of the capillary loops is never observed and crescentic extracapillary proliferation is rare, suggesting that the vasculitic damage is limited to arterial vessels of larger size.

In the case of MPGN with intraluminal deposits, immunofluorescence microscopy reveals intense staining with antisera directed against the immunoglobulins in the mixed cryoglobulins, namely, IgM, IgG, and C3, usually associated with faint irregular segmental subedothelial staining of some peripheral loops. In more chronic stages, when intraluminal deposits are absent, the pattern is that of intense diffuse, granular, subendothelial staining of peripheral loops, very similar to that of type I idiopathic MPGN.

Pathogenesis

It appears that hepatitis C virus directly infects circulating peripheral blood mononuclear cells and bone marrow cells in the majority of patients with types II and III MC, and even some patients without concomitant cryoglobulinemia, although the occurrence of viral replication within cells is still controversial. It has been hypothesized that HCV infection may stimulate the B lymphocytes to synthesize the cryoprecipitating polyclonal rheumatoid factors responsible for type III MC, but the factors that cause this shift are as yet uncharacterized. Factors potentially responsible include duration of the HCV infection as well as superimposed infection with other viruses, such as hepatitis B virus or Epstein–Barr virus. Clonal expansion of IgM-producing cells has been reported, and its reversibility after interferon α (IFN-α) therapy in some patients has also been documented. This hypothesis, which considers MC to be a benign lymphoproliferative disorder, may explain why overt B-cell malignancy occurs during its course in a minority of patients. The induction in mice of an MPGN very similar to human cryoglobulinemic GN by injecting solubilized type II mixed cryoglobulins from patients with this renal disease and HCV infection suggests a role of circulating cryoglobulins rather than host-specific factors in the pathogenesis of nephritis. The monoclonal IgM κ RF isolated from such mixed cryoglobulins is devoid of viral antigenic components. Nonetheless when injected separately into these animals, it was able to deposit in the glomerulus, suggesting a specific affinity of the IgM κ RF component of the cryoglobulins for some glomerular structure. Data demonstrate that the same purified IgM κ binds to cellular fibronectin, a known constituent of mesangial matrix. In contrast, purified monoclonal IgM from patients with Waldenström's macroglobulinemia as well as polyclonal IgM from patients with rheumatoid arthritis or polyclonal IgM from normal subjects lacks this affinity.

Host factors may be responsible for initiating disease once cryoglobulins are present; peripheral blood monocytes isolated from patients with cryoglobulinemic MPGN are less effective in removing cryoglobulins *in vitro* and release excess amounts of cathepsin D precursors in response to cryoglobulins. These cathepsin precursors could then be activated locally to induce tissue injury.

Thus, the prevalent pathogenetic mechanism seems to be the deposition in the glomerulus of a monoclonal IgM RF with particular affinity for the glomerular matrix. This IgM RF is produced by permanent clones of B lymphocytes infected by HCV. We do not yet know whether the IgM RF deposits in the glomerulus: (1) alone, with subsequent *in situ* binding of IgG (perhaps bound already to viral antigens); (2) as a mixed IgG–IgM cryoglobulin, not bound to HCV antigens; or, (3) as a complex composed of HCV antigens, IgG anti-HCV antibodies, and IgM κ RF. Demonstration of HCV RNA or virus antigens in glomeruli has remained elusive, and only recently have specific HCV-related proteins been detected in glomerular and tubulointerstitial vascular structures by indirect immunohistochemistry. Evidence that immune complexes containing intact virion are the main component of the glomerular deposits is scanty, while complexes containing HCV capsular antigens cannot be excluded.

Clinical Features and Outcome

Cryoglobulinemic GN is a disease of individuals in the fifth and sixth decade of life. Extrarenal symptoms include purpura, arthralgias, leg ulcers, systemic vasculitis, Raynaud's phenomenon, and peripheral neuropathy. Renal symptoms are usually a late manifestation of type II MC, and they typically do not appear until a few years after the extrarenal signs. However, the simultaneous appearance of renal and systemic signs of the disease is rather frequent. In some patients, renal involvement may be the main manifestation of the disease, before the appearance of the more suggestive purpura.

The most frequent renal syndrome is isolated proteinuria with microscopic hematuria, sometimes associated with signs of moderate chronic renal failure or, less frequently, proteinuria in the nephrotic range. The corresponding histologic picture is that of MPGN, although patients with isolated urinary abnormalities occasionally present with the nonspecific findings of mild segmental mesangial proliferation.

An acute nephritic syndrome, characterized by macroscopic hematuria, severe proteinuria, hypertension, and rapid development of azotemia is present at the onset of renal disease in 25% of cases, and is complicated by acute oliguric renal failure in 5%. In these individuals, the biopsy shows the typical cryoglobulinemic GN, that is, a severe MPGN characterized by intense monocyte infiltration and massive intraluminal deposits filling many capillary lumens. Hypertension is very frequent (more than 80%) at the time of presentation with renal disease, even in patients without the nephritic syndrome. Hypertension is often severe and difficult to control.

The renal disease has a variable course. In nearly one-third of patients, a remission of renal symptoms, partial or complete, has been described, even if an acute nephritic syndrome or severe nephrotic syndrome was present. Remission after acute nephritic syndrome may occur before any treatment is started, and is associated with the disappearance of the massive intraluminal deposits which characterize this disorder. In another third of patients, the renal disease is indolent, taking several years to progress to renal failure, in spite of the persistence of urinary abnormalities. In 20% of patients, reversible clinical exacerbations, such as nephritic syndrome occur, sometimes associated with flare-ups of systemic signs of the disease. The new episodes of nephritic syndrome can be accompanied by recurrence of massive intraluminal deposits and monocyte infiltration. Repeated exacerbations may occur in a single patient. A moderate degree of renal failure, if not already present at clinical onset, frequently develops at later stages. Terminal renal failure requiring dialysis is relatively rare, even after many years of cryoglobulinemic GN. In the large series of patients with cryoglobulinemic GN studied in Milan, only 15% required regular dialysis after a mean follow up of 131 months. Of these 105 patients, 42 patients died during the period of follow up because of extrarenal complications. Cardiovascular disease (12 patients), infections (nine patients), liver failure (eight patients), and neoplasms, usually of hematological origin (four patients) were the most important causes of death. The 10-year probability of being alive without dialysis was 49%. Older patients and patients with recurrent purpura, high serum cryocrit, low serum C3 levels, and high serum creatinine at presentation were more like to die or to reach end stage renal failure.

The amount of circulating cryoglobulins may vary between patients, and in the same patient over time. These laboratory parameters do not correlate with the degree of activity of the disease, but higher cryoglobulin concentrations appear to be associated with a poor prognosis. The serum complement pattern demonstrates characteristic abnormalities in cryoglobulinemic GN. Concentrations of the early complement components (C1q, C4) and CH50 are usually greatly reduced; C4 can be undetectable. Variably, a moderate decrease in the level of C3 is also observed. Consumption of the early serum complement components, with characteristic sparing of C3, may be attributable to a change in the C4-binding protein that controls activity of classic pathway C3 convertase. Serum complement values do not change very much with clinical evolution of the disease. In addition, RF can be detected, and the Waaler Rose test is usually positive. Serum protein elecrophoresis frequently shows a monoclonal band (IgM κ), and in some cases a monoclonal light chain (usually κ) is evident in the urine.

Treatment

Before the recognition of the etiologic role of HCV infection, when most cryoglobulinemia was considered "essential," acute flare-ups of the renal disease were treated with glucocorticoids, plasmapheresis, and frequently also with cyclophosphamide. High-dose steroid therapy, including initial treatment with intravenous boluses of methylprednisolone (0.5–1.0 g/day), was useful for controlling acute exacerbations of the disease associated with a rapidly progressive deterioration of renal function, especially when given in combination with plasmapheresis and cyclophosphamide. The former was used to remove circulating cryoglobulins during stages of massive deposition in the glomeruli and vessel walls and the latter to limit vasculitic injury and inhibit production of monoclonal RF by the B lymphocytes. Despite the potential of these modalities to increase viral titers, no consistent evidence of a detrimental effect on hepatic disease accompanied their use. Oral steroids were also used, at lower doses, to control the systemic signs of mixed cryoglobulinemia.

With recognition of the association between cryoglobulinemic GN and HCV infection, the rationale for treatment of the systemic disease and its renal complication has shifted to use of antiviral therapy. Interferon α (IFN-α), has become the most extensively employed antiviral agent. Despite its frequent use, the efficacy of IFN-α in cryoglobulinemic GN is still controversial. The three controlled trials that used IFN-α were performed in patients with clinically active mixed cryoglobulinemia associated with HCV infection, but without clearly established renal involvement.

Based on these trials and a review of the literature on IFN-α treatment of patients with HCV infection (with or without mixed cryoglobulinemia and cryoglobulinemic GN), the following conclusions can be drawn:

Sustained virologic response (defined as undetectable serum HCV RNA levels 6 months after completion of treatment) is obtained in no more than 15–20% of patients after an initial 12 months course of IFN-α at the standard dose of 3 million units three times a week.

More intensive treatment courses of IFN-α (6–10 million units three times a week, or each day for the first 4–6 weeks) give only marginally better results.

Combined treatment with IFN-α at the standard dose and ribavirin (1000–1200 mg/day), for at least 6 months, increases the sustained virologic response to 40–45% of patients.

Sustained virologic response to IFN-α, alone or in combination with ribavirin, interrupts the progression of the hepatic damage, and can control the clinical signs of the renal complications in less severe cases, but it does not prevent progression of the renal damage in the presence of the acute exacerbations of cryoglobulinemic GN (characterized by an acute nephritic syndrome with rapidly developing renal insufficiency or a nephrotic syndrome with slower deterioration of renal function), usually associated with recurrence of the systemic signs of mixed cryoglobulinemia. Combination therapy with the inflammatory and cytotoxic drugs, used in the past, is still necessary. In this clinical setting, our current policy is to give:

IFN-α: 3–5 million units three times/week for 6–12 months.
Ribavirin: (1000–1200 mg/day) for 6 months.
Steroids: Methylprednisolone (0.75–1.00 g/day intravenous for three consecutive days), followed by oral prednisone for 6 months (0.5 mg/kg of body weight/day, tapered over a few weeks until small maintenance doses of 10 mg/day or 20 mg/alternate days are achieved).

In the most severe cases, especially if signs of systemic and renal vasculitis are present, we add:

Cyclophosphamide: 2 mg/kg of body weight/day, for 2–4 months
Plasmapheresis: exchanges of 3 L of plasma three times a week, for 2–3 weeks

A controlled trial is needed to verify that the benefits of the addition of steroids and cyclophosphamide outweigh their potential to increase infectious or hepatic complications.

Bibliography

Agnello V, Chung RT, Kaplan LM: A role for hepatitis C virus infection in type II cryoglobulinemia. *N Engl J Med* 327: 1490–1495, 1992.

Brouet JC, Clauvel JP, Danon F, Klein M, Seligman M: Biological and clinical significance of cryoglobulins. A report of 86 cases. *Am J Med* 57:775–778, 1974.

Cacoub P, Lunel Fabiani F, Musset L, Perrin M, Franguel L, Leger JM, Huraux JM, Piette JC, Godeau P: Mixed cryoglobulinemia and hepatitis C virus. *Am J Med* 96:124–132, 1994.

Cameron JS, Turner DR, Heaton J, Williams DG, Ogg CS, Chantler C, Haycock GB, Hicks J: Idiopathic mesangio-capillary glomerulonephritis: Comparison of type I and II in children and adults and long-term pronosis. *Am J Med* 74:175–192, 1983.

D'Amico G: Influence of clinical and histological feature on actuarial renal survival in adult patients with idiopathic IgA nephropathy, membranous nephropathy, and membranoproliferative glomerulonephritis: Survey of the recent literature. *Am J Kidney Dis* 20:315–323, 1992.

D'Amico G, Ferrario F: Mesangiocapillary glomerulonephritis. *J Am Soc Nephrol* 2:S159–S166, 1992.

Dammacco F, Sansonno D, Han JH, Shyamaia V, Cornacchiulo V, Iacobelli AR, Lauletta G, Rizzi R: Natural interferon-α versus its combination with 6-methyl-prednisolone in the therapy of type II mixed cryoglobulinemia: A long-term, randomized, controlled study. *Blood* 84:3336–3343, 1994.

Ferri C, Marzo E, Longobardo G: Interferon-α in mixed cryoglobulinemia patients: A randomized, crossover-controlled trial. *Blood* 81:1132–1136, 1993.

Fornasieri A, Armelloni S, Bernasconi P, Li M, Pinerolo de Septis C, Sinico RA, D'Amico G: High binding of immunoglobulin Mk rheumatoid factor from type II cryoglobulins to cellular fibronectin: A mechanism for induction of *in situ* immune complex glomerulonephritis? *Am J Kidney Dis* 27:476–483, 1996.

Habib R, Kleinknecht C, Gubler MC, Levy MC: Idiopathic membranoproliferative glomerulonephritis in children. Report of 105 cases. *Clin Nephrol* 1:194–214, 1973.

Habib R, Gubler M-C, Loirat C, Ben Maiz H, Levy M: Dense deposit desease: A variant of membranoproliferative glomerulonephritis. *Kidney Int* 7:204–215, 1975.

Holley KE, Donadio JV: Membranoproliferative glomerulonephritis. *In* Tisher CC, Brenner BM (eds) *Renal Pathology: Clinical and Functional Correlates*, pp. 294–329. Lippincott, Philadelphia, 1994.

Johnson RJ, Gretch DR, Couser WG, Alpers CE, Wilson J, Chung M, Hart J, Willson R: Hepatitis C virus-associated glomerulonephritis. Effect of α-interferon therapy. *Kidney Int* 46:1700–1704, 1994.

Meltzer M, Franklin EC, Elias K, McCluskey RY, Cooper N: Cryoglobulinemia: A clinical and laboratory study. II Cryoglobulins with RF activity. *Am J Med* 40:837–856, 1966.

Meyers KEC, Strife CF, Witzleben C, Kaplan BS: Discordant renal histopathologic findings and complement profiles in membrano-proliferative glomerulonephritis type III. *Am J Kidney Dis* 28:804–810, 1996.

Misiani R, Bellavita P, Fenili D, Vicari O, Marchesi D, Sironi PL, Zilio P, Vernocchi A, Massazza M, Vendramin G, Tanzi E, Zanetti A: Interferon α-2a therapy in cryoglobulinemia associated with hepatitis C virus. *N Engl J Med* 330:751–756, 1994.

Tarantino A, De Vecchi A, Montagnino G, Imbasciati E, Mihatsch MJ, Zollinger HU, Barbiano di Belgioioso G, Busnach G, Ponticelli C: Renal disease in essential mixed cryoglobulinemia. Long-term follow-up of 44 patients. *Q J Med* 50:1–30, 1981.

Tarantino A, Campise M, Banfi G, Confalonieri R, Bucci A, Montoli A, Colasanti G, Damilano I, D'Amico G, Minetti L, Ponticelli C: Long-term predictors of survival in essential mixed cryoglobulinemic glomerulonephritis. *Kidney Int* 47: 618–623, 1995.

West CD, McAdams AJ: Paramesangial glomerular deposits in membranoproliferative glomerulonephritis type II correlate with hypocomplementia. *Am J Kidney Dis* 25:853–861, 1995.

FOCAL SEGMENTAL GLOMERULOSCLEROSIS

GERALD B. APPEL AND ANTHONY VALERI

Focal segmental glomerulosclerosis (FSGS) is a clinical and histopathologic entity with a pattern of glomerular injury which may be idiopathic or secondary to a number of etiologies (see Table 1). The most common manifestation is proteinuria which may range from minor amounts to nephrotic levels. FSGS accounts for only 7–20% of cases of idiopathic nephrotic syndrome in children, but as many as 35% of cases in adults. Recent studies performed at several large institutions have documented an increased incidence of FSGS in biopsies of adult patients that is especially noteworthy among nephrotic patients. FSGS is the most common pattern of idiopathic nephrotic syndrome among African-Americans, and in some series it is now the most common pattern among all races. Untreated idiopathic FSGS frequently progresses to end stage renal failure (ESRD). Patients with remissions of nephrotic range proteinuria typically have improved renal survival. However, the ideal type and duration of immunosuppressive therapy as well as adjunctive therapy for idiopathic FSGS remains controversial.

PATHOLOGY

The histopathologic diagnosis of FSGS depends on identifying areas of glomerular scarring in some glomeruli (focal lesions) in only some parts of the glomerular tufts (segmental lesions) (Fig. 1). In addition, fusion or effacement of foot processes is found to some extent in all of the glomeruli including those unaffected by areas of segmental sclerosis. The diagnosis of "idiopathic" FSGS on renal biopsy requires the absence of lesions of other types of focal glomerulonephritis that could heal as focal sclerosing lesions and the absence of immune complex deposition by electron microscopy (EM). Focal areas of IgM and C3 localization isolated to the areas of segmental sclerosis are felt to result from entrapment of immunoglobulin and complement components rather than from true immune complex deposition. The remainder of the glomerular tuft and the glomeruli unaffected by glomerulosclerosis typically have some degree of foot process effacement noted by EM, but they do not have evidence of immune complex deposition by immunofluorescence (IF). Although large amounts of proteinuria and uniform foot process fusion may be present, biopsies taken early in the course of FSGS, when renal function is still normal, show few glomeruli with segmental sclerosing lesions and almost no global sclerosis. At a later stage, as renal function deteriorates, many glomeruli will show segmental or global sclerosis. Some investigators feel the segmental sclerosing lesions are initially present in the juxtamedullary glomeruli and spread outward with time to involve the rest of the renal cortex. Interstitial fibrosis is also a common finding in biopsies with significant glomerulosclerosis. The mechanisms of this damage are unclear but may relate to changes in the postglomerular circulation, absorption of filtered proteins and lipoproteins across tubular epithelia, or incitement of cytokine and growth factors by abnormally filtered substances.

TABLE I

Etiologies of Focal Sclerosis

Primary idiopathic
    Focal segmental glomerulosclerosis
    Variants of minimal change disease
        IgM nephropathy
        Diffuse mesangial hypercellularity
    Variants of FSGS
        Glomerular tip lesion
        Collapsing FSGS
Secondary
    Unilateral renal agenesis or dysplasia
    Renal ablation—remnant kidney
    Sickle cell disease
    Morbid obesity (with or without sleep apnea)
    Congenital cyanotic heart disease
    Heroin nephropathy
    HIV nephropathy
    Aging kidney
    Reflux nephropathy
    Healed focal proliferative or necrotizing GN

The presence of increased tubulointerstitial damage correlates with a poor renal prognosis.

Several variants of FSGS deserve comment. The glomerular tip lesion is characterized by swelling, vacuolation, and proliferation of epithelial cells and later sclerosis and hyalinosis in the segment of the glomerulus adjacent to the origin of the proximal tubule. The remainder of the glomerulus has changes similar by light microscopy (LM) and EM to those seen in minimal change nephrotic syndrome. Another variant of FSGS is associated with focal or global glomerular capillary collapse and sclerosis with visceral epithelial cell swelling similar to that seen in HIV glomerulopathy. This so-called "collapsing" or "malignant" variant of glomerulosclerosis is more common in African-Americans and has a distinctive and more ominous clinical course than other forms of idiopathic FSGS. In addition, there are a number of le-

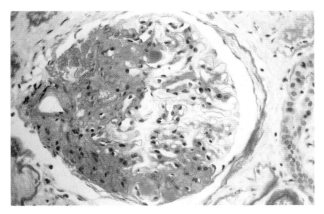

FIGURE I Glomerulus from a patient with focal segmental glomerulosclerosis showing perihilar sclerosis with adhesion to Bowman's capsule (periodic acid–Schiff stain, ×300). Courtesy of Dr. J.C. Jennette.

sions often considered variants of minimal change nephrotic syndrome which may evolve into FSGS, including IgM nephropathy (a picture of minimal change by LM but with IF positivity for IgM and EM mesangial dense deposits), and diffuse mesangial hypercellularity (mild proliferation of cells limited to the glomerular mesangium).

PATHOGENESIS

The pathogenesis of idiopathic FSGS, by definition, is unknown. Some patients who initially appear on biopsy to have minimal change disease evolve into FSGS on repeat biopsy over time. While the initial biopsy in some of these patients may have missed segmental lesions present in only a few juxtamedullary glomeruli, other patients with repeated relapses of the nephrotic syndrome and serial renal biopsies seem more convincingly to have experienced evolution of the lesion. Moreover, all the glomeruli in classic FSGS have fusion of foot processes and are responsible for the proteinuria. As in minimal change nephrotic syndrome, the loss of the charge barrier of the glomerular capillary wall may allow negatively charged albumin to pass through the altered capillary wall into Bowman's space. These alterations appear to be in response to a circulating permeability factor which promotes *in vitro* the permeability of glomeruli to albumin and other plasma proteins. The presence of this permeability factor, which appears to be a 50 kDa anionic protein which is not an immunoglobulin, has been used to predict the rapid development of recurrent proteinuria in the allograft of some FSGS patients who reach ESRD and undergo transplantation. Moreover, some patients with recurrent FSGS in the allograft respond to plasmapheresis or use of a protein absorption column with a reduction in proteinuria.

The proteinuria in FSGS is often less selective than in minimal change disease (vide infra), implying leakage of larger macromolecules through "larger pores" in the glomerular basement membrane. Drug-induced minimal change lesions in some animals (e.g., puromycin nephrosis, adriamycin nephrosis) can develop a picture of FSGS with nonselective proteinuria. In one such model the lifting off of the visceral epithelial cells from the glomerular basement membrane has been correlated with the nonselective proteinuria.

The pathogenesis of the sclerosing lesions and their progressive nature is also debated. Humans with idiopathic FSGS or remnant kidney FSGS initially have a high glomerular filtration rate (GFR) and evidence of hyperfiltration, suggesting that hyperfiltration and increased intracapillary glomerular pressure may be mediators of FSGS. Likewise, patients with glomerulomegaly, as seen in remnant kidneys or due to obesity or hypoxemia in sleep apnea, also have a high incidence of the nephrotic syndrome and FSGS. FSGS without increased glomerular capillary pressure or glomerulomegaly may relate to hyperlipidemia or intraglomerular coagulation.

It is possible and even likely that the pattern of FSGS seen on biopsy represents a common pathway for a number of distinct entities with different pathogenetic mechanisms and clinical courses.

CLINICAL FEATURES

Most patients with idiopathic FSGS present with either asymptomatic proteinuria or the full nephrotic syndrome. In children 90% present with the nephrotic syndrome as opposed to only 60–75% of adults. The 10–30% with asymptomatic, subnephrotic, proteinuria are most commonly detected in children by routine pediatric checkups, and camp or sports physicals; in adults detection of asymptomatic cases occurs most often at military induction examinations, routine gynecologic or obstetric checkups, and insurance or employment physicals. Patients with the nephrotic syndrome present with edema.

Hypertension is found in 30–50% of children and adults with FSGS. Microscopic hematuria is found in 45–55% of these patients, and a decreased GFR is noted at presentation in from 20 to 30%. Daily urinary protein excretion ranges from less than 1 g to 20–30 g/day. Proteinuria is typically nonselective, that is, it contains not only albumin but also higher molecular weight proteins as well. Nevertheless, albumin still comprises the largest component of the urine protein. Complement levels and other serologic tests are normal. Occasional patients will have glycosuria, aminoaciduria, phosphaturia, or a concentrating defect indicating tubular damage as well as glomerular injury.

DIAGNOSIS

The diagnosis of FSGS requires a renal biopsy. Early on, only a minority of the glomeruli will have segmental sclerosing lesion. Even these lesions may show a predilection for the juxtamedullary region of the kidney, so the renal biopsy may look identical to that of minimal change nephrotic syndrome. This is especially likely when a very superficial biopsy contains only a small number of glomeruli. Likewise, a small sample of glomeruli in a biopsy in an older adult may show some glomeruli identical to minimal change disease and one or two globally sclerotic glomeruli. They may be the result of FSGS or merely the obsolescent glomeruli that are found in the kidneys of older individuals due to the aging process. The finding of tubulointerstitial damage in such biopsies should suggest the possibility of unobserved scarred glomeruli and FSGS, but in neither situation can the diagnosis of FSGS be firmly established. Clinically, patients thought to have a minimal change pattern nephrotic syndrome with a poor response to corticosteroids or other immunosuppressive agents are likely to have FSGS. The biopsy may also provide clues to a secondary form of FSGS. In heroin nephropathy there is often more severe tubulointerstitial disease than in idiopathic FSGS. In HIV nephropathy there is often a collapsing variant of glomerulosclerosis with global rather than segmental involvement, and tubuloreticular inclusions are commonly found on EM. In patients with remnant kidneys and hyperfiltration-induced FSGS there is often less effacement of the foot processes than in idiopathic FSGS.

THERAPY AND OUTCOME

Although variable in the individual patient, the course of untreated FSGS is usually one of progressive proteinuria and declining GFR. Patients with asymptomatic proteinuria typically develop the nephrotic syndrome over time. Only a small minority of patients (5–10%) experience a spontaneous remission of proteinuria or the nephrotic syndrome. Both children and adults have a similar course, most develop ESRD 5–20 years from presentation. Several features which have been associated with a more rapid progression to renal failure in idiopathic FSGS include the presence of nephrotic range proteinuria (>3–3.5 g/day as opposed to asymptomatic proteinuria of <3–3.5 g/day), massive proteinuria (>10–15 g daily), a higher serum creatinine at time of biopsy (>1.3 mg/dL), and more tubulointerstitial damage on renal biopsy. Patients with the collapsing variant (or so-called malignant FSGS) will have a more rapid course to ESRD over 2–3 years as well.

Idiopathic FSGS may recur in the transplanted kidney with severe proteinuria and the nephrotic syndrome. Patients who present with more severe degrees of proteinuria, a more rapid course to renal failure, or those who have lost a prior allograft to recurrent FSGS are at greater risk for recurrence in the allograft.

The therapy of FSGS remains controversial with few randomized, controlled trials on which to base judgment. In general, those patients with a sustained remission of proteinuria and the nephrotic syndrome are unlikely to progress to ESRD, while those with unremitting nephrotic syndrome are likely to have progression. In most studies reported before 1980 only 10 to 30% of patients appeared to respond to a course of corticosteroids with a remission of proteinuria. Moreover, only a low response rate to other immunosuppressive agents such as azathioprine, cyclophosphamide, and chlorambucil was recorded, and the relapse rate after treatment was also high. As a result most American nephrologists considered FSGS to be unresponsive to therapy and did not advocate immunosuppressive treatment.

A seminal Canadian study in 1987 noted that 44% of children with FSGS responded to immunosuppressive therapy with a remission of proteinuria. Although the response rate for *treated* adults was similar (39%) to the treated children, most adults did not receive any immunosuppressive therapy. Other studies of the use of immunosuppressives in FSGS have confirmed initial response rates of 25–60%. In children, 20–25% will have a complete remission with a short course of corticosteroids, and up to 50% will remit with a more prolonged course of treatment. A collaborative Italian study (in adults) using much longer courses of prednisone, cyclophosphamide, and/or azathioprine found 60% of FSGS patients to have a complete remission of the nephrotic syndrome. Those patients with a complete remission had an excellent long-term renal survival without the occurrence of ESRD. An uncontrolled trial in children using combined pulse steroids and long-term immunosuppression with corticosteroids and cytotoxics has also found a 60% complete remission rate and a 16% partial remission rate of the nephrotic syndrome and a low rate of progression to renal failure. An American study of over 50 nephrotic adults with nephrotic syndrome due to FSGS also showed a better than 50% response rate as well as long-term improvement in renal survival in the steroid treated group. The median duration of steroid treatment in FSGS to achieve a complete remission is 3–4 months with most patients responding by 6 months. Thus, initial therapy should be at least 4–6 months of daily or alternate day steroids which may be tapered along the course of treatment. Although there are few trials using cytotoxic and other immunosuppressives in steroid resistant or dependent FSGS, some have been successful. The duration of therapy with cyclophosphamide and other agents necessary to achieve remission may lead to untoward side effects.

Several trials have used low-dose cyclosporine (4–6 mg/kg/day for 2–6 months) to treat steroid resistant FSGS patients. Three trials have had complete plus partial remission rates of 60 to >70% with use of cyclosporine versus 17–33% in the placebo group. The largest of these studies, The North American Collaborative Study of Cyclosporine in Nephrotic Syndrome is a double-blinded, randomized, placebo controlled trial in steroid resistant FSGS using low-dose cyclosporine and low-dose prednisone for 6 months. It found 12% complete remission and >70% complete and/or partial remission with the use of cyclosporine despite the fact that some FSGS patients were also even unresponsive to cytotoxic agents. While there is some potential for increased renal damage from the cyclosporine itself, the trial found that cyclosporine treatment resulted in less progression to renal failure and worsening of the GFR than did the placebo group. There are only sparse anecdotal data on the use of other agents such as tacrolimus and plasmapheresis to treat FSGS in native kidneys. Mycophenolate mofetil has been tried with varied success in several small series.

At the present, the ideal regimen to treat idiopathic FSGS is unknown. Many clinicians would not use immunosuppressives to treat patients with subnephrotic levels of proteinuria and little damage on their renal biopsies since these patients have a very favorable prognosis. Adjunctive therapy with angiotensin converting enzyme (ACE) inhibitors and/or angiotensin II receptor blockers to reduce proteinuria and its side effects, and other measures as suggested for patients with secondary FSGS should be used. For patients at increased risk of renal failure such as those with nephrotic range proteinuria, elevated serum creatinines, and interstitial scarring on biopsy, many would treat with a prolonged course (6–9 months) of daily or every other day corticosteroids (starting with 60 mg of prednisone daily or 120 mg every other day and tapering to lower doses after several months) or other immunosuppressive medication in the hopes of inducing a remission of the nephrotic syndrome and preventing eventual ESRD.

For patients with secondary forms of FSGS, treatment of the primary etiology, although rarely possible, is the first step in management. There have been patients with FSGS secondary to obesity and heroin nephropathy who have had remissions of proteinuria after weight reduction, or cessation of drug use, respectively. Use of ACE inhibitors or angiotensin II receptor blockers is probably beneficial. Immunosuppressive medications have not been proven to be consistently effective in any form of secondary FSGS. In those patients with either primary idiopathic or secondary forms of FSGS who remain nephrotic, control of fluid retention and edema can be managed with salt restriction and diuretics. In addition, attention should be given to control of hypertension with antihypertensive medication, control of hyperlipidemia with diet and antihyperlipidemic medications, and perhaps to prevention of hyperfiltration with low protein diets.

Bibliography

Arturo M, Sharma R, Savin VJ, Vincenti F: Plasmapheresis reduces proteinuria and serum capacity to injure glomeruli in patients with recurrent focal glomerulosclerosis. *Am J Kidney Dis* 23:574–581, 1994.

Banfi G, Moriggi M, Sabadini E, Fellin G, D'Amico G, Ponticelli C: The impact of prolonged immunosuppression on the outcome of idiopathic focal-segmental glomerulosclerosis with nephrotic syndrome in adults. *Clin Nephrol* 36:53–59, 1991.

Barisoni L, Valeri A, Radhakrishnan J, Nash M, Appel GB, D'Agati V: FSGS: A 20 years epidemiologic study. *J Am Soc Nephrol* 5:347, 1994.

Briggs WA, Choi MJ, Gimenez LF, Scheel PJ: Treatment of primary glomerulonephritis with mycophenolate mofetil. *J Am Soc Nephol* 9:84(A), 1998.

Cattran D, Appel GB, Hebert LA, Hunsicker LG, Pohl MA, Hoy WE, Maxwell DR, Kunis CL: A randomized trial of cyclosporine in patients with steroid-resistant focal segmental glomerulosclerosis. *Kidney Int* 56:2220–2226, 1999.

D'Agati V: Nephrology forum. The many masks of FSGS. *Kidney Int* 46:1223–1241, 1994.

Dantal J, Bigot E, Bogers W, Testa A, Kriaa F, Jacques Y, Hurault De Ligny B, Niaudet P, Charpentier B, Soulillou JP: Effect of plasma protein absorption on protein excretion in kidney transplant recipients with recurrent nephrotic syndrome. *N Engl J Med* 330:7–14, 1994.

Detwiler RK, Falk RJ, Hogan SL, Jennette JC: Collapsing glomerulopathy: A clinically and pathologically distinct variant of FSGS. *Kidney Int* 45:1416–1424, 1994.

Feld S, Figueroa P, Savin V, Nast CC, Sharma R, Sharma M, Hirschberg R, Adler SG: Plasmapheresis in the treatment of steroid-resistant FSGS in native kidneys. *Am J Kidney Dis* 32:230–237, 1998.

Haas M, Meehan SM, Karrison TG, Spargo BH: Changing etiologies of unexplained adult nephrotic syndrome: A comparison of renal biopsy findings from 1976–1979 and 1995–1997. *Am J Kidney Dis* 30: 621–631, 1997.

Korbet S: Primary focal segmental glomerulosclerosis. *J Am Soc Nephrol* 9:1343–1340, 1998.

Korbet SM, Genchi R, Borok RZ, Schwartz M: The racial prevalence of glomerular lesions in nephrotic adults. *Am J Kidney Dis* 27:647–651, 1996.

Lieberman KV, Tejani A, for the NY–NJ Pediatric Nephrology Study Group: A randomized double-blind placebo-controlled trial of cyclosporine in steroid resistant FSGS in children. *J Am Soc Nephrol* 7:56–63, 1996.

Pei Y, Cattran D, Delmore T, Katz A, Lang A, Rance P: Evidence suggesting under-treatment of adults with idiopathic focal segmental glomerulosclerosis. *Am J Med* 82:938–944, 1987.

Ponticelli C, Rizzoni G, Edefonti A, Altieri P, Rivolta E, Rinaldi S, Ghio L, Lusvarghi E, Gusmano R, Locatelli F, Pasquali S, Castellani A, Casa-Alberighi OD: A randomized trial of cyclosporine in steroid-resistant idiopathic nephrotic syndrome. *Kidney Int* 43:1377–1384, 1993.

Radhakrishnan J, Wang MM, Matalon A, Cattran D, Appel GB: Mycophonlate mofetil treatment of idiopathic FSGS. *J Am Soc Nephrol* 10:114(A), 1999.

Savin VJ, Artero M, Sharma R, Sharma M, et al.: Circulating factor associated with increased glomerular permeability to albumin in recurrent focal segmental sclerosis. *N Engl J Med* 334: 878–882, 1996.

Tune BM, Kirpekar R, Sibley RK, Reznik VM, Griswold WR, Mendoza SA: Intravenous methylprednisolone and alkylating agent. Therapy of prednisone-resistant pediatric FSGS: A long-term follow-up. *Clin. Nephrol* 43:84–88, 1995.

Valeri A, Barisoni L, Appel GB, Seigle R, D'Agati V: Idiopathic collapsing FSGS: A clinicopathologic study. *Kidney Int* 50:1734–1746, 1996.

20

MEMBRANOUS NEPHROPATHY

DANIEL C. CATTRAN

Membranous nephropathy remains the most common histologic entity associated with adult onset nephrotic syndrome. This histologic pattern is more properly called nephropathy than nephritis since there is rarely any inflammatory response in the glomeruli or interstitium (i.e., no nephritis). In 70 to 80% of membranous glomerulopathy (MGN) cases the etiological agent is unknown, and the disorder is termed idiopathic. In the other 20 to 30% a defined agent can be determined, and the disease is categorized as secondary (see Table 1).

This list of known causes is not complete but gives an indication of the variety of disorders that have been seen in association with this histologic pattern. In many cases such as hepatitis B or thyroiditis, the specific antigen has been identified as part of the immune complex within the deposits in the glomeruli. In others, the association is less well defined, but the designation remains because treatment of the underlying condition or removal of the putative agent results in disappearance of the clinical and histologic features of the disease.

The renal manifestations of both the primary and secondary types are very similar by clinical, laboratory, and histologic features, and hence a careful initial history, with attention to potential secondary causes is necessary as is ongoing vigilance because the causative agent may not be obvious for months to years after presentation. This histologic pattern is rare in children and when found, careful and repeated screenings, especially for immunologically mediated disorders such as systemic lupus erythematosus (SLE), is necessary. In the older patient, neoplasms become the most common cause of secondary MGN. There are also marked geographic differences in etiology. In Europe and North America, by far the most common etiological designation is idiopathic, but infectious agents account for a higher percentage in other geographic areas for instance in Africa, malaria, and in the Far East, hepatitis B.

CLINICAL FEATURES

Membranous nephropathy presents in 60 to 70% of cases with features associated with the nephrotic syndrome, including edema, heavy proteinuria, hypoalbuminemia, and hypercholesterolemia. The other 30 to 40% of cases present with asymptomatic proteinuria, usually in the subnephrotic range of ≤3.5 g/day detected on urine testing completed as part of a routine physical examination or an insurance policy requirement. The majority of patients present with normal glomerular filtration rate, that is, a normal serum creatinine and creatinine clearance, but about 10% will have renal insufficiency. The urine sediment is often bland, but 30–40% will have microhematuria and 10–20% will have granular casts. Hypertension is uncommon at presentation, occurring in only 10 to 20% of cases. The clinical features associated with nephrotic range proteinuria in membranous nephropathy can be very severe. The patient almost always has ankle swelling, but ascites

TABLE I
Secondary Causes of Membranous Nephropathy

Etiology	Examples
Neoplasm	Carcinomas (especially solid organ tumors of the lung, colon, breast, and kidney) leukemia, lymphoma (non-Hodgkin's)
Infections	Malaria, hepatitis B and C, secondary or congenital syphilis, leprosy
Drugs	Penicillamine, gold
Immunological	Systemic lupus erythematosus, mixed connective tissue disease, thyroiditis, dermatitis herpetiformis
Postrenal transplant	Recurrent disease, *de novo* membranous nephropathy
Miscellaneous	Sickle cell anemia

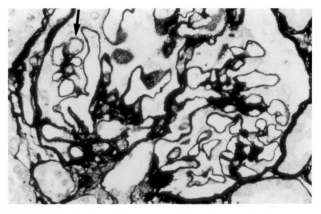

FIGURE 2 Classic spike pattern along glomerular basement membrane (GBM) as it grows around deposits (arrow) (PASM × 400).

pleural, and rarely pericardial effusions may also be present. Complications of this disorder include thromboembolic phenomena and hyperlipidemia. Renal vein thrombosis has been found in between 10 and 30% of cases at some time during the course of this disorder, and subsequent embolic events from this and other origins have been reported in up to 30% of patients. Secondary hyperlipidemia is also common and is characterized by both an increase in total and low density lipoproteins (LDL) cholesterol and often a decrease in high density lipoproteins (HDL). This is a profile known to be associated with accelerated atherogenesis.

PATHOLOGY

Idiopathic

In early membranous nephropathy, the glomeruli appear normal by light microscopy. Increasing size and number of immune complexes in the subepithelial space produce a thickening and apparent straightening or stiffening of the normally lacey looking glomerular basement membrane on light microscopy (Fig. 1). As the complexes accumulate there is also new basement deposition around the deposits producing the classic "spike" pattern on light microscopy (Fig. 2). On immunofluoresence microscopy these immune complexes stain most commonly with antihuman IgG and complement (Fig. 3). This produces a beaded appearance along the glomerular basement membrane pathognomonic of membranous nephropathy. In the most extreme cases, this beading can become so intense that careful examination is required to distinguish it from a linear pattern. On electron microscopy, these deposits are determined to be in the subepithelial space (Fig. 4). A classification system has been developed based on their specific location; stage I is when the deposits are located only on the surface of the glomerular basement membrane (GBM) in the subepithelial location, stage II when the deposits are partially surrounded by new basement membrane, stage III when

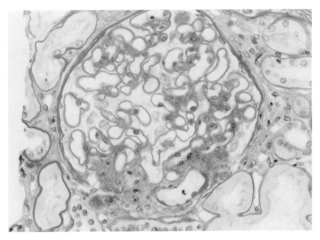

FIGURE 1 Glomerulus from a patient with membranous nephropathy. Capillary walls are diffusely thickened and there is no increase in mesangial cells or matrix (PAS × 250).

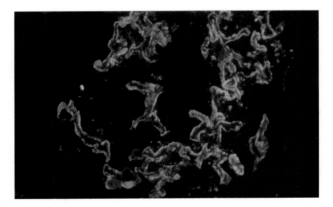

FIGURE 3 Glomerulus with diffuse granular capillary wall staining with anti-IgG antibody (immunofluorescence microscopy × 250).

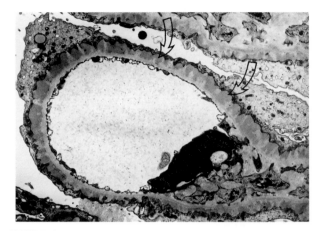

FIGURE 4 Electron photomicrograph of capillary loop with multiple election dense deposits along subepithelial side of GBM (arrows) (×7500).

they are incorporation into the basement membrane, and stage IV when the capillary walls are diffusely thickened but rarefaction (lucent) zones are seen in intramembranous areas previously occupied by the deposits. Unfortunately the clinical and laboratory correlation with these stages is poor. In some cases the pattern appears as if there had been waves of complex deposition with all of the above stages seen in the same patient while in others they appear as if there had been a continuous deposition of complexes with each deposit growing in size over time producing lesions that are all the same stage.

A specific etiology cannot usually be determined by standard pathology. A hint that there is a specific underlying cause can sometimes be suspected. In a patient with SLE for instance, more mesangial cell proliferation and increased matrix formation may be present, and on immunofluorescence staining all the immunoglobulins rather than just IgG may be seen. In rare cases, a specific cause can be confirmed by the use of antibody staining for the suspected causative agent. An example would be the finding of the carcinoma embryonic antigen in the glomeruli of a patient with bowel cancer.

PATHOGENESIS

The precise pathogenesis of human membranous nephropathy is still unclear. In experimental animal models, lesions identical to human MGN have been produced using known antigens by a variety of techniques. However, the identification of the causative antigen in the majority of human cases has remained elusive. The complexing of antigen and antibody in the subepithelial space is unique because the binding occurs on the urinary side of the glomerular basement membrane. The subsequent activation of complement and cytokine factors is therefore reduced because the reaction site is remote from the bloodstream. The reduced response produces a lesion that looks benign on microscopy, that is, no inflammatory cells in the glomeruli or interstitium. The detection and amount of the terminal complement attack component C5b through 9 complex in the urine (because complement activation occurs in the urinary space) has been reported to mirror prognosis and therapeutic efficacy. This has yet to be confirmed in prospective studies in humans.

It is possible that there are susceptibility genes and-genes associated with the more progressive variants, but both are probably polygenic traits, and the effect of hereditary factors versus environmental ones remain largely undetermined.

DIAGNOSIS

Membranous nephropathy is a diagnosis based on histology. The idiopathic designation is made by exclusion. Secondary membranous nephropathy is usually diagnosed by careful history, physical, and laboratory examinations aided by features on pathology. The great majority of cases in the 20- to 55-year old age range are idiopathic. In patients that have clinical features suggestive of a secondary cause, investigations should include the appropriate screening tests such as a complement profile, assays for antinuclear antibodies, rheumatoid factor, hepatitis B surface antigen and hepatitis C antibody, thyroid antibodies, and cryoglobulins. Although idiopathic MGN remains the most common cause in all age groups, a malignancy has been found in association with it in up to 20% of cases presenting over the age of 60. Patients in this category should have a focused history and physical looking for an occult tumor. Laboratory tests should include a chest X ray, examination for occult blood in the stools and perhaps mammography in women and a prostate specific antigen assay in men. The precise cost benefit of this additional screening in the absence of symptoms remains controversial.

TREATMENT OF SECONDARY TYPES

In the secondary types, attention should be focused on removing the putative agent or treating the underlying cause. If this can be done successfully both the histopathology and the clinical manifestations will largely resolve with time.

NATURAL HISTORY AND TREATMENT OF IDIOPATHIC MGN

The natural history of Idiopathic membranous glomerulopathy nephropathy (IMGN) has been documented in several studies and must be understood before considering specific treatment. Overall spontaneous remissions occur in 20 to 30% of IMGN patients and progressive renal failure develops in 20 to 40% of cases. In the remaining patients, mild to severe proteinuria persists through 5 to 10 years of observation. A summary review of 11 large studies demonstrated a 10-year renal survival between 65 and 85%, and a more recent pooled analysis of 32 reports indicated a 60% 15-year renal survival. Complicating the understanding of the natural history is that IMGN often follows a spontaneous remitting and relapsing course.

Spontaneous complete remission rates have been reported in between 20 and 30% of long-term (>10 years) follow-up studies with 20 to 50% of these cases having at least one relapse. A complete remission and a reduction in relapse rate are more common in those patients with persistent low grade (subnephrotic) proteinuria and in females. In contrast, male gender, age greater than 50, high levels of proteinuria (>6 g/day), abnormal renal function at presentation, and tubulo-interstitial disease on biopsy have all been associated with a poor outcome.

PREDICTING OUTCOME

A semiquantitative method of predicting outcome has been developed and validated. It utilizes the clinical parameters of proteinuria and creatinine clearance estimates over fixed periods of time. In its simplest form it demonstrated that the overall accuracy of predicting outcome when proteinuria values over 6 month time frames were persistently ≥4 g/day was 71%, when ≥6 g/day was 79%, and when ≥8 g/day was 84%. If the patient had a below normal creatinine clearance at the beginning of these periods or deteriorating function during the 6 months of observation, the odds of progressing were even higher. The advantages of the algorithm are its reliance on standard measurements of renal function and its dynamic nature, that is, the risk can be calculated and recalculated over time. The issues of age, gender, degree of sclerosis, and hypertension are relevant but are not required in this model because they do not add to its predictive ability.

It is on this natural history background that our current therapies must be evaluated. One helpful framework would be to establish risk of progression categories based on the above algorithm. We could then examine the entry laboratory data of the major clinical trials and segregate the patients into these risk groups. The balance of benefits of treatment to risk both of progression and of medication would then be easier to assess. This is important because most of our current immunosuppressive routines have potentially significant adverse effects, and these are often the overriding concern of both physicians and patients.

RISK OF PROGRESSION CATEGORIES

1. Low risks of progression patients have normal serum creatinine and creatinine clearance values and proteinuria <3.5 g/day.
2. Medium risk patients have normal or near normal creatinine and creatinine clearance values and persistent proteinuria over 6 months of ≥3.5 g/day to <6 g/day.
3. High risk patients include those with moderate to high grade proteinuria (≥6 g/day) persistent over 6 months plus creatinine values either above normal or rising during the observation period. Additional features in this group may include hypertension and interstitial disease or glomerular obsolescence on renal biopsy.

TREATMENT

Treatment can be considered in four broad categories

A. Immunosuppressive therapy aimed at slowing or stopping the immune mediated component of the disease.
B. Nonspecific, nonimmunosuppressive therapy to reduce proteinuria and perhaps secondarily slow the progression of the renal failure.
C. Treatment of the secondary effect of the disease on other systems.
D. Treatment aimed at reducing the complications of the immunosuppressive drugs.

Specific Immunosuppression Treatment

Low Risk of Progression Patients

The prognosis of patients with this level of proteinuria and function [Asymptomatic proteinuria (≤3.5 g/day with normal renal function)] is excellent. In a series of over 300 cases from three distinct geographical regions followed for more than 5 years, less than 8% went on to develop renal insufficiency. Normalization of the blood pressure and reduction of the protein excretion through the use of agents such as angiotensin converting enzyme inhibitors should be utilized. Since the percentage that progresses is not zero, long-term follow-up should include regular measurements of blood pressure and renal function, including protein excretion. Immunosuppression therapy is not recommended provided the patients remain in this low risk category.

Medium Risk of Progression Patients

Corticosteroids such as prednisone alone have been shown to be ineffective in inducing remission of proteinuria in all controlled trials done to date, and in preventing progression in all but one study. Although the follow-up periods were limited to less than 4 years and the dose and duration of corticosteroid treatment varied, it is generally held that these drugs alone should not be used in IMGN treatment. This view is supported by a meta-analysis of studies using this agent.

There is evidence for a benefit when corticosteroids are combined with a cytotoxic agent. In a series of randomized trials from Italy, a significant increase in both partial and complete remission in proteinuria and a reduction in the frequency of renal failure were seen at 10 years after an initial 6-month course of corticosteroids and chlorambucil. Therapy consisted of 1 g of methylprednisolone IV on the first 3 days of months 1, 3, and 5 followed by 27 days of oral methylprednisolone at 0.4 mg/kg alternating in months 2, 4, and 6 with chlorambucil at 0.2 mg/kg/day. This therapeutic routine has been compared by this same group to placebo, to methylprednisolone alone, and to cyclophosphamide substituted for chlorambucil. In their first study comparing the chlorambucil/prednisone routine to no treatment, 40% of untreated patients reached end stage renal disease compared to only 8% of treated patients after 10 year. Proteinuria also improved with the non-nephrotic state maintained during 58% of the follow-up time in the treatment group compared to 22% in the control group. When this routine was compared to methylprednisolone alone there was a significant initial benefit in the combination treated patients but this was nonsignificant by the end of 4 years of follow-up. The original regimen was remarkably safe with only four out of 42 treated patients stopping therapy. All adverse events were reversed after stopping the drugs. When cyclophosphamide, 2.5 mg/kg/day orally, was substituted for chlorambucil and compared to their original regimen, similar results in terms of complete and partial remission rates of proteinuria were seen. However, a substantial relapse rate of approximately 30% was seen within 2 years in both treated groups. Fewer patients had to discontinue their cyclophosphamide (5%) compared to the chlorambucil (14%). Renal function was equally well preserved in both groups for up to 3 years. These results are in contrast to other uncontrolled studies where cyclophosphamide alone has been used. These authors found the frequency of remission was similar to untreated patients.

High Risk of Progression Patients

This group includes those with initial renal insufficiency or persistent high grade proteinuria. The percentage of IMGN patient in this category is small, and very few have been the subject of randomized controlled trials. In a subgroup analysis of patients with initial renal insufficiency from one of the corticosteroid alone trials, there was no difference in the rate of deterioration over 4 years of follow-up between the treated and the control group. One small uncontrolled trial using pulse methylprednisolone for 5 days followed by a tapering dose of prednisone did show initial stabilization in 15 patients with renal failure and IMGN but at follow-up, two had died and five had gone on to end stage renal disease, suggesting only a transient benefit. These data would indicate that corticosteroids alone are not efficacious in slowing the progression rate in this type of patient. Three groups have used a modification of the Italian regimen (prednisone alternating monthly with chlorambucil) in patients with membranous nephropathy and progressive renal insufficiency. In a total of 34 patients approximately 50% showed sustained improvement in renal function, but the adverse effects rate was high even with the appropriate reduction in dosage of chlorambucil. Cyclophosphamide combined with pulse methylprednisolone and oral prednisone has been compared to alternate day prednisone alone in a randomized trial in IMGN patients with documented renal disease progression. It failed to show any significant benefit of the addition of the cytotoxic agent.

The use of cyclosporine in patients with severe disease unresponsive to other immunosuppressive routines has been reported. Early uncontrolled studies suggested an initial benefit but a high relapse rate. In a randomized controlled trial, cyclosporine was compared to placebo in patients with high grade proteinuria and documented progressive deterioration in renal function. It showed a significant reduction in proteinuria in the eight treated patients compared to the eight untreated patients which was sustained for up to 2 years in 50% of cases. As well, the rate of progression as measured by the slope of creatinine clearance was slowed compared to the predrug period by >60% during treatment. This drug is expensive and has substantial nephrotoxic potential. Monitoring for this and other adverse events must be part of any routine that includes this agent.

Two smaller nonrandomized trials have shown a benefit to long-term oral cyclophosphamide with and without prednisone. However, the risks of prolonged cytotoxic therapy such as infertility, infection, and cancer were significant and have limited this approach.

In this category there may be the rare case where deterioration in filtration occurs during the 6-month observation period, and specific treatment and therapy directed toward secondary effects of the disease may need to be started early.

Nonimmunological Treatment

Other nonspecific measures to reduce proteinuria and perhaps slow the rate of renal disease progression have been studied. Although dietary protein restriction has never been associated with a complete remission of the nephrotic syndrome, it does have its biggest impact in reducing proteinuria and slowing progression in patients with the highest grades of proteinuria. Certainly many IMGN patients fulfill this criterion. Blood pressure reduction has also been shown to reduce proteinuria, and drugs of the angiotensin converting enzyme inhibition class have produced improvement in this area beyond that expected by their antihypertensive action alone. This additional benefit has been demonstrated in IMGN patients, but the studies have been small, uncontrolled, and with limited follow-up. The mechanism underlying this action is not fully understood, but it is not solely related to a reduction in the intraglomerular pressure from lowering systemic hypertension. The effect on progression has also been examined using these conservative measures. Stabilization of function may occur because the decrease in tubular reabsorption of proteinuria reduces interstitial toxicity. Patients with IMGN have been included in these studies but not as the sole subjects, and it is therefore difficult to determine a specific benefit in this glomerular disease category.

Treatment of the Secondary Effects of the Disease

In addition to efforts to reduce proteinuria and prevent renal failure, attention must be paid to the associated hyperlipidemia and the increased risks of thromboembolism in patients with IMGN. Patients with the nephrotic syndrome have elevated serum cholesterol and triglycerides and normal or low levels of HDL and increased LDL. This lipidemia probably plays a role in the increased risk of cardiovascular disease, in patients with prolonged high grade proteinuria. Although no trial has been conducted to determine if cholesterol lowering reduces the risk of cardiovascular disease in such patients many clinicians apply evidence from nonrenal patients to advocate the use of HMG CO-A reductase inhibitors in patients with IMGN and persistent high grade proteinuria.

Studies of the risk of thrombotic disease in IMGN have shown a wide variation in prevalence partly related to the rigor of screening (all patients versus selection of high risk groups) and partly to the detection methods used. Deep venous thrombosis in a review were reported in 11%, clinically significant pulmonary emboli in 11%, and renal vein thrombosis in 35% of IMGN patients. Certainly if these figures of thromboembolic events are viewed in the light of data from patients receiving anticoagulants in other populations the benefits would appear to outweigh the risks. However, other studies have reported a lower incidence rate and a higher than average risk to long-term anticoagulant therapy given the hypoalbuminemic state. No consensus has emerged whether prophylactic anticoagulation should be used in this disease. The majority of physicians use this therapy as primary prevention only in high risk cases and reserve its general use until after documentation of a thromboembolic event. The precise mechanism of this hypercoaguable state is unclear although a variety of factors do converge that heighten the thrombotic risk, including a local (renal vein) decrease in perfusion pressure from the lowered oncotic pressure, loss of protein clotting factors in the urine, increased hepatic production of clotting factors, and perhaps even a genetic predisposition to clot.

Treatment Prophylaxis

Many large studies in the renal transplant field and in postmenopausal women have indicated that agents such as bisphosphonates reduce bone loss during long-term use of corticosteroids. Certainly the utilization of such agents in the IMGN patient should be considered when a course of therapy includes prolonged prednisone treatment.

Trimethoprim-sulfamethoxazole has reduced the incidence of pneumocystitis carinii pneumonia infection in patients on prolonged immunosuppressive therapy in both the transplant field and in certain autoimmune diseases. Its use when the IMGN patients are exposed to prolonged cytotoxic agents seems prudent.

MANAGEMENT PLAN

Figure 5 gives a graphic display of a treatment framework for patients with idiopathic membranous nephropathy. In addition the following general rules should be applied.

1. Establish whether the disease is primary or secondary and take appropriate actions for known causes.

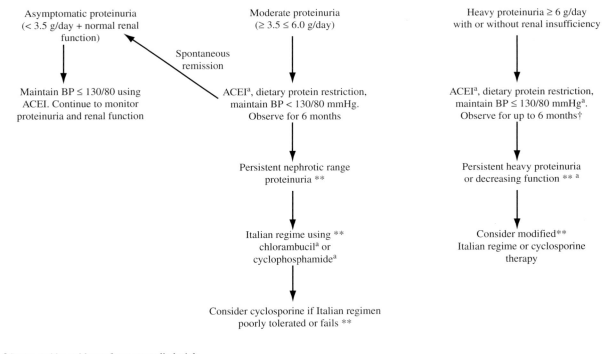

[a] Supported by evidence from controlled trials.
ACEI = Angiotensin converting enzyme inhibiting drug.
** = Introduction of risk reduction strategies for both secondary effects of disease and adverse effects of immunotherapy.
† May initiate treatment early in the rare rapidly progressive case.

FIGURE 5 Guideline for the treatment of idiopathic membranous nephropathy. Patients may change from one category to another during the course of follow-up.

2. For IMGN patients, monitor renal function over a 6-month period and establish a risk of progression score.

3. If persistent nephrotic range proteinuria or deterioration in renal function occurs despite maximum conservative therapy introduce treatment for the secondary effects of the disease, that is, a lipid lowering agent and possibly anticoagulants.

4. Introduce risk reduction strategies such as bisphosphonates or other agents when long-term corticosteroids are used and trimethoprim–sulfamethoxazole if long-term immunosuppressive drugs are employed.

5. First choice as specific therapy for medium risk of progression patients—chlorambucil or cyclophophamide/prednisone routine for 6 months.

6. Specific therapy for high risk patients should be either the modified chlorambucil/prednisone routine or cyclosporine for 6 to 12 months.

7. If both fail and the clinical status warrants further attempts at treatment, consider cyclophosphamide alone for 6 to 12 months.

Bibliography

Adachi JD, Benson WG, Brown J, *et al.:* Intermittent etidronate therapy to prevent corticosteroid induced osteoporosis. *N Engl J Med* 337:382–387, 1997.

Branten AJ, Reichert LJ, Koene RA, *et al.:* Oral cyclophosphamide versus chlorambucil in the treatment of patients with membranous nephropathy and renal insufficiency. *Q J Med* 91:359–366, 1998.

Burnstein DM, Korbet SM, Schwartz MM: Membranous glomerulonephropathy and malignancy. *Am J Kidney Dis* 22:5–10, 1993.

Cameron JS, Healy MJ, Adu D: The Medical Research Council trial of short-term high-dose alternate day prednisolone in idiopathic membranous nephropathy with nephrotic syndrome in adults. The MRC Glomerulonephritis Working Party. *Q J Med* 74:133–156, 1990.

Cattran DC, Greenwood C, Ritchie S, *et al.:* A controlled trial of cyclosporine in patients with progressive membranous nephropathy. Canadian Glomerulonephritis Study Group. *Kidney Int* 47: 1130–1135, 1995.

Cattran DC, Pei Y, Greenwood CM, *et al.:* Validation of a predictive model of idiopathic membranous nephropathy: Its clinical and research implications. *Kidney Int* 51:901–907, 1997.

Falk RJ, Hogan SL, Muller KE, Jennette JC, and the Glomerular Disease Collaborative Network: Treatment of progressive membranous glomerulopathy. A randomized trial comparing cyclophosphamide and corticosteroids with corticosteroids alone. The Glomerular Disease Collaborative Network. *Ann Intern Med* 116:438–445, 1992.

The GISEN Group: Randomized placebo-controlled trial of the effect of ramipril on decline in glomerular filtration rate and risk of terminal renal failure in proteinuric, non-diabetic nephropathy. (*Gruppo Italiano di Studi Epidemiologici in Nefrologia*). *Lancet* 349:1857–1863, 1997.

Haas M: Changing etiologies of unexplained adult nephrotic syndrome: A comparison of renal biopsy findings from 1976–1979 and 1995–1997. *Am J Kidney Dis* 30:621–631, 1997.

Hogan SL, Muller KE, Jennette JC, *et al.:* A review of therapeutic studies of idiopathic membranous glomerulopathy. *Am J Kidney Dis* 25:862–875, 1995.

Honkanen E, Tornroth T, Gronhagen-Riska C: Natural history, clinical course and morphological evolution of membranous nephropathy. *Nephrol Dial Transplant* 7 (Suppl 1):35–41, 1992.

Laluck BJ, Jr, Cattran DC: Prognosis after a complete remission in adult patients with idiopathic membranous nephropathy. *Am J Kidney Dis* 33:1026–1032, 1999.

Ponticelli C, Zucchelli P, Passerini P, *et al.:* A 10-year follow-up of a randomized study with methylprednisolone and chlorambucil in membranous nephropathy. *Kidney Int* 48:1600–1604, 1995.

Ponticelli C, Altieri P, Scolari F, *et al.:* A randomized study comparing methylprednisolone plus chlorambucil versus methylprednisolone plus cyclophosphamide in idiopathic membranous nephropathy. *J Am Soc Nephrol.* 9:444–450, 1998.

Rabelink TJ, Zwaginga JJ, Koomans HA, *et al.:* Thrombosis and hemostasis in renal disease. *Kidney Int* 46:287–296, 1994.

Schieppati A, Mosconi L, Perna A, *et al.:* Prognosis of untreated patients with idiopathic membranous. *N Engl J Med* 329:85–89, 1993.

Wheeler DC, Bernard DB: Lipid abnormalities in the nephrotic syndrome: Causes, consequences, and treatment. *Am J Kidney Dis* 23:331–346, 1994.

21

IgA NEPHROPATHY
AND RELATED DISORDERS

BRUCE A. JULIAN

In 1968 Berger and Hinglais in France described the unique renal immunohistologic features of IgA nephropathy, now recognized as the most common form of primary glomerulonephritis worldwide. It accounts for about 10% of patients reaching end stage renal failure in many countries. Because of enthusiasm of its champion and evolving controversies about the pathogenesis, the eponym Berger's disease has gained increasing favor. The same renal immunohistologic features may be found in patients with nephritis due to Henoch–Schönlein purpura, perhaps the systemic form of the disease process causing IgA nephropathy. These two entities have been grouped as *primary* IgA nephropathy, in distinction to *secondary* IgA nephropathy in patients with other disorders with IgA deposits in renal mesangia: alcoholic cirrhosis, dermatitis herpetiformis, psoriasis, ankylosing spondylitis, celiac disease, inflammatory bowel disease, carcinoma at various sites, and mycosis fungoides.

PATHOLOGY

Immunohistology

The diagnosis of primary IgA nephropathy requires immunofluorescence examination of cortical kidney tissue. IgA is the predominant or sole immunoglobulin and is in the mesangium of all glomeruli, even those with a normal histologic appearance (Fig. 1). In occasional patients, IgA deposits are found in peripheral capillary loops. The IgA is exclusively of the IgA1 subclass, and likely contains monomeric and polymeric forms of the antibody. The intensity of staining for λ light chains often exceeds that for the κ isotype. In about three-fourths of patients, IgG, IgM, or sometimes both, may be detected with staining intensity equal to or less than that for IgA. Staining for C3 (the third component of complement) is usually observed in areas with IgA, although the deposits do not always coincide. Other components of the alternative complement pathway, including properdin and factor H (β1H), as well as the membrane attack complex (C5b-9) are often detected. C4 binding protein is detected in about one-third of patients, sometimes accompanied by a second complement protein of the classical pathway. In renal biopsy specimens with IgG, the minimal or no staining for C1q is a useful criterion to distinguish primary IgA nephropathy from lupus nephritis.

IgA may deposit in dermal capillaries of some patients with Berger's disease without clinically apparent skin lesions. By contrast, IgA within cutaneous vessels affected by a leukocytoclastic process is typical for Henoch–Schönlein purpura. These histologic findings are often cited as support for the hypothesis that the two disorders constitute the spectrum of one disease. However, a skin biopsy does not replace a renal biopsy for diagnosis.

Light Microscopy

The characteristic light microscopic finding of Berger's disease is mesangial enlargement due to proliferation of mesangial cells, increased mesangial matrix, or both (Fig. 2). The abnormalities may be focal (not all glomeruli) and segmental (only a portion of a glomerulus). Most patients exhibit mesangial changes in all glomeruli, whereas a few patients show no significant glomerular abnormality. Segmental sclerosing lesions are found in many patients. Proliferation of glomerular epithelial cells causing crescents is observed occasionally and is more common when IgA deposits are present in the glomerular basement membranes, or in patients with acute renal insufficiency and macroscopic hematuria. Circumferential crescents are rare. Focal necrosis of a glomerular capillary, indicative of vasculitis, may be found in patients with Henoch–Schönlein purpura.

The severity of the findings in the interstitium [fibrosis, tubular damage, infiltration of inflammatory cells (generally lymphocytes), and vascular sclerosis] usually correlates with the extent of the glomerular pathology. A few patients with Berger's disease undergoing renal biopsy at the time of macroscopic hematuria with acute renal insufficiency show sloughing of the tubular epithelial cells ("acute tubular necrosis") with red blood cell casts.

Electron Microscopy

The mesangium is enlarged by proliferation of mesangial cells with abundant cytoplasm, often with increased extracellular matrix. Electron-dense deposits in the mesangial and paramesangial areas correspond to the immune deposits. Deposits in subendothelial areas of the glomeru-

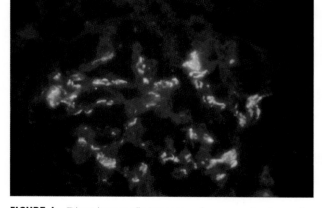

FIGURE 1 Direct immunofluorescence microscopy of a glomerulus with normal architecture by light microscopy using fluorescein-5-isothiocyanate (FTIC) conjugated antihuman IgA. Staining is limited to the mesangial areas (×350).

lar basement membrane are more common in patients with Henoch–Schönlein purpura nephritis than in those with Berger's disease; subepithelial and intramembranous areas are rarely involved. About a third of patients exhibit abnormalities of glomerular basement membranes: focal thinning, splitting, and lamination. The focal distribution of these changes distinguishes primary IgA nephropathy from the diffuse patterns in Alport's syndrome and thin basement membrane syndrome.

CLINICAL FEATURES

Epidemiology

Primary IgA nephropathy affects individuals of all ages, but is most commonly diagnosed in children and young adults. Males outnumber females by two- to threefold. The frequency of disease varies substantially between countries. In southern Europe, Asia, and Australia, Berger's disease accounts for 20

to 40% of patients with primary glomerular disease. Japan has the highest frequency, probably due to widespread screening of school children for urinary abnormalities. The United States and Canada have the lowest frequencies, and primary IgA nephropathy is rare in central Africa.

The wide range in disease prevalence may reflect varying criteria for performing the requisite renal biopsy, as well as genetically determined differences in development of renal disease. In the United States, primary IgA nephropathy is common in some Native American groups and not as rare in African-Americans as previously thought. Several large families with multiple members with IgA nephropathy have been described. The clinical features may vary widely among these relatives; some have Berger's disease while others have Henoch–Schönlein purpura nephritis. Familial IgA nephropathy has been linked to 6q22–23 under a dominant model of transmission with incomplete penetrance in some kindreds from southeastern Kentucky and Italy.

Clinical Presentation

Patients with primary IgA nephropathy usually present with one of three syndromes (Table 1). About half of the patients with Berger's disease have the distinctive history of an episode of macroscopic hematuria concurrent with an infection of the upper respiratory tract. In contrast to a 10- to 14-day delay for macroscopic hematuria in patients with poststreptococcal glomerulonephritis, the urine becomes red or tea-colored 1–2 days after the onset of symptoms; this feature has been labeled "synpharyngitic" hematuria. Patients are usually asymptomatic, but sometimes describe malaise, fatigue, or myalgia. Hypertension and peripheral edema of the nephritic syndrome, common in poststreptococcal glomerulonephritis, are rare. Some patients, especially children, experience loin pain. Macroscopic hematuria may last hours to many days; episodes may recur months or years later with pharyngitis, a febrile illness of another cause, or extreme exercise. This bleeding is more common in children than adults, and intervals between episodes lengthen with increasing age.

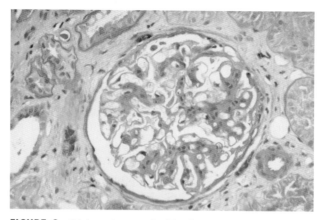

FIGURE 2 Light microscopic histology of glomerulus with increased mesangial cells and matrix (periodic acid–Schiff, ×350).

TABLE 1
Clinical Presentations of Primary IgA Nephropathy

Common
Synpharyngitic macroscopic hematuria
Stable renal function (frequent)
Acute renal dysfunction (infrequent)
Crescentic glomerulonephritis
Acute tubular necrosis
Asymptomatic microscopic hematuria
Proteinuria—variable
Henoch–Schönlein purpura nephritis
Less common
Chronic renal insufficiency
Hypertension
Nephrotic syndrome
Renal dysfunction
"Minimal-change" features on renal biopsy

A second presentation of Berger's disease is asymptomatic microscopic hematuria with proteinuria. Such patients are often adults undergoing routine urinalysis testing for insurance, employment, or annual examinations. They rarely experience macroscopic hematuria after ascertainment. Proteinuria is variable, but many patients excrete less than 1 g/day.

Henoch–Schönlein purpura is a third common presentation, and develops much more often in children than adults. Patients manifest a systemic vasculitis that involves arterioles, capillaries, and venules. This vasculitis is distinct from microscopic polyangiitis (microscopic polyarteritis) due to the presence of IgA-containing immune complexes in the vascular walls. Affected sites frequently include skin, joints, intestinal tract, and kidneys, although some young children never exhibit nephritis. Skin lesions are characteristically more numerous on the legs and lower trunk, and frequently begin as a morbiliform rash that rapidly becomes purpuric. In some patients the skin lesions are quite transient. A skin biopsy shows a leukocytoclastic angiitis with IgA immune complexes. Joint findings may include swelling of the knees and ankles that is nonmigratory and nondamaging. Gastrointestinal symptoms can be striking, with severe abdominal pain, ileus, or bloody diarrhea. Nephritis often develops after initial symptoms subside; therefore, a urinalysis should be checked at a 1-month follow-up visit.

A less common presentation of Berger's disease is the nephrotic syndrome. These patients usually have advanced glomerular disease with hypertension and renal insufficiency. Alternatively, the nephrotic syndrome rarely is the initial clinical feature of patients with normal renal function and normal blood pressure. Proteinuria in the latter setting is often selective, composed of primarily smaller proteins such as albumin. Renal biopsy shows histologic features similar to minimal-change glomerulonephritis, but with diffuse staining for IgA in all mesangia. Whether this entity comprises a variant of Berger's disease or a separate disease is controversial. Chronic renal insufficiency and hypertension (occasionally malignant) are initial manifestations for a minority of patients.

Laboratory Findings

Because the glomerular IgA is apparently derived from the circulation, much attention has focused on circulating IgA or IgA-containing immune complexes. Serum IgA concentrations are increased in about 50% of patients. However, this finding is neither unique nor consistent when multiple samples are obtained from an individual patient over several months. Levels of circulating IgA-containing immune complexes are frequently increased. The complexes may contain C3, IgG, or both, but a microbial or dietary antigen has not been identified. Discovery of circulating IgA–fibronectin complexes in some patients sparked interest as a possible screening test, but the specificity and sensitivity are too poor. Renal biopsy remains the standard for diagnosis. Serum concentrations of complement components are usually normal.

Natural History

Berger's disease is a chronic disease. Although clinical remission (resolution of microscopic hematuria and proteinuria with a normal serum creatinine concentration) may develop in as many as a third of patients several years after renal biopsy, disappearance of the IgA from glomeruli has been documented only rarely. Renal function progressively worsens in about 40% of patients, about half of whom reach end stage renal failure after 20 years of clinically apparent disease. For patients with modest proteinuria at biopsy, an increase in magnitude of proteinuria portends a rise in serum creatinine concentration. About 10% of patients with renal insufficiency develop nephrotic syndrome. In contrast, as many as a third of patients exhibit a benign course with chronic microscopic hematuria, normal serum creatinine concentration, and proteinuria generally less than 1 g/day.

Hypertension in patients with Berger's disease is at least as common as in patients with membranous or membranoproliferative glomerulonephritis, but probably less frequent than in patients with idiopathic focal segmental glomerulosclerosis. Hypertension is more common in patients whose biopsy specimens show vascular sclerosis. Malignant hypertension develops in about 1–2% of patients. Among patients whose urinalysis becomes normal with prolonged observation, half remain hypertensive.

While the purpuric skin lesions in patients with Henoch–Schönlein purpura nephritis may be transient, it is likely that the glomerular lesions persist, as in Berger's disease. Over the longer term, about 15% of patients diagnosed in childhood or adulthood reach end stage renal failure 10 years after renal biopsy. However, the risk of progressive disease differs between clinical presentations. Less than 5% of patients with microscopic hematuria and modest proteinuria develop end stage renal failure in this interval, compared with 40% of patients with nephrotic syndrome and more than 50% of patients with a nephritic urinalysis and nephrotic syndrome.

Prognostic Markers

Several clinicopathological parameters have been shown by multivariate analysis in studies at separate centers to predict a poor long-term clinical outcome in primary IgA nephropathy (Table 2). A history of macroscopic hematuria in patients with Berger's disease confers a better long-term outlook than a history of microscopic hematuria alone. Macroscopic hematuria is more common in pediatric patients who may have had a shorter duration of disease than adults, but it remains a marker for a better course even after taking age into account. In patients with Henoch–Schönlein purpura nephritis, the intensity of extrarenal vasculitis does not correlate with long-term renal outcome; that is, a purpuric relapse does not predict worse proteinuria or hematuria, or loss of renal clearance function. The prognosis in primary IgA nephropathy differs between some ethnic groups, perhaps reflecting varied methods of ascertainment, differences in criteria for performing renal biopsies, or genetically determined

TABLE 2

Clinical and Laboratory Features of Primary IgA
Nephropathy That Portend Loss of Renal
Clearance Function over the Long Term

Clinical
    Hypertension
    Absence of history of macroscopic hematuria
Laboratory
    Renal dysfunction at diagnosis, in absence of acute tubular
        necrosis
    Proteinuria >2 g/day
Renal histology
    Glomerular sclerosis
    Vascular sclerosis
    Interstitial fibrosis
    IgG deposits
    IgA deposits in periphery of glomerular basement membranes

influences on the pathogenesis. The prognostic value of other variables, including older age at diagnosis (with an unknown duration of disease), male gender, and postulated genetic markers is less clear. All of these features are more useful for a group of patients than an individual. Serum IgA concentration and intensity of immunofluorescence staining for IgA in biopsy specimens do not correlate with clinical outcome.

PATHOGENESIS

The pathogenesis of primary IgA nephropathy is not fully understood. However, there is no evidence that the process in Berger's disease differs significantly between patients with macroscopic hematuria or familial disease and those without these clinical features. Multiple mechanisms likely play a role in the primary and secondary forms of IgA nephropathy. Research has focused on characteristics of the IgA molecules in the mesangium, site of synthesis of this antibody, mechanism of the deposition in the mesangium, and the ensuing inflammatory response that culminates in glomerular damage.

Primary IgA Nephropathy

Immunofluorescence and electron microscopic findings of granular mesangial deposits of IgA and C3 in primary IgA nephropathy resemble the pattern of an experimental immune-complex glomerulonephritis. However, it is uncertain whether IgA and C3 deposit from the circulation as a complex or they combine locally through an *in situ* mechanism. Several observations support the hypothesis that the mesangial IgA is derived from the circulation: recurrence of disease after transplantation, clearance of renal IgA from an allograft from a donor with subclinical IgA nephropathy, restriction of mesangial IgA to the IgA1 subclass, and increased circulating levels of IgA1 (with normal levels of IgA2) and IgA1-containing immune complexes.

Several pathogenetic mechanisms have been postu-

lated as the basis to initiate IgA nephropathy. Increased circulating IgA1 levels could result from overproduction of the antibody, either in bone marrow or tonsils. However, this mechanism is not likely to be the sole explanation because patients with high IgA1 levels due to IgA1 myeloma or infection with human immunodeficiency virus rarely exhibit glomerular deposits. Some investigators have proposed that circulating IgA1 binds to a mesangial antigen, either intrinisic to the kidney or extrinsic (e.g., "planted" from the circulation, such as a lectin). The transplantation experience that the IgA disappears within a few weeks after engraftment from a donor with subclinical disease is strong evidence against an intrinsic antigen. Others have postulated that an altered interaction of IgA1 with Fcα receptors on circulating neutrophils or monocytes causes glomerular damage: either increased binding releases cytokines that cause proliferation of mesangial cells, or, alternatively, decreased binding leads to greater mesangial accumulation of IgA1. Mesangial cells may directly bind IgA1 via a Fcα receptor that has not been fully characterized but differs from CD89. Another postulate has been the subject of intense study: a qualitative abnormality of circulating IgA1 enhances mesangial deposition. An increased fraction of circulating IgA1 in patients with Berger's disease are deficient in galactose residues in the O-linked glycans in the hinge region. The pathogenetic features of these molecules are uncertain, but the abnormal glycan moiety may serve as an antigenic focus for IgG or other IgA1 molecules that bind to form immune complexes. Such complexes in the circulation would be too large to enter the space of Disse in the liver to reach hepatic asialoglycoprotein receptors. This complexed IgA1 would thereby escape its normal degradation, allowing greater amounts to overflow into renal mesangia. It is also possible that the galactose deficiency may enhance binding of IgA1 to mesangial cells, by an unknown mechanism. In any event, the pathogenetic importance of these abnormal hinge region glycans in Henoch–Schönlein purpura is underscored by their presence in the circulation of patients with nephritis, and absence in those without renal disease. Other investigators found fibronectin in some circulating IgA1-containing complexes and postulated that it facilitates attachment of the IgA1 to collagen in the mesangial matrix; however, this finding is not specific for primary IgA nephropathy.

The process by which mesangial IgA1 deposits damage glomeruli has not been elucidated. Activation of complement is important, as in other types of glomerulonephritis. Immunohistologic findings suggest involvement predominantly of the alternative pathway, although the classical complement pathway participates in some patients. Cells infiltrating glomeruli from the circulation may accentuate the inflammatory response by secreting cytokines. Furthermore, mesangial cells produce an array of inflammatory mediators and express receptors for some of them. On activation, mesangial cells proliferate and secrete extra matrix. Proteinuria resulting from this glomerular damage may itself be toxic to the kidney. Increased tubular uptake of these filtered proteins may augment inflammatory processes that cause interstitial scarring.

Secondary IgA Nephropathy

The pathogenetic mechanisms of secondary IgA nephropathy are uncertain. Decreased hepatic clearance of IgA-containing immune complexes has been postulated for patients with alcoholic cirrhosis. Increased systemic exposure to dietary antigen leading to increased production of IgA has been proposed for patients with celiac disease, inflammatory bowel disease, and dermatitis herpetiformis. However, the basis for glomerular deposition of IgA in patients with various other diseases, such as carcinoma of the respiratory or gastrointestinal tract, is unknown.

TREATMENT

Treatment of secondary IgA nephropathy is generally directed toward the associated medical condition. Clearance of mesangial IgA deposits has been described in patients whose principal disorder resolved. There is no disease-specific therapy for patients with primary IgA nephropathy, and their management is more controversial. Unfortunately, relatively few controlled trials have been conducted. One approach to treatment is to divide patients into two clinical categories: acute and chronic disease.

Acute Disease

Acute renal dysfunction affects a small minority of patients. The renal biopsy specimen may show focal necrotizing lesions, and sometimes glomerular epithelial crescents. No consensus has been reached about the approach to these patients, but treatment has included glucocorticoids, cytotoxic agents (most often cyclophosphamide), anticoagulants, or plasmapheresis, alone or in combination. Assessment of apparent benefit may be complicated by spontaneous resolution of renal dysfunction in some patients and early treatment-associated improvement in renal function is frequently short-lived. Many centers favor high-dose glucocorticoid therapy, often as methylprednisolone 0.5–1.0 g given intravenously daily for three to five doses, followed by an oral prednisone regimen for several months, combined with cyclophosphamide 0.8–1.25 mg/kg/day for 2–4 months (Fig. 3). For patients with renal dysfunction and macroscopic hematuria whose renal biopsy specimen shows acute tubular necrosis, renal function often returns to baseline with supportive therapy with control of blood pressure and dialysis as necessary.

Chronic Disease

It is of paramount importance to understand that the glomerular deposition of IgA is a chronic ongoing process in primary IgA nephropathy. Abbreviated therapeutic approaches are not likely to succeed, and the potential for cumulative toxicity must always be borne in mind. Many patients are hypertensive, and control of their blood pressure

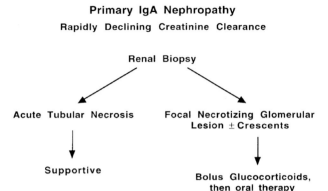

FIGURE 3 Treatment of IgA nephropathy with rapidly declining creatinine clearance. Adapted from Julian BA: *Semin Nephrol* 20:277–285, 2000, and reproduced with permission.

is the cornerstone of therapy. An angiotensin converting enzyme inhibitor is the agent of choice. Not only is blood pressure usually well controlled, but the rate of decline of creatinine clearance is frequently slowed or stopped, possibly due to better control of intraglomerular capillary hypertension or decreased cytokine-induced glomerular sclerosis. Proteinuria often improves, heralding a more stable clinical course. Enthusiasm for this class of agents has increased because of treatment-induced decrement of proteinuria and stabilization of renal function of patients with several types of chronic renal diseases. Treatment of normotensive proteinuric patients has also gained favor (Fig. 4). Patients unable to tolerate an angiotensin converting enzyme inhibitor may benefit from treatment with an angiotensin II receptor antagonist. Titrating the dose of these agents, alone or combined, to achieve a protein excretion rate of less than 0.5 g/day seems reasonable. If the blood pressure remains elevated after reaching this therapeutic goal, additional antihypertensive agents should be given.

Because macroscopic hematuria in patients with Berger's disease frequently coincides with an upper respiratory tract illness, some investigators have postulated that infection may accentuate glomerular damage, perhaps by increasing synthesis of IgA1 or various cytokines that augment the inflammatory process. Nevertheless, chronic antibiotic prophylaxis has not proven to preserve renal clearance function. Alternatively, others have advocated tonsillectomy after noncontrolled, retrospective studies showed that magnitude of hematuria and proteinuia decreased and creatinine clearance stabilized. However, a large retrospective analysis found no benefit of tonsillectomy on long-term renal function. This surgical approach has not yet been tested in a controlled randomized trial and currently can not be endorsed. Phenytoin decreases serum IgA concentrations and treatment may decrease the frequency of macroscopic hematuria, but the renal histologic features do not improve.

In the absence of a disease-specific therapy, investigators have tried various other approaches for Berger's disease. In a randomized study of the efficacy of high-dose glucocorti-

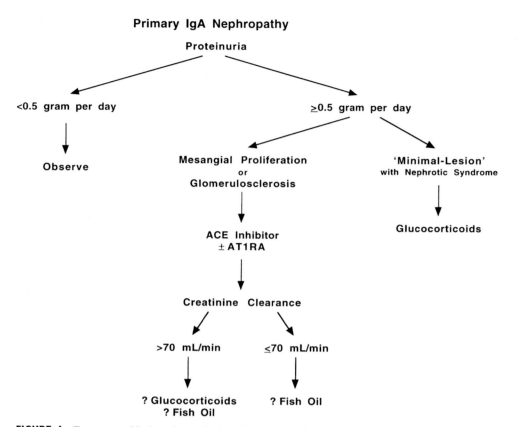

FIGURE 4 Treatment of IgA nephropathy based on quantitative proteinuria. It is not yet clear whether glucocorticoids or fish oil offer additional benefit for preservation of renal clearance function if proteinuria has been reduced to less than 0.5 g/day by using an angiotensin converting enzyme (ACE) inhibitor, angiotensin II type 1 receptor antagonist (AT1RA), or both. Blood pressure should be controlled with additional medications, as needed. Adapted from Julian BA: *Semin Nephrol* 20:277–285, 2000, and reproduced with permission.

coids (intermittent intravenous methylprednisolone combined with alternate-day oral prednisone) over 6 months, treatment preserved renal function and decreased proteinura in adults with creatinine clearance greater than 70 mL/min before treatment. However, the benefit of glucocorticoid therapy was not statistically significant after reduction in proteinuria was added to the multivariate analysis as a covariate. In a separate nonrandomized trial, daily prednisone for 2 years maintained renal function in adults with similar pretreatment renal function. In children with histologic features associated with progressive disease, treatment with alternate-day prednisone in a case-control study maintained renal function with resolution of proteinuria and hematuria. Fish oil rich in omega-3 fatty acids (to provide a daily dose of 1.9 g eicosapentanoic acid and 1.4 g docosahexanoic acid) given for 2 years slowed renal progression in patients with proteinuria at least 1 g/day in a multicenter, placebo-controlled, randomized study. Unlike the recent studies with glucocorticoids, proteinuria was not altered. Therapy was well tolerated: no bleeding complication or increase in plasma cholesterol or triglyceride concentration was observed. Prior results with fish oil had been more controversial; only two of four trials showed a bene-

ficial effect. It is not yet clear whether either glucocorticoid or fish oil therapy will have a marked benefit on renal clearance function if proteinuria has been previously reduced to less than 0.5 g/day by an angiotensin converting enzyme inhibitor or an angiotensin II type 1 receptor antagonist. Treatment with several immunosuppressive or antiinflammatory agents, alone or in combination, have not consistently shown benefit: azathioprine, cyclos-porine, aspirin, dipyridamole, dapsone, and danazol.

Two general treatment options may be helpful. Moderate salt restriction usually enhances an antihypertensive regimen. Also, restriction of dietary protein intake to 0.6 g/kg body weight/day may slow loss of renal function in patients with various chronic renal diseases such as primary IgA nephropathy, but patients should be monitored to avoid protein malnutrition.

A few patients with normal renal function develop nephrotic syndrome with light microscopic histologic features of minimal-change glomerulonephritis. After achieving a glucocorticoid-induced remission of proteinuria, the IgA1 deposits sometimes disappear. Figure 4 outlines an approach to therapy, based on the magnitude of proteinuria.

For patients reaching end stage renal failure due to primary IgA nephropathy, transplantation affords an excellent option. However, disease recurs in about 50 to 60% of patients by 2–5 years after transplantation, and, unfortunately, loss of the kidney is not uncommon. Nonetheless, overall survival rates of the patients and allografts are excellent. Recurrence in some patients with Henoch–Schönlein purpura nephritis is limited to the kidney, without systemic manifestations of a vasculitis. No consensus has been reached whether a laboratory or clinical parameter predicts a greater risk of recurrent disease.

Although several transplant centers have shown a higher rate of recurrence in kidneys from living-related donors than cadaveric donors, survival of the allografts did not differ by donor source. Donation from a living donor remains a desirable choice for renal transplantation.

Bibliography

Berger J, Hinglais N: [Intercapillary deposits of IgA–IgG] Les depots intercapillaires d'IgA–IgG. *J Urol Nephrol* 74:694–695, 1968.

Cameron JS: Henoch–Schönlein purpura: Clinical presentation. *Contrib Nephrol* 40:246–249, 1984.

Cattran DC, Greenwood C, Ritchie S: Long-term benefit of angiotensin-converting enzyme inhibitor therapy in patients with severe immunoglobulin A nephropathy: A comparison to patients receiving treatment with other antihypertensive agents and to patients receiving no therapy. *Am J Kidney Dis* 23:247–254, 1994.

Chauveau D, Droz D: Follow-up evaluation of the first patients with IgA nephropathy described at Necker Hospital. *Contrib Nephrol* 104:1–5, 1993.

Coppo R, Amore A, Gianoglio B for the Italian Group of Renal Immunopathology: Clinical features of Henoch–Schönlein purpura. *Ann Med Interne* 150:143–150, 1999.

Donadio JV Jr, Grande JP, Bergstralh EJ, *et al.* for the Mayo Nephrology Collaborative Group: The long-term outcome of patients with IgA nephropathy treated with fish oil in a controlled trial. *J Am Soc Nephrol* 10:1772–1777, 1999.

Floege J, Burg M, Kliem V: Recurrent IgA nephropathy after kidney transplantation: Not a benign condition. *Nephrol Dial Transplant* 13:1933–1935, 1998.

Freese P, Svalander C, Norden G, *et al.*: Clinical risks for recurrence of IgA nephropathy. *Clin Transplant* 13:313–317, 1999.

Galla JH: IgA nephropathy. *Kidney Int* 47:377–387, 1995.

Ghavani AG, Yan Y, Scolari F, *et al.*: IgA nephropathy, the most common cause of glomerulonephritis, is linked to 6q 22–23. *Nature Genet.* 26:354–357, 2000.

Jennette JC, Falk RJ, Andrassy K, *et al.*: Nomenclature of systemic vasculitides. Proposal of an international conference. *Arthritis Rheum* 37:187–192, 1994.

Julian BA, Tomana M, Novack J, *et al.*: Progress in the pathogenesis of IgA nephropathy. *Adv Nephrol* 29:53–72, 1999.

Julian BA: Treatment of IgA nephropathy. *Semin Nephrol* 20: 277–285, 2000.

Kincaid-Smith P: Treatment of mesangial immunoglobulin A glomerulonephritis. *Semin Nephrol* 19:166–172, 1999.

Locatelli F, Pozzi C, del Vecchio L, *et al.*: New therapeutic approaches in primary IgA nephropathy. *Adv Nephrol* 29:73–91, 1999.

Mustonen J, Pasternack A: Associated diseases in IgA nephropathy. In: Clarkson AR (ed) *IgA Nephropathy*, pp. 47–65. Martinus Nijhoff, Boston, 1987.

Nolin L, Courteau M: Management of IgA nephropathy: Evidence-based recommendations. *Kidney Int* 55(Suppl 70): S56–S62, 1999.

Pozzi C, PierGiorgio B, GlanBattista F, *et al.*: Corticosteroids in IgA nephropathy: A randomised controlled trial. *Lancet* 353:883–887, 1999.

Rasche FM, Schwarz A, Keller F: Tonsillectomy does not prevent a progressive course in IgA nephropathy. *Clin Nephrol* 51:147–152, 1999.

Ruggenenti P, Perna A, Gheradi G, *et al.*: Renoprotective properties of ACE-inhibition in non-diabetic nephropathies with non-nephrotic proteinuria. *Lancet* 354:359–364, 1999.

Schmidt S, Ritz E: Genetic factors in IgA nephropathy. *Ann Med Intern* 150:86–96, 1999.

22

GOODPASTURE'S SYNDROME AND OTHER ANTI-GBM DISEASE

CHARLES D. PUSEY

The term Goodpasture's syndrome was first used by Stanton and Tange in 1957 in their report of nine patients with pulmonary renal syndrome, which referred back to the original patient described by Goodpasture in 1919. It was not until the 1960s that the development of immunofluorescence techniques led to the detection of immunoglobulin deposited along the glomerular basement membrane (GBM) in this condition. Today "Goodpasture's syndrome" is often used to describe the combination of rapidly progressive glomerulonephritis (RPGN), pulmonary hemorrhage, and anti-GBM antibodies. However, some authors use the term Goodpasture's syndrome to describe the characteristic clinical features from any cause, and the term Goodpasture's disease to describe those who in addition have anti-GBM antibodies. The term anti-GBM disease is also widely used to describe any patient with the typical autoantibodies, regardless of clinical features.

CLINICAL FEATURES

There is a bimodal age distribution with peak incidence in the third and sixth decades, and a slight excess of males. Most patients present with RPGN and lung hemorrhage, although about a third may present with isolated glomerulonephritis. Rarely, patients present with isolated lung hemorrhage without renal failure, although many of these have hematuria and proteinuria. General malaise, fatigue, and weight loss are the commonest systemic features and may relate to anemia.

Pulmonary Disease

Pulmonary hemorrhage occurs in around two-thirds of patients and is commoner in young men. It may precede the development of renal disease. Patients often complain of breathlessness and cough, which may be accompanied by minor or massive hemoptysis. Hemoptysis can be triggered by cigarette smoking, inhaled toxins, sepsis, or fluid overload. Clinical signs include tachypnoea, respiratory crackles, and eventually cyanosis, but these are often indistinguishable from those of pulmonary edema or infection. Radiographic features are nonspecific, but usually involve patchy or diffuse alveolar shadowing in the

central lung fields (Fig. 1). The most sensitive test is an elevation in the corrected carbon monoxide transfer factor (Kco) due to the presence of hemoglobin in the alveolar spaces. Bronchoscopy may reveal diffuse hemorrhage, but is perhaps of more importance in excluding infection.

Renal Disease

Patients may present with isolated hematuria or mild renal impairment, but most commonly present with acute renal failure due to RPGN. The clinical features are not distinguishable from those of any other cause of RPGN. Urine microscopy reveals numerous erythrocytes of glomerular origin, red cell casts, and mild to moderate proteinuria (nephrotic range proteinuria is rare). Hypertension and oliguria are late features. Renal ultrasound usually reveals normal sized kidneys and is helpful in excluding other renal disorders.

PATHOLOGY

Light microscopy of the renal biopsy usually reveals a diffuse crescentic glomerulonephritis, with most of the crescents at the same stage of evolution (Fig. 2). There is often segmental necrosis of glomeruli, and some cellular proliferation. Blood vessels are usually normal, but rarely vasculitis has been reported. There is usually a prominent interstitial cellular infiltrate. The immunohistology is characteristic, with linear deposits of IgG (sometimes accompanied by IgA or IgM) and complement C3 along the GBM (Fig. 3). Less intense linear staining with IgG may occasionally be seen in diabetes, systemic lupus erythematosus (SLE), myeloma, and transplanted kidneys. Lung histology is rarely obtained, because transbronchial biopsy does not provide adequate specimens. Open lung biopsy can reveal alveoli full of red cells, hemosiderin-laden macrophages, and fibrin. Immunofluorescence is technically difficult, but may reveal linear deposits of IgG along the alveolar basement membrane.

DIFFERENTIAL DIAGNOSIS

It is important to distinguish anti-GBM disease from other causes of pulmonary renal syndrome and RPGN, because treatment and prognosis are different. Primary

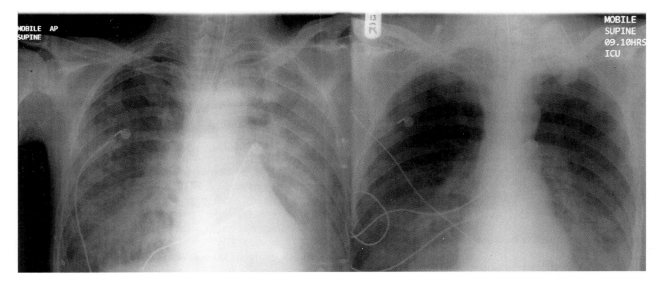

FIGURE 1   Chest radiographs of a patient with Goodpasture's disease showing alveolar hemorrhage (left) and resolution after 4 days of treatment (right).

systemic vasculitis associated with antineutrophil cytoplasm antibodies (ANCA) is the commonest cause of Goodpasture's syndrome and is the main differential diagnosis. Occasional patients have both anti-GBM antibodies and ANCA (see later). Other conditions to consider include systemic lupus erythematosus, cryoglobulinemia, Henoch–Schönlein purpura, and various causes of pulmonary renal syndrome (Table 1). The diagnosis of anti-GBM disease can be made by renal biopsy and by the detection of circulating anti-GBM antibodies. Various ELISAs are available for serological testing, but may vary in their specificity and sensitivity. A screen for other relevant antibodies, for example, ANCA and anti-DNA antibodies, is usually performed at the same time.

ASSOCIATED DISEASES

Anti-GBM disease is rarely associated with other autoimmune disorders, except for systemic vasculitis. Up to 30% of patients have been shown to have ANCA, most commonly perinuclear ANCA (P-ANCA) specific for myeloperoxidase. Conversely, relatively few patients with ANCA-associated vasculitis also have anti-GBM antibodies (5–10%). There is some evidence that these "double positive patients" behave more like those with systemic vasculitis. Several patients with membranous nephropathy have been reported to develop anti-GBM disease. It has also been reported following lithotripsy and urinary tract obstruction. Anti-GBM disease may also develop in the transplanted kidney in patients with Alport's syndrome. Patients with X linked Alport's

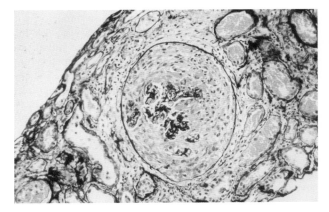

FIGURE 2   Renal biopsy from a patient with Goodpasture's disease showing acute crescentic glomerulonephritis (silver stain).

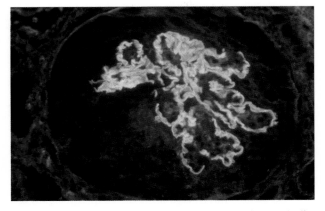

FIGURE 3   Renal biopsy from a patient with Goodpasture's disease: immunofluorescence showing linear deposition of IgG along the GBM.

TABLE I
Causes of Pulmonary Renal Syndrome

More common	Microscopic polyangiitis
	Wegener's granulomatosis
	Goodpasture's disease
	Systemic lupus erythematosus
Less common	Churg–Strauss syndrome
	Henoch–Schönlein purpura
	Hemolytic uremic syndrome
	Behcet's disease
	Essential mixed cryoglobulinemia
	Rheumatoid vasculitis
	Penicillamine therapy

syndrome inherit a defect in the $\alpha5$ chain of type IV collagen, but also lack the $\alpha3$ chain which contains the Goodpasture antigen. Transplantation of a normal kidney therefore exposes the immune system to an antigen to which tolerance has not developed, and an immune response is provoked. The antibodies may be against either the $\alpha5$ or the $\alpha3$ chain. While many patients show antibody deposition along the GBM of the allograft, only a minority develop severe glomerulonephritis.

EPIDEMIOLOGY

Limited epidemiological studies suggest that anti-GBM disease has an incidence of 0.5–1.0 case per million population per year. It is found in up to 2% of kidney biopsies and may account for up to 7% of patients with end stage renal failure. It is predominantly a disease of Whites and is less common in those of African or Asian origin.

Genetic Predisposition

Goodpasture's disease has been reported in siblings and in two sets of identical twins. However, discordant twins have also been documented. As in other autoimmune diseases, there are associations with the major histocompatibility complex. There is a strong association with HLA DR2, which is carried by around 85% of patients with Goodpasture's disease. Molecular analysis of HLA class II alleles has confirmed the association with DRB1*1501 and 1502, and a weaker association with DRB1*04. There are negative associations with DRB1*07 and DRB1*01. Because of linkage disequilibrium, there are also positive associations with DQ genes DQA1*01 and DQB1*06.

Environmental Factors

Several case reports document exposure to hydrocarbons prior to the onset of clinical disease, and case control studies show a higher incidence of anti-GBM antibodies (usually borderline levels) in those exposed to inhaled industrial hydrocarbons. Cigarette smoking undoubtedly precipitates pulmonary hemorrhage, but is of uncertain relevance to the etiology. Several clusters of cases have been reported, and there are suggestions of associations with viral infection. However, no clear association with any specific infectious agent has been proved.

PATHOGENESIS

There is good evidence that anti-GBM disease is due to the development of autoimmunity to a component of the GBM known as the Goodpasture antigen. The GBM is formed from a network of type IV collagen molecules, of which the $\alpha1$ and $\alpha2$ chains are widespread in vascular basement membranes, whereas the $\alpha3$, $\alpha4$ and $\alpha5$ chains are restricted to the GBM and certain other specialized basement membranes. The Goodpasture antigen is present in the noncollagenous 1 (NC1) domain of the $\alpha3$ chain of type IV collagen [$\alpha3(IV)NC1$]. Recent work shows that the main antibody epitope is localized to the amino terminus of the molecule. The antigen is also found in basement membranes of the alveoli, choroid plexus, cochlea, and eye.

Autoimmunity

In Goodpasture's disease, the presence of anti-GBM antibodies is very closely linked to the development of clinical features. There is a broad correlation between anti-GBM antibody levels at presentation and severity of disease, and the disease recurs immediately in renal transplants if the recipient still has circulating antibodies. Importantly, the transfer of anti-GBM antibodies from patients to squirrel monkeys has confirmed that the antibodies are directly pathogenic. However, T cells are also involved in pathogenesis, both by providing help for autoreactive B cells and probably by contributing to cell mediated glomerular injury.

TREATMENT

Untreated anti-GBM disease is usually rapidly fatal, and renal function does not recover. However, the introduction in the 1970s of treatment with plasma exchange, cyclophosphamide, and corticosteroids (together with dialysis when required) now allows the great majority of patients to survive. The rationale behind this treatment regimen is that plasma exchange rapidly removes circulating anti-GBM antibodies, while cyclophosphamide prevents further antibody synthesis. There has only been one small trial of plasma exchange compared with drug treatment alone, and this suggested a trend toward improved outcome. However, the widely reported improvement in mortality and in renal function following introduction of the treatment regimen described above has led to its widespread use. A suggested protocol treatment is shown in Table 2. Some patients have been treated with intravenous methyl prednisolone, but there is no convincing evidence for a benefit, and it may be associated with a greater risk of infection. Cyclosporine has been used in occasional patients unre-

TABLE 2
Initial Treatment of Goodpasture's Disease

Plasma exchange	Daily, 4-L exchange for 5% human albumin solution. Use 300–600 mL fresh plasma within 3 days of invasive procedure (e.g., biopsy) or in patients with pulmonary hemorrhage. Continue for 14 days, or until antibody levels are fully suppressed. Withhold if platelet count <70 × 10^9/mL, or Hb < 9 g/dL. Watch for coagulopathy, hypocalcemia, and hypokalemia.
Cyclophosphamide	Daily oral dosing at 2–3 mg/kg/day (round down to nearest 50 mg; use 2 mg/kg/day in patients over 55 years). Stop if white cell count <4 × 10^9/mL, and restart at lower dose when count >4 × 10^9/mL.
Prednisolone	Daily oral dosing at 1 mg/kg/day (maximum 60 mg). Reduce dose weekly to 20 mg by week 6, and then more slowly. No evidence for benefit of intravenous methylprednisolone and may increase infection risk (possibly use if plasma exchange not available).
Prophylactic treatments	Oral nystatin and amphotericin (or fluconazole): oropharyngeal fungal infection. Ranitidine or proton-pump inhibitor: steroid promoted gastric ulceration. Low-dose cotrimoxazole: Pneumocystis carinii pneumonia.

sponsive to other therapy, but its role is not yet clear. In general, long-term treatment is not necessary, and patients can stop cyclophosphamide after 3 months. Some authors then change to azathioprine, but there is little evidence that this is necessary. Steroids may be tailed off after about 6 months.

PROGNOSIS

Most patients now survive the acute disease, although pulmonary hemorrhage and infection remain important causes of death. In recent series, 1-year patient survival was 75–90%, but only around 40% of survivors recovered independent renal function. Serum creatinine usually starts to fall within 1 or 2 weeks of starting treatment, and most of those with a creatinine <6.8 mg/dL at presentation will recover renal function. However, those with a creatinine >6.8 mg/dL or who are oliguric, rarely recover renal function. Cresent scores of greater than 50% are also associated with a poor renal prognosis. Patients presenting with dialysis dependent renal failure may therefore not benefit from immunosuppression, unless they also have pulmonary hemorrhage. This is in marked contrast to the outcome in patients with ANCA-associated RPGN, in whom the majority should recover renal function, even if presenting with creatinine >6.8 mg/dL. Exacerbations of pulmonary hemorrhage and worsening renal function may occur early in the disease, in the presence of anti-GBM antibodies, and are often triggered by infection. True late recurrence after anti-GBM antibodies have become undetectable is rare. Renal transplantation may be performed once anti-GBM antibodies are undetectable, but it is advisable to delay this until at least 6 months after disappearance of antibodies.

Bibliography

Herody M, Bobrie G, Gouarin C, Grunfeld JP, Noel LH: Anti-GBM disease: Predictive value of clinical, histological and serological data. *Clin Nephrol* 40:249–255, 1993.

Johnson JP, Moore JJ, Austin HJ, Balow JE, Antonovych TT, Wilson CB: Therapy of anti-glomerular basement membrane antibody disease: Analysis of prognostic significance of clinical, pathological and treatment factors. *Medicine* 64:219–227, 1985.

Kluth DC, Rees AJ: Anti-glomerular basement membrane disease. *J Am Soc Nephrol* 11:2446–2453, 1999.

Lerner RA, Glassock RJ, Dixon FJ: The role of anti-glomerular basement membrane antibodies in the pathogenesis of human glomerulonephritis. *J Exp Med* 126:989–1004, 1967.

Levy JB, Pusey CD: Still a role for plasmapheresis in rapidly progressive glomerulonephritis? *J Nephrol* 10:7–13, 1997.

Lockwood CM, Rees AJ, Pearson TA, Evans DJ, Peters DK, Wilson CB: Immunosuppression and plasma exchange in the treatment of Goodpasture's syndrome. *Lancet* 1:711–715, 1976.

Merkel F, Pullig O, Marx M, Netzer KO, Weber M: Course and prognosis of anti-basement membrane antibody mediated disease: A report of 35 cases. *Nephrol Dial Transplant* 9:372–376, 1994.

Phelps RG, Rees AJ: The HLA complex in Goodpasture's disease: A model for analyzing susceptibility to autoimmunity. *Kidney Int* 56:1638–1653, 1999.

Saus J, Wieslander J, Langeveld JPM, Quinones S, Hudson BC: Identification of the Goodpasture antigen as the $\alpha3$(IV) chain of collagen IV. *J Biol Chem* 263:13374–13380, 1988.

Savage COS, Pusey CD, Bowman C, Rees AJ, Lockwood CM: Anti-GBM antibody mediated disease in the British Isles 1980–1984. *Br Med J* 292:301–304, 1986.

Turner N, Mason PJ, Brown R, Fox M, Povey S, Rees A, Pusey CD: Molecular cloning of the human Goodpasture antigen demonstrates it to be the alpha 3 chain of type IV collagen. *J Clin Invest* 89:592–601, 1992.

Wilson CB, Dixon FJ: Anti-glomerular basement membrane antibody-induced glomerulonephritis. *Kidney Int* 3:74–89, 1973.

SECTION 4

THE KIDNEY IN SYSTEMIC DISEASE

RENAL FUNCTION IN CONGESTIVE HEART FAILURE

C. HALLER AND E. RITZ

Congestive heart failure (CHF) is the only major cardiovascular disease with an increasing incidence and prevalence in industrialized countries. Despite considerable progress in the clinical management of heart failure, its prognosis continues to be worse than in many common cancers. The kidney is the principal organ affected by the decline of cardiac function. At the same time, the kidney contributes to the development of the clinical syndrome of heart failure. Its characteristic hemodynamic and neuroendocrine abnormalities determine the pathophysiology, clinical presentation, and prognosis of this disorder. In this context, the kidney has a dual role: activation of the renin–angiotensin–aldosterone system and regulation of sodium excretion. Generally the kidney is intact in heart failure, but extrarenal stimuli alter its function to a point where mechanisms which are initially homeostatic become maladaptive.

PATHOPHYSIOLOGY

The Role of Effective Arterial Volume in CHF

The kidney senses cardiac dysfunction and responds with functional alterations, including salt and volume retention. Initially adaptive, these changes become maladaptive, causing further cardiac compromise by increasing preload and afterload through activation of the sympathetic nervous system and the renin–angiotensin–aldosterone system which leads to volume expansion and increased vascular tone. The primary lesion, a decrease in cardiac pump function, reduces the filling of the arterial vasculature and tends to lower blood pressure in the aorta. In response, the sympathetic nervous system is activated and the peripheral resistance increases to maintain blood pressure.

Information on filling of the arterial tree and blood pressure is conveyed from vascular baroreceptors to the kidney via the sympathetic nervous system. The impaired cardiac pump function is perceived as a decrease in effective arterial volume irrespective of the actual blood volume, which may be normal, but in CHF is frequently increased. The perceived decrease in arterial volume stimulates renal mechanisms which are ideally suited to counteract hemorrhage, but are less useful to compensate for a chronic reduction of effective arterial volume (see Fig. 1). The

counterregulatory responses include an increase in preload through the renal retention of sodium and an increase afterload as vascular resistance rises. Although renal plasma flow is reduced, the fall in glomerular filtration rate (GFR) is initially not as marked and the filtration fraction is increased. Ultrafiltration of a larger than normal fraction of plasma increases the oncotic pressure in the plasma that reaches the postglomerular renal capillaries and results in increased sodium reabsorption in the proximal tubule. The net effect of the renal responses to a decreased effective arterial volume is sodium and water retention, decreased urine output, and the stimulation of salt and water intake. Many of the clinical signs and symptoms as well as prognostic indicators of CHF are in fact not directly related to the impaired cardiac performance, but rather to the renal counterregulatory mechanisms. Correction of such maladaptive responses of the kidney is therefore an important part of patient management.

Neuroendocrine Activation and Renal Mechanisms

Catecholamines

Arterial underfilling due to cardiac pump failure is sensed by arterial baroreceptors in the large vessels. Their activation results in increased sympathetic tone which raises cardiac output by stimulating heart rate and cardiac contractility via adrenergic β-receptors. Sympathetic activation causes arterial constriction and results in an increased peripheral vascular resistance or afterload, an action mediated by adrenergic α-receptors. Sympathetic venoconstriction can increase cardiac filling, or preload. While these effects are useful for maintaining blood pressure and arterial filling in the short run, they are counterproductive in the failing heart; they increase cardiac work and oxygen consumption and may contribute to unfavorable cardiac remodeling. The primary sympathetic transmitter is norepinephrine which acts predominantly as a vasoconstrictor. In the kidney, efferent sympathetic nerves induce renal vasoconstriction and stimulate the intrarenal renin–angiotensin system.

Renal vessels also have receptors for dopamine, but the contribution of endogenous dopamine to the physiological regulation of renal blood flow and function is not clear. The infusion of exogenous dopamine in low doses induces a

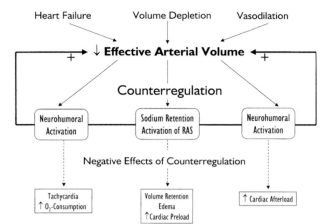

FIGURE 1 Cardiorenal volume regulation: counterregulatory adaptive mechanisms may have negative, maladaptive effects. Heart failure or any other decrease in effective arterial volume activates several counterregulatory cardiorenal mechanisms to increase the effective arterial volume by stimulating renal sodium and volume retention and by increasing vascular resistance. In heart failure, the chronic activation of these counterregulatory mechanisms has a multiplicity of negative effects that characterize the clinical syndrome of CHF. See text.

renal vasodilation and natriuresis whereas high doses cause renal arterial constriction.

Renin–Angiotensin–Aldosterone System

Sympathetic activation changes intrarenal hemodynamics and stimulates the secretion of renin by the juxtaglomerular apparatus of the kidney. As a consequence, angiotensin II is generated. In concert with the sympathetic nervous system, this hormone induces vasoconstriction in the systemic circulation in an effort to increase or at least maintain blood pressure. At the same time, the intrarenal renin angiotensin system is activated. Locally generated angiotensin II has two principal effects: (i) it directly stimulates sodium reabsorption in the proximal tubule; (ii) it preferentially constricts the efferent arteriole, leaving the afferent arteriole relatively unaffected. This differential regulation of afferent and efferent arteriolar resistance increases intraglomerular capillary pressure and filtration fraction and maintains GFR despite decreased overall renal blood flow.

In addition to its hemodynamic effects, angiotensin II stimulates proximal tubular epithelial cells directly to absorb sodium from the tubular fluid. It also induces the synthesis and secretion of aldosterone in the zona glomerulosa of the adrenal cortex. Thus angiotensin II acts in different ways to reduce salt and water excretion. At the same time it increases fluid intake, since it is also a potent dipsogen.

Angiotensin II and aldosterone are the predominant mediators of renal volume retention in CHF affecting, respectively, proximal and distal tubular sodium reabsorption. Angiotensin II increases the portion of proximal tubular absorption of sodium which is linked to proton secretion. The protons are generated from CO_2 by the action of car-

bonic anhydrase. In contrast, aldosterone acts on the distal nephron. In response to aldosterone, more sodium channels are inserted into the luminal membrane of aldosterone responsive tubular cells. Because these sodium channels mediate the electrogenic absorption of sodium in this nephron segment, the tubular lumen becomes more negatively charged relative to the peritubular fluid. The negative luminal potential is a strong stimulus for the secretion of K^+ and H^+. The net effect of aldosterone is therefore the reabsorption of sodium and the secretion of protons and potassium ions.

Antidiuretic Hormone (Vasopressin)

A decrease in effective arterial volume stimulates the secretion of antidiuretic hormone (ADH) from the posterior pituitary. Normally, the secretion of this peptide hormone is regulated by hypothalamic osmoreceptors, and ADH secretion rises with increasing serum osmolality. However, in heart failure ADH secretion occurs despite a normal or even low serum osmolality. The signal for the nonosmotic secretion of ADH arises in the arterial baroreceptors which override the osmotic control of ADH. ADH stimulates a specific subtype of vasopressin receptors (V2) in renal collecting duct cells. As a consequence, the hydraulic permeability of these cells increases due to the insertion of specific water channels, or aquaporins, into their plasma membrane. Water can thus flow down its concentration gradient from the hypotonic urine into the hypertonic interstitium of the renal medulla. The net result is the retention of osmotically "free" water as a counterregulatory response to the reduction of effective arterial volume. Human ADH is also termed arginine vasopressin, a name that emphasizes its potent vasoconstrictor properties. Furthermore, arginine vasopressin is also an effective dipsogen.

Natriuretic Peptides

Under physiological conditions of balance, ingestion or administration of salt results in a prompt natriuresis until the excess sodium is excreted. Such fine-tuned control results from tubuloglomerular feedback mechanisms and the action of atrial and brain natriuretic peptides (ANP and BNP) on distal tubular segments. ANP is secreted by the cardiac atrium in response to increased wall stretch as a consequence of volume expansion. Another natriuretic peptide called urodilatin is elaborated within the kidney and acts in a paracrine manner as a potent natriuretic agent. All of these hormones increase the glomerular filtration rate through afferent arteriolar vasodilatation and efferent arteriolar vasoconstriction. In addition, they reduce sodium reabsorption in the renal collecting duct. Together, these effects lead to a natriuresis. The natriuretic peptides are also systemic vasodilators; in total, their effects counter the increase in effective arterial volume.

In CHF, the plasma concentration of natriuretic peptides is usually increased due to cardiac dilatation and increased wall stretch. Although some evidence suggests that natriuretic peptides limit the salt and water retention in CHF, the other sodium retentive mechanisms previously mentioned override the effects of the natriuretic peptides and render the kidney relatively resistant to their action. Moreover, the therapeutic effects of pharmacological doses of exogenous natriuretic peptides is often limited by a decrease in blood pressure.

Acute Renal Failure in CHF

Patients with intrinsically normal kidneys may develop prerenal azotemia, a reversible decline in renal function due to inadequate perfusion. As heart failure begins to develop, the GFR initially remains normal. It is maintained by an increased filtration fraction despite the reduced cardiac output and renal plasma flow. The glomerular afferent arteriole remains dilated despite concurrent efferent arteriolar constriction. These opposite hemodynamic changes result from different vasoactive mediators. Afferent arteriolar dilatation is mediated by renal prostaglandins, whereas the efferent vasoconstriction is an effect of intrarenal angiotensin II. As cardiac output falls further, these compensatory mechanisms are no longer sufficient to maintain GFR, and it falls in parallel with the decline in renal perfusion. These alterations in glomerular hemodynamics also explain why patients with heart failure are at increased risk for acute renal failure after administration of nonsteroidal antiinflammatory drugs or angiotensin converting enzyme (ACE)-inhibitors. The former class of agents inhibit prostaglandin synthesis, and the latter reduce generation of angiotensin II. Angiotensin receptor blockers have a similar effect on the glomerulus.

Hyponatremia in CHF

In addition to the nonosmotic stimulation of vasopressin release that results from the decrease in effective arterial volume, additional factors may reduce water excretion in CHF. Elaboration of a maximal amount of dilute urine occurs only when three conditions are satisfied. ADH must be completely suppressed, solute and fluid delivery to the diluting sites must be unimpaired, and the diluting sites (the loop and distal convoluted tubule) must function normally. With the decrease in effective circulating volume, augmentation of proximal sodium reabsorption results from the increased angiotensin II levels and the increased peritubular capillary oncotic pressure. These effects diminish sodium delivery to the diluting sites. In addition, the use of loop or distal convoluted tubule diuretics to treat CHF interferes with the action of the diluting sites. Development of hyponatremia is associated with a poor outcome. Hyponatremia is a marker for severe CHF, and it is unclear that the increased mortality results from the reduction in serum sodium concentration itself.

MANAGEMENT OF THE PATIENT WITH CHF

The heart and the kidney are both targets and mediators in CHF. Renal homeostatic mechanisms play a central role in the clinical presentation and the prognosis of CHF. Therapeutic strategies to reverse the renal abnormalities in this condition are not limited to the reduction of volume over-

load by diuretics, but also include efforts to reverse the neuroendocrine derangements.

Management of Edema

Most patients with CHF have edema, that is, sodium and volume overload. Establishing negative sodium balance is therefore a central goal of all CHF treatment strategies (Table 1). A moderate decrease in dietary sodium intake is always appropriate. A 4 g Na^+ daily intake is feasible and can be generally recommended. Some patients can follow tighter restrictions. One potential source of increased sodium intake is sodium containing intravenous fluid or medications. The fluid prescription and drug list should be reviewed with this in mind. Additional benefits of sodium restriction include the reduction of thirst and the limitation of urinary potassium loss during diuretic treatment. Urinary potassium loss is lower when less sodium is delivered to the sodium/potassium exchange site in the distal renal tubule.

Bed rest has traditionally been an ancillary therapeutic measure, because it reduces the hydrostatic work of the

TABLE I
Management of the Edematous Patient with Congestive Heart Failure[a]

Ancillary measures	
Bed rest	Decreased cardiac work
Anticoagulation	Prevention of thromboembolic complications during aggressive diuresis
Sodium restriction	Negative sodium balance, decreased kaliuresis, decreased diuretic requirement, decreased thirst
Diuretic therapy	
Proximal tubule	ACE inhibition: indirect effect; acetazolamide: metabolic acidosis
Henle's loop	Furosemide, bumetanide, torsemide, ethacrynic acid: most effective, but rebound effect (repeated/continuous administration is necessary)
Distal tubule	Thiazides/metolazone: high risk of hypokalemia with relatively small natriuretic effect, not applicable in patients with renal failure
Collecting tubule	Potassium sparing agents, spironolactone: little diuretic effect, but potassium sparing effect useful in combination with other diuretics; spironolactone: prognostic benefit? (RALES trial, see text)
Collecting duct	Vasopressin (V2) antagonists: aquaresis, rather than natriuresis (these currently investigational agents may be useful for the treatment of hyponatremia in CHF in the future)

[a]See text for details.

failing heart and thus improves renal perfusion. The aggressive mobilization of edema fluid increases the risk of venous thromboembolic events during this period of bed rest. Patients who are not already anticoagulated because of cardiac dysfunction should receive appropriate prophylactic measures, that is (low-dose), anticoagulation and elastic or compression stockings.

In the majority of patients with heart failure, these measures are not sufficient to reduce the markedly increased extracellular volume. Hence most patients require diuretics. Diuretic therapy is discussed in detail in Chapter 15, but several points bear emphasis here. Although a significant proportion of sodium absorption occurs in the proximal tubule in exchange for protons which derive from CO_2 via the action of carbonic anhydrase, carbonic anhydrase inhibitors such as acetazolamide play only a limited role in the treatment of heart failure, as distal nephron segments compensate for the reduced proximal sodium absorption. Distal tubule diuretics, such as thiazides, are not very effective as monotherapy, since 90% of the filtered sodium load will already have been absorbed proximal to this site. The potassium-sparing agents (amiloride, triamterene, and spironolactone) are very weak natriuretic agents at best and act even further "downstream" than the thiazides. Their principal role is in combination with other diuretics to reduce K^+ and H^+ secretion. Furthermore, spironolactone has been shown, in a large-scale randomized trial, to be effective in reducing mortality in patients with CHF, perhaps through additional mechanisms besides their diuretic effect. Loop diuretics are the most effective agents available for the treatment of volume overload. They inhibit a specific Na^+–K^+–$2Cl^-$ symporter in the thick ascending limb of Henle's loop which accounts for the reabsorption of some 20% of the filtered sodium load. However, even their efficacy may be reduced by a compensatory increase in the sodium avidity at distal nephron sites.

In mild heart failure, fluid retention may respond to thiazide diuretics (e.g., hydrochlorothiazide 25–50 mg/day), but thiazides can cause severe hypokalemia. Therefore, the use of low doses and their combination with a potassium sparing diuretic (e.g., triamterene 50 mg/day) are preferred. Most patients with advanced CHF require loop diuretics in doses titrated to the clinical response. Because of a rebound increase in renal sodium retention after the loop diuretic action has worn off, repeated administration or the use of a longer acting compound, such as torsemide is necessary. Intravenous administration is preferred in emergency situations or in patients with massive fluid overload. In severe cases, the continuous infusion of a loop diuretic can be helpful. When even high doses of intravenous loop diuretics fail to achieve a negative sodium balance, combination of different classes of diuretics is required. A rational approach is the combination of agents that act on different sites of the nephron, that is, the combination of a loop diuretic with a distally acting compound such as metolazone or chlorothiazide. The addition of a potassium sparing agent is useful to reduce diuretic-induced hypokalemia. Close clinical and biochemical monitoring of the patient is essential during this intensive diuretic therapy. Potassium-

sparing agents are more effective than oral or intravenous potassium supplementation, but one must be aware of the potential risk of life-threatening hyperkalemia, especially during concomitant treatment with high doses of ACE-inhibitors and when renal function is decreased. The risk of hyperkalemia is further increased by a high intake of potassium supplements or potassium-containing salt substitutes.

ACE-Inhibition and Aldosterone Antagonism

ACE-inhibitors have become the cornerstone of the modern treatment of CHF for a variety of reasons. ACE-inhibitors reduce cardiac afterload thereby improving cardiac function by lowering cardiac energy requirements and allowing the heart to perform on a more favorable point of the Starling curve. The resulting improvement in cardiac function reduces sympathetic drive. This is in contrast to the administration of pure vasodilators or diuretics which cause a more pronounced reflex activation of the sympathetic nervous system, partially obviating their cardiac benefits. Apart from these systemic effects, ACE-inhibitors also inactivate the local renin–angiotensin systems in the cardiovascular system. Inhibition of the renin–angiotensin system in the heart and blood vessels has favorable effects on cardiovascular remodeling in hypertensive heart disease or after myocardial infarction. The inactivation of the renin–angiotensin system by ACE-inhibitors (and more recently by angiotensin II antagonists) reduces morbidity and mortality in patients with heart failure.

Because activation of the sympathetic system and the renin–angiotensin–aldosterone system plays a key role in the development of the renal sodium avidity that characterizes CHF, antagonism of this system should reduce renal sodium retention. Consequently, inhibition of the converting enzyme may lower the diuretic requirement in some patients. Usually this effect is obscured, however, by a decrease in blood pressure which stimulates sodium retention. Therefore most patients with advanced CHF require diuretics despite adequate inhibition of the renin–angiotensin system.

Heart failure is characterized by secondary hyperaldosteronism which persists despite treatment with ACE-inhibitors, because aldosterone secretion by the adrenal cortex may "escape" from control by angiotensin II. The mechanisms for this persistent secretion of aldosterone are still unknown. Blockade of the renin–angiotensin system is insufficient to achieve a lasting reduction of the serum concentration of aldosterone. Persistent secondary hyperaldosteronism explains the propensity of many patients with cardiac failure to develop hypokalemia. The latter increases the risk of life-threatening dysrhythmias and is an adverse prognostic factor in CHF. In addition to its mineralocorticoid effects on the kidney and extrarenal epithelial organs, aldosterone also acts on cardiovascular tissues and has been associated with myocardial and vascular fibrosis.

Because of the adverse effects of aldosterone in heart failure, aldosterone antagonism makes sense, although its combination with ACE inhibition entails the potential risk of inducing life-threatening hyperkalemia in patients with reduced renal function. However, this risk is small with low doses of the aldosterone antagonist spironolactone; the addition of spironolactone (up to 25 mg/day) to a baseline regimen of digoxin, ACE inhibitors, and diuretics can effectively and relatively safely reduce the risk of hypokalemia in patients with moderate heart failure (NYHA Classes II–III). The Randomized Aldactone Evaluation Study (RALES), a large, multicenter trial involving more than 1600 patients with severe CHF (NYHA Classes III–IV), compared low doses of spironolactone with placebo. The trial was terminated early because the patients receiving spironolactone in addition to ACE-inhibitors, diuretics, and digoxin had a 30% reduction of mortality and a 35% lower rate of CHF-related hospital admissions. Moreover, there was a significant symptomatic improvement in the spironolactone group. Therefore spironolactone appears to be a very useful addition to the therapeutic armamentarium of heart failure. However, moderate renal dysfunction (serum creatinine concentration >2.5 mg/dL) was an exclusion criterion in RALES. Thus, the impressive results of RALES cannot necessarily be extrapolated to patients with greater reductions in the GFR, as the higher incidence of hyperkalemia with life-threatening cardiac dysrhythmia may outweigh the benefits of aldosterone antagonism in this group of patients.

Prevention and Treatment of Acute Renal Failure in CHF

Nonsteroidal antiinflammatory agents should be avoided in patients with decreased effective arterial volume. If they are indispensable for the treatment of comorbid conditions, they should not be employed unless the intravascular volume is replete.

When used in patients who have undergone an aggressive diuresis with a decrease in intravascular volume, ACE-inhibitors may be associated with a reversible decrease in GFR. Similarly, patients with CHF due to ischemic cardiomyopathy from coronary artery disease may also have renal artery stenosis. Patients with bilateral renal artery stenosis are at risk for ACE-inhibitor induced reductions in GFR. It is often necessary to discontinue these drugs when acute renal failure develops. Cautious reinitiation at a reduced dose after repletion of any intravascular volume depletion may permit their use.

Dopamine infusion in low doses has been advocated in an effort to increase renal blood flow and to induce a natriuresis by stimulating vasodilatory dopamine receptors in the renal arteries and restoring favorable glomerular hemodynamics. However, the clinical benefits of such "renal dose" dopamine therapy are unproved, and the use of this agent in CHF solely to improve renal function cannot be endorsed.

Management of Hyponatremia

Except in rare circumstances, hyponatremia indicates an excess of body water rather than a lack of sodium. Administration of high doses of sodium in this setting is thus inappropriate. Because of its complex pathophysiology, the hyponatremia of CHF is notoriously difficult to treat. The mainstay of therapy is the restriction of free water intake. Limitation of fluid intake to 500 mL in addition to the measured daily fluid output is appropriate. Reduction of diuretic therapy allows partial correction of any element of central hypovolemia and permits restoration of function of the diluting mechanism. Rarely, in patients with advanced prerenal azotemia and hyponatremia, it may be necessary to administer loop diuretics and normal saline simultaneously. The loop agent interferes with urinary concentration, resulting in a fall in the inappropriately elevated urine osmolality and an increase in excretion of electrolyte-free water. Normal saline, which has a higher sodium concentration than the serum of the hyponatremic patient, is administered in an amount matching urinary sodium losses, and intravascular volume is thus maintained. Meticulous monitoring of urinary urine sodium concentration, urine output, and intravascular volume is essential in these patients. Finally, ultrafiltration or even hemodialysis may be required, if renal osmotic and volume regulation is severely impaired in patients with cardiac insufficiency and severe prerenal failure. Specific vasopressin receptor (V2) antagonists are currently undergoing therapeutic trials. They interfere with the effect of vasopressin on the renal collecting tubule, thereby eliminating the major cause of hyponatremia. These agents have additional beneficial extrarenal effects and may prove beneficial in the future.

Bibliography

Schrier RW, Abraham WT: Hormones and hemodynamics in heart failure. *N Engl J Med* 341:577–585, 1999.

Andreoli TE: Pathogenesis of renal sodium retention in congestive heart failure. *Miner Electrolyte Metab* 25:11–20, 1999.

Ichikawa I, Pfeffer JM, Pfeffer MA, Hostetter TH, Brenner BM: Role of angiotensin II in the altered renal function of congestive heart failure. *Circ Res* 55:669–675, 1984.

Eiskjaer H, Bagger JP, Danielsen H, Jensen JD, Jespersen B, Thomsen K, Sorensen SS, Pedersen EB: Mechanisms of sodium retention in heart failure: Relation to the renin–angiotensin–aldosterone system. *Am J Physiol* 260:F883–F889, 1991.

Blazer-Yost BL, Liu X, Helman SI: Hormonal regulation of ENaCs: Insulin and aldosterone. *Am J Physiol* 274:C1373–C1379, 1998.

Schulz-Knappe P, Forssmann K, Herbst F, Hock D, Pipkorn R, Forssmann WG: Isolation and structural analysis of "urodilatin", a new peptide of the cardiodilatin (ANP) familiy, extracted from human urine. *Klin Wochenschr* 66:752–759, 1988.

Dormans TP, Gerlag PG, Russel FG, Smits P: Combination diuretic therapy in severe congestive heart failure. *Drugs* 55:165–172, 1998.

Lee WH, Packer M: Prognostic importance of serum sodium concentration and its modification by converting enzyme inhibition in patients severe congestive heart failure. *Circulation* 73:257–267, 1986.

Schrier RW, Martin PY: Recent advances in the understanding of water metabolism in heart failure. *Adv Exp Med Biol* 449:415–426, 1998.

The SOLVD investigators: Effect of enalapril on survival in patients with reduced left ventricular ejection fractions and congestive heart failure. *N Engl J Med* 325:293–302, 1991.

Pitt B: "Escape" of aldosterone production in patients with left ventricular dysfunction treated with an angiotensin converting enzyme inhibitor: Implications for therapy. *Cardiovasc Drugs Ther* 9:145–149, 1995.

Siscovick DS, Raghunathan TE, Psaty BM, Koepsell TD, Wicklund KG, Lin X, Corb L, Rauaharju PM, Copass MK, Wagner EH: Diuretic therapy for hypertension and the risk of primary cardiac arrest. *N Engl J Med* 330:1852–1857, 1994.

Weber KT, Brilla CG: Pathological hypertrophy and cardiac interstitium: Fibrosis and renin–angiotensin–aldosterone system. *Circulation* 83:1849–1865, 1991.

Duprez DA, Buyzere MLD, Rietzschel ER, Taes Y, Clement DL, Morgan D, Cohn JN: Inverse relationship between aldosterone

and large artery compliance in chronically treated heart failure patients. *Eur Heart J* 19:1371–1376, 1998.

The RALES investigators: Effectiveness of spironolactone added to an angiotensin-converting enzyme inhibitor and a loop diuretic for severe chronic congestive heart failure (The randomized aldactone evaluation study (RALES)). *Am J Cardiol* 78:902–907, 1996.

Pitt B, Zannad F, Remme W, Cody R, Castaigne A, Perez A, Palensky J, Wittes J: The effect of spironolactone on morbidity and mortality in patients with severe heart failure. *N Engl J Med* 341:709–717, 1999.

24

RENAL FUNCTION IN LIVER DISEASE

VICENTE ARROYO AND WLADIMIRO JIMÉNEZ

Renal dysfunction is an important event in cirrhosis. In addition to playing a critical role in the pathogenesis of ascites, it is a highly sensitive prognostic marker in these patients and, therefore, an important selection criterion for liver transplantation. This chapter describes the clinical features and mechanisms of renal dysfunction in cirrhosis.

SODIUM RETENTION

Sodium retention is the most common renal function abnormality in cirrhosis. It is always present in patients with ascites and plays a major role in the pathogenesis of this complication. Ascites disappears in most patients when sodium retention is inhibited by diuretics. Conversely, diuretic withdrawal or a high sodium diet leads to the reaccumulation of ascites. The degree of sodium retention in cirrhosis with ascites varies considerably from one patient to another, being practically nonexistent in some patients and very avid in others. The observation that ascites may disappear when the latter patients reduce sodium intake below sodium excretion is a further argument for the importance of sodium retention in the pathogenesis of ascites. Experimental studies have shown that sodium retention precedes ascites formation in cirrhosis. Thus, the predominant mechanism for sodium retention in these patients is increased tubular sodium reabsorption.

IMPAIRED FREE-WATER EXCRETION

The oral or intravenous administration of a water load to a normal individual is followed by the excretion of hypotonic urine. The volume of water excreted per minute by this individual can conceptually be divided into two parts. The first is the volume of water needed to contain the excreted solute in a solution that is isosmotic with respect to plasma (osmolar clearance, or C_{Osm}). The second is any excess water which is free of solute (free water clearance, or C_{H_2O}).

C_{H_2O} after a water load is normal in cirrhotics without ascites and reduced in most patients with cirrhosis and ascites. The degree of impairment of water excretion in cirrhosis with ascites varies markedly from patient to patient. Patients with very low or negative C_{H_2O} retain most of the water ingested, causing a dilution of the interior milieu, with hyponatremia and hypo-osmolality. Hyponatremia in cirrhosis with ascites is secondary to an excess of water and not to sodium deficiency. This concept is important from a therapeutic point of view. The incidence of hyponatremia in cirrhotic patients with ascites is approximately 35%.

HEPATORENAL SYNDROME

Hepatorenal syndrome (HRS) is a peculiar type of functional renal failure that occurs in patients with acute liver failure and cirrhosis with ascites. It is due to reduced renal perfusion, and in most cases the renal histology is normal or shows only minor abnormalities. HRS can be defined as a syndrome occurring in patients with chronic liver disease, advanced hepatic failure, and portal hypertension that is characterized by impaired renal function and marked abnormalities in the arterial circulation and the activity of the endogenous vasoactive systems (see Table 1). In the kidney, marked renal vasoconstriction results in a reduced glomerular filtration rate (GFR). In the extrarenal circulation there is a predominance of arteriolar vasodilation that results in a reduction of systemic vascular resistance and arterial hypotension. A similar syndrome may also occur in the setting of acute liver failure. HRS is present in approximately 17% of patients admitted to the hospital with ascites and in more than 50% of the cirrhotics who die. The probability of developing HRS, 2 and 5 years after the onset of ascites in patients with cirrhosis is 32 and 41%, respectively. Most patients with HRS die within weeks or months after the onset of the syndrome regardless of the degree of hepatic insufficiency.

There are two distinct types of HRS in cirrhosis. Type-1 HRS is characterized by a rapid increase in blood urea nitrogen (BUN) and serum creatinine, which reach extremely high levels within days after the onset of renal failure (over 100 mg/dL and 5 mg/dL, respectively). Most of these patients also present with progressive oliguria, dilutional hyponatremia (often below 120 mEq/L), and hyperkalemia. The rapidly progressive renal impairment is limited to patients with extremely poor hepatic function who, in addition to ascites, often have other complications

TABLE I
Diagnostic Criteria for Hepatorenal Syndrome[a]

Major criteria
  Chronic or acute liver disease with advanced hepatic failure and portal hypertension
  Low glomerular filtration rate, as indicated by serum creatinine >1.5 mg/dL or 24-hr creatinine clearance <40 mL/min
  Absence of shock, ongoing bacterial infection, and current or recent treatment with nephrotoxic drugs. Absence of gastrointestinal fluid losses (weight loss >500 g/day for several days in patients with ascites without peripheral edema or 1000 g/day in patients with peripheral edema)
  No sustained improvement in renal function (decrease in serum creatinine to 1.5 mg/dL or less or increase in creatinine clearance to 40 mL/min or more) following diuretic withdrawal and expansion of plasma volume with 1.5 L of isotonic saline
  Proteinuria <500 mg/dL and no ultrasonographic evidence of obstructive uropathy or parenchymal renal disease

Additional criteria
  Urine volume <500 mL/day
  Urine sodium <10 mEq/L
  Urine osmolality greater than plasma osmolality
  Urine red blood cells <50 per high-power field
  Serum sodium concentration <130 mEq/L

[a]Reproduced with permission from Arroyo, et al.: Definition and diagnostic criteria of refractory ascites and hepatorenal syndrome in cirrhosis. *Hepatology* 23:164–176; 1996.

of the underlying cirrhosis, such as jaundice or hepatic encephalopathy. Type-1 HRS is commonly observed in alcoholic cirrhotics with superimposed severe alcoholic hepatitis or in any etiologic type of cirrhosis with ascites in which hepatic function deteriorates rapidly as a consequence of a serious bacterial infection, gastrointestinal hemorrhage, or a major surgical procedure. There is limited information on the incidence and the factors that predict development of type-1 HRS after these events. This type of HRS may develop in 15–30% of cirrhotic patients during or after an episode of spontaneous bacterial peritonitis. Type-1 HRS occurs in 10% of cirrhotic patients treated with large volume paracentesis without plasma volume expansion, whereas it is extremely infrequent in patients treated with albumin as plasma expander. The development of type-1 HRS carries an ominous prognosis, since most of these patients die within days or weeks after the onset of the syndrome, regardless of the therapy used (hemodialysis, plasma volume expansion, peritoneovenous shunt, vasoactive agents). Death results from a combination of hepatic and renal failure and the precipitating cause of the syndrome.

Type-2 HRS is characterized by a moderate increase in BUN and serum creatinine (usually lower than 60 mg/dL and 2 mg/dL, respectively) which remains steady for months. It is important to realize, however, that in cirrhosis a small increase in BUN or serum creatinine represents a marked fall in GFR. In fact, GFR in patients with type-2 HRS is reduced by more than 50%. Type-2 HRS usually occurs in cirrhotics with relatively preserved hepatic function whose main clinical problem is ascites refractory to diuretic treatment. The survival for these patients, however, is considerably less than that of nonazotemic cirrhotics with ascites.

The renal impairment that characterizes HRS is functional in nature and related to disturbances in splanchnic and systemic hemodynamics and renal perfusion. HRS in cirrhosis occurs in the setting of circulatory dysfunction characterized by high cardiac output and marked overactivity of the renin–angiotensin–aldosterone (RAS) and sympathetic nervous systems (SNS) and high plasma levels of antidiuretic hormone (ADH) and endothelin (ET), which are powerful arterial vasoconstrictors. Arterial pressure, however, is decreased indicating the existence of an intense arteriolar vasodilation. As a functional form of renal dysfunction, HRS is typically associated with a bland urinalysis that shows only hyaline casts, although a few bilirubin-stained tubular cells or granular casts may be seen when jaundice is severe. Marked sodium avidity, with a urine sodiumion concentration (U_{Na}) less than 10 mEq/L and typically less than 5 mEq/L, and a fractional sodium excretion well below 1% is indicative of preserved renal tubular absorptive capacity. Indeed, even when diuretics that might ordinarily be expected to increase the U_{Na} have been administered, the U_{Na} may be below 5 mEq/L. Nevertheless, HRS associated with relatively high urinary sodium concentration (>20 mEq/L) has been reported in cirrhotic patients with ascites and high serum bilirubin levels. HRS must be distinguished from prerenal azotemia due to volume depletion resulting from variceal hemorrhage, diarrhea from lactulose administration, or diuretic treatment that reverses after modest volume resuscitation. Central venous pressure and cardiac output will be low and systemic vascular resistance high in these disorders, whereas systemic vascular resistance is low and cardiac output high in HRS. In addition, HRS must be distinguished from other causes of renal failure in patients with advanced cirrhosis such as acute tubular necrosis from sepsis or nephrotoxic antibiotics as well as obstructive jaundice. This is an extremely difficult diagnosis since, contrary to what occurs in other clinical conditions, in patients with cirrhosis and ascites acute tubular necrosis is usually associated with low urinary sodium excretion and reduced fractional sodium excretion. Measurement of β_2-microglobulin (or other markers of tubular necrosis) is the only way to differentiate HRS from acute tubular necrosis in cirrhosis with ascites.

HRS may disappear after the expansion of circulating blood volume that follows the insertion of a peritoneovenous shunt, following the correction of portal hypertension by a surgical side-to-side or a percutaneous transjugular intrahepatic portacaval shunt, or after successful liver transplantation. Finally, other studies provide evidence that type-1 HRS may also be reversed by the simultaneous administration of intravenous albumin and vasoconstrictors, such as ornipressin or terlipressin, which have powerful activity on the splanchnic circulation but little vasoconstrictor effect in the renal circulation.

PATHOPHYSIOLOGY OF RENAL FUNCTION ABNORMALITIES IN CIRRHOSIS

Several neurohumoral systems and endogenous substances with sodium or water-retaining activities, or vasoactive properties, have been implicated in the pathogenesis of renal dysfunction in cirrhosis, including the RAS and the SNS, ADH, metabolites of arachidonic acid, natriuretic peptides, nitric oxide (NO), and ET. Although the systems and substances cited above represent only a fraction of the numerous factors that may affect renal function in cirrhotics with ascites, they have been the most extensively investigated. Despite the activation of these vasopressor systems, renal dysfunction in cirrhosis occurs in the setting of arterial circulatory dysfunction characterized by peripheral arterial vasodilation, mainly in the splanchnic circulation, that causes arterial hypotension and a high cardiac output.

Renin–Angiotensin–Aldosterone System

The RAS is activated in most cirrhotics with ascites with marked sodium retention (urinary sodium excretion lower than 5 mEq/L) and in all patients with HRS. In many of these patients, the plasma levels of renin and aldosterone reach extraordinarily high values. In cirrhotic patients with ascites and moderate sodium retention, the plasma levels of renin and aldosterone may be normal or only slightly el-

evated. Plasma renin activity and aldosterone are normal or reduced in cirrhotics without ascites. Several lines of evidence indicate that aldosterone plays a major role in the pathogenesis of sodium retention in cirrhosis. Urinary sodium excretion in cirrhotics with ascites correlates closely with the degree of hyperaldosteronism, plasma aldosterone levels being higher in cirrhotics with marked sodium retention. In addition, sodium retention can be reversed in most of these patients following blockade of the renal tubular effect of aldosterone with spironolactone. The observation that cirrhotics with ascites may present sodium retention in the absence of hyperaldosteronism is generally considered an indication that factors other than aldosterone are involved in the excessive tubular sodium reabsorption.

The use of saralasin, a specific antagonist of angiotensin II (AII), or angiotensin converting enzyme inhibitors to inhibit the endogenous RAS in cirrhotic patients with increased plasma levels of renin is associated with a further decrease of the already reduced arterial pressure and peripheral resistance; this may be striking in patients with marked overactivity of the RAS. Renin release in cirrhotics with ascites is, therefore, a homeostatic mechanism to maintain systemic hemodynamics, with arterial hypotension being the most likely mechanism of hyper-reninism in these patients.

Plasma renin activity is particularly elevated in patients with HRS. Plasma renin activity in nonazotemic cirrhotic patients with ascites is an independent predictor of HRS development. Therefore, it is reasonable to presume that endogenous AII is involved in the pathogenesis of the active vasoconstriction causing HRS in cirrhosis.

Sympathetic Nervous System

The most commonly used method to assess sympathetic nervous activity in humans is measurement of plasma levels of norepinephrine (NE), because most NE circulating in plasma is derived from that released as a transmitter at postsynaptic sympathetic nerve terminals. The plasma NE concentration in peripheral venous samples is normal in cirrhosis without ascites and usually increased in patients showing sodium retention and ascites. Several studies have shown that elevation of plasma NE in cirrhosis is due to increased release and not to impaired degradation. Direct evidence of generalized overactivity of the SNS in cirrhosis has been provided by measuring the sympathetic nerve discharge rates from peripheral muscular nerve. Muscle sympathetic nerve activity is markedly increased in patients with ascites, is normal in patients without ascites, and correlates directly with plasma NE. Since the sympathetic nervous activity stimulates sodium reabsorption and renal vasoconstriction, the suggestion has been raised that it could be involved in the pathogenesis of sodium retention and HRS in cirrhosis. Supporting this concept are data demonstrating that plasma NE and total NE spillover are normal in cirrhotic patients without ascites and usually increased in patients with ascites and sodium retention.

Moreover, in this latter group of patients, sodium excretion, renal perfusion, and GFR correlate inversely with these measurements. Finally, anesthetic blockade of sympathetic nervous activity improves sodium excretion and creatinine clearance in patients with cirrhosis and ascites. These effects have also been observed after acute inhibition of renal sympathetic outflow with clonidine.

Factors other than sympathetic nervous activity and aldosterone are also involved in sodium retention in cirrhosis. In nonazotemic patients with ascites, moderate to intense sodium retention, and normal recumbent levels of plasma renin activity, aldosterone, and NE, these parameters were measured in the upright position and during moderate physical exercise and com- pared with results in normal subjects and cirrhotic patients without ascites. There were no significant differences among the three groups in plasma renin activity, aldosterone, and NE in any of the study conditions. Interestingly enough, the cirrhotic patients with ascites showed high circulating levels of atrial natriuretic peptide, indicating that sodium retention may occur in cirrhosis in the absence of detectable activation of the RAS and SNS and despite increased circulating levels of natriuretic peptides.

Antidiuretic Hormone

ADH plays a major role in the impairment of free-water excretion in cirrhosis. Plasma levels of ADH are increased in most cirrhotics with ascites and correlate closely with the reduction in free-water excretion. Longitudinal studies in rats with experimental cirrhosis and ascites have shown that impairment of water excretion appears in close chronological relationship with the onset of ADH hypersecretion. The blockade of V_2 receptors with specific peptide and nonpeptide ADH antagonists returns the impaired renal water excretion to normal in cirrhosis. This effect has also been observed following the administration of niravoline (RU-51599), a κ opioid agonist that inhibits ADH release. Plasma levels of ADH in patients with cirrhosis and ascites also correlate with renal perfusion and GFR, patients with HRS having the highest levels of ADH. Therefore, ADH might contribute to the active renal vasoconstriction in HRS.

The increased plasma ADH concentration in cirrhosis is due to increased hypothalamic synthesis and not to reduced systemic clearance of the peptide and is related to a nonosmotic hemodynamic stimulus. Most patients with high plasma levels of ADH have a degree of hyponatremia that would be sufficient to suppress the release of this hormone in normal subjects. Moreover, ADH in cirrhotic patients with ascites correlates with plasma renin activity and NE and is supressed by maneuvers that increase effective arterial blood volume such as head-out water immersion or peritoneovenous shunting. Finally, blockade of V_1 receptors with specific ADH antagonists in cirrhotic rats is followed by a further decrease in arterial pressure. This indicates that ADH hypersecretion contributes to the maintenance of arterial pressure in cirrhosis.

Arachidonic Acid Metabolites

Prostaglandins (PGs) play an important role in the homeostasis of renal blood flow and GFR in cirrhotic patients with ascites. The urinary excretion of PGE_2 and 6-keto-$PGF_{1\alpha}$ (a stable metabolite of PGI_2), which are thought to be indicative of renal production of PGE_2 and PGI_2, respectively, are increased in nonazotemic cirrhotics with ascites, whereas they are reduced in patients with HRS.

Nonazotemic cirrhotics with ascites also show high urinary excretion of thromboxane B_2 (a stable metabolite of thromboxane A_2) and $PGF_{2\alpha}$, suggesting that the stimulus promoting synthesis of PGs in these patients acts at the initial step of the arachidonic acid cascade, thus increasing the synthesis of all PGs.

The administration of nonsteroidal antiinflammatory drugs induces a profound decrease in renal blood flow and GFR in nonazotemic cirrhotics with increased activity of the RAS and SNS and marked sodium retention. In contrast, PG inhibition with these drugs in patients with ascites and normal plasma renin activity and plasma NE is not associated with significant changes in renal perfusion and GFR. These findings are the most persuasive arguments indicating that renal PGs are important factors in the maintenance of renal blood flow and GFR in nonazotemic cirrhotics with ascites.

Natriuretic Peptides

Among the different natriuretic peptides, the most extensively studied is atrial natriuretic peptide (ANP). Plasma levels of ANP are increased in nonazotemic cirrhotics with ascites as well as in patients with HRS. In patients without ascites, ANP levels may be either normal or increased. The high plasma ANP in these patients is clearly related to increased production and release, and not to impaired splanchnic and peripheral extraction of the peptide.

Administration of pharmacological doses of synthetic human ANP to patients or animals with cirrhosis and ascites results in a significantly smaller increase in GFR, urine volume, and sodium excretion than in controls. In most patients with marked sodium retention and elevated levels of plasma renin activity, aldosterone, and NE, the renal response to high doses of ANP may be completely blunted. Increased activity of endogenous antinatriuretic factors and enhanced renal degradation of cyclic GMP, the second messenger for natriuretic peptides, have been implicated in the renal resistance to ANP.

The natriuretic peptide family also comprises brain natriuretic peptide, C-type natriuretic peptide, and urodilatin. Circulating plasma levels of brain natriuretic peptide are increased in cirrhotic patients with ascites with and without HRS, and these individuals also have a blunted natriuretic response to pharmacological doses of this peptide. The urinary excretion of urodilatin, which probably reflects the renal production of this peptide, is normal in cirrhotic patients with and without ascites. The circulating natriuretic peptides (atrial and brain natriuretic peptide) and urodilatin are, therefore, independently regulated in patients with cirrhosis and ascites.

Nitric Oxide

NO is a vasodilator substance first detected in the vascular system, but currently recognized as a multifunctional molecule widely distributed in many other tissues, such as the immune and the neuronal system. NO is produced from L-arginine by the enzyme NO synthase. Much evidence supports a role for NO in the pathogenesis of arterial vasodilation in cirrhosis. Cirrhotic patients have increased serum concentrations of nitrite and nitrate, which are metabolites of NO oxidation. Increased NO-dependent vasorelaxation has been described in cirrhotic patients, and several investigations have shown higher expression of one of the NO synthase isoenzymes, NOS III, and its mRNA in vascular tissue from cirrhotic rats than in control animals.

The increased activity of NO in the systemic vasculature of both cirrhotic patients and rats with experimental cirrhosis is not a generalized phenomenon. Results indicate that NOS III activity is decreased in the hepatic sinusoids of both rats and patients with cirrhosis and that gene transfer of NOS III reduces portal pressure in rats with experimental cirrhosis. Therefore, reduced intrahepatic NOS III could be involved in the pathogenesis of sinusoidal portal hypertension in cirrhosis.

Experimental evidence indicates that NO plays a major role in homeostasis of renal hemodynamics in cirrhosis. The administration of L-arginine, the natural substrate for NOS, to cirrhotic patients significantly increases urine volume and sodium excretion despite also producing a decrease in mean arterial pressure, thus raising the hypothesis that this amino acid may have a direct renal effect in these patients. More recently, experimental studies demonstrated that the renal vasodilator effect of L-arginine is greater in cirrhotic than in control rats, a consequence of both reduced renal availability of this amino acid and increased renal NOS III activity. These findings suggest that doses of L-arginine lacking systemic hemodynamic effects could be effective in cirrhotic patients to improve renal perfusion.

Endothelins

Endothelial cells produce ET on stimulation by several procontractile stimuli such as distention of the vascular wall, shear stress, and hypoxia. ET is the most potent *in vivo* and *in vitro* vasoconstrictor known. The term endothelins, however, refers to an isopeptide family of 21 amino acids namely ET-1, ET-2, and ET-3.

Circulating levels of immunoreactive ET are elevated in cardiovascular, renal, and respiratory disorders associated with increased vascular resistance. Under these conditions, endothelial damage or increased shear stress, both enhancing ET secretion and/or leakage into the circulation, would be the main mechanisms responsible for the ele-

vated plasma ET levels. Because cirrhotic patients with ascites have a reduced effective arterial volume secondary to arteriolar vasodilation, the increased plasma ET-1 levels observed in these individuals could be a compensatory response to maintain arterial pressure. Several lines of evidence fail to support this contention. Whereas the activity of the RAS, SNS, and ADH in cirrhotic patients changes in parallel with alterations in effective extracellular volume, ET levels do not. Moreover, no changes in arterial pressure were observed when a specific ET-A receptor antagonist was given to cirrhotic patients with HRS.

Nonetheless, the highest circulating values of ET-1 and ET-3 occur in patients with cirrhosis, ascites, and HRS, and there is a significant relationship between ET-1 plasma concentration and renal function. The putative role of ET-1 in the pathogenesis of HRS has been explored by administering the ET-A receptor antagonist, BQ-123, to three patients with a GFR lower than 30 mL/min/1.73 m^2, sodium retention, and urinary osmolality higher than 420 mOsmol/L. In all three patients, ET blockade resulted in a marked improvement in GFR and renal plasma flow without concomitant changes in heart rate, mean arterial pressure, or systemic vascular resistance.

The "Forward" Theory of Renal Dysfunction and Ascites Formation in Cirrhosis

The considerable amount of data collected during the last two decades has substantially improved our knowledge of the pathogenesis and treatment of ascites and renal dysfunction in cirrhosis. Two pathogenic hypotheses attempted to explain the renal function abnormalities occurring in cirrhotic patients. The "underfilling" hypothesis considered sodium retention to be a consequence of the contraction of the effective plasma volume produced by the formation of ascites. Thus, this theory suggested that renal sodium retention is a secondary event. In contrast, the "overflow" hypothesis postulated that primary plasma volume expansion would result in increased cardiac index and reduced systemic vascular resistance in order to accommodate the excess intravascular volume. The existence of portal hypertension and hypervolemia would lead to overflow of fluid within the peritoneal cavity. More recently, these two classic hypotheses have been replaced by the "forward" theory of ascites. This theory considers renal dysfunction and ascites formation to be the result of arterial vasodilation in the splanchnic circulation that results from portal hypertension and leads to two different sequences of events. First, the secondary increase in inflow of blood into the splanchnic microcirculation causes an increase in capillary pressure and permeability and lymph formation. Second, the decrease in arterial blood pressure produces compensatory activation of the RAS, the SNS, and ADH with fluid retention by the kidneys. The simultaneous occurrence of both these perturbations would lead to continuous accumulation of fluid within the abdominal cavity. The impairment in free water excretion and the development of HRS are extreme expressions of the circulatory dysfunction which deteriorates in parallel with the progression of the hepatic insufficiency and portal hypertension.

Impact of the New Pathophysiological Concepts on the Therapy of Ascites and HRS

The traditional treatment of ascites based on sodium restriction and diuretics and peritoneovenous shunting for patients with refractory ascites (those who do not respond to a maximal diuretic dosage, that is, spironolactone 400 mg/day plus furosemide 160 mg/day) has considerably changed during the last two decades. Sodium restriction (<2 g/day, 90 mmol/day) and diuretics given orally continue to be the treatment of choice in patients with moderate ascites. The core diuretic is spironolactone, which should initially be given alone at a dose of 100–200 mg/day. The diuretic dosage should be increased if there is insufficient diuretic response. Most clinicians add a loop diuretic (furosemide, 25–40 mg/day). The dose of spironolactone and furosemide should be increased to a maximum of 400 mg and 160 mg/day, respectively, for those who fail to respond. However, in patients with tense ascites, therapeutic paracentesis has become the treatment of choice. Diuretic treatment in patients with tense ascites is frequently associated with complications (30% of patients develop renal impairment, hyponatremia, or hepatic encephalopathy). In contrast, paracentesis is a very effective and rapid means of mobilizing ascites and is associated with a much lower incidence of complications. Paracentesis should be performed in association with intravenous albumin infusion (8 g/L of ascitic fluid removed) to prevent intravascular volume depletion. In most centers, total paracentesis (complete mobilization of ascites within 1–2 hr with the aid of a suction system) is preferred over repeated large paracentesis (4–6 L of ascites/day until complete mobilization of ascites).

Once ascites has been mobilized, patients should receive diuretics to prevent its reaccumulation. Therapeutic paracentesis is also the treatment of choice in patients with refractory ascites, since it is associated with less serious adverse effects than peritoneovenous shunting. Preliminary data suggest that transjugular intrahepatic portocaval shunts (TIPS) may be a good treatment for those very few patients with refractory ascites and relatively good hepatic function (Child–Pugh score <12).

It has been shown that type-1 HRS can be reversed by the simultaneous administration of splanchnic vasoconstrictors (terlipressin and ornipressin) associated with plasma volume expansion with albumin. Interestingly enough, HRS does not recur following discontinuation of treatment, and some patients may reach liver transplantation with normal creatinine concentration. Plasma volume expansion at the time of diagnosis of spontaneous bacterial peritonitis drastically reduces the incidence of type-1 HRS.

Liver transplantation is the only definitive treatment for patients with cirrhosis and ascites. Patients who have recovered from an episode of spontaneous bacterial peritonitis and those with marked sodium retention, dilutional hyponatremia, increased plasma renin activity and aldosterone concentrations, arterial hypotension, and renal failure have a lower probability of survival. They should be listed for liver transplantation. Finally, in the near future, aquaretic drugs will be available to manage patients with impaired free-water excretion and dilutional hyponatremia.

Bibliography

Angeli P, Jiménez W, Veggian R, *et al.:* Increased activity of cGMP phosphodiesterase in the renal tissue of cirrhotic rats with ascites. *Hepatology* 31:304–310, 2000.

Arroyo V, Clària J, Saló J, *et al.:* Antidiuretic hormone and pathogenesis of water retention in cirrhosis with ascites. *Semin Liver Dis* 14:44–58, 1994.

Arroyo V, Ginés P, Gerbes AL, *et al.:* Definition and diagnostic criteria of refractory ascites and hepatorenal syndrome in cirrhosis. *Hepatology* 23:164–176, 1996.

Arroyo V, Ginés P, Jiménez W, Rodes J: Renal dysfunction in cirrhosis. In: Bircher J, Benhamou JP, Mc Intyre N, Rizzetto M, Rodés J (eds) *Oxford Textbook of Clinical Hepatology,* 2nd Ed., pp. 733–761. Oxford Medical, Oxford, 1999.

Bosch-Marcé M, Poo JL, Jiménez W, *et al.:* Comparison between two aquaretic drugs (niravoline vs OPC-31260) in cirrhotic rats with ascites and water retention. *J Pharmacol Exp Ther* 289:194–201, 1999.

Esler M, Dudley F, Jennings G, *et al.:* Increased sympathetic nervous activity and the effects of its inhibition with clonidine in alcoholic cirrhosis. *Ann Intern Med* 116:446–455, 1992.

Ginès P, Jiménez W, Arroyo V, *et al.:* Atrial natriuretic factor in cirrhosis with ascites: Plasma levels, cardiac release and splanchnic extraction. *Hepatology* 8:636–642, 1988.

Ginés P, Berl T, Bernardi M, *et al.:* Hyponatremia in cirrhosis: From pathogenesis to treatment. *Hepatology* 28:851–864, 1998.

Guevara M, Ginés P, Férnandez-Esparrach G, *et al.:* Reversibility of hepatorenal syndrome by prolonged administration of ornipressin and plasma volume expansion. *Hepatology* 27:35–41, 1998.

Jiménez W, Poo JL, Leivas A: Endothelin and systemic, renal and hepatic hemodynamic disturbances in cirrhosis. In: Arroyo V, Ginès P, Rodés J, Schrier RW (eds) *Ascites and Renal Dysfunction in Liver Disease,* pp. 291–303. Blackwell Science, Malden, Massachusetts, 1998.

Martin PY, Ginés P, Schrier RW: Nitric oxide as a mediator of hemodynamic abnormalities and sodium and water retention in cirrhosis. *N Engl J Med* 339:533–541, 1998.

Moore K, Ward PS, Taylor GW, *et al.:* Systemic and renal production of thromboxane A2 and prostacyclin in decompensated liver disease and hepatorenal syndrome. *Gastroenterology* 100:1069–1077, 1991.

Schrier RW, Arroyo V, Bernardi M, *et al.:* Peripheral arteriolar vasodilation hypothesis: A proposal for the initiation of renal sodium and water retention in cirrhosis. *Hepatology* 8:1151–1157, 1988.

Soper CPR, Latif AB, Bending MR: Amelioration of hepatorenal syndrome with selective endothelin-A antagonist. *Lancet* 347:1842–1843, 1996.

Sort P, Navasa M, Arroyo V, *et al.:* Effect of intravenous albumin or renal impairment and mortality in patients with cirrhosis and spontaneous bacterial peritonitis. *N Engl J Med* 341:403–409, 1999.

25

POSTINFECTIOUS GLOMERULONEPHRITIS

ALAIN MEYRIER

Infection remains a common cause of proliferative glomerulonephritis (GN). Renal biopsies demonstrate that the same agent may induce more than one histologic type of GN and that a given glomerular lesion may be the consequence of a wide array of pathogens. Thirty years ago, this chapter would have been almost entirely devoted to poststreptococcal acute glomerulonephritis (AGN). However, the epidemiology of postinfectious GN has considerably evolved in the Western world. In fact, what is now true in industrialized countries is not entirely applicable to all parts of the world, and poststreptococcal AGN remains a significant public health problem in Latin America, in Africa, and most probably in eastern Europe. Any proliferative GN whose etiology is unclear should prompt consideration of an infectious origin, even if this etiology is not readily suggested by the clinical context.

CLINICAL APPROACH

The clinical presentation of postinfectious GN spans a large spectrum. A bacterial etiology should be considered in any patient with the acute nephritic syndrome, acute or rapidly progressive GN, or nephrotic syndrome with progressive renal insufficiency. An infectious cause is readily suggested when any of these glomerular syndromes follows or accompanies evident bacterial infection. However, the infection may be covert, or overlooked in the patient's history. These considerations justify wide indications for renal biopsy, as it may be the renal pathologist who alerts the clinician to the presence of a possible infectious cause. One such example is a biopsy done in the course of a febrile episode which discloses glomerular lesions strongly suggestive of infective endocarditis.

Acute Nephritic Syndrome

This is the typical clinical presentation of AGN, irrespective of the offending organism; *Streptococcus* and *Staphylococcus* are the most common agents. However, this syndrome is not pathognomonic of postinfectious GN and can be observed in IgA nephropathy, Henoch–Schönlein purpura, idiopathic membranoproliferative GN (MPGN), and occasionally vasculitis, among others.

The illness is characterized by rapid onset of edema, hypertension, and oliguria, with heavy proteinuria, micro- or macroscopic hematuria, and low urinary sodium as well as a concentrated urine. In contrast to nephrotic syndrome, volume expansion involves both the intravascular and the interstitial compartments. Thus hypertension, cardiac enlargement, and pulmonary edema may be present. The clinical presentation in children can be fulminant, with abdominal pain, acute cerebral edema, and seizures. In the elderly, volume overload may lead to a presentation with acute pulmonary edema. Renal function ranges from normal to oliguric acute renal failure. Contrary to IgA nephropathy, where macroscopic hematuria follows immediately after an upper respiratory infection (synpharyngitic hematuria), in postpharyngitic forms the episode of bloody urine is delayed until 10 to 20 days after infection (see Chapter 21).

Acute or Rapidly Progressive Renal Insufficiency

Postinfectious GN can manifest itself as rapidly progressive or even acute renal insufficiency that is not necessarily correlated with the type of the glomerular lesions. Some cases with purely proliferative and exudative GN may be oliguric at onset but resolve completely. However, severe renal insufficiency may also indicate the presence of extracapillary proliferation. A renal biopsy is almost always required in this setting, both to establish the diagnosis and to guide therapy.

Nephrotic Syndrome and Progressive Renal Insufficiency

Hypertension, usually edema, abundant proteinuria, and microscopic hematuria point to a chronic form of glomerular disease. Except when the initial infectious focus is identified, as in shunt nephritis (described later) or following a clearly identified clinical episode, the date of onset is generally not known. The membranoproliferative variant of postinfectious GN usually leads to chronic renal insufficiency and end stage renal disease (ESRD). Chronic GN with nephrotic proteinuria is an indication for renal biopsy.

PATHOLOGY

The glomerular lesions found in postinfectious GN fall into three patterns: acute endocapillary exudative GN, endo- plus extracapillary (crescentic) GN, and MPGN.

Acute Endocapillary Exudative Glomerulonephritis

This is the classic appearance of acute poststreptococcal GN. However, no routine markers are available for histologic identification of the offending microorganism, and the lesions are the same in AGN due to *Staphylococcus*, other bacteria, and viruses. Many pediatricians would defer a biopsy when the clinical picture is typical. This approach is certainly arguable in adults.

Cell Proliferation

By light microscopy (LM), diffuse hypercellularity involves all glomeruli, so that the diagnosis can be made on a renal sample comprising just a few or only a single glomerulus. The glomerular tufts are greatly enlarged with minimal urinary space remaining and few open capillaries (Fig. 1). Hypercellularity results both from proliferation of resident glomerular cells, mainly mesangial, and the influx of polymorphonuclear leukocytes, monocytes/macrophages, and plasma cells. The term exudative refers to the presence of abundant polymorphonuclear cells, some of which may be eosinophils. It is possible, although unusual, to find small focal regions of necrosis with fibrin in some glomeruli. Overall, cell proliferation may range from massive infiltration obstructing virtually all capillary lumina to mild inflammation with a moderate increase in mesangial cellularity and greater than normal ($n < 5$/glomerulus) numbers of polymorphonuclear leukocytes.

Glomerular Basement Membrane Changes

The most characteristic change in acute GN is the postinfectious subepithelial hump. It is usually easily detected on silver staining (Fig. 2) and appears as a triangular structure on the outer aspect of the glomerular basement membrane (GBM) overlain by a continuous layer of podocyte cytoplasm. The rest of the GBM is normal. Humps are not absolutely pathognomonic of postinfectious GN, but LM and immunofluorescence (IF) easily eliminate other etiologies

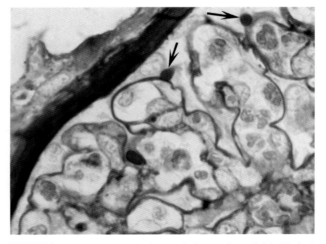

FIGURE 2 Acute poststaphylococcal glomerulonephritis. Typical humps on the outer aspect of the glomerular basement membranes (arrows). Silver methenamine staining.

such as Henoch–Schönlein purpura and MPGN. Humps are especially prominent within the first weeks of disease.

Immunofluorescence

Specific antisera disclose granular IgG and C3 deposits along the capillary wall and within the mesangium (Fig. 3). Humps appear brightly fluorescent. Two IF patterns have

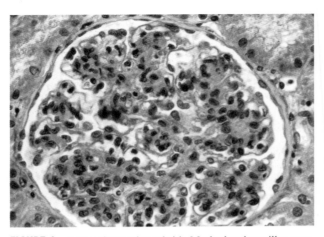

FIGURE 1 Acute glomerulonephritis. Marked endocapillary proliferation. Few capillary lumens remain open. Masson's trichrome staining.

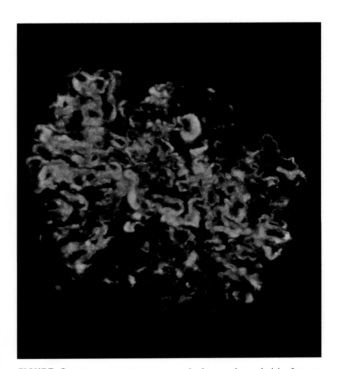

FIGURE 3 Acute poststreptococcal glomerulonephritis. Immunofluorescence with an anti-C3 antiserum discloses widespread "garland type" C3 labeling, mostly along the glomerular basement membranes.

been described. The "garland" type mainly follows the outline of capillary walls. IF shows numerous humps. This type is often associated with heavy proteinuria. The "starry sky" pattern consists of coarser deposits with mesangial predominance and comprises fewer humps. Proteinuria is less abundant than in the garland type. It should be stressed that absence of complement components on IF preparations casts strong doubt on the infectious origin of a glomerulopathy.

Endo- Plus Extracapillary (Crescentic) GN

The classic picture of GN associated with systemic bacterial infection consists of focal GN with cellular and necrotic lesions in some of the glomerular tuft lobules. This was described a century ago as "embolic" GN in the course of subacute bacterial endocarditis. However, the most common picture complicating endocarditis and other forms of septicemia as well as visceral abscesses with negative blood cultures consists of endo- plus extracapillary proliferation (Fig. 4). Crescent formation is an ominous finding that is often accompanied by interstitial edema, inflammation, and tubular atrophy. Crescents appear as layers of inflammatory cells comprising parietal (Bowman's capsule) cells and macrophages. Necrosis is characterized by presence of fibrin. The size and distribution of crescents varies from one glomerulus to another. Circumferential crescents anticipate glomerular obsolescence. The spared lobules show the same proliferative changes as previously described. IF shows IgG and C3 deposits, and fibrin within crescents.

Membranoproliferative Glomerulonephritis

That MPGN may be the consequence of infection has been demonstrated in the case of shunt nephritis. The lesions comprise mesangial proliferation, exudative polymorphonuclear cell infiltration, and characteristic GBM changes consisting of double contours due to inter-

position of mesangial cells beneath the basement membrane elaborating an additional layer of silver-stained mesangial matrix (Fig. 5). Humps and abundant C3 deposits are strongly suggestive of a postinfectious origin of this type of glomerulopathy, and help to differentiate it from the more common idiopathic variety.

ETIOLOGY AND EPIDEMIOLOGY

Acute Postinfectious Glomerulonephritis

Acute poststreptococcal GN due to nephritogenic strains of *Streptococcus pyogenes,* group A remains common in tropical and subtropical regions. It mostly affects children and otherwise healthy adults, including the elderly. The illness can be epidemic. The nephropathy is characterized by the rapid onset of acute nephritic syndrome 10 to 20 days after pharyngeal or cutaneous infection. The offending microorganism is not always identified, but serologic markers usually confirm that the etiologic agent is *Streptococcus.* The complement profile is characterized by hypocomplementemia with activation of both the classic and the alternative pathways and depressed C3 and C4 levels, followed by normalization within approximately 6 weeks. Persistently low C3 levels weeks and months following the initial episode indicate that the disease is not following its usual self-limited course and is progressing to chronic GN. Progression to crescentic GN is uncommon and spontaneous recovery the rule. Proteinuria wanes over weeks. Microscopic hematuria can last a few months before disappearing.

In general, poststreptococcal AGN is a benign disease, although some reports suggest that a remission of overt symptoms is sometimes followed by late development of hypertension, renal vascular lesions, and renal insufficiency. However, it is difficult to determine the actual long-term outcome of AGN, as in many early publications, biopsies were not performed. The reported rate of recovery varied from 28 to 100%. The course appears to be more benign

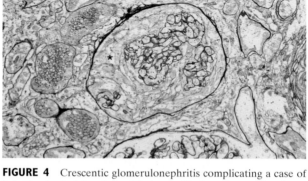

FIGURE 4 Crescentic glomerulonephritis complicating a case of infective bacterial endocarditis in an elderly patient with urinary tract infection due to *Enterococcus faecalis.* A circumferential crescent (asterisk) surrounds the remaining glomerular tuft. Silver methenamine staining.

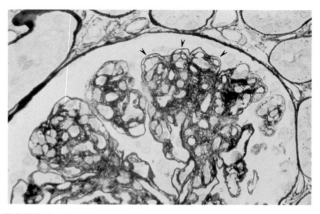

FIGURE 5 Membranoproliferative glomerulonephritis in a 50-year-old male with a life-long history of acne. Typical GBM double contours (arrowheads). Silver methenamine staining.

in children than in adults. Studies carried out during epidemics of streptococcal infection have determined that in a substantial number of affected children, the renal disease is clinically silent with GN detectable only with screening urinalyses, which demonstrate proteinuria and microscopic hematuria. How many of these clinically silent cases might later eventuate in chronic GN is an unsettled issue. This ascertainment bias may account for the impression that the disease is less severe in children. It has never been clearly established whether cases that are clinically mild and detected only by screening have a better long-term prognosis than the sporadic adult cases that come to attention because renal involvement is more severe.

AGN can follow infection with a host of microorganisms. AGN complicating staphylococcal infection is virtually indistinguishable from poststreptococcal AGN. This is also true of AGN due to most of the etiologic agents found in Table 1. In the Western world, the incidence of classic poststreptococcal AGN has steadily declined over the last decades. It has become rare in children. On the other hand, microorganisms other than *Streptococcus* are increasingly recognized as etiologic agents for AGN. Thus, the overall incidence of postinfectious GN has remained the same but with a different distribution of glomerular lesions. In adults, an immunocompromised background is emerging as a predisposing factor, especially in alcoholic, cirrhotic, and diabetic patients. However, individuals with HIV infection, AIDS, and those receiving immunosuppressive medications do not seem to be at increased risk for AGN.

Postinfectious GN with Rapid or Subacute Development

As previously noted, the typical endocapillary exudative AGN does not always resolve spontaneously. However, an unfavorable course is now mainly restricted to patients whose renal involvement consists of endo- plus extracapillary (crescentic) GN. This variety of postinfectious GN is not new; crescentic GN following septicemia such as infective endocarditis has been known for nearly a century. Nevertheless, its relative frequency, as previously indicated, at least in industrialized countries, has grown in inverse proportion to that of acute poststreptococcal GN. Its mode of onset and clinical features are more varied. The onset may be heralded by acute nephritic syndrome or rapidly progressive renal insufficiency, or alternatively, the disorder may not be detected until chronic renal failure has developed. The initial focus of infection is not always easy to identify. Most cutaneous, dental, and visceral infections can be complicated by endo- and extracapillary GN. Several candidate foci may be found in a given patient growing both gram-positive and gram-negative organisms. In contrast to acute poststreptococcal GN, extrarenal manifestations, especially purpura, may be present. In a febrile patient with GN and purpura, a search for endocarditis by ultrasound examination and repeated blood cultures is mandatory. In our experience, low serum complement levels were found in only 24% of 25 cases with crescentic GN.

Risk factors for this form of postinfectious GN include alcoholism, drug addiction, malnutrition, and low socioeconomic level, because of poor dental and cutaneous hygiene and delayed access to medical care. The prognosis depends on the severity of infection, the immunologic status and age of the host, and the findings on renal biopsy. The extent of crescentic proliferation on a biopsy comprising a sufficient number of glomeruli is the best predictor of development to ESRD. Early recognition and eradication of the infectious focus or foci by antibiotic treatment and, if necessary, by visceral or dental surgery, is probably the best means of preventing progression of renal disease.

Postinfectious Membranoproliferative GN

MPGN was long considered idiopathic in a majority of cases. However, some forms were evidently postinfectious, such as shunt nephritis. Ventriculoatrial shunting was devised three decades ago to relieve hydrocephalus, mostly in children. It consists of a silicon catheter and a valve connecting the cerebral ventricle to the right atrium. This prosthetic material can become colonized with *Staphylococcus epidermidis* or, more rarely, other organisms. Nearly 160 cases have been published. The disease is characterized by fever, arthralgias, wasting, purpura, and severe anemia. Laboratory findings are suggestive of immune complex disease, with low serum complement levels, complement-driven hemolytic anemia, antinuclear antibodies, rheumatoid factor, and cryoglobulins. Renal signs and symptoms consist of proteinuria, microhematuria, and renal insufficiency that can be rapidly progressive. Renal biopsy usually discloses type I MPGN, often with numerous endocapillary polymorphonuclear cells and abundant C3 deposits. Endo- and extracapillary GN has also been observed. Removal of the shunt and antibiotic treatment may be followed by stabilization and even regression of

TABLE I
Infectious Agents Associated with Glomerulonephritis

Bacteria	Viruses
Streptococcus	Hepatitis B
Staphylococcus	Hepatitis C
Pneumococcus	Echovirus
Enterobacteriaceae	Adenovirus
Salmonella typhi	Coxackie virus
Meningococcus	Cytomegalovirus
Treponema pallidum	Epstein-Barr virus
Brucella	Enteroviruses
Leptospira	Measles
Yersinia	Mumps
Rickettsia	Varicella
Legionella	Rubella

the glomerular lesions, a demonstration that type I MPGN is not invariably irreversible. Nevertheless, only half of the patients experience a complete remission.

Several observations are consistent with the theory that some cases of "idiopathic" MPGN also are of infectious origin. These include the presence of C3 by IF and epidemiologic studies demonstrating the striking simultaneous decrease in incidence of both AGN and MPGN in western Europe.

PATHOGENESIS

The Offending Microorganisms

A host of microorganisms, including microbes, viruses, and parasites, can be responsible for postinfectious GN. For historical reasons, the most consistent data deal with streptococci. It has been established that only certain strains of group A streptococci lead to acute GN, especially Lancefield type 12, although not all strains of type 12 are nephritogenic. An episode of poststreptococcal infection confers immunity, and AGN does not recur during subsequent infectious episodes; this contrasts with rheumatic fever where the risk of recurrence is lifelong. The main sites of streptococcal infection are the throat, especially in the winter and early spring, and the skin in the late summer and early fall. Tropical or subtropical climate favors skin infection, whereas in temperate climates, a pharyngeal origin is more common. In highly populated areas with low socioeconomic status, poststreptococcal GN is often epidemic. Studies from both the United States and western Europe have documented a decline in poststreptococcal AGN incidence in recent decades in urban areas, contrasting with a stable incidence in rural areas. The same has been observed in the Shanghai area. In fact, the sharply declining incidence of poststreptococcal AGN as well as acute rheumatic fever in industrialized countries contrasts with a continuing high incidence in the tropical regions of Africa, Latin America, and the Caribbean. Its prevalence remains high in the countries of Mediterranean Africa, which have a dry climate but a low per capita income.

Is this declining incidence just the consequence of better socioeconomic conditions? A French government-sponsored study that focused on eradication of rheumatic heart disease employing the systematic free distribution of oral phenoxymethylpenicillin in the French Caribbean was immediately followed by a dramatic decrease in the annual incidence of both rheumatic fever and acute glomerulonephritis. Thus, the weight of the evidence is that early eradication of *Streptococcus pyogenes,* group A infection is effective in preventing AGN. The same is likely true for staphylococcal and other etiologic agents.

The Complex Issue of Postinfectious Glomerular Inflammation

Acute postinfectious GN is an immunologic disease. A good clinical argument for this contention is the latent in-

terval between clinical signs of infection and the onset of GN, at least when the onset of infection can be identified. This interval is usually easy to determine in acute GN, but less readily discerned in endo- and extracapillary forms, and rarely apparent in cases of MPGN. Overall, all forms of proliferative GN appear to follow a triphasic course: (1), induction, depending on an antigen, (2), transduction, characterized by immunoglobulin deposits, and (3), mediation. This last phase involves a host of cytokines that originate from monocytes and macrophages, glomerular mesangial cells, platelets, and endothelial cells, including the C5a and C3a complement fractions, and γ-interferon as well as interleukin 2 (IL-2). Activation of these mediators leads to generation of IL-1, tumor necrosis factor α (TNF-α), and γ-interferon, platelet-derived growth factor (PDGF), and transforming growth factor β (TGF-β). The role of C5b-9 in inducing arachidonic acid, free oxygen radicals, and IL-1 release is probably important. The initial event might be deposition of circulating immune complexes including a bacterial component, or fixation of bacterial antigens with *in situ* immune complex formation. In human disease, the nephritogenic bacterial antigens are seldom identified within the glomeruli, except in some studies dealing with streptococcal or staphylococcal infections. In this respect, it is noteworthy that hepatitis B (HB) viral epitopes have been identified within the glomeruli of HBs carriers having various types of GN. However, considering the diversity of microorganisms and viruses capable of inducing postinfectious GN, identification of specific antigens appears to be a formidable task. Whatever the triggering mechanism, the usual course of poststreptococcal and poststaphylococcal endocapillary exudative AGN is that of a self-limited disease. This is not the case for crescentic GN. Crescent formation in various conditions seems to be related to segmental destruction of the GBM by polymorphonuclear and macrophagic enzymes. Through these gaps immune cells, plasma, fibrin, and inflammatory mediators gain access to Bowman's space and induce an intense proliferative reaction of Bowman's capsule parietal epithelial cells. The natural history of untreated crescentic GN is evolution to fibrosis and glomerular obsolescence. Why other forms of postinfectious GN produce the chronic form of MPGN is not readily apparent. The fact that the incidence of acute poststreptococcal GN and of MPGN have diminished in parallel suggests that, at least in some cases, the latter might be a mode of progression of an initial occult streptococcal glomerular injury.

PROGNOSTIC INDICATORS AND OUTCOME

Prognostic indicators stem from both the background of the patient and the severity of the infectious focus, as well as from features of the glomerulopathy. Patients with poor general health due to malnutrition or cirrhosis are more likely to follow an unfavorable course. Patients with septicemia and those having such sites of infection as visceral abscesses, empyema, meningitis, or endocarditis are more likely to die from the primary disorder than from the consequences of their glomerulopathy. Risk of death is significantly higher in older patients and in those with purpura. Initial presentation with nephrotic syndrome or a serum creatinine above 2.7 mg/dL, and the presence of crescents and interstitial fibrosis on renal biopsy usually herald irreversible renal damage. Two factors at presentation apparently predict a favorable prognosis: the upper respiratory tract as initial site of infection, and pure endocapillary proliferation with an IF starry sky pattern. Proteinuria below 1.5 g/day is well correlated with recovery in patients with pure endocapillary proliferation, whereas nephrotic syndrome at presentation is often followed by persistent chronic GN.

TREATMENT

In the cases of pure endocapillary GN from three decades ago, the course was considered nearly uniformly favorable. More recent experience indicates that the location of the infectious focus is much more varied than the throat and the skin, and it is often still present at the time of renal biopsy. When repeat renal biopsy is carried out months and even years after the initial one, it discloses ongoing inflammatory lesions in patients whose infection persists, whereas in those in whom infection had been eradicated, the glomerular lesions are mainly inactive and fibrous. This reinforces the need to eradicate any persistent infection with appropriate antibiotic therapy and if necessary by a surgical or dental procedure.

Definitive treatment recommendations for the crescentic form of postinfectious GN are not available. Anecdotal experience with glomerular complications of endocarditis suggests that corticosteroid therapy, cyclophosphamide, or plasmapheresis have a favorable effect on renal function. Such observations are uncontrolled. However, they suggest that the prognosis of postinfectious crescentic GN is not necessarily disastrous when an aggressive antiinflammatory and possibly immunosuppressive regimen is utilized after achieving eradication of infection. In addition, postinfectious GN is a public health problem with significant cost implications. In this respect, early, easy access to medical and dental care, control of drug addiction, and the same prophylactic measures that have proven effective in preventing bacterial endocarditis should also be implemented to reduce the incidence of the renal disease.

GLOMERULONEPHRITIS RELATED TO VIRAL INFECTION

Viral infections can be complicated by various types of glomerulopathies, both proliferative and nonproliferative. This confirms that the same agent can induce different histologic types of glomerular diseases.

Hepatitis B Virus-Related Glomerulopathies

The main type of hepatitis B virus (HBV)-related glomerulopathy is membranous glomerulopathy (MGN). It is endemic in Asia and usually affects children infected via maternal–fetal transmission. In the United States, its occurrence is essentially limited to immigrant children from endemic areas and adult drug addicts. The second most common form of GN reported with HBV infection is MPGN. The clinical picture consists of nephrotic syndrome. A history of recent acute hepatitis is usually found in adults. The patients carry HBsAg, HBcAg, and HBeAg. Hypocomplementemia and circulating immune complexes are frequent. Viral antigens can be identified in the glomeruli by immunohistochemistry. Electron microscopy shows virus like particles incorporated into the GBM. Some forms of HBV infection are accompanied by vasculitis in the form of polyarteritis nodosa. Vasculitic lesions may be found in renal arteries. The natural history of HBV-MGN in children is usually characterized by spontaneous clinical remission with only rare progression to ESRD. Corticosteroid treatment is contraindicated. Specific antiviral therapy is indicated for the liver disease, as it has the potential to eventuate in cirrhosis and hepatocellular carcinoma. Ongoing studies on the effect of lamivudine to suppress HBV replication in chronic active hepatitis B might lead to new approaches for treatment of the renal disease.

Hepatitis C Virus-Related Glomerulopathies

That hepatitis C virus (HCV) infection is related to cryoglobulinemia and renal disease was recognized in 1993. Athralgias, peripheral neuropathy, and purpura are common and indicate that the cryoglobulinemia induces a generalized vasculitis. The patients may have elevated serum aminotransferase levels, but this laboratory indication of liver involvement waxes and wanes and may be negative at times. The glomerulopathy is characterized by moderate to nephrotic proteinuria and impaired renal function. In rare cases, the renal biopsy shows membranous glomerulopathy. Typically, it discloses a particular form of MPGN comprising diffuse thickening of the glomerular capillary walls and double contours, but also massive glomerular infiltration by macrophages and eosinophilic thrombi in some capillary loops that are characteristic of cryoglobulinemia. IF shows glomerular capillary wall and mesangial deposition of large amounts of IgG, IgM, and C3, especially on the thrombi. Cryoglobulins are present in serum. They contain HCV RNA and IgG anti-HCV antibodies to the nucleocapsid core antigen (c22-3). Circulating IgM rheumatoid factors are usually present. Treatment is based on antiviral therapy. Interferon γ-2b may suppress viremia and simultaneously ameliorate the course of the glomerulopathy. The combination of interferon and ribavirin may be more effective than interferon alone in preventing the frequent relapses that occur after conclusion of a treatment course, but to date no data are available. Regarding the treatment of the glomerulopathy, reports employing plasmapheresis, methylprednisolone pulses, and cyclophosphamide provide encouraging results, but large, long-term controlled studies are required before such treatments can be endorsed. Hepatitis C related cryoglobulinemia is covered in Chapter 18.

Glomerulonephritis Associated with Other Viruses

Numerous publications report anecdotal cases of virus-associated GN. They are listed in Table 1. In children, viral glomerulopathies may be accompanied with the hemolytic–uremic syndrome.

Bibliography

Bach JF, Chalons S, Forier E, Elana G, Jouannelle J, Kayemba S, et al.: 10-year educational programme aimed at rheumatic fever in two French Caribbean Islands. *Lancet* 347:644–648, 1996.

Beaufils M, Gibert C, Morel-Maroger L, Sraer JD, Kanfer A, Meyrier A, et al.: Glomerulonephritis in severe bacterial infection with and without endocarditis. In: Hamburger J, Crosnier J, Maxwell MH (eds) *Advances in Nephrology*, pp. 217–234. Yearbook Medical Publishers, Chicago, 1977.

Daimon S, Mizuno Y, Fujii S, Mukai K, Hanakawa H, Otsuki N, et al.: Infective endocarditis-induced crescentic glomerulonephritis dramatically improved by plasmapheresis. *Am J Kidney Dis* 32:309–313, 1998.

Gallo GR, Neugarten J, Baldwin DS: Glomerulonephritis associated with systemic, bacterial and viral infections. In: Tisher CC, Brenner BM (eds) *Renal Pathology*, 2nd Ed., pp. 564–595. Lippincott, Philadelphia, 1994.

Haffner D, Schindera F, Aschoff A, Matthias S, Waldherr R, Schärer K: The clinical spectrum of shunt nephritis. *Nephrol Dial Transplant* 12:1143–1148, 1997.

Lai KN, Ho RTH, Tam JS, MacMoune Lai F: Detection of hepatitis B virus DNA and RNA in kidneys of HBV-related glomerulonephritis. *Kidney Int* 50:1965–1977, 1996.

Montseny JJ, Meyrier A, Kleinknecht D, Callard P: The current spectrum of infectious glomerulonephritis. Experience with 76 patients and review of the literature. *Medicine* 74:63–73, 1995.

Parra G, Rodriguez-Iturbe B, Batsford S, Vogt A, Mezzano S, Olavarria F, et al.: Antibody to streptococcal zymogen in the serum of patients with acute glomerulonephritis: A multicentric study. *Kidney Int* 54:509–517, 1998.

Roy SI, Stapleton FB. Changing perspectives in children hospitalized with poststreptococcal acute glomerulonephritis. *Pediatr Nephrol* 4:585–589, 1990.

Silva FG: Acute postinfectious glomerulonephritis and glomerulonephritis complicating persistent bacterial infection. In: Jennette JC, Olson JL, Schwartz MM, Silva FG (eds) *Heptinstall's Pathology of the Kidney,* 5th Ed., pp. 389–453. Lippincott-Raven, Philadelphia and New York, 1998.

26

RENAL INVOLVEMENT IN SYSTEMIC VASCULITIS

J. CHARLES JENNETTE AND RONALD J. FALK

The kidneys are affected by many system vasculitides (Fig. 1), which cause a wide variety of sometimes confusing clinical manifestations. Large vessel vasculitides, such as giant cell (temporal) arteritis and Takayasu arteritis, can narrow the abdominal aorta or renal arteries, resulting in renal ischemia and renovascular hypertension. Medium-sized vessel vasculitides, such as polyarteritis nodosa and Kawasaki disease, also can reduce flow through the renal artery, and may affect intrarenal arteries, resulting in infarction and hemorrhage. Small vessel vasculitides, such as microscopic polyangiitis, Wegener's granulomatosis, Henoch–Schönlein purpura, and cryoglobulinemic vasculitis, frequently involve the kidneys and especially glomerular capillaries.

PATHOLOGY

As depicted in Fig. 1 and described in Table 1, different types of systemic vasculitis affect different vessels within the kidney. In addition, each type of vasculitis has different histologic and immunohistologic features.

Giant cell arteritis and Takayasu arteritis predominants affect the aorta and its major branches. Takayasu arteritis is an important cause of renovascular hypertension, especially in young patients. Giant cell arteritis only rarely causes clinically significant renal disease, although asymptomatic pathologic involvement is more common. Giant cell arteritis often involves the extracranial branches of the carotid arteries, including the temporal artery. Some patients, however, do not have temporal artery involvement,

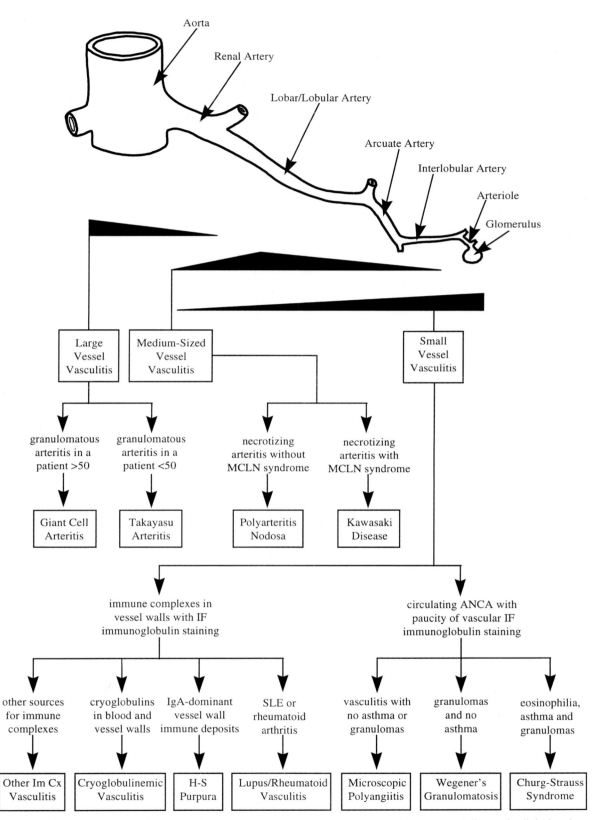

FIGURE I Predominant distribution of renal vascular involvement by systemic vasculitides, and diagnostic clinical and pathologic features that distinguish among them. The width of the black triangles indicates the predilection of small, medium-sized and large vessel vasculitides for various portions of the renal vasculature. Note that medium-sized renal arteries can be affected by large, medium-sized, and small vessel vasculitides, but arterioles and glomeruli are affected by small vessel vasculitides alone based on the definitions in Table 1. MCLN, mucocutaneous lymph node syndrome; H-S, Henoch–Schönlein; IF, immunofluorescence; SLE, systemic lupus erythematosus.

TABLE I

Names and Definitions of Vasculitis Adopted by the Chapel Hill Consensus Conference
on the Nomenclature of Systemic Vasculitis[a]

Large vessel vasculitis[b]	
Giant cell (temporal) arteritis	Granulomatous arteritis of the aorta and its major branches, with a predilection for the extracranial branches of the carotid artery. Often involves the temporal artery. Usually occurs in patients older than 50 and often is associated with polymyalgia rheumatica.
Takayasu arteritis	Granulomatous inflammation of the aorta and its major branches. Usually occurs in patients younger than 50.
Medium-sized vessel vasculitis[b]	
Polyarteritis nodosa (classic polyarteritis nodosa)	Necrotizing inflammation of medium-sized or small arteries without glomerulonephritis or vasculitis in arterioles, capillaries, or venules.
Kawasaki disease	Arteritis involving large, medium-sized, and small arteries, and associated with mucocutaneous lymph node syndrome. Coronary arteries are often involved. Aorta and veins may be involved. Usually occurs in children.
Small vessel vasculitis[b]	
Wegener's granulomatosis[c,d]	Granulomatous inflammation involving the respiratory tract, and necrotizing vasculitis affecting small to medium-sized vessels, e.g., capillaries, venules, arterioles, and arteries. Necrotizing glomerulonephritis is common.
Churg–Strauss syndrome[c,d]	Eosinophil-rich and granulomatous inflammation involving the respiratory tract and necrotizing vasculitis affecting small to medium-sized vessels, and associated with asthma and blood eosinophilia.
Microscopic polyangiitis (microscopic polyarteritis)[c,d]	Necrotizing vasculitis with few or no immune deposits affecting small vessels, i.e., capillaries, venules, or arterioles. Necrotizing arteritis involving small and medium-sized arteries may be present. Necrotizing glomerulonephritis is very common. Pulmonary capillaritis often occurs.
Henoch-Schönlein purpura[d]	Vasculitis with IgA-dominant immune deposits affecting small vessels, i.e., capillaries, venules, or arterioles. Typically involves skin, gut, and glomeruli, and is associated with arthralgias or arthritis.
Essential cryoglobulinemic vasculitis[d]	Vasculitis with cryoglobulin immune deposits affecting small vessels, i.e., capillaries, venules, or arterioles, and associated with cryoglobulins in serum. Skin and glomeruli are often involved.
Cutaneous leukocytoclastic angiitis	Isolated cutaneous leukocytoclastic angiitis without systemic vasculitis or glomerulonephritis.

[a]Modified from Jennette JC, Falk RJ, Andrassy K, *et al.*: Nomenclature of systemic vasculitides: The proposal of an international consensus conference. *Arthritis Rheum* 37:187–192, 1994. Copyright © 1994 John Wiley & Sons, Inc. Reprinted by permission of John Wiley & Sons, Inc.

[b]Large artery refers to the aorta and the largest branches directed toward major body regions (e.g., to the extremities and the head and neck); medium-sized artery refers to the main visceral arteries (e.g., renal, hepatic, coronary and mesenteric arteries), and small vessel refers to the distal arterial radoclar that connect with arterioles (e.g., renal arcuate and interlobular arteries), as well as arterioles, capillaries, and venules. Note that some small and large vessel vasculitides may involve medium-sized arteries; but large and medium-sized vessel vasculitides do not involve vessels smaller than arteries.

[c]Strongly associated with antineutrophil cytoplasmic autoantibodies (ANCA).

[d]May be accompanied by glomerulonephritis and can manifest as nephritis or pulmonary–renal vasculitic syndrome.

and patients with other types of vasculitis (e.g., microscopic polyangiitis and Wegener's granulomatosis) may have temporal artery involvement. Therefore, temporal artery disease is neither a required nor sufficient pathologic feature of giant cell (temporal) arteritis.

Histologically, both giant cell arteritis and Takayasu arteritis are characterized by focal granulomatous inflammation, often with multinucleated giant cells. With chronicity, the inflammatory injury evolves into fibrosis and frequently results in vascular narrowing, which is the basis for renovascular hypertension when a renal artery is involved.

Polyarteritis nodosa and Kawasaki disease affect medium-sized arteries (i.e., main visceral arteries), such as the mesenteric, hepatic, coronary, and main renal arteries. Polyarteritis nodosa often involves the renal arteries,

whereas Kawasaki disease only rarely affects them. These diseases also may involve small arteries, such as arteries within the parenchyma of skeletal muscle, liver, heart, pancreas, spleen, and kidney. By the definitions in Table 1, these vasculitides affect arteries exclusively and do not affect capillaries or venules. Thus, they do not cause glomerulonephritis. The presence of arteritis with glomerulonephritis indicates some form of small vessel vasculitis, such as microscopic polyangiitis.

Histologically, the acute arterial injury of Kawasaki disease and polyarteritis nodosa is characterized by focal vessel wall fibrinoid necrosis and infiltration of inflammatory cells. Fibrinoid necrosis results from plasma coagulation factors spilling into the necrotic areas where they are activated to form fibrin. Early in the inflammatory process, neutrophils predominate, but later mononuclear leukocytes are most numerous. Thrombosis may occur at the site of inflammation, resulting in infarction. Focal necrotizing injury to vessels erodes into the vessel wall and adjacent tissue producing an inflammatory aneurysm, which may rupture and cause hemorrhage. Thrombosis of the inflamed arteries causes downstream ischemia and infarction.

Although small vessel vasculitides may affect medium-sized arteries, these disorders favor small vessels such as arterioles, postcapillary venules (e.g., in the dermis), and capillaries (e.g., in glomeruli and pulmonary alveoli) (Fig. 1). As described in Table 1, there are a variety of clinically and pathogenetically distinct forms of small vessel vasculitis that have in common focal necrotizing inflammation of small vessels. In the acute phase, this injury is characterized histologically by segmental fibrinoid necrosis and leukocyte infiltration (Fig. 2), sometimes with secondary thrombosis. The neutrophils often undergo karyorrhexis (leukocytoclasia). With chronicity, mononuclear leukocytes become predominant and fibrosis develops.

The various forms of small vessel vasculitis differ from one another with respect to the presence or absence of distinctive features, as summarized in Table 1 and Fig. 1. For example, Wegener's granulomatosis has necrotizing granulomatous inflammation, Churg–Strauss syndrome has eosinophilia and asthma, Henoch–Schönlein purpura has IgA-dominant vascular immune deposits, and cryoglobulinemic vasculitis has cryoglobulins. Microscopic polyangiitis has none of these features.

The glomerular lesions of microscopic polyangiitis, Wegener's granulomatosis and Churg–Strauss syndrome are identical pathologically, and are characterized by segmental fibrinoid necrosis, crescent formation (Fig. 3), and a paucity of glomerular staining for immunoglobulin. Patients with these three vasculitides often have antineutrophil cytoplasmic autoantibodies (ANCA). The glomerulonephritis of Henoch–Schönlein purpura is identical to IgA nephropathy. The glomerulonephritis of cryoglobulinemic vasculitis usually is a secondary form of type I membranoproliferative glomerulonephritis (mesangio-

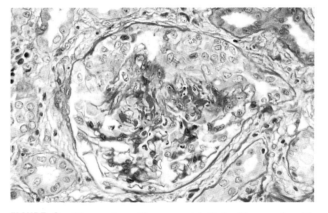

FIGURE 3 Glomerulus with segmental fibrinoid necrosis with red (fuchsinophilic) fibrinous material and an adjacent cellular crescent from a patient with ANCA-small vessel vasculitis (Masson trichrome stain).

capillary glomerulonephritis), although other patterns of proliferative glomerulonephritis occur less often.

Leukocytoclastic angiitis of medullary vasa recta (Fig. 4) also occurs in the ANCA vasculitides, and rarely is severe enough to cause papillary necrosis.

PATHOGENESIS

Vasculitides are caused by the activation of inflammatory mediator systems in vessel walls. The initiating event (i.e., the etiology), however, is unknown for most vasculitides. An immune response to heterologous antigens (e.g., hepatitis B or C antigens in some forms of immune complex vasculitis) or autoantigens (e.g., endothelial antigens in Kawasaki disease) is presumed to be the etiologic event in many vasculitides, but this can be documented in only a few patients. Table 2 categorizes vasculitides based on putative immunologic mechanisms.

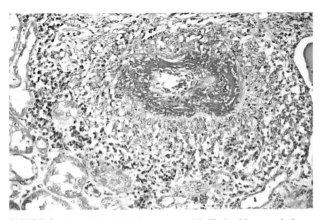

FIGURE 2 Renal interlobular artery with fibrinoid necrosis from a patient with microscopic polyangiitis (Masson trichrome stain).

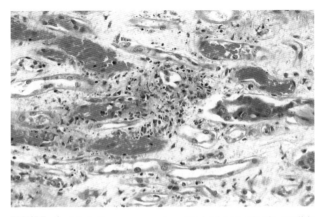

FIGURE 4 Medullary vasa recta with leukocytoclastic angiitis from a patient with Wegener's granulomatosis (Hematoxylin and eosin stain).

Immune complex mediated
   Henoch–Schönlein purpura[a]
   Cryoglobulinemic vasculitis[a]
   Lupus vasculitis[a]
   Serum sickness vasculitis[a]
   Rheumatoid vasculitis
   Polyarteritis nodosa
   Infection-induced immune complex vasculitis[a]
      Viral (e.g., hepatitis B and C virus)
      Bacterial (e.g., streptococcal)

Direct antibody attack mediated
   Goodpasture's syndrome (anti-basement membrane
      antibodies)[a]
   Kawasaki disease (antiendothelial antibodies)

ANCA-associated and possibly ANCA-mediated
   Wegener's granulomatosis[a]
   Microscopic polyangiitis[a]
   Churg–Strauss syndrome[a]

Cell mediated
   Allograft cellular vascular rejection
   Giant cell (temporal) arteritis
   Takayasu arteritis

[a]May be accompanied by glomerulonephritis and can manifest as nephritis or pulmonary–renal vasculitic syndrome.

Primarily because of the pattern of inflammation, T-cell mediated inflammation has been incriminated in the pathogenesis of giant cell (temporal) arteritis and Takayasu arteritis. Several mechanisms of antibody-mediated injury are thought to be important in the pathogenesis of necrotizing small vessel vasculitides, but there also is evidence that T cells play an important role.

The vasculitides listed in the immune complex mediated category in Table 2 all have immunohistologic evidence for vessel wall immune complex localization, that is, granular staining for immunoglobulins and complement. Antibodies bound to antigens in vessel walls activate humoral inflammatory mediator systems (e.g., complement, coagulation, plasmin, and kinin systems), which attract and activate neutrophils and monocytes. These activated leukocytes generate toxic oxygen metabolites and release enzymes that cause matrix lysis and cellular apoptosis, resulting in necrotizing inflammatory injury to vessel walls.

This same final pathway of inflammatory injury also can be reached if antibodies bind to antigens that are integral components of vessel walls. The best documented example is anti-glomerular basement membrane (GBM) antibody mediated glomerulonephritis and Goodpasture's syndrome. A less well-documented example of direct antibody attack is Kawasaki disease. There is evidence that patients with Kawasaki disease have antiendothelial antibodies that react with antigens expressed on the surface of stimulated endothelial cells. T cells with specificity for basement membranes or cells also may participate in the mediation or regulation of glomerular injury.

A very important group of necrotizing systemic small vessel vasculitides, which frequently involve the kidneys, occurs without immunohistologic evidence for vascular immune complex localization or direct antibody binding. This paucity of immune deposits has fostered the designation pauciimmune for this group of vasculitides, which includes microscopic polyangiitis, Wegener's granulomatosis, and Churg–Strauss syndrome. The pathogenesis of these vasculitides is unknown, but their close association with ANCA has lead to speculation that they result from ANCA-induced leukocyte activation and vascular injury.

ANCA are specific for proteins within the granules of neutrophils and lysosomes of monocytes. They often are detected in patient serum by indirect immunofluorescence microscopy using alcohol-fixed normal human neutrophils as substrate. Using this assay, two patterns of neutrophil staining discriminate between the two major subtypes of ANCA; cytoplasmic staining (C-ANCA) and perinuclear staining (P-ANCA). Using specific immunochemical assays such as enzyme-linked immunosorbent assays or radioimmunoassays, most C-ANCA are specific for a neutrophil and monocyte proteinase called proteinase 3 (PR3), and most P-ANCA are specific for myeloperoxidase (MPO).

One hypothesis about the pathogenesis of ANCA-associated vasculitides proposes that ANCA react with cytoplasmic antigens (e.g., PR3 and MPO) that are released at the surface of cytokine-stimulated leukocytes, causing the leukocytes to adhere to vessel walls, degranulate, and generate toxic oxygen metabolites. The interaction of ANCA with neutrophils involves Fc receptor engagement, perhaps by immune complexes formed between ANCA and ANCA-antigens in the microenvironment surrounding the leukocyte. ANCA binding to ANCA-antigens on the surface of neutrophils also may be involved in neutrophil activation. ANCA antigens also may become planted in vessel walls or even produced by endothelial cells, thus providing a nidus for *in situ* immune complex formation in vessel walls. If such *in situ* formation is present, it must be at a level that cannot be detected by immunofluorescence microscopy; ANCA-vasculitides are characteristically pauciimmune.

CLINICAL FEATURES

The diagnosis and management of systemic vasculitides can be very challenging. The clinical features are extremely varied, and are dictated by the category of vasculitis, the type of vessel involved, and the organ system distribution of vascular injury. Irrespective of the type of vasculitis, most patients will have accompanying constitutional features of inflammatory disease, such as fever, arthralgias, myalgias, and weight loss. These are probably caused by increased circulating levels of proinflammatory cytokines.

Giant cell arteritis and Takayasu arteritis typically present with evidence for ischemia in tissues supplied by involved arteries. Patients with Takayasu arteritis often develop claudication (especially in the upper extremities), absent pulses, and bruits. Approximately 40% of patients with Takayasu arteritis develop renovascular hypertension, a feature that only rarely complicates giant cell arteritis.

Giant cell arteritis can affect virtually any organ in the body, but signs and symptoms of involvement of arteries in the head and neck are the most common clinical manifestations. Superficial arteries, for example, the temporal artery, may be swollen and tender. Arterial narrowing causes ischemic manifestations in affected tissues, such as headache, jaw claudication, and loss of vision. About half of the patients with giant cell (temporal) arteritis have polymyalgia rheumatica, which is characterized by aching and stiffness in the neck, shoulder girdle, or pelvic girdle.

Medium-sized vessel vasculitides, such as polyarteritis nodosa and Kawasaki disease, often present with clinical evidence for infarction in multiple organs, such as abdominal pain with occult blood in the stool, and skeletal muscle pain and cardiac pain with elevated serum muscle enzymes. Laboratory evaluation often demonstrates clinically silent organ damage, such as liver injury with elevated liver function tests and pancreatic injury with elevated serum amylase.

Polyarteritis nodosa frequently causes multiple renal infarcts and aneurysms. Unlike microscopic polyangiitis, polyarteritis nodosa typically does not cause severe renal failure. Rupture of arterial aneurysms with massive retroperitoneal or intraperitoneal hemorrhage is a life-threatening complication of polyarteritis nodosa.

Kawasaki disease almost always occurs in young children and has a predilection for coronary, axillary, and iliac arteries. Kawasaki disease is accompanied by the mucocutaneous lymph node syndrome, which includes fever, nonpurulent lymphadenopathy, and mucosal and cutaneous inflammation. Although the renal arteries frequently are affected histologically, clinically significant renal involvement is very rare in patients with Kawasaki disease.

The small vessel vasculitides often present with evidence for inflammation in vessels in multiple organs, but may initially manifest with involvement of only one organ, followed by development of disease in other organs. Hematuria, proteinuria, and renal insufficiency caused by glomerulonephritis are frequent clinical features of all of the small vessel vasculitides listed in Table 1. Other manifestations include purpura caused by leukocytoclastic angiitis in dermal venules and arterioles, abdominal pain and occult blood in the stool from mucosal and bowel wall infarcts, mononeuritis multiplex from arteritis in peripheral nerves, necrotizing sinusitis from upper respiratory tract mucosal angiitis, and pulmonary hemorrhage from necrotizing alveolar capillaritis.

In addition to these features, which are common to patients with any type of small vessel vasculitis, patients with Wegener's granulomatosis and Churg–Strauss syndrome have distinctive clinical features that set them apart. Patients with Wegener's granulomatosis have necrotizing granulomatous inflammation in the upper or lower respiratory tract, and rarely in other tissues (e.g., skin, orbit). In the lungs, this inflammation produces irregular nodular lesions that can be observed by radiography. These lesions may cavitate and hemorrhage, but massive pulmonary hemorrhage in patients with Wegener's granulomatosis is usually caused by capillaritis rather than granulomatous inflammation. By definition, patients with Churg–Strauss syndrome have blood eosinophilia and a history of asthma. They also develop eosinophil-rich tissue inflammation, especially in the lungs and gut.

DIAGNOSIS

Multisystem disease in a patient with constitutional signs and symptoms of inflammation, such as fever, arthralgias, myalgias, and weight loss, should raise suspicion of systemic vasculitis. Data that will assist in resolving the differential diagnosis include the age of the patient, organ distribution of injury, concurrent syndromes (e.g., mucocutaneous lymph node syndrome, polymyalgia rheumatica, asthma), type of vessel involved (e.g., large artery, visceral artery, small vessel other than an artery), lesion histology (e.g., granulomatous, necrotizing), lesion immunohistology (e.g., immune deposits, pauci-immune), and serologic data (e.g., cryoglobulins, hepatitis C antibodies, hypocomplementemia, ANCA) (Fig. 1).

Signs and symptoms of tissue ischemia along with angiography demonstrating irregularity, stenosis, occlusion, or, less commonly, aneurysms of large and medium-sized arteries should suggest giant cell arteritis or Takayasu arteritis. A useful discriminator between giant cell arteritis and Takayasu arteritis is age. The former is rare in individuals less than 50 years of age, and the latter is rare in patients older than 50. The presence of polymyalgia rheumatica is a clinical marker for giant cell arteritis.

Polyarteritis nodosa and Kawasaki disease cause visual ischemia, particularly in the heart, kidneys, liver, spleen, and gut. Arteritis in skeletal muscle and subcutaneous tissues causes tender nodules that can be identified on physical examination. Angiographic demonstration of medium-sized artery aneurysms (e.g., in renal arteries) indicates that some type of vasculitis is present, but it is not disease-specific because giant cell arteritis, Takayasu arteritis, polyarteritis nodosa, Kawasaki disease, Wegener's granulomatosis, microscopic polyarteritis, and Churg–Strauss syndrome all can produce aneurysms. Kawasaki disease occurs almost always in children under 5 years old and is always accompanied by the mucocutaneous lymph node syndrome.

A small vessel vasculitis should be suspected when there is evidence for inflammation of vessels smaller than arteries, such as glomerular capillaries (hematuria and proteinuria), dermal postcapillary venules (purpura), and alveolar capillaries (hemoptysis). To discriminate among the small vessel vasculitides, evaluation of serology data, vessel immunohistology, or concurrent nonvasculitic disease (e.g., asthma, eosinophilia, lupus) is required (Fig. 1).

Evaluation of vessels in biopsy specimens, such as glomerular capillaries in renal biopsies or alveolar capillaries in a lung biopsies, can be helpful, especially if immunohistology is performed. The pauci-immune vasculitides will lack immune deposits, anti-GBM disease will have linear immunoglobulin deposits, and the immune complex vasculitides will have granular immune deposits.

Serology, especially ANCA analysis, is useful in differentiating among the small vessel vasculitides. Wegener's granulomatosis, microscopic polyangiitis, and Churg–Strauss syndrome are strongly associated with ANCA. As depicted in Fig. 5, most patients with active untreated Wegener's granulomatosis have C-ANCA (PR3-ANCA). A minority of patients will have P-ANCA (MPO-ANCA). Therefore, C-ANCA is a very sensitive serologic marker for active Wegener's granulomatosis; however, C-ANCA is not completely specific for Wegener's granulomatosis because some patients with C-ANCA will have systemic small vessel vasculitis without granulomatous inflammation (i.e., microscopic polyangiitis), and others will have pauci-immune necrotizing and crescentic glomerulonephritis alone. Approximately 80% of patients with microscopic polyangiitis have either C-ANCA or P-ANCA, with most having P-ANCA (MPO-ANCA). Patients with Churg–Strauss syndrome usually have either P-ANCA or C-ANCA. A minority of patients with immune complex mediated vasculitis or anti-GBM disease will have concurrent ANCA-associated disease.

Diagnostic serologic tests for immune complex mediated vasculitides include assays for circulating immune complexes (e.g., cryoglobulins in cryoglobulinemic vasculitis), assays for antibodies known to participate in immune complex formation or to mark the presence of a disease that generates immune complexes (e.g., antibodies to hepatitis B or C, streptococci, DNA), and assays for consumption or activation of humoral inflammatory mediator system components (e.g., assays for reduced complement components or for activated membrane attack complex).

THERAPY AND OUTCOME

All of the vasculitides discussed in this chapter respond to antiinflammatory or immunosuppressive therapy. The aggressiveness of treatment should match the aggressiveness of the disease.

Takayasu arteritis and giant cell arteritis usually respond well to high-dose corticosteroid treatment (e.g., 1 mg/kg body weight/day prednisone) during the acute phase of the disease, followed by tapering and low-dose maintenance for several months to a year depending on disease activity. Occasional patients with severe disease or steroid toxicity benefit from cytotoxic agents (e.g., cyclophosphamide). If present, renovascular hypertension should be controlled.

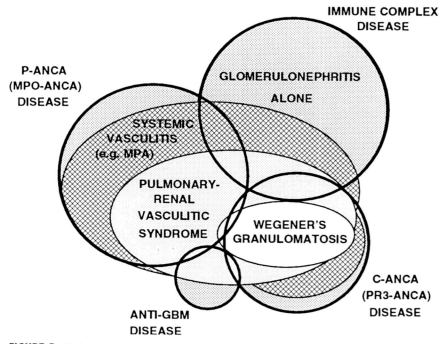

FIGURE 5 Relationship of vasculitic clinicopathologic syndromes to immunopathologic categories of vascular injury in patients with crescentic glomerulonephritis. The circles represent the major immunopathologic categories of vascular inflammation that affect the kidneys, and the shaded ovals the clinicopathologic expressions of the vascular inflammation. Note that clinical syndromes can be caused by more than one immunopathologic process, for example, pulmonary–renal vasculitic syndrome can be caused by anti-GBM antibodies (i.e., Goodpasture's syndrome), immune complex localization (e.g., lupus erythematosus), or ANCA-associated disease (e.g., microscopic polyangiitis and Wegener's granulomatosis). Reproduced with permission from Jennette JC: Anti-neutrophil cytoplasmic autoantibody-associated disease: A pathologist's perspective. *Am J Kidney Dis* 18:164–170, 1991.

After the inflammatory phase is past and the sclerotic phase has developed, reconstructive vascular surgery may be required to improve flow to ischemic tissues, especially in patients with Takayasu arteritis.

Many patients with polyarteritis nodosa have a persistent viral infection, especially hepatitis B virus infection. These patients are usually ANCA negative. In these cases antiviral therapy with or without plasma exchange is recommended. Patients with no evidence for infection usually are managed with corticosteroids with or without cytotoxic drugs.

Corticosteroid treatment is not recommended for Kawasaki disease because it appears to worsen coronary artery disease, which is the most life-threatening aspect of Kawasaki disease. The preferred treatment is a combination of aspirin and high-dose intravenous γ-globulins. This controls the inflammatory manifestations of the disease (e.g., the mucocutaneous lymph node syndrome), prevents thrombosis of injured arteries, and retards the frequency of coronary artery involvement. With appropriate treatment, over 90% of patients with Kawasaki disease have complete resolution of the disease.

Most patients with Henoch–Schönlein purpura have mild self-limited disease that requires only supportive care (Chapter 21). Arthralgias are relieved by nonsteroidal antiinflammatory drugs. Corticosteroid treatment is beneficial in patients who have severe abdominal pain caused by intestinal vasculitis. The treatment of severe glomerulonephritis in patients with Henoch–Schönlein purpura is controversial. There is anecdotal evidence that aggressive crescent glomerulonephritis should be treated with high-dose corticosteroids, cytotoxic agents, and/or plasmapheresis, but this has not been documented in controlled trials. Data from a large pediatric population suggest that corticosteroid treatment may decrease the risk of developing renal involvement in those patients with severe abdominal pain and rash.

The course and treatment of cryoglobulinemic vasculitis depends in part on the presence of associated diseases (Chapter 18). In patients with multiple myeloma or other lymphoproliferative diseases, treatment should be directed at these primary disease. Cryoglobulinemic vasculitis caused by hepatitis C may respond to α-interferon treatment in up to 25% of patients. In patients with severe vascular inflammation, treatment with corticosteroids, cytotoxic drugs, and plasmapheresis may be required.

High-dose corticosteroids (e.g., pulse methylprednisolone) and cytotoxic agents (e.g., cyclophosphamide) are the treatments of choice for necrotizing and crescentic glomerulonephritis associated with microscopic polyangiitis, Wegener's granulomatosis, the Churg–Strauss syndrome or for renal-limited vascular inflammation. Patients with pulmonary–renal vasculitic syndromes in whom hemoptysis is a major clinical feature require emergent treatment.

Induction therapy includes pulse methylprednisolone at 7 mg/kg/day for 3 days followed by daily oral prednisone. Prednisone treatment is typically converted to alternate day treatment during the second month of treatment. Corticosteroid treatment is terminated by the fourth or fifth month after diagnosis. Cyclophosphamide is administered intravenously at a starting dose of 0.5 g/m² and adjusted upward to 1 g/m² based on the leukocyte count. Alternatively oral cyclophosphamide can be initiated at a dose of 2 mg/kg/day and adjusted on the basis of the leukocyte count. The optimal duration of cyclophosphamide treatment has not been defined, but in our practice we plan to stop therapy within 6 months if the patient is in clinical remission or continue for a total of 1 year if signs and symptoms of vasculitis persist.

As many as 80% of ANCA-vasculitis patients will enter remission with aggressive immunosuppression, but approximately 40% will have a relapse within 2 years. There is controversy over how best to treat relapses. One approach is to retreat overt vasculitic relapses with a repeat course of corticosteroids and cyclophosphamide.

Bibliography

Agnello V, Chung RT, Kaplan LM: A role for hepatitis C virus infection in type II cryoglobulinemia N Engl J Med 327:1490–1495, 1992.

Falk RJ, Hogan S, Carey TS, Jennette JC: Clinical course of antineutrophil cytoplasmic autoantibody-associated glomerulonephritis and systemic vasculitis: The Glomerular Disease Collaborative Network. Ann Intern Med 113:656–663, 1990.

Guillevin L, Lhote F, Gherardi R: The spectrum and treatment of virus-associated vasculitides. Curr Opin Rheumatol 9:31–36, 1997.

Guillevin L, Durand-Gasselin B, Cevallos R, Gayraud M, Lhote F, Callard P, Amouroux J, Casassus P, Jarrousse B: Microscopic polyangiitis: Clinical and laboratory findings in eighty-five patients. Arthritis Rheum 42:421–430, 1999.

Hagen EC, Ballieux Be, van Es LA, Daha MR, van der Woude FJ: Antineutrophil cytoplasmic autoantibodies: A review of the antigens involved, the assays, and the clinical and possible pathogenetic consequences. Blood 81:1996–2002, 1993.

Hoffman GS, Kerr GS, Leavitt RY, et al.: Wegener's granulomatosis: An analysis of 158 patients. Ann Intern Med 116:488–498, 1992.

Hunder GG, Arend WP, Bloch DA, Calabrese LH, Fauci AS, Fries JF, Leavitt RY, Lie JT, Lightfoot RW, Jr, Masi AT, McShane DJ, Michel BA, Mills JA, Stevens MB, Wallace SL, Zvaifler NJ: The American College of Rheumatology 1990 criteria for the classification of vasculitis. Arthritis Rheum 3:1065–1067, 1990.

Jennette JC, Falk RJ: The pathology of vasculitis involving the kidney. Am J Kidney Dis 24:130–141, 1994.

Jennette JC, Falk RJ, Andrassy K, Bacon PA, Churg J, Gross WL, Hagen EC, Hoffman GS, Hunder GG, Kallenberg CGM, McCluskey RT, Sinico RA, Rees AJ, van Es LA, Waldherr R, Wiik A: Nomenclature of systemic vasculitides: Proposal of an international consensus conference. Arthritis Rheum 37:187–192, 1994.

Jennette JC, Falk RJ: Pathogenesis of the vascular and glomerular damage in ANCA-positive vasculitis. Nephrol Dial Transplant 13(Suppl 1):16–20, 1998.

Jennette JC, Falk RJ: Small vessel vasculitis. N Engl J Med 337:1512–1523, 1997.

Kaku Y, Nohara K, Honda S: Renal involvement in Henoch–Schönlein purpura: A multivariate analysis of prognostic factors. Kidney Int 53:1755–1759, 1998.

Leung DYM, Collins T, Lapierre LA, et al.: Immunoglobulin M antibodies present in the acute phase of Kawasaki syndrome lyse cultured vascular endothelial cells stimulated by gamma interferon. J Clin Invest 77:1428–1435, 1986.

Lie JT: Systemic and isolated vasculitis: A rational approach to classification and pathologic diagnosis. *Pathol Annu* 24(Pt 1): 25–114, 1989.

Nachman PH, Hogan SL, Jennette JC, Falk RJ: Treatment response and relapse in ANCA-associated microscopic polyangiitis and glomerulonephritis. *J Am Soc Nephrol* 7:23–32, 1996.

Niles JL, Pan GL, Collins AB, *et al.*: Antigen-specific radioimmunoassays for antineutrophil cytoplasmic antibodies in the diagnosis of rapidly progressive glomerulonephritis. *J Am Soc Nephrol* 2:27–36, 1991.

Rieu P, Noel LH: Henoch–Schönlein nephritis in children and adults. Morphological features and clinicopathological correlations. *Ann Med Intern* 150:151–159, 1999.

Ronco P, Verroust P, Mignon F, *et al.*: Immunopathological studies of polyarteritis nodosa and Wegener's Granulomatosis: A report of 43 patients with 51 renal biopsies. *Q J Med* 206:212–223, 1983.

Serra A, Cameron JS, Turner DR, *et al.*: Vasculitis affecting the kidney: Presentation, histopathology and long-term outcome. *Q J Med* 53:181–207, 1984.

Smith DL: Spontaneous rupture of a renal artery aneurysm in polyarteritis nodosa: Critical review of the literature and report of a case. *Am J Med* 87:464–467, 1989.

RENAL MANIFESTATIONS OF SYSTEMIC LUPUS ERYTHEMATOSUS AND OTHER RHEUMATIC DISORDERS

LEE A. HEBERT

Rheumatologic diseases that involve the kidney frequently result in glomerular and tubulointerstitial injury. In general, the degree of systemic inflammation is paralleled by the degree of renal inflammation, although in some cases the kidney may be more or less involved as the target organ. The clinical manifestations of glomerular and tubulointerstitial inflammation are that of hematuria, proteinuria, and renal insufficiency. Usually these clinical features correlate well with the histologic findings on renal biopsy (see Fig. 7 in Chapter 16). The spectrum of clinicopathologic correlation extends from patients with normal glomeruli with no clinical evidence of hematuria or proteinuria to examples of crescentic glomerulonephritis and rapidly progressive glomerular disease resulting in an accelerated loss of renal function. All too often, patients present at the end of their disease process with glomerular and tubulointerstitial scarring, resulting in chronic glomerulonephritis and end stage renal disease. The renal manifestations of rheumatologic conditions such as systemic lupus erythematosus (SLE), systemic sclerosis, Henoch–Schönlein purpura, and rheumatoid arthritis are many. Nonetheless, the most common presentation is that of hematuria and proteinuria with or without renal insufficiency and hypertension. Not only can the disease process itself induce damage, but some of the therapies used in rheumatologic conditions, including nonsteroidal antiinflammatory agents (NSAID), penicillamine, and gold salts are also capable of inducing renal disease. The following discussion highlights the manner in which these diseases injure the kidney and also presents the potential therapeutic options.

SYSTEMIC LUPUS ERYTHEMATOSUS

SLE is an autoimmune, multisystem disease that presents in a myriad of ways. About 25% of SLE patients develop substantial renal manifestations.

Microscopic hematuria is generally present in patients with SLE and renal disease. Glomerular hematuria is characterized by acanthocytes (dysmorphic red cells), and urinary red cell casts, or mixed casts (Chapter 4). It is uncommon for patients with SLE to present with gross hematuria. When observed, it usually is the consequence of cystitis or bacterial infections, or cyclophosphamide therapy. SLE patients with red or brown urine without the presence of red blood cells in the urine may have an autoimmune hemolytic anemia causing hemoglobinuria.

Proteinuria results from an increase in glomerular capillary permeability to both large (immunoglobulins) and small (albumin) plasma proteins. Albumin is the most common plasma protein found in the urine. Proteinuria is the consequence of glomerular inflammation (proliferation) as well as glomerular scarring. Renal insufficiency is most commonly the result of both glomerular and tubulointerstitial inflammation and scarring. In most cases in which there is renal insufficiency, systemic hypertension occurs as well.

In patients with SLE and renal disease, the examining physician should determine whether the patient has a disease process that is limited to the kidney or part of a systemic disease process. It is unusual for SLE patients to present with renal manifestations alone, although it does occur. Usually, signs and symptoms of the systemic disorder accompany the renal disease and include a range of clinical and physical exam findings, and laboratory evaluations that result in a diagnosis of lupus.

The diagnostic approach to lupus has been formalized by the American College of Rheumatology (ACR) revised criteria (Table 1). At least four of these criteria are needed to classify the disorder as SLE. These criteria need not be contemporaneous. Some of the most common findings include constitutional symptoms such as fever, malaise,

or anorexia; dermatologic conditions including skin rash or oral ulcers; cardiopulmonary symptoms including pleurisy or pericarditis; abdominal pain from peritoneal serositis; and neurologic manifestations including seizures or psychosis. Common coexisting laboratory findings are the presence of hematologic abnormalities including anemia, leukopenia, or thrombocytopenia. Serological tests including antinuclear antibody and the more specific double-stranded DNA or anti-SM (anti-Smith antibody) tests are frequently positive. The ACR criteria for SLE do not include low serum complement C3 and C4 levels. However, low C3 and C4 levels suggest activation of the classic complement pathway, which is characteristic of SLE.

Table 2 shows the frequency of the major clinical manifestations of SLE. Note that nephropathy affects only a minority of SLE patients. However, those with moderate to severe renal manifestations generally have worsened outcomes than those with minor or no renal manifestations. Thus, the presence of renal manifestations in the SLE patient is grounds for especially attentive management. Patients with other forms of rheumatoid disease share many of the clinical systemic features. An aid to the differentiation of these conditions is the finding of characteristic autoantibodies in these renal rheumatologic diseases (see Table 3).

Indications for Renal Biopsy in SLE

The presence of SLE glomerulonephritis can generally be assumed when a patient who meets the diagnostic criteria for SLE also manifests proteinuria or hematuria. Nev-

TABLE I

1982 Revised Criteria for Classification of Systemic Lupus Erythematosus[a]

Criterion	Description
Malar rash	Erythema of malar eminences
Discoid rash	Erythematous, scaling plaques with variable skin atrophy
Photosensitivity	Rash in response to sun exposure
Oral ulcers	Oral or nasopharyngeal ulcerations (usually painless)
Arthritis	Nonerosive, nondeforming arthritis of two or more joints
Serositis	Pleuritis, or pericarditis (rub or effusion)
Renal disease	Persistent proteinuria (>0.5 g/dL or 3+ dipstick) or cellular casts
Neurologic disease	Seizures or psychosis (without other etiology)
Hematologic disease	Hemolytic anemia or leukopenia (<4000/μL on two or more occasions), or lymphopenia (<1500/μL on two or more occasions), or thrombocytopenia (<100,000/μL)
Immunologic disease	LE cell prep, or anti-DNA antibody, or antiSm antibody, or false positive serologic test for syphilis (STS)
Antinuclear antibody	Abnormal titer (in absence of associated drugs)

[a]Systemic lupus erythematosus is said to be present if four or more criteria are present or have been present at some time. From Tan EM, Cohen AS, Fries JF: *Arthritis Rheum* 25:1271–1277, 1982.

TABLE 2

Clinical Manifestations Related to SLE in the Total Cohort of 1000 Patients, 1990–1995[a]

SLE manifestations	Number	%	CI
Malar rash	264	26.4	23.7–29.1
Discoid lesions	54	5.4	4.0–6.8
Subacute cutaneous lesions	46	4.6	3.2–6.0
Photosensitivity	187	18.7	16.3–21.1
Oral ulcers	89	8.9	7.1–10.7
Arthritis	413	41.3	38.2–44.4
Serositis	129	12.9	10.7–15.1
Nephropathy	222	22.2	19.7–24.7
Neurologic involvement	136	13.6	11.4–15.8
Thrombocytopenia	95	9.5	7.7–11.3
Hemolytic anemia	33	3.3	2.1–4.5
Fever	139	13.9	11.7–16.1
Raynaud's phenomenon	132	13.2	11.0–15.4
Livedo reticularis	55	5.5	4.1–5.9
Thrombosis	72	7.2	5.6–8.8
Myositis	40	4	5.6–8.8

[a]Reprinted with permission from: Cervera R, Khamashita MA, Font J, *et al.: Medicine* 78(3):167–175, 1999.
[b]CI, 95% confidence interval.

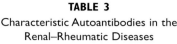

TABLE 3

Characteristic Autoantibodies in the
Renal–Rheumatic Diseases

Disorder	Autoantibodies
Systemic lupus erythematosus	Antinuclear antibodies (ANA) diffuse pattern, anti-DNA, anti-SM, anti-phospholipid (cardiolipin)
Henoch–Schönlein purpura	None
Systemic sclerosis	ANA (speckled), anti-Scl-70 (topoisomerase 1), anticentromere
Mixed connective tissue disease	ANA, anti-RNP (ribonucleoprotein)
Sjögren's syndrome	ANA, anti-Ro (anti-SS-A), anti-La (anti-SS-B)
Rheumatoid arthritis IgM	Rheumatoid factor (mostly antibody to IgG)
Behçet's syndrome	None
Relapsing polychondritis	None (occasional antibodies to type 2 collagen or ANCA)
Familial Mediterranean fever	None

ertheless, renal biopsy is usually recommended if the patient has major renal manifestations, such as proteinuria >2 g/24 hr or increased serum creatinine. The type of renal manifestation can profoundly influence SLE management.

The mildest histopathologic expression of lupus nephritis is that of a mesangial proliferative lupus glomerulonephritis categorized by the World Health Organization (WHO) as class II. With an increasing degree of immune deposits localized in the subendothelial zones of the glomerular capillary, the resultant inflammation causes a focal or diffuse proliferative lupus glomerulonephritis designated as class III or IV lupus nephritis, respectively (Fig. 1). As the degree of inflammation increases, necrosis and crescent formation may ensue. Class V lupus nephritis is also known as lupus membranous glomerulonephritis. In this condition, immune complexes are in the subepithelial portion of the glomerular basement membrane where they are not in contact with the cellular inflammatory mediators available in the blood (Fig. 2). These classes of lupus glomerular disease are not static in nature. There may be transition from one class of lupus nephritis to another (see Fig. 4 in Chapter 16).

A renal biopsy to confirm the presence or absence of lupus nephritis is highly valuable. Several conditions resemble SLE nephritis, either in clinical presentation or renal biopsy findings. Among these are type I or type II membranoproliferative glomerulonephritis (MPGN). In these cases there is a decrease in the serum C3 and sometimes C4 level, but typically no evidence of antinuclear antibodies (ANA) or antibodies directed against double-stranded DNA. Atheroembolism can also cause reduced complement levels and impaired kidney function with

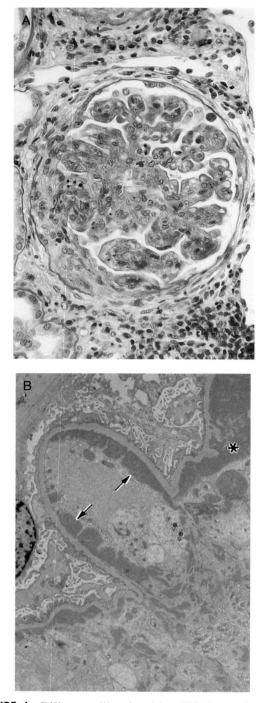

FIGURE 1 Diffuse proliferative (class IV) lupus glomerulonephritis. (A) Light microscopy showing global endocapillary hypercellularity, marked thickening of capillary walls including "wire loops" (upper right), obliteration of some capillary lumens, and a small crescent (lower left) (PAS stain). (B) Electron microscopy showing large subendothelial (arrows) and mesangial (asterisk) electron dense immune complex deposits. The large subendothelial deposits would correspond to "wire loop" lesions by light microscopy. (Courtesy Dr. J.C. Jennette.)

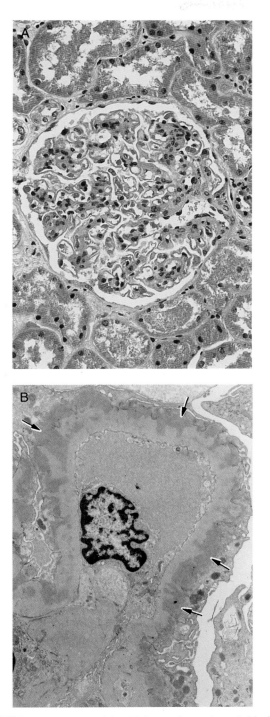

FIGURE 2 Membranous (class V) lupus glomerulonephritis. (A) Light microscopy showing global capillary wall thickening and slight segmental mesangial hypercellularity (hematoxylin and eosin). (B) Electron microscopy showing numerous subepithelial electron dense immune complex deposits (arrows). (Courtesy Dr. J.C. Jennette.)

what looks like a nephritic urine. On renal biopsy, emboli will be found, and ANA are not usually present.

Drug-induced SLE may present in a similar fashion to idiopathic SLE, but drug-induced SLE rarely involves the kidney.

Conditions not related to SLE may also be present on renal biopsy, and these could critically influence management. These include interstitial nephritis of NSAID use, glomerulopathy of infection (visceral abscess), idiopathic focal glomerulosclerosis, or minimal change disease nephrotic syndrome. Each of these conditions has previously been reported in SLE patients. In addition to the diagnostic importance of the renal biopsy, therapeutic decisions rest on the biopsy findings. Therapy for lupus membranous disease may differ from class IV lupus nephritis. Furthermore, the renal biopsy describes the activity (inflammation) of the glomerular and tubulointerstitial lesion, as well as the degree of chronicity (scarring) in the glomerular and tubulointerstitial compartments.

Renal biopsy is not generally indicated in SLE patients with chronic renal insufficiency when it is likely that advanced irreversible disease is present. This is usually the case when small, scarred (echogenic) kidneys are detected by ultrasonography or when moderate or severe renal insufficiency (serum creatinine >3.0 mg/dL) has been present for 6 months or more.

PATHOGENESIS OF SLE

SLE is a multisystem, autoimmune disease that is genetically determined, but its clinical expression is strongly influenced by clinical (environmental) interactions. Both epidemiology and molecular genetic studies provide evidence that SLE is genetically determined. The incidence of SLE in the general population is about 0.1%. However, in first degree relatives of SLE patients (including dizygotic twins), the SLE incidence is 2 to 4%. In monozygotic twins, the concordance rate for SLE is 24 to 58%. Molecular genetic studies have localized candidate susceptibility gene(s) to the 1q41–q42 region of chromosome 1. The discovery of additional SLE susceptibility genes is likely because the epidemiological evidence favors a multigenetic mode of SLE inheritance.

Additional evidence suggests that SLE is also determined by specific interactions with the patient's environment. First, monozygotic twins are not always concordant for SLE. Presumably, the twin with SLE has interacted with an environmental factor(s) causing SLE to be expressed. Those factors are poorly understood. A few are discussed later. Second, estrogens appear to favor the expression of SLE. For example, when SLE has its onset in childhood, the female/male ratio is approximately 1:1. However, when SLE has its onset in adulthood, the female/male ratio is 9:1. In addition, pregnancy—which is characterized by marked increases in estrogen secretion—is a common trigger for SLE relapse, particularly in women with renal involvement. Furthermore, estrogen replacement therapy in postmenopausal women is associated with an increased incidence of new-onset SLE, and estrogen-containing oral contraceptives in SLE patients may be associated with an increased risk of SLE relapse. The mechanism by which estrogens may induce or exacerbate SLE is not clear. However, estrogens suppress immune tolerance (increase autoimmunity) and the ability of the mononuclear phagocyte system to clear circulating immune complexes. One or both of these events could explain the effects of estrogen in SLE. Third, sun exposure is a well-established trigger for SLE onset or SLE relapse. The mechanism is unclear. However, sun damage to the skin may cause autoantigens to be exposed, resulting in immune activation. Finally, infection or psychological stress may be involved in the induction or exacerbation of SLE. For example, Epstein-Barr virus (EBV) infection occurs in nearly 100% of children and young adults with SLE, but in only 70% of controls. EBV "molecular mimicry" of DNA might account for the association of prior EBV infection with the development of anti-DNA antibodies, which leads to SLE. Numerous anecdotal reports link activation of SLE to psychological stress, as well as to environmental exposures such as hair dyes, dusty environments, and cigarette smoking. However, there is still a great deal to be learned about the clinical and environmental triggers of SLE. Knowledge of those triggers could help control SLE and perhaps prevent its onset.

There is solid evidence that hyperactivity of B and T cells is responsible for the excessive production of SLE autoantibodies. The autoantibodies are directed at approximately 30 different cellular antigens. The autoantibodies most characteristic of SLE are those directed at double-stranded DNA in the context of nucleosome (the basic unit of nuclear chromatin). There are also autoantibodies to cell surface antigens such as those on platelets, red cells, and neurons.

The characteristic lesion in SLE is the accumulation of immune complexes. These are identified as electron dense deposits (by electron microscopy) that contain immunoglobulin and complement (by immunofluorescent microscopy). Immune complexes activate the complement system (Fig. 2) by the classic pathway, causing the deposition of the activated form of C3 (C3b). This results in opsonization (adherence of the immune complex to inflammatory cells via their C3b receptors), induction of inflammation by release of the potent chemokines, and cell damage by formation of the membrane attack complex (MAC), which can create lethal pores in cell membranes. Immune complexes also promote inflammation when the Fc regions of the antibodies engage Fc receptors expressed on resident cells (mesangial cells). Certain Fc receptors activate inflammation mechanisms, for example, induction of monocyte chemotactic protein-1, which promotes the influx of inflammatory cells. Finally, immune complexes can cause tissue injury by their sheer physical presence (as when immune complexes disrupt the glomerular basement membrane or podocyte to cause proteinuria).

The autoantibodies that bind to cell surface antigens can lead to cell destruction by complement activation on the cell surface, or by Fc receptor-mediated ingestion of the cell by the resident phagocyte cells of liver and spleen. Autoimmune thrombocytopenia and hemolytic anemia are examples of the latter process.

Autoantibodies, particularly antiphospholipid antibodies (aPL) can induce arterial or venous clotting. These phenomena cause severe encephalopathy, acute or chronic progressive renal failure, bowel infarction, and the nonbacterial verrucous endocarditis of Libman and Sacks (especially on the aortic valve). This often leads to systemic emboli or venous thromboses that, in turn, leads to pulmonary embolism. Not all SLE patients with thrombotic events manifest aPL, suggesting that other pathways also cause thrombosis in SLE.

Therapy of Mild to Moderate Renal Manifestations of SLE

If a patient with SLE has a normal serum creatinine level and minor proteinuria (<1 g/24 hr), it may be sufficient simply to treat with oral prednisone or long-term azathioprine (75 to 125 mg daily, depending on body weight) and sufficient prednisone to control the nonrenal manifestations of SLE. Generally, 6 to 12 months of such therapy is needed to resolve mild to moderate renal manifestations. The therapy of lupus membranous nephropathy is still unclear. Some have regarded SLE membranous nephropathy as an indolent and relatively therapy-resistant disease. However, others have shown that the combination of prednisone and cytotoxic drugs usually induce remission of the nephrotic syndrome. Mycophenolate mofetil and cyclosporine may also be effective in inducing remission of nephrosis in these patients.

Therapy of Severe Renal Manifestations of SLE

In patients with active diffuse proliferative glomerulonephritis with hematuria, aggressive immunosuppressive treatment is indicated. Proteinuria usually exceeds 3 g/24 hr, with or without renal insufficiency. In brief, these patients generally require high-dose prednisone therapy (1 mg/kg/ideal body weight/day, maximum 80 mg daily) for a period of 2 to 4 weeks. In severe SLE, glucocorticoid therapy is often initiated by bolus infusion of methylprednisolone 1 g daily for each of 3 days, followed by oral prednisone therapy. After 2 to 4 weeks of high-dose prednisone therapy, the dose is decreased to 0.75 mg/kg of ideal body weight for a period of another 2 to 4 weeks. Thereafter, the prednisone can be tapered to ensure the adequate treatment of the extrarenal manifestations of SLE.

Cytotoxic drugs are also required for severe SLE renal manifestations. The most prevalent form of therapy is that of the monthly administration of intravenous cyclophosphamide given at a starting dose of 0.5 to 1.0 mg/kg/M^2 of body surface area for at least 6 months. Some authorities suggest that the cyclophosphamide therapy should then begin every 3 months for a total duration of therapy of 2 years. Alternatively, cyclophosphamide can be provided orally at 1.5 to 2.0 mg/kg/ideal body weight (maximum 150 mg) for 8 to 12 weeks, followed by azathioprine at 1.5 to 2.0 mg/kg/ideal body weight (maximum 150 mg) until the patient has been in remission for 1 year.

There are several experimental approaches to the treatment of systemic lupus erythematosus, including cyclosporine, mycophenolate mofetil, antibodies to CD40 ligand, antibodies to C5, and other drugs that impair cytokine or chemokine responses. These drugs are still in experimental trials, with the hope that they will improve the long-term care of SLE.

KEY ISSUES IN THE MANAGEMENT OF SLE NEPHRITIS

The kidney is just one of the organs typically involved with SLE. Thus, the management of the nonrenal manifestations of SLE is important. The most severe extrarenal manifestations of SLE are lupus pneumonitis, cerebritis, and vasculitis. Nonrenal manifestations of SLE that are moderate in severity, such as pleuritis, pericarditis, rash, arthritis, and mild to moderate thrombocytopenia are usually controlled with oral corticosteroids. Other therapies, including hydroxychloroquine and NSAIDs may also be useful. The following are general recommendations.

1. Early treatment of renal relapse may prevent severe renal relapse. Patients who have experienced severe renal manifestations of SLE and then undergo remission should be closely monitored so that if they relapse, which is likely, they can be treated promptly. Early treatment of patients with SLE relapse may decrease the amount and duration of therapy needed to control the SLE.

2. Close monitoring is important and depends on when the patient last experienced a relapse. Within 6 months of a relapse, monthly follow-up is usually indicated. If the most recent relapse occurred more than 6 months ago, testing at 2-month intervals is appropriate. The recommended testing regimen includes urinalysis, determination of serum creatinine level, complete blood count (CBC), and 24-hr urine collection to determine protein and creatinine excretion. Serum C3 and anti-DNA antibody levels are useful in assessing SLE disease activity and should ideally be performed at 2- to 4-month intervals in patients with recently active SLE. Perhaps the most cost-effective test in assessing SLE renal activity is the urine sediment analysis. The appearance of erythrocyte or leukocyte casts, or both, has a high degree of sensitivity and specificity for predicting SLE renal relapse.

3. Fever that develops in a patient with SLE who is receiving high-dose corticosteroid therapy is usually the result of infection, not active SLE. The fever associated with SLE is generally easily suppressed by the administration of prednisone at 20 to 30 mg daily. If fever develops during prednisone therapy at doses greater than 20 to 30 mg daily, infection is the likely cause. Continued use of high-dose glucocorticoid therapy in the febrile SLE patient carries a high risk of fatal outcome from sepsis.

4. If fever develops in a patient with SLE who is receiving high-dose corticosteroid and immunosuppressive therapy, administration of cytotoxic drugs should be stopped and the prednisone dose reduced to 20 to 30 mg daily. A search for infection or other cause of fever should then be undertaken. If infection is present, prednisone 20 to 30 mg daily, should not prevent successful treatment of the infection. At the same time, this dose of prednisone should be sufficient to prevent a severe flare of SLE.

5. Close follow-up is particularly warranted in African-Americans, who are at increased risk for adverse outcomes.

6. If overt proteinuria is present (more than 1 g daily), it is especially important to use adjunctive measures to slow progression of renal disease. These measures include strict control of blood pressure, use of an angiotensin converting enzyme (ACE) inhibitor, control of blood lipids, and reduced dietary salt and, perhaps, protein intake.

Some nonrenal manifestations of SLE do not respond to intense immunosuppressive therapy. These include thrombotic glomerulopathy and clotting disorders that may be associated with antiphospholipid antibodies. In these patients, anticoagulation therapy may be in order. With central nervous system abnormalities, anticonvulsants may be necessary. In rare circumstances, plasma exchange is employed to remove antiphospholipid antibodies and limit a fulminant antiphospholipid syndrome. Severe thrombocytopenia, thrombotic nonbacterial endocarditis, vesicular skin eruptions, and fibromyalgia may all require alternative modes of treatment.

SYSTEMIC SCLEROSIS

Systemic sclerosis (scleroderma) is characterized by progressive fibrosis and dysfunction of the skin and internal organs, principally the heart, gastrointestinal tract, and kidney. Systemic sclerosis is listed with "rheumatic diseases" because these patients commonly complain of joint discomfort, principally the small joints of the hands and wrists. Systemic sclerosis is also listed among autoimmune disorders because these patients often manifest antinuclear antibodies, including ANA (in about 70% of patients), and a highly specific antinuclear antibody Scl-70, topoisomerase 1 (in about 20% of patients). It seems unlikely, however, that systemic sclerosis is primarily the result of autoimmunity because, among other evidence, scleroderma is not improved by immunosuppressive therapy, as are known disorders of autoimmunity. The pathogenesis of systemic sclerosis is unknown, but a primary defect in collagen biosynthesis is suspected.

The clinical presentation of systemic sclerosis is varied. Patients complain of chronic progressive arthralgias of the hands accompanied by thickening of the digits and loss of elasticity of the skin over the phalanges (sclerodactyly). Raynaud's phenomenon is common. Most patients who develop renal disease related to scleroderma have evident skin manifestations when the renal disease develops. However, patients with systemic sclerosis can also present with malignant hypertension or renal failure in the absence of skin or rheumatic findings. The disorder may resemble a primary thrombotic microangiopathy (hemolytic-uremic syndrome) or malignant hypertension from any cause. The patient with systemic sclerosis who presents with renal manifestations but no skin manifestations may develop the skin manifestations 6 months or more afterward.

The renal biopsy can be useful in differentiating primary thrombotic microangiopathy from systemic sclerosis renal involvement. In systemic sclerosis, the arterioles show marked arteriolar sclerosis (multiple reduplications of the internal elastic lamina, indicating multiple episodes of endothelial damage and repair) along with variable amounts of thrombi in arterioles and glomeruli. In acute primary thrombotic microangiopathy, the major findings are those of fibrin thrombi within arterioles and glomeruli (Fig. 3). A biopsy is not needed when skin manifestations and other features of scleroderma precede the onset of typical scleroderma renal crisis. A "nephritic" urine sediment (red cell casts, white cell casts, abundant hematuria, and acanthocytes) is unusual in scleroderma, where the urine sediment can be quite "bland." Proteinuria is often <1.0 g/24 hr. Renal disease typically occurs in the first 5 years of the onset of the disease. Several risk factors for the development of renal disease have been elucidated, including the increased incidence of scleroderma renal crisis in African-Americans, presence of diffuse skin involvement, use of high-dose corticosteroids, and exposure to cold.

Treatment of scleroderma renal disease is primarily that of aggressive blood pressure control. An ACE inhibitor is the agent of choice. Use of an agent in this class leads to an improvement in blood pressure in over 90% of patients. ACE inhibitor therapy has dramatically improved the outcome of patients with scleroderma, including regression of skin changes and improvement in Raynaud's phenomenon. This effect appears to be more than that of blood pressure control. ACE inhibitors suppress angiotensin II formation, which may suppress fibrogenic mechanisms, particularly through transforming growth factor β (TGF-β). When compared to other antihypertensive agents, ACE inhibitors have not only an increased antihypertensive efficacy, but they are also associated with improved survival, preservation of renal function, and an improved opportunity for recovery of renal function that sometimes results in discontinuation of dialysis. With ACE inhibitor therapy, systemic sclerosis patients with acute renal failure have a relatively good short-term prognosis. Most regain kidney function sufficient to discontinue dialysis. Renal disease may remain clinically quiescent during many years of follow-up. Other forms of therapy, including nifedipine (which may help in Raynaud's phenomenon), intravenous prostacyclin, fish oil, and penicillamine may be useful adjuncts.

RHEUMATOID ARTHRITIS

Renal involvement in rheumatoid arthritis is unusual. In rare instances, patients with rheumatoid arthritis may develop an immune complex-mediated renal disease from cryoglobulins formed when rheumatoid factors (IgM antibody with specificity against IgG) form circulating immune complexes. These patients are benefited by prednisone and cytotoxic therapy. NSAID use in rheumatoid arthritis may also induce renal disease. The most common NSAID renal manifestation is an acute decrease in glomerular filtration rate that is probably hemodynamically mediated. NSAID use can also cause the nephrotic syndrome associated with either membranous nephropathy or interstitial nephritis. These conditions resolve when the NSAID is discontinued. Chronic NSAID therapy can also cause progressive renal failure because of direct nephrotoxicity. Rarely, patients with rheumatoid arthritis develop secondary amyloidosis from the deposition of serum protein A, the acute phase reactant. This is termed AA amyloidosis, and its prognosis is poor.

HENOCH–SCHÖNLEIN PURPURA

Henoch–Schönlein purpura is a multisystem disorder in which vasculitis involves the skin (particularly of the lower extremities), gastrointestinal tract (with gastrointestinal bleeding and pain), joints (causing arthritis), kidneys (causing glomerulonephritis), and, rarely, the lungs. Diagnosis depends on the identification of IgA deposits in the affected tissues, usually skin or kidney. Because Henoch–Schönlein purpura is a vasculitis, it must be differentiated from other forms of vasculitis, including the vasculitis associated with antineutrophil cytoplasmic autoantibody (ANCA), SLE, cryoglobulinemia (type I, II, or III), or drug hypersensitivity. Note that types II and III cryoglobulinemia can be associated with SLE, chronic bacterial infections, or

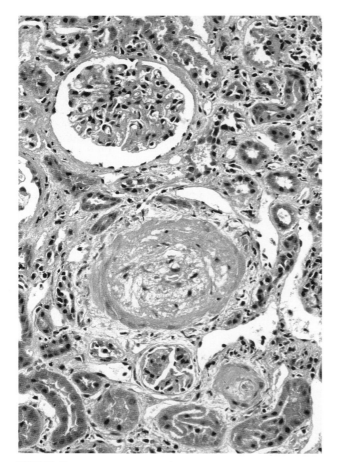

FIGURE 3 Systemic sclerosis (scleroderma) renal crisis. Light microscopy showing obliteration of an interlobular artery by a combination of fibrinoid necrosis and sclerosis. Note the absence of vascular inflammation and the glomerulus with no hypercellularity. (hematoxylin and eosin). (Courtesy Dr. J.C. Jennette.)

infections with hepatitis B, hepatitis C, Epstein-Barr, or human immunodeficiency viruses.

High-dose corticosteroid therapy may benefit patients with the inflammatory manifestations of skin vasculitis and gastrointestinal bleeding. Short-term, high-dose corticosteroid therapy may also benefit patients with the severe crescentic glomerulonephritis of Henoch–Schönlein purpura. Results of uncontrolled studies suggest that long-term prednisone and azathioprine therapy may be useful in inducing remission in patients with chronic disease with heavy proteinuria.

BEHÇET'S SYNDROME

Behçet's syndrome is a multisystem disorder characterized by recurrent aphthous oral and genital ulceration. In addition, erythema nodosum or other rash, nondeforming arthritis, and ocular inflammation may occur. The central nervous system and gastrointestinal tract can also be involved. Arterial or venous occlusive disease due to a thrombotic diathesis is common. Rarely, a rapidly progressive crescentic glomerulonephritis may be observed. Mesangial IgA deposition in the kidney has also been reported. As renal involvement in this disorder is infrequent, definitive treatment recommendations are not available. Prednisone, azathioprine, and cyclosporine have been used as therapy for systemic involvement.

RELAPSING POLYCHONDRITIS

Relapsing polychondritis is characterized by recurrent inflammation of cartilage. Sites of involvement include the ears, nose, respiratory tract, and joints. Uveitis, scleritis, and retinitis may also be observed. The kidneys are affected in up to 22% of patients, although this figure may be skewed by referral bias. Renal involvement includes mesangial cell proliferation as well as focal segmental necrotizing glomerulonephritis with crescent formation. Anticollagen antibodies and antineutrophil cytoplasmic antibodies have been noted. Owing to the rarity of this condition, definitive treatment recommendations for renal involvement are lacking.

FAMILIAL MEDITERRANEAN FEVER

Familial Mediterranean fever is an autosomal recessive disorder that occurs primarily in individuals of Turkish, Armenian, Sephardic, or Arab descent. Recurrent episodes of serositis, fever, and arthritis are associated with secondary (AA) amyloidosis, and the latter may lead to proteinuria and renal failure. Colchicine treatment prevents acute episodes of fever and development of proteinuria. Once nephrotic syndrome is established, however, colchicine is ineffective in preventing development of end stage renal disease.

SJÖGREN'S SYNDROME

Sjögren's syndrome is a chronic inflammatory disorder whose primary manifestations are that of diminished salivary and lacrimal gland secretion. This results in the "sicca complex" with dry eyes and dry mouth. Sjögren's syndrome may also be associated with vasculitic skin lesions, interstitial lung disease, and gastrointestinal involvement with dysphagia, nausea, epigastric pain, and dyspepsia. Hepatic disease resembling primary biliary cirrhosis and cranial neuropathy are also seen.

When the kidney is involved in Sjögren's syndrome, a chronic interstitial nephritis ensues. This picture leads to tubular dysfunction, including renal tubular acidosis and polyuria due to nephrogenic diabetes insipidus. Glomerulonephritis in Sjögren's syndrome is rare.

Few data provide guidance on the appropriate management of renal insufficiency in Sjögren's syndrome. Treatment is typically empirical and includes the use of corticosteroids, with or without immunosuppressive drugs such as azathioprine and cyclophosphamide.

Acknowledgments

Supported in part by National Institutes of Health Grants RR00034, DK48621, and AI41729.

Bibliography

Bansai VK, Beto JA: Treatment of lupus nephritis: A meta-analysis of clinical trials. *Am J Kidney Dis* 29(2):193–199, 1997.

Berden JHM: Lupus nephritis. *Kidney Int* 52:538–558, 1997.

Boumpas DT, Austin III HA, Vaughn EM, Klippel JH, Steinberg AD, Yarboro CH, Balow JE: Controlled trial of pulse methylprednisolone versus two regimens of pulse cyclophosphamide in severe lupus nephritis. *Lancet* 340:741–745, 1992.

Boumpas DT, Fessler BJ, Austin III HA, Balow JE, Klippel JH, Lockshin MD: Systemic lupus erythematosus: Emerging concepts. Part 2: Dermatologic and joint disease, the antiphospholipid antibody syndrome, pregnancy and hormonal therapy, morbidity and mortality, and pathogenesis. *Ann Intern Med* 123:42–53, 1995.

Dooley MA, Hogan S, Jennette C, Falk R, for the Glomerular Disease Collaborative Network: Cyclophosphamide therapy for lupus nephritis: Poor renal survival in black Americans. *Kidney Int* 51:1188–1195, 1997.

Dooley MA, Cosio FG, Nachman PH, Falkenhain ME, Hogan SL, Falk RJ, Hebert LA: Mycophenolate mofetil therapy in lupus nephritis: Clinical observations. *J Am Soc Nephrol* 10:833–839, 1999.

Hebert LA, Middendorf DF, Dillon JJ, Lewis EJ, Peter JB: Relationship between appearance of urinary red cell/white cell casts and the onset of renal relapse in systemic lupus erythematosus. *Am J Kidney Dis* 26(3), 1995.

Hebert LA, Cosio FG, Birmingham DJ: Complement and complement regulatory proteins in renal disease. *In:* Neilson EG, Couser WG (eds) *Immunologic Renal Diseases,* Chap. 18, pp. 377–395. Lippincott-Raven, Philadelphia, 1997.

James JA, Kaufman KM, Farris AD, Taylor-Albert E, Lehman TJA, Harley JB: An increased prevalence of Epstein-Barr virus infection in young patients suggests a possible etiology for systemic lupus erythematosus. *J Clin Invest* 100(12):3019–3026, 1997.

Vercauteren SB, Bosmans J-L, Elseviers MM, Verpooten GA, DeBroe ME: A meta-analysis and morphological review of cyclosporine-induced nephrotoxicity in auto-immune diseases. *Kidney Int* 54:536–545, 1998.

Wallace DJ, Hahn BH (eds): *Dubois' Lupus Erythematosus,* 5th Ed. Williams & Wilkins, Baltimore, 1997.

28

DIABETIC NEPHROPATHY

MARIA LUIZA CARAMORI AND MICHAEL MAUER

Diabetic nephropathy is the single most common disorder leading to renal failure in adults. In the United States, 44% of patients entering end stage renal disease (ESRD) programs are diabetic, most of whom (80% or more) have type 2 diabetes. The annual cost of caring for these patients, in the United States alone, exceeds $6 billion. The mortality rate of patients with diabetic nephropathy is high, and a marked increase in cardiovascular risk accounts for more than one-half of the mortality rate among these patients. Once overt diabetic nephropathy, manifest as proteinuria, is present, ESRD can be postponed, but in most instances it is not prevented by effective antihypertensive treatment and by careful glycemic control. Thus, in the last 10–15 years, there has been intensive research into early predictors of diabetic nephropathy risk, pathophysiologic mechanisms of diabetic renal injury, and early intervention strategies.

EPIDEMIOLOGY

About 0.5% of the population in the United States and central Europe have type 1 diabetes. The prevalence is higher in the northern Scandinavian countries and lower in southern Europe and Japan. Diabetic nephropathy will develop in 25–35% of these patients, with a peak in the incidence after approximately 20 years of diabetes. Type 2 diabetes is about nine times more prevalent than type 1 diabetes, accounting in part for the greater contribution of type 2 diabetic patients to ESRD incidence. Studies in type 2 diabetic patients from western Europe and in Pima Indians from Arizona showed rates of progression to nephropathy similar to those of type 1 diabetic patients. The rate of development of ESRD is much higher in African-American compared to White type 2 American diabetic patients. Glycemic control and genetic factors seem to be very important in determining diabetic nephropathy risk. Systemic blood pressure levels may be important in the *genesis* of diabetic nephropathy, but this is less clear than is the role of blood pressure in the *progression* of established diabetic nephropathy.

DIAGNOSIS OF DIABETIC NEPHROPATHY

The diagnosis of diabetic nephropathy is usually based on the presence of urinary protein loss exceeding 0.5 g/24 hr in a patient with long-term (10 or more years) of diabetes and without indications of other forms of renal disease. The onset of overt proteinuria is often associated with hypertension and declining glomerular filtration rate (GFR). In long-term type 1 diabetic patients, especially if retinopathy is also present and other causes of clinical proteinuria can be excluded, there may be no need for a renal biopsy, as our studies indicate that approximately 95% of these patients will have diabetic nephropathy. Biopsy, however, is clearly indicated in an atypical course (e.g., if the onset of clinical renal disease is within the first 10 years of diabetes or if the decline in renal function is rapidly progressive). In these cases, other nephropathies are more likely to occur, and a patient might benefit from more specific diagnostic, prognostic, and therapeutic options. Proteinuric type 2 diabetic patients with retinopathy also have a very high likelihood of typical diabetic nephropathy. However, often the time of onset of type 2 diabetes is uncertain and retinopathy commonly minimal or absent. Under these circumstances, greater diagnostic uncertainty exists. In these patients, renal biopsy may be helpful and may reveal minor renal changes or atypical forms of diabetic renal injury (see later) or, less likely, other renal diseases.

Years before the development of proteinuria, increased amounts of albumin can be detected in the urine by sensitive measurement methods before being detectable by standard urine dipstick tests and this is termed microalbuminuria (Table 1). Compared to normoalbuminuric patients, patients with persistent microalbuminuria have at three- to four fold increased risk of progression to proteinuria and ESRD. Current studies indicate that about 30–45% of microalbuminuric type 1 diabetic patients will progress to proteinuria after about 10 years of follow-up, while 20–25% will return to normoalbuminuric levels, and the rest will remain microalbuminuric.

SCREENING

The National Kidney Foundation and the American Diabetes Association (ADA) recommend that type 1 patients with diabetes duration of 5 or more years and all type 2 diabetic patients should be tested for proteinuria (dipstick) and, if proteinuria is not present, should be screened for microalbuminuria then and yearly thereafter. Screening for microalbuminuria can be performed by measurement of albumin-to-creatinine ratio in a random spot collection, by 24-hr collection, or by timed (e.g., overnight) collections. The latter is the preferred test be-

TABLE I

Categories of Urinary Albumin Excretion

Category	Timed collection (μg/min)	24-hr collection (mg/24 hr)	Spot collection (μg/mg creatinine)
Normoalbuminuria	<20	<30	<30
Microalbuminuria	20–200	30–300	30–300
Proteinuria	>200	>300	>300

cause of its greater accuracy than spot urines and greater patient acceptance than 24-hr collections. Because of the high day-to-day variability in albumin excretion rate (AER), two out of three specimens done in a 3 to 6 month period need to be in a same category for diagnosis of microalbuminuria or low grade proteinuria (Table 1). AER measurements should not be interpreted in the presence of confounding factors such as urinary infection, fever, marked hyperglycemia, severe hypertension, or congestive heart failure. It should be noted, however, that in a minority of patients, especially in women, the first clinical manifestations of serious underlying renal lesions of diabetes may be declining GFR and, sometimes, rising blood pressure. Thus, all diabetic patients should have careful and repeated blood pressure measures and normoalbuminuric patients, especially women, with diabetic retinopathy or rising blood pressure should be considered for formal GFR measurements and, if GFR is low, for renal biopsy. If formal GFR measurements are not available, GFR can be estimated by using the mean of two to three carefully collected 24-hr creatinine clearances.

NATURAL COURSE OF DIABETIC NEPHROPATHY

For simplicity, the progression of renal involvement in type 1 diabetes can be divided in five stages. Stage I, present at diagnosis, is that of renal hypertrophy–hyperfunction. At this stage, patients at risk and not at risk of diabetic nephropathy cannot be clearly separated. Although some studies suggest that the presence of GFR above the normal range (glomerular hyperfiltration) is an important risk factor, this remains controversial. Stage II is defined by the presence of detectable glomerular lesions in patients with normal AER and normal blood pressure levels. Microalbuminuria defines stage III, typically occurring after 7 or more years of diabetes. At this stage, glomerular lesions are generally more severe than in the previous stages and blood pressure tends to be increasing, often into the hypertensive range. Other laboratory abnormalities, such as increased levels of cholesterol, fibrinogen, Von Willebrand factor, and prorenin can be detected in some patients. Stage IV occurs after 10–20 years of diabetes and is characterized by the presence of dipstick positive proteinuria. Hypertension is present in about 75% of these patients, and reduced GFR is also common. Progression to ESRD (stage V) will occur 5–15 years after the development of proteinuria.

Type 2 diabetic patients can have proteinuria at diagnosis. In these patients, diabetes duration is usually not precisely known, and they can be diabetic for 5–10 years before diagnosis. Interestingly, in studies of Pima Indians where type 2 diabetes duration was known, the clinical course of diabetic kidney disease was similar to that of type 1 diabetic patients.

It is important to keep in mind that these categories are general and that progression is highly variable and is often not linear. The expression and natural history of these overlapping stages may be influenced by complex genetic, environmental, and treatment interactions, which may greatly affect outcome. Thus, the scheme presented here can serve as a useful general guide, but not as an accurate predictor of the course of individual patients.

PATHOGENESIS

Although important modulating factors may exist, diabetic nephropathy is a consequence of the long-term metabolic aberrations found in diabetes. Exposure to elevated glucose levels is necessary for the expression of this disorder. Thus, glomerular lesions are absent at onset, but they can be demonstrated after diabetes has been present for a few years. The same is true when a normal kidney is transplanted into a diabetic patient. Moreover, the development of the earliest diabetic renal lesions can be slowed or prevented by strict glycemic control, as was demonstrated in a randomized clinical trial in type 1 diabetic kidney transplant recipients. Also, intensive insulin treatment decreased the progression rates of glomerular lesions in a controlled trial in microalbuminuric type 1 diabetic patients. Finally, regression of established diabetic glomerular lesions has been demonstrated in the native kidneys of type 1 diabetic patients with prolonged normalization of glycemic levels after successful pancreas transplantation.

The pathogenesis of renal lesions appears to be mainly related to extracellular matrix (ECM) accumulation. ECM accumulation occurs in the glomerular (GBM) and tubular (TBM) basement membranes, is the principal cause of mesangial expansion, and also contributes to interstitium expansion.

The ECM accumulation is probably secondary to an imbalance between synthesis and degradation of ECM components. Many regulatory mechanisms have been proposed to explain the linkage between a high ambient glucose concentration and ECM accumulation. Increased levels of growth factors, particularly transforming growth factor β (TGF-β), can be associated with increased production of ECM molecules. TGF-β can also downregulate the synthesis of ECM degrading enzymes and upregulate the inhibitors of these enzymes. Angiotensin II can also stimulate ECM synthesis through TGF-β activity. High glucose can directly activate protein kinase C (PKC), stimulating ECM production through the cyclic AMP pathway. The accumulation of glycosylation products (generated by nonenzymatic reactions between reducing sugars, such as glucose, with free amino groups, lipids, or nucleic acids) may also contribute to the development of diabetic complications. These products may then influence ECM dynamics. In diabetic patients, oxidative or nonoxidative products of glycated proteins or lipids could accumulate in the vascular wall and induce cytokine and growth factor release, contributing to vascular injury. Other mechanisms that could be involved in the organ damage caused by diabetes include abnormalities of the aldose-reductase, endothelin, and prostaglandin pathways.

Hemodynamic mechanisms may be also involved in the pathogenesis of diabetic nephropathy. Glomerular hyperfiltration could directly promote ECM accumulation, by mechanisms such as increased expression of TGF-β, modeled *in vitro* by the mechanical stretching of mesangial cells. Glomerular hyperfiltration could also be a marker of other process such as increased activity of the renin–angiotensin, TGF-β, and PKC systems. However, patients with other causes of hyperfiltration, such as patients with uninephrectomy, do not develop diabetic lesions. Thus, glomerular hyperfiltration alone cannot fully explain the genesis of the early lesions of diabetic nephropathy. However, clinical observations suggest that hemodynamic factors may be more important in modulating the rate of progression of already well-established diabetic lesions.

Genetic predisposition to diabetic nephropathy appears to be the most important determinant of diabetic nephropathy risk in both type 1 and type 2 diabetic patients. Differences in the prevalence of microalbuminuria, proteinuria, and ESRD in different patient populations support this view. Moreover, only about one-half of patients with decades of poor glycemic control will develop diabetic nephropathy, while some patients will develop lesions despite relatively good control, findings consistent with genetically modulated susceptibility or resistance factors. Genetic predisposition to diabetic nephropathy has been suggested by studies in type 1 and type 2 siblings concordant for diabetes. These studies show extremely high concordance in diabetic nephropathy risk. Diabetic patients with family history of hypertension or cardiovascular disease also have higher risk of diabetic nephropathy thus linking the pathogenesis of diabetic nephropathy to factors also favoring the development of atherosclerosis. The genetic determinants of diabetic nephropathy risk are still not fully understood. However it is reasonable to hypothesize that a single gene with a major effect or several genes with lesser effects that interact with the metabolic abnormalities of diabetes are responsible for the susceptibility to diabetic nephropathy. The ongoing search to identify the genetic loci responsibles has not yet yielded definitive results.

PATHOLOGY

Type I Diabetes

The changes in kidney structure caused by diabetes are specific, creating a pattern not seen in any other disease. The severity of these diabetic lesions is related to the functional disturbances of the disease and also to diabetes duration, degree of glycemic control, and genetic factors. However, the relationship between duration of type 1 diabetes and extent of glomerular pathology is not precise. This is consonant with the marked variability in susceptibility to this disorder such that some patients may be in renal failure after having diabetes for 15 years while others escape complications despite having type 1 diabetes for many decades.

Light Microscopy

The earliest renal structural change in type 1 diabetes, renal hypertrophy, is not reflected in any specific light microscopy (LM) changes. In many patients, glomerular structure remains normal or near normal even after decades of diabetes. Others develop progressive diffuse mesangial expansion seen mainly as increased periodic acid–Schiff (PAS) positive ECM mesangial material (Fig. 1). In about 40–50% of patients developing proteinuria there are areas of extreme mesangial expansion called Kimmelstiel–Wilson nodules or nodular mesangial expansion. Mesangial cell nuclei in these nodules are palisaded around masses of mesangial matrix material with compression of surrounding capillary lumina. Nodules are thought to result from earlier glomerular capillary microaneurism formation. About half of patients with severe diabetic nephropathy do not have these nodular lesions. Thus Kimmelstiel–Wilson nodules are diagnostic of diabetic nephropathy, but they are not necessary for severe renal dysfunction to develop. Early changes often include arteriolar hyalinosis lesions involving replacement of the smooth muscle cells of afferent and efferent arterioles with PAS positive waxy homogenous material (Fig. 1). The severity of these lesions is directly related to the frequency of global glomerulosclerosis, perhaps as the result of glomerular ischemia. One may also detect GBM and TBM thickening by LM, although this is often easier seen by electron microscopy (EM). Finally, usually quite late in the disease, there is tubular atrophy and interstitial fibrosis, common to most chronic renal disorders. Light microscopy changes with monoclonal light chain deposition might resemble diabetes but the mesangial expansion is not fibrillar as in diabetic nephropathy and the vascular hyalinosis absent. Moreover, clinical and laboratory features and immunofluorescence and electron microscopy studies can easily differentiate these entities.

Immunofluorescence

Diabetes is characterized by increased staining of GBM, TBM, and Bowman's capsule especially for IgG (mainly IgG$_4$) and albumin in a linear pattern. This staining is removed only by strong acid conditions, consistent with strong ionic binding. The intensity of staining is not related to the severity of the underlying lesions, and it is important to avoid confusing these findings with the pattern seen in anti-basement membrane antibody disorders.

Electron Microscopy

Using morphometric techniques, the first measurable nephropathy change is thickening of the GBM, which can

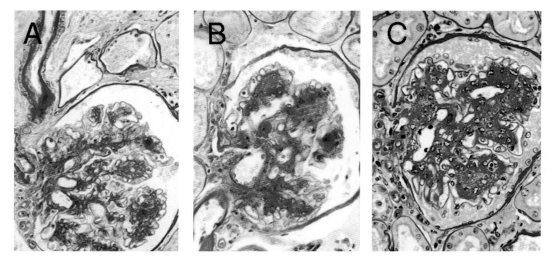

FIGURE I Light microscopy photographs of glomeruli in sequential kidney biopsies performed at baseline and after 5 and 10 years of follow-up in a long-standing normoalbuminuric type 1 diabetic patient with progressive mesangial expansion and renal function deterioration. (A) Note the diffuse and nodular mesangial expansion and arteriolar hyalinosis in this glomerulus from a patient who was normotensive and normoalbuminuric at the time of this baseline biopsy, 21 years after diabetes onset [periodic acid–Schiff (PAS) × 400]. (B) Five-year follow-up biopsy showing worsening of the diffuse and nodular mesangial expansion and arteriolar hyalinosis in this now microalbuminuric patient with declining GFR (PAS × 400). (C) Ten-year follow-up biopsy showing more advanced diabetic glomerulopathy in this now proteinuric patient with further reduced GFR. Note also the multiple small glomerular (probably efferent) arterioles in the hilar region of this glomerulus (PAS × 400), and in the glomerulus in Fig. 1A.

be detected as early as 1 1/2 to 2 1/2 years after onset of type 1 diabetes. TBM thickening can also be detected, and it is parallel to GBM thickening. Increases in the relative area of the mesangium becomes measurable by 4–5 years. The fraction of the volume of the glomerulus that is mesangium increases from about 0.2 in the normal state to about 0.4 when proteinuria begins and 0.6–0.8 in patients with GFRs about 40–50% of normal. Immunohistochemical studies indicate that these changes in mesangium, GBM, and TBM represent expansion of the intrinsic ECM components at these sites, most likely including types IV and VI collagen, laminin, and fibronectin.

Type 2 Diabetes

Glomerular structure in type 2 diabetic patients is less well studied, but appears to be more heterogeneous than in type 1 patients. Between one-third and one-half of type 2 patients have typical changes of diabetic nephropathy, including diffuse and nodular mesangial expansion and arteriolar hyalinosis. Other patients, despite microalbuminuria or even proteinuria, may have no or only mild glomerulopathy. Some patients have disproportionately severe tubular and interstitial or vascular lesions or an increase in globally sclerosed glomeruli. There are reports that type 2 diabetic patients have increased incidence of nondiabetic lesions, such as proliferative glomerulonephritis and membranous nephropathy, but this is most likely because biopsies were done to investigate atypical cases. When biopsies are performed for research purposes,

the incidence of other definable renal diseases is very low (<5%).

STRUCTURAL–FUNCTIONAL RELATIONSHIPS IN DIABETIC NEPHROPATHY

The progression rates vary greatly between individuals. Type 1 diabetic patients with proteinuria always have advanced glomerular, and usually vascular, tubular, and interstitial lesions. Microalbuminuric patients usually have well established lesions, but these vary from mild to levels of pathology bordering on those regularly seen in proteinuric patients. There is a considerable overlap in glomerular structure between long-standing normo- and microalbuminuric patients because normoalbuminuric patients with long-standing type 1 diabetes can have quite advanced renal lesions. On the other hand, many long-standing normoalbuminuric diabetic patients have structural measurements within the normal range.

Expansion of the mesangium, mainly due to ECM accumulation, is believed ultimately to reduce or obliterate glomerular capillary luminal space, decreasing glomerular filtration surface and GFR. The fraction of the glomerulus occupied by mesangium is also related to AER levels and hypertension. Thickness of GBM is also directly related to AER. Percent global glomerulosclerosis (GS) and interstitial expansion are also correlated with the clinical manifestations of diabetic nephropathy (proteinuria, hypertension, and declining GFR). Progressive tubular atrophy, interstitial fibrosis, renal glomerular arteriolar hyalinosis, arteriosclerosis, and

GS may also contribute to the reduction in GFR. Finally, larger vessel atherosclerosis, perhaps especially in type 2 diabetes, may lead to ischemic renal tissue damage.

In type 1 diabetic patients, glomerular, tubular, interstitial, and vascular lesions tend to progress more or less in parallel, whereas in type 2 diabetic patients this is often not the case. Preliminary observations suggest that long-standing normoalbuminuric type 1 diabetic patients who progress to diabetic nephropathy have more advanced glomerular lesions than patients that remain normoalbuminuric after long-term follow-up, but these findings are, as yet, unconfirmed. In type 2 diabetes, current evidence suggests that microalbuminuric patients with typical diabetic glomerulopathy have higher risk of progressive GFR loss than those with less glomerular changes.

MANAGEMENT OF DIABETIC NEPHROPATHY

Principles of ESRD management are covered elsewhere in this text, and thus this chapter will focus on some ESRD issues of special importance to diabetic patients. The management of diabetic nephropathy will be discussed at the various stages of the disease, but some overlap of treatment strategies is inevitable.

Normoalbuminuria

Ideally, specific preventive interventions should focus on patients at increased risk of diabetic nephropathy. Currently, no marker can precisely separate normoalbuminuric patients at risk of diabetic nephropathy from patients not at risk. Thus, all diabetic patients should be oriented to pursue the best glycemic control possible, aiming to prevent not only diabetic nephropathy, but also other long-term complications, such as retinopathy and neuropathy. Strict glycemic control has been proven to prevent clinical and structural manifestations of diabetic nephropathy. The Diabetes Control and Complications Trial (DCCT), evaluating a large number of normoalbuminuric patients, demonstrated that patients randomized to strict glycemic control had a lower incidence of microalbuminuria and proteinuria than patients on conventional treatment. Patients with glycated hemoglobin lower than 7.5% had a low risk of progression. Intensive insulin treatment was also able to prevent development of important early structural glomerular lesions in normal kidney transplanted into type 1 diabetic patients. Intensified glycemic control can also prevent diabetic renal complications in type 2 diabetic patients.

Microalbuminuria

It is not yet established whether the institution of strict glycemic control at the stage of persistent microalbuminuria can prevent progressive renal insufficiency and ESRD. The DCCT study did not established a benefit of glycemic control on progression of microalbuminuric patients to proteinuria, however, larger numbers of microalbuminuric type 1 diabetic patients followed for many years would be necessary to fully answer this question. Two studies from

Japan showed benefits from strict glycemic control in type 2 diabetes but these are not yet confirmed in large White populations. However, intensive glycemic control is highly recommended, because benefits have been shown for normoalbuminuric and proteinuric patients (see later), and because strict glycemic control can slow the rate of development of some diabetic glomerular lesions in microalbuminuric type 1 diabetic patients. Hypertension should be aggressively treated, as this reduces AER and may slow the rate of decline of GFR in microalbuminuric patients (this latter finding may be better established in type 2 diabetic patients). These effects appear to be related to the degree of blood pressure reduction, irrespective of the antihypertensive agent used. In normotensive microalbuminuric type 1 diabetic patients, the evidence for antihypertensive therapy is less clear. Normotensive microalbuminuric patients receiving angiotensin converting enzyme (ACE) inhibitors have decreased AER levels when compared with patients on placebo. Interestingly, when the antihypertensive is withdrawn, AER levels increase quickly, reaching values no longer different from the placebo group, suggesting a masking effect of the treatment on progressive albuminuria. Whether GFR is preserved by this treatment in normotensive microalbuminuric patients requires further documentation. Currently, the ADA and the Canadian Diabetes Associations (CDA) recommend ACE inhibitor therapy for microalbuminuric patients even in absence of hypertension, and it is reasonable to follow these recommendations pending more complete long-term studies. However, it should be kept in mind that spontaneous normalization of AER is not uncommon, and many patients will remain stable without treatment.

Proteinuria

Antihypertensive therapy has been clearly demonstrated to have a strong beneficial effect in reducing the rate of decline of GFR in proteinuric type 1 and type 2 diabetic patients. Type 1 diabetic patients with serum creatinine of 1.5 mg/dL or higher may have an additional beneficial effect when ACE inhibitors are included in the therapeutic plan, but this is not yet documented for patients with lesser degrees of renal insufficiency. In fact, British studies in type 2 diabetes suggested that blood pressure control per se rather than the type of drug used is the key to reducing progression. The goal should be to achieve blood pressures of 130/80 mm Hg or less in these proteinuric patients. In fact this goal should be generalized to all diabetic patients because studies show a reduced risk of cardiovascular mortality in diabetic patients maintained with diastolic blood pressures ≤80 versus ≤85 or ≤90 mm Hg. The value of a low-protein diet on the rate of decline of GFR in proteinuric diabetic patients is less well established. Patients should be instructed to stop smoking, and hyperlipidemia should be treated. Even at this late stage of disease, glycemia remains an independent predictor of the rate of GFR decline, and strict glycemic control should be instructed. When daily urinary protein exceeds 3.5 g, nephrotic syndrome, hypoalbuminemia, anasarca, and more marked hyperlipidemia, often develop. Sodium restriction and diuretic therapy are advised. Diabetic patients are particularly susceptible to episodes of acute renal failure with intravascular contrast injections and, if possible, these should be avoided in patients whose serum creatinine exceeds 2.0 mg/dL.

End Stage Renal Disease

As renal function declines, azotemia develops and renal replacement therapy needs to be started. Renal deterioration occurs faster in type 2 diabetic patients, perhaps due to preexisting hypertension and age-related glomerulosclerosis. Uremic diabetic patients often feel much worse than uremic nondiabetic patients with the same levels of serum creatinine, and this warrants earlier institution of ESRD care for some of these patients. Selection of ESRD therapy needs to be made on an individual basis, with appreciation of the patient's family, social, and economic circumstances. In general, irreversible renal failure in diabetes is managed similarly to that in nondiabetic ESRD patients, but there are differences in several important details and these are discussed in other chapters. Briefly, the options are hemodialysis, peritoneal dialysis, kidney transplantation, and additionally, simultaneous kidney and pancreas transplantation. Hemodialysis is the renal replacement regimen employed for more than 70% of diabetic patients with ESRD in the United States. Only about 10% of diabetic patients are placed on peritoneal dialysis, whereas only 18% ever receive a kidney transplant. The outcome of diabetic patients on hemodialysis is poor, with 50% mortality within the first 2 years. Vascular disease often creates special hemodialysis access problems. Chronic ambulatory peritoneal dialysis (CAPD) and continuous cyclic peritoneal dialysis (CCPD) are also good options for some patients, especially those with severe hemodialysis-associated hypotension or vascular access problems. Although peritonitis is the most common reason for discontinuation of CAPD, the overall risk of peritonitis is no greater in diabetic patients. Perhaps because healthier diabetic patients are selected for kidney transplantation, higher survival rates are noted when they are compared to diabetic patients on dialysis. In some centers, the survival rates of diabetic recipients of a kidney transplant are not different from that of age- and gender-matched nondiabetic recipients over the first 2 years. However, late complications of cardiovascular disease, amputations, blindness, and progressive neuropathy ultimately take a heavy toll on quality of life and survival in these patients as they do in diabetic patients remaining on dialysis. Type 1 diabetic patients can receive a simultaneous cadaver kidney and pancreas transplant, and the success rate of this treatment now rivals that of kidney transplantation alone. This strategy may provide improved survival, although this remains uncertain. This treatment does clearly provide quality of life advantages. However, it is not yet certain that this strategy is superior to initial kidney transplantation using a well-matched living related donor with or without subsequent pancreas transplantation. Many comorbid conditions, including severe diabetic retinopathy, cardiovascular and pe-

ripheral vascular disease, and peripheral and autonomic neuropathy are frequently present in these patients and should be properly evaluated and aggressively treated. There is a high incidence of significant angiographically demonstrable coronary artery lesions in even asymptomatic uremic type 1 diabetic patients. When these asymptomatic patients were randomized to intervention with angioplasty or bypass surgery their survival after subsequent kidney transplantation was improved compared to patients randomized to no preemptive treatment. More than most ESRD patients, the uremic diabetic needs a concerted team approach. The nephrologist should ensure adequate involvement of diabetologists, cardiologists, ophthalmologists, podiatrists, and other specialists as necessary to meet the special needs of these highly complex patients.

Bibliography

1999 United States Renal Data System Annual Report: National Technical Information Service.

American Diabetes Association: Diabetic Nephropathy. *Diabetes Care* 23:S69–72, 2000.

Baynes JW, Thorpe SR: Role of oxidative stress in diabetic complications: A new perspective on an old paradigm. *Diabetes* 48:1–9, 1999.

Bennet PH, Haffner S, Kasiske BL, *et al.*: Screening and Management of Microalbuminuria in Patients with Diabetes Mellitus: Recommendations to the Scientific Advisory Board of the National Kidney Foundation from an Ad Hoc Committee of the Council on Diabetes Mellitus of the National Kidney Foundation. *Am J Kidney Dis* 25:107–112, 1995.

Bilous RW, Mauer SM, Viberti GC: Genetic aspects of diabetic nephropathy. In: Morgan SH, Grünfeld J-P (eds) *Inherited Disorders of the Kidney, Investigation and Management*, pp. 427–448. Oxford Univ Press, Oxford, 1998.

Caramori ML, Fioretto P, Mauer M: The need for early predictors of diabetic nephropathy risk: Is albumin excretion rate sufficient? *Diabetes* 49:1399–1408, 2000.

Fioretto P, Steffes MW, Mauer SM: Glomerular structure in nonproteinuric insulin-dependent diabetic patients with various levels of albuminuria. *Diabetes* 43:1358–1364, 1994.

Fioretto P, Mauer M, Brocco E, *et al.*: Patterns of renal injury in NIDDM patients with microalbuminuria. *Diabetologia* 39:1569–1576, 1996.

Hansson L, Zanchetti A, Carruthers SG, *et al.*: Effects of intensive blood-pressure lowering and low-dose aspirin in patients with hypertension: Principal results of the Hypertension Optimal Treatment (HOT) randomised trial. *Lancet* 351:1755–1762, 1998.

Krolewski AS: Genetics of diabetic nephropathy: Evidence for major and minor gene effects. *Kidney Int* 55:1582–1596, 1999.

Lewis EJ, Hunsicker LG, Bain RP, Rohde RD: The effects of angiotensin-converting-enzyme inhibition on diabetic nephropathy. The Collaborative Study Group. *N Engl J Med* 329:1456–1462, 1993.

Mauer M, Mogensen CE, Friedman EA: Diabetic nephropathy. In: Schrier RW, Gottschalk CW (eds) *Diseases of the Kidney*, pp. 2019–2061. Little, Brown, Boston, 1996.

Mauer SM, Steffes MW, Ellis EN, *et al.*: Structural–functional relationships in diabetic nephropathy. *J Clin Invest* 74:1143–1155, 1984.

Meltzer S, Leiter L, Daneman D, *et al.*: 1998 Clinical practice guidelines for the management of diabetes in Canada. Canadian Diabetes Association. *Can Med Assoc J* 159(Suppl 8): S1–S29, 1998.

Mogensen CE: Microalbuminuria, blood pressure and diabetic renal disease: Origin and development of ideas. *Diabetologia* 42:263–285, 1999.

Østerby R: Glomerular structural changes in type 1 (insulin-dependent) diabetes mellitus: Causes, consequences, and prevention. *Diabetologia* 35:803–812, 1992.

The Diabetes Control and Complications Trial Research Group: Effect of intensive therapy on the development and progression

of diabetic nephropathy in the Diabetes Control and Complications Trial. *Kidney Int* 47:1703–1720, 1995.

United Kingdom Prospective Diabetes Study Group: Tight blood pressure control and risk of macrovascular and microvascular complications in type 2 diabetes: UKPDS 38. *Br Med J* 317:703–713, 1998.

United Kingdom Prospective Diabetes Study Group: Intensive blood-glucose control with sulphonylureas or insulin compared with conventional treatment and risk of complications in patients with type 2 diabetes (UKPDS 33). *Lancet* 352:837–853, 1998.

DYSPROTEINEMIAS AND AMYLOIDOSIS

PAUL W. SANDERS

LIGHT CHAIN-RELATED RENAL DISEASES

Overview

Bence Jones proteins, which were found by Dr. William Macintyre in the urine of an ill patient, were characterized by Dr. Henry Bence Jones in 1847. Bence Jones proteins are now known to consist of immunoglobulin light chains, and the multiple renal lesions associated with deposition of these proteins have been studied extensively. Plasma cells synthesize light chains that become part of the immunoglobulin molecule. Each light chain possesses two independent globular regions, termed constant and variable domains. The variable domain forms part of the antigen-binding site and derives from rearrangement of more than 20 gene segments. Thus, despite similar biochemical properties, no two light chains are identical. Disulfide bonding among two light chains with higher molecular weight proteins (heavy chains) occurs during or shortly after heavy chain synthesis and forms the classic immunoglobulin G (IgG) molecule that is then secreted by plasma cells. A slight excess production of light, compared to heavy, chains appears to be required for efficient immunoglobulin synthesis, but may result in release of free light chains. Light chains can also form homodimers through disulfide bonding to another light chain before secretion.

Once in the circulation, light chains are handled similarly to other low-molecular-weight proteins, which are cleared by the kidney. Unlike albumin, monomers (molecular mass ~22 kDa) and dimers (~44 kDa) are readily filtered through

the glomerulus and reabsorbed by the proximal tubule. In the proximal tubule, endocytosis of light chains occurs through a single class of receptors with relative selectivity for these proteins. The isoelectric point of light chains does not influence reabsorption rate. After endocytosis, lysosomal enzymes hydrolyze the proteins and the amino acid components are returned to the circulation. Reabsorption is saturable and allows delivery of light chains to the distal nephron and appearance in the urine as Bence Jones proteins.

Urinary Bence Jones proteins possess unusual heat solubility properties. When heated to 60°C, the proteins precipitate, but on further heating to 100°C, the proteins resolubilize. Although this distinctive thermal property was initially used as a screening test for the presence of urinary Bence Jones proteins, it is very insensitive and positive only when significant quantities are excreted in the urine. The qualitative urine dipstick test for protein also has a low sensitivity for detection of light chains. While some Bence Jones proteins react with the chemical impregnated onto the strip, other light chains cannot be detected; the net charge of the protein may be an important determinant of this interaction. In healthy adults, the urinary concentration of light chain proteins, which are polyclonal because of escape into the circulation of small amounts of free light chain produced during normal immunoglobulin assembly, is about 2.5 μg/mL. Urinary light chain concentration is generally between 20 and 500 μg/mL in patients with monoclonal gammopathies of undetermined significance, and is often much higher (range 0.02–11.8 mg/mL) in patients with multiple myeloma or Waldenström's macroglobulinemia. The amount of monoclonal light chain excreted is often insufficient for detection using turbidimetric and heat tests. In addition, because of the insensitivity of routine serum protein electrophoresis (SPEP) and urinary protein electrophoresis (UPEP), these tests are no longer recommended as screening tools. Identification therefore rests with antibody detection assays (immunofixation electrophoresis or immunoelectrophoresis) using serum and urine. Immunofixation electrophoresis is very sensitive and detects monoclonal light chains and immunoglobulins even in very low concentrations. Causes of monoclonal light chain proteinuria, a hallmark of plasma cell dyscrasias, are listed (Table 1). The most common cause of light chain proteinuria is multiple myeloma.

Virtually every compartment of the kidney can be damaged from monoclonal light chain deposition (Table 2). Histologic examination of necropsy specimens from 57 patients demonstrated renal lesions in ~48%. Sixty-five percent of those patients with renal lesions had cast nephropathy, or "myeloma kidney," whereas 21% had AL-amyloidosis, and 11% had monoclonal light chain deposition disease (LCDD). The simultaneous occurrence of two or more of these lesions in the same patient is unusual. Light chains take the center stage in the pathogenesis of these renal lesions. The type of renal lesion induced by light chains depends on the physicochemical properties of these proteins.

Cast Nephropathy

Pathology

Cast nephropathy is a noninflammatory tubulointerstitial renal lesion. Characteristically, multiple intraluminal proteinaceous casts are identified mainly in the distal portion of the nephrons (Fig. 1). Casts may also be seen in the proximal tubule, or even in glomeruli when they are abundant. The casts are usually acellular, homogeneous, and eosinophilic with multiple fracture lines. Immunofluorescence and immunoelectron microscopy confirm that the casts contain light chains and Tamm–Horsfall glycoprotein. Persistence of the casts produces giant cell inflammation and tubular atrophy that typify myeloma kidney. Glomeruli are usually normal in appearance.

TABLE I
Causes of Bence Jones Proteinuria

Multiple myeloma

AL-amyloidosis

Light chain deposition disease

Waldenström's macroglobulinemia

Monoclonal gammopathy of undetermined significance

Polyneuropathy, organomegaly, endocrinopathy, monoclonal gammopathy, and skin changes (POEMS) syndrome (rare)

Heavy (μ) chain disease (rare)

Lymphoproliferative disease (rare)

Rifampin therapy (rare)

TABLE 2
Light Chain-Related Renal Lesions

Glomerulopathies
  Light chain deposition disease
  AL-amyloidosis
  Cryoglobulinemia

Tubulointerstitial lesions
  Cast nephropathy ("myeloma kidney")
  Fanconi syndrome
  Proximal tubule injury (acute tubular necrosis)
  Tubulointerstitial nephritis (rare)

Vascular lesions

Asymptomatic Bence Jones proteinuria

Hyperviscosity syndrome

Neoplastic cell infiltration (rare)

Clinical Features

Renal failure from this lesion may present acutely or as a chronic progressive disease and may develop at any stage of myeloma. Diagnosis of multiple myeloma is usually evident when chronic bone pain, pathologic fractures, and hypercalcemia are complicated by proteinuria and renal failure. However, many patients present to nephrologists primarily with symptoms of renal failure or undefined proteinuria; further evaluation then confirms a malignant process. Cast nephropathy should therefore be considered when proteinuria (often more than 3 g/day), particularly without concomitant hypoalbuminemia or albuminuria, is found in a patient who is in the fourth decade of life or older. Hypertension is not a common consequence of cast nephropathy. Diagnosis may be confirmed by finding monoclonal immunoglobulins or light chains in the serum and urine and typical intraluminal cast formation on kidney biopsy. Virtually all patients

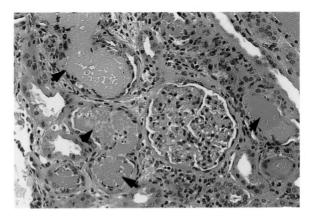

FIGURE I Renal biopsy tissue from a patient who had cast nephropathy. The findings include tubules filled with cast material (arrows) and presence of multinucleated giant cells. Glomeruli are typically normal in appearance (20× magnification, hematoxylin and eosin stain).

with cast nephropathy have detectable monoclonal light chains in the urine or blood.

Pathogenesis

Intravenous infusion of nephrotoxic human light chains in rats elevates proximal tubule pressure and simultaneously decreases single nephron glomerular filtration rate; intraluminal protein casts can be identified in these kidneys. Myeloma casts contain Tamm–Horsfall glycoprotein and occur initially in the distal nephron, which provides an optimum environment for precipitation of light chains. Casts occur primarily because light chains coaggregate with Tamm–Horsfall glycoprotein. Tamm–Horsfall glycoprotein, which is synthesized exclusively by cells of the thick ascending limb of the loop of Henle, comprises the major fraction of total urinary protein and is the predominant constituent of urinary casts. Cast-forming Bence Jones proteins bind to a site on the peptide backbone of Tamm–Horsfall glycoprotein; binding results in coaggregation of these proteins and subsequent occlusion of the tubule lumen by precipitated protein complexes. Intranephronal obstruction and renal failure ensue. Light chains with high affinities for Tamm–Horsfall glycoprotein are potentially nephrotoxic.

Coaggregation of Tamm–Horsfall glycoprotein with light chains also depends on the ionic environment and the physicochemical properties of the light chain, because not all patients with myeloma develop cast nephropathy, even when the urinary excretion of light chains is very high. Increasing concentrations of sodium chloride or calcium, but not magnesium, facilitate coaggregation. The loop diuretic, furosemide, augments coaggregation and accelerates intraluminal obstruction in vivo in the rat. Finally, the lower tubule fluid flow rates of the distal nephron allow more time for light chains to interact with Tamm–Horsfall glycoprotein and subsequently to obstruct the lumen. Conditions that further reduce flow rates, such as volume depletion, can accelerate tubule obstruction or convert nontoxic light chains into cast-forming proteins.

Treatment and Prognosis

The principles used to treat cast nephropathy include decreasing the concentration of circulating light chains and preventing coaggregation of light chains with Tamm–Horsfall glycoprotein (Table 3). Prompt and effective chemotherapy should start on diagnosis of multiple myeloma. Standard treatment employs alkylating agents and steroids. Intermittent treatment with melphalan and prednisone decreases circulating levels of light chains and stabilizes or improves renal function in two-thirds of patients who present with renal failure. Fanconi syndrome may also resolve with this therapy. Because the primary route of elimination of melphalan is through the kidneys, renal failure complicates dosing. An alternative chemotherapeutic regimen that includes vincristine, adriamycin, and either methylprednisolone (VAMP) or dexamethasone (VAD) has been used successfully. VAD can induce a remission more rapidly than melphalan and prednisone and

TABLE 3
Standard Therapies for Cast Nephropathy

Chemotherapy to decrease light chain production

Increase free water intake to 2–3 L/day as tolerated

Treat hypercalcemia aggressively

Avoid exposure to loop diuretics, radiocontrast agents, and nonsteroidal antiinflammatory agents

Alkalinize urine

allows faster reduction in the amount of circulating light chains. Often only two courses of treatment are necessary to determine whether a patient will respond to this chemotherapy, and the physician can rapidly determine the efficacy of such an approach. Other therapeutic options include myeloablative therapy with allogeneic or autologous bone marrow transplantation, but their associated mortality is high. Plasmapheresis removes light chains from the bloodstream effectively over a short period and is useful primarily in the setting of acute renal failure or hyperviscosity syndrome.

Prevention of aggregation of light chains with Tamm–Horsfall glycoprotein is a cornerstone of therapy. Volume repletion, normalization of electrolytes, and avoidance of complicating factors such as loop diuretics and nonsteroidal antiinflammatory agents are helpful in preserving and improving renal function. While not all patients with light chain proteinuria develop acute renal failure following exposure to radiocontrast agents, predicting who is at risk for this complication is difficult, suggesting caution in the use of radiocontrast agents in all patients with multiple myeloma. Daily fluid intake up to 3 L in the form of electrolyte-free fluids should be encouraged, although serum sodium concentration should be monitored periodically. Alkalinization of the urine with oral sodium bicarbonate (or citrate) to keep the urine pH >7 may also be beneficial, but should be avoided in patients who have symptomatic extracellular fluid volume overload.

Hypercalcemia occurs in more than 25% of patients with multiple myeloma. In addition to being directly nephrotoxic, hypercalcemia enhances the nephrotoxicity of light chains. Treatment of volume contraction with the infusion of saline often corrects mild hypercalcemia. Loop diuretics also increase calcium excretion, but furosemide, because it may facilitate nephrotoxicity from light chains, should not be administered until the patient is clinically euvolemic. Glucocorticoid therapy (prednisone, 60 mg/day) is helpful for acute management of the multiple myeloma as well as hypercalcemia. However, clinical response to the latter is often not dramatic. Bisphosphonates, such as pamidronate and etidronate, are used to treat moderate hypercalcemia (serum calcium >3.25 mmol/L, or 13 mg/dL) unresponsive to other measures. Bisphosphonates lower serum calcium by interfering with osteoclast-mediated bone resorption. While hypercalcemia of myeloma responds to bisphosphonates, these agents can be nephrotoxic and should be administered only to euvolemic patients. Therapy with pamidronate allows outpatient management of mild hypercalcemia. Besides controlling hypercalcemia, bisphosphonates appear to inhibit growth of plasma cells and are therefore becoming part of the standard treatment of multiple myeloma.

Dialysis should be used as indicated. Perhaps 5 to 10% of patients who are dialysis-dependent because of cast nephropathy regain sufficient renal function to stop dialysis, so intensive efforts to reverse this lesion, including plasmapheresis, should be considered, especially in suitable patients who present with acute renal failure. Renal transplantation has also been successfully performed in selected patients with multiple myeloma in remission.

Renal failure decreases survival in multiple myeloma. Median survival for patients with renal failure is 20 months, compared with a median survival of 20 to 40 months for the general population of patients with myeloma. Major predictors of survival include the stage of the disease, decline in serum creatinine concentration at 1 month into treatment to less than 3.4 mg/dL, and response to chemotherapy. Response to chemotherapy is important: median survival time for responders is 36 months, but only 10 months for nonresponders.

Other Tubulointerstitial Renal Lesions

Proximal tubule injury, including Fanconi syndrome, and tubulointerstitial nephritis can also rarely occur. Fanconi syndrome may precede overt multiple myeloma. Plasma cell dyscrasia should therefore be considered in the differential diagnosis when this syndrome occurs in adults. More severe damage to proximal tubule epithelium can produce clinical manifestations of acute renal failure. The mechanism of damage to the proximal epithelium is related to accumulation of toxic light chains in the endolysosomal system. An inflammatory tubulointerstitial nephritis with cellular infiltrates including eosinophils and active tubular damage has also been described. A careful search usually detects subtle light chain deposits along the tubular basement membranes almost exclusively in the areas of interstitial inflammation. This interstitial inflammatory pattern is sometimes associated with glomerular involvement, and cast formation is rare. Without detection of the deposits of light chains along the basement membrane, this lesion may be mistakenly considered to be a hypersensitivity reaction to drugs, most notably nonsteroidal antiinflammatory agents.

Light Chain Deposition Disease

Light chain deposition disease (LCDD) is a systemic disease, but typically presents initially with isolated renal injury related to a glomerular lesion associated with non-amyloid electron-dense granular deposits of monoclonal light chains with or without heavy chains. Isolated deposition of heavy chains, termed heavy chain deposition disease, is extremely rare. LCDD may be accompanied by the other clinical features of multiple myeloma or another lymphoproliferative disorder, or may be the sole manifestation of a plasma cell dyscrasia.

Pathology

Nodular glomerulopathy with distortion of the glomerular architecture by deposition of amorphous, eosinophilic material is the most common pathologic finding observed with light microscopy (Fig. 2). These nodules, which are composed of light chains and extracellular matrix proteins, begin in the mesangium. This appearance is reminiscent of diabetic nephropathy. Less commonly, other glomerular morphologic lesions besides nodular glomerulopathy can be seen in LCDD. Immunofluorescence microscopy demonstrates the presence of monotypical light chains in the glomeruli. Under electron microscopy, deposits of light chain proteins are present in a subendothelial position along the glomerular capillary wall, along the outer aspect of tubular basement membranes, and in the mesangium. Tubular cell damage is also notable and obvious even in the early stage of the disease in some patients.

Clinical Features

The clinical presentation is typical of a progressive glomerulonephritis. The major symptoms of LCDD include proteinuria, sometimes in the nephrotic range, microscopic hematuria, and renal failure. Albumin and monoclonal light chains are the dominant proteins in the urine. The presence of albuminuria and other findings of nephrotic syndrome are important clues to the presence of a glomerular lesion and not cast nephropathy. The amount of excreted light chain is usually less than that found in cast nephropathy. Development of renal failure in untreated patients is common. Because renal manifestations generally predominate and are often the sole presenting features, it is not uncommon for nephrologists to diagnose the plasma cell dyscrasia. Renal biopsy is generally necessary to establish the diagnosis. Other organ dysfunction, especially liver and

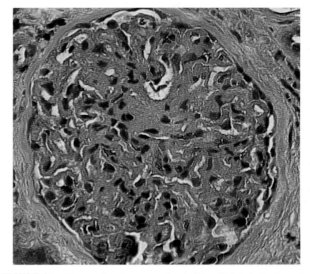

FIGURE 2 Glomerulus from a patient with κ light chain deposition disease showing expansion of the mesangium, related to matrix protein deposition, and associated compression of capillary lumens (40× magnification, hematoxylin and eosin stain).

heart, can develop and is related to deposition of light chains in those organs. Although extrarenal manifestations of overt multiple myeloma can manifest at presentation or over time, a majority (~74%) of patients with LCDD will not develop myeloma or other malignant lymphoproliferative disease.

Pathogenesis

The pathogenesis of LCDD differs from that of cast nephropathy. The response to light chain deposition includes expansion of the mesangium by extracellular matrix proteins to form nodules and eventually glomerular sclerosis. Experimental studies have shown that mesangial cells exposed to light chains obtained from patients with biopsy-proven LCDD produce transforming growth factor-β, which serves as an autacoid to stimulate these same cells to produce matrix proteins, including type IV collagen, laminin, and fibronectin. Thus, transforming growth factor-β plays a central role in glomerular sclerosis from LCDD.

Although light chains play an important pathogenetic role in these glomerular lesions, heavy chains, along with light chains, can be identified in the deposits, prompting some authors to suggest the term monoclonal light and heavy chain deposition disease. In those specimens, the punctate electron-dense deposits appear larger and more extensive than those deposits that contain only light chains, but it is unclear whether the clinical course of these patients differs from the course of isolated light chain deposition without heavy chain components.

Treatment and Prognosis

The treatment of LCDD is difficult. Randomized controlled trials are unavailable, but patients appear to benefit from the same chemotherapy as that given for multiple myeloma, particularly if renal failure is mild at presentation. Early diagnosis is therefore important. Five of eight patients with serum creatinine concentrations less than 4.0 mg/dL at the time of diagnosis did not progress with chemotherapy, while nine of 11 patients with higher creatinine concentrations at presentation progressed to end stage renal failure despite therapy. Caution should be exercised to limit the total dose of the alkylating agent that is used. The role of plasmapheresis in this disease has not been determined and cannot currently be recommended. The 5-year survival is approximately 70%, but is reduced by coexistent myeloma.

AL-Amyloidosis

Amyloid represents a family of proteins. Fifteen different types of amyloid have been identified and are named according to the precursor protein that polymerizes to produce amyloid. AL-amyloidosis, which is also known as "primary amyloidosis," represents a plasma cell dyscrasia that is usually characterized by systemic deposition of amyloid and a mild increase in monoclonal plasma cells in the bone marrow. However, about 20% of patients with AL-amyloidosis have overt multiple myeloma or other lymphoproliferative disorder. In AL-amyloidosis, the amyloid deposits are composed of immunoglobulin light chains. AA-Amyloidosis, or secondary amyloidosis, refers to a disorder that occurs in the course of chronic inflammatory conditions, such as rheumatoid arthritis or connective tissue diseases. The amyloid precursor protein in secondary amyloidosis is serum AA protein, which is an acute phase reactant.

AL-amyloidosis is a systemic disease that typically involves multiple organs (Table 4). Cardiac infiltration frequently produces congestive heart failure and is a common presenting manifestation of primary amyloidosis. Infiltration of the lungs and gastrointestinal tract is also common, but often produces few clinical manifestations. Dysesthesias, orthostatic hypotension, diarrhea, and bladder dysfunction from peripheral and autonomic neuropathies can occur. Amyloid deposition can also produce an arthropathy that resembles rheumatoid arthritis, a bleeding diathesis, and a variety of skin manifestations that include purpura. Kidney involvement is common in primary amyloidosis.

Pathology

Glomerular lesions are the dominant renal features of AL-amyloidosis, and are characterized by the presence of mesangial nodules and glomerular sclerosis (Fig. 3). In the early stage, amyloid deposits are usually found in the mesangium and are not associated with an increase in mesangial cellularity. Deposits may also be seen along the subepithelial space of capillary loops in more advanced stages. Immunohistochemistry demonstrates that the deposits consist of light chains. On electron microscopy, the deposits are characteristicly randomly oriented, non-branching fibrils 7 to 10 nm in diameter. In some cases of early amyloidosis, glomeruli may appear normal on light microscopy. Careful examination, however, will identify scattered monotypic light chains on immunofluorescence microscopy. Ultrastructural examination with immuno-electron microscopy to reveal the fibrils of AL-amyloid

TABLE 4

Relative Frequency of Organ Infiltration by Light Chains in LCDD and AL-Amyloidosis

	Isotype	Renal	Cardiac	Liver	Neurologic	GI	Pulmonary
		\multicolumn{6}{c}{Organ Involvement[a]}					
LCDD	$\kappa > \lambda$	++++	+++	+++	+	rare	rare
AL-amyloid	$\lambda > \kappa$	+++	++	+	+	+++	++++

[a] +, Uncommon but occurs during the course of the disease; ++++, extremely common in the course of the disease.

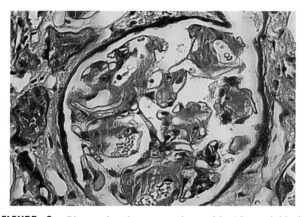

FIGURE 3 Glomerulus from a patient with AL-amyloidosis showing segmentally variable accumulation of amorphous acidophilic material that is effacing portions of the glomerular architecture (40× magnification, PASH stain).

may be required to establish the diagnosis early in the course of renal involvement. As the disease advances, mesangial deposits progressively enlarge to form nodules that compress the filtering surfaces of the glomeruli and cause renal failure. Epithelial proliferation and crescent formation are rare in AL-amyloidosis.

There are significant differences between amyloidosis and LCDD. For amyloid deposition to occur, amyloid P glycoprotein must also be present. The amyloid P component is not part of the amyloid fibrils, but binds them. This glycoprotein is a constituent of normal human glomerular basement membrane and elastic fibrils. In contrast to AL-amyloid, in LCDD the light chain deposits are punctate, granular, and electron-dense and are identified in the mesangium and/or subendothelial space; amyloid P component is absent. Amyloid has characteristic tinctorial properties and stains with Congo red, which produces an apple-green birefringence when the tissue section is examined under polarized light, and with thioflavins T and S. These special stains are not taken up by the granular light chain deposits of LCDD. Another difference between these lesions is the tendency for κ light chains to compose the granular deposits of LCDD, while usually λ light chains constitute AL-amyloid. Both diseases can involve organs other than the kidney (Table 4). Amyloidosis more commonly involves the gastrointestinal tract and lungs, whereas deposits of LCDD infiltrate the liver more frequently than amyloidosis.

Clinical Features

Proteinuria and renal insufficiency are the two major renal manifestations of AL-amyloidosis. Proteinuria ranges from asymptomatic non-nephrotic proteinuria to nephrotic syndrome. More than 90% of patients have monoclonal light chains in urine or blood. Renal insufficiency is present in 58 to 70% of patients at the time of diagnosis. Isolated microscopic hematuria is not common in AL-amyloidosis. Ultrastructural and immunohistochemical examination of biopsies of an affected organ establish the diagnosis. Scintigraphy using ^{123}I-labeled P component, which binds to amyloid, can

often diagnose the degree of organ involvement from amyloid infiltration, but this test is not currently widely available.

Pathogenesis

The pathogenesis of AL-amyloidosis is not completely understood. Internalization and processing of light chains by mesangial cells produce amyloid *in vitro*. The finding that N-terminal sequences of light chain fragments in amyloid are identical to the sequence of soluble light chains suggests that proteolytic cleavage of light chains may play a role in causing amyloid. Presumably, intracellular oxidation or proteolysis of light chains allows formation of amyloid, which is then extruded into the extracellular space. With continued production of amyloid, the mesangium expands, compressing the filtering surface of the glomeruli and producing progressive renal failure.

Treatment and Prognosis

A randomized trial compared colchicine therapy alone (0.6 mg twice daily) to colchicine plus melphalan and prednisone in doses used for multiple myeloma. A 1-year course of intermittent melphalan and prednisone along with colchicine increased survival from 6.7 to 12.2 months, thus supporting the use of chemotherapy in AL-amyloidosis not associated with multiple myeloma. Colchicine should probably be continued indefinitely, but the total dose of melphalan should be limited to 600 mg, because alkylating agents can promote the development of myelodysplastic syndromes or leukemia. In another retrospective study, patients with nephrotic syndrome, a normal serum creatinine concentration, and no echocardiographic evidence of cardiac amyloidosis had the best response rate (39%) to melphalan and prednisone. Response in this subset required 11.7 months of treatment, but the median survival was 89.4 months, with 78% surviving 5 years. Eleven of 17 patients who responded to treatment had complete resolution of nephrotic syndrome and six others had a 50% reduction in urinary protein excretion; only three of the 17 had persistent nephrotic-range proteinuria. Toxicity of treatment in this series was significant; acute leukemia or myelodysplasia developed in seven of the responders. Survival for patients with AL-amyloidosis averages 12.2 months with chemotherapy. At present, there are no controlled trials showing that patients who do not respond to melphalan and prednisone will respond to more aggressive chemotherapeutic regimens. The therapeutic role of bone marrow transplantation in primary amyloidosis is under investigation.

FIBRILLARY GLOMERULONEPHRITIS AND IMMUNOTACTOID GLOMERULOPATHY

Fibrillary glomerulonephritis is a rare disorder characterized ultrastructurally by the presence of amyloid-like, randomly arranged, fibrillary deposits in the capillary wall. Unlike amyloid, these fibrils are thicker (18 to 22 nm) and Congo red and thioflavin T stains are negative (Fig. 4). Most patients with fibrillary glomerulonephritis do not have a plasma cell dyscrasia; however, occasionally a plasma cell

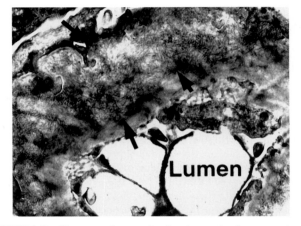

FIGURE 4 Electron micrograph of a glomerulus from a patient with fibrillary glomerulonephritis. Note the randomly arranged relatively straight fibrils with a diameter of approximately 20 nm (arrows). The overall ultrastructural appearance resembles amyloid except that the fibrils are approximately twice as thick (30,000× magnification, uranyl acetate and lead citrate).

dyscrasia is present so screening is advisable. Patients typically manifest nephrotic syndrome and varying degrees of renal failure; progression to end stage renal failure is the rule. No standard treatment for the idiopathic variety is currently available.

Immunotactoid, or microtubular, glomerulopathy is even more uncommon than fibrillary glomerulonephritis and is usually associated with a plasma cell dyscrasia. The deposits in this lesion contain thick (>30 nm), organized, microtubular structures that are located in the mesangium and along capillary walls. Cryoglobulinemia, which is covered in Chapter 18, should be considered in the differential diagnosis and ruled out clinically. Treatment of the underlying plasma cell dyscrasia is indicated for this rare disorder.

WALDENSTRÖM'S MACROGLOBULINEMIA

This disorder constitutes about 5% of monoclonal gammopathies and is characterized by the presence of a monoclonal population of lymphocytoid plasma cells. This condition clinically behaves more like lymphoma, although the malignant cell secretes IgM (macroglobulin). IgM is not excreted and accumulates in the plasma to produce hyperviscosity syndrome. Lytic bone lesions are uncom-

mon, but hepatosplenomegaly and lymphadenopathy are frequently identified. Hyperviscosity syndrome produces neurologic symptoms, visual impairment, bleeding diathesis, renal failure, and symptoms of hypervolemia. Renal failure is usually mild but occurs in about 30% of patients. Hyperviscosity syndrome and precipitation of IgM in the glomerular capillaries are the most common causes of renal failure. About 10 to 15% of patients develop AL-amyloidosis, but cast nephropathy is rare. Because of the typically advanced age at presentation (sixth to seventh decade) and slowly progressive course, the major therapeutic goal is relief of symptoms. All patients with monoclonal IgM levels above 3 g/dL should have serum viscosity determined. Plasmapheresis is indicated in symptomatic patients and shouldbe continued until symptoms resolve and serum viscosity normalizes. Severe renal failure requiring renal replacement therapy is uncommon. Median survival is about 3 years and is related to the advanced age at onset of this disorder.

Bibliography

Ganeval D, Rabian C, Guérin V, et al.: Treatment of multiple myeloma with renal involvement. Adv Nephrol 21:347–370, 1992.

Gertz MA, Kyle RA, Greipp PR: Response rates and survival in primary systemic amyloidosis. Blood 77:257–262, 1991.

Heilman RL, Velosa JA, Holley KE, et al.: Long-term follow-up and response to chemotherapy in patients with light-chain deposition disease. Am J Kidney Dis 20:34–41, 1992.

Preud'homme J-L, Aucouturier P, Touchard G, et al.: Monoclonal immunoglobulin deposition disease (Randall type). Relationship with structural abnormalities of immunoglobulin chains. Kidney Int 46:965–972, 1994.

Sanders PW, Herrera GA: Monoclonal immunoglobulin light chain-related renal diseases. Semin Nephrol 13:324–341, 1993.

Sanders PW, Herrera GA, Kirk KA, et al.: Spectrum of glomerular and tubulointerstitial renal lesions associated with monotypical immunoglobulin light chain deposition. Lab Invest 64:527–537, 1991.

Skinner M, Anderson JJ, Simms R, et al.: Treatment of 100 patients with primary amyloidosis: A randomized trial of melphalan, prednisone, and colchicine versus colchicine only. Am J Med 100:290–298, 1996.

Solomon A, Weiss DT, Kattine AA: Nephrotoxic potential of Bence Jones proteins. N Engl J Med 324:1845–1851, 1991.

Tagouri YM, Sanders PW, Pickens MM, et al.: In vitro AL-amyloid formation by rat and human mesangial cells. Lab Invest 74:290–302, 1996.

Zhu L, Herrera GA, Murphy-Ullrich JE, et al.: Pathogenesis of glomerulosclerosis in light chain deposition disease: Role for transforming growth factor-β. Am J Pathol 147:375–385, 1995.

30

HEMOLYTIC UREMIC SYNDROME/THROMBOTIC THROMBOCYTOPENIC PURPURA

RICHARD L. SIEGLER

The hemolytic uremic syndrome (HUS) and thrombotic thrombocytopenic purpura (TTP) are both characterized by a thrombotic microangiopathy (TMA) in target organs. However, the epidemiology, pathophysiology, clinical expression, response to therapy, and natural history of Shiga toxin (Stx) mediated HUS (previously referred to as classic or postdiarrheal HUS) and TTP are sufficiently different to warrant viewing them as distinct, but similar, disorders. It must be acknowledged, however, that in some cases of non-Stx HUS (i.e., nondiarrheal or atypical HUS), especially as seen in adults, clinical features may be indistinguishable from TTP. This has led to the suggestion by some that they both be viewed as variable expression of a single disorder. TTP was first described by Moschowitz in 1925 when he reported a 16-year-old female who succumbed to anemia and multiorgan TMA. Although Gasser is credited with first describing childhood HUS 30 years later, we owe much of our understanding of the clinical features and natural history of the disease to the observations of Gianantonio in the 1960s and 1970s. A major contribution was also made by Karmali in 1983 when he recognized the syndrome's association with Stx producing *Escherichia coli* (e.g., *E. coli* O157:H7).

HEMOLYTIC UREMIC SYNDROME

Epidemiology

Ninety percent of childhood HUS, but less than 50% of adult cases, is preceded by diarrhea that is usually bloody (Table 1). Classic postdiarrheal (Stx-mediated) HUS is the most common cause of acute renal failure in infants and young children. A second episode of Stx HUS can occur in the same individual, but is very rare. There is persuasive evidence that the disease is caused by *E. coli* that produce potent cytotoxins known as Shiga toxins (previously known as Shiga-like toxins) due to their similarity to the prototypic toxin produced by *Shigella dysenteriae* type I. About 90% of Stx producing *E. coli* in the United States are of the O157:H7 serotype, but dozens of other Stx producing serotypes exist.

Cattle intestines are natural reservoirs for the bacteria, but it is sometimes carried by birds and other mammals.

Fecal contamination of any ingestable substance can lead to hemorrhagic colitis that in 5–10% of cases progresses to HUS. Vectors for the *E. coli* include not only meat, especially beef hamburger, but also contaminated water, fruits, and vegetables as well as unpasteurized apple juice or cider and dairy products. Person to person spread has been responsible for numerous outbreaks. Classic Stx HUS occurs predominately during the warmer months of the year; there is no clear-cut gender predilection. The median age for children is 2 years (mean age 4 years), but it also occurs in adolescents and adults. The incidence varies between different regions of the United States and is generally higher in the more northern latitudes. There is evidence that this may be related to a higher bovine *E. coli* O157:H7 carrier rate in these regions. The overall annual incidence is probably about 1–1.5 cases for every 100,000 children less than 18 years of age. The incidence rises dramatically in infants ages 1 to 2 years (e.g., seven cases/100,000). There are few incidence data available for Stx HUS in adults. A study of *E. coli* O157:H7 associated HUS in Washington State, however, demonstrated an annual incidence of approximately one case/100,000 population for those ages 20–49 years, 0.5 cases/100,000 population for those 50–59 years of age, and close to two cases/100,000 population for those 60 years of age and older. Washington experiences more cases than most regions of the country, so the overall national incidence in adults is probably lower.

Ten percent of childhood HUS and more than one-half of adult cases are not preceded by diarrhea. Although some of these may be caused by Stx (see Pathogenic Cascades section later), nondiarrheal, or atypical HUS, is usually secondary to drugs or other conditions or disorders (Table 2). For example, approximately 10% of patients with systemic sclerosis (scleroderma) experience rapid onset of acute renal failure with clinical and histological features of HUS. Most also have malignant hypertension. Although secondary HUS accounts for the majority of non-Stx cases in adulthood, it is uncommon in children. Most of the non-Stx cases in children, and a few in adults, are idiopathic. Some of these are familial.

TABLE I
Epidemiology and Clinical Features

	Stx HUS	TTP
Antecedents	Diarrhea	Varied
Age (mean)	4 years	35 years
Gender	Equal	70% women
Race	Whites	African-Americans
Seasonally	Warm months	All year
Incidence	1–1.5/100,000 (<18 yrs age)	.37/100,000 (all ages)
Severe colitis	Usually	Rarely
Fever	Mild	Prominent
Encephalopathy	20%	>90%
Thrombocytopenia	Moderate	Severe
Hemorrhage, multiorgan	Rarely	Usually
Hematuria/proteinuria	100%	75%
Oligoanuric renal failure	Usually	Occasionally
Multiorgan involvement	Occasionally	Usually
Death[a]	5%	15%
Recurrences	<1%	20%

[a]With optimal therapy.

Pathogenic Cascades

The pathogenic cascade for Stx mediated HUS is becoming better understood. Ingested Stx producing *E. coli* colonize the distal ileum and large intestines via poorly understood mechanisms and cause a severe (hemorrhagic) colitis that facilitates the entry of Stx and lipopolysaccharides (LPS) into the circulation. There is evidence that severe bowel inflammation may not be a requirement for the systemic absorption of Stx, since some documented Stx mediated cases are not preceded by diarrhea. Stx's are 71-kd protein subunit toxins comprised of five B subunits and one A subunit; they exist in several forms (i.e., SLT-1, SLT-2, SLT-2 variants). Following absorption into the circula-

TABLE 2
Secondary TTP/HUS

Pregnancy (pre-eclampsia and postpartum)	Medications
	Oral contraceptives
Systemic disorders	Cancer chemotherapy
Collagen vascular diseases	(especially mitomycin C,
(especially scleraderma	Bleomycin, CDDP)
and SLE) Malignant	Cyclosporine/FK 506
hypertension	Ticlopidine
Infections	Interferon α
Streptococcus pneumoniae	Quinine
AIDS	Miscellaneous
Stx *E. coli*	Pancreatitis
Cancer	Coronary artery bypass surgery
Bone marrow transplant	Glomerulonephritis

tion, the Stx B subunits rapidly attach to neutral glycolipid (GB$_3$) receptors in the gut and kidneys. The toxin is then internalized where the A subunit inhibits protein synthesis thereby causing cell injury or death. Even though microvascular endothelial cell injury is central to the TMA that characterizes HUS, it is not clear that the endothelial cell is the initial renal target for the toxin. There is some evidence that the renal tubular epithelial cell is initially injured in Stx HUS.

Endothelial cell injury results in diminished glomerular capillary patency due to endothelial cell swelling, detachment from the underlying basement membrane, and accumulation of fluffy material between the endothelial cells and basement membrane. The endothelial cell injury and detachment also results in activation of platelets, and to a lesser extent the coagulation cascade, which in concert further impair the renal microcirculation, causing renal ischemic injury and dysfunction.

The pathogenesis for non-Stx (nondiarrheal) HUS is less well understood, but is presumably caused by drugs or conditions (Table 2) that either damage endothelial cells, or promote microvascular thrombosis. It is sometimes familial (autosomal dominant or recessive) and recurrent. A low serum complement (C3) concentration that is associated with a deficiency of the alternate pathway regulatory protein, factor H, is common in these families. Many other cases are idiopathic with no recognizable antecedent factor.

Prodrome

Stx mediated HUS is preceded by colitis that becomes bloody about 75% of the time. Most children also experience vomiting. Abdominal pain can be severe and is sometimes initially misdiagnosed as acute appendicitis or ulcerative colitis. Rectal prolapse, intussusception, and bowel necrosis with perforation can occur.

Children with non-Stx HUS usually have vomiting without diarrhea. Low-grade fever occurs in almost one-half, and upper respiratory infection in about one-fourth.

Clinical Features

After about a week of diarrhea (range 1–14 days), the onset of HUS (Table 1) is heralded by pallor, oligoanuria, lethargy, and irritability and, in some cases, seizures. Jaundice, petechiae, or purpura occur occasionally. Mild cases, with little or no renal failure, and examples of a partial syndrome (i.e., lacking the triad of hemolytic anemia, thrombocytopenia, and acute renal failure) have been reported. Most children experience oliguric renal failure that lasts on average about 1 week. Close to one-half have a period of anuria that on average lasts about 3 days. Prolonged oligoanuria occurs occasionally.

Hypertension is present in the majority of cases, but is usually mild to moderate, and labile. It usually resolves by the time of discharge from the hospital.

Seizures and other forms of severe central nervous system involvement used to be seen in close to 50% of cases.

Now, however, as a result of more timely diagnoses, greater attention to fluid and electrolyte management, and earlier initiation of dialysis, metabolic encephalopathy (e.g., seizures, coma, semicoma) is seen in only about 20% of cases. There continues to be, however, a 3 to 5% incidence of stroke or generalized cerebral edema.

Pancreatic involvement is seen in approximately 20% of cases. It is usually expressed as elevated serum amylase and lipase enzyme concentrations, with or without pain, tenderness or vomiting; pseudocysts or necrosis have not been reported. Of greater concern is insulin dependent diabetes mellitus that has been reported to occur in up to 10% of cases; on occasion it can be permanent. On rare occasions the TMA can involve the heart, lungs, eyes, parotid gland, skin, or muscle.

Although the clinical features of non-Stx HUS in children can be very similar to those of classic Stx mediated disease, there is a subset of non-Stx HUS patients who present with the insidious onset of nonoliguric renal failure and malignant hypertension that often leads to congestive heart failure. The clinical expression of non-Stx HUS in adults is generally severe. Cases associated with pre-eclampsia are usually characterized by fetal distress, liver involvement, and in about one-third of cases, disseminated intravascular coagulation (DIC). Postpartum HUS typically includes severe renal failure and hypertension. Fever and neurological involvement is frequent. Cancer (especially gastric and metastatic carcinoma) and mitomycin associated HUS is associated with a malignant and rapidly progressive clinical course.

Laboratory features include microangiopathic hemolytic anemia, thrombocytopenia, and azotemia. The anemia, that is largely due to mechanical fragmentation of red blood cells (RBC) as they pass through partially occluded renal microvessels, is characterized by fragmented RBC (e.g., burr cells, shistocytes) on blood smear, and elevated serum lactic dehydrogenase concentrations. A low platelet count can be documented in about 95% of cases, but severe thrombocytopenia ($<10 \times 10^9$/L) occurs infrequently. Prothrombin times and partial thromboplastin times are usually normal. Increased serum concentrations of hepatic enzymes, uric acid, triglycerides, and bilirubin are commonly seen.

Management

Supportive therapy continues to be the cornerstone in managing children with classic Stx HUS. Numerous innovative therapies including heparin, antiplatelet agents, fibrinolytic agents, vitamin E, prostacyclin, intravenous IgG, and infusion of fresh frozen plasma (FFP), have been tried, but have been found to be either too risky, or of no, or only marginal benefit. High doses of intravenous furosemide may decrease the need for dialysis in some patients.

The value of plasma exchange in Stx HUS is unclear (Table 3). Although there are anecdotal reports suggesting benefit, there is only one prospective controlled clinical trial in children; it included both Stx and non-Stx patients. The results of this study suggest that it may be helpful in certain high-risk patients. The response, if any, to plasma exchange is certainly not dramatic, however, and in no way

TABLE 3
Therapeutic Response

	Stx HUS	TTP
Plasma exchange	Marginal benefit	80%
Plasma infusion	No	65%
Vincristine	Unknown	Usually
Immunoabsorption	Unknown	Usually
Steroids	No	Occasionally
Splenectomy	Unknown	Usually
Antiplatelet agents	Marginal benefit	Occasionally
IV γ globulin	No	Occasionally

approaches the response seen in most cases of TTP. Moreover, the difficulty in obtaining vascular access in small infants, the high volume of blood required for operation of some systems, the expense, and the risk of infection when infusing fresh frozen plasma, coupled to the usual good outcome for those treated conservatively, argue against its use. There is a temptation to initiate plasma exchange for those doing poorly, especially for those with severe central nervous system (CNS) dysfunction. Even so, it should be used only with the understanding that it is of unproven value.

There is greater enthusiasm for using plasma exchange in children with non-Stx (atypical or nondiarrheal) HUS, and some reports suggest benefit compared to historical controls who did not receive plasma exchange. There are no published prospective controlled studies to support its recommended use, however. Plasma manipulation (infusion or exchange) is commonly used to treat non-Stx HUS in adults, especially if there is neurological involvement or a relapsing course. Anecdotal reports suggest benefit, but its efficacy has not been tested in large prospective trials. HUS occurring during pregnancy usually resolves following delivery; cases secondary to scleroderma and associated malignant hypertension benefit from treatment with angiotensin converting enzyme (ACE) inhibitors.

Meticulous attention to fluid and electrolyte balance, control of any seizures or hypertension, blood transfusion [using leukocyte filtered packed red blood cells (PRBC)] for severe (Hct <15–20%) anemia, the appropriate use of dialysis, and aggressive nutritional support constitute appropriate management. Maintaining the hematocrit between 33 and 35% may improve CNS oxygen delivery in those with severe encephalopathy. Platelet administration should be discouraged since it may provide substrate for additional microthrombus formation. Total parenteral nutrition (TPN) is necessary for those with severe colitis. Because most children with HUS have severe hypertriglyceridemia, it may not be possible to administer lipid preparations. Pancreatic TMA with subsequent insulin-dependent diabetes mellitus can occur. Frequent blood sugar measurements are therefore necessary, especially in those receiving peritoneal dialysis with 2.5–4.25% dextrose, or those receiving high concentrations of dextrose in TPN fluid.

Outcome

Approximately 5% of children die during the acute phase of Stx HUS, usually from extrarenal disease. Brain involvement (e.g., infarction, hemorrhage, generalized edema) accounts for the majority of fatal complications, but bowel infarction, as well as heart or lung TMA can be fatal. An additional 5% are left with chronic brain damage or end stage renal disease (ESRD). The remaining 90% experience functional recovery, though about 5% are left with chronic hypertension and 30–50% have either proteinuria and/or below normal glomerular filtration rate (GFR). Chronic abnormalities sometimes appear after a period of apparent recovery.

Approximately 10% are left with both chronic proteinuria and low GFR, and are therefore at substantial risk for eventually developing ESRD due to hyperfiltration injury. Those who experience prolonged anuria (i.e., $\geq$10 days) or oliguria (i.e., $\geq$15 days) are at very high risk for chronic renal damage. Additional sequelae include rectal stricture (1–3%), diabetes mellitus (5–10%), that can be permanent, and neurological deficits (e.g., hemiparesis) from stroke (2–4%). Sequelae secondary to involvement of the retina, heart, or lungs are rare (<1%). HUS reoccurs in approximately 10% of those with end stage renal disease who receive renal grafts. Although recurrence may not result in graft loss, graft survival, independent of recurrent HUS, is reported to be lower than normal in some series.

Children with non-Stx HUS, however, experience about a 20% recurrence rate. Moreover in many parts of the world, those with non-Stx HUS experience greater mortality and more ESRD than those with Stx disease.

The outcome is worse in adults. Overall mortality is approximately 15–30%, chronic renal failure occurs in 20–30% of survivors, and recurrence is seen in about 25% of cases. This difference in outcome appears to be largely, but not entirely, due to the much higher incidence of non-Stx cases in the adult population. Adults who have familial HUS experience a high incidence of ESRD, and postpartum, cancer, and mitomycin associated HUS patients experience a 50% or greater mortality rate.

THROMBOTIC THROMBOCYTOPENIC PURPURA

Epidemiology

TTP is largely a disease of adult women and is uncommon in the very young and the elderly (Table 1). It occurs more frequently in women of African-American decent than in Whites. TTP may occur *de novo* without any recognizable antecedent factor or event (idiopathic or classic TTP), and may be familial. Some cases, especially familial, are characterized by multiple relapses that may begin in childhood, and are classified as chronic relapsing TTP. Recent observations shed light on the pathogenesis of classic TTP (see later).

Other cases can be classified as secondary, since they are preceded by such things as pregnancy, systemic disorders, cancers, AIDS, and medications (Table 2).

TTP has been reported to occur once per 25,000 pregnancies. It can present prior to mid-pregnancy, but is usu-

ally seen peripartum; postpartum cases (within several weeks of delivery) also occur. Relapse occurs in about 50% of women, sometimes during subsequent pregnancies.

Systemic disorders including malignant hypertension, collagen vascular disease, especially systemic lupuss erythematosus (SLE), but also systemic sclerosis, dermatomyositis or polymyositis, Wegener's granulomatosis, and Still's disease, account for some cases.

Many reports of TTP occurring during the later stages of AIDS have appeared in the literature. Other infectious causes (e.g., Stx producing *E. coli*) have been reported infrequently.

The association of TTP with cancers, especially metastatic cancer, has been known for decades and can be the presenting feature. Most cases are seen in association with adenocarcinoma, especially gastric tumors, but also occur with cancers of the colon, breast, and lung (small cell carcinoma). There have been numerous reports of TTP following allogeneic bone marrow, and more recently, autologous bone marrow and peripheral blood stem cell transplantation.

The list of drugs associated with episodes of TTP continues to grow (Table 2). It seems ironic that TTP sometimes follows the administration of the platelet antiaggregating agent ticoplidine. The quinine association has been known for a number of years, but is not understood. There are single case reports associating TTP with numerous other medications.

Pathogenesis

The pathogenic cascade of TTP has not been studied to the same extent as that of Stx HUS, but recent observations have substantially increased our understanding of classic TTP. Adults with classic TTP, but usually not those with HUS, have very large von Willebrand's factor (vWF) multimers in their circulation during the acute phase of their disease; multimers tend to persist in those with chronic relapsing TTP. These very large multimeric forms of vWF strongly react with platelets and promote their aggregation. It was more recently discovered that vWF-cleaving protease, that normally degrades the multimeres, is deficient in adult TTP, but not adult HUS patients. In familial cases the defect is congenital and persistent. In nonfamilial cases the cleaving protease defect appears to be transient and is associated with an IgG protease inhibitor autoantibody.

Prodrome

TTP is only rarely preceded by diarrhea, but may follow a viral flulike syndrome characterized by fatigue, fever, abdominal pain, nausea, and vomiting.

Clinical Features

In contrast to classic Stx HUS, patients with TTP generally present with fever (Table 1), bleeding and, in about one-half of the cases, CNS dysfunction. Brain involvement eventually occurs in approximately 90% of cases and is usually the dominant feature of the syndrome. Headache, somnolence, confusion, aphasia, focal neurological deficits, hemiparesis, and minor motor irritability (e.g., tremor, jerkiness) are very common. Seizures occur in about one-third of patients, and coma in approximately 10%. The neurological findings often fluctuate and can be fleeting.

Hemorrhage, in the form of gastrointestinal bleeding, is seen in the majority of cases; epistaxis, menorrhagia, and purpura are also common. Retinal lesions occur in close to 20% of cases.

Although the majority of patients show signs of renal involvement (i.e., hematuria, proteinuria, and azotemia), in contrast to Stx HUS, oliguric renal failure with severe azotemia is uncommon. However, life-threatening involvement of other vital organs (e.g., brain, heart, lungs) is seen much more frequently than in Stx HUS.

Laboratory findings are similar to those described for HUS except that the thrombocytopenia tends to be more severe. This may explain the higher incidence of bleeding.

Management

When secondary TTP is present, efforts should be made to stop the drug or treat the underlying condition. The previously cited supportive therapy guidelines for HUS also apply to treatment of TTP. But in contrast to Stx HUS, available specific therapies are usually of value (Table 3). It is difficult to determine the relative efficacy of the various specific therapies, however, since in most reported series two or more therapies were administered concurrently.

Even so, there is a consensus that, with the probable exception of bone marrow transplant (BMT) TTP, plasma therapies offer the greatest benefit and should be initiated as soon as the diagnosis is established. Plasma exchange is probably the most effective modality with good response in 70–90% of cases. Its efficacy is assumed to result from removal of harmful mediators (e.g., IgG inhibitors of vWF cleaving protease) coupled with the replacement of missing beneficial factors (e.g., vWF cleaving protease). The lack of efficacy in cases of BMT TTP is probably because BMT patients are not deficient in vWF cleaving protease. Commercially available fresh frozen plasma (FFP) has been shown to contain normal protease activity and should be the initial replacement solution. Those who fail to respond can sometimes be salvaged by changing the replacement solution to cryosupernatant, which lacks the very largest vWF multimers. There is no consensus as to frequency and duration of therapy, but seven consecutive daily treatments followed by alternate day exchanges in those showing improvement, using a total exchange volume/ treatment of 1 to 1.5 times the predicted plasma volume of the patient is reasonable. Treatment should be continued until remission is achieved. It is not certain that plasma exchange is superior to the infusion of fresh frozen plasma alone. The better results reported with plasma exchange may be because plasma exchange allows the infusion of much larger volumes of fresh frozen plasma, especially in those with oligoanuria. Periodic infusion of fresh frozen plasma (without plasma exchange) is often effective in preventing relapses in those with recurrent TTP.

Vincristine or protein A immunoabsorption (PAI) is probably of value in those who fail to respond to plasma exchange. Corticosteroids, intravenous immunoglobulins (γ globulin), and antiplatelet agents (e.g., dipyridamole, dextran 70, ticlopidine, cyclosporine) have all been used, usually in combination with other modalities. This makes it difficult to evaluate their efficacy.

Splenectomy may be helpful for those who fail to respond to plasma manipulation and Vincristine and PAI, or who continue to experience recurrences in spite of prophylactic infusions of fresh frozen plasma.

In summary, plasma exchange is the treatment of choice and should be instituted promptly. Those who do not respond can be treated with Vincristine or PAI. Splenectomy should be reserved for those who fail to benefit from less extreme therapies.

Outcome

Both mortality and recurrence are higher in TTP than in childhood Stx HUS (Table 1). Without treatment, the death rate approaches 90%; even with modern plasma therapy there is approximately a 15% mortality rate. Mortality is higher for African-American women. Uncontrollable multisystem involvement (e.g., brain, heart, lungs) accounts for most deaths. Recurrence occurs in approximately 20% of cases. The relative infrequency of TTP compared to Stx HUS, has hampered the acquisition of long-term outcome information.

Bibliography

Bell WR, Braine HG, Ness PM, Kickler TS: Improved survival in thrombotic thrombocytopenic purpura—hemolytic uremic syndrome. Clinical experience in 108 patients. *N Engl J Med* 325:398–403, 1991.

Furlan M, Robles R, Galbusera M, *et al.*: Von Willebrand factor-cleaving protease in thrombotic thrombocytopenic purpura and the hemolytic–uremic syndrome. *N Engl J Med* 339:1578–1584, 1998.

Gordon L, Kwaan HC: Cancer- and drug-associated thrombotic thrombocytopenic purpura and hemolytic uremic syndrome. *Semin Hematol* 34:140–147, 1997.

Hayward CPM, Sutton DMC, Carter WH, Jr, *et al.*: Treatment outcomes in patients with adult thrombotic thrombocytopenic purpura—hemolytic uremic syndrome. *Arch Intern Med* 154: 982– 987, 1994.

Melnyk AMS, Solez K, Kjellstrand CM: Adult hemolytic–uremic syndrome. A review of 27 cases. *Arch Intern Med* 155:2077–2084, 1995.

Remuzzi G, Ruggenenti P: The hemolytic uremic syndrome. *Kidney Int* 47:2–19, 1995.

Rock GA, Shumak KH, Buskar NA, *et al.*: Comparison of plasma exchange with plasma infusion in the treatment of thrombotic thrombocytopenic purpura. *N Engl J Med* 325:393–397, 1991.

Ruggenenti P, Remuzzi G: The pathophysiology and management of thrombotic thrombocytopenic purpura. *Eur J Haematol* 56:191–207, 1996.

Siegler RL: Management of hemolytic–uremic syndrome. *J Pediatr* 112:1014–1020, 1988.

Siegler RL: Spectrum of extrarenal involvement in postdiar-rheal hemolytic–uremic syndrome. *J Pediatr* 125:511–518, 1994.

Siegler RL: The hemolytic uremic syndrome. *Pediatr Clin North Am* 42:1505–1529, 1995.

Siegler RL: Atypical hemolytic–uremic syndrome: A comparison with postdiarrheal disease. *J Pediatr* 128:505–511, 1996.

Siegler RL, Milligan MK, Burningham TH, Christofferson RD, Chang S-Y, Jorde LB: Long-term outcome and prognostic indicators in the hemolytic–uremic syndrome. *J Pediatr* 118:195–200, 1991.

Siegler RL, Pavia AT, Christofferson RD, Milligan MK: A 20 year population-based study of postdiarrheal hemolytic uremic syndrome in Utah. *Pediatrics* 94:35–40, 1994.

Siegler RL, Pavia AT, Cook JB: Hemolytic–uremic syndrome in adolescents. *Arch Pediatr Adolesc Med* 151:165–169, 1997.

31

RENAL DISEASES ASSOCIATED WITH HIV INFECTION

MARIANNE MONAHAN AND PAUL E. KLOTMAN

Renal complications occur frequently in the course of HIV disease and can be subdivided into several categories, including disturbances of fluid and electrolyte metabolism, disturbances in acid–base balance, acute renal failure, chronic progressive renal failure, particularly HIV associated nephropathy (HIVAN), and immune-mediated glomerulopathies (Table 1). Many of these disorders are similar to those seen in the non-HIV+ population. Others, such as HIVAN, are attributable to HIV infection itself or are the side effects of therapeutic agents used commonly in the treatment of AIDS related illnesses. Many of these complications are preventable or treatable, making early recognition and intervention essential.

FLUID AND ELECTROLYTES

Sodium

Electrolyte and acid–base abnormalities are common in AIDS patients. Of these, hyponatremia is the most common. Approximately 30% of hospitalized patients with AIDS develop a serum sodium less than 130 mM/L. Most cases can be attributed to volume depletion from diarrhea, emesis, poor oral intake, or increased insensible losses from fever or pulmonary disease. Other causes of low serum sodium include the syndrome of inappropriate antidiuretic hormone secretion (SIADH) which is a frequent complication of pulmonary infection and central nervous system lesions, adrenal insufficiency, and renal sodium wasting due to nephrotoxic medications like amphotericin and pentamidine. Common drug-related toxicities are listed in Table 2.

Hypernatremia, while much less common, can also be observed in AIDS patients. This also occurs in the setting of volume depletion from impaired oral intake and may be associated with acquired nephrogenic diabetes insipidus from medications such as amphotericin or foscarnet.

Potassium

Hyperkalemia has been reported in 16 to 21% of hospitalized AIDS patients. Similar to seronegative patients with hyperkalemia, increased serum potassium levels may be due to renal failure, adrenal insufficiency, and acidemia. Medications used commonly in the treatment of opportunistic infections like *Pneumocystis carinii* pneumonia have been shown to increase potassium blood levels through more direct mechanisms. Trimethoprim's effect on the distal nephron is similar to that of the potassium-sparing diuretics; it inhibits sodium reabsorption and thereby limits potassium secretion. Pentamidine has been shown to act on the distal tubule in a similar manner. Unexplained hyperkalemia has been attributed to hyporeninemic hypoaldosteronism in some AIDS patients. In addition to increased serum potassium, these patients also develop a metabolic acidosis. In these patients, fludrocortisone has been efficacious in the treatment of hyperkalemia.

TABLE 1
Renal Disorders in Patients with HIV Infection

Fluid–electrolyte and acid–base disturbances

Hypo- and hypernatremia
Hypo- and hyperkalemia
Hypo- and hypercalcemia
Hypomagnesemia
Hypo- and hyperphosphatemia
Syndrome of inappropriate ADH[a]
Nephrogenic diabetes insipidus
Renal tubular acidosis
Lactic acidosis
Fanconi syndrome

Acute renal failure syndromes
Acute tubular necrosis
Acute interstitial nephritis
    Allergic
    Infectious
Hemolytic uremic syndrome and thrombotic thrombocy-
    topenic purpura
Crystalluria/obstructive uropathy

Glomerular syndromes
HIVAN
Membranoproliferative glomerulonephritis (GN)
Minimal change disease
Membranous glomerulopathy
Post infectious GN

[a]ADH, antidiuretic hormone.

Hypokalemia, like hyponatremia, occurs most often in the setting of volume depletion. Amphotericin nephrotoxicity can also present with hypokalemia, often associated with magnesium depletion. More recently, hypokalemia has been observed as a complication of the Fanconi syndrome associated with the antiviral nucleotide analog adefovir.

Calcium

Abnormal serum calcium levels are frequently observed in hospitalized AIDS patients; hypocalcemia occurs in approximately 18% and hypercalcemia in approximately 3%. In many patients, hypocalcemia can be attributed to hypoalbuminemia, a highly prevalent condition in AIDS patients. Medications including foscarnet, pentamidine, and didanosine (ddI) have also been implicated in hypocalcemia. Severe, symptomatic hypocalcemia manifested by paraesthesias and Trousseau's or Chvostek's signs has been reported in patients treated concurrently with pentamidine and foscarnet. Increased serum calcium levels are seen in patients with granulomatous disease and in patients with disseminated cytomegalovirus.

Magnesium

Renal magnesium wasting, resulting in hypomagnesemia, occurs as a complication of treatment with both pentamidine and amphotericin. Drug-induced tubular injury is the proposed mechanism.

TABLE 2
Drug-Induced Nephrotoxicity in HIV-1 Infected Patients

Drug	Toxicity
Acyclovir	Acute tubular necrosis Crystalluria Obstructive nephropathy
Adefovir	Fanconi syndrome
Aminoglycosides	Acute tubular necrosis Renal tubular acidosis
Amphotericin	Acute tubular necrosis Hypokalemia Hyperkalemia Hypomagnesemia Renal tubular acidosis
Cidofovir	Proximal tubular damage Bicarbonate wasting Proteinuria
Foscarnet	Hypocalcemia Hypercalcemia Hypomagnesemia Hyperphosphatemia Hypophosphatemia Nephrogenic diabetes insipidus
Indinavir	Crystalluria Urinary tract obstruction
Nonsteroidal antiinflammatory drugs (NSAIDS)	Acute tubular necrosis Allergic interstitial nephritis
Pentamidine	Acute tubular necrosis Hyperkalemia Hypocalcemia
Rifampin	Allergic interstitial nephritis
Sulfadiazine	Crystalluria Urinary tract obstruction Allergic interstitial nephritis

ACID–BASE BALANCE

Non-anion gap metabolic acidosis from bicarbonate loss in the stool is not unusual. Many AIDS patients develop acute or chronic diarrheal syndromes given their increased susceptibility to opportunistic enteric pathogens, including *Cyclospora cayetanensis*, *Cryptosporidium parvum*, cytomegalovirus, and disseminated *Mycobacterium avium-intracellulare* (MAI). Lactic acidosis can occur in the setting of sepsis from bacterial or fungal infections or severe hypoxemia due to overwhelming pulmonary infection. Type B lactic acidosis, which is lactic acidosis not associated with hypoxia or hypoperfusion, has been reported in some AIDS patients. In these cases, the presumed mechanism of lactic acid accumulation was mitochondrial dysfunction which, in a few cases, was thought to be associated with the use of 3′-azido-3′-deoxythymidine (AZT). Mitochondrial dysfunction has been reported with other antiretrovirals as well.

Pulmonary infections can induce a respiratory alkalosis due to hyperventilation or, later in the course of illness, a respiratory acidosis as the ability of the patient to adequately ventilate decreases secondary to fatigue or acute pulmonary decompensation.

Several medications have also been implicated in the generation of acid–base disturbances. Renal tubular acidosis complicates treatment with gentamicin, amphotericin B, and adefovir. A series of patients who developed unexplained renal tubular acidosis while receiving high-dose trimethoprim-sulfamethoxazole (Bactrim) has also been reported.

FANCONI SYNDROME

Nephrotoxicity is the dose limiting side effect of cidofovir and adefovir, two nucleotide analogs with potent antiviral activity. Toxicity is related to renal uptake through an organic acid secretory pathway. Cidofovir is available for the treatment of cytomegalovirus retinitis and has activity against many of the other herpes viruses. In clinical trials, patients taking cidofovir develop signs of proximal tubule damage in approximately 5–7% of cases manifested as an elevated creatinine concentration, glucosuria, and bicarbonate wasting. Toxicity can be reduced by coadministration of probenecid which decreases renal cellular uptake. A related nucleotide analog adefovir has demonstrated antiretroviral activity against HIV-1 and hepatitis B. Adefovir has activity against HIV isolates that have developed resistance to other antiretrovirals, particularly AZT. Unfortunately, adefovir has been reported to induce Fanconi syndrome in up to 30% of patients on treatment for longer than 6 months. Manifestations include a proximal renal tubular acidosis (RTA) with bicarbonate wasting, hypophosphatemia, glucosuria, aminoaciduria, and hypokalemia. This usually resolves with discontinuation of the drug.

ACUTE RENAL FAILURE

The etiologies of acute renal failure (ARF) in AIDS patients are similar to those identified in patients without AIDS and can be subdivided into prerenal, intrarenal, and postrenal causes. Patients with AIDS are at increased risk of developing ARF from many prerenal causes. Hospitalized AIDS patient are often volume depleted due to complications of their underlying illness including vomiting, diarrhea, fever, and poor oral intake. In addition, patients with AIDS may have a true salt wasting syndrome, although the mechanism is unclear. As a result, AIDS patients are particularly sensitive to many potentially nephrotoxic therapeutic and diagnostic agents as well as changes in hemodynamic status. Not surprisingly, ARF is attributed to ischemic renal injury from sepsis in about 50%, to nephrotoxic agents, including aminoglycosides, amphotericin, pentamidine, and intravenous radiocontrast materials in about 25%, and to other causes, including acute interstitial nephritis, rhabdomyolysis, massive GI bleeding, cardiac failure, and hepatic failure in the remaining 25%.

Acute interstitial nephritis is not unusual in the HIV-infected patient and can be caused by infection or by a hypersensitivity drug reaction from virtually any medication. Infectious agents associated with interstitial disease in the immunocompromised include cytomegalovirus, candida, tuberculosis, and histoplasmosis. Medications used frequently in the treatment of AIDS-related illness that are associated with acute interstitial nephritis include penicillins, cephalosporins, ciprofloxacin, cotrimazole, rifampin, and nonsteroidal antiinflammatory drugs. Treatment requires discontinuation of the medication.

Vascular causes of acute renal failure, particularly hemolytic uremic syndrome/thrombotic thrombocytopenic purpura (HUS/TTP), are increasingly recognized in the HIV infected patient. In 25% of seropositive patients with HUS/TTP, the hematologic disturbance is the presenting manifestation of HIV infection. Centers located in areas with a high prevalence of HIV infection have reported that up to one-third of patients diagnosed with HUS/TTP are HIV positive. The clinical manifestations and pathologic findings of HIV-related HUS/TTP are similar to the idiopathic forms. Patients present with constitutional symptoms of fever and malaise, signs of a bleeding diathesis including mucosal bleeding and easy bruising, and a variety of neurologic signs and symptoms. Laboratory examination reveals a microangiopathic hemolytic anemia and renal insufficiency. Kidney biopsy reveals platelet and fibrin thrombi in renal and glomerular vessels, interstitial fibrosis, and acute tubular necrosis. Treatment with plasmapheresis and fresh frozen plasma (FFP) replacement may be effective.

Postrenal causes of acute renal failure are also common in the seropositive patient. Crystal induced obstructive nephropathy from various drugs should be considered when evaluating acute renal failure in HIV+ patients. The drugs most commonly implicated in seropositive patients are sulfadiazine, intravenous acyclovir, and indinavir. Treatment consists of discontinuation of the drug and vigorous hydration. Indinavir therapy is associated with asymptomatic crystalluria in up to 20% of patients. Symptoms of dysuria and renal colic and signs of mildly elevated serum creatinine occur in approximately 8%. Most patients improve with hydration or discontinuation of the drug.

Finally, many seropositive patients are enrolled in clinical trials with investigational drugs whose side effect profiles are poorly characterized. A high index of suspicion for drug toxicity should be maintained and explored whenever evaluating a seropositive patient for acute renal failure.

CHRONIC PROGRESSIVE RENAL DISEASE

HIVAN is a disease with unique clinical, pathologic, and epidemiologic features that progresses rapidly to end stage renal disease (ESRD). HIVAN was first described in the early 1980s but was rarely reported as a complication of HIV infection even as late as 1990. Since then, however, HIVAN has increased in incidence each year and is now the third leading cause of ESRD in African-Americans between the ages of 20–64. The salient features of HIVAN are indicated in Table 3.

TABLE 3
Clinical Presentation of HIV-Associated Nephropathy

Epidemiology	Third leading cause of ESRD in African-Americans ages 20–64
	Incidence increased each year until introduction of HAART[a]
Presentation	Proteinuria
	Azotemia
	Normal or large, echogenic kidneys on sonogram
	CD4+ cells usually <200
Pathology	Focal segmental glomerulosclerosis, collapsing variant
	Microcystic dilatation of tubules
Pathogenesis	Direct effect of HIV infection or viral proteins on renal epithelium
	Race cofactor
Treatment	HAART
	ACE[b] inhibition

[a]HAART, Highly active antiretroviral therapy.
[b]ACE, Angiotensin converting inhibition.

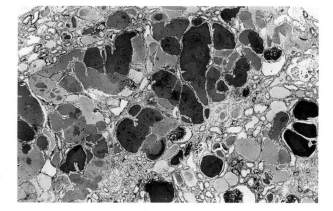

FIGURE 1 Renal biopsy of a patient with HIV associated nephropathy. The classic features of HIVAN are present in this biopsy with microcystic tubular dilatation, proteinaceous casts, modest interstitial infiltrate, and collapsing glomerulosclerosis. Periodic acid–Schiff stain; magnification 50×; photomicrographs kindly provided by Dr. Vivette D'Agati.

Presentation

The morphologic diagnosis of HIVAN is remarkably restrictd to Black patients; almost 90% of cases occur in African-Americans. The remaining 10% of cases are almost exclusively observed in mixed heritage or Hispanic patients. The disorder is only very rarely seen in seropositive White patients. Patients with HIVAN usually present with azotemia and proteinuria. Most patients are normotensive, and on renal sonogram kidneys are typically normal or slightly increased in size. By ultrasound, the kidneys are often described as echogenic. HIVAN is usually a late complication of HIV-1 infection. In 114 patients with biopsy proven HIVAN, all but six patients had CD4 counts less than 200. According to the case definitions of AIDS as revised in 1993 by the Centers for Disease Control, a CD4 count under 200 is an AIDS-defining condition. Thus, the high mortality of HIVAN patients must be viewed in the context of other patients with AIDS.

Pathology

The histopathologic features of HIVAN include focal segmental glomerular sclerosis (FSGS) in combination with microcystic distortion of the tubulointerstitium (Fig. 1). Collapsing glomerulosclerosis is a common variant in patients with HIVAN (Fig. 2A,B), although patients who are seronegative have also been reported with this form of FSGS. Microcysts are often filled with proteinaceous casts, and in some patients there is modest interstitial infiltration by lymphocytes, plasma cells, and monocytes. Immunofluorescence is generally nonspecific. Electron microscopic examination may reveal tubuloreticular arrays, but the prevalence of this finding has been decreasing more recently, probably due to more effective antiretroviral ther-

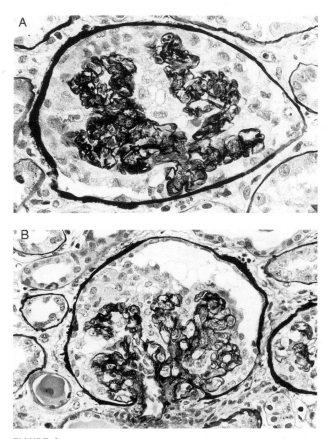

FIGURE 2 Focal segmental glomerulosclerosis of the collapsing variant. Both focal (A) and global collapse can be seen in association with HIV infection. Jones methenamine silver stain; A, 500× and B, 325×.

apy. Biopsy confirmation of HIVAN is extremely important. Even when HIVAN is suspected, 40% of biopsied patients will be found to have another diagnosis on pathologic examination. The relationship of HIV-1 infection to pathogenesis of other glomerular lesions is not as well understood as it is for the constellation of findings present in HIVAN.

Pathogenesis

The exact cellular mechanisms responsible for the pathogenesis of HIVAN have not been clearly established. From both clinical and animal studies, increasing evidence supports a more direct role for HIV-1 in inducing HIVAN. Renal glomerular and tubular epithelial cells, in particular, appear to be sensitive to the effects of HIV-1. Proliferation of glomerular and epithelial cells contributes to microcyst formation and may explain why kidneys are normal to enlarged in size. Collapsing FSGS likely results from pathologic involvement of the glomerular epithelial cell or podocyte. Direct infection of the renal epithelium by HIV-1 appears likely, but whether the epithelial cell can support a productive viral life cycle has yet to be determined.

Treatment

Approaches to the treatment of HIV-related renal diseases can be divided into three categories (1) management of the ESRD patient who is seropositive (2) treatment of HIVAN directed at slowing progression to ESRD, and (3) treatment of the HIV-1 infection.

Management of ESRD

Treatment options for the seropositive patient with ESRD are similar to those when HIV-1 is not the cause of renal failure. Options include hemodialysis, peritoneal dialysis and, more recently, renal transplantation. Studies to evaluate renal transplantation in HIV-1 infected patients are currently underway. The candidate population will be end stage renal patients with undetectable viral burden on a stable HAART (highly active antiretroviral therapy) regimen, who have no evidence of neoplasms or opportunistic infections, CD4 counts >200, and an available living donor. The use of cadaveric transplants in this population has not been considered yet. Transmission of HIV-1 in dialysis units is very unlikely if standard blood precaution practice guidelines are followed. The Centers for Disease Control does not recommend special machines or isolation for HIV-1 seropositive patients undergoing hemodialysis.

Treatment of HIVAN

Studies have suggested that ACE (angiotensin converting enzyme) inhibitors or immune modulators, including prednisone and cyclosporine may be efficacious in slowing progression of HIVAN to ESRD. Fosinopril, an ACE inhibitor, administered at 10 mg po qd, seems to be particularly effective when initiated early in the clinical course, when serum creatinine is still under 2 mg/dL. The mechanism by which ACE inhibition slows progression of HIVAN is unknown. In addition, studies demonstrating efficacy were not randomized or controlled, and the findings must be viewed in this context. Because therapy with ACE inhibitors is likely to be of little risk to the patient, as long as potassium is carefully monitored, it may be a reasonable approach, in the absence of more definitive evidence. ACE inhibitors cannot be viewed as standard therapy, however, until additional studies are completed. They should not detract from an aggressive antiviral strategy.

The use of immunosuppression in the treatment of late stage HIVAN has also been explored in a small prospective study. Treatment with prednisone 60 mg/day for up to 11 weeks, reduced serum creatinine and lowered proteinuria. Long-term outcome, however, was not substantially different from historical controls, and serious opportunistic infections were observed in 30%. Cyclosporine has been used in a small number of seropositive children with FSGS; in some, the nephrotic syndrome resolved.

Treatment of the HIV-1 Infection

No randomized clinical control trials to evaluate HAART in HIVAN have been completed. Preliminary data, however, suggest that the rate of progression of HIVAN to ESRD has been slowed by the introduction of protease inhibitors and HAART. In addition, the incidence of HIVAN in general has begun to decline with the inflection point of the incidence curve occurring at 1995, the time of introduction of HAART therapy with protease inhibitors.

HIVAN in Children

Many of the clinical, demographic, and pathologic features of childhood HIVAN are similar to those seen in the adult disease. HIVAN appears to be a late complication of HIV infection in children as well with 97% of patients having a low CD4 count at the time of HIVAN presentation. Clinical presentation is also similar to that in adults with proteinuria and large echogenic kidneys visible on sonogram.

In contrast to adults, children with HIVAN are more likely to have mesangial involvement or microangiopathic hemolytic anemia at the time of renal biopsy. Perhaps the most striking difference between childhood and adult HIVAN is the slower progression to ESRD observed in children. The average time from first detection of proteinuria to development of renal failure or the nephrotic syndrome is approximately 20 months. In addition, a higher incidence of dilated cardiomyopathy has been reported in children, approaching 65% of children with HIVAN.

OTHER FORMS OF GLOMERULAR/RENAL DISEASE ASSOCIATED WITH HIV INFECTION

Although FSGS secondary to HIVAN is the most common glomerular lesion seen in HIV positive patients, biopsy series have revealed a wide spectrum of lesions in seropositive patients, including membranoproliferative glomerulonephritis, minimal change disease, membranous glomerulopathy, IgA nephropathy, amyloidosis, and a variety of parenchymal infections. Coinfection with hepatitis B or C is common in HIV positive patients, especially in those with a history of intravenous drug use. Because hepatitis B and C are also associated with immune mediated renal disease independent of HIV infection, the specific etiology of the renal disease should be addressed in an individual patient. With the exception of the few cases of IgA nephropathy in HIV seropositive patients, the importance of immune complex disease in the pathogenesis of HIV-related renal disease remains unclear.

Bibliography

Burns GC, Paul SK, Toth IR, Sivak SL: Effect of angiotensin converting enzyme inhibition in HIV-associated nephropathy. *J Am Soc Nephrol* 8:1140, 1997.

Carbone LG, Bendixen B, Appel GB: Sulfadiazine-associated obstructive nephropathy occurring in a patient with the acquired immunodeficiency syndrome. *Am J Kidney Dis* 12:72–75, 1988.

Chattha G, Arieff AI, Cummings C, Tierney LM, Jr: Lactic acidosis complicating the acquired immunodeficiency syndrome. *Ann Intern Med* 118:37–39, 1993.

Cusano AJ, Thies HL, Siegal FP, Dreisbach AW, Maesaka JK: Hyponatremia in patients with acquired immune deficiency syndrome. *J Acquir Immune Defic Syndr* 3:949–953, 1990.

D'Agati V, Appel GB: Renal pathology of human immunodeficiency virus infection. *Semin Nephrol* 18:406–421, 1998.

Ingulli E, Tejani A, Fikrig S, Nicastri A, Chen C, Pomrantz A: Nephrotic syndrome associated with acquired immunodeficiency syndrome in children. *J Pediatr* 119:710–716, 1991.

Kahn J, Lagakos S, Wulfsohn M, et al.: Efficacy and safety of adefovir dipivoxil with antiretroviral therapy: A randomized controlled trial. *JAMA* 282:2305–2312, 1999.

Kimmel PL, Bosch JP, Vassalotti JA: Treatment of human immunodeficiency virus (HIV)-associated nephropathy. *Semin Nephrol* 18:446–458, 1998.

Klotman PE: HIV-associated nephropathy. *Kidney Int* 56:1161–1176, 1999.

Kopp JB, Miller KD, Mican JA, et al.: Crystalluria and urinary tract abnormalities associated with indinavir. *Ann Intern Med* 127:119–125, 1997.

Rao TK, Friedman EA: Outcome of severe acute renal failure in patients with acquired immunodeficiency syndrome. *Am J Kidney Dis* 25:390–398, 1995.

Ray PE, Rakusan T, Loechelt BJ, Selby DM, Liu XH, Chandra RS: Human immunodeficiency virus (HIV)-associated nephropathy in children from the Washington, D.C. area: 12 years' experience. *Semin Nephrol* 18:396–405, 1998.

Stokes MB, Chawla H, Brody RI, et al.: Immune complex glomerulonephritis in patients coinfected with human immunodeficiency virus and hepatitis C virus. *Am J Kidney Dis* 29:514–525, 1997.

Winston JA, Burns GC, Klotman PE: The human immunodeficiency virus (HIV) epidemic and HIV-associated nephropathy. *Semin Nephrol* 18:373–377, 1998.

Winston J, Klotman ME, Klotman PE: HIV associated nephropathy is a late, not early, manifestation of HIV-1 infection. *Kidney Int* 55:1036–1040, 1999.

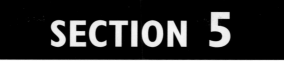

SECTION 5

ACUTE RENAL FAILURE

PATHOPHYSIOLOGY OF ACUTE RENAL FAILURE

MAHENDRA AGRAHARKAR AND ROBERT L. SAFIRSTEIN

The syndrome of acute renal failure (ARF) is defined as a reduction of glomerular filtration rate (GFR) that is often reversible. The syndrome may occur in three clinical settings: (1) as an adaptive response to severe volume depletion and hypotension with structurally and functionally intact nephrons; (2) in response to cytotoxic insults to the kidney when both renal structure and function are abnormal; and (3) when the passage of urine is blocked. Thus ARF may be classified as prerenal, intrinsic, and postrenal. Although this classification is useful in establishing a differential diagnosis see Chapter 33, it is now evident that many pathophysiologic features are shared among the different categories. The intrinsic form of the syndrome may be accompanied by a well-defined sequence of events: an initiation phase characterized by daily increases in serum creatinine and reduced urinary volume; a maintenance phase, where GFR is relatively stable and urine volume may be increased; and a recovery phase in which serum creatinine falls and tubule function is restored. This sequence of events is not always apparent, and oliguria may not be present at all. The reason for this lack of uniform clinical presentation is most probably a reflection of the variable nature of the injury. It is also useful to classify ARF as oliguric or nonoliguric based on the daily urine excretion. Oliguria is defined as a daily urine volume of less than 350 to 400 mL/day. Stratification of the renal failure along these lines helps in decision making, such as the timing of dialysis, and seems to be an important criterion for response to therapy (see later). This chapter considers the pathophysiology of the syndrome, focusing especially on the intrinsic form of the disease, and introducing newer concepts of what causes the syndrome based on more recent observations in human and animal forms of the disease. This better understanding of ARF has led to newer approaches to treatment.

MORPHOLOGY OF ARF

The changes in renal epithelial morphology that accompany ARF are subtle. At least four cellular fates can be identified in ARF: cells may die either by frank necrosis or by apoptosis; they may replicate and divide; or they may appear indifferent to the stress (Fig. 1). Frank necrosis, as is often seen experimentally, is not prominent in the vast

majority of human cases. Necrosis is usually patchy, involving individual cells or small clusters of cells, sometimes resulting in small areas of denuded basement membrane. Less obvious injury is more often noted, including loss of brush borders, flattening of the epithelium, detachment of cells, intratubular cast formation, and dilatation of the lumen. Although proximal tubules show many of theses changes, injury to the distal nephron can also be demonstrated when human biopsy material is closely examined. The distal nephron is also the site of obstruction by desquamated cells and cellular debris.

Apoptosis has been noted in ischemic and nephrotoxic forms of ARF. This form of cell death differs from frank necrosis in that it requires the activation of a regulated program that leads to DNA fragmentation, cytoplasmic condensation, and cell loss without precipitating an inflammatory response (Table 1). In contradistinction to necrosis, the principal site of apoptotic cell death is the distal nephron.

Disruption of the cell cytoskeleton seems to be an important determinant of many of the early morphologic changes, especially in ischemic injury. Loss of the integrity of the actin cytoskeleton leads to flattening of the epithelium, with loss of the brush border, loss of focal cell contacts, and subsequent disengagement of the cell from the underlying substratum. Membrane proteins, including the integrins and the Na^+,K^+-ATPase, redistribute in the plasma membrane as cells lose their polarity. The functional impact of these changes is great as cells lose their capacity to achieve vectorial transport, and the redistribution of the adhesion molecules from the basolateral membrane sites provokes intratubular obstruction. These sublethal changes contribute considerably to the severe impairment of function (see section later on Treatment of ARF), and may help explain the often disproportionate decline in renal function when compared to the minor morphologic changes observed.

Molecular Responses to Renal Injury: Implications for Cell Fate

In sections of the kidney taken from patients with ARF, regeneration and necrosis coexist, so that injury and repair are closely linked. Even in its most severe form, few

Copyright © 2001 by the National Kidney Foundation.
All rights of reproduction in any form reserved.

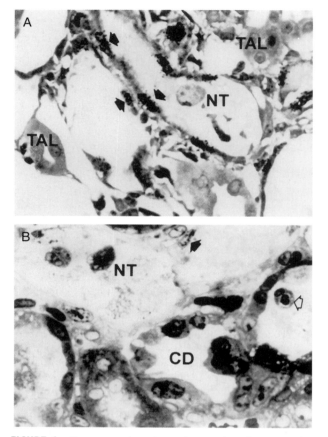

FIGURE I Representative photomicrographs of outer stripe of outer medulla of rat kidney 5 days after cisplatin injection (5 mg/kg body weight) demonstrating cell fate during acute renal failure. (A) Necrosis of the S3 segment of the proximal convoluted tubule is apparent (NT). The solid arrows show regenerating tubules, indicated by the uptake of [3H] thymidine. (B) The open arrow shows an apoptotic body. Thick ascending limbs (Tal) and collecting ducts (CD) are without apparent morphological damage (original magnification ×400).

patients who survive initial dialysis require long-term dialysis, indicating how effective this repair process is. The regeneration process is accompanied by increased renal DNA synthesis and is preceded by prominent changes in gene expression. The changes in renal gene expression can be grouped in at least three major categories (Table 2).

Many of the genes that are expressed after renal injury are involved in cell cycle regulation and are similar to those expressed when growth factors are added to cells to stimulate them to enter the growth cycle. Although the endogenous growth factors that serve this response have not been identified with certainty, administration of growth factors exogenously has been shown to ameliorate and hasten recovery from ARF (see section later on Treatment of ARF). Another group of genes are proinflammatory and chemotactic and may be responsible for the apparent inflammatory aspects of ARF. Depletion of neutrophils, and blockade of neutrophil adhesion each reduce renal injury following ischemia, indicating that the inflammatory response is in part responsible for some features of ARF. This mechanism may be especially prominent in posttransplant ARF. This proinflammatory state may also be important in the prescription of dialysis, especially in sepsis where consideration should be given to whether the procedure will enhance or reduce cytokine production (see later).

These two aspects of the renal molecular response to injury—the increases in protooncogene and chemokine expression—resemble what is observed in cells exposed to adverse environmental conditions such as ionizing radiation, oxidants, and hypertonicity. This response to adversity has been termed the stress response, and is a major determinant of whether cells survive the insult or not. In some circumstances, the stress response leads to apoptosis rather than survival. Whether a cell survives or not is probably a function of the duration of the stress response, its degree, and the specific cell in which the response takes place. In the ischemia–reperfusion model of renal injury these genes are expressed for the most part in the distal nephron, a site of both cell survival and apoptosis (see earlier).

A summary of these important features of the renal stress pathway and its possible consequences is given in

TABLE I
Comparison between Apoptotic and Necrotic Cell Death

	Apoptosis	**Necrosis**
Stimuli	Physiologic	Pathologic
Occurrence	Single cells	Groups of cells
Adhesion between cells	Lost (early)	Lost (late)
Nucleus	Convolution of nuclear outline and breakdown (karyorrhexis)	Disappearance (karyolysis)
Nuclear chromatin	Compaction in uniformly dense masses	Clumping not sharply defined
DNA cleavage	Internucleosomal, "laddering" appearance of distinct fragments on agarose gels	Random: "smear" pattern on agarose gels
Phagocytosis by other cells	Present	Absent
Inflammation	Absent	Present

TABLE 2

Molecular Responses to Renal Ischemia

Increased gene expression
　Genes involved in cell fate determinations: regeneration,
　　apoptosis
　　Transcription factors: c-jun, c-fos
　　Cyclin dependent kinase inhibitors: p21
　Genes involved in inflammation
　　Chemokines: MCP-1,[a] IL-8[b]
　　Adhesion molecules: ICAM-1,[c] integrins

Decreased gene expression—loss of mature phenotype
　Prepro epidermal growth factor
　Tamm–Horsfall protein
　Aquaporin-2
　Sodium proton exchanger 3 (NHE3)

[a] MCP-1, monocyte chemotactic protein 1.
[b] IL-8, interleukin 8.
[c] ICAM-1, intercellular adhesion molecule 1.

Fig. 2. It can be seen that initiation of the stress response may ultimately determine much of the proinflammatory, reparative, cytoreductive, and functional aspects of renal failure. Particular limbs of the response can be targeted for up- or downregulation to limit injury or improve function. Experiments using growth factors (presumably to tip the balance between cell gain and cell loss), as well as the use of antiadhesion molecules to reduce inflammation, support the notion that the renal stress response is an appropriate target for therapy (see discussion on treatment of ARF).

The last group of changes involves what appears to be a loss of the mature phenotype of the kidney, because many of the changes in gene expression involve the loss of proteins that are only expressed maximally during the maturation of the kidney. These include the prepro epidermal growth factor and Tamm–Horsfall protein genes, whose functions are unknown in the kidney, but also include the downregulation of important membrane transporter genes, such as *Aquaporin-2*, and *NHE3*. The loss of these latter proteins may be responsible, in part, for the tubular reabsorptive defects typical of ARF (see later).

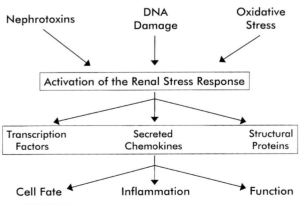
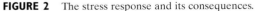

FIGURE 2　The stress response and its consequences.

Pathophysiology of the Cell Injury

The mechanisms of the changes in cell viability during renal injury are complex and incompletely understood. Most of the experimental data have been derived from the ischemia–reperfusion model of acute renal failure and have focused on necrotic cell death. Because as many as 50% of patients have ischemia-induced ARF, the observations should be relevant to a large portion of the patients at risk.

As previously mentioned, different stresses initiate common biochemical events, so that understanding the relevant pathways of one stress will most likely be applicable to others. Such studies have focused on several biochemical pathways: intracellular calcium homeostasis, reactive oxygen species, phospholipases, and executioners of cell death.

The depletion of intracellular ATP that accompanies ischemia increases the cytosolic concentration of calcium. Such increases in intracellular calcium can damage epithelial cells by activating proteases and phospholipases, and can disrupt cellular integrity.

Restoration of renal blood flow after ischemia produces a burst of reduced oxygen species from a variety of processes. Resultant lipid, protein, and DNA damage could lead to cell death. Direct tests of their role in human ARF by the use of oxygen scavengers have been disappointing so far, however.

Members of the phospholipase family, which hydrolyze membrane lipids, could contribute to ischemic renal injury as they appear to do in other organs injured by ischemia. Several products of phospholipid breakdown are vasoconstrictive and chemotactic and could participate in the functional and cytotoxic events of renal failure. Adequate assessment of their role in the cytotoxicity of ischemia awaits the availability of effective inhibitors of the various members of the family.

Activation of endonucleases, which cleave DNA, and caspases, which are cysteine proteases that activate endonucleases to induce cell death, each serve apoptosis and necrosis during cell stress. The use of specific inhibitors of these executioners of cell death shows promise in mitigating the effects of oxidant injury in renal cells. Future studies of the regulation of these pathways are likely to reveal new insights into mechanisms of cell death during acute renal failure.

PATHOPHYSIOLOGY OF ABNORMAL FUNCTION

Reduced GFR

From a consideration of the forces and flows at the glomerular capillary vascular bed it is possible to form a conceptual framework in which to analyze the causes of reduced GFR in ARF (Table 3).

Intrarenal vasoconstriction is the dominant mechanism for the reduced GFR in acute renal failure. Increased preglomerular vascular resistance will have especially devastating effects as glomerular capillary pressure will fall along with the fall in renal blood flow. The reduction in renal

TABLE 3
Determinants of Glomerular Filtration Rate

$$GFR = L_pA \times P_{net}$$

L_pA is the ultrafiltration coefficient, consisting of the hydraulic permeability and area of the glomerular membrane

$P_{net} = \Delta P - \Delta \pi$ is the net ultrafiltration pressure across the entire glomerular capillary

$\Delta P = P_{GC} - P_{PT}$ is the hydrostatic pressure difference between the glomerular capillary and Bowman's space. P_{GC} is the glomerular capillary hydrostatic pressure, and P_{PT} is the intratubular hydrostatic pressure

$\Delta \pi$ is the net glomerular oncotic pressure, the difference between glomerular oncotic pressure (π_{GC}) and tubule oncotic pressure (π_{PT})

blood flow also reduces glomerular filtration by increasing the rate of rise of π_{GC} along the length of glomerular capillary, thus reducing net ultrafiltration pressure further. The mediators of this vasoconstriction are unknown, but tubule injury seems to be an important concomitant finding. There is some evidence experimentally that a low ultrafiltration coefficient may also play a role in reducing GFR during acute renal failure, presumably due to mesangial cell contraction and consequent reduction in the area available for filtration. Although obstruction to the outflow of urine into the collecting system is an obvious cause of reduced net ultrafiltration, less obvious is the intratubular obstruction that results from sloughed cells and cellular debris that evolves in the course of renal failure. The importance of this mechanism is highlighted by the improvement in renal function that follows relief of such intratubular obstruction. Also, when obstruction is prolonged (longer than a few hours), intrarenal vasoconstriction is prominent. Damaged renal epithelium is also abnormally permeable to marker, like inulin; and thus backleak of glomerular filtrate may be an additional mechanism of renal failure. Each of these mechanisms—vasoconstriction, mesangial cell contraction, tubular obstruction, and back-leak contribute individually or in combination to the fall in GFR during the course of ARF.

Apart from the increase in basal renal vascular tone observed during ARF, it is also true that the stressed renal microvasculature is more sensitive to the introduction of potentially vasoconstrictive drugs and otherwise tolerated changes in systemic blood pressure. For example, the use of nonsteroidal antiinflammatory drugs in patients with severe liver disease may precipitate ARF. As a result, a prerenal state may progress to an intrinsic form of renal failure and thus reduce GFR further. Prolonged vasoconstriction may evolve into intrinsic ARF especially when there is concomitant large vessel arterial disease. This latter form of renal failure is often induced by the use of angiotensin converting enzyme inhibitors and/or diuretics. The vasculature of the injured kidney has an impaired vasodilatory response and loses its autoregulatory behavior. This latter phenomenon has important clinical relevance as the frequent reduction in systemic pressure during inter-

mittent hemodialysis may provoke additional damage that could delay recovery of ARF.

PATHOPHYSIOLOGY OF THE CONCENTRATING DEFECT

Another physiologic hallmark of intrinsic ARF is the failure to concentrate urine maximally. The defect is not responsive to pharmacologic doses of vasopressin and is postreceptor in nature. The injured kidney fails to generate and maintain a high medullary solute gradient. Because the accumulation of solute in the medulla depends on normal distal nephron function, this is yet another example of the role of the distal nephron in the pathophysiology of ARF. The mechanism of this defect is not simply a function of lethally injured cells, because necrosis is not prominent in the distal nephron, but rather may involve more subtle effects on function, such as the observed loss of Aquaporin 2 expression following renal ischemia. The failure to excrete a concentrated urine even in the face of oliguria is a helpful diagnostic tool to distinguish prerenal from intrinsic renal disease.

DIAGNOSTIC INDICES OF GLOMERULAR AND TUBULAR FUNCTION USED IN THE DIFFERENTIAL DIAGNOSIS OF ARF

A rapid rise in serum creatinine, which is sometimes associated with a reduced urine volume defines ARF. Given the conceptual framework previously discussed, determination of whether the cause of the renal failure is prerenal, intrinsic, or postrenal usually requires only a few noninvasive tests, in addition to detailed history and a thorough physical examination.

If a prerenal cause of ARF is suggested by history, confirmation of the adaptive nature of the response can be obtained by examining the urine and searching for evidence of enhanced renal water and solute reabsorption. The findings of a highly concentrated urine with a low pH in the absence of cellular elements are suggestive of an adaptive response to volume depletion. These findings, combined with a disproportionate rise of blood urea nitrogen as compared to creatinine and an elevated serum uric acid concentration, all point to prerenal causes. A widely used aid to discriminate between prerenal and intrinsic ARF is the determination of the fractional excretion of sodium ion,

$$FE_{Na} = (U_{Na}/P_{Na})/(U_{Cr}/P_{Cr}) \times 100.$$

Low (<1%) fractional excretion indicates salt and water avidity and is consistent with prerenal causes of renal failure. The fractional excretion of other substances such as urea and uric acid has also been used (Table 4). Lethal and sublethal renal cell injury, on the other hand, would lead to diminished salt reclamation and failure to reach maximum urine concentration, and, as a result, FE_{Na} rises and exceeds 1%. This index is most helpful when the patient is oliguric, and the finding of high FE_{Na} under such circumstances is indicative of intrinsic causes of acute renal failure.

A reliance on any of these determinations alone is hazardous because the regulation of salt and water metabo-

TABLE 4
Urinary Findings in Acute Renal Failure

Measure[a]	Prerenal	Intrinsic
U_{osm} (mOsmol/kg)	>500	<350
U_{Na}	<20	>40
U_{urea}/P_{urea}	>8	<3
U_{Cr}/P_{Cr}	>40	<20
FE_{Na} (%)	<1	>1
FE_{urea} (%)	<35	>50
$FE_{uric\ acid}$ (%)	<7	>15
Urine microscopy	Nonspecific	May show muddy brown granular casts, tubular cell casts

[a]Fractional excretion (FE) of substance X is given by the formula

$$\langle [(U_X/P_X) \div (U_{Cr}/P_{Cr})] \times 100 \rangle$$

where U_X and P_X represent the urine and plasma concentration of X in the same units.

lism is complex and other factors besides the fullness of the intravascular space may be present. For example, the fractional excretion of sodium may be low in intrinsic ARF when there are other comorbid events that enhance salt reabsorption. Coexistent heart and liver disease enhance renal sodium absorption even in the diseased kidney. An accurate history and thorough physical examination are a great help in this regard.

Postrenal causes are detected by renal sonography. Renal perfusion scans do not usually help distinguish among the various causes of reduced renal perfusion except when there is asymmetric perfusion suggestive of renal vascular lesions. In this case, the presence of such lesions should be corroborated by magnetic resonance angiography (MRI) and ultimately confirmed by renal angiography.

TREATMENT OF ARF: IMPLICATIONS DERIVED FROM NEWER UNDERSTANDING OF ITS PATHOPHYSIOLOGY

The mortality of ARF is still high, especially in those patients who require dialysis. This high mortality is in part due to a sicker and older population of patients receiving potentially nephrotoxic medical and surgical therapies. Recent insights into the pathophysiology of ARF have provided newer targets for therapy with the hope of improving outcome in these patients. Such approaches are summarized in Table 5.

Therapeutic Interventions Directed at Renal Vasodilation

A variety of therapeutic approaches have been used to limit the fall in renal blood flow (RBF) and renal vasoconstriction. Calcium channel blockade to relax the renal

vasculature and ameliorate renal failure may be useful in ARF seen after renal transplantation, and after cyclosporine, and radiocontrast dye exposure. It has not been effective in most other forms of renal failure. Dopamine, which vasodilates the normal renal vasculature and increases sodium excretion, is not effective clinically and is associated with significant side effects, especially in the critically ill patient. Atrial natriuretic peptide may improve renal function in oliguric ARF patients, but not in those who are nonoliguric. Isotonic saline infusion at relatively modest rates has been shown to ameliorate radio-contrast-induced ARF in patients with modest reduction of renal function before exposure. Antagonism of the potent renal vasoconstrictive effects of endothelin shows promise experimentally in ischemic renal failure, but there is no clinical experience at present. Newer studies documenting amelioration of experimental ischemic renal failure using specific antagonists of the renal adenosine system also show early promise. Finally, modifying nitric oxide production has also been shown to protect kidneys experimentally. Identification of the effector pathways responsible for the renal vasoconstriction offers the hope of more successful therapy.

Approaches Based on Modifying the Inflammatory Aspects of ARF

Several aspects of the renal stress response are proinflammatory in nature, including the increased expression of the potent monocyte and neutrophil chemotactic chemokines, monocyte chemotactic protein 1 (MCP-1) and interleukin-8 (IL-8), respectively. Overproduction of cytokines may be a factor in many aspects of renal failure, including vasoconstriction and leukocyte invasion.

TABLE 5
Therapeutic Targets of Treatment

Offsetting vasoconstriction	Calcium channel blockage
	Atrial natriuretic factor
	Endothelin blockade
	Adenosine-receptor blockade
	Nitric oxide regulation
Limiting inflammation	α-melanocyte stimulating hormone (α-MSH)
	Antiadhesion strategies,
	Anti-ICAM (intercellular adhesion molecule)
	Anti-integrins
	Biocompatible membranes
	Cytokine absorbing biomembranes
Altering cell outcome	Growth factors and "survival" factors
Dialysis prescription	Hi flux membranes
	Continuous arteriovenous hemodialysis (CAVHD)
	Continuous venovenous hemodialysis (CVVHD)
	hemofiltration (CVVH)

The salutary effect of α melanocyte stimulating hormone (α-MSH) may be mediated by inhibition of chemokine production. Blockade of intracellular adhesion molecule I and integrin-mediated adhesion is a promising new approach, which is mediated perhaps by interfering with inflammation. Strategies directed against the integrins may also operate by reducing intratubular obstruction, as stated above. Additional insight into how these chemokines work in the kidney will most likely yield additional approaches.

Survival Factors

As previously discussed, renal stress initiates a transcriptional program that is intimately involved in cell fate. Some cells participating in this response will survive and repair, whereas others will die by apoptosis. What determines whether a cell will recover from such injury or undergo cell death by necrosis or apoptosis is probably a function of the severity of the stress, specific changes in gene regulation, and the availability of survival factors in the cell's external milieu. For example, cells may be made more vulnerable to otherwise tolerated doses of radiation by disabling a critical DNA repair enzyme or pathway. The survival of bone marrow cells damaged by cancer chemotherapeutic agents may be prevented by addition of growth factors essential to their survival even under normal conditions. Recently, manipulation of the signal transduction pathways responsive to renal ischemia ameliorates cell death and improves renal function. Figure 3 provides the conceptual framework for this approach. The provision of survival factors, such as trophic cytokines and growth factors, in addition to accelerating entry of cells into replicative phases of the cell cycle and hence increasing the rate at which cells reline injured tubules, may also alter an apoptotic or even necrotic outcome to one of survival and repair. Early success with exogenously administered growth factors such as epidermal growth factor (EGF) and insulin-like growth factor (IGF) (among others) show promise in this regard. Survival factors identified during early morphogenesis of the kidney are also likely to be used in treatment of the injured kidney or be used prior to exposure to mitigate the injury.

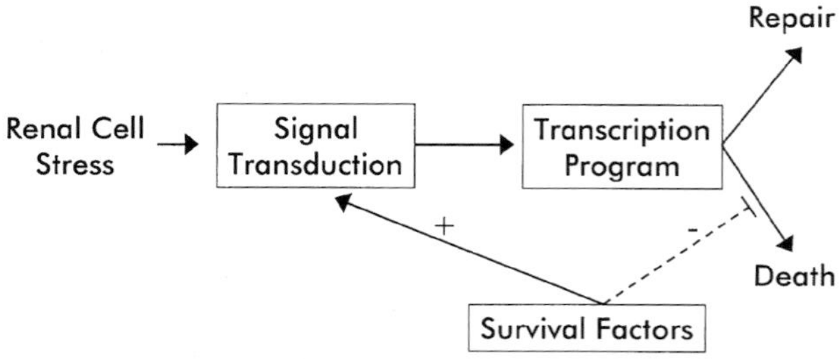

FIGURE 3 Survival factors and cell fate during renal cell stress.

Renal Replacement Therapy

The decision to offer renal replacement therapy should be made cautiously, given the instability of the renal vasculature, the hypotension acute intermittent hemodialysis provokes, and the proinflammatory state of the injured kidney. For these reasons, modifications in the hemodialysis prescription to limit the frequency of hypotensive episodes and diminish cytokine production are currently being pursued.

Bibliography

Chan L, Chittinandana A, Shapiro JI, Stanley PF, Schrier RW: Effect of an endothelin-receptor antagonist on ischemic acute renal failure. Am J Physiol 266:F135–F138, 1994.

Chertow GM, Christiansen CL, Cleary PD, Munro C, Lazarus JM: Prognostic stratification in critically ill patients with acute renal failure requiring dialysis. Arch Intern Med 155:1505–1511, 1995.

Conger J, Robinette JB, Hammond WS: Differences in vascular reactivity in models of ischemic acute renal failure. Kidney Int 39:1087–1097, 1991.

Di Mari JF, Saggi S, Aronson P, Safirstein R: Renal ischemia reperfusion injury reduces Aquaporin-2 and NHE3 expression. J Am Sec Nephrol 7:1823, 1996.

Donohoe JF, Venkatachalam MA, Bernard DB, Levinsky N: Tubular leakage and obstruction after renal ischemia: Structural–functional correlations. Kidney Int 13:208–222, 1978.

Goligorsky MS, Lieberthal W, Racusen LC, Simon EE: Integrin receptors in renal tubular epithelium: New insights into pathophysiology of acute renal failure. Am J Physiol 264:F1, 1993.

Hakim RM: Clinical implications of hemodialysis membrane biocompatibility. Kidney Int 44:484–494, 1993.

Holbrook NJ, Fornance AJ, Jr: Response to adversity: Molecular control of gene activation following genotoxic stress. New Biol 3:825–833, 1991.

Kelly KJ, Williams LWW, Colvin RB, Bonventre JN: Antibody to intracellular adhesion molecule-I protects the kidney against ischemic injury. Proc Natl Acad Sci USA 91:812, 1994.

Noiri E, Peresleni T, Miller F, Goligorsky MS: In vivo targeting of inducible NO synthase with oligodeoxynucleotides protects rat kidney against ischemia. J Clin Invest 97:2377–2383, 1996.

Nouwen E, Verstrepen W, Buyssens N, Zhu M, De Brow M; Hyperplasia, hypertrophy, and phenotypic alterations in the distal nephron after acute proximal tubular injury in the rat. Lab Invest 70:479–493, 1994.

Paller MS: Effect of neutrophil depletion on ischemic renal injury in the rat. J Lab Clin Med 113:379–386, 1989.

Safirstein R, Miller P, Dikman S, Lyman N, Shapiro C: Cisplatin nephrotoxicity in rats: Defect in papillary hypertonicity. Am J Physiol 241:F175–F185, 1981.

Safirstein R, Bonventre JV: Molecular response to ischemic and nephrotoxic acute renal failure. In: Schlondorff D, Bonventre JV (eds) Molecular Nephrology: Kidney Function in Health and Disease, pp. 839–854. Dekker, New York, 1995.

Schumer M, Colombel MC, Sawczuk IS: Morphologic, biochemical, and molecular evidence of apoptosis during the reperfusion phase after brief periods of renal ischemia. Am J Pathol 140:831–838, 1992.

Solez K, Finckh ES: Is there a correlation between morphologic and functional changes in human acute renal failure? Data of Finckh, Jeremy, and Whyte re-examined twenty years later. In:

Solez K, Whelton A (eds) *Acute Renal Failure: Correlations between Morphology and Function.* Dekker, New York, 3–12, 1984.

Solomon R, Werner C, Mann D, E'Elia J, Silva P: Effects of saline, mannitol, and furosemide to prevent acute decreases in renal function induced by radiocontrast agents. *N Engl J Med* 331:1416–1420, 1994.

Star RA: Treatment of acute renal failure. *Kidney Int* 54:1817–1831, 1998.

Thadhani R, Pascual M, Bonventre JV: Acute renal failure. *N Engl J Med* 334:1448–1460, 1996.

Ueda N, Kaushal GP, Shah SV: Recent advances in understanding mechanisms of renal tubular epithelial injury. *Adv Renal Replace Ther* 4:1–8, 1997.

Van Bommel E, Bowry N, So K, *et al.:* Acute dialytic support for the critically ill: Intermittent hemodialysis versus continuous arteriovenous hemodiafiltration. *Am J Nephrol* 15:192–200, 1995.

CLINICAL APPROACH TO THE DIAGNOSIS OF ACUTE RENAL FAILURE

JEAN L. HOLLEY

Acute renal failure is a sudden reduction in glomerular filtration rate that is expressed clinically as the retention of nitrogenous waste products (urea, creatinine) in the blood. The accumulation of these nitrogenous waste products is termed azotemia. In most cases of acute renal failure, the serum creatinine rises 1–2 mg/dL/day. Depending on the clinical circumstances and the symptoms of the patient, renal replacement therapy (dialysis) may be required. Despite the widespread availability of dialysis, the mortality of patients who develop acute renal failure remains high, from 10 to 50% depending on the patient's comorbidities and the medical setting in which the renal failure occurs (e.g., intensive care unit, obstetric, surgical). At least half of all episodes of acute renal failure are iatrogenic and related to medications or procedures. In most cases, by following a basic algorithm that focuses on the patient's history, physical exam, urinalysis, review of basic laboratory results, and, in some instances, radiologic imaging of the kidneys and determination of urine sodium and fractional excretion of sodium, the cause of acute renal failure can be determined. The patient's history (especially medications, procedures, changes in blood pressure), findings on physical exam (particularly assessment of volume status), blood urea nitrogen (BUN): creatinine ratio, and urinalysis results will usually provide the information necessary to determine if the acute renal failure is a prerenal, intrinsic renal, or postrenal event. In some cases, a spot urine sodium concentration or ultrasound of the kidneys may also be needed in the initial evaluation. Once the appropriate classification (prerenal, intrinsic renal, or postrenal) has been determined, the need for additional diagnostic tests as well as therapeutic interventions will be clear.

ACUTE VERSUS CHRONIC RENAL FAILURE

Because acute renal failure usually resolves and chronic renal failure often progresses to end stage renal disease and the need for chronic dialysis, it is useful to determine if a patient's elevated creatinine is the result of an acute insult or a progressive loss of functioning nephrons. When past serum creatinine values are not available, it may be difficult to distinguish acute from chronic renal failure. In such cases, a renal ultrasound to document the size of the kidneys may be helpful. The kidneys will often be small (<10 cm longitudinally in a person of normal stature) and echogenic if the renal failure is chronic and slowly progressive. Normal sized kidneys on ultrasound do not absolutely exclude chronic renal failure, but small, echogenic kidneys are not consistent with acute renal failure alone. Clearly, an individual may have concomitant acute renal failure and chronic renal failure, and in such cases of acute renal failure superimposed on chronic renal failure, the kidney size is less helpful. Laboratory features suggestive but not diagnostic of chronic renal failure include a normocytic anemia, hyperphosphatemia, and hypocalcemia.

The presence of nonspecific symptoms of uremia (e.g., nausea and vomiting, pruritus, fatigue) may also suggest chronic rather than acute renal failure, but there is no single factor other than kidney size or serial elevated creatinine values over time that conclusively establishes that the renal failure is chronic and not acute. Patients with chronic renal failure may also develop episodes of acute renal failure. In such cases, the kidneys are usually small and the baseline creatinine is elevated. An abrupt and unexpected rise in the baseline creatinine in such patients should prompt an evaluation for superimposed, potentially reversible acute renal failure.

CLASSIFICATION OF ACUTE RENAL FAILURE

All cases of acute renal failure can be classified into prerenal, intrinsic (or intrarenal), and postrenal causes (Table 1). Classifying each episode of acute renal failure directs appropriate diagnostic and therapeutic strategies. Acute renal failure is also clinically described as oliguric (<400 mL urine output/24 hr), nonoliguric (>400 mL urine output/24 hr), or anuric (<100 mL urine/24 hr). These categories are helpful to establish cause and predict prognosis. Anuria is uncommon and suggests either complete obstruction, a major vascular event such as bilateral renal infarction or renal vein thrombosis, cortical necrosis, or acute tubular necrosis. Prerenal, intrinsic renal, and postrenal acute renal failure may each present clinically with oliguria or nonoliguria. Nonoliguric acute renal failure is common in intrarenal acute renal failure (e.g., nephrotoxin-induced acute tubular necrosis, acute glomerulonephritis, and acute interstitial nephritis), and oliguria more commonly characterizes obstruction and prerenal azotemia. Regardless of the cause of renal failure, the patient who is oliguric is more difficult to manage because volume overload will occur earlier. Moreover, patients with nonoliguric acute renal failure have a more favorable prognosis and reduced mortality.

PRERENAL ACUTE RENAL FAILURE

Prerenal abnormalities include physiologic responses that lead to decreased renal function (decreased glomerular filtration rate) manifested clinically as an elevated BUN and creatinine because of decreased perfusion of the kidney. The reduced renal perfusion that results in prerenal acute renal failure may occur as a consequence of inadequate volume (e.g., due to blood loss or overly aggressive diuresis), inadequate cardiac output owing to impaired myocardial function (e.g., cardiogenic shock following an acute myocardial infarction or, more commonly, progressive cardiomyopathy), or significant vasodilatation as may occur with sepsis. In each of these situations, the underlying renal function is usually normal, but acute renal failure occurs because the primary problem (volume depletion or reduced cardiac output) compromises renal blood flow enough to reduce glomerular filtration rate. In cases of depleted intravascular fluid volume and congestive heart failure (the two most common causes of prerenal azotemia), the kidney will initially compensate for the diminished perfusion to preserve filtration function. Mechanisms of self-

TABLE I
Classification of Acute Renal Failure

Prerenal (reduced renal perfusion)
Volume depletion
  Renal loss—diuretics, osmotic diuresis (DKA[a]), Addisonian crisis
  Extrarenal loss—vomiting, diarrhea, skin losses (burns, sweating)
Hypotension (regardless of cause)
Cardiovascular
  Congestive heart failure, reduced myocardial function, arrhythmias
Hemodynamic (intense intrarenal vasoconstriction)
  Radiocontrast
  Prostaglandin inhibition (NSAID[b])
  Cyclosporine and tacrolimus
  ACE[c] inhibitors
  Amphotericin B
Hypercalcemia
Hepatorenal syndrome (bland urinary sediment, oliguria, low urine Na^+, not reversed with volume repletion—reversible with successful liver transplant)

Intrinsic or intrarenal
Vascular
  Renal infarction, renal artery stenosis, renal vein thrombosis
  Malignant hypertension, scleroderma renal crisis, atheroemboli
Tubular
  Ischemic—prolonged prerenal state, sepsis syndrome, systemic hypotension
  Nephrotoxic—aminoglycosides, methotrexate, cisplatinum, myoglobin (rhabdomyolysis), hemoglobin
Glomerular
  Acute glomerulonephritis
  Vasculitis (Wegener's, polyarteritis)
  Thrombotic microangiopathy (hemolytic uremic syndrome, TTP[d])
  Myeloma kidney
Interstitium
  Medications—penicillin and cephalosporin antibiotics, phenytoin
  Tumor infiltration (lymphoma, leukemia)

Postrenal (obstruction)
Prostate hypertrophy, neurogenic bladder
Intraureteral obstruction—crystals (uric acid, acyclovir, indinavir), stones, clots, tumor
Extraureteral obstruction—tumor (cervical, prostate), retroperitoneal fibrosis

[a]DKA, diabetic ketoacidosis.
[b]NSAID, nonsteroidal antiinflammatory drugs.
[c]ACE, angiotensin converting enzyme.
[d]TTP, thrombotic thrombocytopenic purpura.

preservation include autoregulatory afferent arteriolar dilation and attenuation of afferent vasoconstriction by intrarenal prostaglandin-mediated vasodilatation. These and other physiologic maneuvers comprise renal compensation or autoregulation and are ultimately an attempt by the kidney to maintain the glomerular filtration rate in the face of hypoperfusion. When the renal compensation is maximized and the factors causing the hypoperfusion remain uncorrected, renal compensation becomes decompensation and acute renal failure occurs. The development of acute renal failure after ingestion of a nonsteroidal antiinflammatory drug (NSAID) by a patient who has congestive heart failure is a common clinical example of this type of hemodynamic insult. In this situation, the protaglandin-mediated compensatory renal vasodilatation that occurs because the kidneys are hypoperfused from poor cardiac output is inhibited by the NSAID, and a consequent reduction in glomerular filtration rate occurs, manifested by a rising BUN and creatinine.

Intense intrarenal vasoconstriction may result in acute renal failure causing reduced renal blood flow and subsequent reduction of glomerular perfusion. This hemodynamically mediated form of acute renal failure resembles prerenal azotemia and is seen with exposure to radiocontrast, cyclosporine and tacrolimus, amphotericin, and nonsteroidal antiinflammatory drugs (Table 1). Uncorrected, such episodes of prerenal azotemia may progress to ischemic acute tubular necrosis. Like other forms of prerenal azotemia, the urinalysis in cases of vasoconstrictor or hemodynamically mediated prerenal azotemia is bland, and urinary sodium is often low.

Evidence of preserved renal functional ability and the kidney's attempt to compensate for the reduced perfusion in prerenal states is the maximum tubular sodium reabsorption that occurs and is reflected in a low urine sodium (<20 mEq/L) and/or low fractional excretion of sodium (<1%, Table 2). The fractional excretion of sodium, unlike the simpler urine sodium, evaluates only the fraction of filtered sodium that is excreted and is therefore not affected by changes in water reabsorption that can affect the simple urine sodium concentration. The fractional excretion of sodium (FE_{Na}) is thus

$$FE_{Na} = (Na^+ \text{ excreted} \div Na^+ \text{ filtered}) \times 100$$
$$= \{\text{urine } [Na^+] \, (V) \div \text{plasma } [Na^+] \, (GFR)\} \times 100,$$

where V is urine volume and GFR is creatinine clearance, which equals urine [creatinine] (V) ÷ plasma [creatinine], or

$$FE_{Na} = (\text{urine } [Na^+] \, (V) \div \{\text{plasma } [Na^+] \times \text{urine [creatinine]} \, (V) \div \text{plasma [creatinine]}\}) \times 100$$
$$= \{(\text{urine } [Na^+]/\text{plasma } [Na^+]) \div (\text{urine [creatinine]}/\text{plasma [creatinine]})\} \times 100.$$

With prerenal azotemia, the kidney's intrinsic ability to function remains intact. Because the renal insult is indirect and results from hypoperfusion, the urinalysis in prerenal acute renal failure is generally unremarkable despite being concentrated (high specific gravity and osmolality). The glomerular basement membrane is intact so there is no proteinuria or blood on dipstick and because there is no tubular, glomerular, or interstitial damage, the urine is bland microscopically and without RBCs, WBCs, or casts with the exception that hyaline casts may be seen. The patient's history will suggest volume loss or cardiac failure (Tables 1 and 3). The most important aspect of the physical exam is to assess the patient's volume status. In terms of renal perfusion, intravascular volume overload (congestive heart failure, cirrhosis) and intravascular volume depletion are identical; each leads to renal hypoperfusion. Thus, in these situations that are clinically quite different, the renal response is the same: maximal sodium retention in an attempt to compensate for the reduced perfusion. Clearly, the appropriate treatment for acute renal failure in this situation is to increase the renal perfusion, and, indeed, rapid reversal of the prerenal azotemia occurs if appropriate treatment is given (e.g., volume repletion). Because, unlike creatinine, urea easily diffuses across tubular membranes, active urea reabsorption occurs when there is reduced urine flow. Therefore, prerenal azotemia is characterized by an elevated BUN:creatinine ratio (BUN:creatinine ratio >20:1). Other causes of a BUN:creatinine ratio >20:1 include postrenal acute renal failure, gastrointestinal blood

TABLE 2
Urinalysis, Urine Na$^+$, and BUN: Creatinine Ratio in Acute Renal Failure[a]

Type of acute renal failure	Urinalysis	U_{Na}	FE_{Na}	BUN:Creatinine
Prerenal	High specific gravity Normal or hyaline casts	<20 mEq/L	<1%	>20:1
Intrarenal				≤20:1
Acute tubular necrosis	Low specific gravity Muddy brown casts Renal tubular epithelial cells	>40 mEq/L	≥1%	
Vascular disorders	Normal or hematuria	>20 mEq/L	(variable)	
Glomerulonephritis	Proteinuria, hematuria RBC casts	>20 mEq/L	<1%	
Interstitial nephritis	Mild proteinuria, hematuria WBCs, WBC casts, eosinophils	>20 mEq/L	≥1%	
Postrenal	Normal or hematuria WBCs, occ granular casts	>20 mEq/L	(variable)	≥20:1

[a] U = urine, Na^+ = sodium, FE_{Na} = fractional excretion of sodium.
Urine sodium and FENa is variable with postrenal, interstitial nephritis, and glomerulonephritis.

TABLE 3
Using the History and Physical Exam as Tools to Categorize Acute Renal Failure

Type of ARF	History	Physical exam
Prerenal	Volume loss (vomiting, diarrhea, diuretics, burns)	Weight, blood pressure (BP), P lying and standing
	Past weights, daily intake/output values	Mucous membranes, axillary moisture
	Cardiac disease, liver disease	Neck veins, S3, lung exam, edema
	Thirst	
	Medications (NSAID, ACE inhibitors, cyclosporine)	
	Radiographic contrast [computed tomography (CT), angiography]	
Intrarenal		
ATN	Medications (aminoglycosides)	Same as above—volume status
	Alcohol abuse, trauma, muscle necrosis (rhabdomyolysis)	Compartment syndrome—extremities
	Episode of hypotension	
Vascular	Trauma, known nephrotic syndrome, flank pain	BP, livedo reticularis
	Vessel catheterization, anticoagulation (atheroemboli)	Funduscopic exam (malignant hypertension)
	Progressive systemic sclerosis	Thickened skin, sclerodactyly, telangectasia
Glomerular	Systemic diseases [systemic lupus erythematosus (SLE), vasculitis]—arthritis, rash	Oral ulcers, arthritis, skin lesions, foot drop
	Uveitis, weight loss, fatigue, IV drug use (hepatitis C)	Pleural and pericardial rubs
	Cough, hemoptysis (Goodpasture's), foamy urine	Edema—periorbital, leg, presacral
Interstitial	Medications (antibiotics, allopurinol, dilantin)	Fever, drug rash
	Arthralgias	
Postrenal	Urinary urgency, hesitancy, gross hematuria	Bladder distension, pelvic masses, prostate
	Intermittent polyuria, history of stones	
	Medications (indinavir, acyclovir, anticholinergics)	

loss (digested protein from an upper gastrointestinal bleed is absorbed and metabolized by the liver), high-dose corticosteroid therapy, and intense catabolism.

POSTRENAL ACUTE RENAL FAILURE—OBSTRUCTIVE UROPATHY

The extent of pathology in postrenal acute renal failure (obstructive uropathy) is determined by the level at which the obstruction occurs. However, the endpoint of all obstructive lesions is the potential destruction of functioning renal parenchyma. The elevated pressures in obstructed conduits results in adaptive dilatation (hydroureter, hydronephrosis) which ultimately progresses to nephron destruction (atrophy of the tubular epithelium, interstitial fibrosis, and ultimately glomerular scarring) if unrelieved. Postrenal causes of acute renal failure necessarily involve obstruction of both kidneys or both ureters unless the patient has only a single functioning kidney. In patients with two functioning kidneys, unilateral obstruction, for example, an obstructing kidney stone, will rarely cause acute renal failure because the glomerular filtration of the unobstructed kidney is not reduced. In postrenal azotemia, the history can identify predisposing factors and symptoms (Tables 1 and 3). Reduced urine output (oliguria) and/or anuria are common in postrenal azotemia. The physical exam, like the history, should focus on the possibility of obstruction (pelvic masses, distended bladder, prostatic enlargement). Because there is reduced urine flow with obstruction, the BUN: creatinine ratio is usually elevated, similar to that seen in prerenal azotemia. The urine sediment and concentration are variable and generally not

helpful in the diagnosis of obstruction. A renal ultrasound will usually show hydronephrosis when obstruction is causing the acute renal failure. Bladder catheterization with significant urine volume or a postvoid residual of >100 mL confirm the presence of postrenal acute renal failure. Rarely, despite the presence of obstruction, hydronephrosis may not be demonstrated on ultrasound. Retroperitoneal fibrosis is often seen in such cases and may be confirmed by computerized tomography (CT) scan or magnetic resonance imaging (MRI). When the clinical suspicion of obstruction is high and hydronephrosis is not seen on ultrasound, additional renal imaging such as a CT scan, MRI, or retrograde nephrograms should be done.

Like the external obstruction that occurs with tumor or prostate enlargement, intraureteral obstruction may also cause azotemia (Table 1). Kidney stones, endogenous (uric acid as in acute tumor lysis) or exogenous crystals (medications such as indinavir, acyclovir), or other material (blood clots, renal papillae as in papillary necrosis, or uroepithelial tumors of the ureter or renal pelvis) can cause postrenal failure by intraureteral obstruction. The acute renal failure caused by obstruction will usually resolve by relieving the obstruction (by placing a Foley catheter or a nephrostomy tube). However, prolonged obstruction may cause irreversible nephron destruction and lead to chronic renal failure.

INTRINSIC OR INTRARENAL ACUTE RENAL FAILURE

Intrinsic acute renal failure can be categorized anatomically by the area of the kidney parenchyma involved: vascular, glomerular, tubular, or interstitial areas. Differences in the clinical setting and presentation, particularly in the history, physical exam, and urinalysis, will distinguish between these types of acute renal failure. Determining if a patient has acute tubular necrosis, acute interstitial nephritis, or acute glomerulonephritis as the cause of acute renal failure is necessary because the treatment and prognosis of each may differ. With all types of intrarenal acute renal failure, the kidney itself is the site of the abnormality. Unlike prerenal and postrenal acute renal failure, the decrement in glomerular filtration rate that occurs with intrinsic acute renal failure is directly linked to renal damage and not the result of reduced renal perfusion or elevated pressures in the renal conduits. For this reason, the BUN:creatinine ratio is usually preserved (remains 10–20:1) in intrarenal acute renal failure. Similarly, because the impaired renal function results from direct renal injury, the urinalysis is usually abnormal in cases of intrinsic acute renal failure. Specific findings on dipstick and microscopic examination of the urine usually provide important clues to the location of the renal parenchymal injury that is causing the renal dysfunction (Table 2). Despite a careful history, physical exam, urinalysis, and additional specific tests, in some cases of acute intrinsic renal failure, the type of the renal failure (tubular, vascular, glomerular, interstitial) remains unclear, and a percutaneous renal biopsy may be needed to determine the cause of the renal dysfunction.

Acute tubular necrosis is the most common type of acute intrinsic renal failure seen in hospitalized patients. Unfortunately, the term acute tubular necrosis, or ATN, is sometimes used interchangeably with acute renal failure. As illustrated in Table 1, ATN is only one form of intrinsic acute renal failure and not synonymous with acute renal failure. By focusing on the details of the history, physical exam, and urinalysis findings, it is usually possible to establish the correct diagnosis and cause for intrarenal acute renal failure (Tables 2 and 3). Additional specific diagnostic or imaging tests or a renal biopsy may be necessary if the initial assessment of a patient with intrinsic acute renal failure does not establish whether the vessels, glomeruli, interstitium, or tubules are the site of the injury.

Acute Tubular Necrosis as a Cause of Intrinsic Acute Renal Failure

At least 45% of the cases of acute renal failure are caused by acute tubular necrosis (ATN). The two major causes of ATN are ischemia and nephrotoxins. Thus, ATN can be characterized as ischemic or nephrotoxic, and important clues to these renal insults are in the patient's history. Ischemia is the most common cause of ATN and often follows a prolonged prerenal state with its associated renal hypoperfusion. The history may reveal systemic hypotension, significant volume depletion, or reduced effective circulating volume. Distinguishing between ongoing prerenal azotemia that is reversible and ATN may be difficult. However, the hallmark of prerenal acute renal failure is its reversibility with restoration of renal perfusion (e.g., appropriate volume repletion); ATN does not im-

prove simply with volume repletion. The point at which a patient moves from prerenal azotemia to ischemic ATN will vary depending on the patient and the clinical situation, but unless the patient is clearly volume overloaded, a fluid challenge will usually be an integral part of the diagnosis as well as the therapy of suspected ischemic ATN to exclude a prerenal state.

Clinical features that may help to distinguish ischemic ATN from prerenal azotemia include the urinalysis and urinary sodium and fractional excretion of sodium (Table 2). As previously discussed, because the kidney is essentially normal in prerenal acute renal failure, the urinalysis is unremarkable. In contrast, with ATN, evidence of the damaged tubules is usually seen in the urinary sediment; renal tubular epithelial cells and granular casts characterize ATN.

The hallmark of ATN is dirty (or muddy) brown casts, a urinalysis finding that is pathognomatic of ATN (see Chapter 4, Fig. 2B). Because the tubules are the only site of renal injury in ATN, urinary findings that typify glomerular (proteinuria, RBCs, RBC casts) or interstitial injury (hematuria, WBCs, WBC casts) are not seen. Unlike ATN, prerenal azotemia is characterized by intact tubular function and reduced renal blood flow and, therefore, maximal tubular reabsorption of sodium (Table 2). Conversely, with ATN there is direct tubular damage and a loss of tubular function manifested by a high urine sodium and fractional excretion of sodium. The findings on urinalysis and the characteristic urinary sodium values with ATN occur with both ischemic and nephrotoxic forms of ATN.

Aminoglycosides are among the most common causes of nephrotoxic ATN. With aminoglycoside-induced ATN, the creatinine usually begins to rise 5–10 days after administration. Other nephrotoxins that may cause ATN include methotrexate, cisplatinum, and endogenous pigments such as hemoglobin and myoglobin (as seen with rhabdomyolysis). As previously discussed, the fractional excretion of sodium is usually high ($\geq 1\%$) in ATN. In most cases, both nephrotoxic and ischemic ATN resolve. However, depending on the level of renal dysfunction that occurs, temporary dialysis may be necessary.

Vascular Damage Resulting in Intrinsic Acute Renal Failure

Acute events involving the main renal arteries or veins can cause acute renal failure. Like with obstruction, bilateral involvement is required for acute azotemia to develop unless at baseline the patient has a solitary functioning kidney. Bilateral renal infarction, renal vein thrombosis, or acute occlusion of the renal arteries may lead to acute intrinsic renal failure. Because the kidney parenchyma itself may not be initially directly injured, some would classify these forms of acute renal failure as prerenal azotemia rather than as cases of intrinsic acute renal failure. Involvement of smaller blood vessels may also cause intrinsic acute renal failure. Examples of this kind of acute renal failure include malignant hypertension, scleroderma renal crisis, and cholesterol atheroembolic disease. In some systems of classification, acute renal failure due to vasculitis will also be included among the vascular types of intrinsic acute renal failure. However, because glomerular involvement with its associated proteinuria and active urinary sediment is common with vasculitis, here vasculitides are classified under glomerular causes of intrinsic acute renal failure (Table 1).

Historical data that suggest an acute vascular event as the cause of acute renal failure include trauma, underlying nephrotic syndrome with significant proteinuria (predisposed to renal vein thrombosis), or acute flank pain with hematuria. Microscopic hematuria, with or without proteinuria, is the most common finding on urinalysis in intrinsic acute renal failure caused by vascular problems. Disease of the renal arteries or veins that results in acute renal failure will generally require imaging to confirm the diagnosis. For example, MRI may reveal renal vein thrombosis or renal artery stenosis, CT scan may show renal infarction, and a radionuclide renal scan or doppler ultrasound study may confirm the presence or absence of renal blood flow. Atheroembolism is the most common vascular problem causing intrinsic acute renal failure. Important historical features of atheroembolic acute renal failure include catheterization of vessels and anticoagulation. The physical exam in atheroembolic acute renal failure may suggest widespread atheroemboli by demonstrating livedo reticularis in the skin of the toes and feet, and Hollenhorst plaques in the retina.

Glomerular Type of Intrinsic Acute Renal Failure

Acute inflammation of vessels and/or glomeruli causing acute renal failure may reflect renal involvement of a systemic illness (e. g., systemic lupus erythematosus, Wegener's granulomatosis, polyarteritis nodosa) that will be suggested by the medical history and physical exam (Table 3). Because proteinuria occurring with glomerular involvement is often in the nephrotic range (>3 g/24 hr), volume overload, and especially edema and hypertension on physical exam, will be common with acute glomerulonephritis. The urinalysis provides the most important clues to intrinsic acute renal failure due to glomerulonephritis. Proteinuria and blood on urine dipstick and microscopic hematuria and RBC casts are characteristic (Table 2). Probably because renin, and thus, aldosterone is stimulated in the setting of glomerulonephritis, the urine sodium may be low. However, the urinalysis and supporting history and physical exam are the diagnostic keys to acute glomeru-

lonephritis. The abnormal urinalysis in acute glomerulonephritis essentially excludes prerenal azotemia and ATN, and thus, urine sodium is rarely a diagnostic key to acute renal failure caused by glomerulonephritis.

Interstitial Type of Intrinsic Acute Renal Failure

Involvement of the interstitium can also cause acute renal failure on an intrarenal basis. Acute interstitial nephritis is associated with a variety of medications (penicillin antibiotics, allopurinol). Thus, the history of exposure to a new medication is the key to the diagnosis of this kind of intrinsic acute renal failure. In about a third of the cases of acute interstitial nephritis, a systemic illness may occur that is characterized by fever, a maculopapular erythematous rash, arthralgias, and eosinophilia. These clinical features have led some to refer to this entity as allergic interstitial nephritis. The urinalysis with acute interstitial nephritis usually shows mild proteinuria, microscopic hematuria, WBCs, and sometimes WBC casts. Eosinophiluria may be present on Hansel or Wright's stain of the urine. However, eosinophiluria is not pathognomatic of acute interstitial nephritis as urine eosinophils may also be seen in cholesterol atheroembolic acute renal failure, glomerulonephritis, and prostatitis. When interstitial nephritis is suspected but the characteristic clinical and urinalysis findings are absent, gallium scan of the kidneys may be positive. Percutaneous renal biopsy may sometimes be needed to distinguish between interstitial nephritis and other forms of acute intrinsic renal failure (notably acute tubular necrosis).

Bibliography

Hou SH, Bushinsky DA, Wish JB, Cohen JJ, Harrington JT: Hospital-acquired renal insufficiency: A prospective study. *Am J Med* 74:243–248, 1983.

Klahr S, Miller SB: Acute oliguria. *N Engl J Med* 338:671–675, 1998.

Liano F, Pascual J: Epidemiology of acute renal failure: A prospective, multicenter community-based study. Madrid Acute Renal Failure Study Group. *Kidney Int* 50:811–818, 1996.

Miller TR, Anderson RJ, Linas SL, Henrich WL, Berns AS, Gabow PA, Schrier RJ: Urinary diagnostic indices in acute renal failure: A prospective study. *Ann Intern Med* 89:47–50, 1978.

Nolan CR, Anderson RJ: Hospital-acquired acute renal failure. *J Am Soc Nephrol* 9:701–718, 1998.

Solomon R: Contrast-medium-induced acute renal failure. *Kidney Int* 53:230–242, 1998.

34

RENAL FAILURE CAUSED BY THERAPEUTIC AGENTS

THOMAS M. COFFMAN

Compounds used for diagnostic and therapeutic purposes are common causes of renal insufficiency. The kidney is a frequent target for injury by therapeutic agents because it is a major route of excretion for a variety of drugs. As a part of the excretory process, these materials may be greatly concentrated in the urinary space and within renal tubular cells, enhancing their potential to cause local toxicity. Also, the rate of blood flow per gram of tissue weight in the kidney is relatively high, resulting in exaggerated exposure of renal endothelial cells and glomeruli to circulating substances. Because most renal functions are dependent on tightly regulated blood flow patterns, agents that impair these hemodynamic relationships may interfere with the ability of the kidney to maintain normal homeostasis.

Drug toxicity in the kidney is manifested through the same clinical syndromes that are associated with kidney diseases of other causes. As depicted in Table 1, these include acute and chronic renal failure, and nephrotic syndrome. Moreover, a single agent may cause more than one of these clinical syndromes. The particular clinical manifestation of nephrotoxicity is determined by the dose and duration of exposure, chemical properties of the agent, as well as factors within the individual patient such as age, volume status, and genetic background. This chapter describes a general approach to nephrotoxicity and reviews the renal effects of some common causative agents. More detailed discussions of individual agents or syndromes associated with toxic renal injury can be found in other chapters (see Chapters 38, 40, 47, and 48).

DIAGNOSIS

The possibility of drug-induced nephrotoxicity should be considered when the serum creatinine concentration rises during administration of a therapeutic agent. Because of the nonlinear relationship between serum creatinine and glomerular filtration rate (GFR), a substantial reduction in GFR is necessary before toxic injury can be appreciated clinically. This point is particularly important to consider in the context of agents that may cause chronic nephropathy. In this case, kidney injury may not be detected until 40 to 50% of kidney function has been irreversibly lost. A number of diagnostic markers, such as urinary excretion of various tubular enzymes, have been evaluated as indicators of renal toxicity that might be more sensitive and specific than serum creatinine. However, none of these have yet found widespread clinical application.

The clinical syndromes caused by drugs mimic those associated with kidney diseases of other causes. Thus, when the etiology of renal failure is being investigated, the possible role of therapeutic agents should always be considered, and a detailed medication history is an extremely important part of the clinical evaluation. Temporal associations between the appearance of a kidney abnormality and medication changes must be documented. In patients who are receiving compounds known to be nephrotoxic, the plan for clinical management should include careful monitoring of renal function, avoidance of clinical risk factors, and, in some cases, monitoring of serum drug levels. Also, the role of nephrotoxins in exacerbating renal failure from other causes should be considered. For example, in the hospitalized patient with acute tubular necrosis, the potentially additive detrimental effects of aminoglycosides, radiocontrast, or other nephrotoxins must be recognized. Renal clearance of some drugs will be substantially reduced in such patients, and doses must be lowered appropriately (see Chapter 41).

ACUTE RENAL FAILURE FROM THERAPEUTIC AGENTS

In approaching any patient with acute kidney dysfunction, a potential causative role for therapeutic agents should always be considered. As illustrated in Table 1, mechanisms of acute renal failure related to drugs can be roughly categorized as prerenal/hemodynamic, intrarenal, or postrenal/obstructive syndromes. As described in Chapter 33, this separation can be extremely helpful in identifying the etiology and directing management of patients with acute renal failure (ARF) from any cause.

Prerenal Azotemia: Hemodynamically Mediated Renal Insufficiency Associated with Drugs

As shown in Table 1, several classes of therapeutic agents including cyclosporine, tacrolimus, radiocontrast, nonsteroidal antiinflammatory drugs (NSAIDS), and angiotensin

TABLE I
Renal Syndromes Caused by Therapeutic Agents

Clinical syndrome	Causative agents
Acute renal failure	
Prerenal/hemodynamic	Cyclosporine, tacrolimus, radiocontrast, amphotericin B, ACE inhibitors, NSAIDs, interleukin 2
Intrarenal	
Acute tubular necrosis	Aminoglycosides, amphotericin B, cisplatin, certain cephalosporins
Acute interstitial nephritis	Penicillins, cephalosporins, sulfonamides, rifampin, NSAIDs, interferon, interleukin 2
Postrenal/obstructive	Acyclovir, analgesic abuse, methysergide, methotrexate
Chronic renal failure	Lithium, analgesic abuse, cyclosporine, tacrolimus, cisplatin, nitrosoureas
Nephrotic syndrome	Gold, NSAIDs, penicillamine, Captopril, interferon

Note: This is a representative, but not exhaustive list of etiological agents. Please refer to individual primer chapters for more complete listings. ACE inhibitors, angiotensin converting enzyme inhibitors; NSAIDs, nonsteroidal antiinflammatory drugs.

converting enzyme (ACE) inhibitors can cause a syndrome of abnormal kidney function that resembles prerenal azotemia. Similar to prerenal azotemia from other causes, hemodynamic renal dysfunction caused by drugs can be associated with low urine sodium excretion. Although such renal dysfunction is usually reversible when the offending agent is discontinued, ischemic damage may result if the insult is prolonged or particularly severe.

Drugs can cause hemodynamically mediated renal dysfunction through several mechanisms. Agents such as cyclosporine, tacrolimus, radiocontrast, and amphotericin cause intense vasoconstriction in the kidney that reduces renal blood flow and glomerular perfusion. These compounds do not seem to affect vascular tone directly but may stimulate production of other vasoconstrictors such as endothelin or thromboxane A_2. Cyclosporine, tacrolimus, and amphotericin can produce renal insufficiency in normal subjects who have no underlying renal circulatory abnormalities.

In contrast, hemodynamic kidney dysfunction associated with NSAIDs generally occurs in patients with preexisting impairment of renal perfusion. NSAIDs inhibit the cyclooxygenase isoenzymes (COX-1 and -2), turning off the synthesis of prostaglandins. In normal subjects, renal prostaglandin production is low, and administration of NSAIDs has very little effect on renal function. However, as an adaptive mechanism, production of vasodilator prostaglandins increases in situations in which renal perfusion is threatened. Inhibiting production of these va-

sodilator compounds by NSAIDs can cause precipitous declines in renal blood flow and GFR. This syndrome is most often seen in patients with volume depletion, heart failure, and preexisting renal disease (see Chapter 40).

Similarly, acute renal failure following administration of ACE inhibitors usually occurs in patients with underlying abnormalities of the renal vasculature and circulation. This syndrome is most commonly seen in patients with congestive heart failure on diuretics, in patients with severe bilateral renal artery stenosis, patients with critical renal artery stenosis in a singe functioning kidney, and in patients with vascular disease and nephrosclerosis. ACE inhibitors lower blood pressure by inhibiting the conversion of angiotensin I to angiotensin II. Angiotensin II is a potent vasoconstrictor that acts to increase peripheral resistance. Within the glomerular circulation, angiotensin II induces preferential constriction of efferent arterioles helping to maintain GFR when renal blood flow is compromised. In the clinical settings previously described, ACE inhibitors cause ARF by reducing systemic blood pressure while simultaneously reducing transglomerular pressure owing to the fall in postglomerular, efferent arteriolar resistance. As with other forms of drug-induced hemodynamic renal insufficiency, kidney function usually returns to baseline when the ACE inhibitor is discontinued. Based on their mechanism of action, type 1 (AT_1) angiotensin receptor blockers would be expected to have similar effects in susceptible patients.

Intrarenal ARF: Acute Tubular Necrosis and Acute Interstitial Nephritis Caused by Drugs

Drug-induced acute renal failure from intrarenal mechanisms can be divided into two entities with distinct clinical and pathophysiologic characteristics: acute tubular necrosis (ATN) and acute interstitial nephritis (AIN). ATN is associated with drug administration and shares many of the clinical features of ATN from other causes. This form of ARF can be seen following administration of agents that are primarily excreted by the kidney, such as aminoglycoside antibiotics, amphotericin B, and chemotherapeutic agents such as cisplatin. Nephrotoxicity often results from direct toxic effects of the compound on renal tubular cells although other hemodynamic mechanisms may play a role. In this setting, the onset of ARF is often nonoliguric and may be slow to develop. If nephrotoxicity is not detected and administration of the causative agent is continued, oliguric ARF may develop. The urinalysis is characteristically bland and may show modest proteinuria, tubular epithelial cells, and noncellular casts. Generally, tubular toxicity will abate when the offending agent is discontinued although there may be a lag before complete recovery of renal function occurs. However, recovery of renal function may not occur following repetitive exposure to tubular toxins. In this case, chronic, irreversible renal impairment may result.

In AIN, drug exposure causes ARF through a syndrome of intrarenal inflammation. This disorder is described in detail in Chapter 38 and is characterized by inflammatory cell infiltration of the renal interstitium with reduced GFR and renal blood flow. Systemic signs of hypersensitivity, including rash, arthralgias, and fever, may also occur. The urinalysis reflects active renal inflammation and usually contains red cells, white cells, and occasional cellular casts with nonglomerular levels of proteinuria. Eosinophiluria can also be observed but is not pathognomonic. Common causative agents include penicillins, cephalosporins, sulfonamide analogs, rifampin, and NSAIDs. AIN usually resolves after the offending agent is removed.

Obstructive Nephropathy Associated with Therapeutic Agents

Drug-associated obstructive uropathy may be caused by intratubular obstruction, intraureteral obstruction, or extrinsic ureteral obstruction from retroperitoneal fibrosis. These obstructive syndromes have been associated with specific causative agents. For example, the antiviral agent acyclovir can cause ARF owing to the precipitation of the drug, which is relatively insoluble, within renal tubular lumens. In analgesic-associated nephropathy (discussed in Chapter 40), patients may present with symptoms of acute ureteral obstruction due to sloughing of necrotic renal papillary tissue. Methysergide has been associated with retroperitoneal fibrosis causing obstructive nephropathy. However, in one survey of patients with retroperitoneal fibrosis, drugs were identified as a cause in less than 3% of cases. Obstructive uropathy has also been reported with the anti-HIV drug indinavir. Although the incidence of this disorder is not clear, indinavir treatment has been associated with crystalluria and nephrolithiasis. Affected patients present with colic and signs of acute urinary tract obstruction. A more chronic and asymptomatic clinical course has also been observed. In both settings, the renal abnormalities regress when the drug is discontinued (also discussed in Chapter 31).

Chronic Renal Failure from Therapeutic Agents

Chronic renal failure caused by drugs is usually manifested as a chronic tubulointerstitial injury. This syndrome of chronic interstitial nephropathy has been associated with a number of structurally diverse agents including lithium, analgesics, cyclosporine, cisplatin, and nitrosureas. Chronic interstitial disease caused by a drug most often presents as an elevation in serum creatinine, which may be slowly progressive. However, abnormalities of renal tubular function may be a predominant feature. Such abnormalities include renal tubular acidosis, concentrating defects, defective potassium secretion, and tubular proteinuria. On histologic examination, interstitial fibrosis, tubular atrophy, and infiltration of the renal interstitium with chronic inflammatory cells are observed. The urinalysis may contain white cells and red cells with modest levels of proteinuria. Although patients with drug-induced chronic interstitial nephropathy may progress to end stage renal disease requiring renal replacement therapy, the course of the disease can usually be stabilized or reversed if the offending agent is identified and discontinued.

Nephrotic Syndrome Associated with Therapeutic Agents

Glomerulopathy with proteinuria may be caused by several drugs, including gold, penicillamine, and NSAIDs. Affected patients often present with proteinuria, edema, and hypoalbuminemia. Pathologically, membranous nephropathy has been associated with all of the agents listed above, whereas minimal change nephropathy has been seen in patients taking certain NSAIDs and penicillamine. In most cases, proteinuria remits when the agent is discontinued. However, in a few cases, renal injury has progressed after the drug is stopped.

SPECIFIC AGENTS THAT CAUSE RENAL FAILURE
Antibiotics

As a class of drugs, antibiotics are the most common cause of clinically recognized drug-induced renal failure. Within this group, aminoglycosides are responsible for the majority of episodes of nephrotoxicity in hospitalized patients. Aminoglycosides most commonly cause an ATN picture, while other antibiotics such as penicillins, rifampin, and sulfonamide more commonly produce AIN. In practice, antibiotics are often administered to patients who are severely ill with other coexistent processes that can independently affect renal function or may aggravate and potentiate nephrotoxicity. Thus, in an individual patient, a causative role for an antibiotic may be difficult to precisely establish.

Aminoglycosides

Aminoglycosides are amphophilic, cationic antibiotics that are used to treat serious gram-negative bacterial infections. They are by far the most common cause of antibiotic-associated renal insufficiency in hospitalized patients. Depending on the criteria used for defining nephrotoxicity, the reported incidence of nephrotoxicity ranges between 7 and 36% of patients receiving aminoglycosides. However, the incidence increases with the duration of therapy and may approach 50% with more than 14 days of therapy. Serum protein binding of aminoglycosides is minimal. They are freely filtered at the glomerulus, and renal excretion is the major route of elimination. Aminoglycosides accumulate within the renal cortex reaching saturation within the first 3 days of treatment. Accumulation of drug within cortical tubular cells probably causes toxicity, although the specific cellular mechanisms of aminoglycoside-induced ARF have not been completely defined. Evidence of tubular cell abnormalities and injury may be seen by both light and electron microscopy.

The usual clinical presentation of aminoglycoside nephrotoxicity is a rising blood urea nitrogen (BUN) and creatinine that typically appears 5 to 7 days into the antibiotic course. Renal insufficiency may occur earlier in the presence of risk factors. Frank azotemia may be preceded by the development of a concentrating defect manifested as polyuria, and the urinalysis most commonly shows modest proteinuria with noncellular casts and occasional tubular epithelial cells. Characteristically, renal function deteriorates progressively, but the process is reversible if the diagnosis is suspected and the aminoglycoside is discontinued. However, there may be a lag time before renal function begins to improve often requiring several weeks for recovery. This is probably related to the kinetics of accumulation of aminoglycosides in renal cortical tissue, since urinary excretion of aminoglycosides has been detected for days to weeks after administration is discontinued.

Although virtually every patient who receives aminoglycosides is at some risk of developing renal toxicity, there is a positive association between the dose and duration of therapy and the risk of developing renal failure. Tailoring aminoglycoside doses to maintain drug levels within a defined therapeutic range serves to minimize the risks of toxicity while maintaining bactericidal concentrations of antibiotic. Single daily dose regimens have been advocated by some authors as an approach to avoid aminoglycoside nephrotoxicity, but the benefits of these regimens have not been clearly demonstrated. Because aminoglycosides are primarily excreted by the kidney, increased aminoglycoside levels can be both a cause and a marker of nephrotoxicity. Monitoring peak and trough drug levels along with serum creatinine every 2 to 3 days is prudent, but daily monitoring may be required in the unstable patient with a serious infection and fluctuating level of renal function.

Several risk factors for aminoglycoside nephrotoxicity have been identified and are illustrated in Table 2. When aminoglycoside therapy is being initiated, these characteristics may be used to identify patient at high risk of developing toxicity for more intensive monitoring and to modify factors such as volume status and electrolyte abnormalities. When possible, alternative antibiotic choices might also be considered in high-risk patients. All members of the aminoglycoside family can potentially cause nephrotoxicity. Although gentamicin is the most extensively utilized, tobramycin has a similar bactericidal profile and exhibits less nephrotoxicity, at least in animal models. Amikacin probably has an intermediate potential for nephrotoxicity between gentamicin and tobramycin.

TABLE 2
Risk Factors for the Development
of Aminoglycoside Nephrotoxicity

Prolonged course of treatment (>10 days)

Volume depletion

Sepsis

Preexisting renal disease

Hypokalemia

Elderly patient

Combination therapy with certain cephalosporins (particularly cephalothin)

Concomitant exposure to other nephrotoxins (i.e., radiocontrast, amphotericin B, cisplatin)

Gentamicin > amikacin > tobramycin

Cephalosporins

Cephalosporins are semisynthetic β-lactam derivatives that have broad spectrum bactericidal activity. Although they are generally tolerated well by patients, renal insufficiency is an infrequent but well-defined complication of cephalosporin therapy. Two forms of renal failure have been described with cephalosporins: ATN and AIN. A profile of tubular toxicity has been best documented with cephaloridine and cephalothin especially when higher doses are used. A rank order potential for cephalosporins to produce proximal tubular toxicity has been defined in animal studies as cephaloglycin>cephaloridine>>cefaclor>cephazolin>cephalothin>>>cephalexin and ceftazidime. Combination therapy with aminoglycosides or furosemide may increase the risk for cephalosporin-associated ATN.

Amphotericin B

Amphotericin B is a polyene antibiotic that is the treatment of choice for the majority of serious fungal infections. Unfortunately, this agent produces a number of side effects with nephrotoxicity being the most clinically problematic. In some series, the degree of nephrotoxicity is roughly proportional to the total cumulative dose received. At least two mechanisms mediate the adverse effects of amphotericin in the kidney. First, the drug produces acute renal vasoconstriction causing reduction in GFR that is hemodynamically mediated. Second, amphotericin is highly bound to cell membranes and causes damage that affects membrane integrity and permeability. In the kidney, this membrane injury is thought to be the basis for characteristic clinical syndromes of potassium and magnesium wasting, inability to maximally concentrate urine, and distal tubule acidification defects. These abnormalities, along with an abnormal urine sediment, usually precede the development of clinically apparent azotemia. Renal failure is frequently nonoliguric and progressive, but will slowly abate when the amphotericin is discontinued. However, high doses and repetitive exposure to amphotericin can cause permanent kidney damage and chronic renal failure. Volume depletion potentiates nephrotoxicity and sodium loading and volume expansion can prevent or ameliorate renal injury. More recently, several formulations of amphotericin in lipid vehicles, including liposomes, have been developed for clinical use. These newer formulations are significantly more expensive than conventional amphotericin. Although they appear to be effective at eradicating invasive fungal infections, the incidence of associated renal toxicity and hypokalemia may be lower than with conventional amphotericin B.

Acyclovir

Acyclovir is an effective and relatively nontoxic antiviral agent that is widely used to treat herpes virus infections. When given by the oral route, acyclovir is essentially devoid of significant renal toxicity. However, nephrotoxicity has been described in a small number of patients who have received intravenous courses of acyclovir, particularly at high doses (>500 mg/m^2). Acyclovir undergoes tubular

255

secretion in the kidney, and renal tissue levels increase substantially during treatment. The mechanism of ARF is thought to be precipitation of the relatively insoluble drug within tubular lumens causing obstruction. The urine sediment may contain red cells and white cells with needle-shaped birefringent crystals. Renal failure generally resolves when the acyclovir is discontinued. Risk factors for toxicity are volume depletion and bolus administration of drug. However, ARF has been observed despite adequate fluid repletion and the use of continuous infusion protocols.

Pentamidine

Approximately 25% of patients treated with pentamidine may experience a fall in GFR that is reversible when the drug is discontinued. Nephrotoxicity with pentamidine may be more common in AIDS patients and has been associated with significant hyperkalemia. Although the incidence of renal problems is reduced with inhaled preparations, renal insufficiency has been reported in association with aerosolized pentamidine use. However, a specific role for pentamidine is often difficult to identify due to the presence of other drugs or comorbid conditions that might also affect renal function.

Radiocontrast

The administration of radiocontrast is a relatively common cause of ARF in hospitalized patients. However, the reported incidence of contrast nephropathy from published studies is quite variable. This variation relates to differences in criteria for defining the syndrome, the period of observation after the contrast administration, and the prevalence of risk factors in the population studied. Preexisting renal insufficiency is the most important and best-documented risk factor, and contrast-induced nephrotoxicity is rare in patients with normal renal function. Other potential risk factors are listed in Table 3. Although animal studies suggested that low osmolality, nonionic contrast agents are less nephrotoxic than conventional high osmolality, ionic

TABLE 3
Risk Factors for the Development of Acute Renal Failure Following Radiocontrast Administration[a]

Preexisting renal dysfunction
Diabetic nephropathy
Severe congestive heart failure
Volume depletion
Elderly patient
Multiple myeloma
Large volumes of radiocontrast
Concomitant treatment with ACE inhibitors, NSAIDs, or exposure to other nephrotoxins

[a]ACE inhibitors, angiotensin converting enzyme inhibitors; NSAIDs, nonsteroidal antiinflammatory drugs.

agents, prospective clinical studies have failed to demonstrate differences in nephrotoxicity in patients treated with ionic or nonionic contrast.

The vasoactive effects of radiocontrast contribute to the pathogenesis of nephropathy. In animals, contrast injection initially causes vasodilatation of the renal circulation, followed by intense and persistent vasoconstriction. The etiology of this vasoconstrictive phase is not clear, but may include reduced production of vasodilator prostaglandins, enhanced endothelin release, or changes in intracellular calcium. Patients with contrast nephrotoxicity typically develop a rise in their serum creatinine within 24 hr after radiocontrast administration, sometimes associated with oliguria. The urinary sediment is unremarkable and the fractional excretion of sodium is typically very low, consistent with the hemodynamic etiology of renal impairment.

Renal failure is usually transient, although occasional patients will require support with acute dialysis. The efforts of the clinician should be directed toward prevention of contrast nephropathy by avoiding unnecessary studies, particularly in patients with risk factors. If contrast administration is unavoidable, the high-risk patient should be given 0.45% saline intravenously at a rate of 1 mL/kilogram of body weight/hour beginning 12 hr before the procedure and continued for an additional 12 hr afterward. This regimen was found to provide better protection against acute decreases in renal function induced by radiocontrast than hydration plus mannitol or furosemide, which in the past had been suggested to be helpful in this setting. Concomitant administration of other nephrotoxic agents should be avoided, and the amount of contrast used during the study should be kept to a minimum. As previously noted, low osmolality, nonionic agents have no clear benefit in preventing nephrotoxicity.

Calcineurin Inhibitor Immunosuppressive Drugs

Cyclosporine and tacrolimus are immunosuppressive agents that inhibit the early events involved in T-cell activation and are extremely effective in suppressing transplant rejection. These agents have distinct chemical structures; cyclosporine is a cyclic peptide and tacrolimus is a macrolide. Despite these marked structural differences, they have identical mechanisms of action. Both compounds produce potent inhibition of calcineurin, an intracellular phosphatase that plays a central role in coordinating T-cell activation by foreign antigens. Based on their efficacy as antirejection therapies, calcineurin inhibitors are the cornerstone of immunosuppressive regimens for patients with virtually every type of organ graft. However, the frequent occurrence of nephrotoxicity and especially concern over the potential for developing chronic, irreversible renal injury have complicated their clinical use.

The clinical manifestations of nephrotoxicity are similar for cyclosporine and tacrolimus, consisting of acute reversible renal dysfunction and chronic interstitial nephropathy. Acute nephrotoxicity is the predominant renal abnormality seen within the first 6 to 12 months after initiating treatment and is characterized by an acute or subacute reduction in renal function that is often dose dependent. Generally, renal dysfunction is nonprogressive and reverses when the dose is lowered or the drug is discontinued. Virtually every patient who receives therapeutic doses of a calcineurin inhibitor will experience a component of persistent, reversible reduction in GFR and renal blood flow. The mechanism of this acute nephrotoxicity is hemodynamic and results from the ability of these agents to induce intense renal vasoconstriction. Calcineurin inhibitors do not cause renal vasoconstriction directly, but may act by stimulating production of other vasoconstrictor compounds such as thromboxane A_2, endothelin, and leukotrienes.

In renal transplant recipients within the first year after transplant, it is often difficult to distinguish acute nephrotoxicity from acute rejection. A stable or slowly progressive increase in serum creatinine that reverses when the cyclosporine or tacrolimus dose is reduced suggests nephrotoxicity. Renal biopsy can be helpful in this setting since aggressive inflammatory cell infiltrates are usually absent in acute nephrotoxicity, and their presence in a biopsy specimen would suggest ongoing rejection. Although serum drug levels are frequently used to monitor therapeutic efficacy and to prevent toxicity, there is only a rough correlation between serum levels and clinical events.

Chronic nephrotoxicity is defined by the development of interstitial fibrosis with reduced levels of GFR in patients receiving long-term treatment with calcineurin inhibitors. The clinical features of the chronic cyclosporine nephrotoxicity are well characterized, although chronic nephropathy also occurs with tacrolimus. Generally, 6 to 12 months of treatment are required before signs of chronic nephropathy become apparent. Because of the irreversible nature of the morphologic abnormalities, this form of toxicity is more ominous than the acute form. Histologically, this chronic nephrotoxicity is characterized by focal or striped medullary interstitial fibrosis. Often these changes are accompanied by tubular atrophy and obliterative arteriolar changes. In more advanced cases, diffuse interstitial fibrosis with focal and segmental glomerular sclerosis can be seen. In renal transplant patients, these changes may be difficult to differentiate from the typical features of chronic rejection. Although the mechanism of chronic nephrotoxicity is not known, it is likely that cumulative dose, arterial hypertension, and immunologic injury contribute to the development of the lesion. Animal studies suggest that severe sodium depletion may potentiate the development of renal fibrosis associated with administration calcineurin inhibitors.

Cyclosporine is metabolized primarily through the action of hepatic P450 microsomal enzymes. Thus, agents that influence the activity of this enzyme system can cause significant changes in cyclosporine metabolism. Generally, drugs that reduce the rate of cyclosporine metabolism, such as erythromycin, ketoconazole, and verapamil, produce increased serum levels and potentiate toxicity. On the other hand, agents that increase the rate of cyclosporine metabolism, such as phenytoin, phenobarbital, and rifampin, may reduce serum levels and thus may blunt therapeutic efficacy.

Antineoplastic Drugs

A number of compounds that are used in the treatment of cancer may be toxic to the kidney. Recognizing and anticipating the potential for renal injury associated with these drugs is critical so that appropriate preventative measures may be implemented. A representative list of antineoplastic agents that affect the kidney is provided in Table 4. The renal effects of three commonly used antitumor drugs are discussed in detail later.

Cisplatin

Cis-diamminedichloroplatin II (cisplatin) is a very effective anticancer agent with a broad range of activity against a number of malignancies. However, administration of cisplatin is associated with a high incidence of nephrotoxicity. The drug is eliminated primarily by the kidney where it is concentrated in glomerular ultrafiltrate accumulating in renal tubular epithelium. Tubular injury seems to be mediated by direct effects on epithelial cell metabolism and through generation of free oxygen radicals. The development of cisplatin nephrotoxicity is dose-related and cumulative. Although the drug can cause reversible acute renal failure, irreversible decline of renal function associated with repeated cisplatin administration is the most common and most disturbing clinical manifestation of toxicity. The development of chronic cisplatin injury may be associated with dense interstitial fibrosis. Another common sequela of cisplatin-induced tubular injury is renal magnesium wasting that often produces clinically significant hypomagnesemia. Hypomagnesemia may be exacerbated by concomitant administration of aminoglycoside antibiotics,

TABLE 4
Nephrotoxicity of Selected Antineoplastic Agents

Drug	Clinical syndrome
Alkylating Agents	
Cisplatin	Tubular injury, acute and chronic renal failure, renal Mg^{2+} wasting
Carboplatin	Less nephrotoxicity than cisplatin
Cyclophosphamide	Hemorrhagic cystitis, hyponatremia
Streptozotocin	Acute renal failure, tubular dysfunction
Antibiotics	
Mitomycin C	Hemolytic uremic syndrome
Mithramycin	Acute tubular necrosis
Antimetabolites	
Methotrexate	Acute renal failure with high-dose therapy
Cytosine arabinoside (Ara-C)	Interstitial nephritis
5-Fluorouracil (5-FU)	Acute renal failure
Biological response modifiers	
Interleukin 2 (IL-2)	Hemodynamically mediated acute renal failure

and it may persist for months after cisplatin has been discontinued.

Maneuvers that increase urine volume during cisplatin administration reduce the risk of nephrotoxicity. Thus, vigorous intravenous fluid administration is indicated for prophylaxis. Increasing urine flow may prevent cisplatin toxicity by limiting the duration of contact between the drug and the renal epithelium. In addition, since increasing the extracellular chloride concentration may inhibit the conversion of cisplatin to a more toxic metabolite, inclusion of isotonic sodium chloride in hydration protocols has been advocated. However, infusions of mannitol also seem to be effective. Fluids should be administered to maintain urine flows of at least 100 mL/hr and preferably above 200 mL/hr for 12 hr before and 12–18 hr after cisplatin is administered. Second generation platinum compounds such as carboplatin appear to have a reduced potential for nephrotoxicity, but renal failure and hypomagnesemia have both been observed with carboplatin.

Cyclophosphamide

Cyclophosphamide is widely used for treating lymphomas and other hematological malignancies. Its common adverse effects are bone marrow suppression, gastrointestinal toxicity, and hemorrhagic cystitis. With high doses of cyclophosphamide (50 mg/kg or more), hyponatremia has been observed. High doses of cyclophosphamide inhibit renal water excretion, and urine osmolality is usually high in the presence of reduced plasma osmolality. Because vasopressin levels are not elevated, the defective water handling appears to be a direct effect of the drug on the distal nephron to promote antidiuresis. Although this defect generally resolves within 24 hr after drug administration, hypotonic fluids should be avoided in the intravenous fluid regimens that are commonly administered to prevent bladder hemorrhage.

Methotrexate

Methotrexate is an antimetabolite that is used to treat a variety of cancers and leukemias. In the absence of preexisting renal dysfunction, nephrotoxicity is uncommon with standard doses of methotrexate. However, significant nephrotoxicity has been observed with high-dose methotrexate regimens. Intratubular precipitation of the drug causing obstruction may contribute to renal dysfunction. In addition, methotrexate has direct toxic effects on

renal epithelial cells. Fluid administration to achieve urine volumes of more than 3 L/day reduces the potential for nephrotoxicity. Because the solubility of methotrexate and its metabolites is increased in alkaline solutions, alkalinization of urine during drug administration is also recommended.

Bibliography

Branch RA: Prevention of amphotericin B-induced renal impairment. *Arch Intern Med* 148:2389–2394, 1988.

DeMattos AM, Olyei AJ, Bennnett WM: Nephrotoxicity of immunosuppressive drugs: Long-term consequences and challenges for the future. *Am J Kidney Dis* 35:333–346, 2000.

Humes HD, Weinberg JM, Knauss TC: Clinical and pathophysiologic aspects of aminoglycoside nephrotoxicity. *Am J Kidney Dis* 2:5–25, 1982.

Kaloyanides GJ: Antibiotic-related nephrotoxicity. *Nephrol Dial Transplant* 9(Suppl 4):130–134, 1994.

Meyer KB, Madias NE: Cisplatin nephrotoxicity. *Miner Electrolyte Metab* 20:201–213, 1994.

Parfrey PS, Griffiths SM, Barrett BJ, *et al.*: Contrast-material induced renal failure in patients with diabetes mellitus, renal insufficiency, or both: A prospective controlled study. *N Engl J Med* 320:143–149, 1989.

Reis F, Klastersky J: Nephrotoxicity induced by cancer chemotherapy with special emphasis on cisplatin. *Am J Kidney Dis* 8:368–379, 1986.

Robinson RF, Nahata MC: A comparative review of conventional and lipid formulations of amphotericin B. *J Clin Pharmacol Ther* 24: 249–257, 1999.

Sawyer MH, Webb DE, Balow JE, Straus SE: Acyclovir-induced renal failure. *Am J Med* 84:1067–1071, 1988.

Schwab SJ, Hlatky MA, Pieper KS, *et al.*: Contrast nephrotoxicity: A randomized controlled trial of a nonionic and an ionic radiographic contrast agent. *N Engl J Med* 320:149–153, 1989.

Solomon R, Werner C, Mann D, D'Elia J, Silva P: Effects of saline, mannitol, and furosemide on acute decreases in renal function induced by radiocontrast agents. *N Engl J Med* 331:1416–1420, 1994.

Tune BM, Hsu C-Y, Fravert D: Cephalosporin and carbacephem nephrotoxicity: Roles of tubular cell uptake and acylating potential. *Biochem Pharmacol* 51(4):557–561, 1996.

US Multicenter FK506 Liver Study Group: A comparison of tacrolimus (FK506) and cyclosporine for immunosuppression in liver transplantation. *N Engl J Med* 331:1110–1115, 1994.

Whelton A: Therapeutic initiatives for the avoidance of aminoglycoside toxicity. *J Clin Pharmacol* 25:67–81, 1985.

Zager RA: Endotoxemia, renal hypoperfusion and fever: Interactive risk factors for aminoglycoside and sepsis-associated acute renal failure. *Am J Kidney Dis* 20(3):223–230, 1992.

35

ACUTE URIC ACID NEPHROPATHY

F. BRUDER STAPLETON

In humans, uric acid is the end product of purine metabolism. Although uric acid provides an efficient means of eliminating nitrogen (containing twice the nitrogen per mole as does urea), uric acid has been retained as the principal source of urinary nitrogen excretion only by birds and some reptiles, most likely because of the low solubility of uric acid in biological fluids. The insoluble nature of uric acid is of particular importance to humans, who unlike other mammals, have a high concentration of uric acid in plasma; therefore, rather modest alterations in urate homeostasis may lead to severe impairment of renal function.

URIC ACID HOMEOSTASIS

Uric acid is a weak organic acid with a pK_a of 5.75. At physiologic pH, uric acid is present almost entirely as monosodium urate. The solubility of monosodium urate is nearly 15 times that of uric acid in aqueous solution. In human plasma, saturation occurs at a monosodium urate concentration of approximately 7 mg/dL. The proton concentration of a solution containing uric acid determines not only the relative amount of monosodium urate, but also the solubility of urate. Thus, in maximally acidified urine, uric acid predominates, with minimal solubility. In addition to pH, the concentrations of other cations affect the solubility of uric acid. Sodium and ammonium decrease urate solubility, whereas potassium increases solubility.

The renal elimination of uric acid involves four components: glomerular filtration, tubular reabsorption, tubular secretion, and reabsorption beyond secretary sites. Uric acid is nearly completely filtered by the glomerular membrane; tubular reabsorption, secretion, and further reabsorption occur along the proximal renal tubule. Excessive excretion of uric acid, to the extent that glomerular filtration is impaired, may be the result of hyperuricemia or altered renal tubular reabsorption or secretion. Fractional excretion of uric acid is less than 10% in healthy adults; however, it is much higher in young children.

URINARY URIC ACID EXCRETION

Approximately 75% of the daily urate excretion is eliminated by the kidneys. The remainder is disposed through the gastrointestinal tract. Normal urinary uric acid excretion in individuals ingesting an unrestricted diet, is less than 700 mg per day in men and less than 600 mg per day in women. In children, uric acid excretion per kilogram of body weight is greater than in adults, with mean values exceeding 20 mg/kg/day in term neonates. In children 3 years of age, the mean urate excretion is 13.5 mg/kg/day and declines during childhood to adult mean values of 6 mg/kg/day. The measurement of uric acid excretion per glomerular filtration rate (GFR) may be a more physiologically relevant assessment of urate elimination. Normal values are less than 0.6 mg/dL × GFR in adults and less than 0.56 mg/dL × GFR in children. This value is calculated as (urine uric acid mg/dL) × (serum creatinine (mg/dL))/urine creatinine (mg/dL).

ACUTE RENAL FAILURE

Acute uric acid nephropathy is an important etiology of oliguric acute renal failure in selected groups of patients in whom the serum rate concentration becomes markedly elevated or in whom a massive uricosuria develops. The most common clinical setting for acute urate nephropathy occurs with rapid turnover of nucleoproteins in patients with leukemia, lymphoma, or other neoplasms, especially during cytotoxic therapy. Called tumor lysis syndrome, acute renal failure with hyperuricemia during therapy for leukemia or lymphomas is associated with hyperkalemia, acidosis, hypocalcemia, and hyperphosphatemia. These metabolic complications develop rapidly and may be life-threatening. Rarely, spontaneous acute urate nephropathy may proceed cytoxic therapy in patients with leukemia or lymphoma. Renal failure from increased serum uric acid and uric aciduria also may complicate inherited disorders of purine metabolism (i.e., Lesch–Nyhan syndrome or hypoxanthine–guanine phosphoribosyl transferase deficiency), hemolysis, rhabdomyolysis, perinatal asphyxia, extreme exercise, and prolonged muscle contractions from status epilepticus. Important risk factors for acute renal failure from hyperuricemia are dehydration and/or acidemia. Many pharmacologic agents increase uric acid excretion. Some, such as the diuretic, ticrynafen, have produced acute renal failure. Radiographic contrast agents also markedly increase uric acid excretion and should be avoided, or used with caution, during hyperuricemia.

Urinary flow drops dramatically in patients with acute uric acid nephropathy. Oliguria results from renal tubular obstruction by the precipitation of uric acid in collecting tubules (Fig. 1). As a result of intraluminal obstruction of

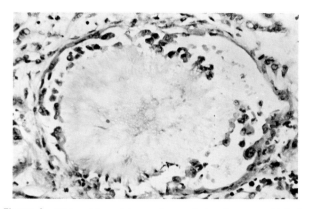

Figure 1 Uric acid crystals are shown obstructing a renal tubule from a child with lymphoma, acute renal failure, and hyperuricemia.

the distal nephron, dilatation of proximal tubules occurs. As discussed previously, uric acid is least soluble in highly concentrated urine of low pH and, predictably, uric acid precipitation occurs in the renal medulla and papilla in acute uric acid nephropathy (Fig. 2). Uric acid precipitation may also occur in the vasa recti supplying the distal nephron. Histologic studies of kidneys during acute urate nephropathy

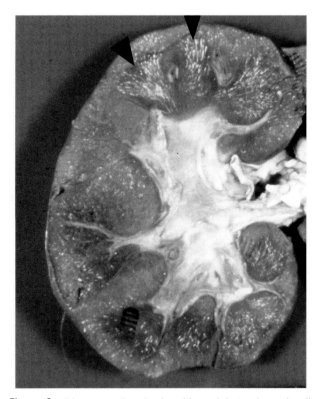

Figure 2 Linear streaks of uric acid precipitates (arrowhead) are seen within the renal medulla in a patient with acute renal failure and a serum uric acid concentration of 34 mg/dL.

show minimal interstitial cellular infiltration; the pathologic changes of acute urate nephropathy are reversible.

Renal function in acute uric acid nephropathy correlates with the rate of urinary excretion of urate, rather than the serum urate level. In patients with hyperuricemia and leukemia, inulin clearances (C_{IN}) is depressed, para-amino hippurate (PAH) clearance is decreased, and the filtration fraction (C_{IN}/C_{PAH}) is decreased. Studies of acute hyperuricemia in laboratory animal models have shown similar alterations in C_{IN} and renal blood flow. Urinary flow is almost always markedly diminished. Precipitation of uric acid in the distal renal tubules and distal renal microvasculature results in increased proximal tubule and distal tubule pressure, and a marked increase in peritubular capillary vascular resistance.

DIAGNOSIS

The clinical diagnosis of acute urate nephropathy should be suspected in high-risk populations when oliguria and decreased renal function (azotemia, hyperkalemia, acidosis, and/or hyperphosphatemia) develop with either an elevated serum uric acid concentration or with copious uric acid or urate crystals in the urinary sediment. Uric acid crystals in the urinary sediment, however, are not a constant finding. Determination of the ratio of urinary uric acid to urinary creatinine concentration may be helpful in the diagnosis of acute urate nephropathy. In adults with acute renal failure, a urinary uric acid/urine creatinine ratio of greater than 1.0 is found in patients with urate nephropathy. This test cannot be applied to infants or children, since the urinary uric acid/urine creatinine ratio normally exceeds 1.0 during childhood. Uric acid excretion is routinely decreased in acute renal failure from etiologies other than urate nephropathy. Serum uric acid concentrations alone are not predictive for acute urate nephropathy.

THERAPY

Although the mortality in acute urate nephropathy was once nearly 45%, current dialysis therapies have dramatically improved survival, so that mortality is now related almost exclusively to the underlying disease process. Medical therapy for patients at risk for urate nephropathy is directed toward reducing intrarenal precipitation of uric acid by maintaining a high urine flow rate with as much hydration as the level of renal function allows. To prevent acute uric acid nephropathy in patients undergoing induction antineoplastic therapy, intravenous fluid administration is begun at 3000 mL/m^2 body surface area per day in both children and adults, when fluid status allows. In patients with extracellular fluid volume depletion, replacement of fluid deficits must precede high volume maintenance. An alkaline urine is maintained with intravenous sodium bicarbonate infusions. When the urine pH cannot be maintained above a pH of 7.0, acetazolamide may also be given orally (provided systemic acidosis is not present). The relative protective roles of urinary flow rate, urine osmolality, and urine pH in the prevention of acute urate nephropathy have been examined in laboratory settings. These studies suggest that a high tubular fluid flow rate, regardless of urine pH or osmolality, offers the maximal protection against urate nephropathy. As mentioned earlier, use of uricosuric drugs, especially radiographic contrast agents, should be avoided in patients with hyperuricemia.

During cytotoxic therapy or in patients with a sustained source of urate overproduction, the filtered urate load is reduced by administering either intravenous or oral allopurinol. Allopurinol is an inhibitor of xanthine oxidase and is extremely effective in reducing the concentration of uric acid in the serum. Urinary oxypurine excretion is increased during allopurinol therapy, however. Renal failure secondary to xanthine precipitation has been observed rarely during allopurinol therapy.

Dialysis or hemofiltration is effective in reducing the serum uric acid concentration and in treating the metabolic consequences of acute renal failure. The clearance of uric acid by hemodialysis is 10 times greater than with peritoneal dialysis; therefore, hemodialysis is the dialysis treatment of choice for acute renal failure from uric acid nephropathy. Occasionally, acute renal failure resolves after one or two dialysis treatments. Due to the tremendous production of uric acid with initial cytotoxic therapy, frequent hemodialysis therapies may be required. For this reason, continuous arteriovenous or venovenous hemofiltration has been shown to be advantageous as renal replacement therapy for patients with acute tumor lysis syndrome. Allopurinol is removed by hemodialysis, and a dose should be given at the conclusion of dialysis treatment.

Uricolysis therapy with the intravenous administration of the enzyme, uricase (uric acid oxidase), appears to hold promise in the prevention of urate nephropathy during cytotoxic therapies. Uric acid is degraded to allantoin in the presence of uricase. Allantoin is extremely soluble, is filtered by the glomerular membrane, and has no known nephrotoxicity. Intravenous administration of a uricase is superior to allopurinol in reducing serum uric acid concentrations in children with leukemia. Peak creatinine concentrations were higher in children treated with allopurinol than in children receiving uricase. Some patients ($<5\%$) receiving the nonrecombinant uricase develop hypersensitivity reactions. Enzymatic uricolysis therapy, although promising for initial induction therapy of lymphoid malignancies, is currently experimental and not available for routine clinical use.

Bibliography

Baldree LA, Stapleton FB: Uric acid metabolism in children. *Pediatr Clin North Am* 2:391–418, 1990.

Cameron JS, Maro F, Simmonds HA: Gout, uric acid and purine metabolism in paediatric nephrology. *Pediatr Nephrol* 7: 105–118, 1993.

Conger JD, Falk SA: Intrarenal dynamics in the pathogenesis and prevention of acute urate nephropathy. *J Clin Invest* 59:786, 1977.

Conger JD, Falk SA, Guggenheim SJ, *et al.:* A micropuncture study of the early phase of acute urate nephropathy. *J Clin Invest* 58:681, 1976.

Jones DP, Stapleton FB, Kawinsky D, *et al.:* Renal dysfunction and hyperuricemia at presentation and relapse of acute lymphoblastic leukemia. *Med Pediatr Oncol* 18:283–286, 1990.

Maesaka JK, Fishbane S: Regulation of renal urate excretion: A critical review. *Am J Kidney Dis* 32:917–933, 1998.

Pui CH, Relling MV, Lascombes F, *et al.:* Urate oxidase in prevention and treatment of hyperuricemia associated with lymphoid malignancies. *Leukemia* 11:1813–1816, 1997.

Rieselbach RE, Steele TH: Influence of the kidney upon urate homeostasis in health and disease. *Am J Med* 56:665, 1974.

Spencer HW, Yarger WE, Robinson RR: Alterations of renal function during dietary-induced hyperuricemia in the rat. *Kidney Int* 9:489, 1976.

Stapleton FB: Urate nephropathy. In: Edelmann CM, Bernstein J, Meadow R, Travis LB, Spitzer A (eds) *Pediatric Kidney Disease,* 2nd Ed., pp. 1647–1661. Little, Brown, Boston, 1992.

Stapleton FB, Strother DR, Roy III S, *et al.:* Acute renal failure at onset of therapy for advanced stage Burkitt lymphoma and B cell acute lymphoblastic lymphoma. *Pediatrics* 82:863–869, 1988.

Tsokos GC, Balow JE, Speigel RJ, *et al.:* Renal and metabolic complications of undifferentiated and lymphoblastic lymphomas. *Medicine* 67:218–227, 1981.

36

CHOLESTEROL ATHEROEMBOLIC RENAL DISEASE

ARTHUR GREENBERG

Cholesterol atheroembolic renal disease results when cholesterol crystals and other debris separate from atheromatous plaques, flow downstream, and lodge in small renal arteries, producing luminal occlusion, ischemia, and renal dysfunction. Depending on the source and distribution of emboli, renal disease may be the sole or predominant manifestation or simply one feature of a systemic illness characterized by multiorgan ischemia or infarction.

Early, autopsy-derived descriptions of renal atheroembolism overemphasized a catastrophic presentation with irreversible renal failure, intestinal infarction, and death from intra-abdominal sepsis. Atheroembolism is now recognized as a cause of occult or reversible renal failure. Recovery of renal function may follow extended survival on renal replacement therapy.

PATHOLOGY

The initial lesion in cholesterol atheroembolism is obstruction of a medium-sized or small artery by atheromatous debris. Arterioles and capillaries are less commonly affected. Lesions may occur in any organ. Cholesterol dissolves in formalin used to process tissue for routine histologic examination; crystals are not seen in tissue sections unless special fixatives are used. However, a characteristic cleft marks the space formerly occupied by the needlelike crystals (Fig. 1). The size of the artery affected is typically around 200 μm, but may range from 55 to 900 μm. The earliest lesion consists of cholesterol crystals and thrombus. After dissolution of the thrombus, macrophages engulf the cholesterol, but the predominant reaction is endothelial. New endothelium covers the crystals. If the vessel wall is eroded by the crystals, an intense perivascular inflammatory response with giant cells is established (Fig. 1). As a late finding, concentric fibrosis, particularly involving the adventitia, occurs. Finally, there is recanalization of small vascular channels. Crystals may reach the glomerular capillary loops (Fig. 2). Crystal dissolution *in vivo* is slow; in experimental models, cholesterol clefts persist as long as 9 months after embolization. The principal glomerular finding is ischemia, with glomerular collapse and basement membrane wrinkling. In some patients, focal segmental glomerulosclerosis with glomerular collapse and epithelial cell prominence occurs. This finding accounts for some of the cases associated with nephrotic range proteinuria.

PATHOGENESIS

The classic autopsy description by Flory noted cholesterol atheroembolism solely in patients with erosive plaques. The prevalence of atheroembolism paralleled the severity of aortic disease. Less severe atherosclerotic lesions or plaques covered by thrombus do not pose a risk of atheroembolism.

Embolization may be spontaneous, particularly with severe aortic disease, but mechanical disruption of plaque during angiographic or surgical procedures usually precedes it. Table 1 lists predisposing factors. Irrespective of the area primarily targeted for imaging, passage of a catheter along the ascending or descending aorta proximal to the renal arteries confers a risk of embolization to the kidneys. Renal artery angioplasty or revascularization may pose a particular risk, and patients who develop atheroembolism in this setting have a worsened outcome. The site of any concurrent nonrenal embolization depends on the path of the catheter.

Thrombus overlying atheromatous plaque can bind and immobilize friable debris. Anticoagulation or thrombolysis removes this protective covering; atheroembolism has been reported after heparin, warfarin, or thrombolytic therapy without angiography.

CLINICAL FEATURES

As expected of a process that complicates severe atherosclerosis, risk factors for atherosclerosis as well as evidence of disseminated atherosclerotic disease are commonly present. The incidence is higher in smokers. Up to 75% of patients are male. The mean age at diagnosis is in the mid seventh decade. Fewer than 5% of patients are below age 50. Table 2 lists other accompanying or predisposing features. Notably, diabetes mellitus is a feature of only 2.5–27% of reported cases.

The severity of cholesterol atheroembolism is highly variable, and manifestations of the disorder depend on both the extent of renal involvement and the extrarenal sites affected. The frequency of organ involvement is

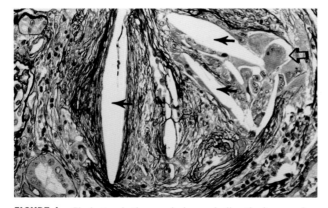

FIGURE 1 Cholesterol atheroembolus occluding the lumen of an interlobular renal artery. Needlelike clefts (solid arrows) are present along with a macrophage/multinucleated giant cell reaction (open arrow). Methenamine silver-trichrome stain, 450×. Figure courtesy of Dr. S.I. Bastacky. Reproduced with permission from Greenberg A, *et al., Am J Kidney Dis* 29:334–344, 1997.

summarized in Table 3. Massive and widespread embolization, in the Multiple Cholesterol Emboli syndrome, presents catastrophically with fever, stroke, acute renal failure, abdominal pain and gastrointestinal bleeding due to bowel infarction, intra-abdominal sepsis, and death. In contrast, spontaneous embolization can have an indolent course.

Autopsy reports are skewed toward patients with severe involvement. In milder disease, renal and cutaneous involvement predominate. Typically, the renal course is characterized by slowly deteriorating renal function. The daily increase in serum creatinine may be as little as 0.1–0.2 mg/dL, and progression to end stage disease may occur over 30 to 60 days or longer. Patients may also present with the insidious development of renal insufficiency over many months. Occasional patients present with heavy proteinuria, with or without associated clinical features of atheroembolism.

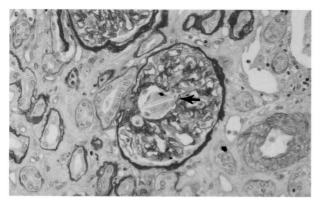

FIGURE 2 Glomerulus with cholesterol clefts at hilum (arrow). The remainder of the glomerulus shows capillary loop thickening and wrinkling due to ischemia. Adjacent tubules show acute ischemic injury. Hematoxylin and eosin stain, 250×. Figure courtesy of Dr. S.I. Bastacky.

TABLE I
Risk Factors for Cholesterol Atheroembolic Renal Disease

Iatrogenic
    Surgery on the aorta proximal to the renal arteries
        Aortic aneurysm repair
        Aortic aneurysm stenting
        Coronary artery bypass grafting
        Cardiac valve surgery
        Other
    Angiography or angioplasty
    Intra-aortic balloon pump circulatory augmentation
    Anticoagulation or thrombolytic therapy
Spontaneous
    Severe ulcerating atherosclerosis

Skin involvement includes livedo reticularis of the lower extremities due to occlusion of small arteries as well as cyanosis of the toes. This classic "blue toes" lesion occurs in spite of preservation of distal pulses. Digital ulceration may occur along with severe pain. Cutaneous involvement may be overlooked unless specifically sought. The livedo may be more prominent with the feet dependent and can be very subtle when the patient is supine.

Features of gastrointestinal involvement include abdominal pain, anorexia, weight loss, and bleeding that can range from a positive stool test for occult blood to brisk hemorrhage. Pancreatitis and acalculous cholecystitis may occur if emboli reach these organs. Bowel infarction and sepsis may also follow an episode of embolization. Central nervous system involvement includes stroke or diffuse cortical dysfunction due to widespread embolization as well as the scotomata, field cuts, or blindness that accompany the classic, but rare, retinal Hollenhorst plaque.

DIAGNOSIS

The diagnosis of atheroembolism relies on a high index of suspicion in patients at risk. During the acute phase, leucocytosis and an elevated erythrocyte sedimentation rate may be present. Eosinophilia is observed in approximately half of affected individuals; hypocomplementemia occurs rarely. Hyperamylasemia suggests pancreatic involvement.

TABLE 2
Associated Findings in 221 Patients with Cholesterol Atheroembolism[a]

Finding	Cases (%)
Hypertension	61
Coronary artery disease	44
Aortic aneurysm	25
Cerebrovascular disease	21
Congestive heart failure	21
Diabetes mellitus	11

[a]Modified from Fine *et al.* (1987).

TABLE 3
Histologic Involvement at Autopsy

Site	Cases (%)
Kidney	75
Spleen	52
Pancreas	52
Gastrointestinal tract	31
Adrenal glands	20
Liver	17
Brain	14
Skin	6

Although nephrotic range proteinuria may occur, proteinuria is typically modest and the urine sediment nonspecific.

Cholesterol atheroembolism is often confused with radiocontrast nephropathy (Chapter 34). The course of the latter is much more rapid, a feature that permits the two to be readily distinguished. In dye nephropathy, renal failure occurs immediately, renal function reaches a nadir within 3 or 4 days, and substantial recovery usually occurs over a similar period. In atheroembolism, the onset of renal failure may be delayed and progression is slower. Recovery occurs after many weeks or months, if at all. Thus, a protracted episode of "radiocontrast nephropathy" occurring after an arteriogram is quite likely due to cholesterol atheroembolism rather than dye-induced. Other disorders that can be mimicked by atheroembolic disease include ischemic acute tubular necrosis, systemic vasculitis, allergic interstitial nephritis, cryoglobulinemia, myeloma, hypertensive nephrosclerosis, and renal artery stenosis.

Most instances of cholesterol atheroembolism are diagnosed clinically, and it is usually not necessary to obtain biopsy confirmation. If a tissue diagnosis is deemed necessary, biopsy of an area of livedo reticularis is the least invasive approach. A muscle biopsy may also be employed. A renal biopsy showing cholesterol atheroemboli is definitive, but alternative means of diagnosis should be considered first.

THERAPY AND OUTCOME

Spontaneous atheroembolism occurs only in patients with more severe vascular involvement. Shedding of atheromatous debris often continues with a progressively declining course. In patients with atheroembolism after vascular surgery or angiography, embolization may be limited to the initial episode. Stabilization and gradual improvement may follow as small vessel inflammation subsides and recanalization with restoration of blood flow occurs. A typical patient will have gradually lessening

anorexia and abdominal and digital pain with subsequent healing of digital ischemic lesions. Management focuses on supportive measures with local care of digital ischemia, analgesia for pain, and digital amputation if tissue is not viable. Anticoagulation should be stopped and repeat angiographic procedures scrupulously avoided. Hemodialysis or peritoneal dialysis may be successfully employed. Some patients recover sufficient renal function to permit discontinuation of dialysis. In others, renal failure is irreversible. Careful attention to supplemental nutrition is beneficial for patients with anorexia due to gastrointestinal tract involvement. Although abdominal or transesophageal ultrasonography may be used to localize diseased areas of aorta, cholesterol atheroembolism occurs in an elderly population with extensive atherosclerotic disease and a high prevalence of hypertensive cardiovascular disease. Such patients present a formidable surgical risk; the role of endarterectomy or resection of diseased aortic segments has not been established.

Bibliography

Belenfant X, Meyrier A, Jacquot C: Supportive treatment improves survival in multi visceral cholesterol crystal embolism. *Am J Kidney Dis* 33:840–850, 1999.

Colt HG, Begg RJ, Saporito JJ, Cooper WM, Shapiro AP: Cholesterol emboli after cardiac catheterization. Eight cases and review of the literature. *Medicine* 67:389–400, 1988.

Fine MJ, Kapoor W, Falanga V: Cholesterol crystal embolization: A review of 221 cases in the English literature. *Angiology* 38:769–784, 1987.

Flory CM: Arterial occlusions produced by emboli from eroded aortic atheromatous plaques. *Am J Pathol* 21:549–565, 1945.

Greenberg A, Bastacky SI, Iqbal A, Borochovitz D, Johnson JP: Focal segmental glomerulosclerosis associated with nephrotic syndrome in cholesterol atheroembolism: Clinicopathologic correlations. *Am J Kidney Dis* 29:334–344, 1997.

Kasinath BS, Corwin HL, Bidani AK, Korbet SM, Schwartz MM, Lewis EJ: Eosinophilia in the diagnosis of atheroembolic renal disease. *Am J Nephrol* 7:173–177, 1987.

Kassirer JP: Atheroembolic renal disease: *N Engl J Med* 280:812–818, 1969.

Krishnamurthi V, Novick AC, Myles JL: Atheroembolic renal disease: Effect on morbidity and survival after revascularization for atherosclerotic renal artery stenosis. *J Urol* 161:1093–1096, 1999.

McGowan JA, Greenberg A: Cholesterol atheroembolic renal disease. Report of 3 cases with emphasis on diagnosis by skin biopsy and extended survival. *Am J Nephrol* 6:135–139, 1986.

Saleem S, Lakkis FG, Martinez-Maldonado M: Atheroembolic renal disease. *Semin Nephrol* 16:309–318, 1996.

Thadhani RI, Carmago CA, Xavier RJ, Fang LST, Bazari H: Atheroembolic renal failure after invasive procedures. Natural history based on 52 histologically proven cases. *Medicine* 74:350–358, 1995.

Tunick PA, Perez JL, Kronzon I: Protruding atheromas in the thoracic aorta and systemic embolization. *Ann Intern Med* 115:423–427, 1991.

37

MYOGLOBINURIC AND HEMOGLOBINURIC ACUTE RENAL FAILURE

DINESH K. CHATOTH AND SUDHIR V. SHAH

Rhabdomyolysis with myoglobinuric acute renal failure (ARF) and hemolysis with hemoglobinuric ARF are collectively termed pigment nephropathy.

RHABDOMYOLYSIS

Rhabdomyolysis is a clinical syndrome that results from skeletal muscle injury and subsequent release of muscle cell contents into the circulation. The earliest reference to rhabdomyolysis is in the Old Testament in the Book of Numbers. The late nineteenth century German literature describes a syndrome of muscle pain, weakness, and brown urine, referred to as Mayer–Betz disease. During the Battle of Britain in World War II, Bywaters and Beall were the first to report a causative link between muscle injury and ARF.

Incidence and Etiology

The exact incidence of rhabdomyolysis induced ARF is unknown, but rhabdomyolysis may account for about 10% of all cases of ARF. Besides crush injuries, several other conditions can cause rhabdomyolysis (Table 1). The causative factors for muscle injury are obvious in most situations but sometimes may be occult.

Intrinsic Muscle Dysfunction

Muscle injury can result from direct trauma, extreme muscular exertion in long distance runners, from contact sports, or in association with seizures, delirium tremens, and status asthmaticus. Exertional muscle injuries in patients who are not sufficiently conditioned before severe physical exertion has been nicknamed white-collar rhabdomyolysis. Volume-depleted individuals or people who exercise in hot, humid weather conditions appear to be susceptible to rhabdomyolysis. Similarly patients who abuse alcohol, especially binge drinkers, appear to have a much lower threshold for muscle injury, presumably because of preexisting muscle injury from ethanol and poor physical conditioning. In contrast, for the same degree of muscle exertion, women have less muscle injury compared to men.

Rhabdomyolysis may result from burns or electric shock, severe hypo- and hyperthermia, and neuroleptic malignant syndrome. Besides direct thermal injury to muscle, hyperthermia can induce increased metabolic demand, cutaneous vasodilatation, intravascular volume depletion, and shunting of blood from the renal circulation. Hypothermia can also cause myoglobinuria by direct muscle injury, as well as by inducing muscle ischemia from vasoconstriction. Rhabdomyolysis can occur in metabolic myopathies such as McArdle's syndrome and carnitine palmitoyltransferase deficiency. McArdle's syndrome results from myophosphorylase deficiency, leading to defective anaerobic glycolysis in muscles, and carnitine palmitoyltransferase deficiency disrupts long-chain fatty acid transport across the muscle mitochondrial membrane. Thus, moderate exercise in these patients can lead to severe muscle necrosis. A few cases of rhabdomyolysis from dermatomyositis and polymyositis have also been reported in the literature.

Acquired Metabolic Muscle Disorders

Hypokalemia impairs muscle synthesis of glycogen, the source of energy during anaerobic work. Importantly, hypokalemia also interferes with the normal increase in muscle blood flow associated with exercise and may cause exertional rhabdomyolysis. Hypophosphatemia can cause depletion of adenosine triphosphate (ATP), the energy source needed to maintain normal cellular functions, leading to membrane injury and muscle necrosis.

Hypoxia

Prolonged external compression of blood supply to a muscle group (comatose states) or decreased oxygen delivery to the muscles (carbon monoxide poisoning) can cause hypoxic myopathy.

Drugs and Toxins

Illicit drugs like heroin, cocaine, amphetamines, and phencyclidine cause rhabdomyolysis by direct toxicity to the muscles. Cocaine and amphetamines can also induce muscle breakdown by hypermetabolism from hyperpyrexia, muscle hyperactivity from seizures and agitation, ischemia and tissue hypoxia from vasoconstriction, as well as from pressure necrosis as a result of coma and immobility. Narcotics like heroin and barbiturates can cause pressure necrosis if they induce prolonged unconsciousness.

TABLE I
Causes of Rhabdomyolysis

Intrinsic muscle dysfunction	Toxins
Traumatic rhabdomyolysis	Ethanol
Muscle injury	Isopropyl alcohol
Burns	Carbon monoxide
Electrocution	Toluene
Exertional rhabdomyolysis	Ethylene glycol
Marathon runners and contact sports	Hemlock
"White-collar" rhabdomyolysis	Snake bites
Status asthmaticus	Spider bites
Delirium tremens	Infections
Seizures	Bacterial
Immunologic disorders	Gas gangrene
Dermatomyositis	Tetanus
Polymyositis	Shigellosis
Genetic disorders	Legionnaires' disease
Myophosphorylase deficiency (McArdle's	Septic shock
syndrome)	Viral
Carnitine palmitoyltransferase deficiency	Epstein-Barr
Glucosidase deficiency	Cytomegalovirus
Phosphohexiosomerase deficiency	Echo
Phosphofructokinase deficiency	Coxsackie
Acquired metabolic muscle disorders	Influenza
Hypokalemia	Hepatitis
Hypophosphatemia	Rickettsial (e.g., Rocky Mountain spotted fever)
Thyroid diseases (thyroid storm, myxedema)	Parasitic diseases
Hyponatremia	Miscellaneous
Hyperosmolar coma	Reye's syndrome
Hypoxic muscle injury	Toxic shock syndrome
Vascular obstruction	Trichinosis
Thromboemboli	Temperature related
Vasculitis	Hypothermia
Vascular dissection	Hyperthermia
External compression	Malignant hyperthermia
Comatose states	Neuroleptic malignant syndrome
Prolonged immobilization	Heat stroke
Sickle cell disease	
Drugs	
Heroin	
Cocaine	
Amphetamines	
Phencyclidine hydrochloride	
Succinylcholine	
Lysergic acid diethylamide	
Theophylline	
Phenylpropanolamine	
Caffeine	
Clofibrate	

Succinylcholine, 3-hydroxy-3-methyl glutanyl coenzyme A (HMG CoA) reductase inhibitors and fibric acid derivatives are some of the important drugs that cause rhabdomyolysis. The cholesterol lowering drugs can cause rhabdomyolysis, especially when combined with cyclosporine, nicotinic acid, or erythromycin. The exact mechanism for this muscle injury remains unclear.

Chronic ethanol abuse is a common cause of myopathy. Ethanol can cause direct sarcolemmal injury and muscle necrosis. Furthermore, alcohol induced seizures, agitation and delirium tremens can cause significant muscle break-down. Chronic alcoholics are also frequently malnourished and have accompanying hypokalemia and hypophosphatemia, which can further aggravate the muscle damage.

Infections

Infections caused by bacterial, rickettsial, viral, or protozoan agents have all been implicated in the etiology of rhabdomyolysis. Infections cause rhabdomyolysis either by direct muscle injury (viral infections) or by releasing toxins (clostridia). Other mechanisms that can cause rhabdomyolysis associated with infections include electrolyte imbalances, hypoxia, hyperthermia, hypotension, and increased metabolic requirements.

Diagnosis and Laboratory Evaluations

Patients with rhabdomyolysis may present with a constallation of feature including severe muscle pain and tenderness, profound weakness, stiffness, swelling, and rarely muscle paralysis. Sometimes, the involved muscles become edematous in confined tissue spaces and result in compartment syndromes and interruption of blood supply causing a "second wave" of rhabdomyolysis. It is easy to overlook the diagnosis because myalgias or weakness may be absent in 50% of the patients with serologically proven rhabdomyolysis. Thus, careful attention to historical information including the drugs ingested in the clinical setting of acute renal failure provide important clues that must be confirmed by laboratory testing.

Examination of the urine often provides the first clue. A dipstick that is markedly positive (3+ to 4+) for blood with a microscopic examination that reveals relatively few red blood cells (RBCs), suggests the presence of heme pigment not present in intact RBCs. In most instances this will be due to myoglobin rather than hemoglobin. This finding in urinalysis raises sufficient suspicion of the diagnosis to seek confirmation to define the presence and extent of muscle injury. Thus specific immunodiffusion, radioimmunoassay, and dipstick tests, which are available for the demonstration of myoglobin in the blood or urine, are often unnecessary in diagnosing rhabdomyolysis. Of course, patients with rhabdomyolysis may also have hematuria due to placement of an indwelling bladder catheter or other cause, so this urinary finding is not always observed. Additional findings include a dark, brown colored urine with an acidic pH and the presence of pigmented brown granular casts in the urine sediment.

Abnormal blood chemistries confirm and define the extent of rhabdomyolysis. Increased levels of serum creatine kinase (CK) frequently accompany rhabdomyolysis and are typically greater than 10,000 IU/L, but can exceed 100,000 IU/L. However, myoglobinuria cannot be characterized by a specific CK level, and some cases of rhabdomyolysis have been reported in the literature with CK below 1000 IU/L. CK is an excellent marker for this disease because it is present in the serum immediately after the muscle injury, is easily measured, peaks in about 12 to 36 hr, and has a half-life of about 48 hr.

Many of the laboratory findings reflect the release of intracellular contents from damaged muscle (Table 2). Creatine in skeletal muscle undergoes dehydration to form creatinine. Rhabdomyolysis leads to the release of large quantities of creatine and then creatinine, so the serum creatinine concentration rises very rapidly and the normal ratio of blood urea nitrogen (BUN) to creatinine of about 10 is reduced, sometimes to approximately 5, early in the course of the ARF. Later, catabolism of muscle protein leads to dramatic increases in urea production and so the BUN:creatinine ratio rises to higher than normal levels.

Muscle damage also leads to the breakdown of intracellular phosphate compounds and release of large quantities of inorganic phosphorus into the circulation to result in hyperphosphatemia. Hyperphosphatemia increases the calcium–phosphorus product, and the damaged muscle tissue serves as the nidus for deposition of calcium phosphate in a process of pathologic calcification. There is resultant hypocalcemia, which is generally asymptomatic and requires no treatment. Later in the course, the soft tissue calcification resolves as the muscle recovers from injury, thereby contributing to the hypercalcemia sometimes observed in the recovery phase of myoglobinuric ARF. Furthermore, secondary hyperparathyroidism from hyperphosphatemia may

TABLE 2
Flow of Solutes and Water across Skeletal Muscle Cell Membrane in Rhabdomyolysis[a]

Condition	Consequences
Efflux from damaged muscle cell	
Potassium	Hyperkalemia and cardiotoxicity aggravated by hypocalcemia and hypotension: peripheral vasodilatation
Release of purines from disintegrating cell nuclei	Hyperuricemia, nephrotoxicity
Phosphate release from cells	Hyperphosphatemia, aggravation of hypocalcemia, and metastatic calcification, including in the kidney
Release of lactic and other organic acids	Metabolic acidosis and aciduria
Myoglobin	Nephrotoxicity, particularly with coexisting oliguria, aciduria, and hyperuricosuria
Thromboplastin	Disseminated intravascular coagulation
Creatinine kinase	Extreme elevation of serum creatinine kinase level
Creatinine	Increased serum creatinine; decreased BUN/creatinine ratio
Influx from the extracellular compartment into muscle cells of water, sodium chloride, and calcium	Hypovolemia and hemodynamic shock, prerenal and later acute renal failure; hypocalcemia aggravating hyperkalemic cardiotoxicity; increased cytosolic calcium with activation of cytotoxic proteases

[a]Modified from Better OS, Rubenstein I, Winaver J: *Semin Nephrol* 12:217–222, 1992.

also contribute to the hypercalcemia. Hyperuricemia results from metabolism of purines released from damaged muscle and can reach extremely high levels. Because most potassium resides within cells and skeletal muscle represent a large part of the total cellular mass, breakdown of even a small volume of skeletal muscle releases a considerable potassium load and may result in life-threatening hyperkalemia.

Hypoalbuminemia is an ominous feature of rhabdomyolysis and indicates capillary damage with leakage of plasma proteins from the vascular space.

HEMOLYSIS AND HEMOGLOBINURIC ACUTE RENAL FAILURE

Hemoglobinemia and hemoglobinuria are associated with conditions that cause massive intravascular hemolysis. Extravascular hemolysis does not usually cause hemoglobinuria because the hemoglobin is released into the tissues and converted to bilirubin, which is promptly taken up by the liver and metabolized.

Etiology and Diagnosis

The causes of hemoglobinuria are listed in Table 3. Transfusion with mismatched blood is the commonest cause of hemoglobinuric ARF. Infections such as mycoplasma, clostridia, and falciparum malaria (Blackwater fever) can cause hemoglobinuria. Furthermore, drugs and chemicals such as aniline, benzene, glycerol, hydralazine, and quinidine can also cause hemolysis with subsequent hemoglobinuria. Diseases such as glucose 6-phosphate dehydrogenase deficiency, paroxysmal nocturnal hemoglobinuria, and "March" hemoglobinuria also cause hemolysis and hemoglobinuric ARF. Other causes include defective or leaking musthetic cardiac values, extracorporeal circulation, and microangiopathic hemolytic anemia. Lastly, absorption of

glycine or distilled water while irrigating the prostatic bed during transurethral prostatectomy can lead to intravascular hemolysis.

As in the case of rhabdomyolysis, a careful history and physical examination is helpful in diagnosing hemoglobinuric nephropathy. Laboratory evaluations of these patients show evidence of intravascular hemolysis that includes elevated lactic dehydrogenase, hyperkalemia, hyperphosphatemia, and mild hyperbilirubinemia. An important distinction is that serum haptoglobin levels are significantly low and plasma hemoglobin levels are usually elevated. Thus, hemolysis and rhabdomyolysis can usually be differentiated by inspection of plasma, which is usually stained pink in hemolysis, but not in rhabdomyolysis. This is because the hemoglobin haptoglobin complex is a large molecule, which is not filtered by the glomerulus. Hemoglobin appears in the urine only after plasma haptoglobin becomes saturated, when total hemoglobin exceeds 100 mg/dL. In contrast, myoglobin is a 17-kDa protein, which has no specific binding protein and is readily filtered by the glomerulus. As previously described, because dipstick tests are exquisitely sensitive for detection of heme pigment in the urine, there is no practical need to perform more sophisticated and expensive tests to either detect or differentiate myoglobin or hemoglobin.

PATHOPHYSIOLOGY OF PIGMENT NEPHROPATHY

The pathological diagnosis in most cases of pigment associated ARF is acute tubular necrosis (ATN). Proximal tubular necrosis and distal tubular pigment casts are the characteristic pathological features of pigment nephropathy. Ischemic, toxic, and intratubular obstructive mechanisms have been implicated in the pathogenesis of pigment induced ARF. These are not mutually exclusive and, indeed, may act in concert. Clinical observations and animal studies

TABLE 3
Causes of Hemoglobinemia and Hemoglobinuria

Transfusion with mismatched blood infections	**Venom**
Mycoplasma	Spider bite
Clostridia	Tarantula
Falciparum malaria (Blackwater fever)	Brown recluse
Drugs and chemicals	Snake bite
Aniline	Rattlesnake
Arsine	Copperhead
Benzene	**Other causes**
Cresol	Mechanical valvular prosthesis
Fava beans	Extracorporeal circulation
Glycerol	Microangiopathic hemolytic anemia
Hydralazine	TURP (Trans urethral resection of the prostate)
Phenol	(distilled water/glycine irrigation)
Penicillin	
Quinidine	
Hematological diseases	
Glucose 6-phosphate deficiency	
Paroxysmal nocturnal hemoglobinuria	
"March" hemoglobinuria	

indicate that neither myoglobin nor hemoglobin is markedly nephrotoxic unless accompanied by volume depletion, hypotension, renal hypoperfusion, and acidic urine supporting ischemic mechanisms. Additionally, heme pigments can induce intrarenal vasoconstriction, at least in part by scavenging the vasodilator nitric oxide and by releasing vasoconstrictors such as endothelin and thromboxane in the renal microcirculation. Studies in experimental animals have shown that ARF from rhabdomyolysis induced by intramuscular glycerol injections can be blunted by saline or mannitol induced volume-expanding maneuvers.

Distal tubular pigment casts formed by the interaction heme with Tamm–Horsfall protein are characteristic features of pigment nephropathy. They may contribute to injury by directly causing intratubular obstruction and indirectly by preventing the egress of heme. The cast formation is enhanced under acidic conditions in keeping with the clinical observation of increased toxicity with acidic urine. Acidic pH also promotes dissociation of these heme proteins to ferrihemates, which are potent inhibitors of tubule transport.

Studies using an animal model have implicated reactive oxygen metabolites and iron in rhabdomyolysis-induced ARF. Thus, the formation of hydrogen peroxide has been shown to be enhanced, and scavengers of reactive oxygen metabolites, the antioxidant glutathione, and iron chelators have all been shown to be protective. Although it has always been assumed that heme is the source of iron, more recent studies indicate that renal cytochrome P450 may serve as the source of iron. Heme oxygenase, which is induced by heme and by oxidant stress, has been shown to increase in an animal model of rhabdomyolysis, and its functional significance as a protective mechanism has been delineated.

MANAGEMENT OF PIGMENT NEPHROPATHY

Early initiation of treatment is critical in the management of pigment nephropathy. In most situations it is advisable to begin treatment as soon as the diagnosis is entertained, even before confirmatory laboratory studies become available. The treatment usually consists of correcting hypovolemia using crystalloid or colloid solutions and using drugs like mannitol and furosemide to promote clearance of myoglobin and hemoglobin. Furthermore, correction of the metabolic complications of pigment nephropathy is an essential component of the effective management of this disorder.

Correction of Hypovolemia

Clinical and experimental data provide compelling evidence for the role of early and aggressive volume repletion in the management of pigment induced ARF. This should be initiated as soon as possible by using isotonic crystalloid solutions, usually normal saline. Hydration should be continued until all clinical signs of dehydration are absent and renal function improves. However, one must be cautious not

to "overhydrate," as these patients are prone to volume overload from accompanying renal failure. Once the diagnosis is confirmed with laboratory evidence, forced alkaline diuresis using a mannitol–bicarbonate cocktail can be instituted. This cocktail, prepared by adding two 12.5-g ampules of mannitol and two 50-mL (100-mEq) ampules of sodium bicarbonate to 800 ml of 5% dextrose solution, is administered at a rate of about 200–250 mL/hr initially for at least 4 hr or until urine output improves (usually 4–6 hr). Then, the solution can be continued at a rate equal to the urine output until all evidence for myoglobinuria has disappeared. Patients with ARF may frequently have difficulty in excreting the bicarbonate load, and therefore close monitoring of electrolytes is warranted to prevent the development of metabolic alkalosis.

Enhancing Elimination of Pigments

Systemic bicarbonate therapy, either in the form of a cocktail (see earlier) or as an intravenous infusion, can be used to achieve a urine pH of >6.5. Alkalization is especially important when severe hyperkalemia and acidosis accompany the ARF. Mannitol has been shown in experimental studies to protect against pigment nephropathy, either because of its proximal diuretic action or because it is a scavenger of reactive oxygen metabolites. Furthermore, mannitol is a volume expander, a potent renal vasodilator, and may help reduce renal ischemia. Furosemide may be beneficial in some clinical situations because of its diuretic action and may assist in the renal elimination of toxic heme proteins.

Management of Complications

Complications associated with rhabdomyolysis require prompt and effective therapy. Whereas hyperkalemia can be initially managed using sodium–potassium exchange resins, intravenous glucose–insulin, intravenous calcium, or β agonists, persistent severe hyperkalemia may require acute dialysis therapy. Severe metabolic acidosis may require prompt intravenous alkalinization using bicarbonate, but emergent dialysis is sometimes required when metabolic acidosis is refractory to medical management. Severe hypocalcemia may result as a complication of pigment nephropathy and can worsen with alkalinization. It is important to realize that treatment of hypocalcemia with intravenous calcium compounds can lead to increased metastatic calcifications; it should be reserved for symptomatic patients. Also, careful attention should be given to the severe hypercalcemia that may develop during early renal recovery from pigment nephropathy. Lastly, one should be vigilant for development of compartment syndromes which may be manifest by a secondary rise of CK in serum, persistent and refractory hyperkalemia, or the appearance of irreversible nerve damage. Measurement of tissue pressure and prophylactic treatment by fasciotomy can prevent secondary tissue necrosis.

In summary, myoglobinuria and hemoglobinuria are important, yet frequently reversible causes of acute renal failure. A high index of suspicion along with prompt diagnosis and early institution of volume expansion can limit the severity of these conditions. Renal failure is a serious complication, and aggressive prophylactic measures should be initiated early to avoid significant morbidity from this complication.

Bibliography

Baker SL, Dodds EC: Obstruction of the renal tubules during the excretion of hemoglobin. *Br J Exp Pathol* 6:247–260, 1925.

Baliga R, Ueda N, Walker, PD, *et al.:* Oxidant mechanisms in toxic acute renal failure. *Am J Kidney Dis* 29(3):465–477, 1997.

Better OS: The crush syndrome revisited (1940–1990). *Nephron* 55:97–103, 1990.

Better OS, Rubenstein I, Winaver J: Recent insights into the pathogenesis and early management of the crush syndrome. *Semin Nephrol* 12:217–222, 1992.

Better OS, Stein JH: Early management of shock and prophylaxis of acute renal failure in traumatic rhabdomyolysis. *N Engl J Med* 322:1417–1422, 1991.

Gabow PA, Kaehny WD, Kelleher SP: The spectrum of rhabdomyolysis. *Medicine* 61:141–152, 1982.

Grossman RA, Hamilton RW, Morse BM, *et al.:* Nontraumatic rhabdomyolysis and acute renal failure. *N Engl J Med* 291:807–811, 1974.

Knochel JP: Catastrophic medical events following exhaustive exercise: "white-collar" rhabdomyolysis. *Kidney Int* 38:709–719, 1990.

Knochel JP: Rhabdomyolysis and myoglobinuria. In: Suki WN, Eknoyan G (eds) *The Kidney in Systemic Disease,* 2nd Ed., pp. 263–284. Wiley, New York, 1982.

Nath KA, Balla G, Vercillotti GM, *et al.:* Induction of heme oxygenase is a rapid, protective response in rhabdomyolysis in the rat. *J Clin Invest* 90:267, 1992.

Nath KA, Grande JP, Croatt AJ, *et al.:* Intracellular targets in heme protein induced renal injury. *Kidney Int* 53:100, 1998.

Odeh M: The role of reperfusion-induced injury in the pathogenesis of the crush syndrome. *N Engl J Med* 324:1417–1422, 1991.

Zager RA: Rhabdomyolysis and myohemoglobinuric acute renal failure. *Kidney Int* 49:314–236, 1996.

ACUTE INTERSTITIAL NEPHRITIS

CATHERINE M. MEYERS

Primary interstitial nephropathies comprise a diverse group of diseases that elicit interstitial inflammation associated with renal tubular cell damage. This process typically spares both glomerular and vascular structures. Traditionally, interstitial nephritis has been classified morphologically and clinically into acute and chronic forms. Acute interstitial nephritis (AIN) generally induces rapid deterioration in renal function, and elicits marked interstitial inflammatory responses characterized by interstitial edema with varying degrees of tubular cell damage, as well as mononuclear cell infiltrates consisting primarily of lymphocytes (Fig. 1). Eosinophils, macrophages, plasma cells, and neutrophils may also be apparent within these infiltrates. In some cases of AIN, interstitial granuloma formation is also observed. Most commonly, this form of granulomatous interstitial nephritis is associated with either drug- or infection-induced renal inflammation. By contrast, chronic tubulointerstitial disease follows a more indolent course and is characterized by tubulointerstitial fibrosis

and atrophy, associated with interstitial mononuclear cell infiltration. AIN is not an uncommon cause of renal dysfunction, and should always be considered in the differential diagnosis of acute renal failure (ARF). Moreover, estimates from large clinical studies suggest that AIN comprises approximately 10–15% of reported cases of ARF.

PATHOGENESIS

Despite the varied inciting factors of tubulointerstitial nephritis in humans (Table 1), the striking similarity of induced interstitial lesions, which consist primarily of T-cell lymphocytes, suggests that immune-mediated mechanisms are important either in initiating the interstitial damage or in amplifying primary interstitial injury from nonimmune causes. Studies from experimental models of interstitial disease suggest that both humoral and cell-mediated immune mechanisms are relevant effector pathways for inducing interstitial injury. Cell-mediated events

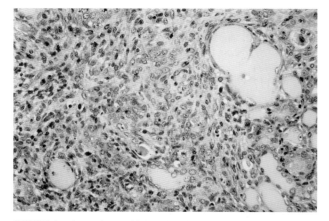

FIGURE I Acute interstitial nephritis. Light microscopic findings demonstrate the loss of normal tubulointerstitial architecture with a dense mononuclear cell infiltrate and some evidence of tubular dilatation and atrophy. Note that the renal tubules are displaced by infiltrating mononuclear cells, edema, and mild interstitial fibrosis (100×).

likely play a prominent role in most forms of human disease, in view of the preponderance of T-cell lymphocytes (CD4$^+$ and CD8$^+$) present within interstitial infiltrates, generally in the absence of antibody deposition. Immunohistochemical studies conducted on biopsies obtained in drug-induced AIN also indicate the importance of cell–cell interactions in intrarenal inflammation, as there is a significant increase in interstitial expression of cellular adhesion molecules. In AIN, increased expression of leukocyte function antigen (LFA)-1 and very late antigen (VLA)-4 cell surface receptors, as well as their respective ligands, intercellular adhesion molecule (ICAM)-1 and vascular cell adhesion molecule (VCAM)-1, is generally observed in areas of mononuclear cell infiltration. Recent studies have extended these observations by examining the role of chemokines, a family of proinflammatory chemotactic mediators, in a number of renal disease mod-

TABLE I
Acute Interstitial Nephritis

Drugs
    Antibiotics (most commonly penicillin analogs, cephalosporins, sulfonamides, and rifampin)
    Nonsteroidal antiinflammatory drugs (NSAIDs)
    Diuretics (most commonly thiazides and furosemide)
Infections
    Direct infection of renal parenchyma
    Associated with a systemic infection
Immunologic disorders
    Systemic lupus erythematosus
    Sjögren's syndrome
    Mixed essential cryoglobulinemia
    Acute allograft rejection
Idiopathic

els associated with marked tubulointerstitial infiltration. RANTES and monocyte chemotactic peptide-1 (MCP-1), chemoattractants for CD4$^+$ T cells and monocytes have been best characterized. Renal expression of RANTES and MCP-1 is markedly upregulated in AIN and correlates directly with the level of monocyte infiltration and interstitial damage. Further support for the cell-mediated hypothesis is also derived from the observation of *in vivo* (delayed-type hypersensitivity responses) and *in vitro* (lymphoblast transformation) activation on repeat exposure to specific inciting agents.

Humorally mediated events may also be important in eliciting some forms of tubulointerstitial injury as occasional patients with drug-induced lesions (rifampin, methicillin, and phenytoin) have revealed IgG and complement deposition along the tubular basement membrane (TBM). Occasional reports of circulating anti-TBM antibodies in such settings have also been reported.

One hypothesis concerning immune recognition of the interstitium suggests that portions of infectious particles or drug molecules may cross-react with or alter endogenous renal antigens. An immune response directed against these inciting agents would theoretically therefore also target the interstitium. Although it is tempting to speculate on the relevance of these cross-reactive antigens in interstitial disease, the nephritogenic potential of such a response has not been tested within an experimental system.

CLINICAL FEATURES

AIN occurs in four distinct clinical settings (Table 1). It may occur as a result of drug therapy, systemic or local infection, as a consequence of immunologic disease, or as an idiopathic lesion without an apparent precipitating cause. AIN is observed in all age groups, however, older patients appear more predisposed to developing ARF. Systemic manifestations of a hypersensitivity reaction, such as fever, rash, and arthralgias, are nonspecific findings that may accompany AIN. In such cases, an erythematous maculopapular rash involves the trunk and proximal extremities. Hypertension and edema are not characteristic of AIN, but have been reported in specific drug-induced lesions. Other nonspecific constitutional symptoms, as well as flank pain with gross hematuria, have been variably reported.

The spectrum of urinary abnormalities (Table 2) consists primarily of microscopic hematuria that at times may be macroscopic, sterile pyuria, and white blood cell casts. Red blood cell casts have also been reported, albeit rarely, in AIN. Eosinophiluria, with greater than 1% of urinary leukocytes positive by Hansel stain is suggestive evidence of AIN, but can be seen in other forms of renal injury and inflammation. In a single-center study, the diagnostic accuracy of eosinophiluria in AIN was examined. Fifty-one patients with various renal diseases, including 15 individuals with a confirmed diagnosis of AIN, were evaluated in this study. The sensitivity of eosinophiluria in this setting was 40% and the specificity was 72%, with a positive predictive value of only 38%. These data illustrate the associ-

TABLE 2
Laboratory Findings in Acute Interstitial Nephritis

Urinary sediment	Erythrocytes, leukocytes (eosinophils), leukocyte casts
Urinary protein excretion	<1 g/day, rarely >1 g/day (NSAIDs)
Fractional excretion of sodium	Usually >1
Proximal tubular defects	Glucosuria, bicarbonaturia, phosphaturia, aminoaciduria, proximal RTA
Distal tubular defects	Hyperkalemia, sodium wasting, distal RTA
Medullary defects	Sodium wasting, urine concentrating defects

ation of eosinophiluria with various morphologic forms of renal inflammation, and demonstrate that it is not a reliable indicator of AIN.

Mild proteinuria, generally less than 1 g/day, is frequently observed in AIN. Nephrotic range proteinuria with acute disease has been reported, however, with nephropathies induced by nonsteroidal antiinflammatory drugs (NSAIDs), and rarely by ampicillin, rifampin, and α-interferon therapy. Serologic studies in AIN, such as anti-DNA antibodies, antinuclear antibodies (ANA), and complement levels, are typically normal, except when AIN occurs in the setting of a systemic autoimmune disorder. Case reports also relate antineutrophil cytoplasmic antibody (ANCA) positivity, a serologic marker for systemic vasculitis, in some patients during the acute phase of interstitial nephritis. Elevated perinuclear (p) ANCA titers have been observed in drug-induced AIN (omeprazole, ciprofloxacin, and cimetidine) and cytoplasmic (c) ANCA in the tubulointerstitial nephritis and uveitis (TINU) syndrome. Of note, two cases of ciprofloxacin-induced AIN also had evidence of necrotizing vasculitis on renal biopsy. The clinical relevance of ANCA titers in AIN is unclear, however, as the overall incidence, antigen specificity, and pathogenicity of these antibodies have not been established.

Urinary fractional excretion of sodium is greater than one in many patients with AIN, but is not a reliable diagnostic indicator. Biochemical abnormalities (Table 2) reflective of the tubular damage induced by the inflammatory process are also observed in these patients. The pattern of tubular dysfunction will vary depending on the principal site of injury. Lesions affecting the proximal tubule result in renal glucosuria, aminoaciduria, phosphaturia, uricosuria, and proximal renal tubular acidosis (type 2 RTA). Distal tubular lesions result in an inability to acidify urine (type 1 RTA), secrete potassium, and regulate sodium balance. Medullary lesions will interfere with maximal urinary concentration and promote polyuria. A considerable degree of overlap in these proximal and distal abnormalities, however, may be apparent clinically. Renal ultrasound in affected patients typically reveals normal or enlarged kid-

neys, depending on the degree of interstitial edema. Renal gallium scanning has been advocated in some centers to distinguish AIN from other causes of ARF, primarily acute tubular necrosis, but this test lacks both sensitivity and specificity. In view of the nonspecific nature of many of these clinical feature of AIN, a definitive diagnosis can therefore only be made through renal biopsy.

CLINICAL COURSE AND THERAPY

The spectrum of renal dysfunction in AIN ranges from mild, self-limited disease to oliguric renal failure requiring dialysis therapy. As this renal lesion is generally reversible, even despite initial severe renal impairment, the overall prognosis is quite favorable. Recovery of renal function may occur over weeks to several months. Some patients have persistent tubular defects and/or residual renal impairment. Progression to end stage renal disease, however, has been reported with all forms of AIN. Moreover, a rapidly progressive fibrosing interstitial nephritis has been described in clusters of patients in weight loss programs who ingested Chinese herbal preparations tainted with nephrotoxic plants (*Aristolochia fangchi*). Renal disease in all affected individuals was irreversible, with many patients requiring dialysis therapy within 1 year of presentation.

Clinical studies suggest that a less favorable prognosis in AIN correlates with extensive interstitial infiltrates, interstitial fibrosis, tubular atrophy, and interstitial granuloma formation on renal biopsy. Other factors that correlate with persistent renal disease are advanced patient age, preexisting renal disease, and a protracted course of oliguric ARF (>3 weeks). In general, chronic renal insufficiency following a bout of AIN is most commonly induced by NSAIDs.

The therapy of AIN consists primarily of supportive measures, after eliminating possible inciting factors such as drugs or infections. Patients with mild renal insufficiency and evidence of recovery of renal function a few days after discontinuing the inciting drug do not require further therapy. The role of corticosteroids in treating more severe cases of AIN has not been clearly elucidated. Rapid improvement and complete recovery of renal function following steroid therapy in several drug-induced lesions, however, have suggested their therapeutic utility in this disorder. Two empirically derived steroid regimens have been employed in drug (primarily antibiotic)-induced AIN, generally when biopsy findings have confirmed the diagnosis. One protocol, for patients with severe renal failure in the setting of AIN, consists of parenteral methylprednisolone (0.5–1.0 g) administration for 1–3 days, followed by daily high-dose oral prednisone (1 mg/kg/day). The other more commonly employed regimen consists of only high-dose daily oral prednisone therapy, or alternate day oral prednisone (2 mg/kg every other day), administered for approximately 4 weeks, with gradual tapering initiated after plasma creatinine levels return to near baseline levels. Anecdotal reports have indicated that steroid unresponsive patients (after 4 weeks of therapy) may respond to cyclophosphamide (2 mg/kg/day). Recognizing that interstitial fibrosis, a lesion unresponsive to current immunotherapy, can begin occurring in AIN as soon as 10–14 days after disease induction, many clinicians are reluctant to expose patients to more potent reagents after steroid treatment failure.

Some clinical investigators have not corroborated the steroid responsiveness of this renal lesion, however, and prospective randomized studies have not been conducted. Steroids are not employed in infection-related AIN, but may be useful in the treatment of nephritogenic responses in systemic immunologic disorders. Although experimental models have suggested a disease-protective role for cyclophosphamide and cyclosporine in interstitial nephritis, similar studies have not been conducted in human disease. Anecdotal reports have also suggested efficacy of adjunctive plasmapheresis therapy, with immunosuppressant therapy, for the rare occurrence of AIN associated with circulating or deposited anti-TBM antibodies.

DISTINCT CAUSES OF ACUTE INTERSTITIAL NEPHRITIS
Drug-Induced Acute Interstitial Nephritis

The list of drugs that reportedly induce AIN is quite extensive (Table 3). Many of these are reports of single cases, however, and have developed in patients exposed to a number of different medications. Drug-induced AIN is a rare idiosyncratic reaction that occurs in a small subset of patients exposed to a particular medication. It is not dose-dependent, and typically recurs on repeat exposure to the same or closely related drug. As seen in Table 3, implicated drugs have diverse chemical structures, although within a class of related drugs, structural similarity can lead to cross-reactive sensitivities. This has been observed particularly with β-lactam drugs, in that penicillin-induced nephropathies have been exacerbated with cephalosporin therapy. A few drugs, most notably penicillins, rifampin, NSAIDs, and sulfonamide derivatives, account for the majority of reported cases of AIN, and their characteristic features will be discussed later.

Penicillins

β-Lactam antibiotics, predominantly penicillins, are the most common cause of drug-induced AIN. The largest number of cases occurred with methicillin, which is no longer used in clinical practice. AIN has been reported with most of the penicillin analogs more routinely prescribed (Table 3), although with much lower incidence than with methicillin. Renal failure in this setting has been observed most commonly in older children and young adults. The classic hypersensitivity triad of fever, rash, and eosinophilia in the setting of ARF may occur in up to 30% of patients with β-lactam-induced AIN. Oliguric renal failure has been reported in approximately 30% of these patients. Clinical studies have suggested a beneficial role for steroids in this patient population, although as previously stated, randomized controlled studies have not been performed. AIN has developed during treatment of a variety of infections, such as endocarditis, osteomyelitis, pneumonia, cellulitis, and abscesses. An underlying infection is clearly not requisite for inducing this reaction, however, as several patients given prophylactic antibiotics have subsequently developed AIN.

NSAIDs

NSAIDs are among the most widely prescribed medications in clinical practice. They mediate a number of adverse renal side effects, largely as a result of their inhibition of renal prostaglandin synthesis, and are extensively discussed in Chapter 40 of this primer. AIN is a less commonly observed side effect of these medications. Propionic acid derivatives appear to cause a disproportionate number of cases (two-thirds of cases have been attributed to fenoprofen, ibuprofen, and naproxen), although AIN has been reported with most NSAIDs currently available (Table 3). Unlike other drug-induced reactions, AIN occurs following long-term exposure to the medication, and has been reported 2 weeks to 18 months after initiating therapy. Patients tend to be nonoliguric females older than 60 years of age, generally lack systemic manifestations of a hypersensitivity reaction, and may present with hypertension, edema, and nephrotic range proteinuria (up to 80% of cases). Interesting histologic features of induced interstitial lesions are the associated minimal change glomerulopathy and occasional interstitial granuloma formation apparent

TABLE 3
Drug-Induced Acute Interstitial Nephritis[a]

Antibiotics
　Penicillin analogs
　　Methicillin, ampicillin, penicillin, nafcillin, carbenicillin, oxacillin, amoxicillin, mezlocillin, flucloxacillin
　Cephalosporins
　　Cephalothin, cefotetan, cephradine, cephalexin, cefoxitin, cefazolin, cefaclor, cefotaxime
　Sulfonamide derivatives
　　Sulfamethoxazole, cotrimoxazole
　Other antibiotics
　　Rifampin, ciprofloxacin, gentamicin, kanamycin, vancomycin, acyclovir, indinavir, aztreonam, erythromycin, azithromycin, ethambutol, tetracyclines, nitrofurantoin

Nonsteroidal antiinflammatory drugs
　Fenoprofen, ibuprofen, naproxen, indomethacin, tolmetin, zomepirac, diflusinal, sulindac, phenylbutazone, aspirin, phenacetin, mefenamic acid, 5-aminosalicylates

Diuretics
　Thiazides, furosemide, triamterene, chlorthalidone

Miscellaneous medications
　Phenytoin, allopurinol, cimetidine, ranitidine, famotidine, phenobarbital, azathioprine, cyclosporine, aldomet, carbamazepine, diazepam, phenylpropanolamine, captopril, clolfibrate, α-interferon, interleukin 2, anti-CD4 monoclonal antibodies, ticlopidine, quinine, propylthiouracil, streptokinase, Chinese herbs, clozapine, phentermine/phendimetrazine, pranlukast

[a]Drugs reported with greatest frequency are shown in italics.

on renal biopsy. Renal disease generally improves after discontinuing the drug, with or without steroid therapy, although chronic renal insufficiency and end stage renal disease are not infrequent complications.

Rifampin

Numerous cases of rifampin-induced AIN have occurred during treatment of tuberculosis. Most of these cases have developed with intermittent therapy or on restarting rifampin after a lapse in uneventful daily therapy. Patients typically complain of flulike symptoms such as fever, chills, malaise, and headache. Unlike other drug-induced lesions, flank pain and hypertension are common in this form of AIN. Moreover, oliguric ARF occurs frequently, and dialysis is required in approximately two-thirds of affected patients. In many cases, this reaction has occurred within hours of a single dose of rifampin. Some patients have developed thrombocytopenia, hemolysis, or abnormalities in liver function in addition to AIN. Histologically, evidence of acute tubular necrosis may be apparent in addition to AIN. In a few cases, an associated proliferative glomerulonephritis has also been observed. Circulating antirifampin antibodies, as well as IgG deposition along the TBM have been reported in some affected patients. As AIN has developed in patients receiving concurrent rifampin and prednisone therapy, there is no evidence to suggest that steroids play a therapeutic role in this disease.

Sulfonamide Derivatives

Drug-induced AIN was first described in the setting of sulfonamide administration. The majority of cases of sulfonamide derivative-induced AIN are reported with combination sulfamethoxazole and trimethoprim therapy. Thiazides and furosemide have also been associated with a few cases of AIN, some of which have developed in patients with preexisting renal disease. The associated hypersensitivity triad of fever, rash, and eosinophilia with renal dysfunction is variably present in affected patients. In addition to the characteristic histologic features of AIN, some biopsies have revealed a predominance of eosinophils within interstitial infiltrates, as well as interstitial granuloma formation. Isolated case reports have suggested beneficial effects of steroid therapy in treating this drug-induced AIN.

Infections Associated with Acute Interstitial Nephritis

AIN was first described in the preantibiotic era in the setting of diphtherial and streptococcal infections. It is now apparent that AIN complicates the clinical course of a number of bacterial, viral, fungal, and parasitic infections, as listed in Table 4. This inflammatory response within the kidney may occur as a result of direct renal infection, that is, pyelonephritis, or as a reaction to a systemic infection. Pyelonephritis, the most common cause of acute infectious interstitial nephritis, typically presents with fever, costovertebral tenderness, dysuria, pyuria, bacteriuria, and leukocytosis. Renal function is unimpaired unless complicated by urinary tract obstruction. Characteristic renal

TABLE 4
Infections Associated with Acute Interstitial Nephritis[a]

Bacterial infections
   Streptococcus, diptheria, brucella, legionella, pneumococcus, *tuberculosis*
Viral Infections
   Epstein-Barr virus, *cytomegalovirus, polyomavirus, Hantaan virus*, measles (rubeola), human immunodeficiency virus, herpes simplex virus type 1
Fungal infections
   Candidiasis, histoplasmosis
Other infections
   Toxoplasmosis, leishmaniasis, schistosomiasis, *Rocky Mountain spotted fever*, ehrlichiosis, malaria, mycoplasma, *leptospirosis*, syphilis, ascaris lumbricoides

[a]Infections associated with direct renal infection are shown in italics.

parenchymal lesions consist of focal areas of neutrophils throughout the interstitium. Pyelonephritis responds well to antibiotic therapy and is discussed more extensively in Chapter 54 of this primer.

Of note, transplant centers have more recently observed human polyoma virus-associated interstitial nephritis occurring in renal allografts. Human polyoma viruses (BK and JC viruses) induce interstitial nephritis in immunosuppressed patients, after reactivation of latent virus in renal epithelium. Histologic features of this lesion are interstitial inflammatory cell infiltration with focal tubular damage, and the typical basophilic or amphophilic intranuclear inclusions. Distinguishing polyoma virus interstitial nephritis from acute rejection is critical in this setting, as therapeutic intervention in these disorders is vastly different. Viral infection-associated graft dysfunction dictates a prudent decrease in immunosuppression, whereas acute rejection indicates more intensive immunosuppression. Further discussion of renal allograft therapeutics can be found in Chapter 68.

In contrast to pyelonephritis, other infection-associated interstitial processes occur in the absence of urinary tract infection. Interstitial infiltrates are frequently perivascular and composed of mononuclear cells, predominantly T-cell lymphocytes. As previously discussed, the pathogenesis of such immune targeting in these infections is not well understood, although cross-reactive determinants may play a role in immune recognition of interstitial structures.

Infection-associated interstitial nephritis is generally transient, and renal function improves with appropriate therapy of the systemic illness, however, chronic progression of renal insufficiency has been reported. Intriguing results of a study examining a series of renal biopsies obtained over 8 years at a single center suggest a prominent role of Epstein-Barr virus (EBV) in cases of chronic interstitial nephritis previously deemed idiopathic. Investigators detected EBV DNA, and its receptor CD21, primarily in proximal tubular cells of all 17 patients with primary idiopathic interstitial nephritis. These findings were not apparent in 10 control renal biopsies. Such observations implicate a more prominent role than previously appreciated for EBV infections in eliciting deleterious cellular immune responses that target the interstitium.

Immune Disorders Associated with Acute Interstitial Nephritis

Although glomerulonephritis is the most common renal manifestation of systemic immunologic disorders, predominant interstitial pathology can be seen in systemic lupus erythematosus, Sjögren's syndrome, and mixed essential cryoglobulinemia. Most affected patients present with nonoliguric renal failure, and biochemical evidence of tubular dysfunction. In addition to the typical pathological features of AIN, biopsies from many of these patients also reveal immune-complex and complement deposition along the TBM, and occasionally within interstitial vessels. Concurrent glomerular pathology may also be apparent. Standard therapeutic modalities in these immunologic disorders consist of corticosteroids and cytotoxic agents. Acute renal allograft rejection, a distinct subset of immunologic disorders, also induces acute interstitial inflammation. These lesions are characterized by marked interstitial mononuclear infiltrates, consisting of recipient T-cell lymphocytes. Allograft rejection is treated with high-dose (pulse) steroids, as well as antibody therapy targeting activated recipient T cells, and is discussed further in Chapter 68 of this primer.

Idiopathic Acute Interstitial Nephritis

In approximately 10–20% of biopsy-proven cases of AIN, no precipitating cause is detected. Systemic manifestations of a hypersensitivity reaction are generally absent in the majority of these idiopathic cases, which often present with nonoliguric renal failure. In accordance with observations previously discussed, one subset of affected patients may have EBV-related interstitial disease. Another subset of these apparently idiopathic lesions, the TINU syndrome, has been described in approximately 40 adolescent or adult females since 1975. Anterior uveitis can precede, accompany, or follow AIN. Bone marrow granuloma formation may be another common feature of this syndrome. Although the cause of TINU syndrome is not known, an autoimmune nature is suggested by occasional positive serologies, such as cANCA, rheumatoid factor, and ANA, in affected patients. A recent report has also revealed that transient hyperthyroidism may be an early feature of TINU syndrome. Both renal and ocular changes typically respond to a brief course of steroid therapy, although a few patients have developed progressive renal disease.

Bibliography

Becker JL, Miller F, Nuovo GJ, et al.: Epstein-Barr virus infection of renal proximal tubule cells: Possible role in chronic interstitial nephritis. J Clin Invest 104:1673–1681, 1999.

Cameron JS: Immunologically mediated interstitial nephritis: Primary and secondary. Adv Nephrol 18:207–248, 1989.

Colvin RB, Fang LST: Interstitial nephritis. In: Tisher CC, Brenner BM, (eds) Renal Pathology with Clinical and Functional Correlations, pp. 728–776. Lippincott, Philadelphia, 1989.

Danoff TM: Chemokines in interstitial injury. Kidney Int 53:1807–1808, 1998.

De Vriese AS, Robbrecht DL, Vanholder RC, et al.: Rifampicin-associated acute renal failure: Pathophysiologic, immunologic, and clinical features. Am J Kidney Dis 31:108–115, 1998.

Dodd S: The pathogenesis of tubulointerstitial disease and mechanisms of fibrosis. Curr Topics Pathol 88:51–67, 1995.

Heptinstall RH: Interstitial nephritis. A brief review. Am J Pathol 83:214–236, 1976.

Kannerstein M: Histologic kidney changes in the common acute infectious diseases. Am J Med Sci 203:65–73, 1942.

Kida H, Abe T, Tomosugi N, et al.: Prediction of the long-term outcome in acute interstitial nephritis. Clin Nephrol 22:55–60, 1984.

Kleinknecht D: Interstitial nephritis, the nephrotic syndrome, and chronic renal failure secondary to nonsteroidal anti-inflammatory drugs. Semin Nephrol 15:228–235, 1995.

Magil AB, Tyler M: Tubulointerstitial disease in lupus nephritis: A morphometric study. Histopathology 8:81–87, 1984.

Markowitz GS, Tartini A, D'Agati VD: Acute interstitial nephritis following treatment with anorectic agents phentermine and phendimetrazine. Clin Nephrol 50:252–254, 1998.

Meyers CM: New insights into the pathogenesis of interstitial nephritis. Curr Opin Nephrol Hypertens 8:287–292, 1999.

Michel DM, Kelly CJ: Acute interstitial nephritis. J Am Soc Nephrol 9:506–15, 1998.

Neilson EG: Pathogenesis and therapy of interstitial nephritis. Kidney Int 35:1257–1270, 1989.

Pusey CD, Saltissi D, Bloodworth L, et al.: Drug associated acute interstitial nephritis: Clinical and pathologic features and the response to high-dose steroid therapy. Q J Med 52:194–211, 1983.

Randhawa PS, Finkelstein S, Scantlebury V, et al.: Human polyoma virus-associated interstitial nephritis in the allograft kidney. Transplantation 67:103–109, 1999.

Ruffing KA, Hoppes P, Blend A, et al.: Eosinophils in urine revisited. Clin Nephrol 41:163–166, 1994.

Shih DF, Korbet SM, Rydel JJ, et al.: Renal vasculitis associated with ciprofloxacin. Am J Kidney Dis 26:516–519, 1995.

Simon AHR, Alves-Filho G, Ribeiro-Alves, MAVF: Acute tubulointerstitial nephritis and uveitis with antineutrophil cytoplasmic antibody. Am J Kidney Dis 28:124–127, 1996.

Vanherweghem JL, Depierreux M, Tielemans C, et al.: Rapidly progressive interstitial renal fibrosis in young women: Association with slimming regimen including Chinese herbs. Lancet 341:387–391, 1993.

MANAGEMENT OF ACUTE RENAL FAILURE

FLORENCE N. HUTCHISON

Morbidity and mortality from acute renal failure (ARF) have improved significantly over past decades due in large part to improved supportive care and early dialysis. Since the kidney usually recovers from an episode of ARF within days or weeks, management of ARF is focused on preventing the consequences of the loss of kidney function and preventing further renal injury. It is important to understand normal kidney function since the symptoms and complications of renal failure derive from the loss of these functions. Homeostasis refers to the process by which the internal body milieu is maintained in a constant state despite marked changes in the external environment and variations in the intake of solute, water, and food. Normal kidney function is critical to the maintenance of volume homeostasis, electrolyte balance, acid–base balance, and for excretion of nitrogenous products of protein metabolism such as urea. Loss of these functions can result in the pulmonary edema, hyperkalemia, acidosis, and uremia which characterize severe renal failure. Although there are numerous causes of ARF, the consequences of ARF can be prevented in most cases by good conservative management, regardless of the etiology.

Therapy for ARF should be initiated as soon as renal injury has been detected. Thus, the first step in management is early recognition that renal failure is present. Because the relationship between serum creatinine concentration and glomerular filtration rate (GFR) is not linear, but hyperbolic, an increase in serum creatinine will not become clinically evident until the GFR is reduced to less than 50 mL/min. Many episodes of ARF with less severe renal dysfunction are not recognized and do not represent clinically significant events. However the relationship between GFR and serum creatinine also implies that *any* increase in serum creatinine above the value previously determined for a given patient represents significant loss of renal function. This point is particularly pertinent in cachectic or elderly patients whose serum creatinine may normally be only 0.8 mg/dL reflecting the smaller amount of creatinine generated from a reduced muscle mass. Although an increase in serum creatinine to 1.5 mg/dL may be within the range of normal values for most clinical laboratories, this represents a significant increase in serum creatinine for these patients and indicates that ARF has occurred. It is also critical to determine the cause of renal dysfunction and to identify reversible causes of renal insufficiency such as prerenal azotemia or urinary tract obstruction. The differential diagnosis of acute renal insufficiency is detailed in Chapter 33.

MANAGEMENT OF VOLUME HOMEOSTASIS

Successful volume homeostasis permits maintenance of a constant internal circulatory and extracellular volume despite variations in water and salt intake and variations in insensible loss of water. The presence of pedal or sacral edema, or overt pulmonary edema in the setting of ARF implies that water and/or salt intake has exceeded the capacity of the injured kidney to excrete the amount of water and salt ingested or admininistered intravenously. This situation can be easily anticipated in the oliguric (<400 mL/day of urine) or anuric (no urine output) patient, but frequently complicates nonoliguric ARF as well.

Most patients with ARF lose the ability to either concentrate or dilute the urine and will excrete a constant volume of urine regardless of fluid intake. Likewise, the ability to excrete a sodium load may be severely curtailed. As a result, urine output and sodium excretion will rarely match spontaneous fluid and salt intake, and either volume overload or volume depletion can result. For example, a patient with acute tubular necrosis whose urine output is fixed at 1200 mL/day who receives parenteral nutrition at a rate of 2000 mL/day along with intravenous antibiotics will gradually develop volume overload and edema unless adjustments are made to the volume of fluid administered. On the other hand, if parenteral nutrition is withheld and he is unable to ingest fluids, urine output will remain at 1200 mL/day, and he will become volume depleted unless parenteral fluids are administered.

Management of volume homeostasis requires that the patient be examined daily to assess the volume status. This is accomplished by measurement of supine and standing blood pressure and pulse to note orthostatic changes suggestive of volume depletion, examination of skin turgor and hydration of mucous membranes, auscultation of the lungs for evidence of pulmonary congestion, a general exam for edema, detailed review of daily input and output records, and accurate measurement of serial daily weight changes.

Each patient with ARF should have a specific individualized prescription for fluid and sodium intake. As a general rule, the patient who is euvolemic on exam should be provided with a volume of fluid equal to daily urine output with an additional 300–500 mL/day to replace insensible water losses. A sodium intake of 2 g/day or less should be prescribed. Patients with increased insensible fluid loss such as those with severe diarrhea and large surface area burns will have a much larger fluid requirement. Because insensible fluid loss cannot be accurately measured, it is imperative that the volume status of the patient be assessed on a daily basis and the fluid prescription modified as necessary. All oral fluid intake as well as intravenous fluids and medications should be included in the patient's fluid prescription. The patient with clinical evidence of volume overload should be restricted to a fluid intake less than the daily urine output. A "fluid restriction" of 1000 mL/day for a patient whose urine output is only 500 mL/day will eventually result in volume overload. A trial of diuretics is worthwhile since some cases of oliguric ARF may be converted to a nonoliguric state. As a rule, nonoliguric ARF has a better prognosis for recovery of renal function than oliguric ARF, and maintenance of a reasonable urine output simplifies fluid management. Low-dose dopamine infusion (0.3 μg/kg/min) has also been advocated to increase urine output in oliguric ARF, but it has not been shown to be efficacious in controlled trials. Patients with clinical evidence of volume depletion should be provided additional volume to achieve a euvolemic state. It should be emphasized that the goal of volume management is to maintain euvolemia. If a patient is allowed to remain hypovolemic because of concern that pulmonary edema might occur, the sustained hypovolemia may worsen renal injury or delay recovery from renal failure. Increased fluid administration may be required during the polyuric recovery phase of ARF.

Hypernatremia and hyponatremia are observed frequently in patients with ARF. Because abnormal serum sodium concentrations are caused by disorders of water metabolism, prevention of hypo- or hypernatremia is linked to volume management. The capacity to modify water excretion is impaired in ARF, as demonstrated by the finding of a persistently isosmotic urine (urine osmolality approximately equal to serum osmolality). Hyponatremia is most common and results from an excess of free water intake relative to solute, whereas hypernatremia results when free water intake is inadequate. Although excessive or deficient oral intake of water can result in hyponatremia or hypernatremia, the most common cause of either disorder in hospitalized patients with ARF is incorrect administration of intravenous fluids. Hypotonic saline solutions are frequently selected to avoid volume overload, but provide a large proportion of electrolyte free water. For example, administering 1000 mL of 0.45% saline (one-half normal saline) is equivalent to giving 500 mL of isotonic (normal) saline and 500 mL of electrolyte free water. In contrast 1000 mL of 0.9% saline is isotonic and provides no electrolyte free water. Most parenteral antibiotics are administered in 5% dextrose in water; their full volume is electrolyte free water. Another source of excess free water intake is from enteral and parenteral feeding solutions, which are formulated with a low sodium concentration. Although prepared enteral solutions may be isosmotic or hypertonic, the solute consists predominantly of carbohydrates and protein that are taken up by cells and

metabolized leaving electrolyte free water behind. Parenteral nutritional solutions are usually hyperosmotic when administered, but again the osmoles consist mainly of dextrose and amino acids which are metabolized leaving a large quantity of solute free water.

The volume of free water required for an individual patient to maintain osmolar balance must be determined empirically and will vary considerably depending on the type and quantity of insensible fluid losses. For example, burn injuries induce large volumes of insensible fluid loss, but the fluid is isosmotic. In contrast, insensible losses from diarrhea and perspiration contain little solute and may dramatically increase the electrolyte free water requirements of the patient. In the absence of abnormally high insensible fluid loss, a patient should be provided either orally or intravenously with 300–500 mL/day of electrolyte free water as part of the total volume prescription. In patients receiving hypotonic enteral nutritional solutions, the serum sodium concentration should be monitored regularly. If it decreases in the absence of volume overload, sodium can be added to the enteral solution as table salt.

In the intensive care unit, clinical assessment of the volume status of a patient may be confounded by surgical wounds, severe pneumonia, or edema due to altered capillary permeability. In this setting, measurements of central venous pressure and pulmonary capillary wedge pressure are important adjuncts to monitor the volume status of the patient. Frequently, these patients are receiving multiple parenteral medications and parenteral nutrition which constitute a large obligatory volume load. Most parenteral medications can be given slowly in a concentrated solution to minimize the volume administered. The parenteral nutrition prescription should be written to provide optimal calories and protein in a minimum volume. Attention should also be given to the solution in which drugs are administered. Most drugs can be administered in normal saline rather than D5W if hyponatremia is a problem.

MANAGEMENT OF ELECTROLYTE HOMEOSTASIS

Hyperkalemia can be a serious consequence of ARF. Normally serum potassium concentration is very tightly regulated by shifts of potassium between the intra- and extracellular compartments. The kidney contributes to overall potassium homeostasis by excreting into the urine the approximately 100 mEq of potassium that is ingested in the average diet so that total body potassium remains constant. Although shifts between intra- and extracellular potassium may contribute to hyperkalemia in ARF, the main cause of hyperkalemia in renal failure is excessive intake of potassium relative to the reduced excretory capacity of the injured kidney.

Prevention of hyperkalemia in the patient with ARF can usually be accomplished by restriction of potassium intake. Because certain types of foods, such as fruits, chocolate, and nuts contain large quantities of potassium, eliminating these foods from the diet is often adequate to prevent hyperkalemia. The potassium content of the diet should be routinely specified for the patient with ARF and typically should be limited to less than 50 mEq/day. Potassium should be omitted from parenteral fluids. It is important not to overlook other nondietary exogenous sources of potassium. These include drugs such as potassium penicillin G, saturated solution of potassium iodide (SSKI), potassium phosphate, dietary additives such as salt substitutes which contain potassium chloride or citrate, and intravenous fluid such as lactated ringers and parenteral nutrition solutions which typically are formulated with potassium chloride or potassium phosphate. Finally, drugs that impair renal potassium excretion, such as potassium sparing diuretics, nonsteroidal anti-inflammatory agents, angiotensin converting enzyme inhibitors, and angiotensin receptor blockers should be avoided.

If dietary restriction of potassium is inadequate to prevent hyperkalemia, potassium binding resins such as sodium polystyrene sulfonate (Kayexalate) can be utilized. The binding resin is usually administered orally as 15–30 g in a solution of 20% sorbitol. It exchanges sodium for potassium in the bowel so that intestinal excretion of potassium can be increased. Potassium binding resins can also be administered rectally as a retention enema. This is particularly valuble if an ileus is present; the time of onset of action will be faster by this route. Although the resins are quite effective in removing potassium, they should not be considered a substitute for dietary potassium restriction. Because sodium is exchanged for potassium, chronic use of these compounds delivers a large sodium load and can worsen volume overload or hypernatremia. Binding resins should never be used orally in patients with intestinal ileus or obstruction due to the possibility of producing or worsening bowel obstruction due to insipation of the resin in the bowel. Diarrhea is a predictable consequence when the binding resin is administered repeatedly with sorbitol and may complicate acidosis by causing intestinal bicarbonate loss. The diarrhea may be intolerable to the patient.

Hyperkalemia that develops despite effective restriction of potassium intake and that cannot be easily corrected with potassium binding resin is an indication for dialysis, but should also be a cue to initiate an investigation for the source of the potassium. If diet or drugs cannot be implicated, one should consider endogenous causes of hyperkalemia such as hyperglycemia and insulinopenia, severe acidosis, hemolysis, rhabdomyolysis, ischemic tissue injury, or other causes of myonecrosis (see Chapter 13). Because potassium lowering therapies, including dialysis, have only a transient effect, appropriate management of hyperkalemia requires identification and specific treatment of the cause of hyperkalemia.

Hypocalcemia frequently complicates ARF, but clinically significant hypocalcemia is rare, as is hypomagnesemia. However, failure to recognize these disorders can produce life-threatening tetany and cardiac arrhythmias. Most reported cases of symptomatic hypocalcemia in patients with ARF have been attributed to hypomagnesemia caused by urinary magnesium wasting in association with cisplatin, amphotericin B, or aminoglycoside antibiotics. Although decreased synthesis of 1,25-dihydroxyvitamin D by the injured kidney may contribute to hypocalcemia by reducing intestinal calcium absorption, hypomagnesemia inhibits

synthesis and release of parathyroid hormone. The resulting functional hypoparathyroidism is a primary mechanism responsible for hypocalcemia. Hypocalcemia may also result as a consequence of transfusion of large quantities of blood products preserved in citrate or as a consequence of phosphorus administration. Prevention and management of this problem can be accomplished by generous supplementation of both electrolytes. Calcium may be supplemented orally, usually 3–4 g/day in divided doses, but symptomatic hypocalcemia should be treated with parenteral calcium. Calcium gluconate and calcium chloride are available as 10% solutions, containing approximately 10 mg/mL and 28 mg/mL, respectively. Either solution should be diluted in saline or 5% dextrose in water and administered slowly through a peripheral vein to avoid cardiac toxicity. Magnesium can be repleted orally as magnesium oxide or parenterally as intramuscular magnesium sulfate, usually 2 g as a single dose.

Phosphorus ingested in the diet and in drugs accumulates in renal failure and may result in hyperphosphatemia. In patients with ARF, this is rarely of clinical consequence except when very high serum phosphorus levels contribute to hypocalcemia, as in rhabdomyolysis, tumor lysis syndrome, and hypercatabolic states. Hyperphosphatemia can be effectively prevented by dietary protein restriction as described subsequently and by oral administration of aluminum hydroxide gels or calcium carbonate or calcium acetate with meals.

MANAGEMENT OF ACID–BASE HOMEOSTASIS

Consumption of a normal American diet by an individual weighing 70 kg produces 60–70 mEq of acid daily which must be excreted by the kidney to maintain normal acid–base balance. Accumulation of these acids in excess of the body's buffering capacity in patients with ARF can produce an anion gap acidosis. However, it is unusual for acidosis to be severe or to occur early in the course of ARF, and acidosis should not be attributed exclusively to ARF until other causes of acidosis such as lactic acidosis or ketoacidosis have been eliminated. The presence of ARF may complicate acidosis of any cause if the kidney is unable to increase acid excretion in response to an acid load or is unable to reclaim bicarbonate filtered into tubular fluid. Acidosis not due specifically to ARF should be treated by removing the source of acid generation or bicarbonate loss as would be done in patients without ARF (see Chapter 9).

Because the majority of the ingested acid load is derived from protein metabolism, dietary protein restriction will slow the development of acidosis in ARF. A diet containing approximately 0.8–1.0 g/kg of body weight of good quality protein usually satisfies the nutritional requirement for protein and minimizes acid production. Administration of protein in excess of metabolic requirements is not beneficial and will worsen uremic symptoms, acidosis, and hyperphosphatemia. Restriction of nonprotein calories may worsen acidosis because body muscle proteins will be catabolized for energy in the absence of other dietary energy sources. Many patients with ARF are anorexic yet have increased caloric requirements due to physiological stress, so inadequate calorie intake is common and should be assessed carefully. The assistance of a skilled dietitian can be invaluble to determine the true calorie and protein requirements of the patient.

If acidosis develops despite dietary protein restriction, or if protein restriction is not desired because of hypercatabolism with sepsis, burn, or a postoperative state, a base equivalent can be administered to buffer the acidosis. Sodium bicarbonate is most commonly used, but sodium acetate can also be used in parenteral solutions. Both compounds have the disadvantage of containing sodium and may worsen volume overload. Bicarbonate can be administered orally as tablets on a regular basis to compensate for continuing acid generation. Parenteral bicarbonate should be administered as an isotonic solution. A solution containing approximately 150 mEq/L can be mixed by adding three ampoules of premixed hypertonic sodium bicarbonate (50 mEq/50 mL) to 1000 mL of 5% dextrose in water. Use of these ampoules which contain 1000 mEq/L sodium bicarbonate without dilution is not recommended unless serum pH is less than 7.1 and then only as a temporizing measure until the cause of the acidosis can be reversed or dialysis initiated since repeated administration will produce hypernatremia. Rapid reversal of acidosis in a patient with hypocalcemia can precipitate tetany.

MANAGEMENT OF UREMIA

Uremia is a syndrome resulting from the accumulation of nitrogenous products of protein metabolism that are normally excreted by the kidney. Early symptoms of uremia are fatigue, lethargy, mental dullness, hiccups, anorexia, and nausea. It may be difficult to determine whether these symptoms are due to ARF or to intercurrent illness. More serious symptoms are myoclonus, confusion, delirium or coma, seizures, and pericarditis. The blood urea nitrogen (BUN) concentration correlates best with symptoms of uremia, but there is considerable variability among patients. As a general rule, few patients have symptoms when the BUN is less than 70 mg/dL, and most patients will experience some symptoms when the BUN is greater than 100 mg/dL.

Because the accumulation of nitrogenous waste products is dependent on dietary protein intake, the degree of loss of renal function, and the duration of renal failure, it is not possible to predict which patients will develop uremic symptoms. In most cases the physican cannot alter either the degree of renal insufficiency or the duration of ARF, and must rely on protein restriction to prevent uremia and on dialysis to ameliorate uremic symptoms. As noted previously, a protein intake of 0.8–1.0 g/kg of body weight is considered the minimum amount adequate to supply nutritional requirements for protein.

NUTRITIONAL MANAGEMENT IN ACUTE RENAL FAILURE

Most episodes of ARF occur as a complication of other serious illness or injury, and studies have clearly demonstrated that adequate nutritional support substantially im-

proves survival in patients in critical care units. Unfortunately, the dietary restrictions required for management of ARF, as well as the anorexia of uremia, may be counterproductive of efforts to optimize nutritional support. For example, very low protein diets (20–40 g protein/day) have been advocated to prevent uremia and avoid dialysis. However, the possible benefits of avoiding short-term dialysis by severe protein restriction must be weighed against the potential increase in morbidity and mortality due to impaired nutrition, and this level of protein restriction is not recommended.

Parenteral nutrition is frequently necessary in seriously ill patients with ARF, but the composition of the parenteral solution must be modified in accordance with the loss of renal function. The *minimum* recommended protein intake in patients with ARF is 0.6–0.8 g/kg of body weight/day and may be considerably higher in very ill hypercatabolic patients. The assistance of an experienced nutritionist to calculate protein catabolic rate and calorie requirements is invalble in estimating actual protein requirements so that excessive or inadequate amino acid administration can be avoided. Carbohydrate and lipid should be maximized with a target of providing 30–35 kcal/kg body weight/day. Provision of adequate carbohydrate and lipid calories will reduce protein requirements and limit symptoms of ARF. Because protein metabolism is the source of endogenous acid generation in renal failure, a base equivalent should be given in an amount adequate to buffer the acid generated from metabolism of the amino acids. Bicarbonate cannot be added to parenteral nutrition solutions without causing precipitation of calcium salts, so sodium acetate is used as a base equivalent. Since approximately 60–80 mEq of acid is generated each day, a similar amount of sodium acetate should be administered on a daily basis. Fluid volume should be limited to the minimum required to deliver adequate caloric intake. The sodium concentration (sodium chloride + sodium acetate) should be adjusted to provide approximately 300–500 mL as electrolyte free water as discussed previously. For example, if a patient is receiving 2000 mL/day of parenteral nutrition, the total sodium concentration should be 100 mEq/L. This is approximately equivalent to 1500 mL of isotonic fluid and 500 mL of free water. If the patient is receiving 1000 mL/day, a sodium concentration of approximately 75 mEq/L will provide the equivalent of 500 mL of isotonic fluid and 500 mL of electrolyte free water. As a rule, potassium, magnesium, and phosphorus should not be added to parenteral nutrition solutions in patients with ARF. If a deficiency of one of these electrolytes exists, it is better to replete that solute specifically than to administer potentially toxic solute on a continuous basis.

DIALYSIS IN ACUTE RENAL FAILURE

In ARF the role of dialysis is to prevent morbidity associated with complications of ARF and provide temporary support until the renal insufficiency resolves. The decision to initiate dialysis and the frequency of dialysis is based on the clinical condition of the patient rather than a particular numerical value of BUN or serum creatinine concentration. Dialysis is indicated in ARF for management of specific problems. Pericarditis and other uremic symptoms can be resolved only with dialysis and are considered absolute indications for dialysis. Other problems, such as volume overload, hyperkalemia, and acidosis are considered relative indications for dialysis; that is, dialysis should be instituted when conservative management has failed or is not practical. For example, an oliguric or anuric patient who requires mechanical ventilation for volume overload pulmonary edema should be dialyzed urgently, because fluid restriction and diuretics will not be effective. The indications for dialysis are summarized in Table 1.

Because dialysis is a temporizing measure in this setting, the dialysis prescription may be considerably different from that typically used for a patient on chronic dialysis. For example, in contrast to the chronic dialysis patient who receives 3 to 4 hr of hemodialysis three times a week, hypercatabolic oliguric intensive care unit patients may require daily dialysis or continuous venovenous ultrafiltration and dialysis (CVVHD) to limit uremic symptoms and to remove the fluid administered daily with parenteral nutrition and medications. Or, a patient who presents with ARF and life-threatening hyperkalemia may require a single dialysis to correct the hyperkalemia and may then be maintained successfully with conservative management. The decision to initiate dialysis must be weighed against the risks associated with large bore dialysis catheter placement and dialysis. Bleeding, infection, and pneumothorax may complicate catheter placement, and dialysis may induce hypotension, mental confusion, and cardiac arrythmias, particularly in unstable critically ill patients.

The details of the dialysis prescription are beyond the scope of this chapter, but it is worthwhile to mention several variations on hemodialysis that are used routinely in patients with ARF. Conventional intermittent hemodialysis is most commonly used. Peritoneal dialysis is also an effective modality for management of ARF and can provide both fluid removal and clearance of solute. Continuous renal replacement therapy, such as CVVHD, may be preferred in patients whose major complication is volume overload, whose medical regimen requires ongoing administration of large volumes of fluid, or whose blood pressure is too unstable to permit hemodialysis. In its simplest form, this procedure provides ultrafiltration only, but variants permit successful diffusive solute clearance (dialysis) as well. It has been proposed that continuous renal replacement therapy might improve the outcome for critically ill patients with ARF by providing more "physiological" control of fluid and electrolyte homeostasis. Unfortunately, the studies performed to date have not demonstrated a difference in morbidity or mortality between continuous therapy and intermittent hemodialysis. The decision to initiate dialysis and the selection of the most appropriate mode of therapy requires the participation of a nephrologist experienced in these procedures. Renal replacement therapies are discussed extensively in Chapters 59 and 60.

TABLE I
Indications for Dialysis

Absolute indications—dialysis is the only possible treatment
  Uremic symptoms
  Uremic pericarditis

Relative indications—dialysis will be required if conservative management of these abnormalities is unlikely to be successful or is contraindicated
  Volume overload
  Hyperkalemia
  Metabolic acidosis
  Other electrolyte abnormalities

TABLE 2
Guidelines to Management of Acute Renal Failure

1. What is the volume status of the patient?
   Normal: Fluid intake = urine output + 300–500 mL/day
            Sodium intake = 2 g/day
   Overloaded: Fluid intake < urine output
            Sodium intake < 2 g/day,
            Try loop diuretic
            Consider dialysis
   Depleted: Restore volume with isotonic saline, then prescribe fluid
            Intake = urine output + 300–500 mL/day
            Sodium intake = 2 g/day

2. Is the patient hyperkalemic?
   No: Potassium intake = 50 mEq/day
   Yes: Look for source of potassium
        Eliminate parenteral potassium
        Reduce dietary potassium intake to < 50 mEq/day
        Potassium binding resin
        Consider dialysis

3. Is the patient acidemic?
   No: Protein intake = 0.8 g/kg/day, 30 kcal/kg/day
   Yes: Look for cause of acidosis
        Reduce protein intake to 0.6 g/kg/day; maintain 30 kcal/kg/day
        Oral bicarbonate or isotonic intravenous bicarbonate
        Consider dialysis

4. Is the patient uremic?
   No: Protein intake = 0.8 g/kg/day, 30 kcal/kg/day
   Yes: Reduce protein intake to 0.6 g/kg/d; maintain 30 kcal/kg/day
        Check for gastrointestinal bleeding
        Consider dialysis

5. Is the patient receiving medication?
   No: Check any new medications for toxicity and adjust doses
   Yes: Stop nephrotoxic drugs
        Adjust medication doses
        Check drug levels

6. Is the nutrition of the patient adequate?
   No: Provide balanced nutrition with 30–35 kcal/kg/day and 0.8–1.0 g/kg/day protein
        Assess need for enteral or parenteral nutrition
   Yes: Reassess periodically

DRUG MANAGEMENT IN ACUTE RENAL FAILURE

Many frequently used drugs are eliminated through the kidney, and doses must be modified in patients with ARF. In the setting of chronic renal failure, the physician can reliably estimate GFR on the basis of the steady state serum creatinine concentration of the patient and make adjustments in drug doses, but this is not the case with ARF. When GFR falls abruptly, the serum creatinine concentration rises as creatinine accumulates in the body until a new steady state level is reached. Thus in ARF, the rate of increase in serum creatinine concentration is a more accurate indicator of the severity of renal failure than the serum creatinine concentration on a given day. Serum creatinine is also dependent on body muscle mass, so an increase of 0.5 mg/dL/day in an elderly patient with reduced muscle mass may indicate that GFR is <10 mL/min, but a similar rate of increase in serum creatinine concentration in a muscular young athlete may indicate that GFR is relatively well preserved at 30–40 mL/min.

A vital component of management of the patient with ARF is a review of all medications to identify those which are excreted in the urine and especially drugs which are toxic at high concentrations, such as digitalis compounds or metformin, or which may cause further renal injury, such as aminoglycoside antibiotics. Compounds containing magnesium and phosphorus are commonly used as antacids and cathartics and can induce hypermagnesemia and hypocalcemia in patients with ARF. Aminoglycoside antibiotics and most vasopressor agents are removed with dialysis, and dosing must be adjusted to compensate for dialytic losses. A variety of texts and handbooks are available which provide modified dosing guidelines for specific drugs for use in patients with renal failure and in dialysis patients. Measurement of creatinine clearance using the average of the serum creatinine concentrations measured before and at the end of the urine collection, and serum drug levels, are also critical adjuncts to appropriate management. Drug prescribing in renal failure is further discussed in Chapter 41.

Table 2 is a checklist providing guidelines for basic management of the patient with ARF. Good management requires early recognition of renal failure, anticipation and prevention of potential problems, and ongoing evaluation of the clinical condition of the patient.

Bibliography

Bellomo R, Cole L, Ronco C: Hemodynamic support and the role of dopamine. *Kidney Int* 53(Suppl 66):S71–S74, 1998.

Denton MA, Chertow GM, Brady HR: "Renal-dose" dopamine for the treatment of acute renal failure: Scientific rationale, experimental studies and clinical trials. *Kidney Int* 49:4–14, 1996.

Feld LG, Cachero S, Springate JE: Fluid needs in acute renal failure. *Pediatr Clin North Am* 37:337–350, 1990.

Gentric A, Cledes J: Immediate and long-term prognosis in acute renal failure in the elderly. *Nephrol Dial Transplant* 6:86–90, 1991.

Joy MS, Matzke GR, Armstrong DK, Marx MA, Zarowitz BJ: A primer on continuous renal replacement therapy for critically ill patients. *Ann Pharmacother* 32:362–375, 1998.

Kierdorf H: Continuous versus intermittent treatment: Clinical results in acute renal failure. In: Siebert HG, Mann H, Stummvoll HK (eds) Continuous hemofiltration. *Contrib. Nephrol.*, Vol. 93, pp. 1–12, 1991.

Leverve X, Barnoud D: Stress metabolism and nutritional support in acute renal failure. *Kidney Int* 53(Suppl 66):S62–S66, 1998.

Manian FA, Stone WJ, Alford RH: Adverse antibiotic effects associated with renal insufficiency. *Rev Infect Dis* 12:236–249, 1990.

Norton DF, Franklin SS: Acute renal failure in the critical care setting. *Acute Care* 13:127–156, 1987.

Pascual J, Orofino L, Liano F, Marcen R, Naya MT, Orte L, Ortuno J: Incidence and prognosis of acute renal failure in older patients. *J Am Geriatr Soc* 38:25–30, 1990.

Schetz M, Lauwers PM, Ferdinande P: Extracorporeal treatment of acute renal failure in the intensive care unit: A critical view. *Intensive Care Med* 15:349–357, 1989.

Schneeweiss B, Graninger W, Stockenhuber F, Druml W, Ferenci P, Eichinger S, Grimm G, Laggnert A, Lenz K: Energy metabolism in acute and chronic renal failure. *Am J Clin Nutr* 52:596–601, 1990.

Schrier RW, Gardenschwartz MH, Burke TJ: Acute renal failure: Pathogenesis, diagnosis, and management. *Adv Nephrol* 10:213–240, 1981.

Speigel DM, Ullian ME, Zerbe GO, Berl T: Determinants of survival and recovery in acute renal failure patients dialyzed in intensive-care units. *Am J Nephrol* 11:44–47, 1991.

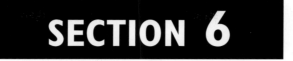

SECTION 6

DRUGS AND THE KIDNEY

40

ANALGESICS AND THE KIDNEY

VARDAMAN M. BUCKALEW, JR. AND RICHARD G. APPEL

The American public consumes billions of doses of over-the-counter (OTC) and prescription analgesics each year. These consist primarily of drugs from two distinct classes: aspirin and other nonsteroidal antiinflammatory drugs (NSAIDs), and acetaminophen and other non-narcotic analgesics. These analgesics are of interest to nephrologists because they are associated with adverse events involving the kidney. Although the absolute event rate is probably low, the renal effects of these drugs are important because of the large numbers of individuals exposed to them.

Adverse renal events fall into two categories: (1) those that occur acutely in individuals taking NSAIDs, and, (2) analgesic nephropathy (AN), a chronic renal disease that occurs in individuals who consume analgesics habitually. It is also possible that chronic analgesic consumption may increase the risk of chronic renal disease due to nephrosclerosis, diabetic nephropathy, and glomerulonephritis. In this chapter, we will discuss the epidemiology, pathophysiology, diagnosis, and treatment of these adverse events.

ACUTE EFFECTS FROM NONSTEROIDAL ANTIINFLAMMATORY DRUGS

Acute Renal Failure

Epidemiology

The incidence and prevalence of acute renal failure due to NSAIDs is not well documented. Available estimates vary widely depending on the methodology used, the setting in which the study was done, and the population observed. According to a study that relied on a data base from a large health maintenance organization in which more than 100,000 outpatients were exposed to NSAIDs over an 11-year period, no patient was hospitalized because of a documented renal complication from NSAID use. Although the methodology used in this study would not have detected adverse events treated without hospitalization, these results must indicate a very low overall rate of acute renal failure or any other serious complication, at least in this urban, largely middle-class population.

The incidence of acute renal failure in two hospital populations was 13 and 18%. In a city hospital that serves primarily an indigent population, acute renal failure occurred in 343 of 1908 inpatients (18%) receiving ibuprofen. In most patients, there was a clinically insignificant rise in serum creatinine, and the incidence of severe acute renal failure was only 0.9%. Furthermore, acute renal failure was no more likely to occur in patients given NSAIDs than in a control group given only acetaminophen. In a multivariate analysis, the only risk factors for NSAID associated acute renal failure were age greater than 65, and coronary artery disease. In a study of an elderly population (mean age 87 years) 15 of 114 patients (13%) given NSAIDs developed a greater than 50% increase in serum urea nitrogen level (but no change in serum creatinine) which was reversible on stopping the drug. Multivariate analysis showed that concomitant use of loop diuretics and higher doses of drug correlated with acute renal failure.

Mechanism

Decreased Renal Blood Flow. The most common type of NSAID-induced acute renal failure is due to decreased synthesis of renal vasodilator prostaglandins (PGs), PGE_2 and PGI_2, leading to decreased renal blood flow and glomerular filtration rate (GFR). Renal blood flow is not dependent on these PGs in normal individuals. However, renal blood flow becomes dependent on their intrarenal production in several clinical states, making individuals with these states susceptible to NSAID-induced acute renal failure (Table 1).

In volume depletion, including decreased effective volume in generalized edema, traumatic or septic shock, and general anesthesia, increased PG synthesis is probably stimulated by the renal vasoconstrictor effects of sympathetic nervous system and renin–angiotensin system activation. The stimulus for PG production is not so clear when renal mass is reduced, as occurs in renal transplantation and other renal diseases. Thus, patients with renal disease of any etiology may develop NSAID-induced renal failure. Those with immune mediated glomerulonephritis and urinary obstruction may be particularly susceptible. In these conditions, increased production of vasodilatory PGs may minimize the effects of intrarenally generated vasoconstrictors such as thromboxane and endothelin.

The well-known decrease in renal blood flow and GFR with age may underlie the increased susceptibility of the elderly to this condition. Other factors that have not yet been identified may also be responsible. The association of NSAID-induced acute renal failure with diuretic use may be related to the edema states for which these drugs are used, or to their ability to stimulate vasodilator PG production. Triamterene may be a more potent stimulator of

TABLE I
Predisposing Factors for NSAID-Induced Hemodynamic
Acute Renal Failure

Decreased effective blood volume
    Congestive heart failure
    Cirrhosis
    Nephrotic syndrome
    Anesthesia
    Shock

Decreased absolute blood volume
    Hemorrhage
    Sodium and water depletion

Chronic renal failure

Acute renal failure due to contrast and obstruction

Drugs
    Diuretics
    Cyclosporine

Advanced age

Renal transplantation

vasodilator PG production than other diuretics, and its use with NSAIDs is not recommended. Cyclosporine increases urinary excretion of vasodilator PGs, probably because of its renal vasoconstrictor effect. As a result, the drug increases the risk of NSAID-induced acute renal failure in both renal and heart transplant patients. In the absence of cyclosporine use, adverse effects of NSAIDs in the setting of renal transplantation may be similar to any setting with reduced renal mass.

In most cases of hemodynamic acute renal failure, the decrease in renal blood flow is purely functional, and recovery is rapid on stopping the drug. In some cases, however, renal biopsy has demonstrated histologic changes of acute tubular necrosis. Its presence may delay recovery.

Interstitial Nephritis and Nephrotic Syndrome. Interstitial nephritis, which appears to be an idiosyncratic reaction particularly to the propionic acid derivatives (ibuprofen, naproxen, fenoprofen), is associated with the nephrotic syndrome in about 90% of cases. In contrast to acute interstitial nephritis (AIN) associated with other drugs, NSAID-induced AIN is associated with a low incidence of hypersensitivity symptoms, eosinophilia, and eosinophiluria and exhibits a predominance of lymphocytes rather than eosinophils in the renal interstitium. The latter phenomenon may explain why nephrotic syndrome is seen almost exclusively with NSAID-induced AIN, because the glomerular lesion is thought to be due to inflammatory mediators such as leukotrienes produced by the interstitial lymphocytes.

In patients with the nephrotic syndrome, minimal change disease is usually found on renal biopsy. A few cases of minimal change glomerulopathy without interstitial nephritis have been observed after long-term (>3 months) use of NSAIDs. This entity has been reported with propionic acid and indoleacetic acid derivatives.

Causative Agents

Several chemical classes of NSAIDs are available in oral form. At this time, only aspirin and the propionic acid derivatives are available OTC (ibuprofen, naproxen, and ketoprofen). All NSAIDs, including aspirin, can potentially cause acute, hemodynamic acute renal failure. The likelihood of an individual drug causing acute renal failure is related to its potential for inhibiting renal PG synthesis. Of the commonly used agents, indomethacin is the most potent, and aspirin the least. All the others are intermediate. Some studies have suggested that sulindac, an indoleacetic acid derivative, may have some renal sparing feature. This drug does have a unique metabolism, in that the active metabolite formed from the prodrug is inactivated by an intrarenal enzyme system. The renal sparing effect of sulindac, if it exists, is not absolute, however, and cases of acute renal failure have been reported. This has been explained as being due to individual differences in the rate at which the metabolite is inactivated, or to high plasma levels of this metabolite which may occur after 10 days of therapy in patients with renal failure.

Selective COX-2 Inhibitors. The antiinflammatory effect of NSAIDs is due mainly to inhibition of the enzyme cyclooxygenase (COX). Two COX isoforms have been identified, COX-1 and COX-2. Most NSAIDs block both COX isoforms. Recently, selective COX-2 inhibitors have become available. No large clinical trials have compared the adverse renal effects of selective COX-2 inhibitors versus older NSAIDs, but renal toxicity has occurred. In this regard, more recent studies indicate that renal medullary interstitial cells constitutively express COX-2 which is important in cell survival. COX-2 inhibition *in vitro* was associated with renal medullary interstitial cell death. Furthermore, upregulation of COX-2 expression in the kidney during sodium and fluid depletion provides additional evidence that the selective COX-2 inhibitors may contribute to NSAID-associated renal injury.

Alterations in Electrolyte and Water Excretion

NSAIDs may cause several alterations in water and electrolyte excretion. These effects are due either directly or indirectly to inhibition of PG synthesis.

Sodium Excretion
PGE_2 and PGI_2 increase renal sodium excretion by a variety of mechanisms, including renal vasodilation and direct inhibition of tubular sodium reabsorption. It is not surprising, therefore, that inhibition of PG synthesis by NSAIDs causes decreased renal sodium excretion. This effect, however, is relatively minor, and is not often clinically significant. Because most diuretics stimulate vasodilator PG production, NSAIDs may interfere with the natriuretic effect of diuretics in both edema states and in hypertension. In the latter, the effect may cause blood pressure to be a few mm Hg higher than usual.

Potassium Excretion

PGE_2 and PGI_2 increase renin release by a direct action on the juxtaglomerular cells. Consequently, NSAIDs have been reported to cause hyperkalemia by inducing hyporeninemic hypoaldosteronism. A secondary mechanism may be a decrease in sodium delivery to the distal tubule and a decrease in urine flow. Risk factors include renal failure, preexisting hypoaldosteronism, advanced age, and the concomitant use of drugs that interfere with potassium excretion such as potassium sparing diuretics and angiotensin converting enzyme inhibitors.

Water Excretion

PGE_2 facilitates water excretion by decreasing Na^+ reabsorption in the loop of Henle, and by inhibiting the hydroosmotic effect of vasopressin. Accordingly, NSAID administration may interfere with water excretion, leading to hyponatremia. Too few cases have been reported to identify the risk factors for this rare complication with certainty. However, two groups which may be at risk are the elderly and infants treated with NSAIDs for patent ductus arteriosus.

Management

In patients presenting with any of these conditions, NSAIDs should be suspected as an etiologic agent. It is important to remember that these drugs may be used either as self-medication or by prescription. The index of suspicion should be especially high in the high-risk groups, particularly the elderly and those with preexisting renal disease, congestive heart failure, and hepatic cirrhosis. A history of use of drugs known to increase the risk of NSAID complications should be sought. Individuals with predisposing factors should be discouraged from taking NSAIDs. Patients known to be taking NSAIDs regularly, especially those with increased risk and those taking large doses, should have their renal function checked frequently. The drugs should be discontinued with the appearance of any of these conditions. Concomitant use of NSAIDs and an orally active PGE_1 analog, misoprostal, has been reported to blunt the decrease in renal blood flow in some patients with renal failure. Misoprostal has also been shown to reduce the renal vasoconstrictor effects of cyclosporine and could reduce the risk of NSAID-induced acute renal failure in transplantation. However, the place of this drug in the long-term management of these conditions has not yet been determined.

Acute renal failure from hemodynamic factors should be differentiated from that due to interstitial nephritis. This can usually be done with a urinalysis, because 90% of those with the latter have heavy proteinuria. Acute renal failure due to hemodynamic factors should reverse rapidly, usually within 3 to 5 days. Occasionally, recovery is delayed by the development of acute tubular necrosis, a condition which may be suspected on the basis of the typical urinary sediment. Recovery will also be slow when acute renal failure is due to interstitial nephritis. Steroids have been reported to improve this condition, but it may also remit spontaneously. No guidelines have yet been developed for steroid use. Renal biopsy may be indicated in patients whose renal failure does not respond quickly to cessation of the drug.

ANALGESIC NEPHROPATHY

It can be argued that the discipline of renal epidemiology began with the studies in the early 1950s of the association between regular consumption of analgesics mixtures and chronic renal failure. These studies, first reported in 1953 in Swiss watchmakers, suggested that the daily ingestion of analgesics containing aspirin and phenacetin caused a syndrome of chronic renal failure due to what was then called chronic pyelonephritis and which today we call chronic tubulointerstitial nephropathy. Later, an association was noted between the habitual use of phenacetin and the development of urinary tract malignancies. Over the intervening 40 years, the literature on (AN) has expanded such that today there is general agreement among nephrologists and epidemiologists about its major features. When the major offending agent was shown to be phenacetin, this popular analgesic was removed from the market in most countries around the world. Despite this attempt to prevent AN, it continues to be a problem even in countries where phenacetin is no longer available, including the United States. This suggests that phenacetin was not the sole cause of the condition and that the spectrum of the disease may be changing, and indicates the need for further investigations and perhaps additional public health measures. In this regard, a National Analgesic Nephropathy Study supported by the National Institutes of Health has been initiated. The objectives of this study are: to determine whether noncontrasted computerized tomography (CT) can be used to identify cases of AN; to determine which analgesics, including combination analgesics, and what dosage and duration of exposure, are associated with the development of AN; to determine the incidence and prevalence of AN as a cause of end stage renal disease (ESRD) in the United States; and to determine the relation of analgesic use to the *de novo* onset of chronic renal failure in general.

Epidemiology

Numerous studies from many countries have documented the existence of a population of individuals who habitually use OTC analgesics for self-diagnosed indications including headache, arthritis, backache, as a sleep aid, and because they just do not feel well. Estimates of the prevalence of habitual analgesic consumption, defined as daily ingestion for at least 1 year, vary widely geographically from as low as 2% to as high as 30%. Highest prevalences are found in industrial workers and hospital patients, with the lowest being found in community-based populations. Within these populations, women are more likely to be habitual users than men.

The type of preparations available for OTC consumption vary with time and location. In the United States, two major changes have been made in the makeup of OTC

TABLE 2
Estimated Prevalence of Habitual Use of Individual Analgesics
in the United States

	1978–1979 (%)	1980–1982 (%)	1991 (%)
Aspirin	55	38	39
NSAIDs	0	22	23
Acetaminophen	19	20	38
Phenacetin	26	20	0

analgesics: phenacetin was removed from the market in late 1983; and the first nonaspirin NSAID, ibuprofen, became available in 1984. These alterations have caused the estimated prevalence of drugs used by habitual consumers to change (Table 2). The prevalence of aspirin use has declined, but total NSAID use (aspirin plus nonaspirin NSAIDs) has actually risen slightly. In addition, the increment in acetaminophen use is almost equal to the prevalence of phenacetin use when it was available.

The relative risk, or odds ratio, of developing either chronic renal failure (CRF) or ESRD in habitual users of analgesics varied between 2.4 and 8 in eight studies spanning the period 1969 to 1992, when the makeup of OTC analgesic preparations was changing. In six of these eight, the risk of CRF or ESRD from individual analgesics could be estimated; phenacetin in five, acetaminophen in three, aspirin in three, and nonaspirin NSAIDs in two (Table 3).

All of these formal epidemiological studies are compromised to some extent by several methodological problems, the most serious of which is "confounding by indication." The association between analgesic use and renal disease could be, at least in part, due to use of analgesics to relieve symptoms caused by renal disease. This problem is closely related to the issue of time order. To document a causal association between exposure to analgesics and renal disease, exposure must be shown to precede onset of disease. Since none of the studies published to date have attempted to deal with this problem, these studies do not distinguish

TABLE 3
Risk of Renal Disease from Individual Analgesics

Drug	Relative risk[a]	
	ESRD	Chronic renal failure
Phenacetin	2.66–19.05 (n = 5)[b]	5.11–8.1 (n = 2)
Acetaminophen	2.1–4.06 (n = 2)	3.21
Aspirin	1.0–2.5 (n = 2)	1.3
NSAIDs	1.0	2.1

[a]All risks greater than 1.3, adjusted for use of other analgesics, are statistically significant except one study in the phenacetin group with a risk of 4.

[b]n = number of studies, if >1.

between the ability of analgesics to cause a specific disease entity, AN, versus their possible effect to accelerate the rate of progression of other chronic renal diseases such as hypertensive nephrosclerosis, diabetic nephropathy, and glomerulonephritis.

Despite their shortcomings, the published studies suggest the following tentative conclusions. First, habitual acetaminophen use may increase the risk of renal disease at a total dose no higher than for phenacetin, but the risk appears to be somewhat less. Second, habitual NSAID use may increase the risk of renal disease, especially in the elderly, but the threshold dose is much higher than that for acetaminophen. Third, the risk of renal disease from habitual aspirin use, if any, may be lower than for either acetaminophen or nonaspirin NSAIDs.

An epidemiological study of AN from Europe suggests that AN occurs only in individuals consuming analgesic mixtures. Based on this and other evidence, the National Kidney Foundation recommended in a recent position paper that analgesic mixtures be made available by prescription only.

The hypothesis that only analgesic mixtures cause renal disease may explain the apparent lower risk of acetaminophen compared to phenacetin (noted earlier). Thus, phenacetin was always marketed as a mixture with other analgesics, usually aspirin plus caffeine, whereas acetaminophen is available both as a single agent and in mixtures with aspirin and other agents. Although the risks calculated from case control studies have been adjusted statistically for the use of other drugs, the question of whether habitual use of single analgesics increases risk of renal disease has not been answered.

The incidence and prevalence of AN in the dialysis population is reported periodically in ESRD registries in Europe, Australia, and now in the United States. In Europe, the average incidence of new cases starting dialysis was 2% in 1990, down from 3% in 1981. However, the rate, although declining, remains high in Switzerland (12%) and Belgium (11%). In Australia, the 1992 rate was 9%, down from over 20% in the early 1970s. The United States Renal Data System (USRDS) indicates that in the period 1993–1997, the diagnosis of AN was made in 0.2% of new dialysis patients, a lower rate than the 0.8% reported in the period 1989–1993. The USRDS does not publish data on geographic variation; however, past reports indicated that AN was more common in the Southeastern United States by a factor of about five. Some of the variability in the reported prevalence of AN may be due to geographical variation, and also to an underdiagnosis or an imprecision in making the diagnosis of AN by nephrologists.

In the United States, AN causing ESRD occurs more commonly in females (63.9%) than males (36.1%). Unlike the major causes of ESRD in the United States, AN is not as significantly over represented in African-Americans (76.9% White, 18.7% African-American).

There are very few estimates of the incidence and prevalence of AN in the population of patients with chronic renal failure not on dialysis. During the phenacetin era in the 1970s, two studies estimated that 7% (in Philadelphia) and

13% (in northwest North Carolina) of patients with chronic renal failure had AN. It is likely that this figure is lower now than 20 years ago.

Pathogenesis

Concepts of the pathogenesis of AN are based primarily on studies in animal models. The results of studies in which single analgesics and various combinations have been fed to rats have, however, been somewhat controversial. In many cases, very large doses have been required to cause renal lesions. In general, combinations of analgesics, especially those that include aspirin, have been more nephrotoxic than single agents. Unlike usuals in humans, aspirin is the most nephrotoxic of all analgesics studied in the rat. Most studies agree that dehydration increases the nephrotoxicity of these agents.

Chronic interstitial inflammation and papillary necrosis are the primary lesions of AN. This is probably due to concentration of the offending agents, especially acetaminophen and salicylates by the countercurrent mechanism. Acetaminophen is metabolized to toxic oxygen radicals by cytochrome P450 mixed function oxidases located in the renal cortex and outer medulla and by prostaglandin endoperoxidase synthases in the renal papilla. Aspirin potentiates the toxicity of these radicals by depleting the kidney of reduced glutathione necessary for their detoxification.

A second proposed mechanism invokes a decrease in renal papillary blood flow in patients consuming analgesics containing aspirin or other NSAIDs which could inhibit renal PG production. In addition, a papillary microangiopathy of unknown pathogenesis has been demonstrated in autopsy studies. It could interfere with the papillary circulation. A lipofuscin pigment in many tissues has been described in autopsies of humans dying with AN. This pigment thought to be an oxidized polymer of unsaturated fatty acids that probably arises from the effect of acetaminophen derived radicals. The role of this pigment in the pathogenesis of AN is not known.

Caffeine is present in many of the analgesic combinations taken by patients with AN. However, its role in the pathogenesis of AN is not known. Most speculation has centered on the possibility that caffeine increases analgesic consumption by causing "caffeine withdrawal" headaches. However, caffeine may also play a role in the nephrotoxicity of acetaminophen as an adenosine antagonist. Adenosine diminishes the transport-associated respiration in the medullary thick ascending limb. Cell necrosis by oxygen radicals might be enhanced if respiration were stimulated by adenosine antagonism.

Urinary tract malignancies have been attributed most often to the N-hydroxylation metabolites of phenacetin which may act directly or indirectly as carcinogens in a urinary tract damaged by analgesics. Since acetaminophen is also metabolized to potential carcinogens, it is not clear why the risk of urinary tract malignancies has been associated to date only with habitual use of phenacetin and not acetaminophen.

The Clinical Syndrome

History and Physical Examination

The clinical syndrome of AN now results from the use of compounds containing or combining acetaminophen (the major metabolite of phenacetin), aspirin, NSAIDs, caffeine, or codeine. The diagnosis of AN is suggested in subjects with chronic renal failure of unknown etiology and a history of daily consumption of analgesic preparations. The key to making the diagnosis is obtaining an accurate history of the type and amount of analgesics consumed. As many as one-third of the patients with AN will deny consuming analgesics, and even those who admit taking them may underestimate the amount taken.

The typical patient with AN is a woman older than 30 with pain, anemia, personality disorders, and gastrointestinal complaints. The pain is usually due to headache or dyspepsia. The anemia, which may be out of proportion to the degree of renal failure, is usually secondary to gastrointestinal bleeding or methemoglobinemia. The best approach is to question the patient about chronic pain such as headache, backache, arthritis, sinus problems, or abdominal pain. Patients are usually willing to describe the pain in great detail and give their favorite analgesic preparation. However, they may be reluctant to disclose how much analgesics they take for the problem. Family members are helpful in determining the amount ingested and determining the total dose of analgesics consumed.

A dose–response relation is evident in most work on AN. The risks associated with phenacetin steadily increased in those who consumed at least 2 kg. Detailed analysis revealed a dose-dependent increase in renal disease after 0.5 to 1.0 kg of analgesic substances in combination (including acetaminophen, aspirin, and/or caffeine-containing drugs). This is equivalent to taking four tablets or powders daily containing 300 mg of analgesics for 3 years. The data regarding single analgesic agents are less clear.

The findings on physical examination in patients with AN are nonspecific. Some investigators have noted a typical personality type in women with this syndrome. They may be excessively dependent and passive–aggressive with a low threshold for pain and features of hypochondriasis. It has also been noted that women with this syndrome appear to be prematurely aged. Generalized atherosclerosis may be found, since this condition may occur with increased frequency in patients with AN compared to patients with other types of renal disease.

Laboratory Findings and Diagnosis

The laboratory findings may be typically those of chronic tubulointerstitial nephritis. Renal functional abnormalities include varying degrees of renal insufficiency, pyuria with/without urinary tract infection, hematuria, proteinuria (<3 g daily), impaired urinary concentrating capacity, urinary acidification defects with serum electrolyte patterns suggestive of renal tubular acidosis, impaired sodium conservation, and hypertension. When the syndrome was caused by phenacetin, an anemia out of proportion to the degree of renal failure was frequently seen. This may not be observed in the syndrome caused by other analgesics.

Are there specific diagnostic criteria for AN? Imaging of the kidney may show a decrease in renal length combined with irregular, bumpy contours of both kidneys. Renal papillary necrosis may be manifest as renal medullary calcification, and this finding has resulted in a positive predictive value of 92%. Other findings such as hypertension, anemia, renal calcifications, sterile pyuria, bacteriuria, and proteinuria, were not sufficiently sensitive or specific enough to be clearly predictive of AN. Renal contours may be difficult to discern on ultrasound in patients with advanced renal disease because of increased echogenicity. Furthermore, it is difficult to precisely localize renal calcium deposits on ultrasound, and papillary calcifications may be incorrectly diagnosed as vascular calcifications or renal calculi. A European study explored the use of computed tomography without contrast to evaluate renal size, contour, and calcifications in subjects with AN.

Renal size was measured as the sum of both sides of a rectangle enclosing the kidney at the level of the renal vessels. Renal volume was considered decreased if this sum was less than 103 mm in males and 96 mm in females. Renal contour was considered bumpy if three or more indentations were observed at the level where the most number of indentations were identified. Calcifications were localized as cortical, papillary, or central. The combination of reduced renal size and either bumpy contours or renal medullary calcification had a sensitivity and specificity of 90% for AN in patients with ESRD and 87% and 100%, respectively, in CRF without ESRD. These findings are illustrated in Fig. 1 which shows CT scans without contrast in two patients with CRF and a history of habitual analgesic ingestion.

Renal papillary necrosis and interstitial nephritis are considered the major pathologic hallmarks of AN. Occasionally, a patient may actually pass a papilla in the urine. The necrosed papillary tissue can calcify and/or slough into

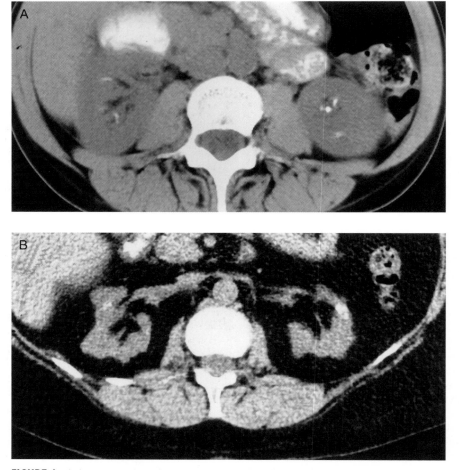

FIGURE 1   (A) CT scan without contrast in a 42-year-old female with a 20-year history of daily analgesic use for headache. Medullary calcifications are prominent without bumpy contours. (B) CT scan without contrast in a 56-year-old female with a 35-year history of habitual analgesic use for headaches. Bumpy renal contours and medullary calcifications are apparent. Renal volume was 61.3 mm on right and 59.2 mm on left (see text).

TABLE 4
Diagnostic Criteria for AN

Major
  History of regular analgesic consumption >1 year, totaling at
    least 1–2 kg
  Small, bumpy kidneys and renal calcification on ultrasound
  Decreased renal volume, bumpy contours and medullary
    calcification on CT without contrast
  Radiologic signs of papillary necrosis
Minor
  Chronic pain syndrome
  History of peptic ulcer disease
  Chronic tubulointerstitial nephritis
  Sterile pyuria
  Bacteriuria

the collecting system, sometimes causing urinary tract obstruction and sometimes mimicking urolithiasis. An increased incidence of renal parenchymal, pelvic, and ureteral carcinoma has been documented in AN. However, this was probably due to phenacetin and may no longer be observed.

Criteria for diagnosing AN, divided into major and minor categories, are summarized in Table 4. A high index of suspicion is indicated in those with CRF or ESRD of unknown etiology and two or three minor criteria, especially if there is a history of a chronic pain syndrome and peptic ulcer disease. Although always inferential, the diagnosis is indicated with a high degree of certainty if two or more major criteria are present, especially if accompanied by some of the minor criteria. In some cases, the diagnosis of AN can only be suspected when the patient has a chronic pain syndrome but denies heavy analgesic consumption.

Treatment

As in patients with renal failure from any cause, treatment of patients with AN should be directed toward slowing or preventing progression, including strict control of blood pressure, dietary protein restriction, and avoidance of nephrotoxic agents. Patients with AN may develop acute papillary necrosis, urinary tract infections, or kidney stones. Therefore, other important management issues include adequate fluid intake, treatment of urinary tract infection, and prevention or alleviation of urinary tract obstruction.

Many patients with AN have chronic pain syndromes and will continue to use analgesics despite advice to the contrary. It is important for nephrologists to monitor the type and amount of analgesics consumed by all patients with chronic renal failure, especially those with AN, and those with other diagnoses whose failure is progressing. Every effort should be made to use single agent analgesic preparations rather than mixtures or combinations. Habitual use of acetaminophen and all NSAIDs should be avoided, although acetaminophen may be used episodically.

One longitudinal study of 57 patients with AN followed for 7 to 150 months showed the progression rate of renal failure was more rapid in 13 patients who continued regular use of analgesics containing acetaminophen or phenacetin than in 44 patients who did not. Although NSAIDs clearly have been shown to reduce GFR of patients with renal failure of any type, and can cause papillary necrosis, there are no data showing that regular use of NSAIDs increases the progression rate of renal failure. Aspirin taken alone may be the safest analgesic in these patients, but strict avoidance of analgesics combining aspirin and acetaminophen is mandatory.

Bibliography

Bennett WM, DeBroe ME: Analgesic nephropathy—a preventable renal disease. *N Engl J Med* 320(19):1269–1271, 1989.

Buckalew VM, Schey HM: Renal disease from habitual antipyretic analgesic consumption: An assessment of the epidemiologic evidence. *Medicine* 11(1):291–303, 1986.

Clive DM, Stoff JS: Renal syndromes associated with nonsteroidal antiinflammatory drugs. *N Engl J Med* 310:563–572, 1984.

Elseviers MM, De Broe ME: Analgesic nephropathy in Belgium is related to the sales of particular analgesic mixtures. *Nephrol Dial Transplant* 9:41–46, 1994.

Elseviers MM, De Broe ME: A long-term prospective study of analgesic abuse in Belgium. *Kidney Int* 48:1912–1919, 1995.

Elseviers MM, De Schepper A, Corthouts R, et al.: High diagnostic performance of CT scan for analgesic nephropathy in patients with incipient to severe renal failure. *Kidney Int* 48:1316–1323, 1995.

Gonwa TA, Corbett WT, Schey HM, Buckalew VM: Analgesic-associated nephropathy and transitional cell carcinoma of the urinary tract. *Ann Intern Med* 93:249–252, 1980.

Henrich WL (ed): Analgesic nephropathy. *Am J Kidney Dis* 28 (Suppl 1):S1–S70, 1996.

Klag MJ, Whelton PK, Perneger TV: Analgesics and chronic renal disease. *Curr Opin Nephrol Hypertens* 5:236–241, 1996.

McLaughlin JK, Lipworth L, Chow W-H, Blot WJ: Analgesic use and chronic renal failure: A critical review of the epidemiologic literature. *Kidney Int* 54:679–686, 1998.

Murray MD, Brater DC, Tierney WM, et al.: Ibuprofen-associated renal impairment in a large general internal medicine practice. *Am J Med Sci* 299:222–229, 1990.

Palmer BF: Renal complications associated with use of nonsteroidal anti-inflammatory agents. *J Invest Med* 43:516–533, 1995.

Perneger TV, Whelton PK, Klag MJ: Risk of kidney failure associated with the use of acetaminophen, aspirin, and nonsteroidal antiinflammatory drugs. *N Engl J Med* 331:1675–1679, 1994.

Sandler DP, Smith JC, Weinberg CR, et al.: Analgesic use and chronic renal failure. *N Engl J Med* 320:1238–1243, 1989.

Sandler DP, Burr R, Weinberg CR: Nonsteroidal anti-inflammatory drugs and the risk for chronic renal failure. *Ann Intern Med* 115(3):165–172, 1991.

Schwarz A, Kunzendorf U, Keller F, Offermann G: Progression of renal failure in analgesic-associated nephropathy. *Nephron* 53:244–249, 1989.

U.S. Renal Data System, USRDS 1999 Annual Data Report, National Institutes of Health, National Institute of Diabetes and Digestive and Kidney Diseases, Bethesda, Maryland, April 1999.

41

DRUG PRESCRIBING IN PATIENTS WITH RENAL FAILURE

WILLIAM M. BENNETT

Patients with renal insufficiency, either acute or chronic, require many pharmaceutical agents to treat a variety of comorbid conditions. Epidemiologic studies have shown that the presence of renal insufficiency per se is a major risk factor for adverse drug reactions since most drugs and chemicals or their metabolites are ultimately excreted by the kidney. When these substances are retained in a patient with renal failure, adverse reactions frequently occur unless dosing adjustments are made. Patients with renal failure are complex; this is magnified by their comorbid diseases such as diabetes, cardiovascular disease, and systemic hypertension. Patient with end stage renal disease (ESRD) on dialysis have the additional factor of the dialysis therapy itself which may remove drugs and chemicals from the body thereby influencing drug pharmacokinetics. This chapter will attempt to elucidate the underlying principles for drug prescribing. Specific recommendations for individual patients are beyond its scope.

GENERAL PRINCIPLES OF DRUG KINETICS

An overall scheme of drug pharmacokinetics is illustrated in Fig. 1. Most drugs are absorbed from the gastrointestinal tract or given parenterally to reach the systemic circulation. Orally administered drugs may be extracted by the liver during their first pass through the portal circulation. The percentage of an orally administered drug that reaches the systemic circulation is the bioavailability of the drug. Once drugs reach the systemic circulation they are bound to plasma proteins, primarily albumin. Renal failure is known to decrease drug protein binding, and patients with renal disease often have low serum albumins as well. The free drug concentration represents the pharmacologically active drug that interacts with tissue receptors. Although there are other minor routes of drug elimination, drug elimination by the kidneys and metabolism by the liver are the two primary routes of drug elimination from the body. Both can be influenced by the presence of renal insufficiency.

PHARMACOKINETIC CHANGES IN RENAL FAILURE

There is a characteristic volume of distribution for most drugs which is the ratio of the dose to the resultant plasma concentration:

$$V_d = \frac{\text{dose}}{\text{blood concentration}}.$$

This apparent volume of distribution does not correspond to a specific anatomical space but is a mathematical construct relating the amount of drug in the body to its corresponding plasma concentration. The volume of distribution for some drugs may be altered by the presence of renal disease. Volume expansion, volume contraction, and plasma protein concentrations are all determinants. Furthermore, renal disease can influence drug absorption and metabolism. Uremia may also influence absorption and thus bioavailability because of nausea with vomiting. Vomiting reduces mucosal contact time for drug absorption. Phosphate binders and other medications may form nonabsorpable complexes with drugs and limit absorption. The ability of the liver to extract drugs from portal blood in renal disease may be impaired, resulting in increased bioavailability. An example of this phenomenon is seen with the β-blocker, propranolol. Thus, it is difficult to make generalizations about absorption, distribution, and bioavailability for individual drugs in renal failure since patients and their physiologic circumstances differ.

Elimination is usually expressed in terms of clearance, which equals the volume of blood or plasma from which a drug is cleared per unit time. This depends on the blood flow to the organ of elimination, in this case the kidney. Total body clearance of the drug equals the drug dose divided by the area under the drug concentration curve. For the kidney, this is the familiar clearance expression:

$$\text{Renal drug clearance} = \frac{\text{urine volume} \times \text{urine drug concentration}}{\text{plasma drug concentration}}.$$

For patients on dialysis, the total clearance of the drug must also reflect the effect of extracorporeal treatment on drug elimination. Drug half-life describes the rate of drug removal from the body and is independent of the drug dose. The two parameters, namely, clearance and half-life, are related by the formula

$$t_{1/2} = \frac{V_d \times e}{\text{Cl}},$$

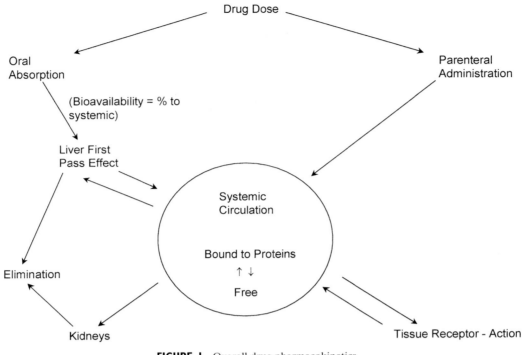

FIGURE I Overall drug pharmacokinetics.

where e is the natural logarithm of 2, or 0.693. If the volume of distribution increases, the half-life increases. If renal clearance is decreased, as by renal failure, half-life increases. Often, increased extrarenal elimination of drugs compensates for the decreased renal clearance in patients with advanced renal failure.

Because only free or unbound drug is pharmacologically active, disease states which reduce the plasma protein binding of drugs may cause pharmacologic effects. In kidney failure, binding of acidic drugs is decreased because of renal retention of binding inhibitors. If protein binding is reduced, the pharmacologic effects of a drug may be seen at lower plasma levels if such levels measure total (bound + unbound) drug. Decreased protein binding may increase the volume distribution of drugs as previously mentioned. Table 1 shows the representative plasma protein binding of various drugs in renal failure categorized by whether they are net acids or bases in body fluids. Sometimes, an increase in metabolism of free drug compensates for the larger V_d leaving $t_{1/2}$ unchanged.

Some drugs have pharmacologically active metabolites that can accumulate in renal failure and cause adverse drug effects (Table 2). Examples of this phenomenon are normeperidine, a metabolite of meperidine which can cause seizures and N-acetyl procainamide, a metabolite of procainamide which has antiarrhythmic properties independent of the parent drug. Hepatic metabolism may be decreased or increased in patients with renal disease, but in sick patients with multiorgan failure hepatic metabolism may be decreased, with impaired liver blood flow resulting in magnification of the tendency for adverse drug reactions. The major pharmacokinetic parameters that determine drug action in patients with renal disease and their implications for drug dosing are summarized in Table 3.

In addition to excretion, the kidney also has a role in drug metabolism. With diminishing kidney function, the renal metabolism of drugs decreases. The prime example of this is exogenous insulin, which is extensively metabolized in the proximal tubular cells of the kidney. With decreasing renal function the insulin requirement for many diabetic patients decreases due to lessened insulin metabolism by the kidney.

TABLE I

Plasma Protein Binding of Drugs in Renal Failure[a]

Acidic drugs	Binding	Basic drugs	Binding
Barbiturates	D	Dapsone	N
Benzylpenicillin	D	Desmethylimipramine	N
Clofibrate	D	Diazepam	D
Dicloxacillin	D	Morphine	D
Furosemide	D	Propranolol	N
Indomethacin	N	Quinidine	N
Phenytoin	D	Triamterene	D
Salicylate	D	Trimethoprim	N
Warfarin	D		

[a]D, decreased; N, normal.

TABLE 2

Example of Parent Compounds and Their Pharmacologically or Toxicologically Active Metabolites

Parent drug	Metabolite	Metabolite activity
Allopurinol	Oxypurinol	Inhibitor of xanthine oxidase
Azathioprine	6-Mercaptopurine	Immunosuppressant
Cephalothin	Desacetylcephalothin	Antibacterial potency 50% of parent compound
Chlordiazepoxide	Oxazepam	Anxiolytic
Clofibrate	Chlorophenoxyisobutyric acid	Hypolipidemic with direct muscle toxicity
Daunorubicin	Daunorubicinol	Cytotoxic
Diazepam	Oxazepam	Anxiolytic
Doxorubicin	Doxorubicinol	Cytotoxic
Meperidine	Normeperidine	Lowers seizure threshold; psychotic changes
Procainamide	N-Acetylprocainamide	Class III antiarrhythmic with possible cardiac toxicity
Propoxyphene	Norpropoxyphene	Narcotic analgesic
Propranolol	4-Hydroxypropranolol	β-Receptor antagonist
Rifampin	Desacetylrifampin	Antimicrobial activity
Sulfadiazine	Acetylsulfadiazie	Nausea, vomiting, rash

Thus the effect of decreased renal function on drug pharmacokinetics can be summarized as follows:

1. Drugs usually excreted by the kidney accumulate.
2. Pharmacologically active drug metabolites that require kidney function for excretion accumulate.
3. Drug distribution changes due to decreased plasma protein binding, low serum proteins, or altered volume of distribution.
4. Renal drug metabolism decreases.

These pharmacologic effects, if not taken into account by the prescribing physician, explain the high incidence of adverse drug reactions in renal patients.

TABLE 3

Effect of Renal Disease on Pharmacokinetic[a] and Pharmacodynamic[b] Variables

Variable	Effect	Examples
Absorption	Decrease in uremia	Edema of gastrointestinal tract Uremic nausea and vomiting Autonomic neuropathy (diabetes, uremia) Peritonitis with reduced peristalsis Drug interactions (phosphate binders)
Distribution	Higher plasma free fraction of drugs in uremia Lower drug concentrations of total drug Loss of binding proteins	Acidic drugs with usual binding greater than 80% Lower "therapeutic" levels of phenytoin Nephrotic syndrome, malnutrition
Metabolism	Decreased rate of metabolism Accelerated drug oxidation Decreased hepatic first-pass effect Decreased renal drug metabolism	Mycophenolate mofetil Induced cytochrome P450 metabolism of phenytoin Propranolol Decreased 1,25-dihydroxyvitamin D hydroxylation Decreased insulin metabolism
Excretion	Decreased excretion of parent drug Decreased excretion of active metabolities	Aminoglycosides, antibiotics Meperidine, morphine
Increased tissue drug sensitivity	Altered drug distribution at tissue receptor sites Metabolic effects of renal disease	Central nervous system drugs Acidemia, hyperkalemia affects cardiac drugs
Altered metabolic loads	Hyperkalemia Hypermagnesemia Sodium loads Nitrogen Impaired water excretion	Salt substitutes, K+ sparing diuretics, B-blockers, ACE inhibitors Antacids, laxatives Antibiotics (penicillins) Steroids, tetracyclines Narcotics, NSAIDs

[a]Mathematical description of drug transit through the body.
[b]The pharmacologic effects of a drug.

DOSIMETRY OF DRUGS IN RENAL FAILURE PATIENTS

The goal of therapy in patients with varying degrees of renal insufficiency is to avoid drug accumulation and therefore toxicities, while maintaining drug efficacy. No simple formula ensures this outcome because of the presence of multiple comorbid conditions, the use of multiple therapeutic agents simultaneously, the potential for drug interactions, and the individual variability of these extremely sick patients. Thus, physicians should go through several steps when prescribing for a patient with renal disease. The best clinicians use their own knowledge and judgement about their individual patients as well as an appreciation of the pharmacology of the prescribed drugs to come to the optimum dosing regimen.

The first step in prescribing for a patient with renal disease is to ascertain the level of renal function. It is customary to express it as the percentage of normal renal function. In a patient with renal disease, the most convenient measurement is the serum creatinine, however, the serum creatinine is particularly insensitive in the elderly patient (see Chapter 3). It is affected by noncreatinine chromogens which accumulate in renal failure. The renal secretion of creatinine is also inhibited by some drugs such as trimethoprim or cimetidine. Furthermore, the relative contribution of creatinine secretion increases as renal function falls making it even less reliable as a marker of glomerular filtration rate (GFR) in severe renal failure. In the absence of an actual measured creatinine clearance, the Cockroft–Gault equation is a very useful estimate of renal function:

$$\text{Estimated } C_{cr} = \frac{(140 - \text{age})(\text{BW in kg})}{72(S_{cr})}.$$

The product is multiplied by 0.85 if the patient is female. It can be made more precise by using the lean body weight for males at 50 kg plus 2.3 kg for each inch over 5 feet and for females 45.5 kg plus 2.3 kg for each inch over 5 feet. Because normal renal function approximates 100 mL/min the formula provides a value that is approximately equal to the percentage of normal renal function demonstrated by the patient. Although useful for the purpose of calculating drug dosing this percentage is only an approximation of renal function and not equal to GFR. It is less reliable with patients who have marked edema or are markedly obese. Furthermore, the formula does not apply to children. In patients with acute renal failure, who have a stable impairment in renal function an accurate 24-hr urine collection should be obtained to assess renal function appropriately and to develop individualized dosing regimens to avoid pharmacologic errors. An isolated serum creatinine value is not reflective of GFR when the creatinine is rising rapidly; for practical dosing purposes it is fair to assume that the GFR is less than 10 mL/min in patients with oliguric acute renal failure.

The next step is to choose the loading dose of the drug. Since the steady state plasma concentration of the drug is usually achieved only after four to five half-lives it may be necessary to give a loading dose if a drug has a long half-life. In a patient with renal dysfunction this loading dose achieves the necessary plasma concentration more rapidly. In most emergency conditions, drugs are administered intravenously to assure that therapeutic drug concentrations are achieved, and usually the loading dose is given as a single dose. In patients with renal dysfunction, the loading dose is usually very similar to the dose used in patients with normal renal function. Loading doses can be calculated if the desired plasma concentration is known:

$$\text{Loading dose} = \text{desired plasma concentration} \times V_d.$$

Use of this formula will requires knowledge of the usual volume of distribution as well as any modifications required because of individual patient factors.

The next step, choosing a maintenance dose for an individual patient, is difficult. Dose adjustment is usually not required in patients with creatinine clearances greater than 50 mL/min or in patients with greater than 50% of normal renal function. For drugs with narrow therapeutic windows or great fluctuations between peak and trough concentrations, dosage adjustment and therapeutic monitoring may be required even with lesser degrees of renal dysfunction. This applies to elderly patients in particular. Maintenance doses are given to sustain the therapeutic plasma concentration after the loading dose. Two different methods may be used to prescribe the maintenance dose: dosage reduction or interval extension. Dosage reduction is usually preferred for drugs with a narrow range between toxic and therapeutic blood levels (low therapeutic index) and disease states that require relatively constant plasma drug concentrations. This is usually the case for antiarrhythmics and anticonvulsants. Interval extension is most useful for agents with long half-lives or for agents associated with toxicities when peak or trough dose levels are exceeded.

In selecting an individual maintenance dosage, the clinician should first decide on the appropriate dose regimen for the patient assuming that renal function were normal. Next, the fraction of drug and pharmacologically active metabolites excreted unchanged by the kidney should be estimated. From this information, a dose adjustment factor can be calculated by taking into account the ratio of the half-life of the drug in the patient to the half-life of the drug in the normal person. This dosage adjusting factor can be used in one of two ways after considering which is most appropriate for an individual drug and patient. The clinician can either divide the dose that is determined for normal renal function by the dosage adjustment factor and continue with the same dosage interval or else continue with the same drug dose but multiply the dosage interval for normal renal function by the dosage adjustment factor. Sometimes these two strategies can be combined. The validity of the dosage adjustment factor depends on a variety of assumptions, including first order pharmacokinetics in the therapeutic range for the drug metabolites and a lack of activity or toxicity of drug metabolites. There must be no difference in the absorption, distribution, and metabolism of the drug in normal and renal failure patients and no change in sensitivity to the drug. Finally, this estimate requires both a fixed relationship assumed between creatinine clearance and the renal elimination of the drug and that renal function be at a relative steady state. To the extent that these assumption are not true, dosimetry may be inaccurate. The dosage adjustment factor is simply an approximation, and each patient must be evaluated individually.

Drug level monitoring should be used when the drug has toxic effects that are serious and which appear at blood levels close to the therapeutic window. Monitoring should only be used when therapeutic endpoints and biologic endpoints are not easily ascertained, since drug level is only a surrogate for the biologic responses. For example, blood levels of antihypertensives and anticoagulants are unnecessary as these drugs are titrated to effect. In patients on chronic drug therapy, drug level monitoring is needed for drugs which demonstrate marked differences in response in individual patients and to exclude drug noncompliance. In clinical practice, drug concentrations are subject to misinterpretation when the timing of the sample in relationship to the dosing of the drug is unknown.

Knowledge of drug–drug interactions and how some drugs can affect the pharmacokinetics and pharmacodynamics of often drugs are particularly important for nephrologists who deal with patients who take many medications concurrents. For example, cytochrome P450 enzymes which are present through the gastrointestinal tract, kidney, and liver play an important role in the metabolism of many exogenous drugs. Cyclosporine is metabolized primarily through the cytochrome P450 3A4 enzyme subfamily. Phenytoin and rifampin induce cytochrome P450, increase the clearance of cyclosporine, and thereby increase the risk of acute rejection. Ketoconazole, deltiozem, and erythromycin may decrease the elimination of cyclosporine and therefore increase the risk of nephrotoxicity. Another type of important interaction is the one resulting from the ability of phosphate binding antacids to impair absorption of drugs such as digoxin, quinoline, antibiotics, and tetracycline.

DOSAGE ADJUSTMENT IN DIALYSIS

The degree to which a drug is removed via dialysis determines whether a supplemental dose is needed. Drug clearance during peritoneal dialysis is usually much lower than hemodialysis primarily due to a substantially reduced dialysate flow rate.

Drug Dosing in Hemodialysis

The amount of drug removed by hemodialysis is approximately equal to the product of drug concentration in the dialysate and the dialysate volume. This value divided by the total body stores of the drug prior to dialysis (product of predialysis serum concentration and volume of distribution) yields the actual fraction of drug removed by dialysis (FDR). In addition, some drugs are adsorbed by dialysis membranes; the eliminated drug will not be reflected in the dialysate concentration. In any event, meas-

TABLE 4
Factors That Increase Dialyzability in Hemodialysis

Drug properties
  Molecular mass <500 Da
  High water solubility
  Small volume of distribution
  No erythrocyte partitioning
  Low nonrenal elimination
Dialysis properties
  Membrane composition and charge
  Large membrane surface area (e.g., high efficiency)
  Large membrane pore size (e.g., high flux)
  High dialysate flow rate or volume
  High blood flow rate

urement of dialysate drug concentrations is not practical in the clinical setting.

Patients may require postdialytic or even interdialytic dosing when the maintenance of serum concentrations within a narrow range is necessary (e.g., anticonvulsants, antiarrhythmics). Accurate information on the dialysis kinetics of drugs is not always readily available. Most clinicians use the guidelines for drug dosing available from the product package insert or standard references. When such recommendations are absent or inadequate, the clinician must use knowledge of certain properties of the drug and the dialysis procedure to make an educated guess regarding how much of the drug has been removed. Factors that favor significant dialysis removal of drugs are listed in Table 4. Water-soluble drugs with molecular weights less than 500 Da and low plasma–protein binding can be expected to be removed by dialysis. The charge characteristics of some drugs favor their adsorption to the hemodialysis membrane (e.g., aminoglycosides binding to polyacrylonitrile membrane). Drugs with smaller V_d are distributed mostly in the intravascular space and hence are more likely to be available for removal by dialysis. Conversely, drugs which partition to the erythrocytes (e.g., cyclosporine) are less available for dialysis removal. Perhaps the two most important dialyzer-related properties for drug removal are membrane pore size and surface area. The use of larger-pore (i.e., high-flux) and/or larger surface-area (i.e., high-efficiency) dialysis membranes increases the dialyzability of drugs. High-flux membranes may remove compounds with molecular masses ranging up to 20,000 Da. As a result, drugs that are not dialyzed by low-flux dialysis membranes will be dialyzed when high-flux membranes are employed. For example, vancomycin (molecular mass, 1442 Da) which has a $t_{1/2}$ of 180 hr with low-flux, low-efficiency dialysis membranes, has a $t_{1/2}$ of 56 hr with high-flux, high-efficiency membranes.

Drugs that are efficiently removed by hemodialysis are administered postdialysis in amounts approximately equal to the amount lost during dialysis. For example, if during a typical hemodialysis session approximately half of the total body amount of a drug is removed, then a dose equal to 50% of the maintenance dose will be required postdialysis. These data on FDR after a typical dialysis session are available from reference sources or they can be assumed based on known drug characteristics.

Drug Dosing in Continuous Ambulatory Peritoneal Dialysis

Factors that increase drug removal by peritoneal dialysis include a low molecular weight, low protein binding, a small V_d, a rapid rate of equilibration between tissue binding sites and blood, and a limited amount of nonrenal metabolism and excretion. As a general rule, if the amount of drug removed by daily peritoneal dialysis is greater than 20–30% of the administered dose, larger doses must be administered. Because of their low clearance by continuous ambulatory peritoneal dialysis (CAPD), in most drugs do not require a dosing regimen different from those for a nondialyzed patient. Drugs with a high V_d, high nonrenal clearance, or high plasma protein binding are not cleared to any significant extent by CAPD.

Pharmacokinetics of Intraperitoneally Administered Drugs

In patients on CAPD, intraperitoneal administration of drugs is the preferred route in some clinical situations: (1) for the administration of antibiotics in patients with CAPD-related peritonitis; and (2) for the administration of insulin. The intraperitoneal administration of a low-molecular-weight drug, such as most antibiotics, rapidly achieves a high local drug concentration within the peritoneal cavity. This concentration gradient leads to rapid diffusion of the drug from the peritoneal cavity into the systemic circulation. The reverse movement from the systemic circulation into the peritoneal cavity is much slower and restricted. As a result, intraperitoneal antibiotics used in the treatment of peritonitis (e.g., aminoglycosides, cephalosporins) are 50 to 80% bioavailable during a 6-hr dwell period. During bouts of peritonitis, the permeability of the peritoneal membrane increases, and as a result, both the rate and extent of intraperitoneal absorption of certain drugs (e.g., vancomycin, gentamicin, various β-lactam antibiotics) increases and remains so for days after the peritonitis episode.

Drug Dosing in Continuous Renal Replacement Therapy

A number of options are available for continuous renal replacement therapy (CRRT) (see Chapter 59.). With continuous hemofiltration techniques such as continuous arteriovenous hemofiltration, or continuous venovenous hemofiltration, dialysate is not reemployed and solute removal occurs exclusively via ultrafiltration (i.e., convective movement). Continuous arteriovenous hemodiafiltration and continuous venovenous hemodiafiltration rely on diffusion as well as convective clearance. As compared to standard hemodialysis, solute clearance per unit time

may be lower during CRRT; however, due to its continuous nature, the overall clearance may be higher. For example, urea clearance during CRRT may be only 15 to 30 mL/min, versus approximately 200 mL/min for intermittent hemodialysis; however, because CRRT occurs 24 hrs/day, the overall weekly clearance of urea for CRRT is 150–300 L versus 90–100 L for intermittent hemodialysis. Most CRRT hemofilters use the same membrane as high-flux hemodialysis filters, and remove molecules with molecular masses of 5000 to 20,000 Da; hence, the molecular weight of the drug is usually not a rate-limiting factor for drug removal. As with hemodialysis, however, highly protein-bound drugs are not significantly removed by CRRT.

Limited data are available for drug dosing in CRRT. Also, the available values in the literature recommend dosing alterations based on a variety of different blood flow settings, filter types, and ultrafiltration rates, which may not be applicable to a specific patient. Because patients who receive CRRT are critically ill, drug dosing adjustments must be made with utmost care. When available, plasma or blood concentrations of drugs should be obtained and monitored, especially for drugs with a narrow therapeutic index (e.g., aminoglycosides, antiarrhythmics). When specific dosing guidelines are unavailable, the amount of drug removed can be estimated from the drug's sieving coefficient (Si). The sieving coefficient of a substance is the relationship between drug concentration in the ultrafiltrate (C_{uf}) and the average drug concentration in the plasma or serum, as calculated from arterial (C_A) and venous (C_V) concentrations, and describes the ability of a drug to pass from the systemic circulation to the ultrafiltrate:

$$Si = \frac{C_{uf}}{(C_A + C_V)/2} = \frac{2C_{uf}}{C_A + C_V}.$$

Si values near 1.0 indicate free drug movement across the membrane, whereas Si values near 0 indicate complete lack of drug movement to the ultrafiltrate. Drugs with a high Si value include aminoglycosides, vancomycin, and some cephalosporins. If no data on Si are available, then the extent of the drug's plasma protein binding can provide a rough estimate, since there is a good correlation between unbound drug (f_u) and Si. Ideally, values for f_u from patients with acute renal failure should be used. If not available, data from with ESRD may be used.

Supplemental dosing may be required during CRRT, if the ratio of extracorporeal clearance to endogenous clearance is greater than 0.25. These data are available in the literature or may be assumed based on known pharmacology of the drug in question.

CONCLUSION

Drug prescribing for patients with renal failure, in particular those with end stage renal disease is difficult. Knowledge of the particular patient and an understanding of pharmacokinetic alterations in renal disease are essential for safe, effective prescribing.

Bibliography

Verpooten GA, Bennett WM: Practical dosing. In: DeBroe ME, Porter GA, Bennett WM, Verpooten GA (eds) *Clinical Nephrotoxins,* pp. 469–478. Kluwer Academic Publishers, Dordrecht, The Netherlands, 1998.

Bennett WM: Guide to drug dosing in renal failure. In: Holford (ed) *Drug Data Handbook,* pp. 49–112. ADIS, Auckland, New Zealand, 1998.

Aronoff GR, Berns JS, Brier ME, Golper TA, Morrison G, Singer I, Swan SK, Bennett WM: *Drug Prescribing in Renal Failure,* 4th Ed., American College of Physicians, Philadelphia, 1999.

Olyaei A, Bennett WM: The effect of renal failure on drug handling. In: Webb AR, Shapiro MJ, Singer M, Suter PM (eds) *Oxford Textbook of Critical Care,* pp. 423–429. Oxford Univ. Press, Oxford, 1999.

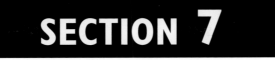

SECTION 7

HEREDITARY RENAL DISORDERS

42

SICKLE CELL NEPHROPATHY

ANTONIO GUASCH

The sickle hemoglobinopathies are caused by the homozygous (Hb SS disease) or heterozygous (Hb AS or sickle cell trait) inheritance of the sickle β globin gene. The substitution of valine for glutamic acid at the 6 position of the β-chain of hemoglobin leads to production of an unstable isoform which, when slowly deoxygenated, can polymerize, leading to the production of sickle cells. These cells lack the fluidity of normal erythrocytes and can impede or block capillary flow. Tissue ischemia results. Other hemoglobin variants (Hb C, D, E, or β thalassemia) may coexist with sickle cell anemia (SCA), producing double heterozygosity. In the United States sickle cell trait occurs in about 8% of individuals of African-American origin, and SS disease is present in about 1 in 500 African-American newborns.

Because of the low pO_2 in the renal medullary interstitium, the kidney is one of the sites vulnerable to vaso-occlusive events. Renal involvement in SCA is very common and is summarized in Table 1.

RENAL HEMODYNAMIC CHANGES

Children with SCA have a high glomerular filtration rate (GFR) (glomerular hyperfiltration) and high renal plasma and blood flows (renal hyperperfusion), both consequences of renal vasodilation. A marked glomerular hypertrophy, present histologically in individuals with no clinical disease, also contributes to the glomerular hyperfiltration. The hypertrophy can be observed in individuals as young as 2 years of age. The elevated GFR is presumed to be a compensation for hypoxia. The supernormal GFR returns to "normal" values after the second or third decade, but renal blood flow rates continue to be higher than in healthy individuals. The mechanisms mediating the renal vasodilation are not known, but some evidence supports a role for vasodilatory prostaglandins or enhanced activity of the nitric oxide system. Treatment of SCA patients with a dose of indomethacin that does not affect GFR or renal plasma flow in normal individuals normalizes GFR and decreases renal plasma flow toward but not completely to normal.

BLOOD PRESSURE IN SICKLE CELL ANEMIA

Despite a higher prevalence of hypertension in the African-American population, hypertension is uncommon in SCA. Blood pressure values are, on average, 5–15 mm Hg lower in SS patients than in healthy African-Americans matched for age and gender, probably as a consequence of a low systemic vascular resistance. However, SCA individuals with blood pressure values higher than the ninetieth percentile of the blood pressure distribution for the SCA population have a higher mortality than other SCA individuals due to an increase in vascular events. In patients with SS disease, this increase in mortality occurs when blood pressure values are higher than 130/84. Relative hypertension in SCA should be identified and appropriately treated.

SICKLE CELL GLOMERULOPATHY

Glomerular involvement is very common in SCA. Proteinuria occurs in 25–30% adult SCA patients, and 14% have proteinuria of 2+ or more. Glomerular damage occurs more frequently in Hb SS than in double heterozygotes (SC, Sβ thalassemia), and is uncommon in sickle cell trait. The proteinuria results from enhanced albuminuria and is not a consequence of tubulointerstitial disease. In a recent series, 27% of adult patients with Hb SS had macroalbuminuria (albumin excretion rate >300 mg/g creatinine) and 41% had microalbuminuria (albumin excretion rate 30–300 mg/g creatinine). The finding of macroalbuminuria in SCA patients indicates the presence of a glomerulopathy, which may be detected before renal insufficiency is clinically apparent. The clinical significance of microalbuminuria in SCA patients is unknown, but those individuals could be at risk for subsequent renal insufficiency. In other sickle hemoglobinopathies (SC, Sβ thalassemia), albuminuria is much less frequent than in SS disease, with prevalences of macroalbuminuria and microalbuminuria of 6 and 36% of adult patients, respectively. A lower prevalence of sickle cell glomerulopathy occurs in SCA patients with concomitant α thalassemia.

Some SCA patients may develop progressive renal insufficiency associated with worsening proteinuria. Detailed studies of glomerular filtration using neutral dextrans of graded size as filtration markers show an increase in glomerular pore size in SCA patients with proteinuria, indicative of impaired membrane permselectivity. Initially, the glomerular capillary ultrafiltration coefficient, K_f, is increased, in keeping with the increase in membrane surface area associated with the glomerular hypertrophy observed. With progression of disease, GFR and renal plasma flow

TABLE I
Renal Involvement in Sickle Cell Anemia

Glomerular
  Glomerular hyperfiltration and hyperperfusion
  Sickle cell glomerulopathy (focal segmental glomerulosclerosis)
    Albuminuria
    Progressive renal insufficiency
    End stage renal disease
  Membranoproliferative glomerulonephritis

Medullary
  Concentrating defects with preserved diluting capacity
  Renal papillary necrosis
  Hematuria

Tubular dysfunction
  Incomplete distal RTA[a]
  Hyperkalemic hyperchloremic acidosis
    Type IV RTA
    Distal RTA with hyperkalemia
    Selective aldosterone deficiency
  Decreased potassium excretion without aldosterone deficiency
  Increased sodium, phosphate reabsorption
  Increased urate secretion

Malignancy
  Renal medullary carcinoma

[a]RTA, renal tubular acidosis.

fall to normal and then subnormal values. Proteinuria increases and K_f falls. At this stage, the histologic findings consist of focal glomerulosclerosis (see Pathology). As sclerosis progresses, glomerular membrane surface area falls, accounting for the decrease in K_f. The prevalence of renal insufficiency in adult patients with SCA has been reported to be between 4 and 7%, based on abnormal serum creatinine values. Renal insufficiency is more common in SS patients than in patients with SC disease. Caution should be employed, however, when the assessment of renal function in SCA patients is based on the serum creatinine norms for healthy individuals. SCA patients have a lower muscle mass than healthy individuals, and serum creatinine values are lower in SCA than in healthy controls. Therefore, serum creatinine values above 1.0–1.1 mg/dL could be abnormal in this population. The determination of the creatinine clearance from a 24-hr urine collection or the estimation of the creatinine clearance from the Cockroft–Gault formula, which integrates serum creatinine along with the age, gender, and weight of the individual, provides a better estimate of renal function than serum creatinine, and could be useful clinically in those circumstances.

CLINICAL PRESENTATION

Sickle cell glomerulopathy occurs more frequently in SS disease than in other sickle hemoglobinopathies and is usually detected by the finding of proteinuria at the time of a routine urinalysis. In the initial stages, the only clinically evident abnormality is proteinuria; serum creatinine and the creatinine clearance are in the normal range. As

disease progresses, renal insufficiency supervenes. Proteinuria is usually between 1.0 and 2.5 g/day, but can be in the nephrotic range. Urinalysis usually reveals no hematuria or pyuria. The presence of hematuria or RBC casts should alert the physician to the possibility of other causes for the glomerulonephritis. Because of their long-term exposure to blood products and higher incidence of infections, other glomerulopathies such as hepatitis-associated glomerulonephritis or HIV nephropathy should be ruled out. Acute glomerulonephritis has been reported in association with parvovirus infection. Because of the lower values of systemic blood pressure in the SCA population, relative hypertension (see earlier) should be identified in patients with sickle cell glomerulopathy and appropriately treated.

PATHOLOGY

Early descriptions of the pathological features of SCA individuals with heavy proteinuria emphasized the occurrence of a membranoproliferative glomerulonephritis, possibly a reflection of an unrecognized infection-related glomerulonephritis. More recently, several reports have described the occurrence of focal segmental glomerulosclerosis (FSGS) in proteinuric SCA individuals. Quantitative morphometric analysis of biopsy specimens obtained in this population show a significant increase in glomerular diameter and cross-sectional area compared with age-matched autopsy controls. These observations are in accord with the conventional histologic findings of FSGS in SCA, which include hypertrophy of unaffected glomeruli, segmental sclerotic lesions which are more prominent in juxtamedullary nephrons and in the perihilar region, global nephrosclerosis, and tubular atrophy with interstitial fibrosis in regions downstream from the affected glomeruli. As with other cases of FSGS, minor deposits of IgM, C1q, and C3 may be found in sclerotic areas on immunofluorescence, but immune complex deposits are absent on electron microscopy. Electron-lucent subendothelial expansion with mesangial interposition is observed in some cases. These findings are suggestive of early non-immune complex–mediated membranoproliferative glomerulonephritis.

TREATMENT

Because of the findings of proteinuria and focal glomerulosclerosis, angiotensin converting enzyme (ACE) inhibitors are a logical choice in patients with sickle cell glomerulopathy. In proteinuric patients with mild to moderate renal insufficiency, low-dose enalapril (5–10 mg/day) given over a 2-week period, has been observed to produce a 50% reduction in proteinuria, without lowering GFR or reducing systemic blood pressure. The efficacy of ACE inhibitors over the long term has not been studied. In patients with microalbuminuria, ACE inhibitors also reduce albumin excretion when given short term, but the long-term use of ACE inhibition in microalbuminuric patients has not been studied.

Hypertension, even in relative terms, should be treated to achieve blood pressure levels below 130/85 mm Hg. Diuretics should be avoided as initial antihypertensive agents because they may cause volume depletion and precipitate sickle cell crises. Patients may also benefit from moderate protein restriction, 0.7–0.8 g/kg/day, although the benefit of protein restriction has not been proved (Chapters 58 and 62). In patients with more advanced renal insufficiency, potassium levels should be followed closely. Many SCA patients have selective tubular excretion defects for potassium, which can be worsened by ACE inhibitor therapy. Other potentially nephrotoxic drugs such as nonsteroidal antiinflammatory drugs should be avoided. Metabolic acidosis can be treated with alkali supplementation. Erythropoietin has been used with moderate success to correct worsening anemia and reduce the need for transfusions.

Patients who develop ESRD can be successfully treated with dialysis or transplantation. The reported survival of SCA on dialysis is very poor, with median survival of only 2 years, although there is the clinical impression that their survival has improved lately. In transplanted patients, data from the United States Renal Data System (USRDS) data base (see Chapter 61) indicate that the 1-year renal allograft survival of SCA individuals is similar to that of non-SCA African-American recipients (78% versus 77%), but their 3-year allograft survival is lower (48% versus 60%, respectively). SCA recipients tolerate immunosuppressive treatment well, but the frequency of sickle pain crises is higher after successful transplantation. Caution should be used with antilymphocyte preparations to prevent or treat acute rejections because they could precipitate acute vaso-occlusive episodes or the acute chest syndrome. Despite these potential drawbacks, USRDS data indicate a trend toward better survival in transplanted patients, as compared to patients who remain on the transplant waiting list. Quite apart from survival data, quality of life is better with transplantation. Thus, patients with SCA related renal failure should be fully informed of the risks but encouraged to undergo transplant evaluation. The high prevalence of stroke, iron overload, and other disorders, however, makes careful screening essential.

RENAL CONCENTRATING DEFECTS

One of the most common renal abnormalities in SCA is an inability to maximally concentrate the urine. The hypertonic and relatively hypoxic environment in the renal medulla is conducive to sickling in the vasa recta. Early on, obstruction of flow and the associated concentration defect can be reversed by transfusion, which reduces the number of sickled cells. By age 15, however, the concentration defect is fixed and associated with fibrosis and obliteration of the medullary vasa recta with papillary shortening, as shown by microangiographic studies. Impairment of vasa recta flow interferes with the formation of the medullary urea and sodium gradient necessary for water reabsorption along those segments of the nephron. Patients with SCA cannot achieve urinary osmolalities above 400 mOsmol/kg and have obligatory water losses of 1.5–2.0 L/day. A

less severe defect occurs in patients with sickle cell trait. Maximal urinary concentration in older children and young adults with Hb AS is 800 mOsmol/kg, and reaches 450–500 mOsmol/kg in older individuals. Therefore, SCA patients should drink 2–3 L of water daily to prevent dehydration which could precipitate sickle cell pain crises. The formation of free water and urinary diluting ability is preserved in SCA.

HEMATURIA

Hematuria is a relatively common manifestation of sickle cell anemia and may occur in both sickle cell trait and Hb SS disease. Hematuria is usually painless and originates from the left kidney in about 70–80% of cases, but can be bilateral in about 10% of cases. It results from sickling in the vasa recta causing microinfarctions or severe stasis in peritubular capillaries with extravasation into the renal parenchyma and collecting system. The differential diagnosis includes glomerulonephritis, nephrolithiasis, renal papillary necrosis, urinary tract infections, and urological malignancies. Initial episodes should be evaluated thoroughly to rule out malignancies. Once the initial workup has been negative, subsequent episodes may be treated without performing imaging studies, but periodic reevaluation may be necessary because of the longer life expectancy of SCA patients and the possibility of a higher frequency of renal medullary carcinoma in this population.

The treatment is bed rest and forced diuresis with hypotonic intravenous fluid administration to decrease the tendency to clot formation in the urinary system. Alkalinization of the urine or diuretics can also be used to reduce medullary sickling. The benign nature and the possible relapsing nature of the condition should be explained to patients to avoid unnecessary procedures. In persistent cases, ϵ aminocaproic acid (EACA) at a dose of 4–12 g/day in four divided doses can be administered. When EACA is used, a high urinary flow rate should be maintained to avoid clot formation in the renal collecting system. Chronic relapsing hematuria can be treated with exchange transfusion, EACA administration, iron supplementation, and the avoidance of strenuous physical activity. Severe cases may require selective embolization, but nephrectomy is only warranted in case of life-threatening hemorrhage because of the tendency to recurrence in the contralateral kidney.

RENAL PAPILLARY NECROSIS

Renal papillary necrosis is a very common manifestation of SCA, as intravenous pyelography demonstrates unilateral or bilateral papillary necrosis in up to 67% of unselected patients without a prior history of urinary symptoms. Papillary necrosis is usually asymptomatic but may present with microscopic hematuria or renal colic. It results from localized medullary ischemia and necrosis of the medullary tip as a result of obliteration of the medullary vessels from sickling. The diagnosis is made with intravenous pyelography or ultrasonographically. Radiographically, there are irregularities in the renal calyces, with formation of a sinus tract that with progress to complete sequestration of the affected area, producing the radiographic "ring sign." In late stages, there is "clubbing" due to the sloughing or reabsorption of the papillae. By ultrasound, there is increased echogenicity of the inner medulla. In more advanced cases, a renal filling defect in the area of the medullary tip can be seen. In symptomatic patients with renal papillary necrosis, an associated urinary tract infection should be ruled out. In contrast to other forms of renal papillary necrosis, the prognosis for long-term renal function is good. Nonsteroidal antiinflammatory drugs should be avoided.

ACIDIFICATION AND POTASSIUM EXCRETION DEFECTS

Under normal conditions, most SCA patients have normal acid–base balance or a mild respiratory alkalosis. Metabolic acidosis may occur when SCA patients are given an acute acid load or when they are stressed by intercurrent illness such as diarrhea that results in gastrointestinal bicarbonate loss. This incomplete form of distal renal tubular acidosis (RTA) results from an inability to lower the urinary pH below 5.3 (normal response <5.0) with a resultant decrease in titratable acid and ammonium excretion. Proximal tubular bicarbonate reabsorption is normal.

Other variants have been described. Some patients with SCA, including sickle cell trait, may develop a hyperkalemic hyperchloremic metabolic acidosis. In some patients, selective aldosterone deficiency or hyporeninemic hypoaldosteronism lead to hyperkalemia, impaired ammoniagenesis, and proton retention despite normal ability to lower urine pH. Other patients have hyperkalemic distal RTA, an inability to generate a tubular transepithelial electrical gradient that permits normal potassium or proton secretion. Treatment is with sodium bicarbonate, a low potassium diet, mineralocorticoids and loop diuretics.

OTHER TUBULAR ABNORMALITIES

Proximal tubular transport processes are typically increased in patients with SCA, but usually with little clinical significance. In some patients, hyperphosphatemia may occur due to increased proximal tubular phosphate reabsorption. Uric acid excretion is increased due to an increased RBC turnover rate and an increase in uric acid production. Even so, gout is uncommon in SCA.

RENAL MEDULLARY CARCINOMA

Recent reports suggest an increased incidence of renal medullary carcinoma in SCA patients. This rare, highly aggressive tumor occurs in young people; the reported age at diagnosis ranges from the second to the fifth decade. The tumor arises in the medulla, but in the reported series, it had already extended beyond the capsule, and metastases were present at diagnosis. Presenting findings are hematuria, abdominal pain, flank mass, or weight loss. Diagnosis requires demonstration by renal imaging studies such as a computerized tomography (CT) scan followed by excision. Chromosomal abnormalities in the tumor tissue have been localized to chromosome 11 and, less often, to chromosome 3. Interestingly, the former is the locus of the gene encoding the hemoglobin β-chain. The latter is the site of the mutation for von Hippel–Lindau syndrome, which is also associated with renal cell carcinoma. Renal medullary carcinoma has a poor prognosis. In one study, mean survival after excision was only 15 weeks (range 2 to 52 weeks). Neither radiotherapy nor chemotherapy has proven useful. The available studies are retrospective, and clinical details were not available for all patients. Thus, these findings require confirmation in more carefully conducted studies. Nevertheless, a urological evaluation should be performed in patients with SCA presenting with hematuria or abdominal pain, but screening asymptomatic SCA patients with CT or ultrasound to uncover urological malignancies is not indicated.

Bibliography

Allon M, Lawson L, Eckman JR, Delaney V, Bourke E: Effects of nonsteroidal antiinflammatory drugs on renal function in sickle cell anemia. *Kidney Int* 34:500–506, 1988.

Battle D, Itsarayoungyuen K, Arruda JA, Kurtzman NA: Hyperkalemic hyperchloremic metabolic acidosis in sickle cell hemoglobinopathies. *Am J Med* 72:188–192, 1982.

Falk RJ, Scheinman J, Phillips G, Orringer E, Johnson A, Jennette JC: Prevalence and pathologic features of sickle cell nephropathy and response to inhibition of angiotensin-converting enzyme. *N Engl J Med* 326:910–915, 1992.

Figenshau RS, Basler JW, Ritter JH, Siegel CL, Simon JA, Dierks SM: Renal medullary carcinoma. *J Urol* 159:711–713, 1998.

Guasch A, Cua M, Mitch WE: Extent and the course of glomerular injury in patients with sickle cell anemia. *Kidney Int* 49:786–791, 1996.

Guasch A, Cua M, You W, Mitch WE: Sickle cell anemia causes a distinct pattern of glomerular dysfunction. *Kidney Int* 51:826–833, 1997.

Guasch A, Zayas CF, Eckman JR, Elsas L: Evidence that microdeletions in the α globin gene protect against the development of sickle cell glomerulopathy, *J Am Soc Nephrol* 10:1014–1019, 1999.

Ojo AO, Govaerts TC, Schmouder RL, Leichtman AB, Leavey SF, Wolfe RA, Held PJ, Port FK, Agodoa LY: Renal transplantation in end-stage sickle cell nephropathy. *Transplantation* 67:291–295, 1999.

Pandya KK, Koshy M, Brown N, Presman D: Renal papillary necrosis in sickle cell hemoglobinopathies. *J Urol* 115:497–501, 1976.

Pegelow CH, Colangelo L, Steinberg M, Wright EC, Smith J, Phillips G, Vichinsky E: Natural history of blood pressure in sickle cell disease: Risks for stroke and death associated with relative hypertension in sickle cell anemia. *Am J Med* 102:171–177, 1997.

Pham PT, Pham PC, Wilkinson AH, Lew SQ: Renal abnormalities in sickle cell disease. *Kidney Int* 57:1–8, 2000.

Powars DR, Elliot-Mills DD, Chan L, Niland J, Hiti AL, Opas LM, Johnson C: Chronic renal failure in sickle cell disease: Risk factors, clinical course, and mortality. *Ann Intern Med* 115:614–620, 1991.

Saborio P, Scheinman JI: Sickle cell nephropathy. *J Am Soc Nephrol* 10:187–192, 1999.

Statius van Eps LW, Pinedo-Veels C, Vries GH, de Koning J: Nature of concentrating defect in sickle-cell nephropathy. Microradioangiographic studies. *Lancet* 1:450–452, 1970.

Zayas CF, Platt J, Eckman JR, Elsas L, Clark WS, Mitch WE, Guasch A: Prevalence and predictors of glomerular involvement in sickle cell anemia. *J Am Soc Nephrol* 7:1401, 1996. (Abstract).

43

POLYCYSTIC AND ACQUIRED CYSTIC KIDNEY DISEASE

GODELA M. FICK-BROSNAHAN

Renal cysts are common; they can be part of congenital disorders or inherited polycystic diseases, or they can present as single or a few "simple" renal cysts unrelated to any disease. The latter are common in the general population; their incidence increases with increasing age. Ultrasound surveys of subjects without renal symptoms and with normal renal function found a prevalence of less than 5% below age 50 years, but 11–16% between age 50 and 70 years and 22% over age 70. The congenital disorders can be consequences of developmental malformations, such as multicystic dysplastic kidney, chromosomal abnormalities, or rare autosomal recessive syndromes in which the renal cysts are only a minor part of the overall clinical spectrum. Four hereditary cystic renal diseases are important because they are more common and often lead to end stage renal disease or other serious complications. They are discussed here in more detail, along with a brief discussion of acquired cystic kidney disease.

AUTOSOMAL DOMINANT POLYCYSTIC KIDNEY DISEASE

Autosomal dominant polycystic kidney disease (ADPKD) is by far the most prevalent of the inherited polycystic kidney diseases, occurring in about 1 in 400 to 1 in 1000 Americans. ADPKD affects people worldwide, but the exact prevalence in African-Americans, Hispanics, and other ethnic group is not known. ADPKD is characterized by the progressive development and enlargement of bilateral renal cysts (Fig. 1), and is accompanied by progressive replacement of normal renal parenchyma with cystic spaces and areas of interstitial inflammation and fibrosis. ADPKD ultimately leads to end stage renal disease (ESRD) in about 50% of patients by age 60 and in 75% by age 70 years. Five to 10% of all ESRD in the United States and Europe is caused by ADPKD. Apart from ESRD, the morbidity is high due to complications of renal and extrarenal manifestations (Table 1).

Genetic Aspects

Mutations in at least two different genes can cause ADPKD. The first, the PKD-1 gene, is on the short arm of chromosome 16, and the second, the PKD-2 gene, is on the long arm of chromosome 4. Disease caused by PKD-2

mutations is in general milder than disease caused by PKD-1 mutations, with an older age at diagnosis and later onset of hypertension and renal failure. In the reported ADPKD2 families to date, onset of renal failure occurred at a mean age of 70–73 years, whereas in ADPKD1 families the mean age at onset of ESRD is 53–56 years. About 85% of Caucasian families are linked to the ADPKD1 gene and 10–15% to the ADPKD2 gene. A few families have been described whose disease is not linked to either PKD-1 or PKD-2. Therefore, a third or possibly more additional gene loci may cause ADPKD.

The PKD-1 gene is a very large gene with 46 exons coding for 4302 amino acids. Exons 1 to 34 are replicated at least three times on a more proximal portion of chromosome 16, which has made mutation detection difficult, because it is necessary to distinguish mutations in the PKD-1 gene from sequence variants stemming from the replicated areas, the PKD homologs. In addition, the PKD-1 gene contains unusually long polypyrimidine tracts, which further complicate gene analysis. In contrast, the PKD-2 gene has no unusual features. It contains 15 exons coding for 968 amino acids. The PKD-2 mutation detection rate is about 80%, compared to 30–50% for ADPKD1. The mutations found so far are scattered throughout both genes and are unique for most families; most mutations are small base pair changes and result in truncated proteins. It is not yet clear whether there are genotype–phenotype correlations within ADPKD1 or 2.

Pathogenesis

The protein products of the PKD-1 and PKD-2 genes are called polycystin 1 and polycystin 2. Polycystin 1 is a membrane-associated glycoprotein with a large extracellular domain, several transmembrane domains, and a short cytoplasmic tail. Polycystin 1 is believed to function as a cell membrane receptor mediating cell–cell and cell–matrix interactions. The intracellular tail has been shown to interact with polycystin 2, which is a membrane protein with six transmembrane domains and two intracellular tails. Polycystin 2 has significant homology with voltage-gated calcium channels, raising the possibility that it functions as an ion channel. Both polycystin 1 and 2 are probably part of a

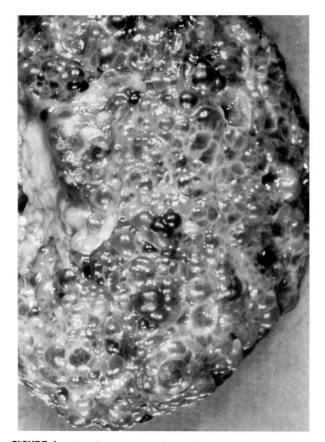

FIGURE 1 A nephrectomy specimen from a patient with autosomal dominant polycystic kidney disease. The kidney is moderately enlarged with cysts of varying size—some of which appear hemorrhagic. Reprinted by permission of *The New England Journal of Medicine,* Gabow PA:329:332-342, 1993. *Massachusetts Medical Society.* All rights reserved.

TABLE I
Clinical Manifestations of ADPKD

Renal
  Cysts, enlarged kidneys
  Hypertension
  Hematuria
  Acute and chronic pain
  Decreased urinary concentrating ability, frequency
Cardiovascular
  Intracranial saccular aneurysms
  Aneurysms of other vascular beds
  Cardiac valvular abnormalities
Other extrarenal
  Liver cysts
  Congenital hepatic fibrosis (rare)
  Pancreatic cysts (usually single cysts)
  Cysts in various organs (usually no clinical sequelae)
Complications
  Nephrolithiasis (hematuria, stone colic, obstruction)
  Cyst infection in kidneys or liver
  Cyst rupture with massive hemorrhage
  Compression of common bile duct, hepatic veins or vena cava
    by liver cysts
  Left ventricular hypertrophy, cardiac disease
  Rupture of intracranial aneurysm, subarachnoid hemorrhage
  End stage renal disease

in interstitial inflammation and ultimately in fibrosis. The interstitial fibrotic process is believed to be the primary mechanism of progression to ESRD. Superimposed is damage from hypertension, as histologic examination of end stage kidneys reveals prominent arteriolar sclerosis and global glomerulosclerosis.

Diagnosis

The diagnosis of ADPKD can be made by gene-linkage analysis or by imaging studies. In clinical practice, ultrasound imaging is the primary tool for diagnosis, because it is sensitive, noninvasive, and relatively inexpensive; it also gives information about the structural severity of the disease (Fig. 2). To make a diagnosis in people with a family history of ADPKD, specific age-dependent criteria have been developed: for someone age 18 to 29 years, at least two renal cysts are required to make the diagnosis of ADPKD, for someone age 30 to 59 years, at least two cysts in each kidney are required, and for someone age 60 years and over, at least four cysts in each kidney are required to make a diagnosis of ADPKD. For a child under 18 years of age, any renal cyst is highly suspicious for the disease. These criteria have been validated by comparison with gene-linkage results for the PKD-1 gene. For ruling out the diagnosis of ADPKD in a person at risk, the age at which 100% of gene carriers have detectable cysts needs to be known. In carriers of a PKD-1 mutation a negative ultrasound has not been observed after age 30 years. A study in five ADPKD2 families also reported a 100% prevalence of ultrasonographically visible

multiprotein complex linking the extracellular matrix with cytoplasmatic signaling proteins and/or the cytoskeleton.

Recently, it was discovered that cysts are monoclonal; some renal and liver cysts have mutations in their second, normal PKD-1 or PKD-2 allele. This suggests that a second, somatic mutation occurs in some tubular and biliary cells, which then proliferate to form tubular outpouchings and cysts. The observation of somatic mutations could explain why only a fraction of nephrons (estimated 1–2%) becomes cystic. The germ line mutation alone may not be sufficient to cause cystic transformation, but a "second hit," a somatic mutation in the other PKD allele, may be necessary. The cyst lining cells are characterized by an immature phenotype. Deficient terminal differentiation results in hyperproliferation, fluid secretion, and production of an abnormal extracellular matrix, all of which are necessary for cyst expansion. Cyst epithelia appear to produce a variety of cytokines, which further stimulate cell proliferation and fluid secretion in an autocrine fashion. Cytokines also diffuse into the interstitium, where they attract macrophages and other inflammatory cells, resulting

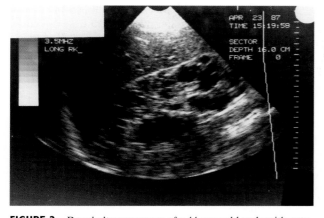

FIGURE 2 Renal ultrasonogram of a 44-year-old male with autosomal dominant polycystic kidney disease. The kidney is moderately enlarged and contains multiple cysts of variable size.

cysts in gene carriers aged 30 years or older. However, the study included only 19 subjects at risk, and it is likely that many ADPKD2 families with mild manifestations remain undiagnosed. In these families the age at first manifestation of cysts could be later. This is important if a person under age 30 years, who has a negative ultrasound, or a person from a known PKD-2 family with a negative ultrasound considers kidney donation for a family member with ESRD.

In these instances gene-linkage analysis should be performed. However, at least two affected family members need to be available to determine the markers that are linked to the ADPKD gene in that family. If the individual in question has the same markers as the affected relatives, the likelihood of being a gene carrier is greater than 99%. Gene-linkage analysis is performed by commercial DNA-diagnostics laboratories, and is also used for prenatal diagnosis. A positive gene-linkage result in the fetus, however, does not predict the severity of the disease, and few parents consider ADPKD a severe enough disease to consider therapeutic abortion. Direct mutation analysis is currently available only on a research basis, but with improved technology this may change in the future.

Clinical Manifestations

In addition to the kidneys, the polycystin proteins are also expressed in virtually all tissues, particularly in liver, pancreas, heart, arteries, and brain. However, only the renal phenotype is observed in 100% of mutation carriers after a certain age, whereas the extrarenal manifestations occur with variable frequency and in various combinations (Table 1). The molecular basis for this variability is not known, but it could relate to the frequency with which "second hits" occur in any individual. The renal disease course is variable as well, with some subjects, including some PKD-1 families, remaining asymptomatic until old age, and some children presenting with enlarged kidneys and hypertension at birth and reaching ESRD as adolescents or young adults.

Renal Manifestations

Renal cysts can be seen on ultrasound in about 60% of affected children under age 5 years, in 75% between age 5 and 18 years, and in 100% of subjects age 30 years or older. After age 30, 95% of affected subjects also have markedly enlarged kidneys, which can reach longitudinal diameters up to 40 cm and weights up to 8 kg. Back and flank pain is a common symptom, occurring in about 60% of adults. If pain occurs acutely, a renal complication has to be considered, such as cyst hemorrhage, infection, or nephrolithiasis. Pain that is chronic, dull, and insidious in onset is believed to be due to stretching of the renal capsule by the enlarging cysts; this chronic pain is more common in patients with large cysts and/or large kidneys, but can also occur in patients with smaller kidneys and can be disabling, leading to narcotic addiction. Before that happens, patients should be referred for a cyst decompression procedure. This can be done percutaneously with alcohol sclerosis if there are only a few large cysts. More often, it will require a laparoscopic or open surgical approach. Renal function is not affected by these procedures.

Cyst bleeding or hematuria are generally treated with bed rest, fluids, and mild analgesics; the bleeding usually resolves within a few days. Urinary tract infections are common in ADPKD patients; if the clinical presentation is that of cystitis or uncomplicated pyelonephritis, treatment is the same as in any other patient. More serious are cyst infections, which are characterized by localized renal tenderness or severe pain, high- or low-grade fevers, malaise and, often, positive blood cultures. Failure to respond to penicillins or aminoglycosides is also suggestive of a cyst infection, because these antibiotics do not penetrate well into the cyst cavities. Therefore, any patient with a severe renal infection or presumed cyst infection should be treated with ciprofloxacin or trimethoprim–sulfamethoxazole, because these antibiotics have demonstrated good cyst fluid accumulation and clinical efficacy. Treatment often needs to be prolonged for 6 weeks or longer to cure a smoldering cyst infection. Rarely cyst drainage or a nephrectomy may be necessary.

Nephrolithiasis occurs in 20–36% of patients with ADPKD and is probably due to metabolic factors and to urinary stasis in a collecting system that is distorted by the cysts. The most common metabolic factor is hypocitriuria, which is found in 50% of ADPKD patients with normal renal function. Evaluation and treatment for metabolic factors is the same as in stone formers of the general population. Hypocitriuria is usually treated with oral potassium citrate in subjects with normal or near normal renal function; it should not be used in the presence of renal failure. Extracorporeal shock-wave lithotripsy has been used successfully in ADPKD patients with symptomatic stones.

Hypertension is an important renal manifestation of ADPKD. About 30% of ADPKD children, 65% of ADPKD adults over age 30 years with normal renal function, and 80% of all ADPKD adults over age 30 years have hypertension. Hypertensive patients have larger kidneys and more severe cystic involvement than normotensive subjects. Hypertension is thought to be caused by stretching of renal arterioles by the cysts and subsequent activation of the renin–angiotensin–aldosterone system. Altered renal sodium handling, release of endothelin, and stimulation of the sympathetic nervous system may also play a role. Hypertensive ADPKD patients progress to ESRD faster than normotensive patients; whether treatment of hypertension or the use of angiotensin converting enzyme inhibitors in particular can slow the progression to renal failure has not been determined. However, the cardiac end-organ effects of hypertension, particularly left ventricular hypertrophy, are common in ADPKD patients. Children and young adults with ADPKD already have higher left ventricular masses than age-matched healthy subjects; frank left ventricular hypertrophy is found in 48% of hypertensive ADPKD patients. Because of the increased cardiovascular morbidity and mortality associated with left ventricular hypertrophy, optimal therapy of hypertension is necessary.

When patients with ADPKD reach ESRD, treatment options are hemodialysis, peritoneal dialysis, or renal transplantation. The latter is the treatment of choice if no contraindications are present. ADPKD patient and graft survival are similar to other primary renal diseases (excluding diabetic patients). Pretransplant native nephrectomy is not generally necessary. Exceptions are patients with a history of recurrent or recent severe renal cyst infections, patients with recurrent gross hematuria, and individuals in whom graft placement is difficult due to the size of the cystic kidneys. Peritoneal dialysis can be offered to patients who do not have extremely large kidneys, diverticulosis, or abdominal wall hernias. Hemodialysis is generally well tolerated by ADPKD patients, and they appear to have a survival advantage over non-ADPKD patients on dialysis, particularly at older ages. This has been attributed to a lower prevalence of severe coronary disease in ADPKD, although cardiac disease remains the most common cause of death among ADPKD patients on renal replacement therapy.

Extrarenal Manifestations

Liver cysts are the most common extrarenal manifestation. They develop later in life than the renal cysts and do not lead to liver failure. Liver cysts are very rare in children; their prevalence increases with age and decreasing renal function, so that by age 60 years at least 75% of ADPKD patients have liver cysts. Women generally have more severe liver involvement than men, particularly women who had multiple pregnancies. Liver cysts often remain asymptomatic; however, complications such as cyst infection, bleeding, or anatomical obstruction of the intrahepatic bile ducts, the vena cava, or hepatic veins (Budd–Chiari syndrome) by the cysts have all been reported and can be life-threatening. A few patients have massive liver enlargement due to the cysts, resulting in abdominal distention and pain, early satiety and, rarely, malnutrition. For such patients, decompression procedures,

such as percutaneous cyst aspiration, laparoscopic fenestration, surgical decompression, and partial liver resection are indicated. In rare instances, orthotopic liver transplantation has been performed.

Cysts have been reported in many other organs, including the pancreas, ovaries, testes, seminal vesicles, prostate, spleen, and arachnoid membranes; usually these cysts have no clinical sequelae. In contrast to previous retrospective reports, a more recent prospective study of non-ESRD ADPKD subjects older than 40 years has not found a higher prevalence of colonic diverticula compared to an age-matched control population.

Noncystic extrarenal manifestations are mitral valve prolapse and intracranial berry aneurysms. Two large studies found mitral valve prolapse in about 25% of ADPKD subjects compared to 2% of a control population. Although mitral valve prolapse can be associated with palpitations and atypical chest pain, it does not appear to contribute to mortality in ADPKD.

Rupture of an intracranial aneurysm can be the most devastating of all ADPKD manifestations. Four prospective studies have shown that 5–10% of asymptomatic ADPKD adults harbor an intracranial aneurysm. However, all aneurysms found by screening were less than 7 mm in diameter, which is usually not considered an indication for elective clipping. Rupture of an aneurysm seems to cluster in certain ADPKD families. The mean age at rupture (~41 years) is younger than aneurysm ruptures in the general population. Multiple aneurysms are found in 20–30% of ADPKD patients with an aneurysm, and in one study recurrent rupture of a second aneurysm occurred in 9% of patients, between 2 days and 14 years after the first rupture. Based on these observations, current recommendations for screening of asymptomatic subjects are: screen all patients with a family history of a ruptured aneurysm, all patients with a previous rupture, patients with high-risk occupations (e.g., pilots), and patients who need screening for peace of mind. The best screening method appears to be magnetic resonance angiography, which is noninvasive and does not use potentially nephrotoxic radio contrast material. Screening of high-risk subjects should start at age 18 years and probably be repeated every 5 to 10 years, unless older age or other conditions limit life expectancy. Other rare vascular manifestations of ADPKD include coronary artery or visceral artery aneurysms, spontaneous cervical or vertebral artery dissections, and cerebral arteriovenous malformations.

AUTOSOMAL RECESSIVE POLYCYSTIC KIDNEY DISEASE

Autosomal recessive polycystic kidney disease (ARPKD) (estimated incidence 1:6000 to 1:55,000) is much less common than ADPKD. Mutations in a single gene on chromosome 6 appear to be responsible. This gene has not yet been cloned. ARPKD affects both the kidneys and the liver. The kidneys are characterized by fusiform cystic dilatations of the collecting ducts. In young children, the kidneys are often grossly enlarged, but with progressive renal insufficiency they tend to regress in size, so that older children and adults can have mildly enlarged, normal sized, or relatively small kidneys. The liver histology shows varying degrees of congenital hepatic fibrosis, which comprises increased fibrous tissue in the portal tracts with proliferation of small bile ducts. Gross cystic dilatation of the intrahepatic bile ducts, called Caroli disease, can also be seen. The diagnosis is made when the child presents with typical clinical and ultrasonographic findings and both parents have a negative ultrasound. However, the clinical and sonographic picture can overlap with ADPKD, and if both parents have a normal renal ultrasound, the question arises whether the child has ARPKD or a new mutation for ADPKD. If clarification of the diagnosis is needed, a kidney or liver biopsy can be performed.

ARPKD usually manifests in childhood, often in the first year of life. In a study of 115 patients, 11% were diagnosed prenatally by linkage analysis or abnormal ultrasound, 41% were diagnosed at less than 1 month old, 23% at less than 1 year old, and 25% at an age older than 1 year. Occasionally, ARPKD is diagnosed for the first time in young adults. The symptoms that most often lead to the diagnosis in neonates and young infants are palpable abdominal masses, hypertension, and urinary tract infections; in older children signs of portal hypertension such as variceal hemorrhage or pancytopenia from hypersplenism may predominate. Both the renal and the liver disease progress with age. Whereas the kidney disease terminates in ESRD, liver function usually remains normal. About 70% of children have hypertension, which begins at a median age of 0.5 years and is sometimes severe. Decreased glomerular filtration rate (GFR) is observed in 72% of children, often starting in the first year of life and slowly progressing to ESRD. If ESRD is present at birth and complicated by oligohydramnios, the infants often die of respiratory failure. Therefore, mortality is relatively high (9–24%) in the first year of life, but by age 15 years survival is still around 80%; many patients now reach adulthood. Renal transplantation is the treatment of choice for those with ESRD. The complications of portal hypertension can usually be controlled with sclerotherapy or shunt surgery.

TUBEROUS SCLEROSIS

Tuberous sclerosis (TS) is an autosomal dominant disorder with a high spontaneous mutation rate and an estimated prevalence of 1:10,000. TS is caused by two different genes, which are located on chromosomes 9 (TSC1) and 16 (TSC2). Both have been cloned and are tumor suppressor genes. The TSC2 gene lies directly adjacent to the PKD1 gene, and contiguous gene deletion syndromes, that is, deletion of the entire TSC2 and PKD1 genes, have been documented in some children with TS and severe early onset polycystic kidney disease. TS is characterized by hamartomas in many organs, including cysts and angiomyolipomas in kidneys and liver, cortical tubers in the brain, astrocytomas, retinal hamartomas, and rhabdomyomas of the heart. Skin manifestations are facial angiofibromas (adenoma sebaceum), hypomelanotic macules (ash-leaf spots), and ungual fibromas. TS shows extreme phenotypic variability. Some patients are severely affected with epilepsy and mental retardation, whereas others are neurologically normal. Renal complications include retroperitoneal hemorrhage due to bleeding angiomyolipomas, ESRD, and occasionally renal cell carcinoma (~1%).

VON HIPPEL–LINDAU DISEASE

Von Hippel–Lindau disease (VHL) is a rare (estimated 1:36,000 to 1:46,000) autosomal dominant disease caused by mutations in a tumor suppressor gene on chromosome 3. It is characterized by the development of multiple tumors, particularly retinal angiomas, cerebellar (80%) and spinal (20%) hemangioblastomas, pheochromocytomas, and renal cell carcinomas. Cysts in kidneys, pancreas, and epididymis are also frequently observed. Occasionally clinical and renal ultrasonographic findings can be indistinguishable from ADPKD. However, the cyst epithelium in VHL is different from that in ADPKD, because it shows a histologic spectrum from normal-appearing single-layered epithelium to multilayered dysplastic epithelium to renal cell carcinoma. Renal carcinomas develop in up to 75% of patients by age 60 years, with 44 years being the mean age at diagnosis; they are often multicentric and bilateral and are the leading cause of death. Annual screening of affected family members with ophthalmoscopy and magnetic resonance imaging of brain, spine, and abdomen is necessary to detect these tumors at a potentially curable stage.

ACQUIRED CYSTIC KIDNEY DISEASE

Acquired cystic kidney disease (ACKD) refers to the development of renal cysts in chronic renal failure (CRF) patients without underlying polycystic disease. ACKD affects both males and females and is found in up to 22% of CRF patients before the start of dialysis. In CRF patients with ACKD, the kidneys are small, whereas they are enlarged in CRF patients due to ADPKD. The frequency of ACKD rises with the duration of hemodialysis or peritoneal dialysis, so that after 4 years 60–80% of chronic dialysis patients have ACKD. After 9 years up to 90% have ACKD.

ACKD is usually asymptomatic. Rarely, cyst bleeding can cause pain or hematuria, or a cyst can become infected. The most serious complication is renal cell carcinoma. The risk for this cancer is significantly higher in ESRD patients, particularly those with ACKD, than in the general population. ACKD-associated renal cell carcinoma occurs most often in males in the fifth or sixth decade of life, is bilateral in 10%, and metastasizes in about 20% of cases. Because the overall mortality of ESRD patients is high due to cardiovascular disease, survival is often not affected. Therefore, screening of asymptomatic patients for renal cell carcinoma with ultrasound or computerized tomography (CT) imaging is not generally recommended; exceptions could be for young, otherwise healthy patients treated with dialysis for more than 3 years, and those awaiting kidney transplantation.

Bibliography

Browne G, Jefferson JA, Wright GD, *et al.:* Von Hippel–Lindau disease: An important differential diagnosis of polycystic kidney disease. *Nephrol Dial Transplant* 12:1132–1136, 1997.

Chauveau D, Pirson Y, Verellen-Dumoulin C, *et al.:* Intracranial aneurysms in autosomal dominant polycystic kidney disease. *Kidney Int* 45:1140–1146, 1994.

Chauveau D, Duvic C, Chretien Y, *et al.:* Renal involvement in von Hippel–Lindau disease. *Kidney Int* 50:944–951, 1996.

Fick GM, Gabow PA: Hereditary and acquired cystic disease of the kidney (review). *Kidney Int* 46:951–964, 1994.

Gabow PA, Kimberling WJ, Strain JD, *et al.:* Utility of ultrasonography in the diagnosis of autosomal dominant polycystic kidney disease in children. *J Am Soc Nephrol* 8:105–110, 1997.

Grantham JJ: Acquired cystic kidney disease (review). *Kidney Int* 40:143–152, 1991.

Grantham JJ: Mechanisms of progression in autosomal dominant polycystic kidney disease. *Kidney Int* 52:S 93–S97, 1997.

Grantham JJ, Schreiner GF, Rome L, *et al.:* Evidence for inflammatory and secretagogue lipids in cyst fluids from patients with autosomal dominant polycystic kidney disease. *Proc Assoc Am Physicians* 109:397–408, 1997.

Gulanikar AC, Daily PP, Kilambi NK, *et al.:* Prospective pretransplant ultrasound screening in 206 patients for acquired renal cysts and renal cell carcinoma. *Transplantation* 66:1669–1672, 1998.

Ivy DD, Shaffer EM, Johnson AM, *et al.:* Cardiovascular abnormalities in children with autosomal dominant polycystic kidney disease. *J Am Soc Nephrol* 5:2032–2036, 1995.

Jamil B, McMahon LP, Savige JA, *et al.:* A study of long-term morbidity associated with autosomal recessive polycystic kidney disease. *Nephrol Dial Transplant* 14:205–209, 1999.

Murcia NS, Sweeney WE, Avner ED: New insights into the molecular pathophysiology of polycystic kidney disease (review). *Kidney Int* 55:1187–1197, 1999.

Nicolau C, Torra R, Badenas C, *et al.:* Autosomal dominant polycystic kidney disease types 1 and 2: Assessment of US sensitivity for diagnosis. *Radiology* 213:273–276, 1999.

Perrone RD: Extrarenal manifestations of ADPKD (review). *Kidney Int* 51:2022–2036, 1997.

Ravine D, Gibson RN, Walker RG, *et al.:* Evaluation of ultrasonographic diagnostic criteria for autosomal polycystic kidney disease 1. *Lancet* 343:824–827, 1994.

Sampson JR, Maheshwar MM, Aspinwall R, *et al.:* Renal cystic disease in tuberous sclerosis: Role of the polycystic kidney disease 1 gene. *Am J Hum Genet* 61:843–851, 1997.

Truong LD, Krishnan B, Cao JTH, *et al.:* Renal neoplasm in acquired cystic kidney disease (review). *Am J Kidney Dis* 26:1–12, 1995.

Watnick T, Germino GG: Molecular basis of autosomal dominant polycystic kidney disease (review). *Semin Nephrol* 19:327–343, 1999.

Watson ML: Complications of polycystic kidney disease (review). *Kidney Int* 51:353–365, 1997.

Zerres K, Rudnick-Schoneborn S, Steinkamm C, *et al.:* Autosomal recessive polycystic kidney disease (review). *J Mol Med* 76:303–309, 1998.

ALPORT'S SYNDROME AND RELATED DISORDERS

MARTIN C. GREGORY

Alport's syndrome is a disease of collagen that affects the kidneys always, the ears often, and the eyes occasionally. Cecil Alport described the association of hereditary hematuric nephritis with hearing loss in a family whose affected males died in adolescence. Genetic advances have broadened the scope of the condition to include optical defects, platelet abnormalities, late-onset renal failure, and normal hearing in some families. At least 85% of kindreds are X-linked, and most or all of those result from a mutation of COL4A5, the gene located at Xq22 that codes for the α5 chain of type IV collagen. Autosomal recessive inheritance occurs in perhaps 15% of cases, and autosomal dominant inheritance has been shown in a few kindreds with associated thrombocytopathy and in rare kindreds without platelet defects.

JUVENILE AND ADULT FORMS

This distinction is fundamental to the understanding of Alport's syndrome. Renal failure tends to occur at a similar age in all males in a kindred, but this age can differ widely between kindreds. Uremia in males occurs in childhood or adolescence in some families, and in the late thirties in others. The families with early onset of renal failure and males are termed "juvenile," and those with renal failure in middle age are called "adult" type nephritis. Extrarenal manifestations tend to be more prominent in the juvenile kindreds. Moreover, because males in juvenile kindreds do not commonly survive to reproduce, these kindreds tend to be small and frequently arise from new mutations. Adult type kindreds are typically large, and new mutations occur infrequently.

CLASSIC GENETICS

In most kindreds, inheritance is X-linked. This was suggested by classic pedigree analysis, strengthened by tight linkage to restriction fragment length polymorphism markers (RFLPs), and proven by identification of mutations.

MOLECULAR GENETICS

Causative mutations of COL4A5, the gene coding for the $\alpha 5$ chain of type IV collagen, appear consistently in many kindreds. Deletions, point mutations, and splicing errors occur. There is poor correlation between mutation type and clinical phenotype, but deletions and some splicing errors cause severe renal disease and early hearing loss. Missense mutations may cause juvenile disease with hearing loss or adult disease with or without hearing loss. Deletions involving the 5' end of the COL4A5 gene and the 5' end of the adjacent COL4A6 gene occur consistently in families with esophageal and genital leiomyomatosis.

Homozygotes or mixed heterozygotes for mutations of COL4A3 or COL4A4 can develop autosomal recessive Alport's syndrome. Heterozygotes for these mutations may account for many cases of benign familial hematuria [familial thin glomerular basement membrane (GBM) disease].

IMMUNOCHEMISTRY

Patients with Alport's syndrome lack a component of the GBM. In most kindreds with Alport's syndrome the GBM of affected males fails to stain in the normal fashion with anti-GBM sera, and the GBM of female heterozygotes stains in an interrupted fashion. Certain sera have in common activity against $\alpha 3$ (IV) and also epidermal basement membrane. The "Alport antigen" that these sera recognize is a 26-kDa monomer belonging to the $\alpha 3$ (IV) chain.

After transplantation, <10% of Alport males develop anti-GBM nephritis, presumably because tolerance to a normal antigen has not been acquired. Recurrences of anti-GBM nephritis are usual but not inevitable after retransplantation. The anti-GBM antibodies developing after transplantation are heterogeneous. All will react with the normal GBM, but only some react with epidermal basement membrane.

BIOCHEMISTRY

The open mesh of interlocking molecules of type IV collagen that forms the framework of glomerular basement membrane is composed of heterotrimers of α chains. In fetal life, these heterotrimers consists of two $\alpha 1$ (IV) chains and one $\alpha 2$ (IV) chain, but early in postnatal development a switch of production to an important minority of $\alpha 3$ (IV), $\alpha 4$ (IV), and $\alpha 5$ (iv) chains occurs. The primary chemical defect in Alport's syndrome most commonly involves the $\alpha 5$ (IV) chain, but faulty assembly of the α 3, 4, 5 heterotrimer produces similar pathology in glomerular, aural, and ocular basement membranes regardless of which α chain is defective. As an illustration of failure of normal heterotrimer formation, many patients whose genetic defect is in the gene coding for the $\alpha 5$ (IV) chain lack demonstrable $\alpha 3$ (IV) chains in GBMs.

PATHOLOGY

In young children, light microscopy may be normal or near normal. An increased number of glomeruli with persisting fetal morphology may be seen. As disease progresses, interstitial and tubular foam cells may become quite prominent, although they can also be found in many other conditions (Fig. 1). Eventually progressive glomerulosclerosis and interstitial scarring develop. Routine immunofluorescence examination is negative. Characteristic features are seen by electron microscopy (Fig. 2). The GBM is thickened and is up to two or three times its normal thickness, is split into several irregular layers, and is frequently interspersed with numerous electron dense granules about 40 nm in diameter. In florid cases of juvenile types of disease the lamellae of basement membrane may branch and rejoin in a complex "basket weave" pattern. Early in the development of the lesion, thinning of the GBM may predominate or may be the only abnormality visible. The abnormalities in chil-

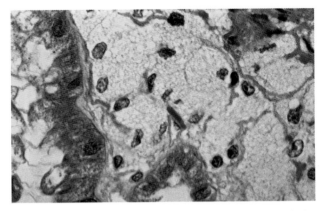

FIGURE I High-power photomicrograph of foam-filled tubular and interstitial cells in a renal biopsy from a patient with Alport's syndrome. Relatively normal proximal tubular cytoplasm stains red in the tubules on the left and at the bottom. The remaining cells appear "foamy" because of the spaces left where lipids have been eluted during processing.

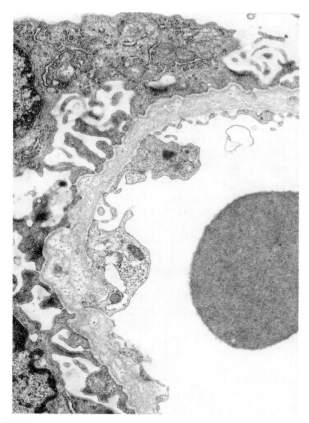

FIGURE 2 High-resolution electron micrograph of glomerular basement membrane from a patient with Alport's syndrome. The glomerular basement membrane varies in thickness. It is split into a number of layers, which in some areas are separated by lucent areas containing small dense granules. Electron micrograph kindly supplied by Dr. Theodore J. Pysher.

dren or adolescents with adult-type Alport's syndrome may be unimpressive or indistinguishable from those of thin GBM disease.

CLINICAL FEATURES

Renal Features

Uninterrupted microscopic hematuria occurs from birth in affected males. Hematuria may become visible after exercise or during fever; this is more common in juvenile kindreds. Microscopic hematuria has a penetrance of approximately 90% in heterozygous females in adult-type kindreds. In juvenile kindreds, the penetrance of hematuria in females has been studied less extensively. Urinary erythrocytes are dysmorphic, and red cell casts can usually be found. Proteinuria is very variable; occasionally it reaches nephrotic levels.

Hemizygous males inevitably progress to end stage renal disease (ESRD). This occurs at widely variable ages that are fairly constant within each family. Heterozygous females are generally much less severely affected. Around one-fifth of them will develop ESRD, usually after the age of 50, but renal failure in girls in their teens and even younger does occur.

In families with autosomal inheritance, females are affected as severely and as early as males. Renal failure often occurs before the age of 20 years in homozygotes for autosomal recessive Alport's syndrome.

Nonrenal Features

Hearing Loss

Bilateral high-frequency cochlear hearing loss is present in many but not all kindreds. Some authors do not use the term Alport's syndrome unless there is substantial hearing loss in the family. Regardless of terminology, the important clinical point is that X-linked nephritis progressing to ESRD can occur in families without overt hearing loss. Expectation of hearing loss causes many missed diagnoses. In families with juvenile type disease, hearing loss is almost universal in male hemizygotes and common in severely affected female heterozygotes.

Hearing loss affects all frequencies but is maximal at 6 through 8 kHz. The loss is also severe at 8 to 20 kHz, but these frequencies are not covered by conventional audiometry. In adult-type Alport's syndrome with hearing loss, there is typically no perceptible deficit until age 20, but loss progresses to 60–70 dB at 6–8 kHz at ages over 40. Hearing loss occurs earlier in juvenile kindreds. The kinetics is not well established in juvenile kindreds, but many grade-schoolers or adolescents require hearing aids.

Ocular Defects

These appear confined to juvenile kindreds. Myopia, arcus juvenilis, and cataracts occur but lack diagnostic specificity. Three changes that are present in a minority of kindreds but that are nearly diagnostic are anterior lenticonus, posterior polymorphous corneal dystrophy, and retinal flecks. Anterior lenticonus is a forward protrusion of the anterior surface of the ocular lens. It results from a weakness of the type IV collagen forming the anterior lens capsule. The resulting irregularity of the surface of the lens causes an uncorrectable refractive error. The retina cannot be clearly seen by ophthalmoscopy, and with a strong positive lens in the ophthalmoscope, the lenticonus can often be seen through a dilated pupil as an "oil drop" or circular smudge on the center of the lens. Retinal flecks are small yellow or white dots scattered around the macula or in the periphery of the retina. If sparse, they may be difficult to distinguish from small hard exudates.

Leiomyomatosis

Several X-linked families show the precocious development of striking leiomyomas of the esophagus and female genitalia in association with Alport's syndrome. These tumors are frequently large and multiple. They may bleed or obstruct, and their resection can be difficult. All families described so far have had a deletion at the 5' ends of the COL4A5 and COL4A6 genes.

DIAGNOSIS

No single feature is pathognomonic. The diagnosis is made by finding hematuria in multiple family members, together with a history of renal failure in related males, and reinforced by biopsy showing characteristic ultrastructural changes in the proband or a relative. Immunofluorescence examination of the biopsy should include staining with fluoresceinated anti-GBM, or anti-α3, or anti-α5 antibodies; this will help distinguish Alport's syndrome from familial thin GBM disease. In large families without a known mutation, segregation analysis can decide whether a particular individual carries a defective gene. In families with a previously defined mutation, molecular diagnosis of affected males and gene carrying females is possible. Molecular diagnosis is nearly 100% sensitive and specific in these families.

The key to diagnosis is to suspect the possibility of Alport's syndrome in any patient with otherwise unexplained hematuria, glomerulopathy, or renal insufficiency. In many cases, the familial nature of the condition will not be immediately apparent. Inquiry into the family must be detailed and insistent. The patient is usually a young male. Chances are that he knows little of his distant relatives, but his mother will likely know more of the family details. Male relatives linked to the patient through one or more females may have renal failure. Check urine samples from the parents of the patient, particularly his mother, for microscopic hematuria. Hearing loss is a helpful clue, but it is crucial to remember that hearing loss is neither a sensitive nor a specific marker of Alport's syndrome; it is neither necessary nor sufficient for the diagnosis. Most patients with hearing loss and renal disease do not have Alport's syndrome, but rather a variety of other disorders, most commonly glomerulonephritis and a banal cause for hearing loss such as noise exposure or aminoglycoside therapy.

TREATMENT

There is no specific treatment for Alport's syndrome. General measures to retard the progression of renal failure, such as effective treatment of hypertension and modest protein restriction appear warranted, but are unproved. As for other forms of progressive renal disease, angiotensin converting enzyme inhibitors may offer a specific advantage. One unconfirmed report claims benefit from cyclosporine in reducing proteinuria and retarding progression of renal insufficiency. Males should wear hearing protection in noisy surroundings. Hearing aids improve but do not completely correct the hearing loss. Tinnitus is generally resistant to all forms of therapy; hearing aids may render it less disruptive by amplifying ambient sounds. Retinal lesions to not appear to affect vision and need no therapy. The serious impairment of vision caused by lenticonus or cataract cannot be corrected with spectacles or contact lenses. Lens removal with reimplantation of an intraocular lens is standard and satisfactory treatment.

RELATED DISORDERS

Familial Thin Basement Membrane Disease

Familial thin basement membrane disease or benign familial hematuria is an autosomal dominant basement membrane glomerulopathy. Some cases result from mutations of the COL4A3 or COL4A4 gene at 2q35–37. Ultrastructurally the GBM is uniformly thinned to about half its normal thickness. There is no disruption or lamellation of the GBM, nor are any other abnormalities of the glomeruli, tubules, vessels, or interstitium visible by light, immunofluorescence, or electron microscopy. Renal insufficiency does not occur. Longevity is unaffected by this condition, and survivors into the ninth decade are recorded. Minor degrees of lamellation of the GBM and hearing loss have been described in some families, but these families could have had unrecognized Alport's syndrome.

Once the precise diagnosis is established, the patient and family can be spared further invasive tests and an appropriate prognosis given to them and to insurers. Unfortunately, the distinction between Alport's syndrome and benign familial hematuria is not always easy to make. To be sure of the pattern of inheritance requires a large pedigree with accurate diagnoses in all the family members. A single mistaken diagnosis from incidental renal disease, inaccurate urinalysis, or incomplete penetrance may vitiate conclusions about the pattern of inheritance in the entire pedigree. Even biopsy evidence is fallible. Early cases of Alport's syndrome may show ultrastructural changes indistinguishable from those of benign familial hematuria. This is particularly likely to occur if a child from an adult-type Alport's kindred is biopsied. Stability of serum creatinine for several years in a child does not exclude adult-type Alport's syndrome. The interpretation is further clouded because homozygous individuals in families with familial thin GBM disease may have Alport's syndrome. In these families, autosomal dominant thin GBM disease and autosomal recessive Alport's syndrome are caused by the same mutations.

Alport's Syndrome with Thrombocytopathy (Epstein's Syndrome)

This uncommon autosomal dominant variant of Alport's syndrome associates moderate thrombocytopenia with severe hearing loss and renal failure in both males and females. The platelets are much larger than normal (about seven μm in diameter), and there is a mild or moderate bleeding tendency. In some families there are inclusion bodies (Fechtner bodies) in leukocytes. Fechtner syndrome is caused by a mutation in nonmuscle myosin heavy chain 9 (MYH9) gene on chromosome 22q12.3–13.1.

Autosomal Recessive Alport's Syndrome

A few children who develop renal disease before the age of 10 years have homozygous or mixed heterozygous mutations of the genes for the α3 or 4 chains of type IV collagen. Boys and girls are equally affected. The heterozygous parents may or may not show hematuria.

APPROACH TO THE PATIENT WITH HEREDITARY NEPHRITIS

Although Alport's syndrome is less common than polycystic kidney disease, it is probably more common than is generally appreciated. Important differential diagnoses of hematuria in young persons are IgA nephropathy or other glomerulonephritis, renal calculi, or medullary sponge kidney. The differential diagnosis of familial renal disease with hematuria includes familial thin GBM disease and familial IgA nephropathy and of course, polycystic disease. Familial renal diseases without hematuria that might be confused include polycystic kidney disease, medullary cystic disease, and some poorly defined forms of inherited glomerular and tubulointerstitial renal disease.

If a patient with unexplained hematuria or renal insufficiency has a family history of hematuria or renal failure, the family history should be extended, concentrating particularly on the male relatives of the mother. Finding hearing losses strengthens, and finding a specific ocular lesion greatly strengthens suspicion for Alport's syndrome. Renal biopsy would generally be indicated in one family member, but once the diagnosis of a basement membrane nephropathy is established in a family, it is hard to justify further biopsies unless there are features that suggest another diagnosis. The extent of investigation will be guided and will relate inversely to the strength of the family history. For example, a young man on the line of descent of a known Alport's family whose urine contains dysmorphic erythrocytes needs minimal investigation. He may need nothing more than a serum creatinine unless there are additional clinical features suggesting a systemic disease. A patient with hematuria and an uncertain family history may merit an intravenous pyelogram or abdominal flat plate and renal sonogram, antinuclear antibodies (ANA), and possibly anti-GBM antibodies, antineutrophil cytoplasmic autoantibodies (ANCA), and renal biopsy.

Genetic testing is presently of limited applicability in sporadic cases and small kindreds because most families have "private" mutations. Patients may wish to enroll in research studies that may eventually identify the mutation in their family. For a hundred or more small families and two very large kindreds in the United States, specific mutation tests are available. In these families, direct mutation analysis can quickly establish whether an individual is a gene carrier and spare the need for a renal biopsy. It is not yet clear whether the two common mutations are sufficiently widespread to justify screening for them in adults with unexplained renal failure or before undertaking a renal biopsy in an adult or child with hematuria.

Patients with any hereditary nephropathy should be informed of the nature of the disease and perhaps given a copy of the genetic analysis or renal biopsy report to avoid unnecessary further investigation. Similar conclusions apply to family members who are potentially gene carriers. Those with Alport's syndrome should be followed for elevation of blood pressure or serum creatinine. The frequency of follow-up will depend on the anticipated age of onset of renal deterioration in the family and will become closer as this age is approached. Those with familial thin basement membrane disease should be checked about every 2 years, because some may ultimately turn out to have Alport's syndrome.

Bibliography

Barker, DF, Hostikka SL, Zhou J, *et al.*: Identification of mutations in the COL4A5 collagen gene in Alport syndrome. *Science* 248:1224–1227, 1990.

Epstein CJ, Sahud MA, Piel CF, *et al.*: Hereditary macrothrombocytopathia, nephritis and deafness. *Am J Med Sci* 52:299–310, 1972.

Gleeson MJ: Alport syndrome: Audiological manifestations and implications. *J Laryngol Otol* 98:449–465, 1984.

Govan JA: Ocular manifestations of Alport's syndrome: A hereditary disorder of basement membranes? *Br J Ophthalmol* 67:493–503, 1983.

Gregory MC, Terreros DA, Barker DF, *et al.*: Alport syndrome—clinical phenotype, incidence, and pathology. In: Tryggvason K (ed) *Molecular Pathology and Genetics of Alport Syndrome*, pp. 1–28. Karger, Basel, 1996.

Gregory MC, Atkin CL: Alport syndrome, Fabry's disease, and nail-patella syndrome. In: Schrier RW, Gottschalk CW (eds) *Diseases of the Kidney*, sixth Ed., pp. 561–590. Little, Brown, Boston, 1997.

Jais JP, Knebelmann B, Giatris I, *et al.*: X-linked Alport syndrome: Natural history in 195 families and genotype–phenotype correlations in males. *J Am Soc Nephrol* 11:649–657, 2000.

Kashtan CE, Kleppel, MM, Gubler, M-C: Immunohistologic findings in Alport syndrome. In: Tryggvason K (ed) *Molecular Pathology and Genetics of Alport Syndrome*, pp. 142–153. Karger, Basel, 1996.

Lemmink HH, Nielsson WN, Mochizuki T, *et al.*: Benign familial hematuria due to mutation of the type 4 collagen gene. *J Clin Invest* 98:1114–1118, 1996.

Tiebosch TA, Frederik PM, van Breda Vriesman PJ, *et al.*: Thin basement membrane nephropathy in adults with persistent hematuria. *N Engl J Med* 320:14–18, 1989.

MEDULLARY CYSTIC DISEASE

ELLIS D. AVNER

Medullary cystic disease is a renal cystic disorder characterized by tubular cystic lesions in corticomedullary regions of the kidney. It is an uncommon, genetically determined tubulointerstitial nephritis that presents in children and young adults and inexorably progresses to end stage renal disease.

DEFINITIONS AND EPIDEMIOLOGY

Medullary cystic disease is a distinct clinicopathological entity that is part of a group of congenital tubulointerstitial nephropathies known as the juvenile nephronophthisis medullary cystic disease (JN–MCD) complex (Table 1). Although genetically heterogeneous, all of the diseases of the JN–MCD complex share common morphologic and functional renal alterations, which lead to similar clinical features and clinical course. Mutations in the *NPHP1* gene on chromosome 2q13 are responsible for autosomal-recessive juvenile nephronophthisis. Genes responsible for autosomal-dominant variants of the complex have been localized by linkage analysis to chromosomes 1q21 and 16p12, but have not yet been identified. The nosology of the diseases comprising the JN–MCD complex has been quite confusing, and they have been presented under a variety of terms, including uremic medullary cystic disease, cystic disease of the renal medulla, familial juvenile nephronophthisis, autosomal-recessive nephronophthisis, autosomal-dominant nephronophthisis, Fanconi nephronophthisis, salt-losing nephritis, and uremic sponge kidney. The overall incidence and prevalence of JN–MCD is unknown. The diseases appear to be uncommon, although more than 300 cases have been reported in the literature, and JN has been reported to cause 10 to 30% of pediatric end stage renal disease in European centers. Pooled data demonstrate a much lower prevalence (less than 5%) in the North American pediatric end stage renal disease population.

PATHOLOGY AND PATHOGENESIS

In general, no significant differences in renal pathology have been demonstrated for the individual conditions that comprise the JN–MCD complex. Early in the course of the disease, there are few renal structural changes which emphasize the functional nature of the renal tubular defects (see later). The characteristic feature of more advanced

cases is severe tubular atrophy with interstitial fibrosis and inflammatory cell infiltration, tubular basement membrane thickening, periglomerular fibrosis, and patchy glomerular obsolescence (Fig. 1). Ultrastructural analysis demonstrates thickening and loss of definition of tubular basement membranes. These changes progress to produce symmetrically small kidneys with severe, diffuse cortical atrophy.

A major feature of diseases of the JN–MCD complex is renal medullary cysts (Fig. 1). Cysts measuring 1 to 2 mm in diameter are generally concentrated along the corticomedullary junctions, and have been localized by microdissection to the distal convoluted and medullary collecting tubules. Although the presence of characteristic cysts has been considered a diagnostic criterion, many cases have been identified in which cysts are absent or detected only late in the course of disease progression. Such cases are otherwise morphologically, genetically, and clinically identical to cases in which medullary cysts are a prominent feature, suggesting that medullary cysts are neither of primary importance in causing clinical manifestations or tubulointerstitial nephritis nor necessary for disease progression to renal failure.

The pathogenesis of tubulointerstitial nephritis and medullary cyst formation in JN–MCD remains unknown. The ultrastructural findings of irregularly thickened and lamellated tubular basement membranes, as well as the decreased or absent expression of certain tubular basement membrane antigens, have suggested a primary biochemical or ultrastructural abnormality of the tubular basement membrane. Studies in the kd/kd murine model of JN–MCD suggest an immunopathogenic basis in which a defect in regulatory T-cell function leads to functional inactivation of suppressor T cells, loss of tolerance to tubular antigens, and facilitated expression of effector T cells that mediate tubulointerstitial injury. Studies in additional murine models of JN–MCD support the hypothesis that a primary defect in tubular cell–matrix interaction triggers disease. Characterization of the protein product of the *NPHP1* gene, nephrocystin, will further delineate the molecular pathophysiology and cell biology of the disease process.

CLINICAL FEATURES

All variants of JN–MCD complex are characterized by the insidious onset of renal failure. The most common symptoms at presentation are polydipsia, polyuria, and

TABLE I
The Juvenile Nephronophthisis–Medullary Cystic Disease Complex[a]

Variant	Genetics	Percentage of JN–MCD cases	Average age at onset of end stage renal disease (years)	Associated features
Juvenile nephronophthisis	AR	50	13	
Renal–retinal dysplasia	AR	15–20	13	Hepatic fibrosis, cerebellar ataxia, neurocutaneous dysplasia, skeletal abnormalities
Medullary cystic disease	AD	15–20	28	Hyperuricemia, gouty arthritis
Nonfamilial sporadic	—	15	17	

[a]AR, autosomal-recessive; AD, autosomal-dominant. Modified from Bernstein J, Gardner KD: In: Contran RS, Brenner BM (eds) *Tubulointerstitial Nephropathies*, pp. 335–358. Churchill-Livingstone, New York, 1983; and Hildebrandt F, Jungers P, Grunfeld J-P: In: Schrier RW, Gottschalk CW (eds) *Diseases of the Kidney*, 6th Ed., pp. 499–520. Little, Brown, Boston, 1996.

enuresis. Additional symptoms include weakness and pallor. Short stature and failure to thrive may be prominent presenting symptoms in children.

Unless at-risk individuals with parents or siblings affected with JN–MCD are monitored for the early symptom of polyuria, most patients present with a reduced glomerular filtration rate (GFR). Anemia is present in most patients at the time of diagnosis and has been considered by some, but not all, investigators to be disproportionately severe relative to the degree of renal dysfunction. Impairment of urinary concentrating ability is the earliest pathophysiological feature of JN–MCD. It has been documented prior to any decrease in GFR and may be present with minimal histological abnormalities. In some families with autosomal recessive variants of the JN–MCD complex, obligatory heterozygotes have demonstrated similar decreases in urinary concentrating ability. Unfortunately, this is not a consistent finding and cannot be utilized to identify

heterozygotes for the autosomal-recessive conditions. Renal salt wasting is another characteristic feature of JN–MCD and has been reported in 20 to 60% of affected patients. Salt wasting presumably reflects the severity and distribution of histological changes, as it does in other tubulointerstitial nephropathies, and may occur with or without the presence of medullary cystic lesions. An additional characteristic clinical feature of JN–MCD is the paucity of urinary abnormalities. Proteinuria and hematuria are exceedingly rare and reported only in some individuals with autosomal dominant variants of the complex. Pyuria and documented urinary tract infection are also uncommon, as is hypertension prior to end stage renal disease. The absence of these clinical features may help to differentiate JN–MCD from the other genetically determined polycystic kidney diseases.

As noted in Table 1, one-fourth to one-third of all patients with autosomal-recessive JN–MCD have associated retinal changes and are clinically classified as the renal–retinal dysplasia variant. Retinal findings are characterized by progressive tapetoretinal degeneration, a specific lesion of the retinal pigmented epithelium. Visual impairment may be present in early infancy or childhood. Fundoscopic alterations are present in all patients with renal–retinal dysplasia by the age of 10 years, and the diagnosis can be confirmed with electroretinography. Some reported patients with this clinical variant also have hepatic fibrosis, cerebellar ataxia, neurocutaneous dysplasia, and various skeletal abnormalities. The sporadic nature of these associations, as well as the irregular clustering in some families, makes these associations difficult to further classify. Retinal findings as well as the noted multiorgan associations have not been reported in the autosomal-dominant or nonfamilial sporadic variants of the JN–MCD complex.

The diagnosis of JN–MCD should be suspected in the child or young adult who presents with progressive renal failure and normal to small kidneys in association with the

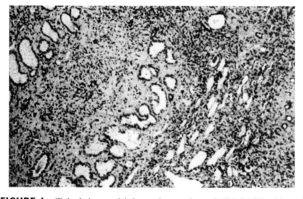

FIGURE I Tubulointerstitial nephropathy of JN–MCD. Noted are tubular atrophy, interstitial infiltration, thickening of tubular basement membranes, and medullary tubular dilatation and cysts. Magnification, 400×.

clinical and laboratory features previously noted. The differential diagnosis may include renal hypoplasia-dysplasia, congenital obstructive uropathies, autosomal dominant- or recessive-polycystic kidney disease, bilateral impairment of the renal circulation, or other forms of chronic tubulointerstitial nephritis. A complete history, with particular attention to family history, physical examination, examination of the urinary sediment, and radiographic imaging (ultrasonography, with computerized tomography and arteriography as indicated) will be adequate to establish the diagnosis of JN–MCD in most cases. On ultrasonography, kidneys are of normal or moderately reduced size, and typically exhibit increased echogenicity and a loss of corticomedullary differentiation. Though variable early in the course, medullary cysts can be demonstrated radiographically in greater than 80% of patients who have reached end stage renal disease. In rare instances, a renal biopsy may be indicated to definitively establish a histopathological diagnosis. However, pathognomonic medullary cysts may not be apparent on needle biopsy specimens. As previously noted, the gene responsible for the autosomal-recessive variant of JN–MCD has been identified, and at least two other genes on human chromosomes 1q and 16p have been linked to some families with autosomal-dominant disease. Thus, in some instances, diagnosis by gene analysis or genetic linkage studies may be possible.

PROGNOSIS AND THERAPY

JN–MCD is characterized by variable, but inexorable progression to end stage renal disease. Regardless of age at diagnosis, the average age at onset of end stage renal disease is 13 years for children with autosomal-recessive disease, and 28 years for adults with autosomal-dominant disease (Table 1). No specific factors have been identified which modify the rapidity of progression or clinical course. Genetic counseling is a cornerstone of therapy for families with genetically defined variants of the complex. If affected individuals are identified prior to the development of end stage renal disease, adequate hydration and sodium supplementation are critical to avoid dehydration and super-imposed prerenal insults. This is particularly true in infants and young children who are subject to episodic febrile illnesses and intercurrent episodes of gastroenteritis. Children with severe polyuria secondary to renal concentrating defects and salt wasting may require nasogastric or gastrostomy tube feedings to maintain hydration and provide adequate nutrition. Anemia is treated with recombinant human erythropoietin, and other manifestations of progressive uremia are treated in standard fashion. Ultimately dialysis and renal transplantation are utilized to treat end stage renal failure. JN–MCD has not, to date, been reported to recur in transplanted kidneys.

Bibliography

Antignac C, Kleinknecht C, Habib R: Nephronophthisis. In: Davison AM, Cameron JS, Grunfeld JP, Kerr DNS, Ritz E, Winearls CG (eds) Oxford Textbook of Clinical Nephrology, 2nd Ed., pp. 2417–2426. Oxford Press, Oxford, 1998.

Avasthi PS, Erickson DG, Gardner KD: Hereditary renal–retinal dysplasia and the medullary cystic disease–nephronophthisis complex. Ann Intern Med 84:157–161, 1976.

Bernstein J, Gardner KD: Hereditary tubulo interstitial nephritis. In: Contran RS, Brenner BM, Stein JH (eds) Tubulointerstitial Nephropathies, pp. 335–358. Churchill-Livingston, New York, 1983.

Hildebrandt F: Nephronophthisis. In: Barratt TM, Avner ED, Harmon WE (eds) Pediatric Nephrology, 4th Ed., pp. 453–458, Lippincott, Williams & Wilkins, Baltimore, 1999.

Hildebrandt F, Jungers P, Grunfeld J-P: Medullary cystic and medullary sponge renal disorders. In: Schrier RW, Gottschalk CW (eds) Diseases of the Kidney, 6th Ed., pp. 499–520. Little, Brown, Boston, 1996.

Hildebrandt F, Otto E, Rensing C, et al.: A novel gene encoding an SH3 domain protein is mutated in nephronophthisis type 1. Nat. Genet. 17:149–153, 1997.

Kelly CJ, Neilson EG: Medullary cystic disease: An inherited form of autoimmune interstitial nephritis? Am J Kidney Dis 10:389–395, 1987.

Mongeau JG, Worthen HG: Nephronophthisis and medullary cystic disease. Am J Med 43:345–355, 1967.

Sibalic V, Sun L, Sibalic A, et al.: Characteristic matrix and tubular basement membrane abnormalities in the CBA/Ca-kdkd mouse model of hereditary tubulointerstitial disease. Nephron 80:305–313, 1998.

SECTION 8

TUBULOINTERSTITIAL NEPHROPATHIES AND DISORDERS OF THE URINARY TRACT

TUBULOINTERSTITIAL DISEASE

WILLIAM F. FINN

DEFINITION AND CLASSIFICATION

Chronic structural abnormalities involving the renal tubules and interstitum develop in two circumstances. In the first, tubulointerstitial nephritis is found as the primary lesion after prolonged exposure to various therapeutic or environmental agents or in association with a number of systemic illnesses (Table 1). Such primary chronic interstitial nephritis accounts for up to 15 to 30% of cases of end stage renal disease. In the second, tubulointerstitial changes occur as a result of progressive glomerular and vascular injury. This has come to be recognized as a significant determinant of the final outcome of these conditions.

HISTOLOGY

The characteristic lesion is composed of an interstitial inflammatory mononuclear cell infiltrate containing lymphocytes—mostly T cells—and occasional plasma cells. This acute cellular infiltrate is generally accompanied by interstitial edema, disruption of the tubular basement membrane, and dissolution of normal interstitial architecture. The transition to a chronic process occurs with the development of interstitial fibrosis, which is accompanied by tubular ectasia, tubular atrophy, and a marked increase in extracellular matrix. Eventually, glomerular and vascular structures are involved, and fibrotic and sclerotic changes occur throughout the kidney.

CLINICAL MANIFESTATIONS

The manifestations of tubulointerstitial nephritis depend on the extent of injury (diffuse or focal), the tubular segments most severely involved (proximal or more distal), and the degree of compensation achieved by the less severely involved nephrons. When proximal tubules are damaged, such substances as sodium, glucose, amino acids, uric acid, and low-molecular-weight proteins, which are ordinarily reabsorbed or metabolized at this site, appear in the urine. A decrease in bicarbonate reabsorption may lead to proximal renal tubular acidosis. Damage to more distal structures, including the loop of Henle, the distal convoluted tubule, and the collecting duct, is accompanied by an inability to maximally concentrate and dilute the urine. The defect in the ability to concentrate the urine may result in polyuria. Damage in this area may decrease excretion of

titratable acid and urinary ammonia excretion, leading to metabolic acidosis. This may be present in conjunction with a defect in the secretion of potassium and result in type IV renal tubular acidosis.

DIAGNOSIS

The clinical diagnosis of tubulointerstitial nephritis is often a diagnosis of exclusion, made when glomerular disease is absent. The histologic diagnosis of tubulointerstitial nephritis requires evidence of an inflammatory infiltrate accompanied by interstitial fibrosis. In the absence of other definable disease, presumptive evidence includes a history of significant exposure to an offending agent or the coexistence of a condition known to be associated with tubulointerstitial disease, the demonstration of abnormalities of tubular function out of proportion to the reduction in glomerular function, and a urinalysis marked by the absence of heavy proteinuria with a tendency for leukocyturia rather than hematuria.

Urinalysis

Evaluation of the urine in patients with chronic interstitial nephritis yields variable results, except that marked proteinuria in uncommon; by quantitative tests, a trace-to-1 + protein may be present; by qualitative analyses, usually less than 1 g of protein/24 hr, and often less than 500 mg is found. Microscopic examination may disclose a preponderance of white blood cells and occasionally white cell casts and granular casts. A general estimate of integrated tubular function may be obtained by determining the capacity of the kidneys to concentrate or dilute the urine in response to water deprivation or administration, the ability to excrete an administered acid load, and the precision with which sodium balance is maintained.

Proteinuria

The normal values of the major urinary proteins are listed in Table 2. In contrast to the high-molecular-weight proteins, a finite amount of low-molecular-weight proteins is normally filtered and then reabsorbed by proximal tubular cells. When the reabsorptive capacity of the proximal tubular epithelium is disrupted, various low-molecular-weight proteins appear in the urine.

TABLE I
Causes of Chronic Tubulointerstitial Disease

Category	Examples
Therapeutic agents/ occupational or environmental agents	Analgesics NSAIDs Chemotherapeutic agents (cisplatin,nitrosoureas) Immunotherapeutic agents (cyclosporine, FK-506) Heavy metals (lead, cadmium) Lithium
Immunologic conditions	Renal allograft rejection Amyloid Vasculitis Cryoglobulinemia Sjögren's syndrome Systemic lupus erythematosus Wegener's granulomatosus
Hematopoietic/neoplastic diseases	Sickle cell disease Multiple myeloma Light chain disease Dysproteinemias Lymphoproliferative disease
Mechanical disorders	Ureteral obstruction
Vascular diseases	Radiation Hypertension Atheromatous emboli
Hereditary/genetic	Karyomegalic interstitial nephritis Medullary cystic disease/ nephronophthis complex Polycystic kidney disease Hereditary nephritis
Miscellaneous conditions	Balkan nephropathy Chinese herb nephropathy Mycotoxins Sarcoidosis
Metabolic disorders	Hypercalcemia Hypokalemia Uric acid nephropathy Oxalate nephropathy Cystinosis
Infections	Systemic Local

TABLE 2
Normal Values for Urinary Proteins in Humans

Urinary protein	MW	Normal value
Tamm-Horsfall glycoprotein[a]		14.3 (5.1–25.5)
Albumin[a]	69,000	5.2 (2.8–15)
α_1-Microglobulin[a]	29,000–33,000	4.20 ± 6
IgG[a]	146,000	1.2 (0.35–2.7)
Transferrin[a]	77,000	0.17 (0.08–0.83)
Cystatin C	13,300	0.113 ± 0.125 mg/L
Protein 1[a]	18,700	0.092 (0.02–0.3)
β_2-Microglobulin[a]	11,800	0.062 (0.021–0.142)
Retinol-binding protein[a]	21,400	0.055 (0.03–0.13)
Lysozyme		0.015 (0.002–0.12) mg/L

[a]mg/g Creatinine.

High-Molecular-Weight Proteinuria

The distinction between "glomerular" proteinuria and "tubular" proteinuria is based on the quantity and quality of the proteins measured in the urine. The appearance in the urine of serum proteins with a molecular mass in excess of 40,000 to 50,000 Da is an early marker of glomerular damage. The commonly measured high-molecular-weight proteins include albumin, transferrin, and IgG.

Low-Molecular-Weight Proteinuria

In contrast, tubular proteinuria is due to excretion of low-molecular-weight proteins. The two most commonly mentioned as potential markers of renal tubular damage are β_2-microglobulin (β_2-m) and retinol binding protein. Other low-molecular-weight proteins include α_1-microglobulin (α_1-m), protein 1, amylase, lysozyme, ribonuclease, and cystatin C. Due to its molecular weight and small radius, β_2-m is readily filtered at the glomerulus. Approximately 99.9% is reabsorbed by the proximal tubular epithelial cells and ultimately catabolized. A very small amount appears in the urine. The urinary excretion of β_2-m is considerably increased in cases of renal tubular impairment. Because β_2-m undergoes degradation at urinary pH of 5.5 or less, accurate measurement demands alkalinization of the urine. Retinol-binding protein is a low-molecularweight protein synthesized in the liver, where it binds to retinol. Once the retinol is released at peripheral sites, the binding protein is rapidly eliminated from plasma by glomerular filtration. It is then reabsorbed and catabolized by proximal tubular cells. Because of its stability in acid urine, the assay of urinary retinol binding protein is preferred over that of β_2-m.

Tamm–Horsfall Protein

Tamm–Horsfall glycoprotein is the most abundant protein of renal origin in normal urine and is the major constituent of urinary casts. Tamm–Horsfall glycoprotein is synthesized by cells of the thick ascending limb of the loop of Henle, and is excreted in the urine at a relatively constant rate. Urinary excretion can increase following injury to the distal tubule.

Enzymuria

The interpretation of urinary enzyme titers is founded on the premise that the sole source of high-molecular-weight enzymes is damaged tubular cells. However, it is hard to correlate specific disease states with the presence or absence of enzymuria. In addition, a relationship between the severity of cellular injury and the magnitude of enzymuria has been difficult to establish. This has been due in part to the observation that urinary enzyme activity is affected by various factors that are independent of cellular

TABLE 3
Some Enzymes Used as an Index of Nephrotoxicity

Enzymes	Cellular location
Alanine aminopeptidase	Brush border
Alkaline phosphatase	
γ-Glutamyltransferase	
Maltase	
Trehalase	
Glutamic oxaloacetic transaminase	Cytosol
Glutamic pyruvic transaminase	
Lactate dehydrogenase	
Malate dehydrogenase	
N-Acetyl-β-D-glucosaminidase	Lysosome
Acid phosphatase	
β-Galactosidase	
β-Glucosidase	
β-Glucuronidase	
Glutamate dehydrogenase	Mitochondria

integrity, that is, urinary pH, osmolarity, and the presence of various enzyme inhibitors or activators. However, in addition to normal cell shedding, enzymes also gain urinary access because of altered cell membrane permeability, increased rate of enzyme synthesis, and frank cell necrosis. Only a limited number of enzymes have been generally accepted as valuable urinary biomarkers. These include N-acetyl-β-D-glucosaminidase, alanine aminopeptidase, and intestinal alkaline phosphatase. It is important to emphasize that the measurement of these enzymes, while of considerable theoretical interest, is of limited clinical utility (Table 3).

N-Acetyl-β-glucosaminidase is found in both the straight (S3) segment of proximal tubular cells and the distal nephron as a lysosomal enzyme. In humans, it has its highest activity in the S3 segment, with less activity in the collecting duct. Elevated urinary levels accompany proximal tubular cell injury. It may also be found in the urine of patients with various forms of glomerular disease, obstructive uropathy, and nephrosclerosis. Other nonspecific increases in urinary activity that limit its usefulness as a diagnostic tool have been described.

Alanine aminopeptidase is restricted to the proximal tubule. Increased excretion has been reported in a variety of renal diseases including pyelonephritis, glomerulonephritis, urologic cancers, and renal transplant rejection. In addition, increased excretion has been reported in association with many well-defined nephrotoxins. Although not specific in discriminating between glomerular and tubular disease, it is very sensitive to acute tubular injury.

Intestinal alkaline phosphatase and nonspecific tissue alkaline phosphatase are two urinary isoenzymes that have elicited interest as potential segment specific markers of the human nephron. Intestinal alkaline phosphatase is expressed on the brush border of the tubuloepithelial cells of the S3 segment of the proximal tubule. The intestinal alkaline phosphatase released in urine has its origin in the kidney and is considered to be a specific and sensitive marker for alterations of the S3 segment. In the kidney, tissue alkaline phosphatase is localized on the brush border in all segments of the proximal tubule. By measuring both enzymes, judgments as to the involvement of S1-S2 versus S3 segments can be achieved in experimental models.

Tubular Antigens

The urinary excretion of specific proximal tubular antigens is increased in a variety of renal diseases. Monoclonal antibodies to membrane and other cellular derived antigens are new, sensitive, specific, and readily available markers of renal cell injury. Increased excretion of tubular antigens occurs in exposure to cadmium, hydrocarbons, cisplatin, and radiographic contrast media. Monoclonal antibodies to human brush-border antigens have been produced and used in investigational studies. Their use may permit detection of site-specific renal damage.

MECHANISM OF FIBROGENESIS

Infiltrating cells stimulate fibrogenesis through the release of various cytokines and growth factors. In response, resident cells in the kidney undergo phenotypic changes and acquire smooth muscle and fibroblastic characteristics. Active in this process may be transforming growth factor β (TGF-β), one of the more potent stimulators of collagen and noncollagen basement membrane components. Examples of the latter include proteoglycans and fibronectin. TGF-β also inhibits matrix degrading enzymes such as collagenase and metalloproteinases. The net result is that for a time the excessive deposition of extracellular matrix can be removed, but eventually complete resolution becomes unlikely. TGF-β also controls the interaction of cells with the extracellular matrix by regulating the expression of various cell adhesion molecules such as integrins. Platelet-derived growth factor also stimulates chemotaxis, influences the production of extracellular matrix, and regulates its subsequent metabolism. Added to this are the interleukins which modulate inflammatory and immune responses by regulating the growth, differentiation, and mobility of effector cells. In an as yet unknown manner, angiotensin II may be linked to the irreversible changes of tubulointerstitial fibrosis.

PRIMARY VASCULAR AND GLOMERULAR RENAL DISEASE

In many forms of renal disease due to primary glomerular injury, there is a remarkable inverse correlation between the extent of tubulointerstitial damage and the glomerular filtration rate. This observation has directed attention to the important role of the tubulointerstitial compartment in the progression of renal disease.

The most obvious explanation to account for the tubulointerstitial injury that occurs with primary glomerular disease is that inflammatory glomerular lesions are accompanied by acute interstitial mononuclear cell infiltrates which later lead to chronic fibrotic changes by mechanisms previously described. Other mechanisms have been suggested. For instance, it is clear that persistent high-grade proteinuria is associated with a progressive loss of renal function and the development of tubulointerstitial disease and renal fibrosis. With the loss of permselectivity that occurs with glomerular injury, various circulating plasma proteins—usually prevented from passing this barrier—may find their way into the glomerular filtrate and tubular fluid where they exert toxic effects on epithelial cells. Some of these proteins may precipitate within the tubular lumen, thereby forming casts and obstructing tubular fluid flow. Preglomerular vasoconstriction follows, with a decrease in peritubular capillary blood flow, eventual tubular atrophy, and further interstitial inflammation. As tubular reabsorptive mechanisms are stimulated, lysosomal degradative enzymes may spill into the cytosol and cause damage. Alternatively, filtered low-molecular-weight cytokines may bind to tubular epithelial cells and lead to activation of the alternate complement pathway.

Without question, immunologic processes involving either the cell-dependent or the humoral pathway may be responsible for the ongoing damage. A release of chemotactic lipids may further the inflammatory response. In addition, changes in tubular oxidative metabolism leading to an increase in renal ammoniagenesis and the generation of reactive oxygen species may contribute to the progressive lesions. Ammonia may interact with the third component of complement with activation of the alternate complement cascade and subsequent immunologic cellular injury. Cytokine-induced generation of nitric oxide and the transferrin-related release of iron with accumulation in tubular cell lysosomes may be associated with oxidative cellular injury. Finally, arachidonic acid metabolites, particularly thromboxane A_2, may stimulate extracellular matrix protein formation and in this way contribute to the progression of renal disease.

Bibliography

Eddy AA: Experimental insights into the tubulointerstitial disease accompanying primary glomerular lesions. *J Am Soc Nephrol* 5:1273–1287, 1994.

Dodd S: The pathogenesis of tubulointerstitial disease and mechanisms of fibrosis. *Curr Top Pathol* 88:117–143, 1995.

Jones CL, Eddy AA: Tubulointerstitial nephritis. *Pediatr Nephrol* 6:572–586, 1992.

Nath KA: Tubulointerstitial changes as a major determinant in the progression of renal damage. *Am J Kidney Dis* 20:1–17, 1992.

Restegar A. Kashgarian M: The clinical spectrum of tubulointerstitial nephritis. *Kidney Int* 54:313–327, 1998.

Sedor JR: Cytokines and growth factors is renal injury. *Semin Nephrol* 12:428–440, 1992.

47

LITHIUM-INDUCED RENAL DISEASE

GREGORY L. BRADEN

Lithium is the best treatment for manic-depressive illness, but therapy with this drug has been associated with side effects in many body systems, including the kidneys. Lithium is freely filtered at the glomerulus, reabsorbed like sodium at several tubular sites, and concentrated in the renal medulla; circumstances that might favor lithium-induced renal disease. Although lithium initially was thought to produce only functional renal abnormalities, such as nephrogenic diabetes insipidus (NDI), additional disorders now attributed to lithium include renal tubular acidosis, chronic interstitial nephritis, and nephrotic syndrome.

NEPHROGENIC DIABETES INSIPIDUS

Polydipsia occurs in up to 40% and polyuria greater than 3 L/day occurs in up to 20% of patients treated with lithium. Despite the high prevalence of polyuria, urine volume is rarely increased enough to require cessation of lithium therapy. Most humans with lithium-induced polyuria are unresponsive to the administration of exogenous antidiuretic hormone (ADH). This could occur either due to abnormalities in the medullary osmotic gradient which drives ADH-mediated water reabsorption or due to direct inhibition of the tubular hydro-osmotic effects of ADH. Chronic administration of lithium diminishes the medullary and papillary osmolar gradients due to depletion of urea without affecting sodium chloride concentrations. However, lithium-induced polyuria is largely due to direct inhibition of the ADH-dependent aspects of water conservation. Only one lithium-treated patient has been reported to have a defect in the pituitary release of ADH indicative of central diabetes insipidus.

Lithium impairs the hydro-osmotic response to ADH by several mechanisms. First, there is abundant physiological and biochemical evidence that lithium directly inhibits the adenylate cyclase system in the mammalian distal nephron, leading to decreased generation of the second messenger, cyclic adenosine-3'5'-monophosphate (cAMP). In addition, lithium has been shown to inhibit transepithelial water movement after the administration of exogenous cAMP, suggesting inhibition of water flow at a site distal to the generation of cAMP. Enhanced water permeability normally occurs as cAMP activates protein kinase A which phosphorylates the water channel protein, aquaporin 2, leading to insertion of these water channels from intracellular vesicles into the apical membrane of collecting duct cells. However, chronic lithium administration can downregulate the expression of aquaporin 2 water channels in collecting ducts, leading to impaired water reabsorption and polyuria.

Although lithium-induced NDI usually improves after lithium withdrawal, some patients have persistent concentrating defects lasting for years. Recently, amiloride has been shown to reduce urinary volume and enhance the concentrating ability of patients with lithium-induced NDI. Amiloride blocks distal tubular reabsorption of lithium, thus lowering the renal tissue lithium level. In addition, amiloride is a diuretic, and the combination of dietary salt restriction and the natriuretic effect of the diuretic induces mild extracellular fluid volume depletion which increases proximal tubular fluid reabsorption, potentially decreases the glomerular filtration rate, and lessens urinary volume. Thiazide diuretics have also been utilized for this, but they may raise serum lithium levels. Interestingly, amiloride has been shown to be effective without inducing any changes in creatinine clearance or serum lithium levels, suggesting that the inhibition of lithium uptake in the distal nephron may be the most important factor accounting for its efficacy. Indomethacin has been effective in a few patients, presumably by inducing a significant fall in the glomerular filtration rate which, similar to diuretics, may lower urinary volume. In addition, indomethacin inhibits synthesis of urinary prostaglandins that inhibit the tubular action of ADH. Finally, a few patients with severe NDI will require cessation of lithium and the substitution of either carbamazepine or valproic acid to treat the manic-depressive illness.

RENAL TUBULAR ACIDOSIS

Lithium impairs distal hydrogen ion secretion in at least 50% of treated patients. During administration of intra-

venous sodium bicarbonate, distal nephron bicarbonate delivery is increased. In normal humans, this stimulates hydrogen ion excretion by the distal nephron proton pumps. The additional protons are buffered by bicarbonate; the carbonic acid formed then dissociates and raises the urinary pCO_2 from 40 to 80 mm Hg or greater. This distal nephron response is impaired in lithium-treated patients; however, there is no evidence for renal bicarbonate wasting, such as in proximal renal tubular acidosis, and the excretion of the urinary buffer, ammonium, is normal. Despite this defect in urinary acidification, the serum bicarbonate and pH remain normal. Taken together, these studies indicate that lithium induces incomplete distal renal tubular acidosis. Thus, patients treated with lithium are prone to systemic acidosis during stressful conditions, such as sepsis or catabolic states.

ACUTE RENAL FAILURE/LITHIUM INTOXICATION

Acute renal failure due to biopsy-proven acute tubular necrosis may occur in lithium intoxicated patients. Nephrotic syndrome due to minimal change disease may occur concomitantly with acute tubular necrosis. Whether lithium can directly cause tubular necrosis or whether tubular necrosis in these patients is secondary to hemodynamic factors is unknown.

Lithium intoxication is classified into three grades of severity based on the blood level (mild, < 2.5 mEq/L; moderate, 2.5–3.5 mEq/L; severe, > 3.5 mEq/L). Toxic effects include nausea, ataxia, tremors, twitching, muscle rigidity, disordered consciousness, seizures, and coma. The pathophysiology of lithium intoxication may be due to its ability to induce dehydration and salt depletion secondary to its inhibitory effect on ADH action and the acute effects of lithium to induce a natriuresis leading to extracellular fluid volume depletion, activation of the renin–angiotensin system, a decrease in glomerular filtration rate and, in turn, increased serum lithium levels. In addition, angiotensin-converting enzyme inhibitors and nonsteroidal, antiinflammatory drugs may cause renal dysfunction leading to lithium intoxication, especially in patients on high therapeutic doses of lithium. Close monitoring of serum lithium levels is warranted after initiation of therapy with these agents.

Patients with lithium intoxication should be admitted to the hospital since seizures can occur at any time. The drug should be discontinued and, if there is an acute ingestion, either gastric lavage or ipecac should be given. Restoration of depleted extracellular fluid volume should be achieved by the administration of intravenous 0.9% normal saline if there is no hypernatremia present. For those patients with mild intoxication with a serum level of 2.5 mEq/L or less, saline diuresis may be enough to enhance renal lithium clearance. If there is no history to preclude vigorous volume expansion, then up to 6 L of saline can be given daily until the lithium level decreases to the nontoxic range. With this therapy, the lithium level should fall approximately 1 mEq/day. However, patients who are euvolemic usually do not respond to saline or forced diuresis. For patients with moderate or severe toxicity, hemodialysis is the therapy of choice and may need to be repeated if serum lithium levels rebound after the first hemodialysis treatment. If hemodialysis is unavailable, continuous veno venous hemodiafiltration is an alternative means of therapy that effectively removes lithium and can prevent posttherapy rebound.

NEPHROTIC SYNDROME

Lithium causes nephrotic syndrome in a small number of patients. Renal biopsy demonstrated focal segmental glomerulosclerosis in the majority of patients and minimal change disease in a smaller number. Several patients with focal segmental glomerulosclerosis and serum creatinine levels >2.0 mg/dL have progressed to end stage renal failure requiring dialysis. Patients with minimal change disease often have complete remission of the nephrotic syndrome on withdrawal of lithium. However, minimal change disease may occur after readministration of lithium.

CHRONIC INTERSTITIAL NEPHRITIS

Lithium was first associated with chronic interstitial nephritis in 1977 when a renal biopsy study described an increase in interstitial fibrosis, focal nephron atrophy, or both, in lithium-treated patients compared to age-matched controls. In this study, 80% of the lithium-treated patients had decreased creatinine clearances. Subsequently, a number of retrospective and uncontrolled studies found the prevalence of renal insufficiency to be 3–20% in patients treated long-term with lithium, but other disorders causing renal insufficiency were not always excluded. In contrast, additional studies compared lithium-treated patients to a more suitable control group, psychiatric patients not receiving lithium, and found no differences in serum creatinine or creatinine clearance, but renal biopsies were not performed.

Prospective studies have shown that chronic lithium therapy in psychiatric patients can significantly impair the glomerular filtration rate compared to similarly matched psychiatric patients who never received lithium. Renal biopsies in lithium-treated patients have demonstrated increased interstitial fibrosis and a unique tubular lesion consisting of microcyst formation due to cystic dilation of the distal tubules lined with enlarged columnar epithelium.

Taken together, these studies indicate that a small number of patients treated with lithium develop progressive renal damage associated with chronic interstitial nephritis. In those patients with mild to moderate chronic renal insufficiency from lithium, withdrawal of lithium may be associated with gradual improvement in glomerular filtration rate. However, several patients have been reported to develop end stage renal failure requiring dialysis therapy de-

spite withdrawal of lithium, particularly if they were treated with lithium for greater than 20 years. Baseline renal function studies, including serum creatinine, blood urea nitrogen (BUN), and creatinine clearance, should be performed prior to the initiation of lithium therapy and thereafter measured yearly. Patients who demonstrate deterioration in renal function should have lithium therapy withdrawn and either carbamazepine or valproic acid initiated. For those patients who can only be managed on lithium due to psychological dependence on this drug, lithium therapy can probably be continued with careful monitoring of renal function by creatinine clearance over time while maintaining the serum lithium level within the lower therapeutic range.

Bibliography

Allen HM, Jackson RL, Winchester MD, Deck LV, Allon M: Indomethacin in the treatment of lithium-induced nephrogenic diabetes insipidus. *Arch Intern Med* 149:1123–1126, 1989.

Batlle D, Gaviria M, Grupp M, Arruda JAL, Wynn J, Kurtzman NA: Distal nephron function in patinets receiving chronic lithium therapy. *Kidney Int* 21:477–485, 1982.

Batlle DC, von Riotte AB, Gaviria M, Grupp M: Amelioration of polyuria by amiloride in patients receiving long-term lithium therapy. *N Engl J Med* 312:408–414, 1985.

Boton R, Gaviria M, Batlle DC: Prevalence, pathogenesis, and treatment of renal dysfunction associated with chronic lithium therapy. *Am J Kidney Dis* 10:329–345, 1987.

Hestbech J, Hansen HE, Amdisen A, Olsen S: Chronic renal lesions following long-term treatment with lithium. *Kidney Int* 12: 205–213, 1977.

Jorkasky DK, Amsterdam JD, Oler J, Braden G, Alvis R, Geheb M, Cox M: Lithium-induced renal disease: A prospective study. *Clin Nephrol* 30:293–302, 1988.

Leblanc M, Raymond M, Bonnardeaux A, Isenring P, Pichette V, Geadah D, Ouimet D, Ethier J, Cardinal J: Lithium poisoning treated by high-performance continuous arteriovenous and venovenous hemodiafiltration. *Am J Kidney Dis* 27:365–372, 1996.

Lehmann K, Ritz E: Angiotensin-converting enzyme inhibitors may cause renal dysfunction in patients on long-term lithium treatment. *Am J Kidney Dis* 25:82–87, 1995.

Marples D, Christensen S, Christensen EI, Ottosen PD, Nielsen S: Lithium-induced downregulation of aquaporin-2 water channel expression in rat kidney medulla. *J Clin Invest* 95:1838–1845, 1995.

Poindexter AE, Braden GL, Honeyman D, Germain M, O'Shea MH, Mulhern JG, Pekow P: Lithium-induced chronic renal failure: Improved renal function after discontinuing lithium vs progression to end stage renal disease with long-term continued use. *J Am Soc Nephrol* 10:86A, 1999.

Rimmer RT, Sands JM: Lithium intoxication. *J Am Soc Nephrol* 10:666–674, 1999.

Tam VKK, Green J, Schwieger J, Cohen AH: Nephrotic syndrome and renal insufficiency with lithium therapy. *Am J Kidney Dis* 27:715–720, 1996.

Walker RG, Bennett WM, Davies BM, Kincaid-Smith P: Structural and functional effects of long-term lithium therapy. *Kidney Int* 21:513–519, 1982.

48

LEAD NEPHROPATHY

HARVEY C. GONICK

HISTORY

Although lead intoxication had been recognized for thousands of years, the relationship between lead exposure and chronic interstitial nephritis was not appreciated until the mid-nineteenth century. In the eighteenth and nineteenth centuries, port wine was heavily fortified ("sweetened") with lead, and the squires of England, heavy ingesters of port wine, were frequently afflicted with gout. Garrod, in 1859 was the first to recognize the association between lead exposure, gout, and renal disease.

In 1897 an "epidemic" of gout and renal disease was reported from Queensland, Australia. Many of the young adults had suffered from childhood lead poisoning, occurring from the ingestion of lead-based paint which flaked off their houses. Later epidemiological tests showed that virtually all had positive CaEDTA lead-mobilization tests and several had elevated bone levels of lead. Subsequently, an outbreak of lead-induced kidney disease associated with gout, and occasionally with hyperkalemic acidosis, was noted in moonshine whiskey drinkers from the Southern United States. In this instance, the lead was derived from the old battery casings in which the whiskey was distilled.

RISK FACTORS

Populations at Risk

Occupational exposure to lead occurs in smelters, miners, painters, and plumbers, and in workers involved in the manufacture of storage batteries, pottery, and pewter. Environmental exposure occurs though the use of lead-glazed pottery, the consumption of moonshine whiskey, and the ingestion of lead-containing food or water. Lead pipes and soldered joints are important sources of lead in drinking water, whereas soil contaminated with lead from industrial activities is an important source of lead in foodstuffs. Lead is most harmful to children under 6 years of age in that they absorb about 50% of the ingested lead. In comparison, adults absorb only 5 to 10%. For children, flaking lead-based paint and dust in old homes are important sources of lead. The removal of lead from gasoline and paint has significantly reduced the lead exposure in children and adults alike.

Susceptibility

In addition to the age at which exposure occurs, the amount of lead absorbed and the severity of the disease may be influenced by the amount of calcium in the diet, the presence of iron deficiency, and exposure to sunlight and vitamin D.

PATHOPHYSIOLOGY

Markers of Effect

Low lead exposure has little definable effect on the creatinine clearance (C_{Cr}), whereas moderate exposure may be accompanied by a slight state of hyperfiltration. However, a negative correlation between blood lead and the C_{Cr} has been found, such that a 10-fold rise in blood lead concentration was associated with as much as a 10 to 13 mL/min reduction in the C_{Cr}. Thus, lead exposure may impair renal function in the population at large, although it is possible that renal impairment itself may lead to an increase in the blood lead concentration.

Proteinuria of either a low- or high-molecular-weight is an inconsistent finding. Albuminuria tends to occur only with advanced disease. With elevated blood lead levels, an increase in urinary retinol binding protein but not β_2-microglobulin may be found. Likewise, elevated blood lead levels may be accompanied by an increase in certain urinary enzymes, such as N-acetyl-β-D-glucosaminidase, intestinal alkaline phosphatase, and ligandin (Table 1).

Mechanism of Toxicity

The nephrotoxicity is due to the renal tubular reabsorption of lead with deposition of lead in the tubules. Nuclear inclusion bodies that form in proximal tubule epithelial cells have a high sulfhydryl group content representing a lead-binding protein that sequesters intracellular lead (Fig. 1). A major toxic effect of the free lead involves the inhibition of cellular respiration and energy production as a result of the accumulation in mitochondria and the ensuing defects in mitochondrial structure and function.

Clinical Manifestations

At least two types of renal impairment may be found in association with lead poisoning. In the first and more acute form, generalized defects in proximal tubular function result. Chronic lead nephropathy, the second type of renal impairment associated with lead poisoning, is an indolent

TABLE I
Clinical and Pathological Abnormalities of Lead Nephropathy

Reduced glomerular filtration rate

Reduced renal blood flow

Proteinuria absent or minimal

Urine sediment normal

Hypertension variable

Hyperuricemia and low urate clearance common

Acidosis and hyperkalemia due to hyporeninemia sometimes seen

Increased urinary enzymes: N-acetyl-β-D-glucosaminidase, ligandin, and intestinal alkaline phosphatase

Increased urinary low-molecular-weight proteins: α-1-microglobulin, retinol binding protein, brush-border antigen

Fanconi syndrome: only in acutely intoxicated children

Renal biopsy: interstitial nephritis and proximal tubular nuclear inclusion bodies (early)

disease difficult to separate from other forms of chronic slowly progressive renal insufficiency with tubulointerstitial disease. In the absence of a history of acute lead nephropathy, the diagnosis is suspected when the course of the renal disease is protracted, without definable cause, and associated with symmetrical contraction of both kidneys. Urine protein excretion tends to be less than 1 g/24 hr and is marked by the presence of low-molecular-weight proteins such as α-1-microglobulin or retinol-binding protein. Urinary β_2-microglobulin, elevated in the presence of cadmium nephrotoxicity, is usually normal. Evidence of ex-

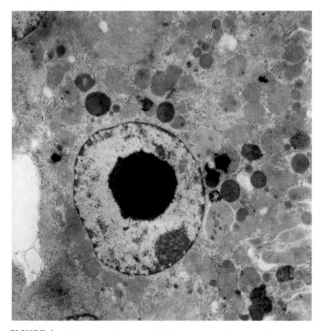

FIGURE I   Electron micrograph of proximal tubular cells demonstrating nucleus with dense inclusion body and outer fibrillary zone ($\times$7500).

cessive lead absorption is supplied by determining urinary lead excretion after administration of the calcium disodium salt of ethylene diamine tetraacetic acid ($CaNa_2EDTA$), a lead chelator, as described later or by use of the bone X-ray fluorescence test for defining the level of lead in bone. Chronic lead nephropathy is generally considered to be irreversible.

Hypertension

Several epidemiologic studies have suggested a weak, but positive, association between blood pressure and blood lead or bone lead levels in humans. There is a definite relationship between development of hypertension and feeding of low lead content ($\sim$100 parts per million) but *not* high lead content, in normal rats. The pathogenesis of this relationship involves an increase in reactive oxygen species, which leads to a decrease in nitric oxide metabolites via inactivation and a compensatory increase in nitric oxide synthase. The elevation in blood pressure may be due to either the increased reactive oxygen species, the diminished nitric oxide, or both. Whether low lead exposure in man is a major cause of essential hypertension remains to be determined.

Saturnine Gout

Chronic lead toxicity is often associated with an increase in tubular urate reabsorption, hyperuricemia, and saturnine gout. Because gout is unusual in other forms of chronic renal failure, chronic lead nephropathy should be considered in a patient with chronic renal failure and symptomatic gout. This is particularly true in women, as there is an overwhelming male predominance of idiopathic gout.

Several studies have demonstrated increases in $CaNa_2EDTA$-stimulated lead excretion in gouty patients without known lead exposure.

DIAGNOSIS

The most useful screening tests for recent, as opposed to remote, excessive lead exposure in adults are blood lead levels and erythrocyte protoporphyrin. Blood lead levels represent exposure within the past 1 to 2 months, along with some degree of equilibration with lead present in soft tissues and bone, the ultimate repository for lead. Erythrocyte protoporphyrin provides evidence of impaired heme synthesis from lead toxicity. Erythrocyte protoporphyrin concentrations are not useful in screening for low-level exposure to lead, and thus blood lead levels should be used as the primary screening method for children, newborns, and lead-exposed workers.

In cases with chronic continuous low-level lead exposure or remote exposure to lead, a lead mobilization test may provide evidence of excessive lead absorption. The test is performed by measuring urinary lead excretion following the administration of EDTA. After baseline determinations, 1 g of EDTA is given twice, 8 to 12 hr apart. During this time, a 24-hr urine specimen is collected. An excessive body lead burden is indicated by excretion of more than

600 μg of lead/day. In cases with renal impairment, 1 g of CaNa$_2$EDTA in 250 mL of 5% glucose solution may be given intravenously over the course of 1 hr. Urine is collected at 24-hr intervals for 3 consecutive days or longer depending on the level of renal function.

Alternatively, tibia, patella, or calcaneus may be subjected to the noninvasive X-ray fluorometry test for lead stores.

Often, the diagnosis of chronic lead nephropathy rests on clinical evidence of indolent, slowly progressive renal failure marked by shrunken kidneys and histologic evidence of renal cortical atrophy, tubular fibrosis, and proliferation of the interstitial tissue. The finding of low-molecular-weight proteinuria, the *de novo* appearance of gout, and an appropriate history of environmental or occupational exposure to lead further support the diagnosis.

PATHOLOGY

The gross pathologic finding of chronic lead nephropathy is that of a granular, contracted kidney. Tubular atrophy and dilation with interstitial fibrosis but minimal cellular infiltration are characteristically seen. Glomeruli become sclerotic secondary to impairment of blood flow, but there is no evidence for a primary glomerulonephritis of immune pathogenesis. Vascular lesions, with intimal proliferation and hyaline degeneration of the media, may be prominent. The eosinophilic proximal tubular nuclear inclusion body, once thought to be pathognomonic of lead nephropathy, is present only during the early years of lead exposure (Fig. 1). Thus, the diagnosis of lead nephropathy is usually inferential, based primarily on a history of lead exposure, evidence of renal impairment by functional testing, and renal biopsy disclosure of a nonimmunologically mediated interstitial nephritis.

TREATMENT

Workers with blood lead levels $\geq$50 μg/dL must be removed from occupational lead exposure until their blood lead levels fall below 40 μg/dL. Workers whose blood lead exceeds 70 to 80 μg/dL may require chelation therapy with CaNa$_2$EDTA or with 2,3-dimercaptosuccinic acid (DMSA), an orally effective agent.

In the absence of marked interstitial fibrosis, patients who have been demonstrated to have an excessive body burden of lead may be treated with long-term, low-dose chelation therapy, 1 g CaNa$_2$EDTA (with procaine) intramuscularly three times a week. CaNa$_2$EDTA is not nephrotoxic when administered at an appropriate dosage even in patients with compromised renal function. Normalizing the EDTA lead mobilization test defines the end point of therapy, although it is questionable whether improved renal funtion actually occurs.

Bibliography

Batuman C: Lead nephropathy, gout, and hypertension. *Am J Med Sci* 305:241–247, 1993.
Chia KS, Jeyaratnam J, Lee J, Tan C, Ong HY, Ong CN, Lee E: Lead-induced nephropathy: Relationship between various biological exposure indices and early markers of nephrotoxicity. *Am J Indust Med* 27:883–895, 1995.
Emmerson BT: Chronic lead nephropathy. *Kidney Int* 4:1–5, 1973.
Fels LM, Herbert C, Perganda M, Jung K, Hotten G, Rosello J, Gelpi E, Mutti A, DeBroe M, Stolte H: Nephron target sites in chronic exposure to lead. *Nephrol Dial Transplant* 4:1740–1746, 1994.
Goering PL: Lead–protein interactions as a basis for lead toxicity. *Neurotoxicology* 14:45–60, 1993.
Gonick HC, Ding Y, Bondy SC, Ni Z, Vaziri ND: Lead-induced hypertension. Interplay of nitric oxide and reactive oxygen species. *Hypertension* 30:1487–1492, 1997.
Hu H, Aro A, Payton M, Korrick S, Sparrow D, Weiss ST, Roznitzky A: The relationship of bone and blood lead to hypertension. The normative aging study. *JAMA* 275:1171–1176, 1996.

49

HYPEROXALURIA

CARLA G. MONICO AND DAWN S. MILLINER

The pathophysiologic properties of oxalate result from the relative insolubility of calcium oxalate in body fluids and tissues. Calcium oxalate crystals form readily in su-

persaturated urine and lead to urolithiasis. Seventy-five percent of stones formed in the upper urinary tract are composed of calcium oxalate. In certain circumstances such as primary hyperoxaluria, oxalate induced renal tubular and parenchymal injury leads to compromise of renal function followed by calcium oxalate deposition in multiple organ systems and severe multisystem disease. Idiopathic hyperoxaluria associated with urolithiasis is the most common of the hyperoxaluric states. Metabolic overproduction of oxalate, as found in the primary hyperoxalurias, accounts for the most severe consequences of hyperoxaluria in individual patients. Secondary forms of hyperoxaluria, including enteric hyperoxaluria and ingestion of drugs and toxins, are also encountered and have variable clinical manifestations.

PHYSIOLOGY OF OXALATE

Oxalate is an end product of metabolism and is not degradable by any known biological system of man. The elimination of oxalate has been shown to be predominantly renal, both in health and disease. However, there has been increasing evidence for an excretory role of the gastrointestinal tract, mainly the large intestine. The daily balance among intestinal absorption, metabolic production, and excretion is such that plasma oxalate values in healthy individuals are much lower than urine concentrations, and are on the order of 0.4 to 3.0 µmol/L (0.04 to 0.26 mg/L). Endogenous metabolic production accounts for 80 to 90% of oxalate that is excreted in the urine. Conversion of precursors with formation of oxalate occurs in the liver, and the relevant metabolic pathways are only partially understood. Primary substrates include glycine and ascorbate. However, exogenous ascorbic acid, even in large amounts, does not result in substantial increases in oxalate production in normal individuals. Hepatic peroxisomal alanine glyoxylate aminotransferase (AGT) is important in converting glyoxylate to glycine, thereby diverting glyoxylate from oxalate production (Fig. 1). Pyridoxine acts as a cofactor in the AGT pathway and can sometimes be of therapeutic benefit. Glycerate dehydrogenase and glyoxylate reductase are also believed to play an important role, although their specific sites in the enzyme pathway are not as well understood.

Ten to twenty percent of oxalate in the urine is of dietary origin. Oxalate is a constituent of many foods, particularly those obtained from plants. Estimates of the oxalate content of the average Western diet range from 80 to 175 mg/day. In healthy subjects, only 2 to 14% of ingested oxalate is absorbed. Bioavailability varies considerably depending on other dietary constituents. Dietary calcium binds to oxalate in the lumen of the intestinal tract and has a large effect on the proportion absorbed. Availability of dietary oxalate for absorption may also be influenced by oxalate degrading bacteria residing in the intestinal tract. Concentrations of oxalate degrading bacteria of up to 10^8/g of stool have been demonstrated in some healthy individuals. The quantitative importance and role of oxalate degrading bacteria in man has yet to be established.

Absorption of oxalate under normal physiologic conditions can occur from gastric mucosa and all segments of the intestine. However, most oxalate from food is absorbed in the small bowel. Patients with total colectomy appear to absorb and excrete the same amount of oxalate as individuals with an intact colon. Oxalate absorption does occur across the normal large intestine, and it is at this site that enhanced oxalate absorption occurs in patients with enteric hyperoxaluria. Absorption of dietary oxalate occurs early after a meal as demonstrated by increases in urine oxalate occurring within 2 to 4 hr following ingestion of high oxalate foods.

Data regarding renal handling of oxalate are limited. Oxalate is freely filtered by the glomerulus and then undergoes bidirectional transport along the renal tubule. In man, the proximal tubule plays a major role, exhibiting both absorption and secretion of oxalate. Whether overall tubular handling of oxalate results in net secretion or reabsorption is not well understood, and may vary with clinical circumstances. Studies in healthy subjects suggest net reabsorption, whereas those in patients with disorders of high oxalate production suggest net secretion.

The upper limit of normal for urine oxalate excretion is approximately 0.45 mmol (40 mg)/24 hrs. Several assays for urine oxalate are currently in use, and normal values vary with the method. Enzymatic and ion chromatographic

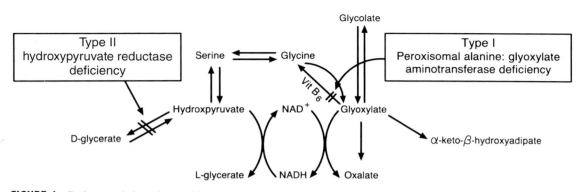

FIGURE 1 Pathways of glyoxylate and hydroxypyruvate metabolism in primary hyperoxaluria. Reproduced from Smith LH: Urolithiasis. In: Schrier RW, Gottschalk CW (eds) *Diseases of the Kidney, 4th edition*, pp. 785–813. Little, Brown, and Co., Boston, 1988.

techniques are the most reliable. There is no difference in urine oxalate excretion between males and females, and during adult life, there is no difference by age. In growing children and adolescents, urine oxalate excretion should be normalized to body surface area and, when expressed in this fashion, is the same as for adults (<0.45 mmol (40 mg)/1.73 m^2/24 hr). Acidification of the urine to a pH of less than 2 during or immediately after the collection is important to ensure accurate results. Acidification prevents precipitation of oxalate and also prevents *in vitro* autoconversion of excreted ascorbate to oxalate.

Colonic excretion of oxalate has been demonstrated in animal models of chronic renal failure. In normal rats, net active absorption occurs across the apical and basolateral surfaces of the large intestine. Within hours of nephrectomy to induce renal failure, net active secretion is observed. The reversal from net absorption to net secretion is accompanied by upregulation of the receptors for angiotensin in the distal colon. This process is blocked by the addition of an angiotensin II receptor antagonist, and suggests a regulatory role of angiotensin II.

METABOLIC OVERPRODUCTION OF OXALATE

The Primary Hyperoxalurias

Two types of primary hyperoxaluria (PH) have been well described. Both are autosomal recessive inborn errors of metabolism.

Type I PH

Type I PH is caused by a deficiency of the enzyme AGT, an enzyme that is both liver and organelle-specific, requiring localization within hepatic peroxisomes for catalytic transamination of glyoxylate to glycine. This transamination diverts glyoxylate to a harmless amino acid, rather than allowing its oxidation to oxalate (Fig. 1). The gene encoding human AGT maps to chromosome 2q36–37. A number of different mutations of AGT as well as normal polymorphisms have been recognized. Patterns of AGT enzyme expression in patients with PH I are varied and include: (1) absence of both AGT immunoreactivity and catalytic activity (approximately 30% of PH I patients), (2) presence of immune reactive AGT without enzymatic activity (approximately 25% of PH I), and (3) presence of both immunoreactive AGT protein and catalytic activity (approximately 40%). In the latter patients, most of the AGT is selectively mistargeted from the peroxisomes to the mitochondria, where it is ineffective in glyoxylate metabolism. Hepatic enzyme activity and subcellular localization profiles do not correlate well with clinical severity and are of limited prognostic usefulness. Furthermore, the levels of AGT activity in the group of patients with peroxisome to mitochondria mistargeting may be indistinguishable from asymptomatic heterozygotes.

Patients with PH I most often present clinically with urolithiasis and demonstrate active stone formation. The diagnosis is strongly suggested by a 24-hr urine oxalate value of greater than 1.2 mmol (105 mg)/1.73 m^2 and an el-evated urine glycolate. In patients with typical features and no other identifiable causes of hyperoxaluria, these findings may be sufficient to establish the diagnosis. As many as 20 to 25% of patients with PH I will have normal urine glycolate excretion. In this circumstance, liver biopsy for AGT analysis may be required to confirm type I PH. DNA analysis, either by mutational analysis for the known mutations in PHI or by linkage studies, can also be of diagnostic value. However, at present less than 50% of patients with PH I can be identified by DNA testing.

Some patients with PH I first come to medical attention due to end stage renal failure and have no antecedent history of urolithiasis. Due to the low GFR, urine studies may not be helpful, but the diagnosis is suggested by markedly elevated plasma oxalate and plasma glycolate concentrations. Interpretation of plasma oxalate values in dialysis patients is complicated by the high plasma values seen in patients with renal failure of other causes. In hemodialysis patients, predialysis plasma oxalate levels are often in the range of 30 to 70 μmol/L (2.6 to 6.2 mg/L) and overlap significantly with the values of 40–120 μmol/L (3.5 to 10.6 mg/L) typically seen in PH patients on dialysis. Most patients with end stage renal disease due to PH will have dense nephrocalcinosis demonstrable on a plain film of the kidneys (Fig. 2). Since this is rarely seen in other clinical settings, it is a valuable clue to the diagnosis. Abundant oxalate deposits will be evident on kidney biopsy (Fig. 3). If renal failure has been present for more than a few months, bone marrow examination may be helpful in showing oxalate deposits. Due to the difficulty in interpreting plasma and urine oxalate concentrations, most patients with end stage renal disease and suspected PH require liver enzyme analysis to confirm the diagnosis, differentiate between PH I and PH II, and provide a basis for decisions regarding renal replacement therapy. As a more complete definition of AGT mutations is developed, DNA analysis may replace enzyme analysis as the definitive diagnostic study.

The diagnosis of PH I is most often made during the first or second decade of life, although the disease may remain

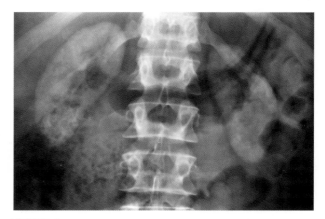

FIGURE 2 Abdominal radiograph showing dense nephrocalcinosis in a patient with primary hyperoxaluria and end stage renal disease.

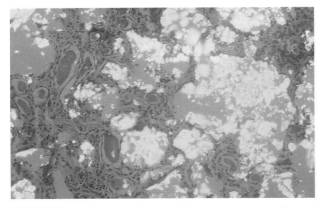

FIGURE 3 Histologic section of a kidney of a patient with end stage renal disease due to primary hyperoxaluria type I. Note the extensive oxalate deposits in the tubules and interstitium.

unrecognized in some patients until the third or fourth decade. As long as renal function is well preserved, the excess oxalate is excreted by the kidneys, the plasma oxalate level remains normal to mildly elevated, and the primary clinical problem is urolithiasis. With time, progressive damage to kidneys related to parenchymal deposition of calcium oxalate as well as renal damage resulting from obstruction, infection, and/or stone removal procedures leads to end stage renal disease. When the glomerular filtration rate (GFR) declines to 20 to 30 mL/min/ 1.73 m^2, plasma oxalate concentration increases, setting the stage for systemic calcium oxalate deposition. Bone marrow, trabecular bone, myocardium, the cardiac conduction system, the vascular system, retina, and soft tissues are the most frequently affected. The calcium oxalate deposits result in serious morbidity and mortality. Dialysis is an inefficient means of removal of oxalate, and most dialysis regimens cannot keep pace with daily production. Patients maintained on standard dialysis regimens almost always continue to accumulate oxalate in multiple organ systems. Prior to the implementation of aggressive treatment regimens, including transplantation, nearly all patients died before the third decade of life. Even with intensive dialysis and transplantation, patients with systemic oxalosis are very ill and present substantial management challenges.

Treatment strategies for PH I must take into account individual patient characteristics, including renal function. Twenty to thirty percent of patients with PH I respond to pharmacologic doses of pyridoxine (a cofactor in the AGT enzyme pathway) with a reduction in oxalate production to normal or near normal. Accordingly, all patients suspected of having PH I should receive a trial of pyridoxine of 5 to10 mg/kg/day for a minimum of 3 months to assess responsiveness. In patients with adequate renal function, serial urine oxalate determinations will confirm a response. In patients with advanced renal failure, assessment of pyridoxine responsiveness is difficult, though plasma oxalate and glycolate are sometimes helpful. In dialysis patients, when the response is uncertain, pyridoxine should be continued. Most pyridoxine responsive patients require no

more than 5 to 7 mg/kg/day. A few appear to respond only to very high-dose pyridoxine (up to 1 g/day in adult patients). Peripheral neuropathy can occur with long-term use of very high- dose pyridoxine (>10 mg/kg/day) although this complication has not been reported in PH I patients.

High oral fluid intake to maintain a urine volume of 3 to 6 L daily (depending on individual oxalate production) is a mainstay of management in all patients other than those with end stage renal failure. Orthophosphate at 30–40 mg/kg/day of elemental phosphorus (in divided doses) has been shown to decrease calcium oxalate crystalluria, decrease calcium oxalate supersaturation, and increase inhibitors of calcium oxalate crystal formation in the urine of PH I patients. Orthophosphate also appears to be beneficial with regard to long-term preservation of renal function. Phosphate therapy should be considered in all patients with adequately preserved renal function (i.e., GFR >30 mL/min/1.73 m^2). It should be used only with caution at lower GFRs due to the liability for hyperphosphatemia and is contraindicated in patients with end stage renal disease. There is evidence of benefit from citrate in patients with PH I as well. Magnesium has been advocated, but to date there have been no intermediate nor long-term studies to substantiate its effectiveness. Low oxalate diets are of limited benefit in primary hyperoxaluria because metabolic overproduction accounts for nearly all the oxalate excreted.

Patients with advanced renal insufficiency pose particular problems, and management is best individualized, ideally with assistance from someone who has experience with this disorder. Since the majority of patients progressively accumulate tissue oxalate while on dialysis, the goal should be early transplantation ideally at a GFR of approximately 20 ml/min/1.73 m^2 and before a large oxalate tissue burden develops. If there is a delay in transplantation, daily hemodialysis or a combination of hemodialysis 3 to 4 days weekly along with daily peritoneal dialysis is necessary to minimize tissue oxalate deposition. Pyridoxine responsive patients and those with minimal tissue oxalate may be best served by kidney transplantation alone. This is particularly true if a living donor is available and transplantation can be done expeditiously. Other patients will have greater benefit from combined liver and kidney transplantation. Loss of renal allografts due to rapid oxalate deposition continues to be a major problem with both kidney only and combined liver/kidney transplantation. This is due to large tissue oxalate stores that typically accumulate before transplantation and continue to be mobilized and excreted for months to years after transplantation. Patients with PH require intensive posttransplant monitoring and treatment interventions specifically directed to minimize damage to the allograft. A transplant center experienced in the management of PH I patients is preferred.

Type II PH

Type II primary hyperoxaluria (PH II) is a rare disorder that is due to deficiency of hepatic hydroxypyruvate reductase (HPR), an enzyme which also has both glyoxylate reductase (GR) and D-glycerate dehydrogenase (D-GDH) activities. The cause of increased oxalate production is unclear. Hydroxypyruvate accumulation may indirectly increase oxalate synthesis from glyoxylate. The reduction of hydroxypyruvate to L-glycerate enhances the oxidation of glyoxylate to oxalate in a coupled reaction catalyzed by lactic dehydrogenase (Fig. 1). The resulting increase in glycerate production appears to account for the hyperglyceric aciduria characteristic of PH II. The gene encoding human hydroxypyruvate/glyoxylate reductase has been localized to chromosome 9 and a specific mutation identified in a small cohort of PH II patients. As in PH I, continued advances in genetics testing will facilitate the diagnosis of this disease in the future.

Patients with PH II typically present in the first two decades of life with urolithiasis. Urine oxalate excretion tends to be lower in PH II patients than PH I but is usually greater than 1.0 mmol (88 mg)/1.73 m^2/24 hr. There is considerable overlap in both the amount of oxaluria and in the clinical features between the two PH subtypes. The diagnosis of PH II is suggested by a markedly elevated urine oxalate without an identifiable secondary cause, elevated urine glycerate, and normal urine glycolate. The diagnosis can be confirmed by hepatic enzyme analysis. With recent identification of a genetic mutation responsible for PH II, DNA analysis may, in the future, provide an alternative to hepatic enzyme analysis. Treatment consists of a high oral fluid intake and, in most patients, orthophosphate therapy. Oral citrate and/or magnesium may be considered. Stone formation is easier to control, and there appears to be better preservation of renal function over time in PH II patients when compared with PH I. However, end stage renal disease is observed in PH II and has been reported in three of 24 published cases.

The term type III primary hyperoxaluria has been used by some authors to describe an as yet unclassified hyperoxaluria which may also be metabolic in origin. The small number of patients described to date have heterogeneous features, and some were evaluated before reliable assays were available for oxalate, glycolate, and glycerate and before hepatic enzyme analysis was available. Until such patients can be well characterized and diagnostic criteria developed, the use of this term is best avoided.

Oxalate Precursors: Drugs and Toxins

Intake of drugs or toxins that are metabolized to oxalate is a rare cause of marked hyperoxaluria and can result in acute renal failure. Ethylene glycol (found in antifreeze) ingestion is encountered more frequently than others. Epidemics of acute renal failure due to diethylene glycol contamination of paracetamol elixirs have occurred in recent years in Bangladesh, Nigeria, and Haiti. Ethylene glycol ingestion should be considered in unexplained acute renal failure accompanied by a severe anion gap metabolic acidosis not attributable to other causes. The acidosis is caused by the accumulation of glycolic acid. The glycolic acid is further metabolized to oxalic acid and formic acid. The symptom complex may include central nervous system

changes, cardiovascular instability, and respiratory insufficiency. As little as 15 mL of concentrated ethylene glycol can be lethal in a young child. Since the initial metabolic degradation step involves alcohol dehydrogenase, early intravenous infusion of ethanol can slow the metabolic degradation and is of therapeutic benefit. Fomepizole, a more potent competitive inhibitor of alcohol dehydrogenase, was recently approved as the antidote of choice for the treatment of ethylene glycol poisoning in adults. Hemodialysis can also be effective in clearing the ethylene glycol as well as its toxic metabolites. Ethylene glycol ingestion is suggested by calcium oxalate crystalluria and can be confirmed by direct measurement of plasma, urine oxalate level or, if the patient is anuric, by measurement of the plasma oxalate. A renal biopsy will show characteristic deposition of calcium oxalate crystals in tubules and interstitium.

Other agents metabolized to oxalate include methoxyflurane anesthetics and xylitol, a bulk sweetener used in sugar-free preparations of various foods. Although oral ingestion of xylitol is considered safe, intravenous preparations previously used in substitution for glucose in parenteral nutrition have been abandoned. Mild hyperoxaluria has also been observed in premature infants receiving parenteral nutrition, although the source of the excess oxalate has not yet been defined.

The potential for ingested ascorbic acid to undergo endogenous metabolism to oxalate is controversial. Oral doses of up to 2 g/day do not produce an increase in urine oxalate. The current adult recommended daily allowance of vitamin C is 60 mg, an amount that achieves a plasma concentration of 0.8 mg/dL (45 μM) and provides body stores of 1500 mg. When daily intake exceeds 200 mg, as is commonly seen in diets supplemented with vitamin C, plasma concentrations can reach 2 mg/dL (110 μM), a level associated with significant renal excretion of ascorbic acid. In recent studies, no urinary excretion of ascorbic acid was observed for vitamin C doses of less than 100 mg/day. However, approximately 25% of 100 mg, and 50% of 200 mg, were excreted. *In vitro* autoconversion of ascorbate to oxalate appears to account for the hyperoxaluria previously reported under such circumstances.

INCREASED ABSORPTION OF OXALATE

Enteric Hyperoxaluria

The bioavailability of oxalate is dependent on a number of intraluminal factors, including calcium concentration, fatty acids, and bile salts. Normally, approximately 2 to 15% of ingested oxalate is absorbed. In "enteric hyperoxaluria," a condition typically seen in association with small bowel disease in the context of a healthy colon, as much as 35% of an ingested oxalate load may be absorbed. Enteric hyperoxaluria is now recognized in a variety of clinical settings characterized by intestinal malabsorption of fat or bile salts with increased oxalate absorption in the large intestine. These include small bowel resection, small bowel bypass for obesity, primary small bowel disease with malabsorption, chronic pancreatitis, liver diseases such as primary biliary cirrhosis or chronic cirrhosis of other causes, and enteric hyperoxaluria has also been reported with external biliary drainage procedures. Factors responsible for colonic oxalate hyperabsorption include: (1) Increased delivery of malabsorbed bile acids to the colon which increases colonic permeability to oxalate; (2) complexation of calcium in the lumen of the intestine by malabsorbed fatty acids which frees oxalate to be absorbed; and (3) increased permeability of the colon to oxalate due to fatty acids. All of these factors are influenced by diet composition. A high oxalate diet, especially if dietary calcium is low or fat content is high, will be particularly disadvantageous and can have a pronounced effect on the amount of oxalate absorbed. The magnitude of the hyperoxaluria generally parallels both the degree of steatorrhea and the total length of bowel resection or extent of disease. A contributory role for the colonic oxalate degrading bacteria, *Oxalobacter formigenes,* which is inhibited by bile salts, has also been suggested. Patients with enteric hyperoxaluria often have very active stone formation, and some patients develop renal calcium oxalate deposition and renal failure. The hyperoxaluria is most often 0.8 to 1.5 mmol (70–132 mg)/1.73 m^2/24 hr. In adults, enteric hyperoxaluria is by far the most common cause of moderate hyperoxaluria.

Malabsorption can cause increased lithogenicity of the urine by a variety of mechanisms. Hyperoxaluria is typically just one component. Others include increased urine concentration due to fluid loss in the gastrointestinal tract, hyperuricosuria, hypomagnesemia, and hypocitric aciduria. The multifactorial aspects of urinary tract stone formation in patients with malabsorption should be taken into account and treatment regimens individualized. Treatment should address as many causative factors as possible. A low oxalate, high calcium diet should be prescribed. Calcium supplements may be recommended. Increased oral fluid intake as tolerated is important in improving the solubility of oxalate in the urine. A low fat diet in those with steatorrhea can be very helpful. Cholestyramine should be considered in patients with bile acid malabsorption. Some patients with difficult stone problems and persistently low urine pH may benefit from citrate or bicarbonate administration. Citrate, a known inhibitor of calcium oxalate crystal growth, also forms a soluble salt with calcium, reducing calcium oxalate supersaturation. Urine alkalinization increases the solubility of uric acid. Potassium or magnesium supplements may be needed.

Dietary Factors

In normal subjects, an increase in dietary animal protein from 55 to 89 g/day results in an increase in urinary oxalate of up to 24%. This is because meat proteins contain amino acids that are partially metabolized to oxalate. Low calcium diets result in higher oxalate excretion due to reduced binding of oxalate to calcium in the intestinal lumen, and there is increased absorption of the unbound oxalate. The contribution of dietary oxalate to urine oxalate excretion is less than that of either protein or calcium but can be a significant factor when the diet is also low in calcium.

HYPEROXALURIA IN IDIOPATHIC UROLITHIASIS

Twenty to thirty percent of patients with idiopathic urolithiasis have hyperoxaluria. Due to the high prevalence of urolithiasis in the general population, this form of hyperoxaluria accounts for a large majority of the patients with hyperoxaluria encountered in any clinical practice. The degree of idiopathic hyperoxaluria is modest (typically in the range of 0.5 to 0.8 mmol (44–70 mg)/1.73 m^2/24 hr) but has an effect on urinary supersaturation of calcium oxalate that exceeds equivalent increases in urine calcium concentrations. There may be more than one cause for the hyperoxaluria. There is evidence to support enhanced gastrointestinal absorption of oxalate, an abnormality of cellular oxalate transport, and alterations in glyoxylate metabolism.

Hyperabsorption of dietary oxalate (up to 16 to 20% of ingested oxalate) has been found in a number of studies of patients with idiopathic urolithiasis. However, most studies involved manipulations of dietary calcium, and it is unclear whether the increased absorption of dietary oxalate was a primary feature or simply a by-product of the lower calcium content of the study diets.

Abnormalities of cellular transport of oxalate may occur in idiopathic urolithiasis and have implications for intestinal absorption and excretion and for renal tubular secretion of oxalate. An abnormal transmembrane flux rate of oxalate in red blood cells (RBCs) has been described; it is characteristic of patients with idiopathic calcium oxalate stone disease and is not present in patients with secondary forms of calcium urolithiasis. Renal and colonic epithelial cells share many features of oxalate transport with RBCs. It has now been shown that the increased RBC oxalate flux found in idiopathic calcium oxalate stone formers is associated with faster intestinal absorption and a higher renal clearance of oxalate. These observations provide a link between the RBC oxalate transport abnormalities and observations that some patients with idiopathic hyperoxaluria have an increased fractional excretion of oxalate that can exceed unity, suggesting secretion. Identification of this transport abnormality may have implications for treatment, since the transport is returned to normal by thiazide diuretics. To date, however, there have been no reports of the effect of thiazides on the urine oxalate of patients with this RBC transport abnormality.

A small number of patients thought to have idiopathic hyperoxaluria have been described to have elevations of urine glycolate, suggesting increased metabolic production of oxalate. Administration of pyridoxine has been reported to reduce both the oxalate and glycolate to normal in these circumstances. Additional studies are needed to more fully characterize glyoxylate metabolism in such patients.

Patients with idiopathic hyperoxaluria are most effectively managed with a high oral fluid intake to reduce the concentration of oxalate in the urine and a low oxalate diet that contains an adequate amount of calcium. Foods and beverages with high oxalate bioavailability such as peanuts, almonds, pecans, chocolate, spinach, rhubarb, tea, and colas should be avoided. If these measures are insufficient to control stone formation, additional treatment is warranted.

Neutral phosphate and potassium citrate have been shown to be effective in idiopathic calcium oxalate urolithiasis. If there is concomitant hypercalciuria, addition of a thiazide may be considered.

Bibliography

Allison MJ, Cook HM, Milne DB, et al.: Oxalate degradation by gastrointestinal bacteria from humans. *J Nutr* 116:455, 1986.

Brinkley LJ, Gregory J, Pak CYC: A further study of oxalate bioavailability in foods. *J Urol* 144:94–96, 1990.

Chlebeck PT, Milliner DS, Smith LH: Long-term prognosis in primary hyperoxaluria type II (L-glyceric aciduria). *Am J Kidney Dis* 23:255–259, 1994.

Cochat P, Schärer K: Should liver transplantation be performed before advanced renal insufficiency in primary hyperoxaluria type 1? *Pediatr Nephrol* 7:212–218, 1993.

Cramer SD, Ferree PM, Lin K, Milliner DS, Holmes RP: The gene encoding hydroxypyruvate reductase (GRHPR) is mutated in patients with primary hyperoxaluria type II. *Hum Mol Genet* 8:2063–2069, 1999.

Danpure CJ, Rumsby G: Enzymology and molecular genetics of primary hyperoxaluria type 1. Consequences for clinical management. In: Khan SR (ed) *Calcium Oxalate in Biological Systems*, pp. 189–205. CRC Press, New York, 1995.

Danpure CJ, Smith LH: The primary hyperoxalurias. In: Coe FL, Favus MJ, Pak CYC, Parks HJ, Preminger GM (eds) *Kidney Stones: Medical and Surgical Management*, pp. 859–881. Lippincott-Raven, Philadephia, 1996.

Hatch M, Freel RW: Oxalate transport across intestinal and renal epithelia. In: Khan SR (ed) *Calcium Oxalate in Biological Systems*, pp. 217–238. CRC Press, New York, 1995.

Hatch M, Freel RW, Vaziri ND: Regulatory aspects of oxalate secretion in enteric oxalate elimination. *J Am Soc Nephrol* 10:S324–S328, 1999.

Hillman RE: Primary hyperoxalurias. In: Scriver CR, Beaudet AL, Sly WS, Valle D (eds) *Metabolic Basis of Inherited Diseases*, 6th Ed, pp.933–944. McGraw-Hill, New York, 1989.

Johnson CM, Wilson DM, O'Fallon WM, et al.: Renal stone epidemiology: A 25-year study in Rochester, Minnesota. *Kidney Int* 16:624–631, 1979.

Lindsjö M: Oxalate metabolism in renal stone disease with specific reference to calcium metabolism and intestinal absorption. *Scand J Urol Nephrol* 119:1–53, 1989.

Marangella M, Fruttero B, Bruno M, et al.: Hyperoxaluria in idiopathic calcium stone disease: Further evidence of intestinal hyperabsorption of oxalate. *Clin Sci* 63:381–385, 1982.

Milliner DS, Eickholt JT, Bergstralh E, et al.: Primary hyperoxaluria: Results of long-term treatment with orthophosphate and pyridoxine. *N Engl J Med* 331:1553–1558, 1994.

Mitwalli A, Ayiomamitis A, Grass L, et al.: Control of hyperoxaluria with large doses of pyridoxine in patients with kidney stones. *Int Urol Nephrol* 20:353–359, 1988.

Robertson WG: Epidemiology of urinary stone disease. *Urol Res* 18(1):S3–S8, 1990.

Smith LH: Enteric hyperoxaluria and other hyperoxaluric states. In: Coe FL, Brenner BM, Stein JH (eds) *Contemporary Issues in Nephrology*, pp. 136–164. Churchill Livingstone, New York, 1980.

Wilson DM, Liedtke RR: Modified enzyme-based colorimetric assay of urinary and plasma oxalate with improved sensitivity and no ascorbate interference: Reference values and sample handling procedures. *Clin Chem* 37:1229–1235, 1991.

50

RENAL PAPILLARY NECROSIS

GARABED EKNOYAN

Necrosis of the renal parenchyma may affect the cortex or the medulla. Unlike cortical necrosis which is a rare, and often catastrophic event, necrosis of the medulla is a relatively common, chronic event which generally pursues an insidious course and is often localized to the inner zone of the medulla and more specifically the papilla. Renal papillary necrosis (RPN) occurs in a selected group of individuals afflicted with an apparently disparate group of diseases (Table 1).

PATHOGENESIS

Restriction of the necrotic lesions to the papilla can be ascribed to the unique structural and functional features of this region. The first is the blood supply to the papilla. The rich vascular plexus formed by the descending and ascending vasa rectae is principally devoted to the countercurrent exchange mechanism necessary to maintain medullary hypertonicity. The small fraction of medullary

Conditions	Frequency
Diabetes mellitus	50–60%
Urinary tract obstruction	10–40%
Analgesic abuse	15–20%
Sickle hemoglobinopathy	10–15%
Renal allograft rejection	<5%
Pyclonephritis	<5%

[a]The figures indicate the frequency with which each cause has been noted in major reviews of RPN cases.

blood flow that serves a nutrient function is provided by capillaries that branch off for this purpose. Hence, total medullary blood flow cannot be equated with tissue supply. Additionally, the number and size of the vasa rectae and their intercommunications and that of their branching nutrient capillaries gradually decrease during the course of their descent to the inner zone such that the tip of the papilla has only small terminal vessels with sparse intercommunications. There is also a three- to fourfold increase in interstitial mass in the inner zone of the medulla compared to that of the cortex and medulla. The net effect is a relatively poor blood supply to the parenchyma of the papilla compared with the remainder of the kidney. Conditions associated with occlusive lesions of the small vasculature of the kidney (diabetes mellitus, sickle hemoglobinopathy, transplanted kidney) therefore predispose to ischemic necrosis of the renal papilla. Furthermore, over 50% of RPN cases are observed in individuals greater than 60 years of age (except in sickle hemoglobinopathies). The propensity of the elderly to arteriosclerosis has been implicated as a further cause of reduced medullary blood flow. Another important feature of the papillary vasculature that predisposes it to necrosis is its apparently greater dependence on vasodilator prostanoids. On a mole per tissue weight basis the ratio of prostaglandin synthetase activity of the papilla to that of the medulla and cortex is 100:10:1. Agents that inhibit cyclooxygenase activity [nonsteroidal antiinflammatory drugs (NSAIDs)] will compromise blood flow sufficiently to result in ischemia of this relatively underperfused region. Patients with chronic arthralgias (rheumatoid arthritis, gouty arthritis, osteoarthritis) who use NSAIDs chronically (more than a cumulative dose of 1000 tablets) have a 12% risk of developing RPN.

A second factor predisposing the papilla to necrosis is the ability of the tubule to concentrate solutes in this region. Although necessary to promote water reabsorption, this has a deleterious effect when potentially nephrotoxic agents are concentrated in the medulla, with the greatest accumulation being in the papillary tip. This explains the prevalence of renal papillary necrosis in individuals who abuse analgesics (phenacetin, acetaminophen, salicylates). Whereas the coadministration of these agents provides a biochemical basis of their cytotoxicity, by producing an ox-

idant stress and blocking its reduction, it is their concentration in the medulla that localizes the initial and major injury caused by analgesic abuse to the papilla. Abolition of medullary hypertonicity by water diuresis results in a reduction in the concentration of analgesics in the papilla and provides protection from RPN.

Another aspect of medullary hypertonicity relevant to papillary necrosis may be its detrimental effect on the normal phagocytic function of polymorphonuclear leukocytes, which would predispose it to infection. Urinary tract infection was once considered a principal cause of papillary necrosis. However, although urinary tract infection is present in most patients with papillary necrosis, it is not a uniform finding. It is more likely a secondary complication superimposed on necrotic foci, particularly when the necrotic tissue causes obstruction. Independent of infection, obstruction of the urinary tract can cause RPN, because of reduced medullary blood flow. Following obstruction, an initial brief period of vasodilatation is followed by significant and persistent vasoconstriction. That this vasoconstriction should exert its most detrimental effect in the papilla is not unexpected given the sparse blood flow of this region and its dependence on vasodilatory prostanoids.

In the clinical conditions which have been associated with papillary necrosis, more than one causative factor (obstruction, infection, diabetes, chronic analgesic or NSAID use) is present in over half of the patients who develop RPN. As such, although each of these clinical conditions (Table 1) alone may cause papillary necrosis, the coexistence of more than one predisposing condition increases the risk of papillary necrosis. Thus, a diabetic who abuses analgesics would be more prone to develop medullary injury, since the papilla injured by diabetic vasculopathy produces less vasodilatory prostanoids and is more prone to further ischemic injury due to NSAIDs. Additionally, the resultant necrotic focus can become the nidus of an infection; if it sloughs it could cause obstruction. Thus, it is usually a vicious cycle of vascular occlusion, vasopasm, infection, and obstruction that leads to full-blown papillary necrosis, whereby RPN would result from the overlap of several detrimental factors operating in concert.

COURSE AND CLINICAL MANIFESTATIONS

The necrotic process may be localized to one or involve several papillae. Both kidneys are involved in 65–70% of cases. Patients who have a unilateral lesion at the time of initial diagnosis will often develop papillary necrosis in the other kidney as well. The process begins with foci of coagulative necrosis, consistent with ischemic necrosis, which coalesce and extend to involve the rest of the tissue. Depending on the localization of the initial necrotic process it may assume the medullary form, in which the necrosis is in the innermost medullary region while the fornices and papillary tip are viable, or the papillary form, in which the fornices and papillary tip are destroyed. The medullary form is more common in sickle cell hemoglobinopathies.

The necrotic lesions have a well-demarcated sharp border and proceed to form a sequestrum which may either calcify, slough, or be resorbed leaving a sinus tract or cavity at its site. Cavity and sinus formation is more common in the medullary form whereas calcification and sloughing is more common in the papillary form. The sloughing is generally associated with hematuria, which can be massive. The passage of sloughed necrotic tissue may be associated with lumbar pain and ureteral colic, which is clinically similar to that of nephrolithiasis. The necrotic tissue or the stagnant urine in the cavities may be the nidus of a urinary tract infection that can be either chronic, smoldering and recurrent, or may present in an acute, fulminant form. With the advent of antibiotics and improved management of superimposed urinary tract infection, the central role once attributed to infection in the development and course of RPN has diminished considerably.

The course of papillary necrosis is variable. Occasionally, it will present as an acute disease with septicemia and rapidly progressive renal failure. Sometimes, it will pursue a protracted but symptomatic course with recurrent episodes of urinary infection or renal colic. Much more commonly, the lesions remain totally asymptomatic, with the papillary RPN detected as an incidental finding on urinary tract visualization or an unexpected discovery at postmortem examination as in over one-half of diabetics, two-thirds of patients with sickle cell disease, and one-tenth of arthritic patients who consume analgesics.

The level of renal insufficiency which develops depends on the number of papillae involved. Although some loss of renal reserve is expected to result from any renal parenchymal necrosis, renal failure does not always occur. Even when several papillae are affected, localization of the necrosis to the papillary tips results in the loss of only the juxtamedullary nephrons whose loops descend to the papillary tip while the cortical nephrons, which terminate in the outer zone of the medulla, are spared. Sufficient functioning nephrons remain to maintain homeostasis. As more of the papillae necrose and cortical scarring develops, renal failure will ultimately occur.

Because it is the deep nephrons which are primarily affected, an inability to concentrate the urine maximally is an early manifestation. Consequently, polyuria and nocturia are common and may be a presenting complaint, can be elicited in the history, or may be demonstrated by appropriate testing.

Proteinuria is common (70 to 80% of cases) but is usually only modest (<2 g/day). Pyuria is also common (60 to 80% of cases). Microscopic hematuria (20 to 40%) and gross hematuria (20%) are less common.

DIAGNOSIS

In symptomatic patients, the diagnosis can be made on finding portions of necrotic tissue in the urine, the pathologic examination of which establishes their papillary origin. A deliberate search for papillary fragments should be made by straining the urine through a filter.

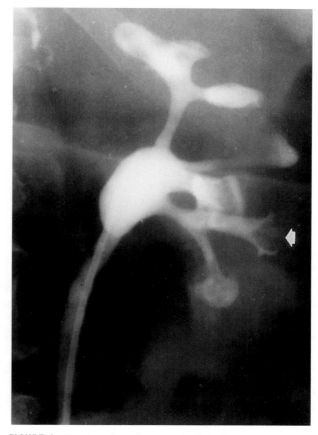

FIGURE 1 Retrograde pyelogram of a diabetic patient with papillary necrosis. The calyces are all blunted. One (arrow) demonstrates a sloughed papilla nearly encircled by contrast—the "ring" sign. (Courtesy Dr. William L. Campbell.)

In the absence of a tissue diagnosis excretory or retrograde urography has been the best method to establish a diagnosis. Unfortunately, the radiologic changes do not become apparent until the lesions are advanced and the papillae are shrunk or sequestered (see Fig. 1). Ultrasonography, technetium scintigraphy, and computerized tomography are less sensitive, but can be helpful, especially in patients with poor renal function.

THERAPY

In the absence of a causative factor which can be avoided (analgesics) or surgically corrected (obstruction), therapy is directed toward associated complications. Control and/or eradication of urinary infection is essential. The blood glucose of diabetics should be well controlled. Analgesic mixtures and NSAIDs should be avoided. Increased fluid intake should be encouraged to avoid the medullary concentration of these potentially nephrotoxic agents if their continued use is necessary. Control of hypertension, as in any other renal disease, is important. Antihypertensive agents which reduce renal blood flow (β-blockers, thiazides) are best avoided. Conversely, angiotensin-converting

enzyme inhibitors can provide protection. Volume depletion, which compromises renal blood flow, and dehydration, which increases blood viscosity, should be prevented.

Bibliography

Bach PH, Nguyen TK: Renal papillary necrosis. . . 40 years on. *Toxicol Pathol* 26:73–91, 1998.

Delzell E, Shapiro S: A review of epidemiologic studies of non-narcotic analgesics and renal disease. *Medicine* 77:102–121, 1998.

Eknoyan G, Qunibi WY, Grissom RT, Tuma SN, Ayus JC: Renal papillary necrosis: An update. *Medicine* 61:55–73, 1982.

Griffin MD, Bergstralh EJ, Larson TS: Renal papillary necrosis—a sixteen year clinical experience. *J Am Soc Nephrol* 6:248–256, 1995.

Groop L, Laasonen L, Edgren J: Renal papillary necrosis in patients with IDDM. *Diabetes Care* 12:198–202, 1989.

Sabatini S, Eknoyan G (eds): Renal papillary necrosis. *Semin Nephrol* 4:1–106, 1984.

Segasothy M, Chin GL, Sia KK, Zulfiqar A, Samad SA: Chronic nephrotoxicity of anti-inflammatory drugs used in the treatment of arthritis. *Br J Rheumatol* 34:162–165, 1995.

Shyan-Yih C, Porush JG, Faubert PE: Renal medullary circulation: Hormonal control. *Kidney Int* 37:1–13, 1990.

OBSTRUCTIVE UROPATHY

STEPHEN M. KORBET

Obstructive uropathy refers to the structural or functional interference with normal urine flow anywhere along
the urinary tract from the renal tubule to the urethra. The
resultant increase in pressure within the urinary tract proximal to the obstruction contributes to a number of structural and physiologic changes. Hydronephrosis, dilatation
of the calyces and renal pelvis, is the anatomic outcome of
an obstructive process that affects the collecting system distal to the renal pelvis (Fig. 1). Hydroureter, the term applied to ureteral dilatation, often accompanies hydronephrosis when the level of obstruction is distal to the
ureteropelvic junction. The functional and pathologic
changes of the kidney that can ensue are termed obstructive nephropathy.

In the United States, approximately 400,000 patients a
year are hospitalized with problems related to obstructive
uropathy. The overall prevalence of obstructive uropathy
as diagnosed at autopsy by the presence of hydronephrosis is approximately 3%, with men and women affected
equally. This obviously underestimates the true prevalence
of the disorder as temporary conditions such as nephrolithiasis would not be included. Differences in the frequency
and causes of obstruction occur between males and females
when evaluated at different times of life. The frequency
of obstruction is similar between males and females up
to the age of 20 years. Strictures of the urethra or ureter,
and neurologic abnormalities account for most causes of

obstruction identified at autopsy in those patients ≤10
years of age. The rate of obstruction in women is greatest
between the ages of 20–60 years, primarily due to obstruction from pregnancy and gynecologic cancers. Above the
age of 60 years, obstructive uropathy is more common
in males due to benign prostatic hypertrophy or prostate
cancer.

Urinary tract obstruction, if left untreated, can result in
progressive, irreversible loss of renal function and end stage
renal disease if both kidneys are affected or a solitary kidney exists. However, obstructive uropathy represents one
of the few potentially curable forms of renal disease, and
should therefore be considered in the differential diagnosis of any patient presenting with unexplained acute or
chronic renal failure. Since the overall success of therapeutic intervention is directly linked to the duration and
degree of obstruction, early identification is crucial.

CLASSIFICATION, CLINICAL, AND LABORATORY MANIFESTATIONS

Urinary tract obstruction is often classified based on the
duration, location, and degree of the obstructive process.
The duration of obstruction is described as acute (hours to
days), subacute (days to weeks), and chronic (months to
years). The location of the obstruction (Tables 1–3) can be
anywhere from the renal tubule to the urethral meatus, and

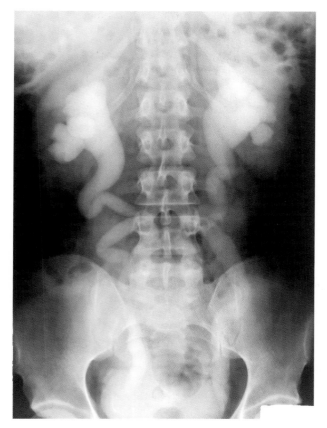

FIGURE I Intravenous pyelogram demonstrating bilateral, severe dilatation of the renal calyces, pelvis, and ureter. (Courtesy of Dr. Suresh K. Patel, Rush Medical College.)

TABLE I
Intrinsic Causes of Obstructive Uropathy

Intraluminal
  Intrarenal
    Tubular precipitation of proteins or crystals
      Bence Jones proteins
      Uric acid
      Medications
  Extrarenal
    Nephrolithiasis, blood clots, papillary necrosis, fungus balls
Intramural
  Anatomic
    Tumors (renal pelvis, ureter, bladder, urethra)
    Strictures (ureteral or urethral)
      Infections
      Granulomatous disease
      Instrumentation or trauma
      Radiation therapy
  Functional disorders of the bladder
    Diabetes mellitus
    Multiple sclerosis
    Spinal cord injury
    Anticholinergic agents

ney) laboratory features of acute renal failure will be observed.

The presenting clinical features associated with subacute or chronic obstruction are generally more subtle and insidious in nature. Instead of severe pain, the development of vague symptoms such as flank or suprapubic fullness may be described depending on the location of the obstruction. In addition, patients may experience frequency,

TABLE 2
Extrinsic Causes of Obstructive Uropathy

Reproductive disorders
  Female
    Uterus (pregnancy, prolapse, tumors)
    Ovary (abscess, cysts, tumor)
    Tubules (pelvic inflammatory disease)
  Male
    Prostate (benign hyperplasia, adenocarcinoma)
Gastrointestinal disorders
  Appendicitis
  Crohn's disease
  Diverticulitis
  Pancreatitis
  Colorectal carcinoma
Vascular disorders
  Aneurysms (abdominal aortic, iliac)
  Venous (ovarian vein thrombophlebitis, retrocaval ureter)
Retroperitoneal disorders
  Fibrosis (idiopathic, drug related, inflammatory)
  Infection
  Radiation therapy
  Tumor (primary or metastatic)
  Iatrogenic complication of surgery

thus can affect one (unilateral obstruction) or both (bilateral obstruction) collecting systems. Finally, the degree of obstruction may be partial or complete.

These basic attributes of the obstructive process ultimately determine the clinical and laboratory manifestations with which a patient presents. The clinical presentation of patients with an acute obstruction is typically that of abrupt pain. If the process is unilateral and at the level of the renal pelvis or ureter, severe flank pain results, often described as colicky in nature when due to an intraluminal process such as nephrolithiasis or papillary necrosis. If this occurs at the level of the bladder outlet, suprapubic pain and fullness may be experienced. This may be accompanied by urinary frequency and urgency if the outlet obstruction is partial, or anuria if the obstruction is complete. On physical exam, flank pain on percussion or a suprapubic mass may be demonstrated in patients with outlet obstruction. In patients with two kidneys, laboratory manifestations of unilateral obstruction will often be limited to abnormalities of the urinalysis. With intrinsic forms of obstruction, microscopic or gross hematuria may be observed, and with either intrinsic or extrinsic processes, secondary infection may result in pyuria and bacteriuria. In conditions leading to bilateral obstruction (or unilateral obstruction in patients with a solitary kid-

TABLE 3
Congenital Causes of Obstructive Uropathy

Ureter
    Ureteropelvic junction obstruction
    Ureteroceles
    Ectopic ureter
    Ureteral valves
    Megaureter
Bladder
    Myelodysplasias
    Bladder diverticula
Urethra
    Prune-belly syndrome
    Urethral diverticula
    Posterior urethral valves

polyuria or nocturia, and may also have difficulty initiating or stopping urination as well an urgency if bladder outlet obstruction is present. The physical findings may include a flank mass from a hydronephrotic kidney or a suprapubic mass, extending to the umbilicus, due to a greatly distended bladder. Laboratory evaluation of the urine can be similar to that seen in acute obstruction but may include proteinuria (often less than 2g/day). Impairment in renal function will also be observed in patients with bilateral disease, as evidenced by laboratory features of chronic renal failure, hyperkalemia, renal tubular acidosis, and an inability to concentrate the urine.

The differential diagnosis of obstructive uropathy is extensive (Tables 1–3). In addition to the features previously described, clinical and laboratory characteristics unique to the individual disorders should be considered and pursued in the evaluation of a patient with obstructive uropathy.

ETIOLOGY

Acquired-Intrinsic

The acquired forms of obstructive uropathy (Tables 1 and 2) are often classified based on the location of the obstructive process as intrinsic (obstruction occurring within the urinary tract) or extrinsic (obstruction resulting from external compression of the urinary tract). Intrinsic disorders leading to obstruction are divided into intraluminal and intramural processes.

Intraluminal obstruction may be the result of renal tubular obstruction, otherwise called intrarenal obstruction. This is most often identified with acute renal failure in multiple myeloma from the precipitation of Bence Jones proteins in the tubules (myeloma kidney), and in the tumor lysis syndrome where the chemotherapeutic treatment of a malignancy (generally a lymphoma) leads to the massive production and subsequent precipitation of uric acid crystals within the tubules. Several drugs are also associated with intrarenal obstruction due to precipitation or crystal formation within the renal tubules, and these include sulfadiazine, sulfamethoxazole, acyclovir, indinavir, and methotrexate. The predisposition for obstruction in these conditions is enhanced in the setting of volume contraction with the excretion of a concentrated, acidic urine. Of the extrarenal causes of obstruction, nephrolithiasis is the most common, particularly in young men. The most common form of stone contains calcium, most often calcium oxalate (see Chapter 53). Papillary necrosis can lead to ureteral obstruction and may be seen in sickle cell disease, diabetes mellitus, amyloidosis, and analgesic abuse (see Chapter 50). In addition, gross hematuria with blood clots resulting from any cause, but including renal trauma, polycystic kidney disease, IgA nephropathy, or sickle cell trait may lead to extrarenal obstruction.

Intramural obstruction can be divided into anatomic or functional causes. Of the anatomic abnormalities that lead to urinary obstruction (tumors and strictures), transitional-cell carcinomas of the renal pelvis and ureter account for the highest proportion. Of particular note, patients with analgesic nephropathy are at increased risk for the development of transitional cell carcinoma of the urinary tract. Ureteral or urethral strictures may result from infection, trauma, or postradiation therapy for pelvic tumors. Worldwide, *Schistosomiasis haematobium* infection is a considerable problem affecting nearly 100 million people. The ova deposit in the walls of the distal ureter and bladder causing inflammation which leads to ureteral stricture, and fibrosis and contracture of the bladder in 50% of chronically infected patients. The incidence of bladder cancer is also increased. Rarely, obstructive uropathy may result from ureteral strictures from granulomatous disease or urethral stricture due to gonococcal and nongonococcal infections. Functional obstruction results from an abnormality (neuromuscular) leading to an alteration in the normal dynamic response of the urinary tract. In neurologic disorders resulting in injury to upper motor neurons involuntary bladder contraction (spastic bladder) results, whereas with lower motor neuron injury the bladder becomes flaccid and atonic. Either condition may lead to abnormalities in the forward flow of urine and an increase in residual urine volume that can result in obstructive uropathy with vesicoureteral reflux. Almost 90% of patients with multiple sclerosis develop bladder dysfunction. This disorder is also common in patients with long-standing diabetes mellitus, and may complicate Parkinson's disease as well as cerebrovascular accidents. A number of medications are known to alter the neuromuscular activity of the bladder resulting in decreased contractility or tone and thus urinary retention, with an incidence of >10% in some instances (levodopa and disopyramide). The use of these agents may be particularly problematic in patients with a preexisting obstructive condition such as benign prostatic hyperplasia in men.

Acquired-Extrinsic

The most common cause of extrinsic obstruction in women is pregnancy. In up to 90% of pregnant women, some degree of ureteral dilatation will be observed by the third trimester. This has been attributed to pressure by the gravid uterus on the pelvic brim and affects the right ureter more than the left. However, ureteral dilatation may be seen as early as the first trimester, and it has been suggested that this may be the result of hormonal (progesterone) effects on peristalsis. This process is often asymptomatic and resolves spontaneously after delivery. Rarely, bilateral ureteral obstruction during pregnancy can lead to acute renal failure (see Chapter 50). The second most common cause of urinary obstruction in women is carcinoma of the cervix, with obstruction seen in 30% of patients, usually a result of direct extension. In older women, uterine prolapse can lead to hydronephrosis, and this may occur in up to 80% of patients if there is total prolapse. In these women the ureters are trapped between the levator muscles and the fundus of the prolapsed uterus. Endometriosis occasionally leads to pelvic inflammation with fibrosis and ureteral obstruction. Pelvic inflammatory disease may result in obstruction in up to 40% of patients if associated with a tubo-ovarian abscess.

Benign prostatic hyperplasia is the most common cause of obstructive uropathy in older men with symptoms of outlet obstruction in 50 to 75% of males over 50 years of age and significant hydronephrosis in 10% of cases. Overall, adenocarcinoma of the prostate is second only to carcinoma of the cervix as the leading form of extrinsic obstruction due to tumors. Obstruction from prostate cancer (or any pelvic malignancy) can be due to either direct extension of tumor to the bladder outlet or ureters, or metastases to the ureters or surrounding lymph nodes.

In addition to colorectal carcinomas (ureteral metastases), a number of gastrointestinal disorders are associated with obstruction (often unilateral) resulting from local infection and/or inflammatory processes. Vascular diseases, the most common of which is abdominal aortic aneurysm, will lead to ureteral obstruction from retroperitoneal fibrosis (inflammatory aneurysms) or from direct pressure of the expanding aneurysm. Rarely, systemic diseases associated with vasculitis (systemic lupus erythematosus, polyarteritis nodosa, Wegener's granulomatous, and Henoch–Schönlein purpura) have been associated with obstruction.

A number of conditions involving the retroperitoneal space may result in ureteral obstruction by fibrosis or direct invasion and compression. Periureteral fibrosis can be a consequence of radiation therapy, trauma, surgery, granulomatous disease, or infection. Retroperitoneal fibrosis has been linked to the use of a number of drugs, including methysergide, bromocriptine, and β-blockers. Patients in whom an obvious cause for retroperitoneal fibrosis cannot be identified have idiopathic retroperitoneal fibrosis, which is predominantly a disease of men (3:1) in the fifth and sixth decade of life. Flank pain which is insidious in onset, dull, and not colicky, is the presenting symptom in 80% of patients. This may be accompanied by fever, weight loss, and nonspecific gastrointestinal complaints. On intravenous pyelography, medial deviation of the ureters is a characteristic feature. The fibrous tissue appears to extend from the aorta, encasing and drawing the ureters medially, and may be up to 6 cm thick. Although the etiology of this entity is unknown, the histologic findings are those of an inflammatory process involving collagen and fibrosis. Sur-

gical release of the ureters (ureterolysis) is often successful in relieving obstruction and pain symptoms.

Primary tumors, such as lymphomas, can involve the retroperitoneal space and can lead to obstruction. In addition, metastatic spread to the retroperitoneum of a number of carcinomas, most commonly cervix (30%) and bladder (20%), but including breast, prostate, colon, and ovary, can also result in ureteral obstruction. The most likely cause of obstruction after pelvic irradiation for malignancy is recurrent tumor if obstruction occurs within 2 years of therapy. Radiation fibrosis is the more common cause after 2 years.

Congenital

Of the congenital causes of obstructive uropathy (Table 3) ureteropelvic junction obstruction, and posterior urethral valves are the most common. If severe enough, obstruction may have its onset *in utero* and may lead to major renal abnormalities in the developing fetus. Early in development, obstruction results in a kidney that appears dysplastic. Obstruction later on leads to a kidney with cortical cysts and a reduced nephron mass. Those fetuses in whom obstruction develops late in gestation have features similar to that seen postnatally, such as hydronephrosis and renal parenchymal thinning. Occasionally, obstruction may not manifest itself until childhood.

Ureteropelvic junction (UPJ) obstruction is the most common cause of hydronephrosis in infancy and early childhood. In childhood, the majority of patients are males, whereas in adults, females dominate. In infancy, UPJ obstruction is bilateral in 30% of cases, an uncommon finding in adults. The presentation in children is that of an abdominal mass with flank pain or abdominal pain and failure to thrive. In adults, the pain is episodic and is often precipitated by high urine flow rates. Abnormal peristalsis due to a derangement in the smooth muscles of the renal pelvis has been proposed as the primary mechanism for UPJ obstruction. Additionally, a hyperdistensible renal pelvis, incapable of draining completely, has been suggested as the cause in some cases. Less often, UPJ obstruction may result from crossing blood vessels, fibrous bands, or strictures.

Posterior urethral valves, leading to outlet obstruction, are seen strictly in males and are best diagnosed by a voiding cystourethrogram. Presentation is infancy is with a palpable bladder and kidneys along with marked renal insufficiency. Older children will often present with urgency or enuresis. One of the more unusual causes of obstructive uropathy is the prune-belly syndrome. Predominantly seen in males, this consists of the triad of deficiency of abdominal muscles (resulting in loose, wrinkled, redundant skin over the abdomen appearing like a "prune"), cryptorchidism, and hydroureteronephrosis. The obstruction is bilateral, with abnormal ureteral peristalsis and prostatic hypoplasia implicated as possible mechanisms.

Nonobstructive Urinary Tract Dilatation

In a number of situations dilatation of the urinary tract may occur without evidence of obstruction. However, these conditions, if chronic, may also result in impaired renal function and atrophy of renal parenchyma. This can be seen with vesicoureteral reflux, acute pyelonephritis, and high flow states (such as diabetes insipidus or primary polydipsia). As already mentioned, ureteral dilatation can be observed in 90% of women during pregnancy, but it usually resolves within a few weeks of delivery and therefore does not result an any functional or pathologic renal impairment unless complicated by infection.

PATHOPHYSIOLOGY

Our understanding of the consequences of urinary tract obstruction on renal function are primarily derived from the effects of short-term (24 hr) complete obstruction in experimental animals. The alterations in renal function that result are divided into those that affect either glomerular or tubular function.

Glomerular Function

Glomerular filtration rate (GFR) declines progressively after complete obstruction. Within the first few hours of acute ureteral obstruction, there is an increase in proximal tubular pressure, the magnitude of which is partially dependent on hydration status (greater with increased hydration). This results in a decrease in net glomerular filtration pressure (net glomerular filtration pressure = glomerular filtration pressure − intratubular pressure) and thus a decrease in GFR. Simultaneously, an increase in the production of prostacyclin and PGE_2 leads to afferent arteriolar dilatation (vasodilative phase) and an increase in renal blood flow which increases glomerular filtration pressure. However, since the increase in glomerular filtration pressure is not as great as the increase in intratubular pressure, the decrease in net glomerular filtration pressure persists, resulting in a GFR that is 80% of the preobstruction value.

At 4 to 5 hr after obstruction, intratubular pressure begins to decline due to ongoing reabsorption of sodium and water by the nephron, dilatation of the collecting system, and lymphatic removal of solute and water. A decrease in renal blood flow due to an increase in afferent arteriolar resistance (vasoconstrictive phase) also ensues, leading to a decrease in glomerular filtration pressure. Since glomerular filtration pressure declines at a faster rate than the intratubular pressure, a further decrease in net glomerular filtration pressure occurs and GFR continues to decline. Thus, the relatively higher intratubular pressure remains a significant factor responsible for the ongoing decrease in GFR which can be as low as 20% of normal by 24 hr.

The vasoconstrictive phase is mediated by angiotensin II (AII), thromboxane A_2, antidiuretic hormone (ADH), and a decrease in endothelium-derived relaxing factor (EDRF) or nitric oxide production. The increase in intrarenal production of AII is a consequence of decreased delivery of sodium and chloride to the macula densa and the effects of vasodilating prostaglandins on renin release. The source for the increased synthesis of thromboxane in the obstructed kidney includes intrinsic glomerular cells and leukocytes (macrophages and T lymphocytes) which infil-

trate soon after obstruction. In addition to their effects on vascular resistance, AII and thromboxane A_2 alter GFR by producing mesangial contraction which leads to a decrease in the ultrafiltration coefficient. Pretreatment with angiotensin converting enzyme inhibitors (ACEi) and inhibitors of thromboxane A_2 synthesis has been shown to counteract the effects of obstruction on GFR and renal plasma flow in experimental models.

The degree of improvement in GFR after release of obstruction in animals is related to the duration of obstruction. Complete recovery of GFR is observed after obstruction of up to 7 days, 70% recovery with 14 days of obstruction, 30% recovery with 28 days of obstruction, and essentially no recovery of renal function after obstruction of 56 days.

Tubular Function

Abnormalities in reabsorption of sodium and water are characteristic of obstructive nephropathy. In the acute phases of obstruction, there is an initial increase in sodium and water reabsorption secondary to underperfusion of the distal nephron. This is evidenced by reductions in urinary sodium concentration, fractional excretion of sodium, and free water clearance. In clinical practice, this results in urinary indices which can have a prerenal pattern, with a urinary sodium of <20 mEq/L, fractional excretion of sodium of <1%, and a urine osmolality of >500 mOsmol (see Chapter 33). With more prolonged or chronic obstruction, subsequent alterations in tubular function result in a decrease in sodium and water reabsorption and indices similar to those seen with ATN.

After the release of chronic obstruction, there is decreased sodium reabsorption by the nephrons, leading to an increased fractional excretion of sodium. The decrease in sodium reabsorption results from a reduction in Na^+,K^+-ATPase activity in the nephron. Additionally, there is an associated increase in excretion of calcium, phosphate, and magnesium which parallels sodium excretion. The ability to concentrate urine is also impaired after release of obstruction, and results in an increased fractional excretion of water. The concentrating defect is due to multiple factors including: (1) decreased medullary tonicity from washout of solute due to an increase in medullary blood flow and decreased sodium chloride reabsorption at the thick ascending limb of Henle, (2) decreased response to ADH, and (3) a decrease in the number of functional juxtamedullary nephrons. The greater natriuresis and diuresis observed after release of bilateral ureteral obstruction (BUO) as compared with unilateral renal obstruction (UUO) is attributed to the accumulation of sodium and water, urea retention, retention of other impermeable solutes, and higher levels of atrial natriuretic peptide which occur in BUO but not UUO.

Abnormalities in potassium and hydrogen excretion are also common in obstructive uropathy. Hyperkalemia results as the fractional excretion of potassium is less in obstructive uropathy than in other forms of renal disease with similar levels of renal insufficiency. The decrease in potassium secretion is attributed to either a reduction in the secretion or response of the distal tubule to aldosterone, or a combination of both. Hyperkalemic–hyperchloremic acidosis is also frequently seen in patients with obstructive uropathy. This may be explained by a defect in hydrogen ion secretion and maximal urine acidification (distal renal tubular acidosis), and/or a defect in secretion of aldosterone secondary to a decrease in renin production (hyporeninemic hypoaldosteronism or type IV renal tubular acidosis). Furthermore, a decrease in sodium reabsorption in the distal nephron has been suggested as an additional factor, which by reducing the degree of intraluminal negativity would decrease the voltage-dependent secretion of both potassium and hydrogen. Finally, reduced levels of H^+-ATPase (a major transport pathway) in the cortical and medullary collecting ducts have been observed in obstructive uropathy and may further explain the problem with hydrogen ion excretion. The acidifying defect is often reversible but may persist in some cases.

RENAL PATHOLOGY

The pathology of hydronephrosis is similar irrespective of the underlying cause of obstruction. In early hydronephrosis, the kidney is enlarged and edematous with an increase in the renal pelvic cavity and blunting of the renal papilla. Later on there is retraction and dimpling of the papilla, and this is most evident at the upper and lower poles. Microscopically the renal cortex appears normal but the tubules may be dilated, and Tamm–Horsfall protein is seen in Bowman's space (characteristic of obstruction or reflux). The principal lesion in the medulla and papilla is ischemic atrophy associated with flattening and atrophy of tubular epithelium and interstitial fibrosis. As the hydronephrosis advances, the atrophy becomes even more pronounced. The kidney transforms into essentially a fluid sac with loss of papillae and marked thinning of the cortex and medulla. The progressive sclerosis and fibrosis results in few renal features that are recognizable.

The morphologic changes in obstructive uropathy are primarily attributed to the ischemia from the marked reduction in renal blood flow. However, another contributing factor which has gained interest is the role played by macrophages and T lymphocytes which invade the interstitium early on in obstruction. Within 4–12 hr after obstruction, there is an increase in interstitial macrophages which continues to increase thereafter. Chemoattractants, such as monocyte chemoattractant peptide-1 and osteopontin, appear to be released from tubular epithelial cells in response to the increase in intratubular pressure from ureteral obstruction. Fibrogenic cytokines, such as transforming growth factor β (TGF-β), produced by the invading macrophages and T lymphocytes become central in the progressive fibrosis observed in obstructive nephropathy. Transforming growth factor-β increases matrix synthesis by interstitial fibroblasts, and decreases matrix degradation by downregulating the production of matrix degradation proteins, and promoting the generation of proteinase inhibitors. It has also been shown that vasoactive compounds such as angiotensin II (which is increased in obstruction) may directly stimulate the production of TGF-β by tubular epithelial cells or macrophages. In experimental obstructive uropathy, the use of ACEi significantly reduces the mRNA levels of TGF-β and type IV collagen, resulting in a marked decrease in the degree of tubulointerstitial fibrosis and preventing further progression of renal disease. The beneficial effects of ACEi were observed even when initiated 1 week after the onset of obstruction. These experimental insights suggest a potentially important role for ACEi in the medical management of patients with obstructive uropathy.

DIAGNOSIS

Dilatation of the urinary tract is the radiographic feature characteristically used to confirm the presence of obstruction (Fig. 1). When the diagnosis of obstructive uropathy is suspected, a careful history, physical exam, and laboratory evaluation (measure of renal function, electrolytes, and urinalysis and culture) is essential in developing a differential diagnosis and diagnostic approach (Fig. 2).

Obstructive uropathy should always be a consideration in patients presenting with renal failure (acute or chronic), especially when the nature of the renal failure is unexplained. Renal failure in obstructive uropathy may come as a result of either bilateral upper tract obstruction or, more commonly, outlet or lower tract obstruction. In the presence of clinical clues to obstruction of the bladder outlet (i.e., difficulty urinating, suprapubic pain, or fullness and a palpable bladder) a postvoid bladder catheterization is initially beneficial both diagnostically and therapeutically. Further diagnostic evaluation with ultrasonography (US) allows a quick, noninvasive way to confirm and assess the cause and severity of obstruction and avoids the possibility of nephrotoxic insult from the use of intravenous contrast required in other imaging procedures such as the intravenous pyelogram (IVP).

The use of ultrasonography to diagnose chronic obstruction when sufficient time has elapsed for the urinary tract to dilate, has a sensitivity of 98% and a specificity of 75%. False-positive results are often due to normal variants such as blood vessels in the renal sinuses, and these can be discerned with the use of duplex doppler evaluation. The use of duplex doppler evaluation in determining the resistive index is also helpful in distinguishing true obstruction (elevated resistive index) from nonobstructive causes (having a normal resistive index of 50–60%) of urinary tract dilatation. A false-negative ultrasound evaluation should be extremely rare in the evaluation of chronic obstruction. Computerized tomography (CT) is also an accurate technique for the detection of urinary tract dilatation and may be more likely than US to identify the obstructing lesion. However, in order to enhance structural identification with conventional CT, contrast is often required. Whether or not unenhanced spiral CT will prove beneficial, over and above conventional CT or US, in the evaluation of chronic obstruction is yet to be seen. Ultimately, with upper tract obstruction, antegrade or retrograde pyelography may be required to further define the site and cause of obstruction. The use of retrograde pyelography may be of particular value in the situation where a nondilated obstructive uropathy due to retroperitoneal

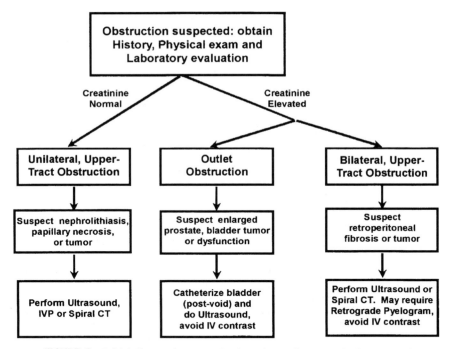

FIGURE 2 Initial diagnostic approach when obstructive uropathy is suspected.

fibrosis or an infiltrating malignancy is suspected. Although these studies can be useful when it is not possible to do an IVP or when the use of intravenous contrast is contraindicated (allergy to contrast or renal failure), the risk of urinary tract infection is of concern particularly with retrograde pyelography. To further evaluate (and treat) causes of lower urinary tract obstruction, cystoscopy and urodynamic studies may be indicated. Urodynamic studies are most worthwhile when a functional abnormality of the bladder (neurogenic bladder) is suspected.

In patients with symptoms of acute, unilateral obstruction (renal function is often normal), such as in nephrolithiasis, sufficient time for identifiable dilatation of the collecting system may not have elapsed, and therefore the IVP has been considered the "gold standard." Whether or not the use of less invasive technology such as US can replace the IVP in detecting acute urinary tract obstruction has been an area of intense interest (Fig. 3A, B). This stems primarily from the small but definite morbidity and mortality associated with the use of radiographic contrast. The success of ultrasound in diagnosing acute obstruction varies substantially (sensitivity reported to be as low as 50% and as high as 90%). In part, the variable success of US is attributed to its subjective nature making it highly operator dependent with most false negatives due to cases of grade 1 hydronephrosis (mild dilatation of the renal sinus central-echo complex) or nondilated obstructive uropathy (i.e., retroperitoneal fibrosis). Because nephrolithiasis is the leading cause of acute renal colic and obstruction, and >90% of renal stones are radiopaque, combining plain abdominal radiography [kidney, ureter, bladder (KUB)] with US increases the sensitivity of detecting obstruction to

>95%. Finally, the use of duplex doppler ultrasound, to demonstrate the presence of a high resistive index (>70%) from increased vascular resistance in obstruction, has been shown to further reduce the false-negative results associated with US (this is helpful in either acute or chronic obstruction). Thus, the combination of US and KUB may be a viable alternative to studies requiring radiographic contrast. A limitation of US remains its inability to determine the level and the cause of obstruction as compared to IVP. Enthusiasm is mounting for the use of unenhanced spiral CT in the evaluation of acute renal colic. The scan takes only 50 sec to obtain images from the top of kidney to the base of the bladder and does not require contrast. Furthermore, it is more sensitive than combined KUB and US in identifying causes of renal colic, and it allows visualization of the obstructive lesion.

Although a chronic condition, UPJ obstruction is often associated with symptoms which are acute in nature and reproduced only during periods of high urine flow rates. Often a diagnosis of UPJ obstruction requires the use of diuresis urography which combines the use of intravenous furosemide with an IVP in order to evaluate for dilatation and abnormal emptying of the upper urinary tract during a state of high urine flow. A similar evaluation can be obtained with diuresis renography using radionuclides (see later).

NONOBSTRUCTIVE URINARY TRACT DILATATION

Nonobstructive urinary tract dilatation may be differentiated from that due to obstruction with diuresis renography or diuresis urography. Diuresis renography utilizes

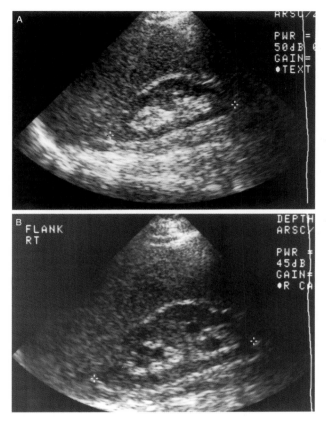

FIGURE 3 (A) Ultrasound of the right kidney, long axis, demonstrating the normal echo-dense central area, the renal sinus central echo-complex. (B) Repeat ultrasound of the right kidney, long axis, in the same patient 3 weeks later after presenting with a 3-day history of right flank pain. Note hydronephrosis (pyelocalyceal dilatation) as demonstrated by a marked separation of the renal sinus central echo-complex.

radionuclide imaging and evaluates the pattern of radionuclide elimination by each kidney before and after intravenous furosemide. Prolonged retention of radioactivity after diuresis is consistent with obstruction. In nonobstructive dilatation, there is a rapid "washout" of radioactivity with diuresis. Similar findings can be demonstrated with the use of diuresis urography (see earlier).

TREATMENT

The treatment of obstructive uropathy is dictated not only by the underlying cause but also by the location. It should be obvious that evidence for renal failure (acute or chronic) resulting from urinary tract obstruction warrants emergent attention as the potential for permanent renal damage increases with the duration of obstruction. The urgency and aggressiveness with which obstructive uropathy must be treated is also determined by the severity of symptoms (flank pain, dysuria, frequency, etc.) as well as the presence of infection.

Nephrolithiasis, the most common cause of acute unilateral obstruction, can most often be treated with conserva-

tive measures such as intravenous fluids and pain medications. As 90% of stones <5 mm pass spontaneously with increased urine flow alone, no addition treatment is required. However, with increasing stone size, the likelihood of spontaneous passage diminishes and the possible need for more aggressive measures arise. These are discussed in detail in Chapter 53. In extreme situations of chronic or recurrent unilateral obstruction of any cause, the obstructive process may lead to advanced hydronephrosis associated with severe pain, recurrent pyelonephritis, or pyonephrosis, in which case a nephrectomy may be indicated especially if the remaining function of the affected kidney is minimal.

The initial treatment approach for patients presenting with bilateral urinary tract obstruction and renal failure is primarily dictated by the location of the obstruction. In patients with a neurogenic bladder or disorders involving the bladder outlet (i.e., prostatic hypertrophy or cancer), the placement of a urethral catheter will often suffice. For patients in whom a urethral catheter cannot be passed into the bladder, a suprapubic cystostomy may be required. Lesions obstructing the ureters require cystoscopy and stent placement. If a stent cannot be passed beyond the ureteral obstruction in a retrograde fashion, a percutaneous nephrostomy tube can be placed and antegrade placement of a stent can be attempted. Placement of a percutaneous nephrostomy is successful in over 90% of patients, resulting in clinical improvement in up to 70% of cases. Major complications (abscess, sepsis, hematomas) occur in less than 5% of patients.

Once an acute solution to relieve the obstruction has been initiated, then specific treatment of the underlying disease becomes the primary focus. For example, in neurogenic disorders of the bladder, timed voiding and pharmacologic agents (in patients with a spastic bladder, anticholinergic agents: oxybutynin or propantheline bromide) may be useful, but in many patients, particularly those with bladder atony, intermittent catheterization of the bladder (four times daily) is necessary. For men with prostatic hyperplasia, the long-term treatment approach is dependent on the severity of the outlet obstruction. If symptoms are minimal, and not associated with infection or upper urinary tract abnormalities, close observation is appropriate. Cases with mild to moderate symptoms of prostatism can be managed medically with either α antagonists or 5-α reductase inhibitors. Alpha antagonists (doxazosin or terazosin) act by relaxing the smooth muscle of the prostate and bladder neck, thus decreasing urethral pressure and outlet obstruction. Hormonal therapy with a 5-α reductase inhibitor (finasteride) inhibits the conversion of testosterone to the active dihydrotestosterone and thereby leads to a reduction in prostate size. The combined use of these agents may be beneficial in some patients, as they are felt to act synergistically. In patients with hyperplasia of the prostate resulting in signs and symptoms of severe obstruction (significant urinary retention or renal failure), surgical intervention [i.e., transurethral resection of the prostate (TURP) or transurethral incision of the prostate (TUIP)] is generally required.

In disease processes which lead to irreparable damage of the lower urinary tract (as in bladder, cervical, or prostate cancer) or ureters, a diversion procedure such as an ileal conduit or percutaneous nephrostomy will be needed. In patients with obstructive nephropathy secondary to malignancy, percutaneous nephrostomy can relieve the obstruction in >75% of cases and resulted in a significant increase in survival (>6 months in 50%) as well as an increase in number of days spent at home as compared to patients in whom the procedure was not performed. Thus, patients with apparently terminal diseases can benefit from this aggressive approach.

Postobstructive Diuresis

Release of bilateral obstruction can result in marked polyuria (postobstructive diuresis). A number of factors, physiologic and pathologic, lead to development of this condition. Physiologic factors contributing to the diuresis include excess sodium and water retention, accumulation of urea and other nonreabsorbable solutes, and accumulation of atrial natriuretic peptide. Pathologic factors including decreased tubular reabsorption of sodium, inability to maximally concentrate urine due to a decreased medullary concentrating gradient and decreased response to ADH, and increased tubular flow reducing equilibration time for absorption of sodium and water. Once the accumulated excess of sodium and water has been excreted, the potential for severe volume contraction as well as hypokalemia exists if patients are not carefully monitored and given appropriate fluid and solute replacement. Urinary output should be measured frequently during the diuresis (at least every 6 hr and in cases with large urine outputs, hourly). Once the patient has diuresed to the point they are euvolemic, fluid replacement (intravenous plus oral) should be administered as needed to prevent volume contraction based predominantly on clinical and laboratory parameters. This is often accomplished by replacement of 75% of the urine losses with intravenous fluids having a solute composition similar to what is excreted (0.45% normal saline). Serum electrolyte levels should also be monitored closely during the diuresis, at least daily if not more often, and replaced as needed. The postobstructive diuresis is self-limited, resolving over several days to a week. Persistence of the polyuria is often due to overzealous hydration (in excess of urinary output) which perpetuates the solute and water diuresis.

Recovery of Renal Function

The likelihood of regaining renal function postobstruction is dependent on the degree and duration of obstruction. The longer the process goes untreated the less likely significant recovery in renal function will occur. In general, the majority of improvement in renal function should be apparent within 2 weeks postobstruction. Complete recovery of renal function is anticipated in patients with acute uncomplicated obstruction of short duration (≤1 to 2 weeks),

and little to no improvement in severe, complete, or partial obstruction which persists for a prolonged period of time (>12 weeks). However, recovery of renal function in patients has been recorded after obstruction for up to 70 days. The use of radionuclide renography has been suggested as one way to predict recovery of renal function. This is usually done several weeks after a temporary procedure to relieve the obstruction (such as a percutaneous nephrostomy) has been performed.

Bibliography

Better OS, Arieff AI, Massry SG, *et al.*: Studies on renal function after relief of complete unilateral obstruction of three months duration in man. *Am J Med* 54:234–240, 1973.

Cronan JJ: Contemporary concepts for imaging urinary tract obstruction. *Urol Radiol* 14:8–12, 1992.

Curhan GC, Zeidel ML: Urinary tract obstruction. In: Brenner BM (ed) *The Kidney*, 5th Ed., pp. 1936–1958. Saunders, Philadelphia, 1996.

Davidson AJ, Hartman DS: The dilated pelvocalyceal system. In: Davidson AJ, Hartman DS (eds) *Radiology of the Kidney and Urinary Tract*, 2nd Ed., pp. 571–780. Saunders, Philadelphia, 1994.

Diamond JR: Macrophages and progressive renal disease in experimental hydronephrosis. *Am J Kidney Dis* 26:133–140, 1995.

Haddad MC, Sharif HS, Shahed MS, Mutaiery MA, Samihan AM, Sammak BM, Southcombe LA, Crawford AD: Renal colic: Diagnosis and outcome. *Radiology* 184:83–88, 1992.

Harrington KJ, Pandha HS, Kelly SA, Lambert HE, Jackson JE, Waxman J: Palliation of obstructive nephropathy due to malignancy. *Br J Urol* 76:101–107, 1995.

Hill GS: Calcium and the kidney, hydronephrosis. In: Jennette JC, Olson JL, Schwartz MM, Silva FG (eds) *Heptinstall's Pathology of the Kidney*, 5th Ed., pp. 891–936. Lippincott-Raven, Philadelphia, 1998.

Hoffman LM, Suki WN: Obstructive uropathy mimicking volume depletion. *JAMA* 236:2096–2097, 1976.

Ishidoya S, Morrissey J, McCracken R, Klahr S: Delayed treatment with enalapril halts tubulointerstitial fibrosis in rats with obstructive nephropathy. *Kidney Int* 49:1110–1119, 1996.

Katz DS, Lane MJ, Sommer FG: Unenhanced helical CT of ureteral stones: Incidence of associated urinary tract findings. *Am J Radiol* 166:1319–1322, 1996.

Klahr S: Pathophysiology of obstructive nephropathy: A 1991 update. *Semin Nephrol* 11:156–168, 1991.

Klahr S: New insight into the consequences and mechanisms of renal impairment in obstructive nephropathy. *Am J Kidney Dis* 18:689–699, 1991.

Klahr S, Purkerson ML: The pathophysiology of obstructive nephropathy: The role of vasoactive compounds in the hemodynamic and structural abnormalities of the obstructed kidney. *Am J Kidney Dis* 23:219–223, 1994.

Klahr S, Ishidoya S, Morrissey J: Role of angiotensin II in the tubulointerstitial fibrosis of obstructive nephropathy. *Am J Kidney Dis* 26:141–146, 1995.

Spital A, Spataro R: Nondilated obstructive uropathy due to a ureteral calculus. *Am J Med* 98:509–511, 1995.

Suki W, Eknoyan G, Rector FC, Jr, Seldin DW: Patterns of nephron perfusion in acute and chronic hydrinephrosis. *J Clin Invest* 45:122–131, 1966.

Vehmas T, Kivisaari L, Mankinen P, Tierala E, Somer K, Lehtonen T, Standertskjöld-Nordenstam C-G: Results and complications of percutaneous nephrostomy. *Ann Clin Res* 20:423–427, 1988.

52

VESICOURETERAL REFLUX AND REFLUX NEPHROPATHY

BILLY S. ARANT, JR.

The urine that emerges from the papillary collecting ducts through ducts of Bellini is collected in the calyces, flows into the renal pelvis and down the ureter to enter the bladder via the ureteral orifice located in the trigone. The intravesical pressure is usually maintained low (<20 cm H_2O) as the smooth muscle of the bladder wall relaxes while the bladder gradually fills with urine. During micturition, the intravesical pressure rises, but it usually does not exceed 35 cm H_2O as the bladder smooth muscle contracts, because the external sphincter relaxes to permit urine to exit the bladder via the urethra. In the normal bladder, urine does not reenter the ureter because the distal end of the ureter forms a flap valve by penetrating the bladder wall in an oblique fashion and following a submucosal course of about 5 cm in the adult before reaching the bladder lumen. The contraction of the bladder smooth muscle and flattening of the mucosa by the increased intravesical pressure assure competence of the ureterovesical junction during micturition.

An incompetent ureterovesical junction permits urine to flow retrograde from the bladder into the ureter, an occurrence termed vesicoureteral reflux (VUR). Often, a shortened submucosal portion does not permit the flap valve to occlude the ureter during micturition—one explanation for the more frequent presence of VUR in infants, as their submucosal ureter may be only 2 cm long. When intravesical pressure is high enough, refluxing urine can fill the ureter and renal pelvis, actually reenter the ducts of Bellini, and even traverse the entire course of the nephron to reach Bowman's space—intrarenal reflux. When there is no other abnormality of the bladder, VUR is primary and may be observed in the fetus or at birth in which case it is congenital or, if identified only at some time after birth, may be acquired. However, in the presence of functional or anatomic obstruction VUR is considered secondary. When VUR is associated with unusually high intravesical pressure or pyelonephritis, any resulting renal parenchymal injury is termed reflux nephropathy.

PREVALENCE

The actual incidence of VUR in the general population has never been described. When adults with no history of a urinary tract infection (UTI) underwent voiding cystourethrography, VUR was identified in $<0.5\%$. On the other hand, VUR could be demonstrated in 20 to 50% of infants and children when they were investigated following their first recognized UTI; VUR was found in only 4% of adults with UTI. In children <6 years of age, the cumulative incidence rate for a first time symptomatic UTI is 6.6% for girls and 1.8% for boys. There is no gender difference in the incidence of VUR following UTI. VUR appears to occur equally among races except for African-American children who, in most reports, have had VUR associated with UTI in $<4\%$. Therefore, based on a current U.S. population of ~25 million children <6 years of age, just over 1 million will have a symptomatic UTI and, on average, 40% or 460,000 will have VUR.

When asymptomatic siblings of children with VUR were screened, VUR was found in about 35–45%. Although a common gene has not been identified, VUR does occur in several generations of the same family, suggesting hereditary factors predispose to primary VUR. There is no such familial pattern among children with secondary VUR.

DIAGNOSTIC STUDIES TO IDENTIFY VUR

Avoiding cystourethrogram (VCUG) is used to identify VUR (Fig. 1). To perform this study, a catheter is inserted through the urethra or a suprapubic needle used to fill the urinary bladder with radiographic contrast material or a solution containing a radionuclide. Observations are made before, during, and after micturition. VUR will be identified most often at peak intravesical pressure generated during micturition. The reported incidence of VUR is based mostly on studies that used contrast VCUG data. This technique may fail to detect VUR—even dilating reflux—in up to 40% of patients with UTI. Although the increased sensitivity of radionuclide testing is desirable, neither the grading of VUR nor identification of anatomical abnormalities can be accomplished by this method. Ultrasound is of no value in detecting VUR, but can identify urinary tract obstruction.

The grading of VUR has had an important role when clinical decisions are considered. In general, higher grades of VUR are associated more often with renal injury and, in the past, were grounds for early recommendation of sur-

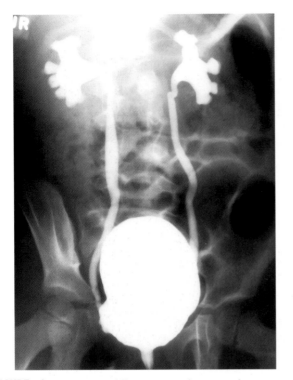

FIGURE I Contrast voiding cystourethrogram demonstrates vesicoureteral reflux when intravesical pressure is highest. Both collecting systems are filled completely and dilated with mild tortuosity of the ureters and blunting of the calyces—grade III VUR (international classification).

gical correction. The five-grade classification proposed by the International Study of Reflux in Children has been adopted almost universally. When contrast enters the ureter but does not reach the renal pelvis, grade I is assigned. If the entire collecting system is filled but not dilated, grade II is assigned. In grades III, IV, and V, progressive dilatation and tortuosity of the ureter are observed. Such a classification is useful when a prospective study is conducted or an individual patient is followed with serial studies to confirm any change in VUR, but its reproducibility depends heavily on the VCUG being conducted in a very standardized fashion. Although it is relatively easy for anyone to assign a grade of VUR on any static image, VUR is an active urodynamic process which depends not only on the competence of the ureterovesical junction but also on the intravesical pressure, the elasticity of the collecting system, rate of ante grade flow of urine, and the timing of the study. The international classification depends on the grade of VUR being assigned at peak voiding pressure, which usually occurs within 30 to 60 sec of initiating the urinary stream. Although relied on heavily in the past, there is probably no clinical relevance to grading VUR other than nondilating (grades I and II) or dilating (grades III, IV, and V), because the resolution rate and the prevalence of renal injury is similar among grades in these two groups.

RENAL SCARRING

When VUR is associated with UTI and pyelonephritis develops, renal injury can result in parenchymal scarring or reflux nephropathy. Similar scarring which follows acute pyelonephritis without VUR has always been termed chronic pyelonephritis. Renal ultrasound can detect only gross parenchymal scarring but can provide accurate measurements of renal size—a discrepancy in length of the two kidneys should raise suspicion of renal scarring. Intravenous urography will not identify acute renal injury, but when performed in a careful fashion, established renal scars or parenchymal thinning overlying an abnormal calyx can be identified (Fig. 2). A radionuclide scan using 99Tc-dimercaptosuccinic acid (DMSA) is the imaging study recommended to detect both acute pyelonephritis and renal scars.

Renal scarring will occur in about 10% of kidneys after the first episode of pyelonephritis. With each subsequent episode, the likelihood of scarring increases, reaching 58% after the fourth episode. Although scarring has been observed most often (25 to 40%) when dilating VUR is present at the time of diagnosis, the total number of kidneys affected by dilating VUR is relatively small. A much larger total number of children with UTI have nondilating VUR with normal appearing kidneys at diagnosis and a lower incidence of renal scarring (10%) identified in follow-up studies. Only half of the children with acute pyelonephritis will exhibit VUR, but many without VUR will also develop renal scarring. Therefore, the total number of kidneys scarred by pyelonephritis is larger when VUR is absent or nondilating. Previously, there has been an opinion, strongly held, that renal scarring occurs only in infants and young children. One study, however, reported renal scarring in 80% of older children and adolescents with acute pyelonephritis, which was nearly identical to the incidence in younger patients.

PATHOLOGY

The gross appearance of a renal scar, either from pyelonephritis or reflux nephropathy, is a cortical depression overlying a calyx. The characteristic histopathologic findings include atrophy of both cortex and medulla in which glomerular remnants and thyroidization of tubular structures may still be identified. Failure to identify glomeruli in segmental scars was once interpreted as renal hypoplasia—the kidney did not develop normally, and, therefore, glomeruli were never formed in the segment. Subsequent studies, however, demonstrated segmental scarring in a previously normal kidney was produced by parenchymal injury that heals by segmental atrophy with progressive glomerular sclerosis. Deterioration of renal function after further acute renal injury has stopped most likely is explained by hyperfiltration, as with any other remnant kidney or untreated arterial hypertension. Proteinuria is a sign of renal injury and may be minimal or heavy. Surgical correction of VUR does not prevent further deterioration of renal function due to prior parenchymal injury but may

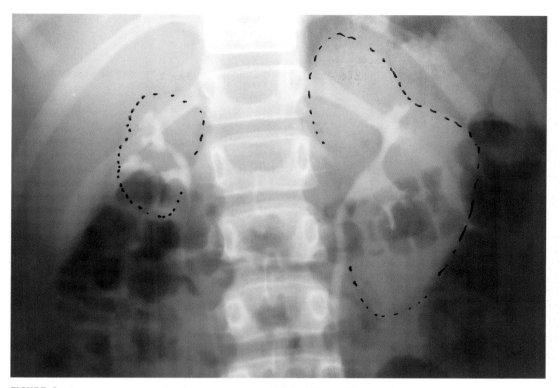

FIGURE 2 Intravenous urography demonstrates a small right kidney with extensive scarring but prompt excretion of contrast material into deformed calyces. The left kidney is larger than normal (compensatory hypertrophy) but has a cortical depression overlying a deformed calyx in the upper pole.

prevent or reduce subsequent episodes of acute pyelonephritis.

CONSEQUENCES OF RENAL SCARRING

The morbidities associated with renal scarring of any degree are hypertension, and, when scarring is more extensive and involves both kidneys, chronic renal insufficiency. In fact, a common cause of hypertension in women under 30 years of age is renal scarring from VUR. It is observed most often in females at puberty, when birth control pills are prescribed, and during pregnancy. This suggests a role for estrogen in raising blood pressure. The hypertension from renal scarring is angiotensin-mediated, and angiotensin converting enzyme (ACE) inhibition or angiotensin receptor (AT-1) blockade are suitable therapeutic approaches. Since hypertension may go undetected for years in this age group, it may follow a malignant course and can be responsible for further renal parenchymal destruction, especially during pregnancy. Once renal scarring is detected, serial measurement of blood pressure and regular assessment of glomerular filtration rate must be performed. When scarring is bilateral and serum creatinine concentration is elevated above normal, consideration should be given to initiating treatment to reduce angiotensin effects, glomerular hyperfiltration, and deterioration of renal function even if blood pressure is normal, in keeping with JNC VI guidelines (<135/80 mm Hg).

PREVENTING RENAL INJURY

Because renal injury is associated with acute pyelonephritis and because scarring occurs rarely in adults, prevention of renal damage must be directed at aggressive management of UTIs in children with or without associated VUR. Prompt treatment of acute pyelonephritis with an effective antibiotic can prevent renal scarring. Every clinician should understand that while most children with acute pyelonephritis will have fever, some, will not. Moreover, a urinalysis is not sufficient to confirm the presence of a UTI. A urine culture is required. Once a diagnosis of UTI is made in a child, with or without a urine culture, there is an obligation to follow through with a complete radiologic evaluation and plan of follow-up.

When patients with a UTI and VUR were treated medically for more than 30 years using a regimen that included daily antibiotic prophylaxis, further renal scarring was prevented. In another study, episodic treatment of UTI without prophylaxis was associated with renal scarring in more than 20% of patients. Therefore, prophylaxis should be considered as part of conservative treatment as long as VUR presists. The drugs recommended for antibiotic prophylaxis are trimethaprim-sulfa and nitrofurantoin. Equally important is establishing a normal pattern of micturition to empty the bladder regularly and completely. This will reduce the number of bacteria that gain transurethral access to the bladder, particularly in females.

Additional treatment may include surgical correction of VUR, but well-designed, prospective studies comparing patients allocated randomly to surgery or medical management alone demonstrated no advantage of one over the other. Clinical guidelines for managing UTI in children have been established more recently by the American Academy of Pediatrics and for VUR by the American Urological Association.

Children with abnormal urodynamics or dysfunctional micturition not only have recurrent UTI, but also may generate high intravesical pressures which may lead to or worsen VUR, risking acute pyelonephritis. Surgical correction of the VUR in these patients is usually unsuccessful. These patients require special attention and management.

Bibliography

American Academy of Pediatrics: Practice parameter: The diagnosis, treatment, and evaluation of the initial urinary tract infection in febrile infants and young children. *Pediatrics* 103:843–852, 1999.

Arant BS, Jr: Vesicoureteric reflux and renal injury. *Am J Kidney Dis* 17:491–511, 1991.

Arant BS, Jr: Medical management of mild and moderate vesicoureteral reflux: Follow-up studies of infants and young children. A preliminary report of the Southwest Pediatric Nephrology Study Group. *J Urol* 148:1683–1687, 1992.

Arar MY, Arant BS, Jr, Hogg RJ, *et al.:* Etiology of sustained hypertension in children in the Southwestern United States. *Pediatr Nephrol* 8:186–189, 1994.

Benador D, Benador N, Slosman D, *et al.:* Are younger children at highest risk of renal sequelae after pyelonephritis? *Lancet* 149:17–19, 1997.

Bernstein J, Arant BS, Jr: Morphologic characteristics of segmental renal scarring in vesicoureteral reflux. *J Urol* 148:1712–1714, 1992.

Elder JS, Peters C, Arant BS, Jr *et al.:* Pediatric vesicoureteral reflux guidelines panel summary report on the management of primary vesicoureteral reflux in children. *J Urol* 157:1846–1851, 1997.

Jacobson SH, Eklof O, Eriksson CG, *et al.:* Development of uraemia and hypertension after pyelonephritis in childhood—27 year follow-up. *Br Med J* 299:703–706, 1989.

Jodal U: The natural history of bacteriuria in childhood. *Infect Dis Clin North Am* 1:713–729, 1987.

Marild S, Jodal U: Incidence rate of first-time symptomatic urinary tract infection in children under 6 years of age. *Acta Paediatr* 87:549–552, 1998.

Martinell J, Jodal U, Lidin-Janson G: Pregnancies in women with and without renal scarring after urinary infections in childhood. *Br Med J.* 300:840–844, 1990.

Noe HN: The long-term results of prospective sibling reflux screening. *J Urol* 148:1739–1742, 1992.

Rushton HG, Majd M, Jantausch B, *et al.:* Renal scarring following reflux and nonreflux pyelonephritis in children. Evaluation with 99m-technetium dimercaptosuccinic acid scintigraphy. *J Urol* 147:1327–1332, 1992.

Wennerstrom M, Hansson S, Jodal U, *et al.:* primary and acquired renal scarring in boys and girls with urinary tract infection. *J Pediatr* 136:30–34, 2000.

53

NEPHROLITHIASIS

ALAN G. WASSERSTEIN

Nephrolithiasis has an annual incidence of 7 to 12 cases per 10,000 persons and lifetime prevalence in White men of about 10% in the United States. The predominant age of onset is the third to sixth decade. Men are affected about three times as often as women.

The most common clinical consequence of nephrolithiasis is stone passage with acute renal colic. Flank pain radiating to the groin, abrupt in onset and extreme in severity, is typical. Gross or microscopic hematuria, dysuria or frequency, and nausea, vomiting, and occasionally ileus can accompany stone passage. Renal failure can be caused by

nephrocalcinosis (primary hyperparathyroidism, renal tubular acidosis) or staghorn formation (struvite, cystine); but in idiopathic calcium nephrolithiasis, it occurs only in the unusual event of bilateral urinary obstruction or obstruction in a solitary kidney. Noncontrast spiral computed tomography (CT) is probably superior to intravenous urography (IVU) in the evaluation of renal colic. Advantages of CT include higher sensitivity for nonobstructing calculi [98–100% versus 64% for intravenous pyelogram (IVP)], rapidity, avoidance of intravenous contrast, and diagnosis of pathology outside the urinary tract. IVU is equally good in detecting obstructing stones and is sometimes required to distinguish distal ureteral stones from phleboliths. For follow up of radio-opaque stones plain abdominal film is usually adequate (though far less sensitive than CT), while follow up of radiolucent (usually uric acid) stones is conveniently done with ultrasound.

Classification and characteristics of renal calculi are given in Table 1. Idiopathic calcium stones are usually comprised of calcium oxalate and calcium phosphate or pure calcium oxalate. Predominant calcium phosphate stones usually occur with alkaline urine and often have specific causes such as primary hyperparathyroidism, renal tubular acidosis, or alkali therapy.

Stone disease tends to recur. After a first calcium stone, 40% of untreated patients have another stone within 5 years, and an additional 40% of individuals will have another stone within the next 25 years.

PATHOGENESIS

Stone formation can be attributed to increased urinary concentration of crystalloids, decreased inhibitors, or increased promoter substances (Table 2). Stone formation begins with nucleation, the association of small amounts of crystalloid to form submicroscopic particles. Nucleation requires urinary saturation and generally occurs on surfaces (heterogeneous nucleation) such as papillary epithelium, renal tubular epithelial cells, or cellular debris. Submicroscopic particles ordinarily wash out in the urine; but if they either are attached to epithelial surfaces or associate rapidly to form larger particles they become too large to wash away (aggregation). Stone growth occurs by aggregation or by crystal growth, the orderly movement of ions out of solution onto growing crystal. A growing body of evidence suggests that stone formation is not only a physicochemical event but also depends crucially on cell-mediated events, possibly beginning with oxalate-induced epithelial cell damage.

Urinary supersaturation with respect to calcium oxalate is found in more than half of the general population. Since stone formation occurs in only a minority, the role of inhibitors must be crucial. Such inhibitors include citrate and magnesium, which form soluble complexes with calcium and oxalate, respectively. These complexes do not participate in nucleation. Macromolecules such as nephrocalcin (an inhibitor of crystal growth) or Tamm–Horsfall protein (an inhibitor of aggregation) may be defective in stone formers, but the clinical significance of these abnormalities has not yet been defined.

Not all stone disease can be attributed to metabolic risk factors. Several conditions predispose to stone formation because of anatomical derangements, including polycystic kidney disease, horseshoe kidney, and medullary sponge kidney. Medullary sponge kidney (MSK) is a congenital disorder occurring predominantly in women (6–25% of female stone formers). Collecting ducts undergo cystic dilatation, predisposing to stagnant fluid flow and, therefore, to calcium stones and recurrent urinary tract infection (but not to renal insufficiency). Many cases are discovered incidentally with intravenous urography, which demonstrates the characteristic papillary striation or brush effect. Medullary nephrocalcinosis may be extensive. Primary hyperparathyroidism and distal renal tubular acidosis may be associated with MSK.

METABOLIC EVALUATION OF NEPHROLITHIASIS

Two kinds of stone activity are distinguished: anatomic activity, the movement of an existing stone (usually into the pelvis or ureter) where it may cause symptoms; and metabolic activity, the formation of a new stone, growth of an existing stone, or formation and passage of multiple tiny stone fragments ("gravel"). As in the evaluation of a pulmonary nodule by comparison with prior radiographs, serial imaging is needed to determine metabolic activity. Figure 3 in Chapter 6 shows an anatomically active stone. It is important that urine be strained to recover stones for analysis during stone passage; the discovery of uric acid, struvite, pure calcium phosphate, or cystine on stone analysis can transform the diagnostic and therapeutic approach. A first calcium stone requires limited evaluation beyond stone analysis: urinalysis, serum calcium, phosphate, uric acid, creatinine, and blood urea nitrogen. Recurrent stone formers should have, in addition, 24-hr urine collections for measurement of calcium, phosphate, oxalate, citrate, uric acid, creatinine, volume, pH, urea nitrogen, and sodium, preferably on several occasions and with the patient following his or her usual diet. The metabolic evaluation and treatment of calcium and uric acid stones are summarized in Table 3. Prospective controlled trials demonstrate the utility of thiazide diuretics or potassium citrate for idiopathic calcium stones regardless of the metabolic profile. One might therefore question the usefulness of detailed metabolic evaluation, but clinicians generally prefer thiazides for hypercalciuria or osteopenia and potassium citrate for hypocitraturia.

TABLE I
Classification and Characteristics of Renal Calculi

Type	Frequency (%)	Sex	Crystals	Radiography
Calcium oxalate	75	M	Envelope	Round, radiodense
Uric acid	10–15	M = F	Diamond	Round or staghorn, radiolucent
Struvite	15–20	F	Coffin-lid	Staghorn, radiodense
Cystine	1	M = F	Hexagon	Staghorn, intermediate

TABLE 2
Urinary Risk Factors for Calcium Nephrolithiasis

Crystalloid concentration
  Hypercalciuria
  Hyperoxaluria
  Low urine volume
Promoters
  Hyperuricosuria
  Alkaline pH
Inhibitor deficiency
  Hypocitraturia
  Hypomagnesuria
  Macromolecules

RISK FACTORS FOR CALCIUM NEPHROLITHIASIS

Calcium oxalate stones are the consequence of a variety of urinary abnormalities, including low urinary volume, hypercalciuria, hyperoxaluria, hypocitraturia, and hyperuricosuria; often more than one is present in an individual case.

Low Urinary Volume

Individuals with newly diagnosed urinary calculi have significantly lower urine volumes (and therefore fluid intakes) than nonstone formers. Saturation of urine with relevant crystalloids falls as water is added to urine, whether *in vitro* or by increased oral intake. The universal advice given to stone formers to increase their fluid intake may account for the so-called stone clinic effect, the observation that that metabolic activity of nephrolithiasis diminishes during treatment regardless of any other specific advice or treatment. The benefit of increased fluid intake has been proven in a prospective controlled trial. Stone formers should strive to excrete at least 2 L of urine daily. Epidemiological evidence suggests that moderate alcohol intake may reduce stone risk by 40%, whereas apple and grapefruit juice increase risk; coffee and tea may reduce risk modestly, presumably because caffeine has some diuretic effect.

Hypercalciuria

Hypercalciuria is defined as daily urinary calcium excretion of more than 300 mg in men or 250 mg in women or 4 mg/kg in either sex. The distribution of calcium excretion in the general population is not normal, and 10% of the stone-free general population has a calcium excretion above these limits. Because hypercalciuria, like hypertension, is a graded risk factor for stone formation, desirable calcium excretion (to limit stone formation) may be lower than the so-called normal range.

Hypercalciuria, usually idiopathic, is present in about 50% of calcium stone formers. A small proportion (5%) has primary hyperparathyroidism. Renal tubular acidosis,

TABLE 3
Metabolic Evaluation and Treatment of Nephrolithiasis

Abnormality	Evaluation	Treatment
Calcium stones	Measure serum and urine calcium, urine oxalate, citrate, uric acid, magnesium, creatinine, and volume on self-selected diet	
Hypercalciuria	Urine sodium and urea nitrogen PTH[a] and ionized serum calcium 1,25-Dihydroxyvitamin D DEXA scan for bone density	Dietary salt and protein restriction, thiazides, potassium citrate, potassium magnesium citrate neutral phosphate
Hypercalcemia	PTH and ionized serum calcium	Parathyroidectomy
Hyperoxaluria	Assess dietary oxalate and calcium, vitamin C, artificial sweetener (xylitol), ileal disease or bypass	Dietary oxalate restriction, magnesium supplements, pyridoxine, calcium supplements (enteric hyperoxaluria) (thiazides or potassium citrate)
Hypocitraturia	Urine pH after acid load (severe hypocitraturia) Serum K, creatinine, urine culture	Potassium citrate
Hyperuricosuria	Assess dietary purine intake	Dietary purine restriction, allopurinol
Low urine volume	Measure 24-hr urine volume	Scheduled fluid intake 16 oz. q 4 hr while awake
Uric acid stones	Measure urinary uric acid and urine pH	Potassium citrate and/or allopurinol

[a]PTH, parathyroid hormone.

sarcoidosis, and various familial hypercalciuric syndromes are rare causes of hypercalciuria. Primary hyperparathyroidism predominantly affects middle-aged and older women; their hypercalciuria is due to excess renal production of 1,25-dihydroxyvitamin D under the influence of parathyroid hormone (PTH). The degree of hypercalcemia is usually mild to moderate. Some of the so-called "normocalcemic" cases of hyperparathyroidism are due to an inappropriately defined normal range of values for serum calcium. The true upper limit of normal serum calcium in women (10.1 mg/dL) is lower than that in men. Moreover, some patients with normal total serum calcium may have elevations of the ionized fraction. In general, the diagnosis of primary hyperparathyroidism is unlikely in the absence of hypercalcemia or high normal serum calcium. On the other hand, stone formers with hypercalcemia are overwhelmingly likely to have primary hyperparathyroidism. Presence of nephrocalcinosis and stone composition exclusively of calcium phosphate should also heighten the suspicion of primary hyperparathyroidism. Parathyroid exploration is indicated in all stone formers with primary hyperparathyroidism, regardless of the level of the serum calcium.

Three inherited hypercalciuric syndromes—Dent's disease, X-linked recessive hypercalciuria, and X-linked hypophosphatemic rickets—have more recently been linked to a common molecular defect, loss of the chloride tranporter CLC-5 in the renal tubule. These disorders share the features of nephrolithiasis, hypercalciuria and low molecular weight proteinuria, but differ in other features such as renal failure, nephrocalcinosis, and rickets. The mechanism by which a defect in chloride transport produces these abnormalities remains to be elucidated.

Idiopathic hypercalciuria (IH) is predominantly a disease of men in the fourth and fifth decade of life. It is associated with obesity, hypertension, and possibly affluence, and it is familial. IH offers a tantalizing array of features that at present defies a unifying explanation. Intestinal calcium absorption is increased out of proportion to the high normal or slightly elevated circulating 1,25-dihydroxyvitamin D that is often observed. Parathyroid hormone is usually low and suppressed by the relatively high serum calcium that results from intestinal calcium hyperabsorption and increased bone resorption. The precise cause of intestinal calcium hyperabsorption is uncertain; increased intestinal vitamin D receptors have been found in the genetic hypercalciuric rat model but not in patients. Evidence of increased bone resorption includes fasting hypercalciuria, negative calcium balance on low calcium diets, and low bone density, including osteoporosis in some cases. The increased bone resorption is apparently mediated by cytokines, including interleukin 1 (IL-1), IL-6, and tumor necrosis factor. A longstanding low dietary calcium intake ingested by individuals in an effort to prevent stones may also contribute to the low bone density. Categorizing hypercalciuria into absorptive and fasting types tends to be a fruitless task as bone density is equally low in both groups. Dietary calcium restriction risks low bone density regardless of category, and treatment with effective drugs such as thiazides or potassium citrate does not depend on such categorization.

Several dietary factors exacerbate idiopathic hypercalciuria. The most important of these is dietary sodium intake, which increases renal calcium excretion. The mechanism is reduction of proximal tubular sodium reabsorption, which in turn reduces reabsorption of solutes that are reabsorbed in parallel with sodium, such as calcium. Another dietary factor is protein intake, which can be assessed by measuring urine urea nitrogen. Dietary animal protein exacerbates calciuria because an acid load inhibits renal tubular calcium reabsorption, and because protein feeding stimulates calciuric factors such as insulin, glucagon, and prostaglandins. Animal protein intake has been convincingly associated with nephrolithiasis in epidemiological studies, but dietary protein restriction has not been proven to ameliorate stone formation in prospective trials. A third factor is dietary calcium. In normal persons, only 6% of dietary calcium appears in the urine; hypercalciuria from dietary calcium excess or calcium supplements alone is therefore unusual. In patients with idiopathic hypercalciuria, the proportion of ingested calcium that is absorbed in the intestine is higher. However, intestinal oxalate absorption in such patients rises disproportionately during dietary calcium restriction. Because urinary oxalate may be at least as important as urinary calcium in the genesis of nephrolithiasis, dietary calcium restriction may be deleterious even in patients with hypercalciuria. In a large prospective study of patients without nephrolithiasis, the risk of developing kidney stones was inversely related to dietary calcium intake. Regardless of the presence of hypercalciuria, patients with nephrolithiasis should be counseled to maintain at least a moderate calcium intake (two to three servings of dairy products or other high calcium foods daily) because of the twin risks of increased urinary oxalate and loss of bone mineral. An even higher level of dietary calcium may be desirable, but optimum calcium intake in calcium stone-formers has not been defined. Refined carbohydrates are also calciuric, and high dietary fiber is anticalciuric. Dietary measures should be tried before drug therapy in the treatment of idiopathic hypercalciuria. The goal is moderate sodium (100 to 125 mEq), moderate protein (60 to 70 g/day), moderate calcium (two dairy servings daily), high fiber, and low refined carbohydrate intakes.

If metabolic activity of nephrolithiasis persists despite high fluid intake and dietary modification, drug treatment is indicated. Thiazides work by two mechanisms: first, by causing extracellular fluid (ECF) volume depletion and thereby increasing proximal tubular calcium absorption; second, by stimulating calcium reabsorption directly in the early distal convoluted tubule. A low-salt diet helps maintain ECF volume contraction. Prospective, controlled trials have confirmed the efficacy of thiazides in reducing stone formation both in hypercalciuric and normocalciuric patients. Thiazides are particularly preferred in patients with low bone density, which can be ameliorated by their long-term use. I recommend measurement of bone density in patients with hypercalciuria, who are at increased risk of osteoporosis. In the genetic hypercalciuric rat (a model of IH) on low calcium diet, alendronate, an inhibitor of bone resorption, reduces urine calcium excretion. This effect, which supports an important role of bone resorption in pathogenesis of IH, has not yet been reported in patients with IH; nevertheless, bisphosphonates or other inhibitors of bone resorption are potentially of benefit to patients with IH and osteoporosis.

Potassium citrate and potassium magnesium citrate have also been proved effective in nephrolithiasis in controlled trials regardless of the level of calciuria. Unlike sodium citrate, potassium citrate may reduce calciuria slightly, but its main benefit is increasing urine excretion of the stone formation inhibitor citrate. Thiazides tend to reduce urine citrate excretion by causing potassium depletion; potassium citrate is the potassium supplement of choice in patients with nephrolithiasis. Adding amiloride to thiazide is another means of preventing hypokalemia, and amiloride has an independent hypocalciuric effect. Triamterene should be avoided, as it has been found in stones on analysis.

Another treatment that inhibits calciuria and stone formation is neutral orthophosphate. It works at bone, intestinal, and renal sites to inhibit calciuria and stone formation. Because it inhibits production of 1,25-dihydroxyvitamin D, orthophosphate should be especially effective in patients with elevated levels of this hormone. A potassium preparation of neutral or alkaline pH is preferred, since both acid and sodium increase calciuria. A sustained release potassium phosphate preparation has been developed. Orthophosphate can cause diarrhea, and it is contraindicated in renal insufficiency and infection stones. Compared to thiazides, orthophosphate it has fewer metabolic side effects, but it has not yet been proven efficacious in a controlled prospective study. Cellulose phosphate is a nonabsorbable form of phosphate that binds calcium in the gut. Its use should be avoided, as it increases urine oxalate excretion and risks bone mineral loss.

Hyperoxaluria

Oxalate is an end product of metabolism that forms a poorly soluble complex with calcium. Normal oxalate excretion is 15 to 40 mg daily; most is derived from endogenous synthesis. Physicochemical considerations suggest that a small increment in urinary oxalate has a larger effect on calcium oxalate saturation than a relatively greater increase in urinary calcium; however, in several studies, the oxalate excretion of stone formers was not greater than that of control individuals. Hyperoxaluria may be caused by increased synthesis or enhanced intestinal absorption. Increased synthesis can be due to congenital enzyme deficiencies (primary hyperoxaluria types I and II), which in some cases produce extreme elevations of urinary oxalate, dense nephrocalcinosis, and renal failure in early adulthood (see Chapter 49). These enzyme deficiencies may also cause urinary calculi at any stage of life. High vitamin C intake (2 g daily) in susceptible persons can also increase oxalate production, as can pyridoxine deficiency. Increased intestinal absorption can be due to high oxalate diet, malabsorption (enteric hyperoxaluria), or calcium restriction (or cellulose phosphate) therapy prescribed for patients with idiopathic hypercalciuria. Patients with Crohn's disease and individuals who have undergone ileal surgery are at highest risk for entric hyperoxaluria; of note, an intact colon is required. Three mechanisms have been proposed: (1) intestinal calcium is bound in soaps and unavailable for calcium oxalate complex formation, so free oxalate is hyperabsorbed in the colon; (2) poorly absorbed bile salts stimulate increased colonic transport of oxalate; and (3) poorly absorbed bile salts inactivate an oxalate-metabolizing bacterium (*Oxalobacter formigenes*) and thereby promote oxalate absorption. Dietary calcium restriction in patients with idiopathic hypercalciuria presumably enhances oxaluria by a similar mechanism, reducing luminal calcium and calcium-oxalate complexation and thereby increasing free oxalate absorption. Specific treatment of hyperoxaluria includes dietary oxalate restriction (tea, citrus juices, colas, spinach, rhubarb, peanuts, and chocolate should be omitted); provision of adequate dietary calcium; magnesium supplements; and pyridoxine in the uncommon cases of oxalate overproduction. Enteric oxaluria is treated with calcium supplements, which also bind intestinal oxalate; urinary calcium excretion is low in these cases, and hypercalciuria is not a concern. Specific treatment of hyperoxaluria is often unsuccessful, and patients with calcium stones and hyperoxaluria may do best with the nonspecific but proven therapy of thiazide and/or potassium citrate.

Hypocitraturia

Normal citrate excretion is 300 to 900 mg daily. Citrate acts as an inhibitor of nucleation by forming soluble complexes with calcium. Urinary citrate is higher in premenopausal women than in men. It is also higher in pregnancy. This is teleologically a useful response, as pregnancy is associated with increased urinary calcium excretion. Idiopathic hypocitraturia is found in 10 to 40% of stone formers. Hypocitraturia also may be due to any cause of intracellular acidosis, including potassium deficiency, renal failure, distal (type I) renal tubular acidosis (RTA), chronic diarrheal states and malabsorption, or acetazolamide therapy. In urinary tract infection, bacteria may metabolize citrate and reduce its urinary excretion.

Distal RTA causes a profound reduction in urinary citrate excretion, usually to less than 50 mg daily; it also causes hypercalciuria and persistently alkaline urine, but hypocitraturia is the most important contributor to the stone diathesis. Measurement of urinary citrate is a useful alternative to acid loading to establish the diagnosis of distal RTA. Nephrocalcinosis and renal failure may occur. The alkali requirement to correct hypocitraturia (4 mEq/kg/day or more) may be higher than that required to correct systemic acidosis or hypokalemia (1 to 2 mEq/kg/day); correction of hypocitraturia may a more relevant guide to alkali dosage in these patients. Potassium citrate is the treatment of choice for idiopathic hypocitraturia and distal RTA. Sodium citrate or bicarbonate are less desirable, as their sodium content tents to increase calciuria.

Uric Acid

Hyperuricosuria, usually due to high dietary purine consumption, is a risk factor for calcium stone formation, probably because uric acid acts as a surface for heterogeneous nucleation. Allopurinol reduces calcium stone formation in patients with isolated hyperuricosuria.

OTHER TYPES OF NEPHROLITHIASIS

Uric acid stones occur in two circumstances: excessive urinary uric acid and persistently acid urine. Only 20% of patients with uric acid stones have hyperuricosuria. Hyperuricosuria is due, with rare exceptions, to dietary purine overconsumption. Persistently acid urine, due to deficient renal ammoniagenesis, is a feature of gout, idiopathic uric acid stones, and chronic diarrheal disease, because of loss of alkali equivalent in the stool. Uric acid is 10 to 20 times more soluble at pH 7 than at pH 5. Hence urine alkalinization is an effective treatment for most patients with uric acid stones; indeed it is more effective than allopurinol, which generally reduces uric acid excretion by about half. The target urine pH is 6.0 to 7.0. It should be monitored by the patient with nitrazine paper; higher urine pH should be avoided because of the risk of promotion of calcium phosphate stones. Allopurinol can be added if uric acid production is excessive (over 1000 mg daily) and if dietary purine restriction is unsuccessful. Unlike calcium stones, uric acid stones may dissolve during medical therapy (if they are not secondarily calcified).

Infection stones are the most severe form of nephrolithiasis. They can cause progressive renal failure, urosepsis or perinephric abscess, intractable urinary tract infection, pain, and bleeding. Infection stones consist of struvite (magnesium ammonium phosphate) and apatite (calcium phosphate). They form only during urinary infection with urease-positive bacteria, usually *Proteus* or *Providencia* species, and almost never with *Escherichia coli*. These bacteria cleave urea to ammonia, elevating the urine pH to 8 or more and favoring precipitation of struvite and apatite. Bacterial infection in stone interstices is difficult to clear. Approximately 40% of patients with struvite stones have an underlying metabolic abnormality that predisposes to nephrolithiasis, which in turn predisposes to recurrent urinary tract infection. In contrast, patients with primary struvite stone formation and no other abnormality often have large staghorn calculi and usually have never passed stones.

Treatment consists first of antibiotics, usually penicillin or ampicillin. Sterile urine is achieved in only about 20% of patients. Because of the large stone burden, stone removal usually requires combined percutaneous and extracorporeal lithotripsy. If stone removal is complete, a cure may be possible. If not, the residual fragments serve as a nidus for intractable infection and recurrent stone formation, and antibiotic suppression is sometimes required indefinitely. The urease inhibitor acetohydroxamic acid can help to prevent stone formation if urinary tract infection persists.

Cystine stones result from an unusual inherited disorder in which renal tubular reabsorption of cystine, ornithine, arginine, and lysine (COAL) is reduced. Cystine is the disulfide reduction product of cysteine. The solubility of cystine is 250 mg/L. In patients with moderate levels of cystinuria, a high urine volume (4 L/day) will be sufficient to reduce the concentration of cystine below this threshold. It is particularly important to continue high fluid intake throughout the night, as there is disproportionate cystine excretion at that time. Those with more severe cystinuria require pharmacotherapy. Penicillamine or tiopronin react with cystine to form a soluble mixed cysteine disulfide; they also reduce total cystine production.

UROLOGICAL MANAGEMENT OF STONES

Most symptomatic renal calculi (90%) pass spontaneously. The probability of spontaneous passage depends on the width, length, and location of the stone. Ureteral stones 4 mm or less in width are likely (more than 70%) to pass within 1 year; stones 8 mm or more in width are unlikely (less than 10%) to pass. Stones that come to clinical attention in the lower ureter are twice as likely to pass as upper ureteral stones. Stones that are judged to be likely to pass and that are not associated with pain or obstruction may be managed expectantly for as long as 1 year. Indications for urological intervention for ureteral stones include obstruction, pain, fever, and observed or anticipated failure of spontaneous passage. On the basis of incomplete animal data, it is believed that complete obstruction requires relief within 2 weeks and partial obstruction within 4 to 6 weeks (depending on the severity of hydronephrosis) to avoid permanent renal injury. Fever requires emergency decompression of the obstructed urinary tract with a retrograde stent or percutaneous nephrostomy; definitive stone removal is deferred until infection resolves. Stones in the renal pelvis or upper ureter are treated with extracorporeal shock wave lithotripsy (ESWL); stents are placed in cases where large stone burden increases the risk of obstruction by pulverized material (*Steinstrasse*) after ESWL. Lower ureteral stones can also be treated with ESWL but the rate of success is only 70 to 80%; ureteroscopy with basket retrieval or ultrasonic or laser lithotripsy (for impacted stones) is successful in 98 to 99% of cases. Recommendations for use of the ESWL for asymptomatic intrarenal calculi vary. With calyceal stones, we reserve ESWL for the classic indications of pain, obstruction, or bleeding. However, a stone of 5 mm or more in the renal pelvis generally should have ESWL to prevent obstruction. Use of ESWL requires that the distal urinary tract be free of obstruction so that fragmented material can pass; ESWL is contraindicated in obstruction, pregnancy, and in patients with an aortic or renal artery aneurysm. In pregnancy, an obstructing stone can be managed with a retrograde stent until after delivery, when ESWL can safely be performed. The success of ESWL begins to diminish as stones exceed 1 cm in size and is poor with stones above 2 cm. In these cases, percutaneous lithotripsy may be combined with

ESWL. Cystine stones are relatively refractory to ESWL, and percutaneous techniques may be necessary. ESWL and percutaneous techniques have dramatically reduced the need for open surgical treatment of nephrolithiasis, which now accounts for less than 5% of urological interventions. Complications of ESWL and percutaneous lithotripsy include transient loss of renal function, bleeding, hematoma, and urosepsis. Early studies suggesting that delayed hypertension may occur as a surgical of ESWL have not been confirmed in more recent trials.

Bibliography

Barcelo P, Wuhl O, Servitge E, *et al.:* Randomized double-blind study of potassium citrate in idiopathic hypocitraturic calcium nephrolithiasis. *J Urol* 150:1761–1764, 1993.

Bataille P, Achard JM, Fournier A, *et al.:* Diet, vitamin D and vertebral mineral density in hypercalciuric stone formers. *Kidney Int* 39:1193–1205, 1991.

Borghi L, Meschi T, Amato F, *et al.:* Urinary volume, water and recurrences in idiopathic calcium nephrolithiasis: A 5-year randomized prospective study. *J Urol* 155:839–843, 1996.

Coe FL, Parks JH, Asplin JR: Pathogenesis and treatment of kidney stones. *N Engl J Med* 327:1141–1152, 1992.

Curhan GC, Willett WC, Rimm E, *et al.:* A prospective study of dietary calcium and other nutrients and the risk of symptomatic kidney stones. *N Engl J Med* 328:833–838, 1993.

Ettinger B, Citron JY, Livermore B, *et al.:* Chlorthalidone reduces calcium oxalate calculus recurrence but magnesium oxide does not. *J Urol* 139:679–684, 1998.

Hosking DH, Erickson SB, van den Berg CJ, *et al.:* The stone clinic effect in patients with idiopathic calcium urolithiasis. *J Urol* 130:1115–1158, 1983.

Lemann J: Composition of the diet and calcium kidney stones. *N Engl J Med* 328:880–882, 1993

Lerner SP, Malachy JG, Griffith DP: Infection stones. *J Urol* 141:753–758, 1989.

Lloyd SE, Pearce SHS, Fisher SE, *et al.:* A common molecular basis for three inherited kidney stone diseases. *Nature* 379:445–449, 1996.

Pahira JJ: Management of the patient with cystinuria. *Urol Clin North Am* 14:339–346, 1987.

Uribarri J, Oh MS, Carroll HJ: The first kidney stone. *Ann Intern Med* 111:1006–1009, 1989.

54

URINARY TRACT INFECTION

LINDSAY E. NICOLLE

Urinary infection is the presence of microbial pathogens within the normally sterile urinary tract. Infections are overwhelmingly bacterial, although fungi, viruses, and parasites may occasionally also be pathogens (Table 1). Urinary infection is the most common bacterial infection in humans, and may be either symptomatic or asymptomatic. Symptomatic infection is associated with a wide spectrum of morbidity, from mild irritative voiding symptoms to bacteremia, sepsis, and occasionally death. Asymptomatic urinary infection is isolation of bacteria from urine in quantitative counts consistent with infection, but without localizing genitourinary signs or symptoms, and with no systemic symptoms attributable to the infection.

The term bacteriuria simply means bacteria present in the urine, although it is generally used to imply isolation of a significant quantitative count of organisms. This term is often used interchangeably with asymptomatic urinary infection. Recurrent urinary infection is frequent and may be either relapse, which is recurrence post-therapy with the pretherapy isolate, or reinfection, recurrence with a different organism. An important aspect in the management of urinary infection is whether it occurs in a normal (uncomplicated urinary infection or acute nonobstructive pyelonephritis) or abnormal (complicated urinary infection) genitourinary tract.

A microbiologic diagnosis of urinary infection requires isolation of a pathogenic organism in sufficient quantitative amounts from an appropriately collected urine specimen. A quantitative count of $\geq 10^5$ cfu/mL of bacteria is the usual standard to discriminate infection from organisms present as contaminants. The use of the quantitative urine specimen has been important in the identification of urinary infection and description of the natural history, but this quantitative standard is not always appropriate.

Primer on Kidney Diseases, Third Edition

TABLE I
Nonbacterial Pathogens Causing Urinary Tract Infection

Fungi	Viruses	Parasites
Candida albicans	JC, BK viruses	Schistosoma hematobium
Candida parapsolosis	Adenovirus types 11,21	
Candida glabrata	Mumps	
Candida tropicalis	Hantavirus[a]	
Blastomyces dermatitidis[b]		
Aspergillus fumigatus[b]		
Cryptococcus neoformans[b]		
Histoplasma capsulatum[b]		

[a] Hemmorhagic fever and renal syndrome.
[b] With disseminated infection.

ACUTE UNCOMPLICATED URINARY INFECTION

Acute uncomplicated urinary infection, or acute cystitis, is infection occurring in individuals with a normal genitourinary tract and no prior instrumentation. It is a common syndrome, and occurs virtually entirely in women. As many as 35% of young, sexually active women will experience at least one urinary infection, and 1–2% will have frequent recurrent infection. The frequency increases with both genetic and behavioral factors. First degree female relatives of women with recurrent acute uncomplicated urinary infection also have an increased frequency of urinary infection, and women who are nonsecretors of blood group substances are more likely to have urinary infection. Sexual intercourse is strongly associated with infection, and the frequency of infection increases with frequency of intercourse. The use of spermicides or a diaphragm for birth control both increase the frequency of infection, but use of the birth control pill or condoms without spermicide do not alter the occurrence of infection. Women with recurrent acute cystitis also have an increased frequency of asymptomatic urinary infection.

Escherichia coli is the most common infecting organism, and occurs in 80–85% of episodes. *Staphylococcus saprophyticus,* a coagulase negative staphylococcus, is isolated from 5 to 10% of episodes. This organism is seldom identified as a pathogen outside the urinary tract and is isolated infrequently from individuals with complicated urinary infection. It has a seasonal predilection with increased occurrence in the late summer and early fall. *Klebsiella pneumoniae* and *Proteus mirabilis* are each isolated in 3–5% of cases. All these organisms originate from the normal gut flora, colonize the vagina and periurethral area, and ascend to the bladder. With selected organism virulence factors, an inflammatory response and symptomatic urinary infection will occur. The vaginal flora in women who experience this syndrome is altered from the normal acidic pH with lacto-bacillus predominant to neutral pH and increased colonization with *Escherichia coli.*

The clinical presentation, diagnosis, and recommended treatment for acute uncomplicated urinary infection is summarized in Table 2. A quantitative count of $\geq 10^5$ cfu/mL is no longer considered a diagnostic microbiologic standard for this syndrome, as 30–50% of women have lower quantitative counts isolated. Any quantitative count of a potential uropathogen with pyuria is considered sufficient for diagnosis in the presence of consistent clinical symptoms. As the bacteriology is predictable and quantitative microbiology is not definitive, it is generally recommended that urine culture not be obtained routinely, and empiric antimicrobial therapy be given. A urine specimen for culture prior to antimicrobial treatment is recommended, however, if there is uncertainty about the diagnosis or early recurrence following therapy. The differential diagnosis includes urethritis due to sexually transmitted diseases such as *Neisseria gonorrhea* or *Chlamydia trachomatis,* yeast vulvovaginitis, or herpes genitalis.

Antimicrobial therapy is selected based on patient tolerance, documented efficacy for treating urinary infection, and local prevalence of resistance of community-acquired *E. coli.* Fosfomycin trometemol and pivmecillinam are antimicrobials with indications virtually limited to treatment of this syndrome, whereas nitrofurantoin is used for treatment of this and other presentations of urinary infection. A 3-day course of antimicrobial therapy is usually effective. A longer course of 7 days may be preferable for individuals treated with nitrofurantoin or a β-lactam antibiotic, for postmenopausal women, for women with symptoms longer than 7 days, or for women with an early recurrence of symptomatic infection (less than 30 days) following prior antimicrobial therapy.

Frequent recurrence of acute cystitis is a disruptive and distressing problem for many women. Antimicrobial prophylaxis, given either as a long-term low-dose regimen or postintercourse will prevent recurrent infection (Table 3). Continuous low-dose prophylaxis is recommended to be taken at bedtime and initially given for 6 to 12 months, but it remains efficacious even when continued as long as 2 to 5 years. Following discontinuation of prophylactic therapy, the frequency of urinary infection is similar to that observed prior to prophylaxis, and approximately 50% of women will have a recurrent infection within 3 months. Postintercourse prophylaxis is, obviously, most appropriate for women who identify sexual intercourse as a precipitating factor for their recurrent symptomatic episodes. An alternate approach preferred by some women is self-treatment. It has been rigorously evaluated only for single-dose trimethoprim/sulfamethoxazole therapy, but is a widely used strategy, and can be considered for compliant women who can reliably identify their symptomatic episodes and wish a role in self-management.

ACUTE NONOBSTRUCTIVE PYELONEPHRITIS

Acute nonobstructive pyelonephritis is symptomatic renal infection occurring in women with an otherwise nor-

TABLE 2
Diagnosis and Management of Common Symptomatic Syndromes of Urinary Infection

Clinical presentation	Microbiologic diagnosis	Treatment
Acute uncomplicated urinary infection Lower tract irritative symptoms; dysuria, frequency, urgency, suprapubic discomfort, hematuria	$\geq 10^3$ cfu/ml of uropathogen with pyuria	First line TMP/SMX[a] 160/800 mg bid Trimethoprim 100 mg bid Nitrofurantoin 50–100 mg qid Fosfomycin trometemol 3 g one dose Pivmecillinam 400 mg bid[b]
		Second line [c]Norfloxacin 400 mg bid [c]Ciprofloxacin 250 mg bid [c]Ofloxacin 400 mg bid [c]Levofloxacin 400 mg bid Amoxicillin/clavulanic acid 500 mg bid Cephalexin 500 mg qid Cefixime 400 mg od
Acute nonobstructive pyelonephritis Costovertebral angle pain and tenderness; +/− fever, +/− lower tract symptoms	$\geq 10^4$ cfu/ml	First line TMP/SMX[a] 160/800 mg bid Trimethoprim 100 mg bid [c]Norfloxacin 400 mg bid [c]Ciprofloxacin 250–500 mg bid [c]Ofloxacin 400 mg bid [d]Gentamicin 3–5 mg/kg/24 hr in one or two doses +/− ampicillin 1 g q 4–6 h
		Second line Amoxicillin/clavulanic acid 500 mg tid Cephalexin 500 mg qid [d]Cefotaxime 1 g tid [d]Ceftriaxone 1–2 g od
Complicated urinary infection Variable, including Asymptomatic Lower tract symptoms; pyelonephritis Systemic symptoms (fever, shock)	$\geq 10^5$ cfu/ml	TMP/SMX[a] 160/800 mg bid [c]Norfloxacin 400 mg bid [c]Ciprofloxacin 250–500 mg bid [c]Ofloxacin 400 mg bid [c]Levofloxacin 400 mg bid Amoxicillin/clavulanic acid 500 mg tid Cephalexin 500 mg tid [d]Gentamicin 3–5 mg/kg/24 in one or two doses +/− ampicillin 1g q 4–6 h or piperacillin 3 g q 4 h
		[d]Ceftazidime 1 g tid [d]Cefotaxime 1 g tid

[a]Trimethoprim/sulfamethoxazole.
[b]Not liscenced in United States.
[c]Quinolones are contraindicated in pregnancy and in children under the age of 16.
[d]Parenteral therapy.

mal genitourinary tract. Women who experience acute uncomplicated urinary infection are also at risk of nonobstructive pyelonephritis, with the frequency of episodes of cystitis relative to pyelonephritis reported to be 18 to 1. The bacteriology is similar to that of acute uncomplicated urinary infection, with *E. coli* isolated in about 85% of episodes. *Escherichia coli* strains are characterized by almost uniform expression of a virulence factor, the p fimbria. This surface antigen attaches to uroepithelial cells within the urinary tract and induces an inflammatory response. Additional organism virulence factors include hemolysin and aerobactin production. Bacteremia, which

occurs in about 10% of episodes, is more frequent in diabetic and elderly women.

Acute pyelonephritis presents classically with fever with costovertebral angle pain and tenderness. There may also be associated lower urinary tract symptoms. Fever may be low grade or, occasionally, absent. A urine specimen for culture and susceptibility testing should be obtained prior to the initiation of antimicrobial therapy from every woman with a suspected diagnosis of pyelonephritis. Growth of $\geq 10^4$ cfu/ml of a uropathogen with pyuria and consistent clinical findings is sufficient for diagnosis. The majority of women can be treated as outpatients with oral

TABLE 3

Prophylactic Antimicrobial Therapy for Women with Frequent
Recurrence of Acute Uncomplicated Urinary Infection

	Regimen	
Agent	**Long-term**	**Postcoital (one dose)**
Trimethoprim/ sulfamethoxazole[a]	80/400 mg daily or 3 × weekly	80/400 mg
Trimethoprim[a]	100 mg	100 mg
Nitrofurantoin[a]	50 mg	50–100 mg
Cephalexin	125 mg	250 mg
Norfloxacin	200 mg every other day	200–400 mg
Ciprofloxacin	—	250 mg

[a]Recommended first line agents.

TABLE 4

Abnormalities of the Genitourinary Tract Consistent
with Complicated Urinary Tract Infection

Metabolic	Medullary sponge kidney
	Nephrocalcinosis
	Malakoplakia
	Xanthogranulomatous pyelonephritis
	Diabetes mellitus
Congenital	Cystic disease
	Duplicated drainage system with obstruction
	Urethral valves
Obstruction	Vesicoureteral reflux
	Pelvicalyceal obstruction
	Papillary necrosis
	Uretheral fibrosis/stricture
	Bladder diverticulum
	Neurogenic bladder
	Prostatic hypertrophy
	Tumors
	Urolithiasis
Instrumentation	Indwelling catheter
	Intermittent catheterization
	Cystoscopy
	Ureteric stent
Other	Immunocompromised
	Postrenal transplant
	Neutropenic

antimicrobial therapy (Table 2). Hospitalization and initial parenteral antimicrobial therapy are recommended for women where oral medication may not be tolerated due to severe gastrointestinal symptoms, where there is hemodynamic instability, or when there is significant systemic signs of illness and concerns about compliance. Parenteral therapy can usually be replaced by oral therapy once clinical improvement has occurred, usually by 48 to 72 hours. The urine culture results are also available by this time and can direct selection of the oral antimicrobial.

If there has not been substantial clinical improvement by 48–72 hours of effective antimicrobial therapy, an abnormality within the genitourinary tract causing urinary obstruction or abscess formation should be excluded. Women with early symptomatic recurrence post-therapy should also be considered to have a potential complicating abnormality of the genitourinary tract. An initial ultrasound examination is helpful to exclude obstruction, although it may not identify small stones. Computed tomography with contrast may be better at delineating small stones or intrarenal abscess. The selection of imaging approaches should be individualized based on initial presentation, clinical course, and access to diagnostic testing.

COMPLICATED URINARY TRACT INFECTION

The most important physiologic host defense against urinary infection is intermittent unobstructed voiding of urine. Any abnormality of the genitourinary tract which impairs voiding may increase the frequency of urinary infection. Urinary infection in individuals with structural or functional abnormalities of the urinary tract, including those who have undergone instrumentation including indwelling urethral catheters, is considered "complicated urinary infection" (Table 4). The occurrence of infection is determined by the underlying abnormality, and is not influenced by gender or age. For some of these groups infection is infrequent, but difficult to manage, as with infected cysts with polycystic kidney disease. In others, such

as indwelling catheters where the infection rate is 5% per day, infection is frequent.

Complicated urinary infection is frequently asymptomatic. The clinical presentation in symptomatic infection presents along a spectrum from mild lower tract symptoms to systemic signs such as fever, and even septic shock. Individuals with complete obstruction or mucosal bleeding are at greatest risk of the most severe clinical presentations. The quantitative count of organisms in the urine of $\geq 10^5$ cfu/mL remains the standard for diagnosis of complicated urinary infection. Two consecutive cultures with the same organism(s) isolated are required for diagnosis of asymptomatic urinary infection. The microbiology of complicated urinary infection is characterized by a greater diversity of organisms and increased prevalence of antimicrobial resistance when compared to uncomplicated infection. Organisms less frequently express virulence factors, as the host abnormality of impaired voiding is sufficient for infection to develop. Increased antimicrobial resistance occurs because of nosocomial acquisition or repeated courses of antimicrobial therapy for recurrent infection. Where repeated broad-spectrum antimicrobial therapy has been given for prolonged periods, reinfection may occur with yeast species or highly resistant strains such as some *Pseudomonas aeruginosa*.

Asymptomatic infection, with or without pyuria, does not usually require treatment. Exceptions, where antimicrobial therapy is recommended, include prophylaxis prior to an invasive genitourinary procedure, suppressive therapy when struvite stones are present and cannot be removed, neutropenic patients, and patients with infection in the early postrenal transplant period. For symptomatic infection, the antimicrobial should be selected based on the known or suspected susceptibilities of the infecting organism. If possible, antimicrobial therapy should not be initiated until urine culture results are available. Patients with moderate to severe symptoms, however, may require empiric therapy. The patient's recent history of antimicrobial use and prior urine culture results are helpful in directing the choice of empiric therapy. Parenteral therapy may initially be required for ill patients with severe systemic manifestations, where oral therapy is not tolerated, or when the infecting organism is suspected or known to be resistant to any available oral therapy. Seven days of therapy is generally adequate when the clinical presentation is of lower tract symptoms. Where fever or other systemic symptoms are present, 10–14 days of therapy is recommended.

Complicated urinary infection is preventable if the underlying abnormality can be corrected. There is a high likelihood of recurrence when the underlying genitourinary abnormality cannot be corrected. For instance, in patients with neurogenic bladders emptied by intermittent catheterization, 50% will experience a recurrence of infection by 4–6 weeks following antimicrobial therapy. Prophylactic antimicrobials are not recommended, as long-term antimicrobial therapy has not been shown to decrease infections, and reinfection will be with organisms resistant to the antimicrobial given. In selected cases with severe symptomatic recurrences and an abnormality which cannot be corrected, long-term suppressive therapy may be considered. This therapy is individualized in every case, but usually initiated with full therapeutic antimicrobial doses, which may be subsequently decreased to one-half the regular dose if the urine culture remains negative and the clinical course is satisfactory.

SPECIAL POPULATIONS

Urinary Tract Infection in Children

Urinary infection occurs more frequently in boys than girls in the first year of life. Infection in boys is often within 3 months of birth, and may be associated with congenital anomalies of the urinary tract or lack of circumcision. The clinical presentation is usually that of neonatal sepsis without localizing signs to the genitourinary tract, and these episodes are treated as neonatal sepsis. Subsequent to the first year of life, urinary infection occurs more frequently in girls than boys, and the clinical presentation is of genitourinary symptoms. Most episodes in girls are acute uncomplicated urinary infection, and these girls will also experience urinary infection more frequently as adults. For girls with recurrent urinary infection, vesicoureteral reflux which may lead to impaired renal function must be excluded. Imaging studies including voiding cystourethrogram, ultrasound, and dimercaptosuccinic acid (DMSA) scan are indicated for any child presenting with pyelonephri-

tis, for a first urinary infection in a boy of any age or a girl less than 3 years, a second urinary infection in a girl over 3 years, and a first urinary infection at any age in a girl with a family history of urinary tract abnormalities, with abnormal voiding, hypertension, or poor growth. (See Chapter 52.)

The recommended duration of treatment of acute lower tract infection in young girls is 3–7 days. Pyelonephritis should be treated for 10–14 days. Generally, the antimicrobials used are similar to those in adults, with appropriate dose adjustments. The quinolones are not recommended for children under the age of 16 years because of potential adverse effects on cartilage. Long-term low-dose prophylactic therapy is indicated for young girls with vesicoureteral reflux and recurrent urinary infection or frequent symptomatic recurrence.

Asymptomatic urinary infection is common in schoolgirls. Treatment of asymptomatic urinary infection does not alter the natural history of renal disease in young girls and does not influence renal scarring. In fact, treatment of asymptomatic bacteriuria with antimicrobials appears to increase the frequency of symptomatic infection. Thus, it is not recommended to screen for or treat asymptomatic bacteriuria in girls.

Urinary Infection in Pregnancy

Hormonal changes in pregnancy produce hypotonicity of the autonomic musculature leading to urine stasis. In addition, obstruction at the pelvic brim, more marked on the right than left side, occurs with the enlarging fetus. These changes are maximal at the end of the second trimester and beginning of the third trimester, and explain the increased risk of pyelonephritis at this stage of gestation. Acute pyelonephritis may precipate premature labor and delivery, as may any febrile illness in later pregnancy. Women who have asymptomatic bacteriuria in early pregnancy have as much as a 30% risk of developing acute pyelonephritis later in pregnancy. About two-thirds of episodes of acute pyelonephritis in pregnancy are prevented by identification and treatment of asymptomatic bacteriuria early in pregnancy.

All pregnant women should have a urine specimen for culture at 12 to 16 weeks gestation. If significant bacteriuria is identified, the urine culture should be repeated. If the presence of infection is confirmed, it should be treated. The antimicrobial is selected on the basis of susceptibilities. A 3-day course of amoxicillin, nitrofurantoin, or cephalexin is usually sufficient. Trimethoprim-sulfamethoxazole has been widely used and is effective, but there remains some reluctance to use it in pregnancy because of theoretical concerns of adverse fetal effects. Quinolones are contraindicated. Women with either symptomatic or asymptomatic infection treated in early pregnancy should be followed with monthly urine cultures throughout the remainder of the pregnancy to identify recurrent infection. If a second episode occurs, it should be treated, and low-dose prophylactic therapy with nitrofurantoin or cephalexin continued until delivery.

URINARY INFECTION IN MEN

Men rarely present with acute uncomplicated urinary infection or acute nonobstructive pyelonephritis. Lack of circumcision, acquisition of infection from a sexual partner, and homosexuality have been identified as potential risk factors in the few cases which do occur. *Escherichia coli* is the usual infecting organism. These clinical presentations, however, are so uncommon in men, that all men who present with urinary infection should be investigated for the possibility of an underlying abnormality. A pelvic and renal ultrasound is the most useful initial test.

Elderly men with prostatic hypertrophy have an increased frequency of urinary infection due to obstruction and turbulent urine flow. They are also prone to develop bacterial prostatitis. Once bacteria are established in the prostate, poor diffusion of antibiotics into the prostate and formation of prostatic stones mean infection is often impossible to eradicate. The prostate then serves as a nidus for recurrent symptomatic or asymptomatic bladder infection. If recurrent symptomatic infection occurs, suggesting prostatic infection, a repeat course of 6–12 weeks of therapy is recommended as this is associated with a greater likelihood of long-term response.

URINARY TRACT INFECTIONS IN THE ELDERLY

Urinary infection is the most common infection occurring in either ambulatory or institutionalized elderly populations. The prevalence of bacteriuria is 5–10% for women and 5% in men over 65 years living in the community, and increases further with age. In long-term care facilities, 25–50% of all elderly residents have asymptomatic bacteriuria at any time. The prevalence increases with increasing functional impairment, including dementia and bladder and bowel incontinence.

Asymptomatic bacteriuria in elderly patients should not be treated with antimicrobials. Antimicrobial treatment does not decrease morbidity or mortality, but is associated with increased adverse effects, cost, and increasing antimicrobial resistance. It follows that asymptomatic elderly populations should not be screened for bacteriuria.

Symptomatic infection in the elderly may have a clinical presentation similar to younger populations. However, the diagnosis may not be straightforward, particularly in the institutionalized or functionally impaired population. Difficulties in communication, comorbid illnesses with chronic symptoms, and the high frequency of asymptomatic bacteriuria may impair diagnostic acumen. In addition, acute confusion may be a prominent presenting symptom, and a lower fever response and lower frequency of leukocytosis occur.

Antimicrobial selection for therapy is similar to younger populations. Dose should be adjusted for renal function, but not for age, per se. The duration of treatment is also similar to that recommended for younger populations, although cure rates with 3-day therapy are lower than in younger women, and it has been suggested that 7-day therapy is preferable to treat postmenopausal women. Post-treatment urine cultures to document microbiologic cure are not recommended unless symptoms persist or recur.

Urinary Infection in Patients with Renal Failure

Treatment of urinary infection requires high concentrations of effective antimicrobials in the urine. There is decreased excretion of antimicrobials into the urine with renal impairment, and adequate urinary antimicrobial levels may not be achieved. With severe bilateral renal impairment, it is difficult to cure urinary infection. Antimicrobials such as nitrofurantoin and tetracyclines other than doxycycline should not be used in the presence of renal failure because of toxicity. Others, such as aminoglycosides, may not penetrate nonfunctioning kidneys sufficiently to provide effective therapy. The penicillins and cephalosporins, as well as quinolones, are effective treatment for most individuals with renal failure. Obviously, appropriate dosage adjustments for renal function are necessary. In some situations, such as infected native kidneys in transplant recipients, infection cannot be eradicated and long-term suppressive therapy may be necessary to manage symptomatic recurrences.

Where renal impairment is unilateral, the functioning kidney will preferentially excrete the antimicrobial. Antimicrobial levels may be high in bladder urine, but not achieve therapeutic levels in the nonfunctioning kidney. If infection is in the nonfunctioning kidney, then, there may not be effective antimicrobial levels at the site of infection despite adequate levels in the excreted urine. This may explain relapsing infection in some individuals.

Fungal Urinary Tract Infection

Fungal urinary infection has been increasing in frequency. It is primarily a nosocomial infection and occurs in the setting of diabetes, foley catheters, and intense broad spectrum antimicrobial therapy. *Candida albicans* is the species most frequently isolated, but other *Candida* species, such as *C. glabrata, C. krusei, C. parapsolopsis,* and *C. tropicalis* also occur. The clinical importance of fungal urinary infection is often difficult to assess, in part because these tend to be complex patients with multiple associated problems. Generally, if there are no symptoms, treatment is not necessary. If an indwelling urethral catheter is in place it should be discontinued. Fungus balls may lead to obstruction and should be excluded in individuals with renal failure or persistence of funguria.

Where repeated cultures have grown yeast $\geq 10^4$ and there are symptoms referable to the genitourinary tract, funguria should be treated. Fluconazole 100–400 mg/day for 7 days is recommended because of good urinary excretion. However, itraconazole (100–400 mg/day), 5-flucytosine (50–150 mg/kg/day for 7 days), and amphotericin B have also been effective. The non-*albicans Candida* are more likely to be resistant to the azole antifungals, and amphotericin B is recommended for treatment. Amphotericin B bladder irrigation (50 mg/L continuous for 5 days) is no longer considered first line therapy, as it is difficult to deliver, requires catheterization, and is not superior to oral therapy. In selected situations, particularly in subjects with renal failure, it may still be appropriate. The success rate with any treatment has been reported to be only 70–75%, but significant accompanying illness frequently limits assessment of outcome.

Bibliography

Cardenas DD, Hooton TM: Urinary tract infection in persons with spinal cord injury. *Arch Phys Med Rehab* 76:272–280, 1995.

Collins TR, Devries CR: Recurrent urinary tract infections in children: A logical approach to diagnosis, treatment, and long-term management. *Comprehensive Ther* 23:44–48, 1997.

Falayas ME, Gorbach SL: Practice guidelines: Urinary tract infections. *Infect Dis Clin Pract* 4:241–257, 1995.

Fisher JF, Newman CL, Sobel JD: Yeast in the urine: Solutions for a budding problem. *Clin Infect Dis* 20:183–189, 1995.

Lipsky BA: Urinary tract infection in men. Epidemiology, pathophysiology, diagnosis, and treatment. *Ann Intern Med* 110:138–150, 1989.

Nickel JC: Prostatitis: Evolving management strategies. *Urol Clin North Am* 26:789–796, 1999.

Nicolle LE: A practical guide to the management of complicated urinary tract infection. *Drugs* 53:583–592, 1997.

Nicolle LE: Asymptomatic bacteriuria in the elderly. *Infect Dis Clin North Am* 11:647–662, 1997.

Pinson AG, Philbrick JT, Lindbeck GH, Schorling JB: Oral antibiotic therapy for acute pyelonephritis: A methodologic review of the literature. *J Gen Intern Med* 7:544–553, 1992.

Rubin RH, Shapiro ED, Andriole VT, Davis RJ, Stamm WE: Evaluation of new anti-infective drugs for the treatment of urinary tract infection. *Clin Infect Dis* 15(Suppl 1): 216–227, 1992.

Stamm WE, Hooton TM: Management of urinary tract infections in adults. *N Engl J Med* 329:1328–1334, 1993.

Warren JW, Abrutyn E, Hebel JR, Johnson JR, Schaeffer AJ, Stamm WE: Guidelines for antimicrobial therapy of uncomplicated acute bacterial cystitis and acute pyelonephritis in women. *Clin Infect Dis* 29:745–758, 1999.

Warren JW: Catheter-associated urinary tract infections. *Infect Dis Clin North Am* 11:609–622, 1997.

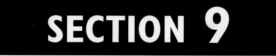

SECTION 9

THE KIDNEY IN SPECIAL CIRCUMSTANCES

THE KIDNEY IN INFANTS AND CHILDREN

R. ARIEL GOMEZ

ANATOMICAL DEVELOPMENT OF THE KIDNEY

In humans, the metanephric or definitive kidney appears during the fifth week of gestation. Nephrogenesis terminates by 32 to 36 weeks of gestation. Renal function and urine production begin about 10 weeks into embryonic life. The kidneys can be detected by ultrasound by the eighteenth week of gestation. Term infants are born with a full complement of nephrons. However, because deeper glomeruli develop earlier than superficial ones (centrifugal maturation), juxtamedullary glomeruli are larger and more mature than outer cortical ones. The glomeruli become equal in size by the fourteenth postnatal month and reach adult size (200 μm) at 3 1/2 years of age. The proximal tubule continues to increase in length well into adult life.

FUNCTIONAL DEVELOPMENT OF THE KIDNEY

Glomerular Filtration Rate

In newborn babies, glomerular filtration rate (GFR) correlates with gestational age. The GFR increases postnatally and doubles by 2 weeks of age. When corrected for surface area, the GFR reaches adult values at 1 to 2 years of age. The normal values of GFR for infants and children are shown in Table 1. Factors responsible for the increase in GFR with maturation include: increase in arterial pressure, increase in renal blood flow, increase in glomerular permeability, and increase in filtration surface area.

Creatinine clearance can be used to measure the GFR after 1 month of age providing that urinary creatinine excretion is between 15 and 25 mg/kg/day. However, in infants it is difficult to obtain 24-hr urine collections. Shorter collections are not adequate because of variations in creatinine excretion throughout the day. The following formula permits estimation of GFR (mL/min/1.73 m^2) without the need for urine collections,

$$\text{GFR} = K\, L/S_{\text{cr}},$$

where K is a constant (0.33 in preterm, 0.45 in term neonates, 0.55 in children and adolescent girls, and 0.70 in adolescent boys), L is the length of the infant or standing height of the child in centimeters, and S_{cr} is serum creatinine (mg/dL). Although this formula is clinically useful, inulin clearance or iothalamate clearance should be obtained if a more accurate value of GFR is needed. Along with changes in GFR, serum creatinine levels vary with age and

degree of maturity. During the first 48 hr after birth, creatinine levels are similar to the maternal values. A week after birth, the fullterm neonate should have a creatinine below 1.0 mg/dL. These levels should continue to decrease to about 0.3 mg/dL by 3 months of postnatal life. In preterm infants, however, creatinine levels can be high (about 1.5 mg/dL) during the first few weeks of postnatal life. These levels progressively decrease to 0.4 to 0.8 mg/dL by 3 to 6 months of postnatal life. When evaluating a neonate with a high creatinine, serial measurements are more meaningful than a single determination; creatinine levels should progressively decrease. An increase in serum creatinine indicates a reduction in GFR, regardless of the gestational age. The normal values for creatinine during childhood are shown in Fig. 1.

Urine Concentration

In human fetuses, urine flow rate increases from 0.1 mL/min at 20 weeks of gestation to 1.0 mL/min at 40 weeks of gestation. In neonates, urine flow rate decreases again to around 0.1 mL/min. Fetal urine flow correlates with (and may be modulated by) fetal arterial pressure. The fetal urine is hypotonic (100 to 200 mOsmol/L), unless stress such as hypoxemia or volume depletion develops. Nevertheless, the urinary concentrating ability is lower in the fetus than in the adult. Several factors contribute to the decreased urinary concentrating ability. In the fetus, the organization and anatomical development of the medulla is delayed with respect to glomerular development. Short loops of Henle and reduced NaCl transport in the ascending loops of Henle are also important factors. In addition, preferential blood flow to the inner portions of the cortex dissipates an already low intrarenal concentration gradient. Although arginine vasopressin (AVP) is secreted properly in response to volume and osmolar challenges, decreased AVP receptor number or coupling to cAMP generation likely contribute to the decreased concentrating ability found in infants.

Maximal urinary concentration increases progressively throughout the first year of life (Table 2). In premature neonates, maximal urine osmolality is about 400 to 500 mOsmol/L. Later in life, infants born prematurely are able to concentrate their urine to levels found in term infants of similar postnatal age. This is probably due to a rapid maturation of the concentration gradient in the premature infant.

TABLE I
Normal Values of GFR[a]

	(mL/min/1.73 m²)
Preterm (25–28 weeks)	
1 week	11.0 ± 5.4
2–8 weeks	15.5 ± 6.2
Preterm (29–34 weeks)	
1 week	15.3 ± 5.6
2–8 weeks	28.7 ± 13.8
Term	
5–7 days	50.6 ± 5.8
1–2 months	64.6 ± 5.8
3–4 months	85.8 ± 4.8
5–8 months	87.7 ± 11.9
9–12 months	86.9 ± 8.4
2–12 years	133 ± 27

[a]From Schwartz GJ, Brion LP; Spitzer A: The use of plasma creatinine concentration for estimating glomerular filtration rate in infants, children and adolescents. *Pediatr Clin North Am* 34:571–590, 1987, and Greene MG: *The Harriet Lane Handbook. A Manual for Pediatric House Officers,* 12th Ed., pp. 1–434. Mosby, St. Louis, 1991. (Adapted from S Meites (ed): *Pediatric clinical chemistry* ed 2 and 3, 1981, The American Association for Clinical Chemistry; NW Tietz: *Textbook of clinical chemistry,* 1986; GD Lundberg et al: *JAMA* 260:73, 1988; and J. Wallach: *Interpretation of diagnostic tests,* Boston 1992, Little Brown and Co.)

Sodium

Sodium metabolism in the newborn period is characterized by: (1) a progressive increase in renal reabsorptive capacity, (2) positive balance in the term infant, and (3) an inability to promptly excrete a solute and volume load.

About 30% of the dietary sodium is retained by the healthy infant receiving formulas containing different sodium concentrations. Although sodium intake varies widely, positive sodium balance is usually maintained, thus allowing the necessary conservation of sodium, a requirement for normal somatic growth. However, premature infants excrete more sodium than full-term infants. In fact, sodium excretion is negatively correlated to gestational age. The fractional excretion of sodium at 31 weeks of gestation is approximately 5% and declines to less than 1% by 2 months after birth. Thus, in contrast to full-term healthy newborns that are able to conserve sodium and maintain a positive sodium balance, preterm infants are at risk of developing a negative sodium balance during the first weeks of life. It is believed that the high sodium excretion in the premature baby is due to a relative inability of the distal tubule to respond to aldosterone. Newly born preterm infants who receive human breast milk or formulas with a composition similar to that of breast milk containing relatively low sodium concentrations continue to excrete large amounts of sodium in the urine and eventually develop a negative sodium balance and hyponatremia. The hyponatremia can be prevented by the addition of supplemental sodium chloride to the formula.

Although sodium retention in the maturing individual is essential for growth, the counterpart of this chronically enhanced sodium reabsorption is that newborns have difficulty in rapidly excreting an acute load of sodium and water. The renal excretory response to a sodium load increases progressively during infancy and is fully developed by the first year of life. In addition to the low GFR, enhanced distal tubular sodium reabsorption is responsible for the retention of sodium.

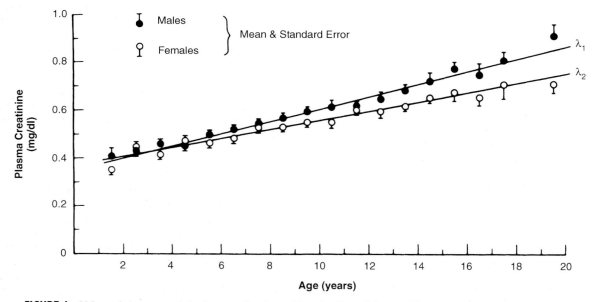

FIGURE I   Values of plasma creatinine in normal males and females. From Schwartz GJ, Haycock MB, Chir B, and Spitzer A: Plasma creatinine and urea concentration in children: Normal values for age and sex. *J Pediatr* 88:828–830, 1976. With permission.

TABLE 2
Maximal Urine Osmolality[a]

	(mOsmol/L)
3 days	515 ± 172
6 days	663 ± 133
10–30 days	896 ± 179
10–12 months	1118 ± 154
14–18 years	1362 ± 109

[a]Means ± SD. Data from Polacek E: The osmotic concentrating ability in healthy infants and children. *Arch Dis Child* 40:291, 1965.

TABLE 3
Calcium Levels According to Age[a]

	(mg/dL)
Premature (<1 week)	6–10
Fullterm (<1 week)	7–12
Child	8.0–10.5
Adult	8.5–10.5

[a]From Greene MG: *The Harriet Lane Handbook. A Manual for Pediatric House Officers,* 12th Ed., pp. 1–434. Mosby, St. Louis, 1991. (Adapted from S Meites (ed): *Pediatric clinical chemistry* ed 2 and 3, 1981, The American Association for Clinical Chemistry; NW Tietz: *Textbook of clinical chemistry,* 1986; GD Lundberg et al: *JAMA* 260:73, 1988; and J. Wallach: *Interpretation of diagnostic tests,* Boston 1992, Little Brown and Co.)

Based on the information previously described, the sodium requirements for a term newborn range from 1 to 1.5 mEq/kg/day, whereas the requirements for a preterm neonate range from 3 to 5 mEq/kg/day. The sodium content of breast milk is appropriate for the feeding of the healthy term infant. It should be remembered, however, that if excess sodium is given, such as feeding undiluted cow's milk, there is a risk of inducing sodium and water retention with extracellular volume expansion and sometimes clinically evident edema.

Oliguria

Most neonates void within the first 24 hr after birth. Any newborn baby, whether term or premature, who has not urinated within the first 24 hr of life should be evaluated for renal disease. Oliguria in infancy is defined as urine flow rate less than 1 mL/kg/hr. This is based on the usual renal solute load (7 to 15 mOsmol/kg/day) contributed by feedings and a maximal urinary osmolality of 500 mOsmol/kg. To maintain solute balance, the newborn will therefore need to urinate about 30 mL/kg/day (1.25 mL/kg/hr). In infants, oliguria can be easily evaluated by calculating the fractional excretion of sodium (FE_{Na}) (see Chapter 1).

Determination of the FE_{Na} is convenient because it does not require a timed urine collection. The FE_{Na} is particularly helpful in distinguishing oliguria due to a prerenal (low FE_{Na}) etiology from that due to a renal (high FE_{Na}) cause. In the oliguric term neonate, a FE_{Na} higher than 2.5% indicates a renal cause (such as acute tubular necrosis), whereas a FE_{Na} of less than 2.5% suggests prerenal causes such as dehydration, hypovolemia, hypoalbuminemia, or decreased effective plasma volume. As previously mentioned, premature babies normally have higher FE_{Na} (around 5%) and, therefore, the cutoff of 2.5% is not useful until after 10 days of postnatal life. In the older child, as in adults, a FE_{Na} of 1% is utilized as the break point (see Chapter 33).

Calcium

Fetal calcium levels are higher than maternal values because of active calcium transport across the placenta toward the fetal side. The fractional reabsorption of calcium by the loop of Henle increases with maturation. There-

fore, infants excrete more calcium in the urine than older children. Most commonly, hypercalciuria in the newborn is seen in neonates with bronchopulmonary dysplasia who have received calciuric drugs such as furosemide or glucocorticoids. Hypercalciuria, in turn, can lead to nephrocalcinosis, urolithiasis, and decreased renal function. When possible, a thiazide diuretic that reduces urine calcium excretion should be used instead of furosemide. Phosphate depletion in preterm infants can also lead to hypercalciuria. With the use of new formulas richer in phosphate, hypercalciuria and other complications of phosphate depletion such as osteopenia are less frequently observed.

Urine calcium excretion in the neonate can be estimated by calculating the calcium/creatinine ratio in a random urine sample. A ratio above 0.8 in preterm and 0.4 in fullterm infants is considered hypercalciuria. In older children, a ratio above 0.2 or a calcium excretion in a timed urine sample of greater than 4 mg/kg/24 hr are used to diagnose hypercalciuria.

Newborn infants are also prone to hypocalcemia, especially when they are sick. Contributing factors include decreased responses to Parathyroid hormone (PTH), high serum phosphate levels, and the rapid bone mineralization characteristic of the newborn period. The normal range for calcium levels in infants and children are shown in Table 3.

Phosphate

Serum phosphate concentration is normally higher in the neonate than in the adult (Table 4). Any neonate with a serum phosphate below 4 mg/dL should be evaluated for tubular wasting of phosphate. This can be easily done by calculating the tubular reabsorption of phosphate (TRP) after measuring the concentrations of creatinine and phosphate both in urine and plasma. The TRP can be envisioned as the complement of the fractional excretion of phosphate:

$$TRP = [1 - FE_{PO4}] \times 100\%$$

TABLE 4
Normal Phosphate Levels[a]

	mg/dL
Newborn	4.2–9.0
1 year	3.8–6.2
2–5 years	3.5–6.8
Adult	3.0–4.5

[a]From Greene MG: *The Harriet Lane Handbook. A Manual for Pediatric House Officers*, 12th Ed., pp. 1–434. Mosby, St. Louis, 1991. (Adapted from S Meites (ed): *Pediatric clinical chemistry* ed 2 and 3, 1981, The American Association for Clinical Chemistry; NW Tietz: *Textbook of clinical chemistry*, 1986; GD Lundberg et al: *JAMA* 260:73, 1988; and J. Wallach: *Interpretation of diagnostic tests*, Boston 1992, Little Brown and Co.)

Since,

$$FE_{PO4} = Clearance_{PO4}/GFR$$

or,

$$FE_{PO4} = (U_{P04}/P_{P04})/(U_{cr}/P_{cr})$$

then,

$$TRP = [1 - (U_{P04}/P_{P04})/(U_{cr}/P_{cr})] \times 100\%$$

where U_{PO4} and P_{PO4} are the urinary and plasma concentrations of phosphate (mg/dL), respectively, and P_{cr} and U_{cr} are the plasma and urinary concentrations of creatinine (mg/dL), respectively. It should be remembered that the normal TRP varies with age. After the first week of postnatal life, the TRP should exceed 95% in full-term and 75% in preterm neonates. After the first month of postnatal life and throughout adulthood, the TRP should be above 85%. Values below those just mentioned should suggest Fanconi syndrome, hyperparathyroidism, or chronic renal failure.

Potassium

The total body potassium (K^+) in infants is 40 mEq/kg, compared with the larger quantity found in adults (50 mEq/kg). Growing infants maintain a positive K^+ balance that is necessary for growth. Conservation of K^+ during infancy is reflected also by higher serum K^+ values (Table 5). In comparison with the adult, the newborn has a low basal rate of K^+ excretion and a decreased ability to rapidly excrete a K^+ load (Table 5). The fractional excretion of K^+ in the newborn is about half of that in the adult (Table 5) in part owing to reduced K^+ secretion by the cortical collecting duct, the main site for K^+ excretion. The factors that limit urinary K^+ excretion by the principal cells during early life are: (1) unfavorable electrochemical gradient (low cellular K^+ concentration, decreased Na^+,K^+-ATPase activity and transepithelial voltage), (2) limited membrane permeability to K^+, (3) low tubular fluid flow rates, and (4) decreased sensitivity to mineralocorticoids.

TABLE 5
Plasma Levels and Excretion of Potassium in Normal Infants and Children[a]

Age (years)	Plasma (K⁺) (mEq/L)	K⁺ clearance (mL/min/1.73 m²)	FEK[b] (%)
0–0.3	5.2 ± 0.8	5 ± 3	8.5 ± 3.8
0.4–1.0	4.9 ± 0.5	14 ± 6	14.6 ± 5.0
3–10	4.2 ± 0.5	20 ± 11	14.5 ± 8.9
11–20	4.3 ± 0.3	21 ± 8	16.2 ± 8.2

[a]Modified from Jones DL, Chesney RW: Tubular function. In: Holliday MA, Barrett TM, Avner FD (eds) *Pediatric Nephrology*, 4th Ed., pp. 59–82. Williams & Wilkins, Baltimore, 1999.
[b]Fractional excretion of potassium:

$$\frac{(urinary\ K^+)(plasma\ creatinine)}{(plasma\ K^+)(urinary\ creatinine)} \times 100\%\ .$$

Also, enhanced K^+ absorption by intercalated cells of the medullary collecting ducts may be a contributory factor. In fact, medullary collecting tubules (which reabsorb K^+) mature earlier than the principal cells of the cortical collecting duct (which secrete K^+), a factor that may be important in the decreased ability to excrete K^+ during early life. In addition, as GFR increases with maturation, fluid delivery to the cortical collecting duct increases, promoting K^+ secretion. Under normal conditions, the reduced ability of the neonate to excrete K^+ is not manifested clinically. However, hyperkalemia can develop if the neonate is exposed to excessive exogenous or endogenous (i.e., cell breakdown) K^+ loads.

Acid–Base Balance

Infants have lower blood pH and HCO_3^- than older children and adults (Table 6). Overall, the newborn kidney is capable of maintaining normal acid–base status. However, infants are prone to the development of acidosis when they are sick or receive inadequate nutrition or in response to an exogenous acid load. The plasma concentration of HCO_3^- increases with age due to an increase in the renal threshold of HCO_3^- with maturation. The approximate renal threshold of HCO_3^- is 18 mEq/L in the premature and 21 mEq/L in the term neonate. Adult values (24 to 26 mEq/L) are reached by 1 year of age. Several factors seem to be responsible for the low renal HCO_3^- threshold observed in infancy: low activity of carbonic anhydrase, extracellular fluid volume expansion contributing to proximal HCO_3^- wasting, immaturity of luminal Na^+–H^+ exchange, and imbalance between filtration and reabsorption of HCO_3^- in newly formed nephrons. Also, HCO_3^- reabsorption in the distal nephron may not compensate for HCO_3^- that escapes the proximal tubule.

Infants have a decreased ability to acidify the urine when compared to adults under basal conditions. Maximal titratable acid and ammonium excretion increase with age and achieve adult values (when corrected by GFR) by 2 months of age. Several factors are responsible for the relative in-

TABLE 6
Acid–Base Measurements as a Function of Age[a]

Age	pH	$paCO_2$ (mm Hg)	HCO_3^- (mEq/L)
Preterm (1 week)	7.34 ± 0.06	31 ± 3[b]	17.2 ± 1.2[b]
Preterm (6 weeks)	7.38 ± 0.02	35 ± 6	21.9 ± 4.4[b]
Term (birth)	7.24 ± 0.05[b]	49 ± 10[b]	20.0 ± 2.8[b]
Term (1 hr)	7.37 ± 0.05	34 ± 9	19.0 ± 2.3[b]
3–6 months	7.39 ± 0.03	36 ± 3	22.0 ± 1.9[b]
21–24 months	7.40 ± 0.02	35 ± 3	21.8 ± 1.6[b]
3.5–5.4 years	7.39 ± 0.04	37 ± 4	22.5 ± 1.3[b]
5.5–12.0 years	7.40 ± 0.03	38 ± 3	23.1 ± 1.2[b]
12.5–17.4 years	7.38 ± 0.03	41 ± 3	24.0 ± 1.0[b]
Adult males	7.39 ± 0.01	41 ± 2	25.2 ± 1.0

[a] Mean $\pm$ 1 SD.
[b] Significantly different from adult males ($p < .05$) by Tukey's test.

ability of the newborn to excrete an acid load, including a limited availability of urinary buffers such as phosphate and ammonium. The low GFR and high TRP prevailing in the neonatal period markedly limit the phosphate available as a urinary buffer. Prior to 2 months of age, ammonia generation and secretion are also limited. Immaturity of the collecting ducts (fewer intercalated cells, fewer proton pumps per cell) and immaturity of carbonic anhydrase activity could also limit distal acidification. In addition to this impairment in renal excretion, infants have an increased exogenous and endogenous proton load in comparison to adults. In prematures, endogenous acid production can be as high as 2 to 3 mEq/kg/day. A large amount of acid is generated during the metabolism of proteins. Accretion of calcium into the growing bone also results in the release of 0.5 to 1.0 mEq/kg/day of H^+ that needs to be excreted by the kidney or neutralized by HCO_3^- absorbed through the gastrointestinal tract. For this reason, during episodes of gastroenteritis, infants are susceptible to metabolic acidosis.

Blood Pressure

The normal blood pressure values vary with age, gender, stature, and degree of maturation. Accepted normal values are based on demographic studies. The reader should consult the report of the "Second Task Force on Blood Pressure Control in Children—1987" and its more recent update in 1996 which provide normative data and guidelines for detection and treatment of children with hypertension. A child is considered hypertensive if the systolic or diastolic blood pressure is above the ninety-fifth percentile for age and sex on at least three occasions. The classification of hypertension by age group is shown in Table 7. The most common etiologies of hypertension vary with the age of the patient population. As a rule, the younger the patient, the more likely it is for hypertension to be secondary. In the newborn period, renal artery thrombosis, congenital renal malformations, coarctation of the aorta, and bronchopulmonary dysplasia are the most common causes. In children between infancy and 6 years of age, renal parenchymal diseases, renal artery stenosis, and coarctation of the aorta are leading causes. Between 6 and 10 years of age, renal parenchymal diseases, renal artery stenosis, and essential hypertension are frequently found. In the adolescent, essential hypertension and renal parenchymal diseases are the two most prominent causes.

TABLE 7
Classification of Hypertension by Age Group[a]

Age group	Significant hypertension	Severe hypertension
Newborn		
7 days	Systolic $\geq$ 96 mm Hg	Systolic $\geq$ 106 mm Hg
8–30 days	Systolic $\geq$ 104 mm Hg	Systolic $\geq$ 110 mm Hg
Infant (<2 years)	Systolic $\geq$ 112 mm Hg	Systolic $\geq$ 118 mm Hg
	Diastolic $\geq$ 74 mm Hg	Diastolic $\geq$ 82 mm Hg
Children (3–5 years)	Systolic $\geq$ 116 mm Hg	Systolic $\geq$ 124 mm Hg
	Diastolic $\geq$ 76 mm Hg	Diastolic $\geq$ 84 mm Hg
Children (6–9 years)	Systolic $\geq$ 122 mm Hg	Systolic $\geq$ 130 mm Hg
	Diastolic $\geq$ 78 mm Hg	Diastolic $\geq$ 86 mm Hg
Children (10–12 years)	Systolic $\geq$ 126 mm Hg	Systolic $\geq$ 134 mm Hg
	Diastolic $\geq$ 82 mm Hg	Diastolic $\geq$ 90 mm Hg
Adolescents (13–15 years)	Systolic $\geq$ 136 mm Hg	Systolic $\geq$ 144 mm Hg
	Diastolic $\geq$ 86 mm Hg	Diastolic $\geq$ 92 mm Hg
Adolescents (16–18 years)	Systolic $\geq$ 142 mm Hg	Systolic $\geq$ 150 mm Hg
	Diastolic $\geq$ 92 mm Hg	Diastolic $\geq$ 98 mm Hg

[a] From the Report of the Second Task Force on Blood Pressure Control in Children—1987. *Pediatrics* 79(1):1–25, 1987.

Bibliography

Al-Dahhan J, Haycock GB, Nichol B, Chatler C, Stimmler L: Sodium homeostasis in term and preterm neonates. III. Effect of salt supplementation. *Arch Dis Child* 59:945–950, 1984.

Barone, MA: *The Harriet Lane Handbook. A Manual for Pediatric House Officers,* 14th Ed. Mosby-Year Book, St. Louis, 1996.

Chevalier RL: Developmental renal physiology of the low birth weight pre-term newborn. *J Urol* 156:714–719, 1996.

Gomez RA: Postnatal regulation of water and electrolyte excretion. In: Brace RA, Ross MG, Robillard JE (eds) *Reproductive and Perinatal Medicine, Volume XI. Fetal and Neonatal Body Fluids: The Scientific Basis for Clinical Practice,* pp. 307–318. Perinatology Press, New York, 1989.

Jones DP, Chesney RW: Tubular function. In: Holliday MA, Barrett TM, Avner ED (eds) *Pediatric Nephrology,* 4th Ed., pp. 59–82. Williams & Wilkins, Baltimore, 1999.

Mathew OP, Jones AS, James E, Bland H, Groshong T: Neonatal renal failure: Usefulness of diagnostic indices. *Pediatrics* 65:5760, 1980.

Polacek E: The osmotic concentrating ability in healthy infants and children. *Arch Dis Child* 40:291, 1965.

Report of the Second Task Force on Blood Pressure Control in Children—1987: *Pediatrics* 79(1):1–25, 1987.

Robillard JE, Guillery EN, Petershack, JA: Renal function during fetal life. In: Holliday MA, Barrett TM, Avner ED (eds), *Pediatric Nephrology,* 4th Ed., pp. 21–37. Williams & Wilkins, Baltimore, 1999.

Schwartz GJ, Brion LP, Spitzer A: The use of plasma creatinine concentration for estimating glomerular filtration rate in infants, children and adolescents. *Pediatr Clin North Am* 34:571–590, 1987.

Update on the 1987 Task Force Report of High Blood Pressure in Children and Adolescents: A Working Group Report from the National High Blood Pressure Education Program. *Pediatrics* 98(4):649–658, 1996.

Woolf, AS: Embryology. In: Holliday MA, Barrett TM, Avner ED (eds), *Pediatric Nephrology,* 4th Ed., pp. 1–19. Williams & Wilkins, Baltimore, 1999.

THE KIDNEY IN PREGNANCY

PHYLLIS AUGUST

An intriguing aspect of reproduction is the close dependency of reproductive function on normal renal function. Pregnancy, in the setting of significant maternal renal disease, is hazardous and frequently unsuccessful. Pregnancy imposes a hemodynamic strain on maternal renal function such that in some cases renal function deteriorates irreversibly in women with preexisting renal disease during or after pregnancy. In general, the closer to normal the glomerular filtration rate (GFR) and blood pressure, the greater the chance of successful pregnancy. Management of gravidas with kidney disease may be complicated, and requires an understanding of the physiologic changes associated with pregnancy, as well as close cooperation between obstetrician and nephrologist.

RENAL ANATOMY AND PHYSIOLOGY IN PREGNANCY

Anatomic and Functional Changes in Urinary Tract

Kidney length increases approximately 1 cm during normal gestation. The major anatomic alterations of the urinary tract during pregnancy, however, are seen in the col-

lecting system, where calyces, renal pelves, and ureters dilate, often giving the erroneous impression of obstructive uropathy. The cause of the ureteral dilation is disputed and has been attributed to hormonal mechanisms as well as mechanical obstruction by the enlarging uterus. These morphologic changes result in stasis in the urinary tract and a propensity of pregnant women with asymptomatic bacteriuria to develop frank pyelonephritis. Because they contain substantial volumes of urine, the dilated widened ureters may lead to collection errors when 24-hr urine specimens are obtained. It has been recommended that pregnant women receive a water load and remain in lateral recumbency for 1 hr before the start of the collection.

Renal Hemodynamics

Pregnancy is characterized by marked vasodilatation, which is detectable early in the first trimester. In fact, more recent studies of the menstrual cycle demonstrate the vasodilation is also present in the late luteal phase, prior to conception. There is lower blood pressure throughout gestation, as well as increased renal plasma flow (RPF) and

GFR. Increases in renal hemodynamics reach a maximum during the first trimester, and perfusion and filtration rate are approximately 50% greater than nonpregnant levels. The basis for the increased GFR and RPF is unknown. Micropuncture studies performed in the gravid rat are consistent with a major role of renal vasodilatation and increased glomerular plasma flow in these changes. Experimental models of nitric oxide synthesis inhibition suggest that hormonally mediated increased nitric oxide generation may be in part responsible for the renal vasodilatation.

Creatinine production is unchanged during pregnancy, thus increments in clearance result in decreased serum levels. One study reported average values of 0.83 mg/dL in nonpregnant women, and 0.74, 0.58, and 0.53 mg/dL in first, second, and third trimester of pregnancy, respectively. The increased GFR and RPF also result in increased excretion of glucose, amino acids, calcium, and urinary protein. The clinical consequences of these alterations are an increase in the upper limit of normal for urinary protein excretion (from 150 mg/day to 300 mg/day).

Acid–Base Regulation in Pregnancy

The bicarbonate threshold decreases, and early-morning urines are more alkaline than in nonpregnant women. Plasma bicarbonate concentration decreases by approximately 4 mmol/L, averaging 22 mmol/L. This is believed to be a compensatory renal response to hypocapnia, which occurs during pregnancy as a consequence of physiologic hyperventilation. pCO_2 averages only 30 mm Hg, and thus, since both pCO_2 and bicarbonate levels are already diminished, pregnant women may be disadvantaged when threatened by acute metabolic acidosis. Finally, it should be appreciated that a pCO_2 of 40 mm Hg signifies considerable carbon dioxide retention in pregnancy.

Water Metabolism

Pregnancy is associated with a decrease in plasma osmolality of 5 to 10 mOsmol/kg below that of nongravid women. This decrease in plasma osmolality is associated with appropriate responses to water loading and dehydration, and suggests a resetting of the osmoreceptor system. Clinical studies demonstrating decreased osmotic thresholds for thirst and arginine vasopressin (AVP) release in pregnant women support this hypothesis. In addition, pregnant women metabolize AVP more rapidly as a consequence of production of placental vasopressinases and may develop syndromes of transient diabetes insipidus due to the increased metabolism of AVP. These syndromes may be treated with D-arginine vasopressin (dDAVP).

Volume Regulation

Total body water increases by 6 to 8 L during pregnancy, 4 to 6 L of which is extracellular. Plasma volume increases 50% during gestation, the largest rate of increment occurring in midpregnancy. There is a gradual cumulative retention of about 900 mEq of sodium during pregnancy, which is distributed between the products of conception and the maternal extracellular space. Despite the increase in plasma volume during pregnancy, there is no evidence for a hypervolemic (i.e., overfilled circulation) state during pregnancy. Indeed, the marked vasodilation which is observed as early as the first trimester may be the stimulus for increased sodium retention and increased plasma volume. The observations that blood pressure is significantly lower, and that the renin–angiotensin system is stimulated during normal pregnancy are consistent with primary vasodilation preceding and causing the increase in plasma volume.

Blood Pressure Regulation

Mean blood pressure decreases early in gestation, with diastolic levels averaging 10 mm Hg less in midpregnancy compared with antepartum levels. Later in pregnancy, blood pressure may increase enough to reach nonpregnant levels near term. The decrease in blood pressure is due to vasodilation, which may be mediated by the effects of placental hormones on vascular endothelium. The role of nitric oxide and other endothelial products in the vasodilation of pregnancy is currently under investigation. In response to the vasodilation and lower blood pressure, the renin–angiotensin system is markedly stimulated in pregnancy.

Increases in plasma renin activity (PRA) are apparent early in pregnancy, and levels increase to reach a maximum of about four times nonpregnant values by mid pregnancy. The increase in PRA is accompanied by increases in aldosterone secretion. Angiotensin II levels have not been studied extensively, but are likely to be increased as well. Despite the increased renin and aldosterone levels, blood pressure and electrolytes are normal during pregnancy. Indeed, normotensive gravidas demonstrate exaggerated responses to acute converting enzyme inhibition, suggesting that the stimulated renin–angiotensin system is an important defense against hypotension during pregnancy.

Mineral Metabolism

Serum calcium levels decrease in pregnancy, as does serum albumin concentration. Ionized calcium remains normal. There are significant increases in circulating levels of 1,25-dihydroxy vitamin D_3 during pregnancy, owing to increased renal production as well as increased placental production. Gastrointestinal absorption of calcium increases, and there is an "absorptive hypercalciuria," with 24-hr urine excretion often exceeding 300 mg/day. Intact parathyroid levels are lower during pregnancy compared with nonpregnant values.

KIDNEY DISEASE IN PREGNANCY

Kidney disease during pregnancy may be due to (1) pre-existing renal disease that was diagnosed prior to conception, (2) chronic renal disease that was unappreciated prior to pregnancy and diagnosed for the first time during pregnancy, or (3) renal disease that develops for the first time during pregnancy. There is some overlap with respect to the different diseases that are typical of the three categories. For example, lupus nephritis may be a chronic condition, or it may develop for the first time during pregnancy.

Chronic Renal Disease: General Principles

Fertility and ability to sustain an uncomplicated pregnancy are related to the degree of renal functional impairment, rather than to the specific underlying disorder. The greater the functional impairment, and the higher the blood pressure, the less likely the pregnancy will be successful. Patients are arbitrarily considered in three categories: preserved or mildly impaired renal function (serum creatinine less than or at 1.4 mg/dL), moderate renal insufficiency (creatinine 1.5 mg to 3.0 mg/dL), and severe renal insufficiency (creatinine greater than or equal to 3 mg/dL). Table 1 summarizes the maternal and fetal prognosis in each category. Women with moderate or severe renal dysfunction should be discouraged from conceiving, since up to 40% of these pregnancies are complicated by hypertension or deterioration in renal function which may be irreversible. The level of blood pressure at the time of conception is an important variable in pregnancy outcome. In the absence of hypertension, there is significantly less chance of irreversible deterioration in renal function during pregnancy. When hypertension is present, and especially when it is severe, pregnancy outcome is rarely uncomplicated. Premature delivery and deterioration in renal function are expected. Urine protein excretion may increase markedly in pregnant women with underlying renal disease. Although the increments in protein excretion during pregnancy may not necessarily reflect worsening of the underlying kidney disease, increased proteinuria is associated with worse fetal prognosis.

Renal Diseases Associated with Systemic Illness

Diabetes is one of the most common medical disorders encountered during pregnancy, and the majority of cases are due to gestational diabetes. Preexisting diabetes poses significant risks to pregnancy. Many younger women with diabetes that antedates pregnancy have type 1 diabetes, and if their disease has been present for 10 to 15 years, they may show early signs of diabetic nephropathy. Women with microalbuminuria, well preserved renal function, and normal blood pressure have a good prognosis for pregnancy, although they are at increased risk for preeclampsia and urinary infection. It is not unusual for urinary protein excretion to increase significantly during pregnancy, and many women with nonnephrotic range proteinuria preconception develop nephrotic range proteinuria during pregnancy. Women with overt nephropathy preconception, particularly those with impaired renal function and hypertension, as in any other renal disease, have a high incidence of premature delivery, and deterioration in maternal renal function. Women with type 1 diabetes with microalbuminuria and normal renal function and normotension should be encouraged *not* to postpone pregnancy because of the worse prognosis once overt nephropathy develops.

The most important aspect of management of diabetes in pregnancy with or without nephropathy is tight glucose control, because of the clear-cut relation between glucose control and fetal outcome. Thus all women with diabetes should be managed by physicians experienced with diabetes in pregnancy. Blood pressure control is also important. However, since angiotensin converting enzyme inhibitors and angiotensin receptor blockers are contraindicated during pregnancy, women should be switched to other agents prior to conception.

Women with lupus nephritis during pregnancy present unique problems. Although similar considerations apply regarding the relationship between level of renal function and blood pressure to pregnancy outcome, in general, lupus is a much more unpredictable illness, because of the tendency of the disease to flare. Whether or not pregnancy per se is a risk factor for lupus flares has been disputed, although a more recent prospective well-controlled study suggests that pregnancy is in fact associated with a greater chance of disease exacerbation. Women with lupus are advised not to conceive unless their disease has been "inactive" for the preceding 6 months. Additional complications associated with lupus and pregnancy include placental transfer of maternal autoantibodies which can cause a neonatal lupus syndrome characterized by heart block, transient cutaneous lesions, or both. Women with lupus are also more likely to have clinically significant titers of an-

TABLE I
Pregnancy and Renal Disease: Functional Renal Status and Prospects[a]

Outcome	Category		
	Mild (Cr < 1.5 mg/dL)	Moderate (Cr 1.5–3.0 mg/dL)	Severe (Cr > 3.0 mg/dL)
Pregnancy complications	25%	47%	86%
Successful obstetric outcome	96% (85%)	90% (59%)	47% (8%)
Long-term sequelae	<3% (9%)	25% (71%)	53% (92%)

[a]Cr, serum creatinine. Estimates are based on 1862 women with 2799 pregnancies (1973–1992) and do not include collagen diseases. Numbers in parentheses refer to prospects when complications develop before 28 weeks' gestation. From Davison JM, Lindheimer MD: Renal disorders. In: Creasy RK, Resnik RK (eds) *Maternal Fetal Medicine*, 4th Ed. Saunders, Philadelphia, 1999. Reprinted with permission.

tiphospholipid antibodies which are associated with spontaneous fetal loss, hypertensive syndromes indistinguishable from preeclampsia, and thrombotic events including deep vein thrombosis, pulmonary embolus, myocardial infarction, and strokes. Thus all women with systemic lupus erythematosis should be screened for antiphospholipid antibodies early in gestation. When titers are elevated (more than 40 GPL), daily aspirin (80 to 325 mg) is recommended. If there is a history of thrombotic events, then heparin in combination with aspirin is recommended. One of the difficulties in managing lupus nephritis during pregnancy is that increased activity of lupus may be difficult to distinguish from preeclampsia. Both are characterized by an increase in proteinuria, a decrease in GFR, and hypertension. Thrombocytopenia may also be observed in both conditions. Hypocomplementemia is not a feature of preeclampsia, whereas abnormal liver function tests, which may be observed in preeclampsia, are not characteristic of lupus activity. If disease activity is present before 20 weeks of gestation, then preeclampsia is not likely. In the latter half of pregnancy, it may be impossible to distinguish between a renal lupus flare and preeclampsia. In fact, frequently both are present simultaneously, and what starts as increased lupus activity appears to trigger preeclampsia. Unfortunately, delivery may be necessary if immunosuppressive therapy and supportive care fails to stabilize the condition. Appropriate therapy for lupus nephritis during pregnancy includes steroids and azathiaprine. Cyclophosphamide is generally not recommended during pregnancy, because of potential fetal toxicity, and should only be used when the life of the mother is in jeopardy.

Chronic Glomerulonephritis

Childbearing women may be afflicted with any of the forms of chronic glomerulonephritis common in this age group. These include IgA nephropathy, focal and segmental glomerulosclerosis, membranoproliferative glomerulonephritis, minimal change nephritis, and membranous nephropathy. There are insufficient data to suggest that histologic subtype confers a specific prognosis for pregnancy. Rather, the previously mentioned principles are applicable to women with chronic glomerulonephritis; when renal function is normal and hypertension absent, prognosis is good.

Polycystic Kidney Disease

Young women with autosomal dominant polycystic kidney disease (ADPKD) are frequently assymptomatic, with normal renal function and normal blood pressure, and indeed may be unaware of their diagnosis. Older women with progressive disease and functional impairment and hypertension are at risk for preeclampsia and premature delivery. There is an increased incidence of urinary tract infection as well. Estrogen is reported to cause liver cysts to enlarge, and repeated pregnancies may result in symptomatic enlargement of liver cysts. Given the association between cerebral aneurysms and ADPKD in some families, screening for such aneurysms should be considered prior to natural labor. All patients should undergo genetic counseling before pregnancy to ensure they are aware that 50% of their offspring are at risk.

Vesicoureteral Reflux

Dilation and stasis in the urinary tract make vesicoureteral reflux in gravidas more prone to exacerbation. These women should have a high fluid intake and should be screened frequently for bacteriuria. Because of their reported adverse prognosis during pregnancy, these high risk women should be treated promptly when infection is documented.

Chronic Renal Diseases That May Be First Diagnosed during Pregnancy

The presence of chronic renal disease may first be appreciated during pregnancy in part because pregnant women are scrutinized more closely, and also because the renal hemodynamic alterations during pregnancy may cause proteinuria to increase and be clinically detectable for the first time. Frequent measurement of blood pressure may also lead to diagnosis of renal diseases accompanied by hypertension. Furthermore, the presence of even mild preexisting renal disease is associated with an increased risk of preeclampsia, thus underlying renal disease may first become apparent after preeclampsia has developed in later pregnancy. Renal diseases that may have been relatively silent preconception that may "present" during pregnancy include IgA nephropathy, focal segmental glomerulosclerosis (FSGS), polycystic kidney disease, and reflux nephropathy. Renal diagnostic testing during pregnancy can include blood and urine testing and ultrasonography. Renal biopsy is usually deferred until after delivery unless an acute deterioration in renal function occurs or morbidity from nephrotic syndrome is significant. The timing of renal biopsy after delivery depends on the clinical circumstances. If renal function is normal, and only proteinuria is present, it is reasonable to delay biopsy by at least 1 to 2 months since proteinuria may improve once the hemodynamic alterations associated with pregnancy have resolved. If renal function is impaired, then biopsy should be considered within a few weeks of delivery.

Renal Diseases That Develop for the First Time during Pregnancy

Pregnant women are at risk for any of the renal diseases that occur in childbearing age women including pyelonephritis, glomerulonephritis, interstitial nephritis, and acute renal failure. Pyelonephritis in pregnant women is more likely to be associated with significant azotemia compared with nonpregnant women, and should be treated aggressively. Glomerulonephritis or interstitial nephritis are not more likely to develop during pregnancy, although they do occur. Acute renal failure in association with pregnancy is becoming less common, and less likely to occur in early pregnancy, largely as a consequence of liberalization of abortion laws and improvement of prenatal care. Recent estimates suggest that the incidence of acute renal failure from obstetric causes is less than 1 in 20,000 pregnancies.

When acute renal failure occurs early in pregnancy (12 to 18 weeks) it is usually in association with septic abortion or prerenal azotemia due to hyperemesis gravidarium. Most cases of acute renal failure in pregnancy occur between gestational week 35 and the puerperium and are primarily due to preeclampsia and bleeding complications. Although most cases of preeclampsia are not usually associated with renal failure, the HELLP syndrome, which is a variant of preeclampsia (*h*emolysis, *e*levated *l*iver enzymes, *l*ow *p*latelet count) may be associated with significant renal dysfunction, especially if not treated promptly. The important clinical entities causing renal failure during pregnancy are as follows:

Thrombotic Microangiopathy

Although rare, thrombotic microangiopathies [thrombotic thrombocytopenic purpura (TTP) and hemolytic uremic syndrome (HUS)] are an important cause of pregnancy associated acute renal failure because they are associated with considerable morbidity. They also share several clinical and laboratory features of pregnancy specific disorders such as the HELLP variant of preeclampsia and acute fatty liver of pregnancy. Thus, distinction of these syndromes is important for therapeutic and prognostic reasons. Features that may be helpful in making the correct diagnosis include timing of onset and the pattern of laboratory abnormalities. Preeclampsia typically develops in the third trimester, with only a few cases developing in the postpartum period, usually within a few days of delivery. TTP usually occurs antepartum, with many cases developing in the second trimester, as well as the third. HUS is usually a postpartum disease. Symptoms may begin antepartum, but most cases are diagnosed postpartum.

Preeclampsia is much more common than TTP/HUS, and it is usually preceded by hypertension and proteinuria. Renal failure is unusual, even with severe cases, unless significant bleeding or hemodynamic instability or marked disseminated intravascular coagulation (DIC) occurs. In some cases, preeclampsia develops in the immediate postpartum period, and when thrombocytopenia is severe, it may be indistinguishable from HUS. However, preeclampsia spontaneously recovers, whereas HUS seldom improves.

In contrast to TTP/HUS, preeclampsia may be associated with mild DIC and prolongation of prothrombin and partial thromboplastin times. Another laboratory feature of preeclampsia/HELLP syndrome that is not usually associated with TTP/HUS is a marked elevation of liver enzymes. The presence of fever is more consistent with a diagnosis of TTP than preeclampsia or HUS. The main distinctive features of HUS are its tendency to occur in the postpartum period and the severity of the associated renal failure. Treatment of preeclampsia/HELLP syndrome is delivery and supportive care. More aggressive treatment is rarely indicated. Some centers have reported the use of steroids in cases of severe HELLP syndrome, although this therapy has not been rigorously evaluated in placebo-controlled clinical trials. Treatment of TTP/HUS includes plasma infusion or exchange and other modalities used in nonpregnant patients with these disorders.

Bilateral Renal Cortical Necrosis

Bilateral renal cortical necrosis may be induced by abruptio placenta or other severe complications associated with obstetric hemorrhage. Both primary DIC and severe renal ischemia have been proposed as the initiating events. Affected patients typically present with oliguria or anuria, hematuria, and flank pain. Ultrasonography or computed tomography may demonstrate hyperechoic or hypodense areas in the renal cortex. Most patients ultimately require dialysis, but 20 to 40% have partial recovery of renal function.

Acute Fatty Liver of Pregnancy

Acute fatty liver of pregnancy is a rare complication of pregnancy that is associated with significant azotemia. Women with this disorder often complain of anorexia, nausea, vomiting, and occasionally abdominal pain in the third trimester. Clinical features suggesting preeclampsia including hypertension and proteinuria are not uncommon, and azotemia is frequently more severe than that observed in HELLP syndrome. Laboratory tests reveal elevations in liver enzymes, hypoglycemia, hypofibrinogenemia, and prolonged partial thromboplastin time. Delivery is indicated, and most patients improve shortly afterward. This disorder was formerly associated with a more ominous outcome, which may have been a consequence of late diagnosis. When diagnosed early, long-term morbidity is rare.

Urinary Tract Obstruction

Pregnancy is associated with dilation of the collecting system, which is not usually accompanied by renal dysfunction. Rarely, complications such as large uterine fibroids that enlarge in the setting of pregnancy can lead to obstructive uropathy. Occasionally, acute urinary tract obstruction in pregnancy is caused by a kidney stone. Diagnosis can usually be made by ultrasonography. Often the stone will pass spontaneously, but occasionally cystoscopy is necessary for insertion of a stent to remove a fragment of stone and relieve obstruction, particularly if there is sepsis or a solitary kidney. Extracorporeal shock wave (ESW) lithotripsy is contraindicated during pregnancy because of the possibility of adverse effects on the fetus.

Management of acute renal failure occurring in pregnancy or immediately postpartum is similar to that in nongravid subjects although there are several important considerations unique to pregnancy. Uterine hemorrhage near term may be concealed, and blood loss underestimated, thus any overt blood loss should be replaced early. Both peritoneal dialysis and hemodialysis have been used successfully in patients with obstetric acute renal failure. Neither pelvic peritonitis nor the enlarged uterus is a contraindication to the former method. In fact, this form of treatment is more gradual than hemodialysis and thus less likely to precipitate labor. Because urea, creatinine, and other metabolites that accumulate in uremia traverse the placenta, dialysis should be undertaken early, with the aim of maintaining the blood urea nitrogen at approximately 50 mg/dL. Excessive fluid removal should be avoided, because it may contribute to hemodynamic compromise, reduction of uteroplacental perfusion, and premature labor. In some cases it may be advisable to perform continuous fetal monitoring during dialysis, particularly after mid pregnancy.

THERAPY OF END STAGE RENAL DISEASE DURING PREGNANCY

Dialysis

Fertility is reduced in dialysis patients, and conception is uncommon in women who have had end stage renal disease for several years. Most pregnancies occur within the first few years of starting dialysis. Although previously the outcomes of such pregnancies were poor, with only approximately 25% resulting in surviving infants, new information suggests that pregnancy in dialysis patients is successful as often as 30 to 50% of the time in those pregnancies that reach the second trimester. Considerable problems exist in such pregnancies, however, and conception should not be encouraged in women on maintenance dialysis. Prematurity is common, and approximately 85% of infants born to women who conceive after starting dialysis are born before 36 weeks gestation. There is a high incidence of very low birthweight and intrauterine growth restriction. Maternal complications include accelerated hypertension and even mortality. The approach to dialysis during pregnancy should include increasing dialysis time in order to minimize the uremic environment. Both the number of sessions per week as well as the time per session can be increased to a minimum of 20 hr of hemodialysis. Heparinization should be minimal to prevent obstetric bleeding. If peritoneal dialysis is being used, decreasing exchange volumes and increasing exchange frequency is recommended. Adequate calorie and protein intake should be encouraged. Antihypertensive therapy should be adjusted for pregnancy. Anemia should be treated with supplemental iron, folic acid, and erythropoietin. There is no evidence that one dialysis modality is superior with respect to pregnancy outcome.

Renal Transplantation

Several thousand women have undergone pregnancy following renal transplantation. As expected, outcome is improved with living related donor transplants. In most pregnancies (greater than 90%) that proceed beyond the first trimester succeed, however, there are certain predictable maternal and fetal complications. These include complications of steroid therapy such as impaired glucose tolerance, hypertension and increased infection, ectopic pregnancy, and even uterine rupture. Fetal complications include a higher incidence of premature delivery, intrau-

terine growth restriction, congenital anomalies, hypoadrenalism, thrombocytopenia, and infection. The following criteria are suggested for transplant recipients for conception.

1. Good health and stable renal function for 2 years after transplantation
2. Absent or minimal proteinuria
3. Normal blood pressure or easily managed hypertension
4. No evidence of pelvicalcyceal distention on ultrasonography prior to conception
5. Serum creatinine less than 2 mg/dL, and preferably less than 1.5 mg/dL
6. Drug therapy: prednisone 15 mg daily or less; azathioprine 2 mg/kg or less; cyclosporine less than 5 mg/kg day.

Transplant registry data support the recommendation that a creatinine below 1.5 mg/dL and absence of hypertension are associated with the best prognosis. Although cyclosporine levels tend to decrease during pregnancy, there is no information regarding whether or not drug dosage should be increased. Experience with tacrolimus is limited. There are several case reports of successful pregnancy in patients receiving this agent, however, there are also reports of fetal growth restriction, and neonatal hyperkalemia and anuria. Mycophenolate mofetil has not been widely used in pregnancy, and has been reported to be embryotoxic in animals. This drug should be discontinued during pregnancy, and women should be switched to azathiaprine if indicated.

HYPERTENSIVE DISORDERS OF PREGNANCY

Hypertensive disorders in pregnancy are one of the most common medical disorders complicating pregnancy. Although maternal death is a rare event in most Western nations where access to prenatal care is adequate, hypertensive disorders are one of the leading causes of maternal death worldwide, accounting for 15–20% of all maternal deaths in the developing as well as the developed world. In the United States, approximately 8–10% of all pregnancies are complicated by hypertension, with half of these cases attributable to the pregnancy specific disorder preeclampsia. In addition to maternal morbidity and mortality, hypertensive disorders in pregnancy are a major cause of fetal morbidity and mortality. Hypertension is one of the leading causes of premature birth, which may be associated with lifelong medical complications. Hypertensive disorders in pregnancy are significantly more common than kidney disease in pregnancy, and although commonly managed by obstetricians alone, the nephrologist is frequently called as a consultant in cases of severe preeclampsia especially when multiorgan system involvement is present. The classification schema of hypertensive disorders in pregnancy is one that has been in use for many years in the United States, and has been endorsed by The National High Blood Pressure Education Program and the American College of Obstetricians and Gynecologists (Table 2).

TABLE 2

Classification of Hypertensive Disorders in Pregnancy

Preeclampsia

Chronic hypertension

Chronic hypertension with superimposed preeclampsia

Transient hypertension

Preeclampsia

This disorder is unique to pregnancy and is a systemic maternal syndrome characterized by hypertension, proteinuria, edema, and at times coagulation and liver function abnormalities, as well as a fetal syndrome characterized by poor placentation, growth restriction, and at times death. Eclampsia is the convulsive form of preeclampsia. Preeclampsia usually develops in the third trimester, less frequently in the second trimester, and extremely rarely as early as 20 weeks gestation. The syndrome is more common in nulliparous women. Preexisting renal disease, hypertension, or diabetes also increase risk. Additional risk factors include multiple gestations, positive family history, extremes of reproductive age, and hydatiform mole. Hypertension in pregnancy is defined as a blood pressure of 140/90 mm Hg or greater (Korotkoff V). When preeclampsia develops close to term in previously healthy nulliparous women it is not likely to recur. However, women with early, severe preeclampsia, particularly those who are multiparous, may have a recurrence rate as high as 50%.

The cause of preeclampsia is not known. It is clearly more than a hypertensive disorder and affects many organ systems including brain, liver, kidney, blood vessels, and placenta. Although the focus may be on hypertension and proteinuria, it is important to recognize that such signs and symptoms may be minimal while other, life-threatening syndromes develop including convulsions and liver failure, both often associated with thrombocytopenia. Current research regarding pathophysiology has focused on the alterations in maternal endothelial cell function that are present, including reductions in nitric oxide and prostacylin, and increased endothelin. There is evidence that the placenta may be critically involved in the genesis of preeclampsia, and failure of trophoblastic invasion of the uterine spiral arteries is one of the earliest changes in this disorder. Failure of trophoblast to invade these vessels results in more constricted spiral arteries, and decreased placental perfusion.

The characteristic renal histologic lesion seen in preeclampsia is called glomerular capillary endotheliosis. The glomerular capillary endothelial cells are swollen, and the appearance is that of a "bloodless glomerulus." There are several alterations in renal function in women with preeclampsia, although as already mentioned, preeclampsia is rarely associated with significant renal failure. Both GFR and RPF decrease in preeclampsia, with decrements on average about 25% in most instances, such that GFR remains above pregravid values in most cases. Changes occur in the renal handling of urate in preeclampsia. There is decreased uric acid clearance, accompanied by an increase in blood levels which

may in fact precede other clinical signs of the disease. In pregnancy, serum urate levels above 4.5 mg/dL are suspect. The level of hyperuricemia has been observed to correlate with the severity of the preeclamptic renal lesion. Increased proteinuria is an important feature of preeclampsia, and the diagnosis is suspect in its absence. The magnitude of the proteinuria (which may range from minimal to massive) does not appear to affect maternal prognosis, although severe proteinuria is associated with greater fetal loss. Calcium handling is also altered in preeclampsia. Marked hypocalciuria is often seen in preeclampsia, possibly due to increased proximal tubular reabsorption, as well as increased distal tubular reabsorption which may be mediated by excess parathyroid hormone.

Management of preeclampsia includes accurate early diagnosis, bed rest, judicious use of antihypertensive therapy, close monitoring of both maternal and fetal condition, prevention of convulsions with magnesium sulfate, and appropriately timed delivery. Once the diagnosis of preeclampsia is suspected, in all but the mildest cases, hospitalization is advisable. Rest is an important aspect of therapy, as it improves uteroplacental perfusion. Delivery should be considered in all cases at term, and in cases remote from term when there are signs of impending eclampsia (hyperreflexia, headaches, epigastric pain) or when blood pressure cannot be controlled. Most obstetricians consider the development of the HELLP syndrome to be an indication for delivery. The rationale for lowering blood pressure is to prevent the adverse consequences of accelerated hypertension in the mother. Lowering blood pressure does not "cure" preeclampsia, and there is even some concern that aggressive lowering of blood pressure will compromise uteroplacental perfusion, which may be hazardous to fetal well-being. Although there is no consensus regarding what level of blood pressure should be treated in women with preeclampsia, levels that exceed 150/100 mm Hg may be hazardous in women who previously had low–normal blood pressures. Parenteral therapy is recommended when delivery is likely to take place in the next 24 hr (Table 3). If it appears that delivery can be safely postponed, an oral agent is advisable. Magnesium sulfate is an effective agent for the prevention of eclamptic convulsions. Although it is not considered to be an antihypertensive agent, it does in fact lower blood pressure to a mild degree in some women. This agent is usually prescribed immediately after delivery,

TABLE 3

Antihypertensive Therapy in Preeclampsia

Imminent delivery	Delivery postponed
Hydralazine (intravenous, intramuscular)	Methyldopa
Labetolol (intravenous)	Labetolol, other β-blockers
Calcium channel blockers	Calcium channel blockers
Diazoxide (intravenous)	Hydralazine α-blockers Clonidine

since convulsions are most likely to occur in the immediate postpartum period. Magnesium is occasionally administered antepartum; however, it may slow the progress of labor, and may complicate anesthesia and intraoperative monitoring during cesarean section.

Prevention of preeclampsia has not been successful so far. Although earlier small studies suggested that either low-dose aspirin or calcium supplementation might be beneficial, subsequent large, placebo controlled trials have all failed to demonstrate a significant benefit of these prophylactic strategies. An exception to this is women with antiphospholipid antibody syndrome or other thrombophilias (e.g., protein S deficiency, protein C deficiency, Factor V Leiden mutation) who are at risk for early, severe recurrent preeclampsia. Anticoagulation has been shown to benefit women with antiphospholipid antibody syndrome (heparin and aspirin throughout pregnancy), and these results have led some to recommend treating other thrombophilias with similar approaches, although there are no published data regarding benefits of treatment. Although calcium supplementation was more recently shown to be ineffective in preventing preeclampsia in low risk nulliparous women ingesting a normal calcium diet, there are no data regarding high risk women. Moreover, there are compelling data that women in developing nations who ingest a calcium supplemented diet experience fewer hypertensive complications in pregnancy than women who follow a low calcium diet.

Chronic Hypertension

Women with preexisting or chronic hypertension may have either essential or secondary hypertension. Most women with stage 1 or 2 essential hypertension do well during pregnancy, although they are at increased risk for the development of superimposed preeclampsia. This risk may be as high as 25%. Preexisting maternal hypertension is also associated with an increased risk of placental abruption, intrauterine growth restriction, and mid trimester fetal death.

Women with chronic hypertension often have reductions in blood pressure by the end of the first trimester, so that their blood pressures may not exceed that observed in normotensive pregnant women. The failure of this decrement to occur, or increases in blood pressure in early or midtrimester pregnancy indicates a guarded prognosis for the pregnancy. Fetal outcome is certainly worse in hypertensive women with superimposed preeclampsia compared to previously normotensive women who develop preeclampsia. Chronic hypertension with superimposed preeclampsia also seems responsible for most cases of cerebral hemorrhage in pregnancy.

The approach to treatment of chronic hypertension during pregnancy differs from the approach in the nonpregnant individual. In the latter case, the primary concern is reducing long-term cardiovascular risk. In the former case the concern is maintaining maternal health during the period of gestation, and maintaining a favorable intrauterine environment to allow fetal maturity, while minimizing fetal exposure to potentially harmful drugs. There are few data to support a target level of blood pressure that should be attained during pregnancy. There are also no data that suggest that maintaining blood pressure levels close to normal prevents the development of superimposed preeclampsia. Thus, a reasonable strategy is to treat maternal hypertension when levels of blood pressure are in excess of 145–150/95–100 mm Hg. The antihypertensive agents that are currently recommended during pregnancy as well as those that are considered contraindicated are listed in Table 4.

TABLE 4
Antihypertensive Drugs and Pregnancy

Alpha 2 adrenergic receptor agonists
Methyldopa is the most extensively used drug in this group. Its safety and efficacy are supported by evidence from randomized trials and a 7.5-year follow-up study of children born to mothers treated with this agent.

β adrenergic receptor antagonists
These drugs appear to be safe and efficacious in late pregnancy, but fetal growth restriction has been reported when treatment was started in early or midgestation. Fetal bradycardia can occur, and animal studies suggest that the ability of the fetus to tolerate hypoxic stress may be compromised

α adrenergic receptor and β adrenergic receptor antagonists
Labetolol is as effective as methyldopa, but there is limited information regarding follow up of children born to mothers given labetolol. Rare cases of hepatotoxicity have been reported.

Arterial vasodilators
Hydralazine is frequently used as adjunctive therapy with methyldopa and β-adrenergic antagonists. Rarely, neonatal thrombocytopenia has been reported. Trials with calcium channel blockers look promising. The experience with minoxidil is limited, and this drug is not recommended.

Calcium channel blockers
Small uncontrolled studies, and a meta-analysis suggests that these agents are safe and effective in pregnancy. There is limited information regarding follow up of children exposed to calcium channel blockers *in utero*.

Angiotensin converting enzyme inhibitors
Captopril causes fetal death in diverse animal species, and several converting enzyme inhibitors have been associated with oligohydramnios and neonatal renal failure when administered to humans. Do not use in pregnancy. Advise women of childbearing age who are taking these agents to inform their physician of their intent to conceive so that alternative therapy can be selected.

Angiotensin II receptor blockers
These drugs have not been used in pregnancy. In view of the deleterious effects of blocking angiotensin II generation, angiotensin II receptor antagonists are also considered to be contraindicated in pregnancy.

Diuretics
Many authorities discourage the use of diuretics, but others continue these medications if they were prescribed before conception or there is evidence of salt sensitivity

Although secondary hypertension is considerably less common than essential hypertension, failure to recognize the presence of these entities can result in adverse pregnancy outcomes. Renal disease is the most common form of secondary hypertension, and has already been discussed. Both pheochromocytoma and renovascular hypertension are associated with poor maternal and fetal prognosis. Accelerated hypertension, superimposed preeclampsia, and fetal demise are more common. Women with primary aldosteronism may have relatively uncomplicated pregnancies, particularly if hypertension is only stage 1. However, if more severe hypertension is present, pregnancy may be complicated and dangerous. It is preferable to diagnose secondary hypertension prior to conception. If women are first seen after conception, then blood and urine tests can be performed to rule out pheochromocytoma, and to screen for primary aldosteronism. However, in view of the normal stimulation of the renin–angiotensin–aldosterone system in pregnancy, plasma renin and aldosterone levels may be difficult to interpret during pregnancy. Renovascular hypertension is also difficult to diagnose during pregnancy. Improved technical results with magnetic resonance angiography can aid in anatomic diagnosis of renal artery lesions. Angioplasty has been performed successfully in early second trimester, and should be considered in women with severe, poorly controlled hypertension, particularly if previous pregnancies have been complicated by severe preeclampsia in association with fetal complications (e.g., early delivery, growth restriction, demise).

Transient Hypertension

This category refers to women with late pregnancy hypertension, without other features suggestive of preeclampsia. Among nulliparas, some patients may be preeclamptics who have not manifested other signs of the disease. Some women develop hypertension in two or more pregnancies and become normotensive after delivery. These women are likely to develop essential hypertension later in life.

Bibliography

Armenti VT, Ahlswede KM, Ahlswede BA, Cater JR, Jarrell BE, Moritz MJ, Burke JF: Variables affecting birthweight and graft survival in 197 pregnancies in cyclosporine-treated female kidney transplant recipients. *Transplantation* 59:476–479, 1995.

August P, Mueller FB, Sealey JE, Edersheim TG: Role of renin–angiotensin system in blood pressure regulation in pregnancy. *Lancet* 345:896–897, 1995.

August P, Lindheimer MD: Chronic hypertension in pregnancy. In: Lindheimer MD, Roberts JM, Cunningham FG (eds) *Chesley's Hypertensive Disorders in Pregnancy,* 2nd Ed., pp. 605–633. Appleton & Lange, Stamford, CT, 1999.

Baylis C: Glomerular filtration and volume regulation in gravid animal models. *Clin Obstet Gynaecol* 1:789, 1987.

Brown MA, Sinosich MJ, Saunders DM, Gallery EDM: Potassium regulation and progesterone–aldosterone interrelationships in human pregnancy. A prospective study. *Am J Obstet Gynecol* 155:349, 1986.

Bucher HC, Guyatt GH, Cook RJ, Hatala R, Cook DJ, Lang JD, Hunt D: Effect of calcium supplementation on pregnancy-induced hypertension and preeclampsia: A meta-analysis of randomized controlled trials. *JAMA* 275:1113–1117, 1996.

Chapman AB, Johnson AM, Gabow PA: Pregnancy outcome and its relationship to progression of renal failure in autosomal dominant polycystic kidney disease. *J Am Soc Nephrol* 5:1178–1185, 1994.

CLASP Collaborative Group. CLASP: A randomized trial of low-dose aspirin for the prevention and treatment of preeclampsia among 9364 pregnant women. *Lancet* 343:619–629, 1994.

Davison JM, Shiells EA, Philips PR, Lindheimer MD: Serial evaluation of vasopressin release and thirst in human pregnancy: Role of chorionic gonadotropin in the osmoregulatory changes of gestation. *J Clin Invest* 81:798, 1988.

Hou S: Pregnancy in chronic renal insufficiency and end-stage renal disease. *Am J Kidney Dis* 33:235–252, 1999.

Jones DC, Hayslett JP: Outcome of pregnancy in women with moderate or severe renal insufficiency. *N Engl J Med* 335:226–232, 1996.

Jungers P, Chauveau D: Pregnancy in renal disease. *Kidney Int* 52:871–885, 1997.

Lim VS, Katz AI, Lindheimer MD: Acid–base regulation in pregnancy. *Am J Physiol* 231:1764, 1976.

Lindheimer MD, Davison JM: Renal biopsy during pregnancy: "To b . . . or not to b . . ." *Br J Obstet Gynecol* 94:932, 1987.

Lindheimer MD, Richardson DA, Ehrlich EN, Katz AI: Potassium homeostasis in pregnancy. *J Reprod Med* 32:517, 1987.

Okundaye IB, Agrinko P, Hou S: A registry for pregnancy in dialysis patients. *Am J Kidney Dis* 31:766–773, 1998.

Saltiel C, Legendre C, Grunfeld JP, Descamps JM, Hecht M: Hemolytic uremic syndrome in association with pregnancy. In: Kaplan BS, Trompeter RS, Moake JL (eds), *Hemolytic Uremic Syndrome and Thrombotic Thrombocytopenic Purpura,* pp. 241–254. Dekker, New York, 1992.

Sibai BM: Drug therapy: Treatment of hypertension in pregnant women. *N Engl J Med* 335:257–265, 1996.

Sibai BM, Kustermann L, Velasco J: Current understanding of severe preeclampsia, pregnancy-associated hemolytic uremic syndrome, thrombotic thrombocytopenic purpura, hemolysis, elevated liver enzymes, and low platelet syndrome, and postpartum acute renal failure: Different clinical syndromes or just different names? *Curr Opin Nephrol Hypertens* 3:436–445, 1994.

57

THE KIDNEY IN AGING

NEESH PANNU AND PHILIP F. HALLORAN

The age-related changes in kidney function are relatively predictable and easily measured, making renal aging an interesting problem in its own right and a general model for the aging process. From middle age onward, the kidney undergoes a series of both structural and functional changes resulting in a rise in renal vascular resistance and a decline in renal plasma flow and glomerular filtration rate (GFR). These changes proceed slowly but in the presence of other diseases such as diabetes, hypertension, and heart disease, the kidney becomes vulnerable to failure. Clinical studies would suggest that the elderly are a heterogeneous population and that people in excellent health can have normal GFRs at age 80. Thus the effects of aging on renal function are often difficult to separate from the effects of the common age-related comorbidities, and the phenotype of the old kidney in a medical population represents a composite of age and age-related disease effects.

MOLECULAR THEORIES OF AGING

The term aging is difficult to define. The term renal senescence describes the phenotype of the aged kidney. The term replicative senescence is applied to the phenotype of somatic cells in culture, which have reached their finite number of replications (Hayflick limit) and have irreversibly stopped cycling. The relationship between the *in vivo* senescence phenotype and the *in vitro* phenotype of replicative senescence is not established.

It is well recognized in humans that senescence is accompanied by a loss of cell mass. This cell loss is result of two processes: continuing stress ("normal" wear and tear as well as abnormal stresses) coupled with a finite capacity to repair. Presumably the senescence phenotype reflects changes in the remaining cells. There are two major theories in the current medical literature that attempt to explain tissue senescence.

Accumulated Damage over Time: Role of Oxidation

Most cells are exposed to oxygen, some forms of which are reactive (reactive oxygen intermediates or ROI) and can damage biological components—DNA, membrane lipids, and proteins. ROI consists of toxic free radicals such as superoxide anion, hydrogen peroxide, and hydroxyl radicals, which are natural by-products of cellular metabolism. Successful organisms have antioxidant mechanisms, but

they are not completely effective, leaving some oxidant injury—a slow burn. Other biochemical changes such as the accumulation of advanced glycosylation end products (AGE) generated by cellular metabolism cumulatively damage postmitotic cells and limit their eventual survival. The proposed role of AGE comes from experimental evidence that the interaction between AGE and cell receptors results in functional changes similar to aging.

Genomic Damage

The "telomere shortening theory" explains the Hayflick limit in culture. Somatic cells in culture cannot replicate the end of each chromosome (the telomere) completely because they lack telomerase. Each cell cycle results in a loss of a number of base pairs. When the telomere is critically short, the cell senses this as DNA damage and shuts itself off, altering gene expression in the process. The senescent cell does not necessarily die: it may survive and compromise the biology of the tissue in still unknown ways. It is not yet clear whether senescent cells accumulate in renal senescence *in vivo*. However, telomere shortening does occur in the human kidney cortex with age. Whether this contributes to the senescence phenotype is not clear. Damage to mitochondrial DNA could also contribute to aging.

Genetic Programs and Programmed Cell Death

Senescence could result from a genetic program inherent in all living organisms. Some cells are programmed to die at a certain time, such as the tadpole tail. However, genetic programming may be less likely than cumulative injury and finite repair as an explanation for renal senescence.

PATHOLOGY OF RENAL AGING

One hallmark of senescence is the loss of renal mass. Renal mass reaches 400 g by the fourth decade, then declines to less than 300 g by the ninth decade. This loss of mass is primarily in the cortex, with relative sparing of the medulla. Sclerosis of the small arteries is presumably the morphological counterpart to the rise in renal vessel resistance. The selective atrophy of the afferent and efferent arterioles in the juxtamedullary glomeruli causes direct channel formation between afferent and efferent arterioles. Global sclerosis (not focal sclerosis) of glomeruli results in nephrons dropping out, presumably reflecting the changes in small vessels. This process accounts for the observation of increased glomerulosclerosis with age, estimated to be 10–30% by age 65, and therefore decreased numbers of functioning glomeruli. The morphological changes observed in apparently disease-free human studies are described in Table 1.

The glomerular changes in humans include an increase in mesangial matrix followed by thickening of the glomerular basement membrane. In a process called glomerular simplification, intraglomerular anastomoses appear and the number of capillary loops decrease. Eventually, the afferent and efferent arterioles atrophy and the glomerular tuft collapses and scleroses. In the medulla, the associated vascular changes, specifically the direct joining of afferent and efferent arterioles, may maintain renal medullary perfusion in the face of ongoing cortical atrophy. Tubular and interstitial changes occur in parallel and are described above.

At a biochemical level, the chemical composition of the glomerular basement membrane appears to change with age with increased glycosylation of proteins and glycosaminoglycans. It is not clear that human glomeruli actually show increased collagen or other basement membrane components relative to their size. The focal sclerosis often seen in aging rats is not seen in human glomeruli.

These structural changes of renal senescence resemble some changes of chronic renal failure, especially those seen in hypertension. Whether this simply reflects the presence of subclinical renal disease, instead of normal aging, is yet to be determined, but renal disease mechanisms (e.g., cyclosporine, diabetes, bacterial infection, hypertension,

chronic vasoconstriction in heart failure) would represent a stress which could accelerate aspects of the senescent phenotype.

FUNCTIONAL CHANGES IN RENAL AGING

Methodological Difficulties in Studying Renal Aging

There are a number of problems inherent in studying senescent changes in aged humans: the selection of patient population, the definition of "normal," and a lack of suitable animal models. Aging will produce the senescence phenotype in healthy humans but age-related diseases can accelerate this phenotype and add additional features, thus each study must identify whether it has included or excluded the age-related diseases. The studies may be cross-sectional or longitudinal. The cross-sectional studies reflect a typical unselected medical population, and show a decline of renal function by about 10%/decade after age 30. This observed decline in renal function may represent the effects of hypertension, heart failure, and subclinical renal disease which accelerate renal senescence.

There has only been one longitudinal study to date that has examined the issue of age-related changes in renal function with exclusion of all renal disease and hypertension—the Baltimore Longitudinal Study of Aging (BLSA). The BLSA studied 884 self-recruited community dwelling men over a 10-year period. These participants were divided into separate study groups on the basis of comorbidity and further stratified by age in decades. Creatinine clearance was determined using 24-hr urine collections. The study found that in the healthy cohort one-third of the study subjects showed no decline in GFR over a 20-year period and displayed normal GFR at age 80. The observed decline in GFR reported in the study was associated primarily with cardiovascular diseases. These observations suggest that the "age-related" decline in GFR that we commonly observe in elderly patients reflects the accelerating effect of comorbid conditions (hypertension, heart failure), and that the intrinsic rate of renal senescence is actually much slower. One illustrative example is the finding of reduced renal function in those with asymptomatic bacteriuria. Table 2 summarizes the functional changes commonly associated with aging.

In addition to the morphological changes that have been described in relation to the aging process, there are also dramatic changes in renal hemodynamics and renal function.

TABLE I
Age-Related Changes in Kidney Morphology

Macroscopic changes	Decreased weight and size Cortical atrophy
Vascular changes	Arterial sclerosis: loss of media, fibrosis of the intima Arterial hyalinosis Obliteration of afferent arterioles in cortex Direct channel between afferent and efferent arterioles in juxtamedullary glomeruli
Glomerular changes	Increased number of sclerosed glomeruli Thickening of basement membrane Mesangial matrix expansion Fusion of foot processes
Tubular changes	Reduction in numbers of tubules Atrophy of tubular epithelium Tubular dilatation Thickening of basement membrane
Interstitial changes	Interstitial fibrosis

Renal Blood Flow

Renal blood flow (RBF) declines by approximately 10% per decade after the age 40, as evidenced by the observation that renal plasma flow (RPF) decreases from 600 mL/min/1.73 m^2 at age 30, to 300 mL/min/1.73 m^2 by age 90. This reduction is accompanied by increased afferent and efferent arteriolar resistance. Xenon washout studies have demonstrated that decreased RBF is not entirely attributable to loss of renal mass. In fact, the decline in RBF with

TABLE 2
Functional Changes Related to Renal Aging

Renal blood flow (RBF)	Decreases by 10% per decade after age 40
Glomerular filtration rate (GFR)	Variable, but generally observed to decline by 7.5% per decade (0.75 ml/min/1.73 m/year) after age 40
Fluid/electrolyte handling	Decreased ability to retain sodium with severe sodium restriction and to excrete sodium when sodium loaded
Concentrating/diluting ability	Decreased concentrating and diluting ability as compared to young controls, of little clinical significance
Acid/base balance	Decreased ammonium excretion, mild metabolic acidosis
Hormonal changes	A 40–60% decline in plasma renin after age 65, decreased aldosterone responsiveness

age results in decreased blood flow per unit of renal mass. In addition, the reduction in RBF is not uniform in the kidney; there is a selective decline in cortical blood flow with sparing of the juxtamedullary glomeruli.

The cause of reduced blood flow and increased vascular resistance has not been identified. Anatomical studies performed using postmortem angiography suggest that over time there is increased irregularity and tortuosity of the preglomerular vessels and tapering of the afferent arterioles. There is also a loss of vasodilator responsiveness to such stimuli as amino acids or to L-arginine. One postulated mechanism is a decrease in nitric oxide production or activity; other potential explanations include impaired baroreflexes, increased renal sympathetic activity, or a derangement in thromboxane/prostacyclin equilibrium.

Functional Changes—GFR

Cross-sectional studies report a slow decline in GFR after the fourth decade of life. The GFR falls more slowly than RBF owing to an increase in filtration fraction. The shunting of renal blood flow to the juxtamedullary glomeruli enhances this phenomenon. As previously discussed, the BLSA is the only published study that has corroborated this finding in both the cross-sectional and longitudinal aspects of the study. Those "normal" patients who had undergone repeated studies of renal function showed a progressive decline in GFR after the age of 50 of approximately 0.75 mL/min/1.73 m²/year. However, it is important to note that 35% of the study subjects had no decline in GFR over the study period, suggesting that there is no predictable relationship between GFR and age. A number of theories have been proposed to explain this observation, and it is likely that part of the decline in GFR with age may be attributable to increased protein intake.

No corresponding increase in serum creatinine was observed in the previous studies because the decline in GFR was accompanied by a proportional decline in lean body mass, resulting in a decreased urinary creatinine excretion rate. This fall in the creatinine excretion rate is important because using serum creatinine alone as an index of renal function will overestimate GFR.

Attempts to express the relationship between GFR, creatinine, and age have led to the development of a number of mathematical equations including the Cockcroft–Gault formula, derived from a cross-sectional study of hospitalized patients.

$$CrCl\ mL/min = \frac{(140 - age) \times weight\ (kg)}{72 \times serum\ Cr\ (mg/dL)}.$$

Although these equations have gained widespread acceptance as a way to predict creatinine clearance, they were developed and validated on selected populations, which may not necessarily represent the patient populations on which they are used. Unfortunately no study has compared the use of a calculated creatinine clearance to the gold standards, inulin or ^{131}I-iothalamate clearance.

Fluid/Electrolyte Balance

No electrolyte abnormalities are specifically associated with aging, however the mechanisms of homeostasis are less able to deal with acute illness and with extremes of loading or depletion, leaving the elderly vulnerable to fluid and electrolyte imbalance.

Although sodium handling is one of the most important functions of the kidney, relatively little is known about how this is affected by age. What has been observed is that aged kidneys appear to have a limited capacity to conserve sodium in the face of sodium restriction, and to excrete sodium in conditions of sodium excess. One possible explanation is that a decrease in the number of functioning nephrons with age leads to an increased solute load per nephron. The clinical consequences of this altered sodium handling may be a slight tendency toward volume depletion in low-salt intake states and a higher frequency of salt sensitive hypertension in those with higher amounts of dietary sodium.

Concentrating/Diluting Ability

Urinary concentrating ability declines with increasing age. Healthy elderly subjects after 12 hr of water deprivation have lower urine concentrations as compared with younger subjects. This decrease in concentrating ability is not due solely to a decline in GFR as no such correlation could be made in one study. The two hypotheses that have been put forward by various investigators include increased medullary blood flow and subsequent solute washout, and inadequate response to antidiuretic hormone (ADH) owing to tubulointerstitial structural changes. At the opposite end of the spectrum, elderly subjects are also less able to decrease their urine osmolality than younger subjects after a 20 mL/kg water load (52 versus 92 mOsmol/kg).

Acid/Base

Despite the substantial changes in the aging kidney, the blood pH, $p\text{CO}_2$, and serum bicarbonate are well preserved. Older patients often have a prolonged response to acid loading, but are able to achieve the same degree of urinary acidification as younger subjects. Ammonium generation may be mildly impaired, and the elderly excrete a greater proportion of acid as titratable acidity. Thus renal senescence results in a mild subclinical metabolic acidosis.

The Renin–Angiotensin–Aldosterone Axis

Age-related changes include a decline in plasma renin activity, resulting in a 40–60% drop in levels by age 65. This fall in renin levels is due to impaired renin synthesis and release. The response to renin may also be blunted in the elderly, as is the case with aldosterone. Angiotensin II levels are not affected by age.

CLINICAL CONSEQUENCES OF AGE-RELATED CHANGE

Drug Pharmacokinetics

Age-related changes in body composition and renal function have important implications for drug dosing. Serum albumin tends to decline, resulting in higher free drug levels, particularly for those that are highly protein bound. The volume of distribution is also substantially different with increasing age. Total body water and lean body mass decrease with age, resulting in a decrease in the volume of distribution, therefore potentially increasing serum levels of drugs such as digoxin that normally distribute in body water. The elderly are less able to clear renally excreted medications due to the age-related decline in GFR. Although drug dosages are routinely altered for increases in serum creatinine to reflect decreased renal excretion, there is often a failure to modify drug dosing in the elderly to account for the 30 to 40% reduction in GFR. From a transplantation perspective, the nephrotoxicity of calcineurin inhibitors is more apparent in both allografts from older renal donors and native kidneys in older patients with nonrenal transplants.

The Interaction between Age and Acute Renal Failure

Acute renal failure (ARF) is most frequent among the aged, mainly due to the comorbidities and the interventions they require. Reports from individual centers indicate that about half of all acute renal failure occurs in persons greater than age 65. This number is disproportionately high compared to the number of patients hospitalized in this age group. The aged are at risk for four reasons: (1) the decline in renal function associated with age, (2) polypharmacy, many medications such as diuretics, laxatives, nonsteroidal antiinflammatory drugs (NSAIDS), antibiotics, and angiotensin converting enzyme (ACE) inhibitors are potentially nephrotoxic, (3) comorbidity and intercurrent illness, and (4) the prevalence of obstructive uropathy.

The etiology of ARF among the elderly is difficult to determine as the available studies vary in terms of definitions of elderly and ARF. Prerenal failure is the most commonly reported cause of ARF among the elderly because of their tendency toward sodium loss and volume depletion. Dehydration, decreased cardiac output, and the use of vasoactive medications in this susceptible population account for the majority of cases of prerenal failure.

Two vasoactive drugs with widespread use in the elderly include ACE inhibitors and NSAIDs. Acute renal failure due to ACE inhibitor use is second only to antibiotics as the most frequent cause of drug-induced renal failure. Several risk factors for the development of ARF during ACE inhibitor treatment include sodium restriction, impaired renal function, renal artery stenosis, heart failure, and diuretic use. Elderly patients are also at risk for developing NSAID-related nephrotoxicity.

Among those elderly patients who are biopsied for ARF, acute glomerulonephritis, acute tubular necrosis (ATN), and vascular disease are the most common findings. Rapidly progressive glomerulonephritis, which makes up half of all cases, is known to be more prevalent in geriatric populations and carries a poor prognosis.

ATN due to antibiotics or radiocontrast dye are also common causes of ARF. Age is a risk factor for both gentamicin and radiocontrast nephropathy. In a prospective study of 183 patients over age 70 who received radiocontrast dye, 11% had an increase in serum creatinine greater than 0.5 mg/dL. ATN due to sepsis or surgery is also more common in this age group.

Urinary obstruction is one of the most important causes of ARF in the elderly because it is reversible. Benign prostatic hypertrophy is extremely common among elderly men affecting 50% by age 50 and up to 90% by the age of 90. All elderly men presenting with ARF should be catheterized and undergo a renal ultrasound to rule out obstruction.

There is considerable controversy as to whether age is an independent predictor of prognosis in ARF. Several studies have identified age as a poor prognostic factor using both univariate and multivariate analysis, whereas others have failed to corroborate this finding. These studies all differ in terms of their definitions of ARF, the setting of ARF, as well as the place of treatment. It should be noted that many of the severity indexes currently used in ICU studies include age as a prognostic factor. The outcome in ARF continues to be disappointingly pessimistic, with mortality rates in the range of 40–50%, and even higher in the ICU setting. Although few studies have looked at long-term renal survival in ARF in the geriatric population, it is generally believed that older patients have a prolonged time to renal recovery and achieve a lower level of renal function.

The High Incidence of ESRD in the Elderly

The elderly are the fastest growing population of patients requiring renal replacement therapy, due both to changing demographics—the aging population—and to changing referral patterns. The European Dialysis and Transplantation

Association (EDTA) registry reported that patients greater that 65 years of age made up 9% of patients in ESRD programs in 1977, 38% of patients in 1992, and 45% of patients in 1995. A similar increase shift is evident in the United States in the U.S. Renal Data System (USRDS), the elderly account for 46% of patients in end stage renal disease (ESRD) programs, of which 20% overall are greater than age 75. This influx of the elderly has influenced the predominance of various forms of renal disease, and diabetes and renovascular disease now account for 66% of all cases. Among the elderly, renovascular disease (including hypertension) is the main cause of ESRD (38%) in patients greater than 65 years of age. Many cases of ESRD in the elderly are not assigned a diagnosis. The interaction of disease mechanisms with the processes of senescence most likely account for the remarkable rise in ESRD in the elderly. This problem represents one of the great public health problems in nephrology in the developed world.

Bibliography

Anderson S, Brenner BM: Effects of aging on the renal glomerulus. *Am J Med* 80:435–442, 1986.

Baylis C, Schmidt R: The aging glomerulus. *Semin Nephrol* 16:265–276, 1996.

Bodnar AG, Ouellette M, Frolkis M, *et al.:* Extension of life-span by introduction of telomerase into normal human cells. *Science* 279:349–352, 1998.

Campo C, Lahera V, Garcia-Robles R, *et al.:* Aging abolishes the renal response to L-arginine infusion in essential hypertension. *Kidney Int* 49:S-126–S-128, 1996.

Cockcroft DW, Gault MH: Prediction of creatinine clearance from serum creatinine. *Nephron* 16:31–41, 1976.

Cortes P, Zhao X, Dumler F, *et al.:* Age-related changes in glomerular volume and hydroxproline content in rat and human. *J Am Soc Nephrol* 2 (12):1716–1725, 1992.

Epstein M, Hollenberg NK: Age as a determinant of renal sodium conservation in normal men. *J Lab Clin Med* 87:411–417, 1976.

Filser D, Zeier M, Nowack R, *et al.:* Renal functional reserve in healthy elderly subjects. *J Am Soc Nephrol* 3:1371–1377, 1993.

Filser D, Franek E, Joest M, *et al.:* Renal function in the elderly: Impact of hypertension and cardiac function. *Kidney Int* 51:1196–1204, 1997.

Halloran PF, Melk A, Barth C: Rethinking chronic allograft nephropathy—the concept of accelerated senescence [review]. *J Am Soc Nephrol* 10:167–181, 1999.

Hollenberg NK, Adams DF, Solomon HS, *et al.:* Senescence and the renal vasculature in normal man. *Circ Res* 34:309–316, 1974.

Johnson FB, Sinclair DA, Guarente L: Molecular biology of aging. *Cell* 96:291–302, 1999.

Jung FF, Kennefick TM, Ingelfinger JR, *et al.:* Down-regulation of the intrarenal renin–angiotensin system in the ageing rat. *J Am Soc Nephrol* 8:1573–1580, 1995.

Kasiske BL: Relationship between vascular disease and age-associated changes in the human kidney. *Kidney Int* 31:1153–1159, 1987.

Lewis WH, Jr, Alving AS: Changes with age in the renal function of adult men. I. Clearance of urea. II. Amount of urea nitrogen in the blood. III. Concentrating ability of the kidneys. *Am J Physiol* 123:500–515, 1938.

Lindeman RD, Lee TD Jr, Yiengst JJ: Influence of age, renal disease, hypertension, diuretics, and calcium on the antidiuretic response to suboptimal infusions of vasopressin. *J Lab Clin Med* 68:206–223, 1966.

Lindeman RD, Tobin J, Shock NW: Longitudinal studies on the rate of decline in renal function with age. *J Am Ger Soc* 33:278–285, 1985.

Luft FC, Grim CE, Fineberg N, *et al.:* Effects of volume expansion and contraction in normotensive whites, blacks and subjects of different ages. *Circulation* 59:644–650, 1979.

Melk A, Ramassar V, Helms LM, *et al.:* Telomere shortening in kidneys with age. *J Am Soc Nephrol* 11:444–453, 2000.

Pascual J, Liano F, Ortuno J: The elderly patient with acute renal failure. *J Am Soc Nephrol* 6:144–153, 1995.

Rowe JW, Shock NW, DeFronzo RA: The influence of age on the renal response to water deprivation in man. *Nephron* 17:270–278, 1976.

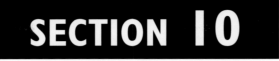

SECTION 10

CHRONIC RENAL FAILURE
AND ITS THERAPY

PATHOPHYSIOLOGY AND MANAGEMENT OF PROGRESSIVE CHRONIC RENAL FAILURE

ROBERTO PISONI AND GIUSEPPE REMUZZI

MECHANISMS OF RENAL DISEASE PROGRESSION

Stages of Progression

Once the glomerular filtration rate (GFR) falls below 25% of normal, renal function inevitably tends to decline even if the initial insult to the kidney has been eliminated. The progression typically moves through four phases: diminution of renal reserve, renal insufficiency, overt renal failure, and uremia with end stage renal disease (ESRD). A diminution of renal reserve happens when GFR is reduced up to 25% of normal. The patient is asymptomatic; azotemia is absent and acid–base, fluid, and electrolyte balance are maintained through an adaptive increase of function in the remaining nephrons. Renal insufficiency implies a reduction in GFR by 75%. The patient usually has no symptoms; azotemia is present and the serum creatinine is increased; levels of hormones such as erythropoietin, calcitriol, and parathyroid hormone (PTH) may be abnormal. Overt renal failure involves a further loss of renal mass. Symptoms, if present, are mild; patients may have anemia, acidosis, hypocalcemia, hyperphosphatemia, and hyperkalemia. This stage rapidly progresses to clinical uremia and to the need for renal replacement therapy through dialysis or transplant. The time when this therapy begins marks the onset of ESRD.

Measurement of Progression

Assessment of GFR continues to be the single most useful quantitative index of renal function in health and disease, and is currently used to determine the effectiveness of therapies designed to slow the progression of renal diseases. Rigorous assessment of GFR requires the measurement of renal clearance of a filtration marker such as inulin. This method, however, is not suitable for routine clinical practice. Radionuclides that are handled by the kidney in a fashion similar to inulin can provide accurate and precise GFR measurement, but their use may be limited for safety reasons. Procedures using minute doses of nonradioactive contrast agents, including iothalamate and iohexol can also be used. However, in everyday practice, the most widely utilized methods to estimate GFR are the serum creatinine concentration and creatinine clearance. Unfortunately, since creatinine metabolism is altered in chronic renal insufficiency, GFR measurements using creatinine are, at best, gross estimates. Thus other methods have been proposed, such as the reciprocal of the serum creatinine. Linear regression of reciprocal creatinine plotted against time produces a straight line in most patients, making it possible to predict the course of progression. Limitations of the reciprocal creatinine plot must, however, be kept in mind. When the GFR is above 60 mL/min/1.73 m^2 spontaneous variations in serum creatinine are large relative to the changes which occur as a result of the fall in GFR, and the slope of reciprocal serum creatinine is unreliable.

Risk Factors for Progression of Renal Disease

The rate of GFR decline varies depending on different factors. The amount of urinary protein strongly correlates with the renal outcome. In 840 patients with nondiabetic renal disease enrolled in the "Modification of Diet in Renal Disease" (MDRD) study, proteinuria was the strongest predictor of renal disease progression. The "Ramipril Efficacy in Nephropathy" (REIN) study showed that, in 352 patients with chronic nondiabetic proteinuric nephropathies, independently of the nature of the underlying disease, baseline urinary protein excretion rate was best single predictor of GFR decline and ESRD. The higher the urinary protein excretion, the faster the subsequent decline in GFR and the quicker the progression to ESRD. Patients with baseline urinary protein excretion <1.9 g/24 hr had the lowest rate of GFR decline and kidney failure over 3 years of follow-up, whereas patients with nephrotic range proteinuria (>3.9 g/24 hr) lost >10 mL/min/1.73 m^2 GFR/year with 30% kidney failure at 3 years.

Besides predicting the rate of renal progression, urinary protein excretion can be used to identify which patients would benefit most from renoprotective treatments. In the MDRD trial, patients with higher baseline proteinuria were those whose rate of GFR decline was reduced most by strict blood pressure control. Among patients with urinary protein excretion ≥3 g/24 hr in the REIN study, the beneficial effect of ramipril, an angiotensin I converting enzyme (ACE) inhibitor, in slowing the GFR decline and in reducing the risk of ESRD increased as the baseline level of proteinuria increased.

385

TABLE I
Risk Factors for Renal Disease Progression

Proteinuria >1.5 g/24 hr
Protein to creatinine ratio >1 g/g
Hypertension
Type of underlying renal disease
African-American race
Male sex
Obesity
Diabetes mellitus
Hyperlipidemia
Smoking
High protein diet
Phosphate retention
Metabolic acidosis

There is also evidence that, in nondiabetic proteinuric chronic nephropathies, the protein-to-creatinine (P/C) ratio in a single spot morning urine closely correlates with 24-hr protein excretion and predicts GFR decline and risk progression to ESRD even better than 24-hr protein excretion. A P/C ratio of more than 1.0 g/g distinguishes progressors from nonprogressors. This easy and inexpensive procedure can establish the severity and prognosis of renal disease and is less time-consuming than 24 hr collection. Furthermore, it avoids any error in urine collection.

Many studies have shown a direct association between hypertension and the rate of progression that is slowed by lowering blood pressure with antihypertensive agents. In the REIN study, mean arterial pressure (MAP) was predictive of GFR decline and kidney survival but to a lesser degree than 24-hr urinary protein excretion.

The type of renal disease also appears to be a risk factor for progression to ESRD: glomerulonephritis, diabetic and hypertensive nephropathies, and polycystic kidney disease, tend to progress faster than tubulointerstitial diseases. Finally, other variables such as race, male sex, diabetes mellitus, obesity, hyperlipidemia, cigarette smoking, metabolic acidosis, and phosphate retention may have some effects on renal disease progression (Table 1).

Pathophysiology of Progressive Renal Diseases

Almost 20 years ago, developments in experimental renal physiology led to the formulation of a unifying hypothesis for the progressive nature of renal disease: the "common pathway" theory. According to this scheme, the reduction in nephron number associated with the initial insult damaged the remaining intact nephrons. This damage was a consequence of the adaptive increases in glomerular pressure and flow that were required to sustain renal function.

In animals with experimental surgical reduction of renal mass, the surviving nephrons undergo sudden hypertrophy after the removal of a critical mass of renal tissue, and the concomitant lowering of renal arteriolar resistance leads to

an increase in glomerular plasma flow. Glomerular capillary pressure rises because the tone of afferent arterioles drops more than the tone in efferent ones, and more filtrate is formed per nephron. These hemodynamic changes help restore GFR in the short term, but they are detrimental in the long term, leading to renal functional and structural damage. Therapies such as dietary protein restriction, ACE inhibitors, and angiotensin receptor antagonists attenuate these maladaptive changes, minimize structural injury, and limit the GFR decline over time.

Animal and human studies have now shown that an essential feature of this process of progressive destruction of nephron units is the impaired glomerular perm-selectivity to proteins, secondary to glomerular capillary hypertension (Fig. 1). Abnormally filtered proteins may have intrinsic renal toxicity; they accumulate in the lumen of the proximal tubules and, after endocytosis into proximal tubular cells, contribute to renal interstitial injury through a complex cascade of intracellular events. Those include upregulation of vasoactive and inflammatory genes such as the endothelin-1 (ET-1) gene, the monocyte chemoattractant protein 1 (MCP-1) gene which encodes for an inflammatory peptide involved in macrophage and T-lymphocyte recruitment, and the RANTES (regulated on activation, normal T-cell expressed and secreted) that encodes for a chemotactic molecule for monocyte and memory T cells. These molecules, formed in excessive amounts, are secreted toward the basolateral side of tubular cells, giving rise to an inflammatory reaction.

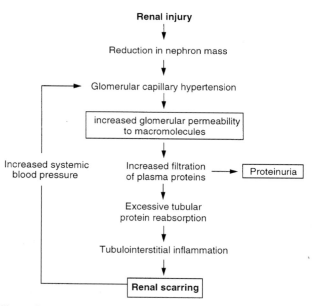

Figure 1 Schematic representation of the events leading to progressive renal damage. Excessive reabsorption of proteins as a consequence of increased glomerular permeability results in the accumulation of proteins in proximal tubular cells which may trigger activation of nuclear factor-κB (NF-κB) dependent and independent genes encoding chemokines, cytokines, and endothelin. Excessive synthesis of inflammatory and vasoactive substances contribute to fibroblast proliferation and interstitial inflammation.

Interstitial inflammation and progression of disease can be limited by drugs such as ACE inhibitors and angiotensin receptor antagonists that decrease glomerular perm-selectivity, reducing proteinuria and filtered protein-dependent signaling for mononuclear cell infiltration and extracellular matrix deposition. Complement components, also filtered across the glomerular barrier, can cause interstitial injury too. Other mechanisms and coexisting factors such as enhanced angiotensin II generation, glomerular hypertrophy, mesangial stretching, and macrophage infiltration are involved in chronic renal disease progression. Excess angiotensin II, besides mediating preferential vasoconstriction of the efferent arteriole and subsequent glomerular capillary hypertension, can directly increase the permeability of the glomerular barrier to proteins, thus enhancing the macromolecular flux into the mesangium, inducing cytokine release, glomerular cell proliferation, and mesangial matrix formation.

TREATMENT OF RENAL DISEASE PROGRESSION

The management of progressive chronic renal failure has several goals: first, to stop or to slow the rate of GFR decline; second, to prevent additional kidney damage caused by superimposed events; finally, to maintain nutritional status and prevent or limit the complications of chronic renal failure (CRF) and uremic syndrome.

ACE Inhibitors in Chronic Nephropathies

Any medication that reduces urinary protein excretion in humans also protects renal function from decline. The control of systemic blood pressure helps slow the progres-

sion of renal disease in diabetic and nondiabetic patients. In human nephropathies, ACE inhibitors are more reno-protective than other antihypertensive at comparable levels of blood pressure control; this appears to be because they lower urinary protein excretion more than other antihypertensive drugs. In patients with insulin-dependent diabetes mellitus (IDD) and overt nephropathy, the ACE inhibitor captopril preserved renal function better than conventional antihypertensive drugs and halved the combined risk of dialysis, transplantation, or death. Systemic blood pressure control was similar in the two treatment groups, but urinary protein excretion decreased with captopril and increased with other antihypertensives.

The same result was found in patients with urinary protein excretion ≥ 3 g/24 hr where ramipril was superior to other antihypertensives in limiting GFR decline and halved the combined risk of doubling serum creatinine or ESRD. These effects were associated with a reduction of the urinary protein excretion rate to below that expected for the degree of blood pressure lowering, indicating that the renoprotection was linked to the reduced protein traffic. Prolonged therapy with ramipril further limited the rate of GFR decline and the progression to ESRD (Fig. 2); GFR could be stablized in patients who continued ramipril therapy for more than 36 months.

The tendency of GFR to decline with time in chronic diabetic and nondiabetic nephropathies cannot only be slowed but also reversed, suggesting that long-term ACE inhibition therapy may even lead to remission of CRF at least in some patients. Ramipril was also renoprotective in patients with non-nephrotic proteinuria where it halved the risk of progression to ESRD or to persistent nephrotic range proteinuria, compared to other antihypertensives.

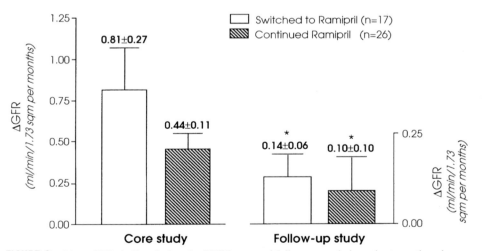

FIGURE 2 Mean GFR decline during the REIN core and follow-up study in patients continued on or switched to the ACE inhibitor ramipril. In the REIN core study, patients were randomized to ramipril or to placebo and other conventional antihypertensive drugs in order to achieve and maintain a comparable blood pressure control. At the end of the core study, patients continued on or shifted to ramipril and were formally enrolled into the follow-up study (12). Mean of the differences of GFR decline between the core and follow-up study was 0.34 (95% confidence interval (CI) 0.08–0.60) and 0.66 (95% CI 0.17–1.15) mL/min/m²/month in patients continued on or switched to ramipril, respectively. *p=0.017 versus core.

Safety of ACE Inhibitors

ACE inhibitors are generally well tolerated, but in patients with impaired renal function, hyperkalemia and acute declines in GFR may be observed. ACE inhibitors lower circulating angiotensin II and consequently the production of aldosterone, impairing potassium excretion which may already be reduced in patients with CRF. Acute renal failure is more likely to arise in patients with significant bilateral renovascular disease or volume depletion. Patients with hypertension, particularly if highly renin-dependent, are often given ACE inhibitors with a diuretic, and the marked fall in blood pressure and renal perfusion pressure may even cause acute renal failure, which is usually reversible on discontinuation of the drug and correction of the volume depletion. Thus, temporary withdrawal of diuretic therapy (for at least 24 hr) is recommended before the first dose of ACE inhibitors is administered in order to limit the risk of acute, symptomatic hypotension.

ACE inhibitors should always be started at lower doses and then progressively uptitrated according to tolerance and action on blood pressure and urinary protein excretion. Close follow-up measurements of serum potassium and creatinine are recommended; an evaluation of these parameters should be made before starting the ACE inhibitor therapy and repeated 7 days after the first administration and subsequent dose titrations. Monitoring of hematocrit is also advisable since long-term ACE inhibition may occasionally worsen the anemia of CRF.

The slight increase in serum creatinine ($<30\%$), which usually occurs early during ACE inhibitor therapy, reflects a hemodynamically mediated reduction in GFR that may be renoprotecive in the long term; thus it is not an indication for drug withdrawal. In contrast, withdrawal of the ACE inhibitor is recommended in patients with sustained hyperkalemia (>5.5 mEq/L), despite dietary potassium restriction, concomitant diuretic treatment, and effective correction of metabolic acidosis. In the REIN study, few patients needed to be withdrawn because of hyperkalemia or acute worsening of renal failure; ramipril was well tolerated even in patients with advanced renal insufficiency. Thus, the practice of avoiding ACE inhibitors in severe renal failure to prevent further renal impairment and hyperkalemia is not justified.

Strict Blood Pressure Control

Recent studies have found that reducing systolic and diastolic blood pressure to less than 130/80 mm Hg can slow the progression of diabetic and nondiabetic renal disease even more effectively than conventional blood pressure control. In the MDRD study, patients with chronic nephropathies of various cause were randomly assigned to a standard or low protein diet and to a conventional or low blood pressure goal. The patients assigned to the lower blood pressure target had a substantially slower mean decline of GFR than those assigned the conventional blood pressure goal. This beneficial effect of blood pressure control was more evident in the patients with higher baseline proteinuria. These findings led the authors to recommend considering the level of proteinuria when blood pressure goals are being set in patients with chronic nephropathy. In particular, they suggested a blood pressure goal of 125/75 mm Hg (MAP 92 mm Hg) or less in patients with >1 g/24 hr urinary proteins and 130/80 mm Hg (MAP 98 mm Hg) or less in those with proteinuria from 0.25 to 1 g/24 hr. This study suggested for the first time that, once close blood pressure goal is achieved and mantained, different antihypertensives may equally reduce urinary protein excretion and slow renal disease progression. This conclusion was biased by the fact that the lower blood pressure goal was achieved by a more liberal prescription of ACE inhibitors, but it is corroborated by a more recent meta-analysis performed in human diabetic nephropathy where the greater the blood pressure reduction the less the antiproteinuric response depends on the class of antihypertensive employed.

Dietary Protein Restriction

In rats with renal mass ablation and in animals with experimental diabetes and adriamycin nephropathy, a low protein diet prevents proteinuria and renal injury. Confirmation of a beneficial effect of dietary protein restriction in clinical trials has been inconclusive because of deficiencies in their design or because changes in renal function were assessed only by measurements of serum creatinine, which may be affected by diet. Recently, the MDRD study found only a nonsignificant trend toward a slower GFR decline in patients following a very low protein diet (0.28 g/kg body weight/day) which was consistent with a moderate effect of very low protein intake or of the keto acid and amino acid mixture that the subjects received. Nonetheless, there was no significant difference between the different diet groups in the time to the occurrence of ESRD. Thus, available data do not support protein restriction as an effective treatment to slow disease progression in chronic nephropathies. It seems, however, prudent to avoid a dietary protein intake in excess of 1 g/kg/day, and the protein intake should ideally be around 0.8 g/kg/day of high biological value proteins in patients with persistent heavy proteinuria and with CRF. Patients for whom a high protein intake is specifically prescribed for short-term management of malnutrition are exceptions. Whether dietary phosphorus reduction slows the progression of renal disease is still uncertain.

Management of Hyperlipidemia

Hyperlipidemia is common in patients with CRF, especially in those with nephrotic syndrome. In addition to accelerating the development of systemic atherosclerosis, experimental studies suggest that hyperlipidemia may enhance the rate of progressive glomerular injury. In animals, cholesterol loading enhances glomerular damage, and reducing lipid levels with a statin slows the rate of progressive renal injury. Moreover, the beneficial effect of lipid lowering may be additive to that of lowering blood pressure. The factors responsible for lipid effects are incompletely understood; it has been shown that hyperlipidemia stimulates mesangial cell proliferation and the synthesis of proinflammatory molecules which could contribute to glomerular injury. However, the clinical evidence on the role of controlling dyslipidemia in preventing the progression of renal disease is still lacking. Thus, the main goal of treatment of hyperlipidemia in CRF is actually the prevention of atherosclerotic disease. Circulating levels of low density lipoproteins (LDL) cholesterol less than 130 mg/dL has been recommended for patients without cardiovascular disease, whereas plasma values less than 100 mg/dL have been the target for those with cardiovascular disease or other forms of atherosclerotic disease. Diet and body weight reduction may help to improve the lipid profile, but often the use of statins, which are generally well tolerated, is necessary. However, potential liver and muscle toxicity, ranging from myalgias to myositis and rhabdomyolysis, possibly associated with myoglobinuric acute renal failure, should be taken into account. ACE inhibitors and angiotensin receptor antagonists often reduce serum lipids, and the magnitude of these changes appears to be related to the degree of fall in protein excretion.

Glycemic Control

In patients with type 1 diabetes mellitus, strict glucose control significantly reduces the rate of onset of micro- and macroalbuminuria as well as the incidence of microvascular complications, although it is associated with increases in the frequency of hypoglycemic crises and body weight. Thus, in these patients good metabolic control is recommended for primary prevention of diabetic nephropathy. Similarly, The UK Prospective Diabetes Study (UKPDS) 33 showed decreased incidence of microvascular complications (retinopathy) in patients with type 2 diabetes mellitus, when improved blood glucose control is achieved. However, in these patients the effect of strict metabolic control on primary and secondary prevention of nephropathy remains ill defined.

Future Aims

At present, close blood pressure control and ACE inhibitors are the most effective treatments to achieve remission in chronic progressive nephropathy. The low blood pressure target of the MDRD study (MAP 92 mm Hg) is recommended. It should be reached through a low sodium diet and an ACE inhibitor as first-choice treatment and as needed a diuretic or a β-blocker. It is important to reduce blood pressure gradually, especially in patients with autonomic neuropathy and arteriosclerosis.

Remarkable advances have been made in strategies aimed at preventing chronic renal disease progression, and avoiding ESRD is now a potentially achievable goal. High-dose ACE inhibitors, angiotensin receptor antagonists, the combination of both at lower dosages, and endothelin receptor antagonists are being evaluated. Questions remain about the renoprotective effects of nondihydropyridine calcium channel blockers and the best levels of blood pressure control (Table 2).

TABLE 2
Treatment Measures in Order to Achieve Remission in Chronic Progressive Nephropathy

Tight blood pressure control (MAP ≤92 mm Hg) using:
Low sodium diet
ACE inhibitors at high dosage
Angiotensin receptor antagonists
Diuretics
Nondihydropyridine calcium channel blockers

Dietary protein restriction

Glycemic control

Treatment of dyslipidemia

PREVENTION OF FURTHER KIDNEY DAMAGE DUE TO CONCOMITANT INJURIES

Beside slowing progression of the primary renal disease, it is important to protect patients with renal impairment from further nephrotoxic insults such as fluid depletion, malignant hypertension, urinary tract infection, obstruction, and drug toxicity. Intercurrent diseases must be treated promptly, and diligence must be applied in avoiding nephrotoxic drugs, if possible. Aminoglycosides are a common cause of acute renal failure and, even though it is usually reversible, residual damage is not rare.

Nonsteroidal antiinflammatory drugs (NSAIDs) inhibit the production of vasodilatatory prostaglandins in the kidney, and this can further impair GFR in patients with chronic renal failure. Drugs such as β-lactam antibiotics, sulfonamides, diuretics, and captopril can cause interstitial nephritis. Medications normally excreted by the healthy kidney can accumulate in the presence of reduced GFR, leading to renal and nonrenal side effects. It is important to adjust the drug dosage in relation to GFR in patients with chronic renal failure (see Chapter 41). Radiographic contrast agents can result in temporary or, occasionally, permanent loss of renal function. They should be avoided in patients at risk, but, if they are indispensable, the patient must be adequately hydrated before and after the procedure (see Chapter 34). Also, decisions to perform invasive procedures in patients with CRF must take into account the risk of renal injury. Arterial catheterization, for example, can cause atheroembolic renal disease which is often irreversible and progresses to ESRD (see Chapter 36). Care is needed in the preoperative management of patients with CRF, and it is important to correct any acid–base, electrolyte, and coagulative abnormalities. In women with CRF, pregnancy involves a risk of acceleration of the GFR decline, worsened hypertension and development of preeclampsia, urinary tract infections, cortical necrosis, intrauterine fetal growth retardation, and preterm delivery. Pregnant women with CRF should be followed closely with periodic serum creatinine tests and blood pressure measurements. Termination of pregnancy should be considered if GFR drops in the absence of clearly reversible causes or in the presence of uncontrolled hypertension. Pregnancy is inadvisable when the serum creatinine is more than 2–3 mg/dL. Pregnancy in renal disease is discussed in Chapter 56.

COMPLICATIONS OF CHRONIC RENAL DISEASE AND THE UREMIC SYNDROME: CLINICAL FEATURES AND TREATMENT

Chronic Renal Disease

In renal insufficiency the kidney progressively loses its regulatory capacity so that both excretion and conservation of water and electrolytes are altered. Thus, in case of sudden loads of fluid or electrolytes, signs of decompensation may occur. These complications of CRF can be divided into water, electrolyte, acid–base, metabolic, and organ–system disorders.

Water

Free water clearance is conserved until late in renal failure. In advanced renal failure, the reduced capacity of the kidney to concentrate or dilute urine may lead to hypernatremia or hyponatremia. Dehydration occurs easily in patients with inadequate fluid intake because of persisting diuresis. The reduced capacity for concentrating the urine is particularly common in patients with diseases affecting the renal medulla such as interstitial nephritis and pyelonephritis. Patients with a normal thirst mechanism and access to fluid will usually ingest an appropriate amount of fluid to match obligate losses. Careful attention to the fluid prescription is necessary when access to water is impaired by intercurrent illness.

Sodium

Maintaining sodium balance is very important in patients with CRF. Both sodium retention, with signs of fluid overload, and sodium depletion, with signs of fluid depletion, are common. In most patients with stable CRF, the total body sodium content is already increased but only slightly; major sodium retention is common when GFR falls below 10 mL/min/1.73 m^2 and in patients with concomitant nephrotic syndrome or cardiac failure. Sodium retention contributes to, or aggravates, hypertension, edema, and congestive heart failure. A sodium-restricted diet (less than 2 g/day) and loop diuretics are often required. On the other hand, sodium conservation may be impaired early in CRF, especially in tubulointerstitial disease.

Extrarenal causes of sodium loss (vomiting, diarrhea, fever) may lead to extracellular fluid volume depletion with thirst, dry mucous membranes, tachycardia, orthostatic hypotension, vascular collapse, dizziness, syncope, and a reversible fall in renal function. Apart from treating the underlying cause of sodium depletion, it may be necessary to give intravenous isotonic saline; diuretics, if used, must be temporarily withdrawn.

Potassium

Because of an adaptive increase in potassium excretion by the remnant nephrons, patients with CRF usually have a normal serum potassium concentration until oliguria occurs. However, in patients with metabolic acidosis, characterized by a shift in potassium from intracellular to extracellular fluids, and in hyporeninemic hypoaldosteronism (seen in tubulointerstitial disease and diabetes mellitus), hyperkalemia may develop early. Hyperkalemia can also arise from an acute potassium load or with drugs that alter potassium secretion such as ACE inhibitors, angiotensin receptor blockers, potassium-sparing diuretics, β-blockers, NSAIDs, cyclosporine, and tacrolimus. Acute management of hyperkalemia is discussed in Chapter 13. Dietary restriction is the mainstay of chronic management of hyperkalemia. Potassium-binding resins can be useful for long-term control but they are seldom necessary.

Spontaneous hypokalemia is uncommon in CRF, but it can be seen in salt-wasting nephropathy, Fanconi syndrome, hereditary or acquired tubulointerstitial diseases, and renal tubular acidosis. In patients with CRF, hypokalemia is usually due to low dietary potassium intake combined with high doses of diuretics, or to gastrointestinal loss.

Acid–Base Disorders

Acid–base balance is normally mantained by renal excretion of the daily acid load both as titratable acid (primarily phosphate) and as ammonium. With advancing renal failure (GFR below 25 mL/min), hydrogen ion excretion by the kidney is not sufficient to balance endogenous acid production or exogenous acid loads and chronic metabolic acidosis develops. As the patient approaches ESRD, the plasma bicarbonate concentration tends to stabilize between 12 and 20 mEq/L and rarely falls below 10 mEq/L. The treatment of mild acidosis (arterial pH >7.25) is desirable to prevent osteopenia and muscle catabolism. In fact, bone buffering of some of the excess hydrogen ions leads to the release of calcium and phosphate from bone which may worsen the bone disease. Moreover, uremic acidosis increases muscle breakdown. This may be exacerbated by a low protein diet and decreased albumin synthesis, leading to loss of lean body mass and muscle weakness. The muscle breakdown is in part due to the stimulated release of cortisol and decreased release of insulin-like growth factor-1 (IGF-1). These abnormalities in muscle function and albumin metabolism may be reversed by alkali therapy. In animals, the local accumulation of ammonia secondary to the increased acid excretion from each remaining nephron, has been shown directly to activate complement and induce tubulointerstitial injury that may be minimized by alkali therapy. However, in humans, the renal protective effect of alkali therapy is unproved. Metabolic acidosis may also induce abnormalities in the growth hormone (GH) axis, such as impaired pulsatile GH secretion and decreased secretion of IGF-1, that may contribute to the inibition of growth in children. Thus, the use of alkali therapy is recommended in patients with CRF in order to maintain a plasma bicarbonate concentration higher than 22 mEq/L. Sodium bicarbonate (in a daily dose of 0.5 to 1 mEq/kg) is the agent of choice; it is well tolerated and generally produces little or no sodium retention or increase in blood pressure. Sodium citrate (citrate is rapidly metabolized to bicarbonate) should be avoided in patients also receiving phosphate binders containing aluminum, because it increases intestinal aluminum absorption and the risk of aluminum intoxication.

Phosphate, Calcium, and Bone

Phosphate retention begins early in renal disease. Even during its initial and mild stage, it contributes to the development of the secondary hyperparathyroidism that plays an important role in the pathogenesis of renal osteodystrophy and in other uremic complications. Moreover, the excess phosphate may contribute to renal failure progression. This is probably due to precipitation of phosphate with calcium in the renal interstitium which may induce an inflammatory reaction leading to fibrosis. In animals, these problems can be minimized by a low phosphate intake, although a similar benefit has not been well documented in humans. Once GFR falls below 25 mL/min, the addition of oral phosphate binders are often necessary to prevent hyperphosphatemia. The agents of choice to bind intestinal phosphate are calcium salts and the most frequently used is calcium carbonate whose dosage has to be gradually increased (2.5 to 20 g/day). The point is to bind dietary phosphorus; intake with meals improves efficacy. Strict monitoring of calcium values is indicated because hypercalcemia is a common complication of this therapy, above all in patients treated with calcitriol to protect against renal osteodystrophy. In order to prevent aluminum intoxication or hypermagnesemia, phosphate binders containing these elements should be avoided. A more recently developed compound which binds phosphate without inducing hypercalcemia and aluminum intoxication is the nonabsorbable agent poly(allylamine hydrochloride), sevelamer. At present, its use is reserved for patients who do not tolerate calcium carbonate and those who have persistent hyperphosphatemia.

The development of CRF is accompanied by abnormalities in bone structure characterized by varying degrees of osteitis fibrosa, osteomalacia, and adynamic bone disease. (see Chapter 1.3) The combined effects of hyperphosphatemia, metabolic acidosis, hypocalcemia, secondary hyperparathyroidism, decreased receptor number for calcitriol, and reduced circulating levels of its active form, lead to the development and progression of the bone injury. Osteitis fibrosa is characterized by an increased bone turnover due to secondary hyperparathyroidism; osteomalacia is characterized by a reduced bone turnover and an increased volume of unmineralized bone (osteoid). Osteomalacia is generally due to aluminum bone deposition. In adynamic bone disease, bone turnover is reduced but there is no increase in osteoid formation. Symptoms of these disorders generally do not occur until after the patient has started dialysis. Prevention and treatment of these abnormalities is based on the administration of phosphate binding antacids and calcitriol that directly suppresses the secretion of PTH, whose increased production is the major cause of osteitis fibrosis. The effect of calcitriol in patients with CRF is debated because it might worsen renal function by causing hypercalcemia, hyperphosphatemia, and hypercal-

ciuria. At the moment, there is no evidence that calcitriol worsens renal function provided that prolonged hypercalcemia is avoided. Thus, a low dose of calcitriol (0.25 μg/day) is safe and probably effective in reducing PTH secretion. It should be given in CRF when plasma PTH levels are increased or hypocalcemia is present despite correction of hyperphosphatemia. It is important to normalize the plasma phosphate levels before giving this vitamin D metabolite.

The Uremic Syndrome

The uremic syndrome is the clinical manifestation of severe renal failure. It is a state of systemic poisoning that affects the cardiovascular, gastrointestinal, hematopoietic, immune, nervous, and endocrine systems. It is partly the result of a reduction in renal excretory function with retention of toxic substances that impair cell regulatory mechanisms. It is also the consequence of derangements in endocrine and metabolic functions regulated by the kidney. The signs and symptoms vary from one patient to another, depending partly on the speed and severity of the loss of renal function (Table 3).

Cardiovascular System

Cardiovascular disorders are the leading cause of death in uremic patients, accounting for over half of the deaths. Hypertension and congestive heart failure (CHF) are common; salt and water retention is very important in the pathogenesis of both. Hypertension is present in more than 80% of patients with ESRD and is presumably a major risk factor for cardiovascular disease, CHF, and cerebrovascular disease. In addition to salt and water retention, in uremia several factors, such as enhanced activity of the renin–angiotensin system, excess aldosterone secretion, increased sympathetic tone, and reduced production of vasodilatory hormones such as prostaglandins and kinins may contribute to the development of hypertension. Even the cause of CHF is multifactorial; anemia and electrolyte alterations such as hyperkalemia, hypocalcemia, and acidosis may contribute to CHF. The introduction of erythropoietin therapy has improved exercise performance and reduced elevated cardiac output and left ventricular mass in dialysis patients. Valvular stenosis and insufficiency, and accelerated atherosclerosis are common during the progression to ESRD. Serious arrhythmias, as a consequence of electrolyte imbalance or coronary artery disease, are frequent in uremia, and their incidence is increased in the presence of left ventricular dysfunction or coronary artery disease. Symptomatic myocardial ischemia usually results from coronary artery-disease, but it is nonatherosclerotic in origin in about 25% of patients. Widespread arterial calcification, probably due to secondary hyperparathyroidism and phosphate retention, is a common complication of CRF. Uremic cardiomyopathy, possibly caused by PTH-induced myocardial calcification and fibrosis, has been described, whereas uremic pericarditis has become rare because of earlier initiation of dialytic therapy. Cardiac complications of renal disease are covered in Chapter 64.

TABLE 3
Major Clinical Abnormalities in Uremia

Water and electrolyte abnormalities
  Volume expansion and depletion
  Hypernatremia and hyponatremia
  Hyperkalemia and hypokalemia
  Metabolic acidosis
  Hyperphosphatemia and hypocalcemia
Cardiovascular abnormalities
  Hypertension
  Congestive heart failure
  Cardiomiopathy
  Pericarditis
  Accelerated atherosclerosis
  Arrhythmias
Gastrointestinal abnormalities
  Anorexia, nausea, and vomiting
  Uremic fetor
  Stomatitis, gastritis, and enteritis
  Peptic ulcer
  Gastrointestinal bleeding
Hematologic and immunologic abnormalities
  Anemia
  Bleeding
  Phagocyte inhibition
  Lymphocytopenia
  Increased susceptibily to infection and neoplasia
Neurological abnormalities
  Malaise
  Headache
  Irritability and sleep disorders
  Muscle cramps
  Tremor
  Asterixis
  Seizures
  Stupor and coma
  Peripheral neuropathy
  Restless legs
  Motor weakness
Endocrine and metabolic abnormalities
  Carbohydrate intolerance
  Hypertriglyceridemia
  Protein malnutrition
  Impaired growth
  Infertility, sexual dysfunction, and amenorrhea
  Renal osteodystrophy
  Secondary hyperparathyroidism
  Hyperuricemia and hypermagnesemia
Dermatologic abnormalities
  Pallor
  Hyperpigmentation
  Pruritus
  Ecchymoses
  Uremic frost

Gastrointestinal System

Gastrointestinal complications are common in CRF and in some cases may be the first or only complaint on presentation. Anorexia, nausea, vomiting, and uremic fetor, with its typical ammoniacal odor on the breath, are common early manifestations of uremia. Vomiting may occur without nausea, often is prominent in the early morning, and is the more aggravating of these symptoms. Stomatitis, gastritis, and enteritis can develop with the progression of renal failure in untreated patients. Mucosal ulcerations can occur at any level of the gastrointestinal tract and, with the bleeding tendency of uremia, they account mostly for the gastrointestinal bleeding seen in untreated uremia. An altered gastric mucosal barrier may contribute to the development of ulcerative lesions. Peptic ulcer occurs in about one-fourth of uremic patients. Parotitis develops in some and may be related to the high salivary urea content in the presence of the low salivary flow rates that characterize renal failure. Pancreatitis is rarely a significant clinical problem. Drugs such as metoclopramide can control nausea and enhance gastric emptying. Ulcerogenic medications, especially NSAIDs, should be avoided.

Red Blood Cells and Hemostasis

Anemia develops early during renal failure and is one of the major causes of malaise and fatigue as renal failure progresses. The anemia is normocytic and normochromic except when complicated by aluminum intoxication linked to phosphate binders containing aluminum (microcytic anemia resistant to iron supplementation), iron deficiency due to gastrointestinal bleeding (microcytic), folate deficiency due to dietary restriction (macrocytic), or fibrosis of the bone marrow due to hyperparathyroidism. It is mainly due to underproduction of red blood cells (RBCs) secondary to reduced erythropoietin production by the diseased kidneys and, to a lesser extent, to the presence of circulating inhibitors of erythropoiesis and to a reduced survival of RBCs. This subject is covered in detail in Chapter 65. In CRF, the management of anemia has radically changed with the advent of recombinant human erythropoietin that stimulates terminal differentiation of the erythroid precursor cells. Correction of anemia improves cardiac function, central nervous system symptoms, appetite, and sexual function. Since the improvement in exercise capacity of individuals with CRF secondary to erythropoietin is only modest, it should be used in predialysis patients only with anemia dependent-angina, easy fatiguability, or severe anemia. The current target hematocrit lies between 30 and 36%. Higher values may worsen hypertension and sometime cause seizures. Although raising the hematocrit may increase systemic and perhaps intraglomerular pressures, in humans, correction of anemia does not seem to affect renal disease progression as long as blood pressure remains well controlled. An adequate response to erythropoietin necessitates the maintenance of sufficient iron stores; thus iron administration is usually required.

Uremic alterations in hemostasis include both a bleeding tendency and hypercoagulability. The uremic tendency to abnormal bleeding develops late and appears to correlate closely with prolongation of the bleeding time, due primarily to impaired platelets. Ecchymoses, epistaxis, and gastrointestinal bleeding are most common; surgery or invasive procedures always increase the risk for bleeding in uremic patients whereas spontaneous organ bleeding is rare. Platelet dysfunction is due to multiple factors such as the retention of uremic toxins, anemia, nitric oxide, and hyperparathyroidism. The importance of uremic toxins is suggested by the beneficial effect of acute dialysis on platelet dysfunction. How uremic toxins might interfere with platelet function is not completely understood. *In vitro* studies suggest that a dialyzable factor might interfere with the binding of fibrinogen to GPIIb-IIIa. The degree of anemia correlate strictly with the degree of prolongation of the bleeding time, and correction of anemia with erythropoietin shortens bleeding time. Rheologic factors have an important role in the relationship between anemia and platelet dysfunction. Uremia induced changes in nitric oxide production may also contribute, as the latter inhibits platelet aggregation produced by endothelial cells and platelets. *In vitro*, PTH inhibits platelet aggregation and induces accumulation of cyclic AMP (cAMP) and calcium in platelets; the increased platelet calcium content in dialyzed patients is reduced by calcitriol. However, the role of PTH in uremic bleeding is incompletely established. No specific therapy is indicated in asymptomatic patients. Correction of the platelet dysfunction is desirable in patients actively bleeding or who undergo surgical procedures. Raising the hematocrit to above 25 to 30% with erythropoietin reduces the bleeding time in many patients, and this is associated with enhanced platelet aggregation and increased platelet adhesion to endothelial cells. Secondary therapeutic procedures include intravenous or intranasal desmopressin, cryoprecipitate, conjugated estrogens, and dialysis. Other coagulation parameters are generally intact in uremia.

Immune Response

Functional and phenotypic alterations in both humoral and cellular immunity have been identified at an early stage in the course of CRF, worsen with the progression of uremia, and are exacerbated by the dialysis procedure. The antibody response to several antigens is impaired, and the serum level of complement may be depressed.

The leukocyte count is normal and increases appropriately in response to infection in uremia, but metabolic and functional abnormalities of polymorphonuclear leukocytes (PMNLs) contribute to an increased susceptibility to infection. They include altered adherence to endothelial cells, altered generation of reactive oxygen species, altered release of microbial enzymes, impaired chemotaxis, phagocytosis, intracellular killing of bacteria, altered carbohydrate metabolism, and impaired ATP generation. Several studies report on correlations between PMNL dysfunction and ferritin content. Deferoxamine therapy improves PMNL function that may be also normalized by correcting anemia with erythropoietin. Increased intracellular calcium is associated with several alterations of PMNL function and metabolism, which improve by normalization of calcium content either by calcium channel blockers or by lowering elevated PTH values. Several compounds, isolated from uremic serum, inhibit the biological activity of PMNLs. Granulocyte inhibitory protein I (GIP I) and II (GIP II) inhibit the uptake of deoxyglucose, chemotaxis, oxidative metabolism,

and intracellular killing by PMNLs. GIP I displays homology with light chain protein and GIP II with β_2-microglobulin, respectively. Degranulation inhibitory protein I (DIP I) and II (DIP II) inhibit spontaneous and stimulated PMNL degranulation and are identical to angiogenin and complement factor D, and immunoglobulin light chains.

Moderate lymphocytopenia with reduced circulating T cells, increased suppressor cell activity, and reduced helper cell activity may be present in uremic patients. The ratio of T4 to T8 cells may be reduced. The response of lymphocytes to mitogens is reduced. Interferon production is decreased, too. Thus, reduced renal clearance of unknown toxins, possible development of nutritional deficiences, and administration of immunosuppressive medications can lead to aberrant immune regulation in CRF. An increased incidence of infections, including tuberculosis, bacteremia, immunological disorders such as systemic lupus erythematosus, cancer, and inadequate antibody production to several antigens, as in response to hepatitis B vaccination, are typical of uremia. Vaccination has an important role in attenuating the infection risk, but impaired humoral and cell-mediated immunity contributes to suboptimal and short-lived antibody responses to vaccines. Reinforced vaccination schedules, increased vaccine dosage, and association of adjuvant immunomodulators have variably improved the defective antibody responses to certain vaccines. Monitoring antibody titers helps to determine the need for booster vaccination. Immunization against hepatitis B virus significantly decreased the prevalence and incidence of this infection in hemodialysis units. The use of influenza vaccine in uremic patients and of polyvalent pneumococcal vaccine in special risk circumstances has reduced the morbidity and mortality due to these infections. On the other hand, *Staphylococcus aureus* vaccine is ineffective in preventing peritonitis or exit side infections in patients receiving continous ambulatory peritoneal dialysis (CAPD). Other killed vaccines have not been comprehensively studied but generally have the same indications for use as in normal individuals. Since the protection given by these vaccines may be inadequate or transient, new infection control strategies are needed.

Neurological System

Central nervous system disorders are seen in severe renal insufficiency (see Chapter 66). The early symptoms are those of disturbances of mentation and cognition due to reduced general cerebral activity, such as apathy, fatigue, confusion, impaired memory, and decreased capacity for prolonged intellectual effort. As the disorder progresses, disorientation and irritability may manifest, followed by hallucinations, anxiety, depression, mania, and occasionally schizophrenia. Finally, lethargy, stupor, and coma occur. Signs of cerebral hyperexcitability may also be present and are characterized by myoclonic seizures. Most of these symptoms are responsive to dialysis, which is indicated when the impairment develops. The normal cyclic course of sleep may be altered in CRF, and patients may have nightmares and insomnia. Deep sleep stages are rarely reached and dream times are reduced. In uremia, the blood–cerebrospinal fluid barrier is altered, and protein and lymphocytes concentrations in the cerebrospinal fluid may be modestly elevated.

Peripheral neuropathy is common in advanced CRF. It is generally symmetrical and slowly progressive, and begins distally and spreads proximally. Since longer axons are affected first, the lower extremities are involved before the the upper extremities. Sensory changes—paresthesias, burning sensations, and pain—often precede the motor impairments. Electrophysiologic studies are the most sensitive way to detect uremic neuropathy. Dialysis can control the progression of peripheral neuropathy. Autonomic neuropathy tends to manifest with orthostatic hypotension, impaired sweating, and impotence.

Metabolic and Endocrine Disorders

Glucose intolerance develops in most patients with CRF, mainly due to resistance to the peripheral action of insulin, but release of insulin in response to hyperglycemia may also be impaired. In patients with GFR less than 10 to 15 mL/min, insulin clearance is reduced so insulin requirements are lower (see Chapter 66).

Alterations in lipid metabolism may be present early in the course of progressive renal disease. They show only a modest correlation with the severity of renal failure, and respond only slightly to dialysis. Plasma levels of triglycerides are elevated with a smaller rise in total cholesterol, the so-called type IV hyperlipoproteinemia pattern. Hyperlipoproteinemia is an important risk factor for coronary artery disease, but its role in the progression of renal disease in humans is still unclear. Hypertriglyceridemia is due to a decreased catabolism of very low-density lipoproteins (VLDL) rather than an increased synthesis.

Protein synthesis gradually decreases with progressive renal failure, and the majority of uremic patients are catabolic, with a negative nitrogen balance. Malnutrition, insulin resistance, metabolic acidosis, and hyporesponsiveness to growth hormone may contribute to the negative nitrogen balance.

Free thyroxinc (T4) and serum thyroxine stimulating hormone (TSH) are usually normal whereas serum triiodothyronine (T3) is low because of decreased peripheral conversion of T4 to T3; the majority of these patients are clinically euthyroid and need no treatment. Basal plasma levels of GH are elevated in uremia in proportion to the degree of renal failure; growth retardation, however, is a serious problem in uremic children and may be partially reversed by high doses of recombinant human GH.

In uremic women, estrogen production is low and prolactin levels are high, leading to disturbances in menstruation and fertility. Men may be impotent, infertile, or oligospermic secondary to low plasma testosterone levels. Asymptomatic hyperuricemia develops frequently but does not require therapy. Symptomatic gout, which is relatively uncommon is an indication for treatment. Hypermagnesemia is common in CRF.

Integument

The cutaneous manifestations of uremia include pallor (anemia), ecchymoses (impaired hemostasis), pruritus, pigmentation, and dehydration. Uremic patients have a characteristic sallow pallor due to anemia, retention of urochrome pigments and urea, and increased melatonin. The skin is generally dry and atrophic. In advanced azotemia, the precipitation of urea crystals secreted in sweat leads to uremic frost. Several factors may contribute to uremic pruritus, including secondary hyperparathyroidism, dry skin, increased calcium phosphate deposition in the skin, anemia, peripheral neuropathy, high aluminum levels, and hypervitaminosis A. Pruritus is probably due to the release of histamines from skin mast cells. Though many of these abnormalities improve with dialysis, pruritus is usually resistant to most systemic and topical therapies. At present, the best therapy for severe pruritus is a combination of erythropoietin, ultraviolet phototherapy (UVB), and, if necessary, an antihistamine.

Uremic Toxins and Hormonal Deficiencies

The retention of several organic and inorganic substances contributes to the uremic manifestations. The search for a specific toxin or toxins responsible for all the clinical manifestations of uremia has been largely frustrating, although PTH is receiving renewed attention. Uremic retention substances are divided according to their molecular masses: low-molecular mass solutes (10 to 3000 Da) such as urea and creatinine, middle molecules (3000 to 15000 Da) including PTH and β_2-microglobulin, and large solutes (more than 15000 Da) such as myoglobin. The metabolized proteins and amino acids have been studied the most.

Urea toxicity has been debated; it causes symptoms only at very high concentrations, especially when its level in the blood rises sharply; thus urea alone is probably not toxic at the concentrations typical of ESRD. However, urea is an extremely useful marker of uremic retention and elimination in dialytic patients. The U.S. National Cooperative Dialysis Study showed a direct correlation between urea turnover and morbidity of patients on dialysis, and this has led to the use of urea kinetic modeling to evaluate protein intake and dialysis adequacy (see Chapter 59).

Guanidine compounds are toxic in animals—they may cause gastritis, polyneuritis, reduced calcitriol synthesis, and coagulation abnormalities, but their toxicity in humans has not yet been convincingly demonstrated. Myoinositol and other polyols are neuronal phospholipids which are retained in uremia and are a possible cause of peripheral neuropathy. In vitro studies showed that FPA (3-carboxy-4-methyl-5-propyl-2-furanpropanoic acid), an organic acid derived from the diet and the breakdown of complex lipids, is an inhibitor of erythropoiesis and a potential toxin.

Parathyroid hormone, a middle molecule of about 9000 Da, is an important uremic toxin; it is oversecreted during ESRD in response to hypocalcemia, hyperphosphatemia, vitamin D_3 deficiency, and metabolic acidosis. Hyperparathyroidism causes the intracellular accumulation of calcium which inhibits mitochondrial oxidative pathways and ATP generation. The increased intracellular calcium uptake may affect the brain, myocardium, pancreas, and platelets. Hyperparathyroidism also induces changes in membrane permeability, integrity, and phospholipid turnover, stimulation of cyclic AMP production, soft tissue calcification, and protein catabolism. It also contributes to glucose intolerance, inhibition of platelet function and erythropoiesis, and cardiomyopathy. In experimental settings, parathyroidectomy or calcium channel blockers may prevent the PTH metabolic effects, but parathyroidectomy does not reverse clinical uremia.

β_2-Microglobulin is a human leucocyte antigen (HLA) class 1 light-chain component, present in all mammalian cells, which accumulates in renal failure; it is responsible for amyloid deposition in the carpal tunnel, synovial membrane, and the ends of long bones. Carpal tunnel syndrome, bone cysts, and destructive arthropathy result (see Chapter 63). Numerous other substances, many known and many as yet unidentified, are retained in uremia. All of them are potential toxins. Furthermore, some nontoxic molecules by themselves, may become toxic if mixed with other compounds. Thus, the uremic syndrome has to be defined as the result of overall retention of solutes.

The uremic syndrome is characterized not only by solute accumulation but also by hormonal alterations such as decreased production (erythropoietin and calcitriol), decreased clearance (insulin), end-organ resistance (insulin and PTH), and excess production (PTH), as previously discussed.

Preparation for ESRD Therapy

Uremic patients inevitably progress to ESRD and require renal replacement therapy in the form of dialysis or transplant. Early identification of patients who will require replacement therapy is important since adequate preparation may decrease morbidity and also permit the evaluation from patient and family members for a living related renal allograft prior the start of dialysis. Dialysis is the most widely used renal replacement therapy; the decision to start dialysis depends more on the severity of uremic symptoms (uncontrolled hyperkalemia and metabolic acidosis, fluid overload, gastrointestinal, and neurological symptoms) than on the serum creatinine concentration. However, many nephrologists prefer to start dialysis early in order to avoid the risk to more serious complications of uremia such as pericarditis and pulmonary edema (Table 4). There is also some evidence that the early initiation of dialysis improves long-term survival. Patients and their families have to be involved in the decision to start renal replacement therapy; the risks and benefits of hemodialytic therapy (in-center or at home), peritoneal dialytic methods (continuous or intermittent), and renal transplantation (living or cadaveric donor) should be clearly explained. A team approach including nurse clinicians, social workers, and other health professionals to assess the home situation and educate the patient and family may be advantageous in this phase.

The patient about to start hemodialysis needs to have an arteriovenuous fistula established at least 6 to 8 weeks in

TABLE 4
Indications for Initiation of ESRD Therapy

Uncontrolled hypertension
Uncontrolled pulmonary edema and fluid overload
pericarditis
Advanced encephalopathy or peripheral neuropathy
Clinical bleeding
Persistent anorexia, nausea, and vomiting
Malnutrition
Uncontrolled hyperkalemia
Uncontrolled metabolic acidosis

advance in order to ensure time for adequate maturation of the vessels. The best place for the access is the nondominant upper extremity. Three principal types of vascular access are used for maintenance dialysis: primary arteriovenous (AV) fistulas, synthetic arteriovenous fistulas (AV grafts), and double-lumen, cuffed tunneled catheters. Primary AV fistulas are preferred. They are constructed with an end-to-side vein-to-artery anastomosis of the cephalic vein and the radial artery. They have good long-term patency and infrequently develop infectious complications. AV grafts are used in patients where endogenous AV fistula placement has failed. They have higher long-term complications than primary fistuals. Cuffed tunneled catheters are central venous catheters that can be used immediately after placement. They are used as intermediate-duration vascular access to allow maturation of primary fistulas or for the long term in patients who have exhausted all available sites. Peritoneal dialysis can be started 1 or 2 days after placement of the peritoneal catheter although some nehrologists prefer waiting for 1–2 weeks in order to minimize the risk of fluid leak. Dialysis can overcome many of the uremic abnormalities associated with ESRD but transplantation is more effective in this regard. A succesful kidney transplant improves the quality of life and reduces the mortality risk when compared with maintenance dialysis.

Bibliography

Abbate M, Zoja C, Remuzzi G, et al.: In progressive nephropathies, overload of tubular cells with filtered proteins translates glomerular permeability dysfunction into cellular signals of interstitial inflammation. *J Am Soc Nephrol* 9:1213–1224, 1998.

Breyer JA, Bain RP, Evans JK, et al.: Predictors of the progression of renal insufficiency in patients with insulin-dependent diabetes and overt diabetic nephropathy. *Kidney Int* 50:1651–1658, 1996.

Dubrow A, Levin NW: Biochemical and hormonal alterations in chronic renal failure. In: Jacobson HR, Striker GE, Klahr S (eds) *The Principles and Practice of Nephrology*, 596–603. Mosby, St. Louis, 1995.

Gaspari F, Perico N, Remuzzi G: Measurement of glomerular filtration rate. *Kidney Int* 52(Suppl 63):S-151–S-154, 1997.

Lakkis FD, Martinez-Maldonado M: Conservative management of chronic renal failure and the uremic syndrome. In: Jacobson HR, Striker GE, Klahr S (eds) *The Principles and Practice of Nephrology*, 614–620. Mosby, St. Louis, 1995.

Lewis EJ, Hunsicker LG, Bain RP, *et al.:* The effect of angiotensin-converting-enzyme inhibition on diabetic nephropathy. *N Engl J Med* 329:1456–1462, 1993.

Loghman-Adham M: Role of phosphate retention in the progression of renal failure. *J Lab Clin Med* 122:16–26, 1993.

Mackenzie HS, Brenner BM: Prevention of progressive renal failure. In: Brady HR, Wilcox CS (eds) *Therapy in Nephrology and Hypertension.* Saunders, Philadephia, 1999.

Maschio G, Alberti D, Janin G, *et al.:* ACE inhibition in progressive renal insufficiency study group: Effect of the angiotensin-converting-enzyme benazepril on the progression of chronic renal insufficiency. *N Engl J Med* 334:939–945, 1996.

Peterson JC, Adler S, Burkart JM, *et al.,* for the Modification of Diet in Renal Disease (MDRD) Study Group: Blood pressure control, proteinuria, and the progression of renal disease. *Ann Intern Med* 123:754–762, 1995.

Remuzzi G, Bertani T: Is glomerulosclerosis a consequence of altered glomerular permeability to macromolecules? *Kidney Int* 38:384–394, 1990.

Remuzzi G, Bertani T: Pathophysiology of progressive nephropathies. *N Engl J Med* 339:1448–1456, 1998.

Remuzzi G: Bleeding in renal failure. *Lancet* 1(8596):1205–1208, 1988.

Roth D, Smith RD, Schylman G, *et al.:* Effects of recombinant human erythropoietin on renal function in chronic renal failure predyalisis patients. *Am J Kidney Dis* 24:777–784, 1994.

Ruggenenti P, Perna A, Remuzzi G, *et al.,* on the behalf of the Gruppo Italiano di Studi epidemiologici in Nefrologia (GISEN): Proteinuria predicts end-stage renal failure in non-diabetic chronic nephropathies. *Kidney Int* 52(Suppl 63): S-54–S-57, 1997.

Ruggenenti P, Gaspari F, Remuzzi G, *et al.:* Cross sectional longitudinal study of spot morning urine protein:creatinine ratio, 24 hour urine protein excretion rate, glomerular filtration rate, and end stage renal failure in chronic renal disease in patients without diabetes. *Br Med J* 316:504–509, 1998.

Ruggenenti P, Perna A, Remuzzi G, *et al.,* on the behalf of the GISEN Group: Renal function requirement for dialysis in chronic nephropathy patients on long-term ramipril: REIN follow-up trial. *Lancet* 352:1252–1256, 1998.

Ruggenenti P, Perna A, Remuzzi G, *et al.,* on the behalf of the GISEN Group: In chronic nephropathies prolonged ACE inhibition can induce remission: Dynamics of time-dependent changes in GFR. *J Am Soc Nephrol* 10:997–1006, 1999.

Ruggenenti P, Perna A, Remuzzi G, *et al.:* Renoprotective properties of ACE-inhibition in non-diabetic nephropathies with non-nephrotic proteinuria. *Lancet* 354:359–364, 1999.

Ter Wee PM: Initial management of chronic renal failure. In: Cameron S, Davison AM, Grunfeld JP, Kerr D, Ritz, E (eds) *Oxford Textbook of Clinical Nephrology,* 1173–1191. Oxford Medical Press, Oxford, 1992.

The GISEN Group: Randomised placebo-controlled trial of effect of ramipril on decline in glomerular filtration rate and risk of terminal renal failure in proteinuric, non-diabetic nephropathy. *Lancet* 349:1857–1863, 1997.

UKPDS 33: Intensive blood-glucose control with sulphonylureas or insulin compared with conventional treatment and risk of complications in patients with type 2 diabetes. *Lancet* 352:837–853: 1998.

Weidmann P, Schneider M, Bohlen L: Therapeutic efficacy of different antihypertensive drugs in human diabetic nephropathy: An updated meta-analysis. *Nephrol Dial Transplant* 10(Suppl 9): 39–45, 1995.

HEMODIALYSIS AND HEMOFILTRATION

ALFRED K. CHEUNG

STRUCTURE OF HEMODIALYZERS AND HEMOFILTERS

Extracorporeal therapy for renal failure refers to the process in which fluid and solutes are removed from or added to the patient's blood outside the body. During this process, blood from the patient is continuously circulated through a hemodialyzer or hemofilter containing an artificial semipermeable membrane and returned to the patient.

A typical modern hemodialyzer is made up of several thousand parallel hollow fibers. The wall of these fibers is the semipermeable membrane separating the blood in the fiber lumen from the dialysate outside. The total internal surface area of all the fibers is usually between 0.5 and 2.0 M^2. Less commonly, the membranes are in the form of flat plates rather than hollow fibers. The blood path either in the lumen of the hollow fibers or between the plates converges into a single inlet on one end and a single outlet on the other end of the dialyzer plastic casing. There is also an inlet and an outlet in the dialyzer casing for the dialysate compartment that are separate from those for the blood. The dialysate is usually circulated in a single-pass fashion, countercurrent to the blood flow. Because hemofiltration (see later) does not utilize dialysate, hemofilters that are specifically designed for hemofiltration have an inlet and an outlet for blood but only a single outlet for the ultrafiltrate compartment.

TYPES OF EXTRACORPOREAL THERAPY FOR RENAL FAILURE

Among the numerous modalities of extracorporeal renal therapy outlined in Table 1, "high efficiency hemodialysis" and perhaps "conventional hemodialysis" are most commonly used, although "high flux hemodialysis" continues to gain popularity in the United States, and hemodiafiltration has become more commonly used in some parts of Europe and Japan in the last few years for the treatment of chronic renal failure. Dialysis removes solutes by diffusion, based on concentration gradients of solutes between the blood and dialysate across the semipermeable membrane (Fig. 1A). For example, urea diffuses from the blood to the dialysate compartment, thereby decreasing the total urea mass in the body as well as the urea concentration in the plasma. Conversely, the concentration gradient of bicarbonate usually favors the diffusion of this ion from the dialysate to the blood compartment. Movement of water carrying solutes across the dialysis membrane is not necessary for solute transport in this modality, although removal of fluid from the patient is often desirable because these patients are usually fluid overloaded. High efficiency hemodialysis refers to hemodialysis using high blood flow rates or large surface area membrane dialyzers in order to remove urea and other small solutes (such as potassium) more rapidly than during conventional hemodialysis. High flux hemodialysis utilizes membranes with large pores which allow for rapid removal of water and solutes that are substantially larger than urea but smaller than albumin (so-called "middle molecules"). For chronic renal failure patients, maintenance hemodialysis is usually performed intermittently, for example, 3–5 hr three times a week either at home or in-center at a dialysis unit. Infrequently, hemodialysis is performed for 8–10 hr three times a week either in the daytime or nighttime (nocturnal hemodialysis), or even for a few hours on a daily basis.

Hemofiltration is another form of extracorporeal therapy which removes fluid by convection, that is, movement of water across the large pore hemofiltration membrane into the ultrafiltrate compartment drags along the solutes that are dissolved in the water (Fig. 1B). A crucial distinction between hemodialysis and hemofiltration is that, in the latter, fluid removal is required for solute removal. Removal of fluid with its accompanying solutes results in a loss in the total body mass of the solute, but not necessarily a decrease in the plasma concentration. In order to achieve a substantial decrease in the concentration, "clean" replace-

TABLE I

Glossary of Various Types of Extracorporeal Therapy for Renal Failure

Hemodialysis (HD)
  Conventional hemodialysis—hemodialysis using a conventional low flux (small pore size) membranes. Solute removal is primarily by diffusion.
  High efficiency hemodialysis—hemodialysis using a low flux (small pore size) membrane with high efficiency (K_oA) for removal of small solutes. It is typically achieved by using a larger surface area membrane.
  High flux hemodialysis—hemodialysis using a high flux (large pore size) membrane. It is more efficient in removing larger solutes, but may or may not be more efficient than conventional hemodialysis in removing small solutes.

Hemofiltration (HF)
  Continuous arteriovenous hemofiltration (CAVH)—removal of small and larger solutes using a high flux membrane and convection rather than diffusion. Blood is accessed from an artery and returned to a vein with the driving force deriving from the systemic arterial pressure. Because it is performed continuously (usually in the intensive care setting), it is also very effective in removing large amounts of fluid.
  Continuous venovenous hemofiltration (CVVH)—similar to CAVH except that blood is accessed from a vein and returned to another vein using a blood pump.
  Intermittent hemofiltration—hemofiltration performed on an intermittent basis for chronic renal failure.

Hemodiafiltration (HDF)
  Continuous arteriovenous hemodiafiltration (CAVHD)—similar to CAVH in that solutes are removed by convection using a high flux membrane in an acute setting. In addition, dialysate flows continuously through the dialysate compartment in order to enhance solute removal by diffusion, i.e., it is a combination of hemodialysis and hemofiltration.
  Continuous venovenous hemodiafiltration (CVVHD)—similar to CAVHD except that blood is accessed from a vein and returned to another vein using a blood pump.
  Intermittent hemodiafiltration—hemodiafiltration performed on an intermittent basis for chronic renal failure.

Hemoperfusion (HP)
  Removal of solutes by adsorption to charcoal or resin, primarily for treatment of acute poisoning.

ment fluid devoid of that solute is infused intravenously to approximately replace the large volume of plasma fluid removed in the hemofilter. This modality is analogous to glomerular filtration, in which plasma solutes are also removed by convection. In the case of the glomerulus, however, the replacement fluid is the water and electrolytes that are selectively reabsorbed from the renal tubules (Fig. 1C).

Hemodiafiltration refers to the combination of hemodialysis and hemofiltration operating simultaneously using a large pore membrane, that is, solutes are removed by both diffusion and convection. Hemofiltration and hemodiafiltration are used in the United States primarily for acute renal failure. Under these circumstances, they are applied continuously for days to weeks, usually in the intensive care

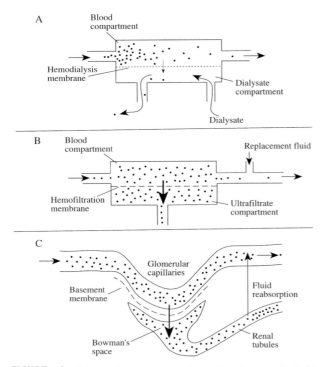

FIGURE 1 Schematic representation of solute and fluid transport across the semipermeable hemodialysis membranes. (A) Hemodialyzer. The plasma concentration of small solutes (solid circles) in the blood inlet is high. Because of the diffusive loss across the semipermeable hemodialysis membrane (dashed line), the plasma concentration in the blood outlet is much lower. The thin arrow across the dialysis membrane represents a small amount of fluid loss (which is not necessary for solute removal). High dialysate flow rate is necessary to maintain the concentration gradient across the dialysis membrane. (B) Hemofilter. Plasma concentration of small solutes in the blood compartment remains unchanged as blood travels the length of the fiber, and is similar to their concentrations in the ultrafiltrate. The hemofiltration membrane (broken line) has relatively large pores, which allow the necessary removal of large volume of fluid (heavy arrow). Replacement fluid is infused into the blood outlet in order to lower the plasma concentration of solutes and compensate for the fluid loss. (C) Glomerulus. Analogous to hemofiltration, plasma concentration of small solutes remains unchanged throughout the length of the glomerular capillary and is similar to that in Bowman's space. Fluid removal across the glomerular basement membrane (broken curve) is large (heavy arrow). Reabsorption of fluid from the renal tubules lowers the plasma concentration of the solutes.

unit, and are therefore termed continuous renal replacement therapy (CRRT). In Europe and Japan, hemofiltration and hemodiafiltration are also utilized on an intermittent basis for treatment of chronic renal failure. During a 4- to 5-hr session of maintenance hemofiltration, 16–20 L of body fluid is typically exchanged.

Hemoperfusion is the removal of solutes (usually toxins) from blood by adsorption onto materials, such as charcoal or resins, in the extracorporeal circuit. Hemoperfusion is primarily used for treatment of acute poisoning.

HEMODIALYSIS AND HEMOFILTRATION MEMBRANES AND MACHINES

Transport and, to a lesser extent, biocompatibility are two characteristics of dialysis membranes that are of interest to clinical nephrologists. Although there are exceptions, commercial hemodialysis membranes that are made from cellulose (a natural substance derived from plants) usually have small pores which restrict the movement of large solutes, and to some extent, the movement of water. In contrast, high flux hemodialysis membranes, which can also used be for hemofiltration, are usually made from synthetic polymers with large pores that facilitate transport of water and middle molecules.

Biocompatibility of dialysis membranes refers to the interactions that occur as a result of contact of blood with the membrane. Examples include the activation of proteins of the coagulation and complement system, as well as various peripheral blood cells. Biocompatibility is relative since, all dialysis membranes induce reactions to a certain extent which can manifest, for example, as thrombosis in the dialyzer and rarely as acute anaphylactoid reactions. Studies in the past few years have suggested that the type of dialysis membrane used influences the outcome of patients with acute renal failure and chronic renal failure. While the results of these studies are inconsistent, they raise the possibility that either the solute removal capabilities or biocompatibility characteristics, or both, are important features of hemodialysis membranes.

The dialysis machine incorporates many important features, such as a pump to deliver blood to the dialyzer at a constant rate up to approximately 500 mL/min, monitors to ensure that the pressures inside the extracorporeal circuit are not excessive, a detector for leakage of red blood cells from the blood compartment into the dialysate compartment, an air detector and shut-off device to prevent air from entering the patient, a pump to deliver dialysate, a proportioning system to properly dilute the dialysate concentrate, a heater to warm the dialysate to approximately body temperature, an ultrafiltration controller to precisely regulate fluid removal, and conductivity monitors to check dialysate ion concentrations. These devices ensure the proper, safe, and reliable delivery of blood and dialysate to the filter where exchange of water and solutes takes place. Some modern machines also incorporate more sophisticated features, such as devices that detect changes in the intravascular volume of the patient, and programs that alter the ultrafiltration rate during the course of the treatment according to parameters preset by the dialysis personnel for individual patient needs.

Machines employed for intermittent hemofiltration are similar to those for hemodialysis, with the additional requirements for precise fluid replacement control, and on-line generation of sterile replacement fluids in some machines. In contrast, continuous arteriovenous hemofiltration (CAVH) does not require any machinery. Blood is delivered to the hemofilter from an artery, such as the femoral artery, via a large bore (~14–15 gauge) catheter and returned to a large vein, with the driving force derived from the systemic arterial blood pressure rather than a mechanical pump. Unfortunately, blood flow and therefore ultrafiltration rates are sometimes erratic in CAVH. Nowadays, it is more customary to employ specially designed machines that pump blood from a vein through the hemofilter and back to a vein, a technique known as continuous venovenous hemofiltration (CVVH). The machines for CVVH are usually simpler in design than conventional hemodialysis machines, because dialysate production and many other devices are absent. One disadvantage of CAVH and CVVH is that they are less efficient than hemodialysis in removing urea, potassium, and other small solutes because there is no dialysate to permit diffusion. In order to improve solute clearance, continuous dialysate flow is sometimes added to these systems; these techniques are known as continuous arteriovenous hemodiafiltration (CAVHD) and continuous venovenous hemodiafiltration (CVVHD). Unfortunately, the addition of dialysate also adds complexity to these systems. As a result, CVVHD machines are in fact quite similar to regular hemodialysis machines. CVVHD is gaining popularity in intensive care units in the United States and many parts of the world.

WATER TRANSPORT AND SOLUTE CLEARANCE PROFILES

The effectiveness of water transport across a dialysis membrane is measured as the ultrafiltration coefficient, which is sometimes imprecisely called the ultrafiltration rate. Ultrafiltration coefficients for conventional hemodialysis membranes are usually 2–5 mL/hr/mm Hg. With a transmembrane pressure of 200 mm Hg, a dialyzer with a coefficient of 2.5 mL/hr/mm Hg will remove 0.5 L of fluid/hr, or 2 L in 4 hr. Ultrafiltration coefficients for high flux dialysis or hemofiltration membranes are much higher, at 15–60 mL/hr/mm Hg. The ultrafiltration coefficients of dialysis membranes are seldom limiting; the most important determinant is usually the ability of the patient to tolerate the rapidity of fluid removal.

The solute transport properties of dialysis membranes are usually expressed as the mass transfer–area coefficient, which is the product of the mass transfer coefficient (K_o) and membrane surface area (A). The clearance profile of solutes by conventional hemodialysis membranes presented in Fig. 2 reflects primarily the K_oA of the membranes and only provides a rough estimation of what might be achieved clinically. The actual solute clearances depend also on the blood flow rate, dialysate flow rate, and fluid removal. Diffusive clearance of solutes by hemodialysis decreases rapidly with increasing molecular size. For small solutes such as urea, however, removal per unit time by high efficiency hemodialysis (180–220 mL/min) is close to two times that achieved by the glomeruli in two native kidneys (90–125 mL/min for adults), which itself is significantly higher than the urinary excretory rate of urea after tubular reabsorption. However, patients spend only 9–15 hr/week on hemodialysis, whereas native kidneys function continuously for a total of 168 hr/week. As a result, the total weekly clearance of urea by hemodialysis

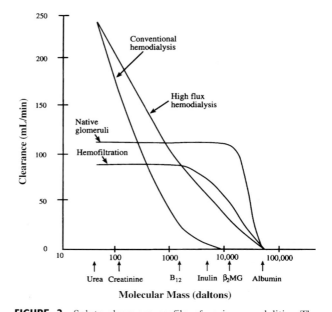

FIGURE 2 Solute clearance profile of various modalities. The curves are constructed based partially on data and partially on theoretical projection. The actual values may vary depending on the surface area of the membrane and operating conditions, such as blood flow rate. Native glomeruli refer to the summation of all the glomeruli in two normal kidneys. "Glomeruli" instead of "kidneys" are used because tubular reabsorption lowers the renal clearance of certain solutes (e.g., urea and glucose) substantially. B_{12}, vitamin B_{12}; $\beta_2 MG$, β_2-microglobulin.

is far lower than that achieved in a patient with normal functioning kidneys.

Clearance of larger solutes, such as β_2-microglobulin (12,000 Da), by conventional hemodialysis is much lower than that for urea. Because of the diffusive nature of transport, clearance by high flux membranes also decreases rapidly with molecular size, albeit less rapidly compared to conventional low flux dialysis membranes. In contrast, clearance by hemofiltration, even using the same membranes as for high flux hemodialysis, is maintained for solutes up to ~1000 Da. This is because the mode of transport in hemofiltration is convection, instead of diffusion. Solute transport by convection is, up to a certain point for a particular membrane, independent of solute size. For solutes with molecular weights higher than that threshold, however, clearances by convection also decline. Clearances of β_2-microglobulin are usually lower than those of urea and creatinine, even for convective transport across hemofiltration membranes.

DIALYSATE

The dialysate creates solute concentration gradients to drive diffusion across the dialysis membrane. The typical composition of dialysate for hemodialysis is shown in Table 2. Sodium is removed primarily by convection such that ultrafiltration of 4 L of isotonic fluid results in ~560 mEq or 13 g of sodium removal without a change in plasma so-

TABLE 2
Composition of Dialysate Commonly
Used in Clinical Hemodialysis

Ions	Concentrations
Na^+	132–145[a] mEq/L
K^+	0–4.0 mEq/L
Cl^-	103–110 mEq/L
HCO_3^-	0–40 mEq/L
Acetate[b]	2–37 mEq/L
Ca^{2+}	0–3.5 mEq/L
Mg^{2+}	0.5–1.0 mEq/L
Glucose	0–200 mg/dL

[a]Higher dialysate sodium concentration is sometimes used in "sodium modeling".

[b]Either HCO_3^- or acetate is used primarily as buffer.

dium concentration. In fact, dialysate sodium must be kept at a concentration similar to or higher than that of plasma, in order to avoid hemolysis from an abrupt decrease in plasma sodium concentration. In contrast, dialysate potassium concentration is often kept low in order to decrease plasma potassium concentration. Because dialysis patients are generally acidemic, base in the form of either bicarbonate or acetate is offered. Acetate dialysate is slightly less expensive but has the disadvantages of inducing hypoxemia and a transient worsening of metabolic acidosis because of the initial loss of bicarbonate from the plasma. It also causes intradialytic hypotension, cardiac arrhythmias, and an ill sensation in some patients. Proportioning systems in modern machines have made delivery of bicarbonate dialysate a relatively easy task. Dialysates containing primarily acetate are seldom used in the United States, although they are still prevalent in some other countries. Calcium concentration in the dialysate varies depending on the specific need of the patient. Dialysate magnesium concentration is sometimes lowered so that the patient can take oral magnesium-containing phosphate binders. Glucose is usually provided at 200 mg/dL to maintain the plasma glucose level stable for both diabetic and nondiabetic patients and to avoid hypoglycemia.

VASCULAR ACCESS

An adequate vascular access for hemodialysis should permit blood flow to the dialyzer of 200–500 mL/min in adults, depending on the size of the patient. The trend in the United States is to increase the blood pump speeds toward 450–500 mL/min for chronic hemodialysis, whereas in Asia, blood pump speeds of 200–250 mL/min are common. For acute hemodialysis, a large vein, such as the femoral vein, is often cannulated with a double lumen catheter. One lumen is for extracting the blood from the patient (so-called arterial side even though it may come from the vein of the patient), and the other returns blood

to the patient (venous side). Femoral catheters are seldom left in place for more than one dialysis session unless the patient is nonambulatory, because they are prone to kinking, dislodgement, and infection.

For usage of 1 to several weeks, an indwelling double lumen catheter is often placed in an internal jugular or subclavian vein percutaneously. These catheters can be infected, dislodged, or occluded by thrombi. In addition, catheters at these sites predispose the vessels to stenosis. Stenosis of these vessels can cause outflow obstruction and severe swelling of the ipsilateral arm, especially if a permanent arteriovenous fistula, with arterialized venous pressure and augmented blood flow, is present in that arm. Subclavian veins appear to be more likely to develop stenosis than internal jugular veins, and therefore should be avoided if at all possible. Stiff catheters are incriminated more frequently than softer ones. Softer catheters with anchoring cuffs offer a good alternative. These catheters are usually tunneled subcutaneously in the upper thorax before entering a proximal vessel or, rarely, inserted via the groin into the femoral vein. They may be used indefinitely. Thrombosis of these catheters can be resolved with local instillation of thrombolytic agents. Several types of cuffed catheters are clinically used. Some have two lumens in a single catheter. Others are twin catheters (one for inflow and the other for outflow) lying side-by-side in the central vein which may be joined at the external end. These twin catheters allow blood flow rates sometimes as high as 450 mL/min. The original form of temporary vascular access was the Scribner shunt, a plastic conduit placed outside the skin with the two internal ends inserted and anchored to an artery and a vein, respectively. The disadvantage of this shunt is that it often destroys a potential site for a future permanent access. Scribner shunts are also prone to infection and thrombosis and carry the potential danger of rapid blood loss if dislodged. They are sparingly used nowadays, but their high blood flow rate is an advantage in selected patients.

Long-term vascular access for hemodialysis is usually established by the creation of an arteriovenous (AV) fistula in an upper extremity, although a lower extremity or even an axillary vessel may sometimes be employed. A fistula is established by connecting an artery to a nearby vein either by direct surgical anastomosis of the native vessels or with an artificial vascular graft, for example, one made of polytetrafluoroethylene (PTFE). Native fistulae are preferred over PTFE grafts because of their relative longevity (~80 versus 50% patency in 3 years) and lower susceptibility to infection. The disadvantages are a need for sufficiently large native veins and a 4–16 week maturation period during which the wall of the fistula thickens and the lumen enlarges before the fistula is ready for use. PTFE grafts can be used earlier, occasionally at 1 week or less, but they tend to elicit acute transient local inflammatory reactions manifested by pain, swelling, and redness which resemble infectious cellulitis. These findings usually subside spontaneously within a few weeks. PTFE grafts are also more prone to thrombosis and infection, but the convenience that they offer has made them a popular choice among many dialysis personnel. PTFE grafts are more common than native fistulae in the United States. Declotting of AV fistulae can be accomplished surgically, with local infusion of thrombolytic agents, or, as more recently, with mechanical devices inserted percutaneously to break up the clot.

Stenosis at the outflow tract of AV fistulae, especially PTFE grafts, occurs frequently. Partial obstruction impedes the flow of cleansed blood from the dialyzer back to the central veins; as a result, the blood recirculates back to the "arterial" (afferent) limb of the fistula and decreases the amount of fresh systemic blood delivered to the dialyzer. Hence, the overall efficiency of the dialysis process is diminished. Obstruction of the fistula outflow tract also leads to an increase in pressure inside the "venous" (efferent) tubing during hemodialysis, which has been used as a clue to the presence of fistula outflow stenosis. Techniques involving noninvasive devices and the dilution principle have been developed to assess the total blood flow through AV fistulae. Monitoring changes in total fistula flow rates over time allows earlier detection of stenosis. In some centers, doppler ultrasound is a well-established procedure for this diagnosis. An angiogram (also called fistulogram in this context) with the injection of contrast dye (or carbon dioxide for patients who are allergic to contrast), however, remains the gold standard for the confirmation and anatomical definition of AV fistula stenosis and the connected blood vessels (e.g., collateral veins). Fistula stenosis is treated surgically by replacing or bypassing the stenotic segment. Alternatively, stenosis may be relieved by angioplasty with or without the placement of a stent to keep the lumen patent. If left untreated, most stenotic fistulae eventually become totally occluded by thrombi. AV fistulae, especially PTFE grafts can become infected. The common infecting organisms are *Staphylococcus* and gram-negative bacteria. Mild infection can be treated with antibiotics; more severe infection is treated by resection of the fistula. Although they are more difficult to treat conservatively, infected PTFE grafts do not invariably require surgical removal.

Spontaneous blood flow through the AV fistula often exceeds 1 L/min and occasionally 2 L/min, accounting for 20–40% of cardiac output, although the blood flow through the dialysis needles inserted into the fistula is considerably lower. This diversion of cardiac output from the capillary beds by the fistula can cause distal ischemia, that is, steal syndrome. Rarely, it can precipitate or exacerbate congestive heart failure. Surgical ligation or banding to decrease the luminal diameter of the fistula is sometimes necessary.

Early planning and placement of a permanent native AV fistula before the chronic renal failure patient requires dialysis is the preferred approach. For patients with poor veins, synthetic (e.g., PTFE) grafts will have to be used. When early placement of an AV fistula is not accomplished, surgical placement of a tunneled soft catheter in the proximal internal jugular vein is a good alternative while waiting for the AV fistula to mature. For patients with a short life expectancy or when sites for placement of fistula are no longer available, cuffed, tunneled catheters are used on a permanent basis. They may remain functional over 2 years, but infection and obstruction typically requires that they be replaced sooner. Percutaneous catheters which are not tunneled under the skin are often used as a temporary measure while waiting for a PTFE graft to become ready. The internal jugular vein on the contralateral side of the planned AV fistula is preferable. The temporary catheter should be removed as soon as the permanent access becomes functional. Repeat catheterization of femoral veins for individual dialysis sessions, especially for short periods, is a reasonable alternative.

ANTICOAGULATION

Exposure of blood to the extracorporeal circuit activates the clotting mechanisms. Heparin is used commonly as the anticoagulant in clinical hemodialysis. It is often given as an intravenous bolus of 1000–5000 units at the beginning of the session, followed by either intermittent boluses or, more commonly, continuous infusion at ~500–2000 units/hr up until the last hour of dialysis. In some dialysis units, the activated clotting time or partial thrombin time is measured periodically for determining heparin requirement and monitoring for individual patients. For patients in whom full systemic anticoagulation is particularly risky, lower dose heparin (sometimes termed tight or minimum heparin) can be used with careful observation of the extracorporeal circuit for clotting. Hemodialysis can sometimes be performed without using any anticoagulants. Underlying coagulation defects, high blood flow rates, and periodic flushing of the blood compartment with saline are helpful to prevent clotting under these circumstances. This technique is most often indicated in patients who are actively bleeding or who have recently had an intracranial bleeding episode.

Regional heparinization is another technique to minimize systemic anticoagulation. In this technique, heparin is infused into the "arterial" blood entering the dialyzer, and then neutralized by infusion of protamine sulfate into the "venous" line. Regional citrate is a similar technique except that citrate and calcium are used to produce and reverse anticoagulation, respectively. These procedures are relatively cumbersome and are employed infrequently, although some have advocated their use in patients with a high risk of bleeding in the acute setting. The antiplatelet agent prostacyclin has also been used successfully, albeit rarely, as a systemic anticoagulant during clinical hemodialysis. Hypotension can be a significant side effect of this medication.

INDICATIONS FOR HEMODIALYSIS AND HEMOFILTRATION

Acute hemodialysis is primarily performed for renal failure and drug overdose. Indications for emergency dialysis in the acute renal failure setting include fluid overload (often with pulmonary edema), hyperkalemia (often with serum potassium >7 mEq/L), and uremic signs and symptoms (see Chapter 39 for more details). Initiation of dialysis prior to onset of these problems is preferable. If reversal of the acute renal failure does not appear to be imminent, dialysis is often instituted when the blood urea nitrogen (BUN) is around 70–80 mg/dL or estimated glomerular filtration rate is 5–10 mL/min, before overt clinical symptoms occur. Maintenance dialysis for chronic renal failure is usually started at glomerular filtration rates (estimated as the mean of urea clearance and creatinine clearance) of 7–10 mL/min, unless the clinical condition dictates earlier intervention. Some have advocated the initiation of chronic dialysis even earlier. Although hemofiltration is more effective in removing larger solutes than hemodialysis, the clinical indications for this form of therapy on a chronic intermittent basis have not been precisely defined.

Continuous extracorporeal therapies, such as CAVH and CVVH, are particularly useful for patients in the intensive care unit whose cardiovascular status is too unstable for rapid fluid removal, as may occur during intermittent hemodialysis. They are also used in patients from whom removal of substantial amounts of fluid on a continuous basis is desired, for example, patients with multiorgan trauma receiving parenteral nutrition, blood products, and various intravenous medications. Clearances of urea and potassium by CAVH and CVVH are sometimes inadequate to maintain plasma concentrations of these solutes in the desirable range. Under these circumstances, continuous dialysate flow is added to the system, that is, CAVHD or CVVHD are employed. The limited available data have not demonstrated a clearly superior clinical outcome associated with continuous therapy compared to intermittent hemodialysis. Peritoneal dialysis is another form of continuous therapy that can be used in patients suffering from acute renal failure with unstable hemodynamics, but for technical reasons it has been largely replaced by continuous extracorporeal modalities in this setting.

QUANTITATION OF HEMODIALYSIS

The amount of chronic hemodialysis that should be delivered to patients has not been well defined. Frequently, an arbitrary duration, blood flow rate, and size of the dialyzer are used based on the experience and intuition of the nephrologist. Removal of fluid to maintain the patient euvolemic, or slightly hypovolemic, after dialysis is often desirable, but this so-called dry weight for individuals is often defined arbitrarily as the weight below which the patient develops symptomatic hypotension or muscle cramps. There are, of course, many imprecisions associated with this approach. For example, the likelihood of developing hypotension depends not only on the amount of fluid removed, but also on the rate of fluid removal.

Normalization of plasma electrolytes, such as potassium and hydrogen ions, is obviously important. Guidelines for removal of other uremic toxins are, however, more difficult to establish. Urea has been widely used as a marker to guide dialysis because it is an index of the production and accumulation of all nitrogenous waste products derived from protein metabolism. In addition, the removal of

urea by hemodialysis appears to correlate with clinical outcome to some extent. In urea kinetic modeling, the index Kt/V is often used for quantitation of the dose of dialysis therapy; K is the hemodialyzer clearance, t is the duration of the dialysis session, and V is the volume of distribution of urea in the body. A Kt/V value of 1.2 for each hemodialysis session is currently considered to be the minimum amount. Because the V as a fraction of total body weight varies significantly among patients, determining Kt/V precisely is a tedious process unless a computer is used. Therefore, the decrease in BUN during dialysis is often used as a simpler and alternative guide. The "urea reduction ratio," or URR, is calculated as:

$$ URR = \frac{\text{predialysis BUN} - \text{postdialysis BUN}}{\text{predialysis BUN}} \times 100 $$

A postdialysis to predialysis BUN ratio of 0.35 or a URR of 65% is roughly equivalent to a Kt/V of 1.2. The relationship between urea reduction ratio and Kt/V, however, varies depending on the ultrafiltration volume. There are some suggestions that a larger dose of hemodialysis, for example, a Kt/V value of 1.6–1.8, is beneficial, although definitive data supporting this notion are lacking. Delivery of large Kt/V values requires an adequate vascular access to provide high blood flow rates, a highly efficient dialyzer, or the willingness of the patient to endure longer dialysis sessions. It must be emphasized that the recommendation Kt/V of 1.2 refers only to the usual 3–5 hr/session thrice weekly as practiced in the United States and may not be applicable to other schedules, for example, 8- to 10-hr dialysis or daily dialysis. Furthermore, the use of urea kinetics does not substitute for frequent and diligent clinical evaluation of the patient. Increasing the amount of dialysis should be considered if the patient exhibits uremic symptoms, regardless of the Kt/V value. The clinical impact of removal of larger solutes (middle molecules) is at present unclear, although limited data suggest that their removal is also important.

Quantitation of acute hemodialysis is even more empirical. The dosage of dialysis provided for the treatment of toxins, for example, salicylates and lithium, is often guided by the plasma levels of the toxin and the clinical status. Dosage of dialysis for acute renal failure has been guided by the plasma chemistries, including BUN, potassium, and bicarbonate, body fluid volume and other clinical markers, with the objective of maintaining the BUN below ~80 mg/dL most of the time. In more recent years, some nephrologists have advocated the quantitation of hemodialysis for acute renal failure using urea kinetics as well, although it is unclear if Kt/V values similar to those targeted for chronic dialysis are also appropriate in the acute setting. The significance of middle molecule removal in acute renal failure has not been carefully studied.

COMPLICATIONS OF HEMODIALYSIS

Although hemodialysis is nowadays a relatively safe procedure, a number of complications may still arise. Some are inherent side effects of the normal extracorporeal circuit;

some result from technical errors, and yet others are due to abnormal reactions of patients to the procedure. Intradialytic hypotension is common and has been attributed variably to body volume depletion, shifting of fluid from extracellular to intracellular space as a result of a decrease in serum osmolality induced by dialysis, impaired sympathetic activity, vasodilation in response to warm dialysate, sequestration of blood in the muscles, as well as splanchnic pooling of blood if the patient eats during dialysis. Treatments including avoidance of large interdialytic fluid gain, administration of normal saline, hypertonic saline, hypertonic glucose, mannitol, or colloids, decreasing dialysate temperature to produce vasoconstriction, and avoidance of eating during dialysis are sometimes useful to reduce the frequency of hypotensive events. Other strategies that are used to minimize intravascular volume depletion include varying ultrafiltration rates during the session ("ultrafiltration modeling"), isolated ultrafiltration, which removes fluid in the absence of dialysate and therefore does not decrease plasma osmolality and cause intracellular fluid shifts, and "sodium modeling," which tailors dialysate sodium concentrations (135–160 mEq/L) during the dialysis session to maintain extracellular volumes.

Cardiac arrhythmias may occur as a result of rapid electrolyte changes, especially in patients taking digitalis and dialyzed against very low potassium dialysate (0–1 mEq/L). The use of acetate dialysate also appears to induce arrhythmias. Arrhythmias can induce or aggravate hypotension and overt or silent myocardial ischemia.

Muscle cramps, nausea, and vomiting occur commonly during hemodialysis, and are often a result of rapid fluid removal. Too rapid removal of urea and other small solutes may lead to the disequilibrium syndrome (see Chapter 58), manifested by headache with nausea and vomiting, altered mental status, seizures, coma, and even death. The pathophysiology of this symptom complex has not been well defined. A prevalent hypothesis is that the rapid decrease in plasma urea concentration and osmolality causes fluid shifts into the brain and cerebral edema. Severe disequilibrium syndrome is now rare because hemodialysis is usually initiated at an early stage when the BUN is not yet very high, and the efficiency of solute removal is often deliberately limited during the first treatment session.

Anaphylactoid reactions during hemodialysis are rare. They are manifested by various combinations of hypertension or hypotension, pulmonary symptoms, chest and abdominal pain, vomiting, fever, chills, flushing, urticaria, and pruritus. Cardiopulmonary arrest and death occasionally follow. The etiologies are probably multifactorial. Among the causes are activation of plasma complement components by dialysis membranes, administration of angiotensin converting enzyme inhibitors concomitant to dialysis using a membrane that intensely activates kinins (e.g., a certain type of polyacrylonitrile membrane), and the release of noxious materials that have contaminated the dialyzers during the manufacturing or sterilization process. Treatment for these anaphylactoid reactions is largely symptomatic. Preventive measures include thorough rinsing of the dialyzer before use and avoidance of the type of dialyzer or medications to which a particular patient is hypersensitive. Dialyzers or dialysates that are contaminated with microorganisms or their toxins can rarely cause fever and infection. Hepatitis B was prevalent in the 1970s, whereas hepatitis C infection is more common in hemodialysis units currently. The mode of transmission of hepatitis C in dialysis units has not been well established.

Hypoxemia occurs commonly during hemodialysis using acetate (instead of bicarbonate) as the dialysate buffer. The primary mechanism appears to be the initial loss of bicarbonate and carbon dioxide by diffusion into the dialysate, with subsequent hypoventilation. Dialysis membrane bioincompatibility may play a role by releasing mediators that impair gas exchange in some instances. A decrease in systemic arterial pO_2 of 10–12 mm Hg is not uncommon. This could be deleterious for patients with underlying cardiopulmonary disease.

An array of technical errors associated with hemodialysis has been described, but fortunately they occur rarely. Inadequate purification of city water prior to use may result in high levels of contaminants in the dialysate, resulting in, for example, aluminum or calcium intoxication. Dialysate contaminated with chloramine and improper proportioning or overheating of dialysate by the dialysis machine also lead to hemolysis. Rupture of the dialysis membrane causes blood loss into the dialysate and entry of microorganisms from the dialysate into the blood. Defective blood circuit and monitoring devices may result in air embolism. Difficult or improper puncture with the dialysis needle may cause a local hematoma around the vascular access or external bleeding, which can be aggravated by intradialytic administration of heparin.

DIALYZER REUSE

Hemodialyzers can be reused repeatedly on the same patient after thorough cleansing and disinfection, employing various agents such as formaldehyde, glutaraldehyde, sodium hypochlorite (bleach), and the combination of hydrogen peroxide and peroxyacetic acid. The blood compartment must be thoroughly rinsed to remove all the disinfectants prior to the next use, because infusion of residual disinfectants into the patient can be harmful. Inadequate disinfection, on the other hand, has been associated with infection by common or rare microorganisms. In general, reused dialyzers can clear small solutes as effectively as new dialyzers unless a substantial portion of the hollow fibers has been occluded by clotted blood; in contrast, middle molecule clearance is sometimes impaired even when small solute clearance is maintained. The total volume of the hollow fiber lumens is usually checked after each processing, and the dialyzer is discarded if the volume is below 80% of that of a new dialyzer. Other contraindications to reuse include a disrupted dialyzer casing and hepatitis B infection. Reports on the effect of reuse on long-term clinical outcome are conflicting. Because of the economic benefits and lack of definite harmful effects when practiced properly, dialyzer reuse is popular in the United States.

CHOICE OF HEMODIALYZERS

There are several considerations when choosing a hemodialyzer for clinical use. One of the most important considerations is the capacity (K_oA) of the membrane to clear urea, because urea removal by dialysis has been shown to correlate with clinical outcome. Increasing amounts of data suggest that the removal of middle molecules is also beneficial. Biocompatibility characteristics of dialysis membrane are taken into account by some, albeit not all nephrologists. Therefore, high flux dialysis membranes, which are more effective in removing middle molecules and are generally considered to be more biocompatible, continue to gain popularity. Purchase cost and reusability of the dialyzer are additional concerns.

DRUG USAGE IN HEMODIALYSIS

The removal of a drug by hemodialysis depends on the properties of the drug as well as the conditions of the dialysis procedure (see Chapter 41). Guidelines for dosing medications in renal failure with or without dialysis have been published. It is imperative to refer to these publications for individual drugs if the physician is unfamiliar with their use in these settings. For example, different types of penicillins behave differently, and the clearance of a drug by hemodialysis can be substantially different from that by hemofiltration or peritoneal dialysis. It is also important to remember that these publications provide only a rough guideline. The information might be derived from conventional hemodialysis and might not be applicable to high flux dialysis. Finally, the efficacy of the particular dialysis session must be taken into account. A short and inefficient dialysis because of vascular access problems would remove only a small amount of aminoglycosides, and the postdialysis supplemental dose should be adjusted accordingly. Frequently, monitoring of drug levels is required.

Bibliography

Ambalavanan S, Rabetoy G, Cheung A: High efficiency and high flux hemodialysis. In: Schrier RW (ed) *Atlas of Diseases of the Kidney*, Vol. 5, pp. 3.1–3.10. Current Medicine, Philadelphia, 1999.

Cheung AK, Leypoldt JK: Evaluation of hemodialyzer performance. *Semin Dial* 11:131–137, 1998.

Hakim RM, Held PJ, Stannard DC, Wolfe RA, Port FK, Daugirdas JT, Agodoa L: Effect of the dialysis membrane on mortality of chronic hemodialysis patients. *Kidney Int* 50:566–570, 1996.

Held PJ, Port FK, Wolfe RA, Stannard DC, Carroll CE, Daugirdas JT, Bloembergen WE, Greer JW, Hakim RM: The dose of hemodialysis and patient mortality. *Kidney Int* 50:550–556, 1996.

Ing TS, Cheung AK, Golper TA, Lang GR, Lazarus JM, Letteri JM, Levin NW, Lundin AP, Molony DA, Mujais SK, Port FK, Ward RA: National Kidney Foundation report on dialyzer reuse. *Am J Kidney Dis* 30:859–871, 1997.

Leypoldt JK, Cheung AK, Carroll CE, Stannard DC, Pereira BJG, Agodoa LY, Port FK: Effect of dialysis membranes and middle molecule removal on chronic hemodialysis patient survival. *Am J Kidney Dis* 33:349–355, 1999.

National Kidney Foundation Dialysis Outcomes Quality Initiative Clinical Practice Guidelines. *Am J Kidney Dis* 30:(Suppl 2 and 3), 1997.

Nissenson AR, Fine RN, Gentile DE (eds): *Clinical Dialysis*, 3rd Ed. Appleton & Lange, Norwalk, Connecticut, 1995.

Pereira BG, Cheung AK: Biocompatibility of hemodialysis membrane. In: Owen WF, Pereira BJG, Sayegh MH (eds) *Dialysis and Transplantation: A Companion to Brenner & Rector's The Kidney*, pp. 32–56 Saunders, Philadelphia, 2000.

Schwab SJ, Beathard G: The hemodialysis catheter conundrum: Hate living with them, but can't live without them. *Kidney Int* 56:1–17, 1999.

Suki WN, Massry SG (eds): *Therapy of Renal Diseases and Related Disorders*, 3rd Ed. Kluwer Academic, Norwell, Massachusetts, 1997.

Vanholder RC, Ringoir SM: Adequacy of dialysis: A critical analysis. *Kidney Int* 42:540–558, 1992.

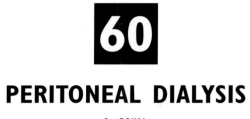

PERITONEAL DIALYSIS

R. GOKAL

In the 1950s and 1960s, peritoneal dialysis (PD) was utilized predominantly to manage patients in acute renal failure. Patients with end stage renal disease (ESRD) were treated almost exclusively by hemodialysis (HD) and occasionally by intermittent PD. However, the introduction in 1976 of continuous ambulatory peritoneal dialysis (CAPD) transformed this situation. There has been a dramatic rise in the use of PD over the last two decades. The rate in the United States is not increasing, but continues to do so in various countries, especially in the developing world. Currently there are over 130,000 patients on PD, comprising roughly 15% of the total world dialysis population. PD is still utilized for managing some cases of acute renal failure.

PRINCIPLES OF PERITONEAL DIALYSIS

Peritoneal dialysis represents solute and fluid exchange between the peritoneal capillary blood and dialysis solution in the peritoneal cavity across the peritoneal membrane. Solute movement follows physical laws of diffusion and convective transport, whereas fluid shifts relate to osmosis created by the addition of appropriate osmotic agents to the PD solutions.

Solute Movement

During PD, solutes such as urea, creatinine, and potassium move from the peritoneal capillaries across the peritoneal membrane to the peritoneal cavity, whereas other solutes such as bicarbonate and calcium move in the opposite direction. Small solute movement is mainly by diffusion and is thus based on the concentration gradient of the solute between dialysate and blood. Solutes also move across the peritoneal membrane by convection—the movement of solutes related to fluid removal. Large solute removal also occurs via the same mechanisms.

Fluid Movement

PD fluid contains a high concentration of glucose. Thus, dialysate is hyperosmolar compared to serum, causing fluid removal (ultrafiltration) to occur. The volume of ultrafiltration depends on the concentration of glucose solution used for each exchange, the length of the dwell, and the individual patient's peritoneal membrane characteristics (see

later). With increasing dwell time, transperitoneal glucose absorption diminishes the dialysate glucose concentration and the osmotic gradient. Ultrafiltration is therefore decreased with long dwell times, for example, with the overnight exchange on CAPD or the daytime exchange on automated PD (APD).

The crucial physiological components of the PD system are, therefore, peritoneal blood flow, the peritoneal membrane (neither amenable to any manipulation on a routine clinical basis) and the dialysate volume, dwell time, and number of exchanges/day (the only factors that can be manipulated to maximize solute and fluid removal). Various techniques and regimens have now emerged in the field of PD based on more recent understanding of the peritoneal membrane transport characteristics or permeability, and the amount of solute and fluid to be removed.

TECHNIQUES OF PERITONEAL DIALYSIS

Continuous Ambulatory Peritoneal Dialysis

CAPD utilizes the smallest volume of dialysate to prevent uremia; this usually means a daily volume of 8–10 L of dialysate to be equilibrated with body fluids. The CAPD technique usually entails three to five daily exchanges of 0.5–3.0 L each, with dialysis occurring continuously and occupying the entire 24-hr period. The prescription (volume, dwell time, number of exchanges) will depend on patient size, peritoneal permeability, and residual renal function.

PD fluid is initially instilled by gravity into the peritoneal cavity and drained out after a dwell period of several hours. The basic CAPD system, which to this day remains unchanged, consists of a plastic bag containing 0.5–3.0 L of PD fluid, a transfer set (tubing between the catheter and the plastic bag), and a permanent, indwelling, silastic catheter, which is implanted such that the intraperitoneal portion lies in the pelvis. The connection between the bag and the transfer set is broken three to five times a day and the procedure must be performed using a strict, semisterile, nontouch technique (about 1500 exchanges/year), which the patient or helper performs at home. The most common connection device currently utilized is based on the "Y"-disconnect system. This entails drainage of the effluent after the connection is made with the new bag, thereby enabling any touch contamination in the tubing to be "flushed" out before new fluid is drained into the peritoneal cavity (Fig. 1). This system reduces the incidence of infection and in addition leaves the patient free from carrying the empty bag and transfer set, thus improving the psychological aspects and quality of life of CAPD patients.

Automated Peritoneal Dialysis

APD is a broad term that is used to refer to all forms of PD employing a mechanical device (called a cycler) to assist in the delivery and drainage of the dialysis fluid. APD variants range from intermittent peritoneal dialysis (IPD) performed in acute or chronic patients three times a week

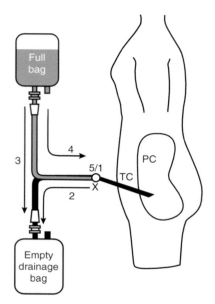

FIGURE I Diagrammatic representation of a CAPD exchange using a Y-set disconnect system. The Y-set consists of tubing with a full bag of dialysate at one end an empty drainage bag at the other, placed on the floor. Fluid flow is by gravity, and the direction is controlled by clamps on the tubing. Between exchanges, the peritoneal cavity (PC) contains dialysate and only a short, capped extension tubing attached to the peritoneal Tenckhoff catheter (TC). The exchange procedure comprises five steps.

1. To begin the exchange the patient connects the Y tubing to the short extension tubing at X.
2. Keeping the clamp on the full bag closed, the clamp on the peritoneal catheter extension tubing is opened to allow the fluid in the PC to drain into the drainage bag by gravity. Time: 10–15 min.
3. The patient closes the clamp on the peritoneal catheter extension tubing and opens the clamp on the full bag, allowing the fresh fluid to "flush" the tubing of air and any contamination into the drainage bag. Time: a few seconds (Count of 5).
4. The patient closes the clamp on the drainage bag and opens the clamp on the peritoneal catheter extension tubing, allowing fresh dialysis fluid into the PC via the TC. Time: 10 min.
5. The final step is to close the clamp on peritoneal catheter extension tubing, disconnect the Y tubing, and cap the short extension tubing.

in sessions of 24 hr exchanging 20–60 L of dialysis fluid to the more sophisticated ones. The latter involve continuous cycling peritoneal dialysis (CCPD—originally entailed three exchanges during the night and one during the day—a reversal of the CAPD regime), nightly intermittent peritoneal dialysis (NIPD—rapid exchanges during the night with the abdomen kept dry during the day—"dry day"), nightly PD plus two exchanges during the day to allow for increased solute and fluid clearance (NIPD with "wet day"), and tidal peritoneal dialysis (TPD)—40–60% of the volume introduced in the first cycle is left in the abdomen, and the exchanges, the tidal volume, replace only the rest of the volume. Continuous fluid–membrane contact improves the efficiency but requires 20–30 L of fluid. These regimes are illustrated in Table 1.

These regimes usually entail an increased number of short dwell exchanges to enhance solute and fluid removal. The cycler delivers a set number of exchanges over 8 to 10 hours, the last fill constituting the long day dwell, which may be necessary to provide additional dialysis to achieve solute and fluid removal targets. The most obvious advantage of APD is that it eliminates the need for intensive manual involvement, with most of the dialysis occurring at night during sleep. In essence, APD entails two procedures only-an initial connection of catheter to the machine and a disconnection at end of dialysis. There is increasing use of APD in the United States at the expense of CAPD. This may be due to the convenience of performing the dialysis connections and to the new cycler models, which are smaller and more attractive to patients.

PD Solutions

PD solutions (Table 2) comprise varying concentration of glucose as an osmotic agent and differing amounts of lactate, sodium, potassium, and calcium. Lactate, in dialy-

TABLE I
Various Regimens Used in Peritoneal Dialysis

Type of dialysis[a]	Number of daytime exchanges	Number of nightime exchanges	Volume of exchanges (L)
CAPD	2–3	1–2[b]	1.0–3.0
CCPD	1	3–4	1.0–3.0
NIPD	0	3–5	2.0–3.0
NIPD "wet day"	1–2	3–5	2.0–3.0
TPD	0	20	1.0–1.5

[a]CAPD, continuous ambulatory peritoneal dialysis; CCPD, continuous cycling peritoneal dialysis; NIPD, nocturnal intermittent peritoneal dialysis; TPD, tidal peritoneal dialysis.
[b]If an additional exchange is needed during CAPD to achieve adequate dialysis, a mechanical exchange device can be used to perform the exchange during the night while the patient is asleep. CAPD is the only regimen that does not use an automated device called a cycler. IPD is an infrequently utilized regime to manage end stage renal failure patients. It cycles 30–40 L fluid over a 48-hr period with 1–2 L exchange volumes, usually twice a week.

TABLE 2
Composition of Peritoneal Dialysis Fluids Including
the Osmotic Agents Used

Sodium (mEq/L)	132
Chloride (mEq/L)	96–102
Calcium (mEq/L)	0, 1.2, 2.5, 3.5
Magnesium (mEq/L)	0.5, 1.25
Lactate (mEq/L)[a]	35, 40
Glucose (g/dL)	1.5, 2.5, 4.25
Amino acid[b]	1.1%
Icodextrin[c]	7.5%

[a]Lactate is to be replaced with bicarbonate or bicarbonate/lactate mixtures, making the base replacement much more physiological.

[b]It is advocated that this be used for management of protein malnutrition, usually one exchange per day. Greater use is associated with a degree of acidosis.

[c]This is a macromolecular osmotic agent, undergoing clinical trials in the US but freely used in Europe for long dwells on a once a day basis. Its use is especially valuable in patients with UF loss and long dwells in APD.

sis solutions, is gradually being replaced by bicarbonate, which is an ideal buffer for PD. Glucose is still the commonest osmotic agent. Other agents ("icodextrin—an isosmotic glucose polymer that produces ultrafiltration by colloid osmosis even at dwell periods of up to 12 hr; and mixtures of amino acids used as a protein supplement in malnourished patients) are now available commercially, and these will be used increasingly to improve outcomes in PD. Peritoneal dialysis solutions are unphysiological in being of low pH and high osmolality, and they contain glucose degradation products which were generated during preparation. All of these factors are potentially harmful to the peritoneal membrane.

Peritoneal Catheters

The access for PD is a catheter, which is inserted into the abdominal cavity by either a surgeon or a nephrologist, generally using local anesthetic with sedation. The catheter can be inserted surgically, or percutaneously or using a peritoneoscope. Although there are numerous newer catheter designs, none offers a significant advantage over the original double cuffed silastic Tenckhoff catheter, which is still the commonest catheter used. The intra-abdominal portion of the catheter has multiple perforations through which dialysate flows. With the deep cuff placed in a paramedian position in the rectus muscle, the catheter is tunnelled through the subcutaneous tissue to exit laterally and downward. The subcutaneous superficial cuff is located about 2–3 cm from the exit site of the catheter. PD can be initiated immediately if exchange volumes are small and the patient is kept recumbent. Alternatively, PD may be deferred until the insertion site is well healed, at which time the patient is trained to perform CAPD or APD. He-

modialysis can be used if necessary as a temporary measure until PD is initiated.

Peritoneal Membrane

The peritoneal membrane is the dialyzing surface. The visceral peritoneal membrane covers the abdominal organs, whereas the parietal peritoneum lines the abdominal cavity. The peritoneal membrane consists of a single layer of mesothelial cells overlying an intersitium in which the blood and lymphatic vessels lie. The mesothelial cells are covered by microvilli that markedly increase the 2-m^2 surface area of the peritoneum.

Measuring Solute and Fluid Transport to Determine Peritoneal Membrane Characteristics

PD effectively removes substances with a low molecular weight such as creatinine, urea, and potassium which are not in the infused dialysate. With increasing dwell time, the ratio of dialysate to serum urea levels approaches one. Because the peritoneal membrane has a negative charge, negatively charged solutes such as phosphate will move across it more slowly than positively charged solutes such as potassium. Macromolecules such as albumin cross the peritoneum by mechanisms not completely understood but probably via lymphatics and through large pores in the capillary membranes.

During a dwell, the osmotic gradient created by the dialysate within the abdominal cavity declines as the glucose is absorbed, resulting in fluid reabsorption into the systemic circulation. In addition, continuous lymphatic absorption diminishes net fluid removal.

The rate of movement of small solutes such as creatinine between dialysate and blood differs from one patient to another. Peritoneal function characteristics have been quantified in the peritoneal equilibration test (PET) (Fig. 2). In this standardized test, 2 L of 2.5 g/dL glucose dialysate are infused and the dialysate: plasma creatinine ratio (D/P) at the end of a 4-hr dwell is measured. Using this test, each patient's membrane can be categorized as having high (D/P >0.81), high average (0.65 to 0.81), low average (0.50 to 0.65), or low (<0.5) peritoneal transport capability.

Removal of fluid and solutes are very dependent on the type of transporter status (Fig. 3). Patients with a high D/P creatinine (high transporters) have rapid clearance of small molecules but poor ultrafiltration owing to rapid glucose absorption and dissipation of the concentration gradient between dialysate and blood. These patients will require short dwell peritoneal dialysis regimes to achieve adequate fluid removal. In addition, because the volume of fluid also dictates the solute clearance of equilibrated dialysate, high transporters will also have reduced solute clearance over long dwells because of low drain volumes. Patients with a low D/P creatinine (low transporters) have low clearances for solutes and generally require increased numbers of dialysis exchanges and/or increased volume per exchange to avoid uremic symptoms once residual renal function is lost. Ultrafiltration in this category of patient is usually excellent.

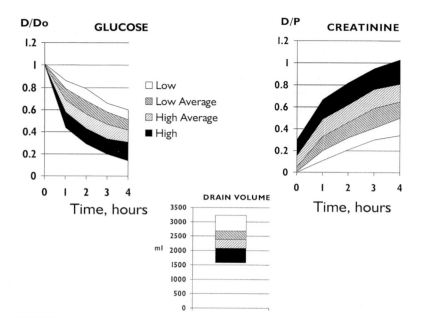

FIGURE 2 The peritoneal equilibration test (PET) measures the transport characteristics of glucose movement from the peritoneal fluid and creatinine movement from plasma. D/Do represents the ratio of dialysate glucose concentration, D, at various times to the dialysate glucose concentration at time 0, D_0 D/P represents the ratio of dialysate, D, to plasma, P, concentrations). The rate of transport of these molecules will depend on the the permeability of the membrane; the higher the permeability (high transporter) the more rapid the transport of glucose, with dissipation of the osmotic gradient and therefore less drain volume. The instillation volume for the PET is 2 L.

The majority of patients have high average to low average peritoneal transport and do well on either CAPD or APD.

MANAGING PATIENTS ON PD

Peritoneal Dialysis Prescription

In arriving at a particular prescription for an individual patient, one needs to take into account the fixed components, including residual renal function, peritoneal membrane permeability, and size of the patient as well as the variable components of dialysate volume, dwell times, concentration of glucose, and the number of exchanges. A prescription will, therefore, entail modifications of the variable components to arrive at a regime which provides for adequate solute and fluid removal to meet clinical as well as patient lifestyle needs and maintain reasonable quality of life. The hope is that the prescription arrived at will enhance outcomes.

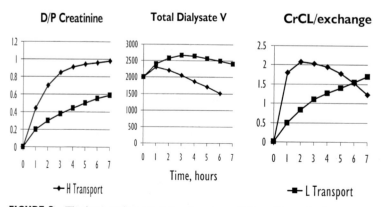

FIGURE 3 The intraperitoneal dialysate volume (V) profiles and solute transport of creatinine (creatinine clearance/exchange) in relationship to dwell time in hours, in high (H) and low (L) transporters. This dictates the need for adjusting dwell times and setting the prescription. For long dwell CAPD, high transporters show both low fluid removal as well as creatinine clearance as compared to low transporters.

The setting of a PD prescription is outlined in Fig. 4, which is a flow diagram used to arrive at a prescription utilizing the various factors (peritoneal permeability, residual renal function, size, dwell times, fill volume, number of exchanges) to meet adequacy and nutritional targets. The prescription is then modified by regular monitoring of dose of dialysis, fluid status, and clinical well-being. The various regimes and methods for daily PD are outlined earlier.

The overall clearance capacity of the peritoneum for small solute clearance is limited by the volume of dialysis fluid that can be prescribed. Many CAPD patients are prescribed four exchanges of 2 L volumes/day. Four 2-L CAPD exchanges/day with 2 L of ultrafiltration/day represents a drain volume of 70 L/week, which is inadequate in the absence of significant residual renal function for most patients, especially large patients (>80 kg). Initially, most patients have residual renal function, contributing to the total clearance. As renal function is lost, patients require larger exchange volumes (2.5 or 3.0 L) and may also need five daily exchanges to avoid uremic symptoms and reach the target values of Kt/V and creatinine clearance (see later). The fifth exchange may be provided by use of a device that will deliver a middle of the night exchange. Larger patients should be started on 2.5 or 3.0 L exchange volumes. APD can achieve higher solute clearance, but it may be necessary for 1- or 2-day dwells (wet day), in addition to three to four nocturnal exchange volumes of 2.5 to 3.0 L.

Peritoneal Dialysis Adequacy

Adequacy of PD is determined by both clinical assessment, solute clearance measurements, and fluid removal.

The well-dialyzed patient has a good appetite, no nausea, minimal fatigue, and feels well. In contrast, the uremic patient is anoretic with dysgeusia, nausea, and complaints of fatigue. In addition to these clinical parameters, the measures utilized to assess adequacy of solute removal include:

1. An index of urea removal, expressed as Kt/V, which is urea clearance (K) per unit time (t) related to total body water (V). Kt is obtained by multiplying the effluent blood urea nitrogen concentration ratio (D/P_{urea}) by the 24-hr effluent drain volume. Renal urea nitrogen clearance is added to this. The daily value is multiplied by seven to provide a weekly value. V can be estimated as 60% of weight in males and 55% of weight in females. A typical calculation is given in Table 3.

2. Creatinine clearance (both peritoneal and residual renal). This is also obtained from a 24-hr collection of dialysate, to which is added the renal creatinine clearance (by tradition the latter is arrived at by averaging creatinine and urea nitrogen clearance as an estimate of glomerular filtration rate—to correct for tubular secretion of creatinine, which overestimates glomerular filtration rate). An adjustment for body surface area is also required.

Various national and international bodies have set minimal targets for these solute clearances. The National Kidney Foundation in the United States has published the Dialysis Outcome Quality Initiative (DOQI) Practice Guidelines, which set a target minimum urea clearance— Kt/V of 2.0 and total weekly creatinine clearance of 60 L. Failure to achieve these guidelines may lead to uremic symptoms, decreased protein intake, and an increase in mortality.

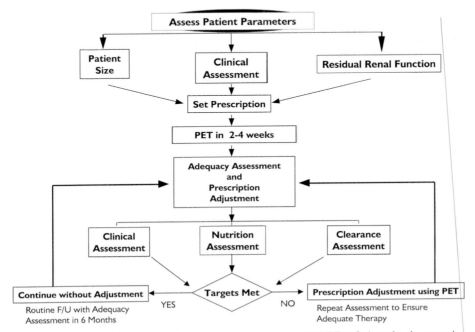

FIGURE 4 The algorithm for prescription setting. After the initial PET at 2–4 weeks, the prescription is altered according to the permeability. For high transporters, short dwell APD is appropriate; for high average and low average transporters, CAPD would suffice.

TABLE 3
An Example of a Kt/V Calculation

Patient
  70 kg female on CAPD (four exchanges/day)

Data to be measured
  24-hr dialysate volume (e.g., 9 L; 4×2 L + 1 L ultrafiltrate), D/P ratio for urea, determined by collecting the total dialysate for 24 hr, (e.g., 0.9)
  24-hr urine collection for urea clearance by dividing the 24-hr urine urea by blood urea (e.g., 2 mL/min which corresponds to 20 L/week)

Calculation

Peritoneal urea clearance/day ($D/P \times$ volume)	$= 0.9 \times 9 = 8.1$ L
Weekly peritoneal urea clearance	$= 8.1 \times 7 = 56.7$ L/week
Residual renal urea clearance	$= 20$ L/week
Total urea clearance (Kt)	$= 56.7 + 20 = 76.7$ L/week
Volume of urea distribution[a] ($0.55 \times$ weight)	$= 38.5$ L
Kt/V	$= 76.7/38.5 = 2.0$

[a]V can be estimated from using 0.60 (male) or 0.55 (female) of body weight. It is more accurate to use the formula of Watson and Watson which takes into account weight, height, gender, and age. For males: $V(L) = 2.477 + [0.3362 \times$ weight in kg] $+ [0.1074 \times$ height in cm] $- [0.09516 \times$ age in years]. For females $V(L) = -2.097 + [0.2466 \times$ weight in kg] $+ [0.1069 \times$ height in cm]. The calculation of creatinine clearance is similar to Kt/V. However, the urinary component of creatinine clearance is usually corrected for creatinine secretion by averaging it with the urinary urea clearance. The peritoneal creatinine clearance is simply measured by dividing the creatinine content of the 24-hr dialysate by serum creatinine. The total creatinine clearance (peritoneal + renal) is normalized to 1.73 m^2 body surface area.

Nutrition in the Peritoneal Dialysis Patient

Forty percent of PD patients are protein malnourished. This is in part due to losses of amino acids and protein in the dialysate, the latter generally being 8 to 10 g/dL. Peritonitis markedly increases dialysate protein losses. The appetite of the patient may be suppressed from the absorbed dialysate glucose as well as from uremia. Both Kt/V and weekly creatinine clearance correlate, albeit weakly, with protein intake, suggesting that a certain minimum dose of dialysis is required for adequate protein intake. The serum albumin level is inversely related to both mortality and hospitalization in PD patients. A protein intake of at least 1.2 g/kg/day is recommended for PD patients, but many patients ingest only 0.8 to 1.0 g/kg/day. Amino acid dialysate (in which amino acids replace the glucose) has been used on a limited basis as a means of correcting protein malnutrition, but proof of its long-term benefit is thus far lacking.

The calories absorbed from dialysate glucose depend on the dextrose concentration used (1.50, 2.50, 4.25 g/dL) as well as on the membrane permeability of the patient. The development of obesity therefore is not unusual in PD patients, especially those already overweight at the start of dialysis. In addition, glucose absorption frequently results in hyperlipidemia, which may contribute to cardiovascular diseases.

COMPLICATIONS OF PD

Peritonitis

Diagnosis of peritonitis requires the presence two of the following criteria in any combination:

- presence of organisms on Gram stain or subsequent culture.
- cloudy fluid (white cell count greater than 100/mm; greater than 50% neutrophils)
- symptoms and signs of peritoneal inflammation.

Cloudy dialysate effluent is almost invariably present, whereas abdominal pain is present in about 80–95% of cases. Gastrointestinal symptoms, chills, and fever are present in up to 25% of the cases, while abdominal tenderness accompanies the symptoms in three-quarters of the cases. Bacteremia is rare. Gram stain of the effluent is seldom helpful, except for fungal peritonitis, but cultures are generally positive. In many centers, 20% of peritonitis episodes result in no growth, predominantly owing to inadequate culture techniques.

The etiologies of peritonitis are given in Table 4, together with the frequency of organisms. Peritonitis rates due to *Staphylococcus epidermidis* have decreased, and *Staphylococcus aureus* and enteric organisms account for a larger proportion of peritonitis episodes than before. Because patients with these organisms are more symptomatic than those with *S. epidermidis* peritonitis, peritonitis has become a less frequent, but more severe complication, often requiring hospital admission.

Peritonitis remains an important cause of hospitalization, catheter loss, and transfer to hemodialysis. Peritonitis

TABLE 4
Microorganisms Causing Peritonitis and Change in Peritonitis Rates for Organisms with Introduction of Y-Set Systems Reported in One Series[a]

Microorganisms	(%)	Peritonitis rates (episodes/patient year) Conventional	Y-set
Gram-positive			
S. epidermidis	30–40	0.34	0.17
S. aureus	15–20	0.15	0.13
Streptococcus	10–15		
Other gram-positive	2–5		
Gram-negative		0.12	0.10
Pseudomonas	5–10		
Enterobacter	5–20		
Other gram-negative	5–7		
Fungi	2–10	0.02	0.01
Other organisms	2–5		
Culture negative	10–30		

[a]Conventional refers to systems prior to the introduction of Y-set incorporating the "flush before fill" concept.

rates, originally very high, have decreased to less than an episode every 2–3 dialysis years, owing to improvements in the procedure for performing the dialysis tubing connections, which have decreased the risk of touch contamination (Fig. 1). As a result, the catheter removal rate for peritonitis depends on the infecting microorganism. Peritonitis with *S. epidermidis* is less likely to result in catheter loss than peritonitis due to *S. aureus* or *Pseudomonas aeruginosa*. Fungal peritonitis generally requires catheter removal, since a medical cure can only rarely be achieved.

The initial treatment of peritonitis is empiric and designed to cover both gram-positive cocci and gram-negative bacilli. A first generation cephalosporin, such as cefazolin or cephalothin may be used in conjunction with an aminoglycoside or a third generation cephalosporin with subsequent therapy tailored to the culture and sensitivity results. This initial empiric approach does have some drawbacks. The use of aminoglycosides can cause a loss of residual renal function (nephrotoxicity), whereas the first generation cephalosporins do not adequately cover methicillin resistant organisms. A listing of antibiotics and the dosing schedule is given in Table 5. Because of the concern about the emergence of vancomycin-resistant organisms, vancomycin use should be restricted to treatment of methicillin-resistant organisms or for patients allergic to cephalosporins. Antibiotics are usually given intermittently once a day and administered intraperitoneally in the long dwell exchange (overnight in CAPD and during the daytime long dwell in APD). They can also be given continuously in every exchange. The dose may need adjustment for residual renal function. Duration of therapy depends on the organisms and the severity of the peritonitis. For *S. epidermidis* infections this is usually 14 days (and 3 weeks for most other infections).

It should be possible, in up to 80% of cases, to achieve complete cure without having to resort to catheter removal. Persistent symptoms beyond 96 hr can occur in about 10–30% of episodes, and cure is effected by removal of the catheter. Cure can be obtained if antibiotics are continued beyond 96 hr, but there is high risk of damage to the peritoneum. Relapsing peritonitis is a feature in about 10–15% of episodes. Catheter removal is necessary in up to 15% of cases, and death is reported in about 1–3% of cases. Peritonitis results in a marked increase in peritoneal protein losses, transient decrease in ultrafiltration and, over time with long-term PD, there can be an increase in solute transport and loss of ultrafiltration with the development of a hyperpermeable membrane. Although the changes in a peritoneal membrane are usually transient and related to peritonitis, peritoneal fibrosis, often referred to as sclerosing peritonitis may result from severe episodes, or a cumulative effect of multiple episodes or episodes later in the course of PD (see later).

Peritoneal Catheter Infection

These include infections of exit site (erythema or purulent drainage from the exit site) and tunnel infections (edema, erythema, or tenderness over the subcutaneous pathway). *Staphylococcus aureus* is responsible for the majority of catheter infections. *Staphylococcus aureus* exit site infections are difficult to treat, with frequent progression to tunnel infections and peritonitis, in which case catheter removal is required for resolution. *Staphylococcus aureus* nasal carriage is associated with an increased risk of *S. aureus* catheter infections. Treatment of nasal carriers with intransal mupirocin twice a day for 5 days each month, mupirocin applied daily to the exit site, or oral rifampin 600 mg every day for 5 days every 12 weeks are all effective in reducing *S. aureus* catheter infections. *Pseudomonas aeruginosa* catheter infections are also difficult to resolve and frequently relapse. Ciprofloxacin is used to treat *P. aeruginosa* catheter infections but if *P. aeurginosa* peritonitis develops, the catheter must be removed to resolve the infection.

Catheter Malfunction, Hernias, and Fluid Leaks

The most important noninfectious complications during PD are abdominal wall related hernias, leakage of dialysis fluid, and inflow and outflow malfunction.

Before PD treatment is started all significant abdominal wall related hernias should be corrected. With the presence of 2–3 L of dialysate in the abdominal cavity, there is an increased intra-abdominal pressure, and a preexisting hernia will worsen during PD treatment. The most frequently occurring hernias during PD are insertional, umbilical, and inguinal. Significant hernias should primarily be repaired surgically, and following repair intermittent PD may be

TABLE 5
Listing of Antibiotics and Dosing Schedules for Intraperitoneal Use Unless Otherwise Stated

Antibiotic	Initial dose (mg/L)	Subsequent dose (mg/L each exchange)	Subsequent doses (mg/L once daily)
Ampicillin	125	125	No data
Aztreonam	1000	250	1000 qd
Cefazolin	500	125	500 qd
Ceftazidime	500	125	1000 qd
Fluconazole	200 mg po		200 mg po qd
Aminoglycosides[b]	20 mg	4	20 mg
Metronidazole	500 mg po/iv		500 mg po/iv tid
Vancomycin	15–30 mg/kg	25	15–30 mg/kg q 5–7 day

[a]po, per oral; iv, intravenous.

[b]This group includes gentamicin, tobramycin, and netilmicin (same dose for all). Once daily antibiotics with the long dwell is preferred to antibiotic addition to each exchange; this has been shown to be efficacious for cefazolin, cephalothin, and ceftazidime. For APD, patients may be changed to a CAPD schedule. If patients stay on an APD schedule, the antibiotics are added to each exchange as per the second column.

continued postoperatively using low volumes in a supine position.

Leakage of peritoneal fluid is related to catheter implantation technique, trauma, or patient-related anatomical abnormalities. It can occur early (less than 30 days) or late (greater than 30 days) after implantation and can have different clinical manifestation depending on whether the leak is external or subcutaneous. Early leakage is usually external, appearing as fluid through the wound or the exit site. Subcutaneous leakage may develop at the site of an incision and entry into the peritoneal cavity. The exact site of the leakage can be determined with computerized tomography after infusion of 2 L of dialysis fluid containing radio contrast material. Scrotal or labial edema can be a sign of fluid leak, usually through a patent processus vaginalis. Therapy usually entails a period off PD during which the patient, if needing dialysis, is maintained on HD or limited small volume supine PD. For recurrent leaks, surgical repair is essential. Leakage of fluid into the subcutaneous tissue is sometimes occult, difficult to diagnosis, and may present as diminished drainage, which might be mistaken for ultrafiltration failure. Computerized tomography and abdominal scintography may identify the leak.

Outflow/inflow obstruction are the most frequently observed early events within 2 weeks of the catheter implantation, although these complications can be seen later during PD-related complications such as peritonitis.

One way outflow obstruction is the most frequent problem and is characterized by poor flow and failure to drain the peritoneal cavity. Both intraluminal factors (blood clot, fibrin) or extraluminal factors (constipation, occlusion of catheter holes from pressure exerted by adjacent organs or omental wrapping, catheter tip dislocation out of the true pelvis, and incorrect catheter placement at implantation) are common causes. A Kidney–ureter–bladder (KUB) X-ray is useful in localizing the PD catheter tip and evaluating for malposition. Depending on the cause, appropriate therapy entails laxatives, heparinized saline flushes, urokinase instillation in the catheter, fluoroscopy, and manipulation (using a stiff wire or stylet manipulation combined with a whiplash technique), revision, or replacement.

Peritoneal Membrane Changes and Loss of Ultrafiltration

The peritoneum undergoing PD reacts to changes in response to the new environment. There is thickening of the peritoneal interstitium and basement membrane reduplication both in the mesothelium as well as in the capillary. Such changes have been identified to occur secondary to the unphysiological composition of the dialysis solutions, and also the direct action of glucose and glucose degradation products, which bring about advanced glycosylation end product (AGE) related changes in the peritoneal membrane. Some of the changes are diabetiform in nature alterations of peritoneal micro vessels and neovascularization as seen in diabetic retinopathy with deposition of type IV collagen. Case controlled studies have also shown that peritoneal damage is related to greater glucose exposure. Other factors that are important in the pathogenesis are acute peritonitis and chronic inflammatory reactions, mediated by activation of peritoneal macrophages, and intraperitoneal production of bioactive substances promoting inflammation and peritoneal fibrosis. To maintain membrane integrity, there is a need to introduce more physiological solutions and to minimize peritonitis.

Changes to the peritoneal membrane have been described with time on dialysis, physiologically reflected in a hyperpermeable membrane, that is, high D/P creatinine ratio on PET. This results in rapid dissipation of the osmotic gradient as previously described. Most of the changes previously described lead to a hyperpermeable membrane. Membrane changes vary but can progress eventually to the rare sclerosing encapsulating peritonitis, a misnomer because this pathologic condition is not actually peritonitis, but characterized by marked thickening of the peritoneum. This occurs late (usually >5 years after onset of PD) and can result in decreased permeability, which can also result from extensive adhesions.

Net ultrafiltration failure is the most important transport abnormality in long-term PD. Based on clinical symptoms, its prevalence has been reported to increase from 3% after 1 year on CAPD to about 30% after 6 years. Ultrafiltration failure is defined as net ultrafiltration of less than 400 mL after a 4 hr dwell using 2 L of 4.25% glucose containing dialysate. This condition is associated with a large vascular peritoneal surface area and impaired aquaporin channel mediated water transport. The former results in a marked increase in the small pores, across which the glucose diffuses rapidly with dissipation of the osmotic gradient.

These patients are best managed with frequent short dwells and elimination of long dwells, such as with nocturnal APD, combined with daytime icodextrin. Icodextrin acts at the level of the small pores, through the process of colloid osmosis and hence can maintain ultrafiltration even when the membrane permeability is increased. Improvement of peritoneal function can be brought about by minimizing glucose exposure, peritoneal rest (use of glucose free dialysate), and use of icodextrin, which has been shown to extend therapy time on PD in patients with loss of ultrafiltration, who would otherwise need hemodialysis. Mortality in this group is higher than in other patients on PD, probably because of poor fluid control and increased protein losses in the dialysate.

Diabetics on Peritoneal Dialysis

Diabetic glomerulosclerosis is the most common cause of renal failure in PD patients. The vast majority of diabetic patients require insulin on PD, even if they did not require insulin prior to the initiation of dialysis. This is partly due to glucose absorption from the dialysate and the associated weight gain. Insulin can be given to PD patients via the intraperitoneal route (thought to be better because it is more physiological, but evidence for this is lacking), the subcutaneous route, or a combination of both. If given intraperitoneally, the dose of insulin required will increase as insulin adsorbs on to the polyvinyl chloride bags. Patients on APD generally require long acting subcutaneous insulin (with or without intraperitoneal regular insulin) for adequate glucose control. The use of intraperitoneal insulin has not been shown to increase the risk of peritonitis. Gastroperesis can be a troublesome complication in patients with autonomic neuropathy. Metoclopramide (10 mg daily) given orally or intraperitoneally is helpful. The overall care of the diabetic patient needs to continue, particularly diligent foot care.

OUTCOMES IN PATIENTS ON PD

The death rate of PD patients in the United States from 1991 to 1993 was 30/100 dialysis years at risk. The leading causes of the death are cardiovascular disease and infections. In the United States, patients over age 55 had a greater risk of death on PD compared to hemodialysis, but these results have not been seen in other countries such as Italy and Canada whose PD patients have lower mortality rates than those in the United States. Outcome results in terms of patient and technique survival are improving. In the 1990s, various single center studies showed that the 5 years actuarial patient survival on PD ranges from 50 to 60%, whereas 5 years technique survival (death and transplantation are censured) ranges from 55 to 70%. Risk factors for death on PD include increasing age, the presence of cardiovascular disease, or diabetes mellitus, decreased serum albumin level, poor nutritional status, and inadequate dialysis. For CAPD patients, a decrease in the Kt/V by 0.1 U/week increases mortality by 6% whereas a decrease in creatinine clearance by 5 L/week/1.73 m^2, increases mortality by 7%.

One of the advantages of PD as compared to hemodialysis is the better preservation of residual renal function. If patient preference and medical conditions allow, PD may well be the preferred dialysis therapy when a patient reaches end stage.

A high proportion of patients transfer off PD to hemodialysis for a multitude of reasons including peritonitis or exit site infection, catheter malfunction, inability to perform the dialysis procedure, and inadequte clearance or ultrafiltration (particularly with loss of residual renal function) (Fig. 5.). In many cases, the patient who loses a catheter owing to either peritonitis or a catheter infection may elect to remain on hemodialysis permanently. The increasing use of the disconnect systems is associated with improved technique survival on CAPD, primarily due to lower peritonitis rates. It is hoped that long-term outcomes will improve with greater emphasis on adequacy, greater use of more physiological PD solutions, and the use of PD in an intergrated renal replacement treatment program, wherein PD is an equally important modality. In this setting, with good initial outcome results, PD may arguably be the first dialytic treatment of choice for most ESRD patients, provided that medical condition and patient preference allow this choice.

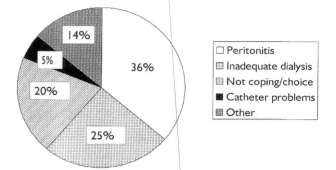

FIGURE 5 Causes of technique failure in long-term PD patients. Data derived from a summation of the data from various reports of outcome in long-term PD patients.

Transplantation is the goal for most patients on dialysis. The allograft and patient survivals of PD patients who are transplanted are similar to those of transplanted hemodialysis patients. If the transplant does not initially function, PD can be continued as long as the peritoneal cavity was not entered. The peritoneal catheter is generally left in place for 2 to 3 months until the graft is functioning well.

PERITONEAL DIALYSIS FOR ACUTE RENAL FAILURE

Intermittent peritoneal dialysis (IPD) may be successfully used to manage patients with acute renal failure. In this case, the peritoneal catheter is often inserted percutaneously using a stylet, without a subcutaneous tunnel (which however, increases the risk of a leak). Rapid exchanges are done to maximize small solute clearance, often one to two exchanges/ hour using a cycler. The patient may be kept on a cycler for 48 hr or even longer, or IPD may be performed daily for 10 to 12 hr. Although extremely effective for volume control and better tolerated in the hemodynamically unstable patient than hemodialysis, clearance of small solutes may be inadequate in catabolic patients or patients on total parenteral nutrition receiving large protein loads. In addition, in the intensive care unit setting there is considerable risk of peritonitis. For these reasons, IPD has been largely replaced by hemodialysis and continuous hemodiafiltration for the management of acute renal failure.

Bibliography

Churchill D, Taylor DW, Kesheviah PR, CANUSA Peritoneal Dialysis Study Group: Adequacy of dialysis and nutrition in continuous peritoneal dialysis: Association with clinical outcome. *J Am Soc Nephrol* 7:198–207, 1996.

Churchill DN, Thorpe KE, Nolph KD, *et al.*: Increased pertioneal membrane transport is associated with decreased patient and technique survival for continuous peritoneal dialysis patients. *J Am Soc Nephrol* 9:1285–1293, 1998.

Coles G: Have we underestimated the importance of fluid balance for survival of PD patients? *Perit Dial Int* 17:321–326, 1997.

Coles G, Williams JD: What is the place of peritoneal dialysis in the integrated treatment of renal failure? *Kidney Int* 54:2234–2240, 1998.

Davies S, Phillips L, Griffiths A, *et al.:* What really happens to people on long-term peritoneal dialysis? *Kidney Int* 54:2207–2217, 1998.

Dinesh KC, Golper T, Gokal R: Adequacy, nutrition and cardiovascular outcome in peritoneal dialysis. *Am J Kidney Dis* 33:617–632, 1999.

Fenton SSA, Schaulbel DE, Desmeules M, *et al.:* Hemodialysis versus peritoneal dialysis: A comparison of adjusted mortality rates. *Am J Kidney Dis* 30:334–342, 1997.

Gokal R: New strategies for peritoneal dialysis solutions. *Nephrol Dial Transplant* 12(Suppl 1):74–77, 1997.

Gokal R, Alexander SR, Ash S, *et al.:* Peritoneal catheters and exit-site practices toward optimum peritoneal access: 1998 update. *Perit Dial Int* 18:11–33, 1998.

Hendriks PM, Ho-dac-Pannekeet MM, van Gulik TM, *et al.:* Peritoneal sclerosis in chronic peritoneal dialysis patients: Analysis of clinical presentation, risk factors, and peritoneal transport kinetics. *Perit Dial Int* 17:136–143, 1997.

Holley JL, Bernardini F, Piraino B: Infecting organisms in continuous ambulatory peritoneal dialysis on the Y-set. *Am J Kidney Dis* 23:569–573, 1994.

Kawaguchi Y, Hasegawa T, Nakayama M, *et al.:* Issues affecting the longevity of continuous peritoneal dialysis therapy. *Kidney Int* 52(Suppl 62):S105–S107, 1997.

Keane WF, Alexander SR, Bailie GR, *et al.:* Peritoneal dialysis-related peritonitis treatment recommendations: 1996 update. *Perit Dial Int* 16:557–573, 1996.

Mistry CD, Gokal R, Peers E, and the Midas Study Group: A randomised multicentre clinical trial comparing isosmolar dextrin 20 with hyperosmolar glucose solutions in Continuous Ambulatory Peritoneal Dialysis (CAPD): A 6 month study. *Kidney Int* 46:496–503, 1994.

Nakayama M, Kawaguchi Y, Yamada K, *et al.:* Immunohistochemical detection of advanced glycosylation end-products in the peritoneum and its possible pathophysiological role in CAPD. *Kidney Int* 51:182–186, 1997.

National Kidney Foundation: Dialysis Outcomes Quality Initiative (DOQI): Clinical practice guidelines: Peritoneal dialysis adequacy. *Am J Kidney Dis* 30(Suppl 3):S67–S136, 1997.

Nissenson A, Prichard SS, Cheng IPS, *et al.:* ESRD modality selection into the 21st century: The importance of non-medical factors. *ASAIO J* 43:143–150, 1997.

The Mupirocin Study Group: Nasal mupirocin prevents *Staphylococcus aureus* exit site infection during peritoneal dialysis. *J Am Soc Nephrol* 11:2403–2408, 1996.

Twardowski ZJ, Prowant BF: Current approaches to exit site infections in patients on peritoneal dialysis. *Nephrol Dial Transplant* 12:1284–1295, 1997.

OUTCOME OF END STAGE RENAL DISEASE THERAPIES

WENDY E. BLOEMBERGEN

The expected outcomes of an end stage renal disease (ESRD) patient remain inferior to those of the general population. This chapter includes an overview of ESRD patient outcomes, assessed in terms of mortality, morbidity, technique survival, quality of life, rehabilitation, and cost. The availability of the U.S. Renal Data System (USRDS), a national data base of all treated ESRD patients, and large cohort studies allows the description of many of these outcome measures.

MORTALITY

The mortality of the ESRD population is high relative to the general population. In 1997, the crude mortality rate of the U.S. ESRD population was 17 deaths/100 patient years. For the dialysis only population, the rate was 22.7 deaths/100 patient years. The expected remaining lifetime of a patient with ESRD is one-third to one-sixth that of the general population for all age and race categories. Figure 1 shows that the diagnosis of ESRD carries with it a prognosis between that for colon and lung cancer.

The failure of currently available "renal replacement" therapies to provide ESRD patients with expected survival similar to the general population is likely due to the high prevalence of comorbid conditions (many of which are already present as patients start ESRD therapy), the inability of dialysis to fully replace all of the functions of native

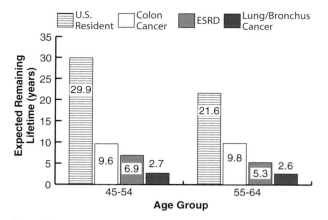

FIGURE 1 Expected remaining lifetime for age groups 45–54 and 55–64 for U.S. resident population (1990), and selected subpopulations with chronic disease, including colon cancer population (1983–1989), ESRD population (1992), and lung/bronchus cancer population (1983–1989). Reproduced from the *U.S. Renal Data System 1995 Annual Data Report*. National Institutes of Health, National Institute of Diabetes and Digestive and Kidney Diseases, Bethesda, Maryland, 1995.

kidneys, and adverse consequences or side effects of the dialysis or transplantation.

Causes of Death

Characterization of causes of death helps to better explain the high mortality of the ESRD population. Figure 2 shows USRDS data on the reported causes of death for the adult ESRD population. Cardiac causes combined account for 48% of all deaths. Infection, cerebrovascular dis-

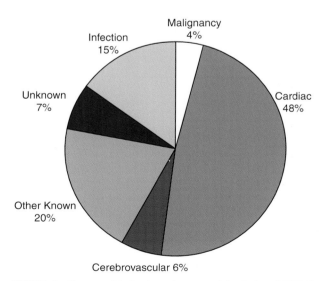

FIGURE 2 Percent distribution of causes of death for all ESRD patients over age 20, 1995–1997. Data from the *U.S. Renal Data System 1999 Annual Data Report*. National Institutes of Health, National Institute of Diabetes and Digestive and Kidney Diseases, Bethesda, Maryland, 1999.

ease, and malignancy are reported to account for 15, 6, and 4%, respectively.

The predominant cause of cardiac deaths is reportedly cardiac arrest or sudden death, accounting for 39%, followed by acute myocardial infarction (24%), atherosclerotic heart disease (9%), cardiomyopathy (10%), and arrhythmia (14%) (Fig. 3). A high prevalence of both coronary artery disease (CAD) and left ventricular hypertrophy (LVH), which is already present among patients starting ESRD therapy, contribute to these cardiac deaths.

Disruption of the skin barrier by the vascular access in hemodialysis (HD) patients and the peritoneal catheter in peritoneal dialysis (PD) patients are factors which are in part responsible for the high risk of death due to infection. Comorbid conditions such as diabetes and peripheral vascular disease also contribute. In addition, there is laboratory evidence that patients with ESRD have defects in cellular immunity, neutrophil function, and complement activation. Figure 3 also shows the reported breakdown of infectious causes. Septicemia owing to the vascular access and due to peritonitis were each reported to account for 8% of deaths. The contribution of vascular access infection may be under estimated, since it is possible that other access infections present as blood borne infections in other organs.

Factors Associated with Mortality

Demographics

Several demographic factors have been shown to be associated with mortality in the U.S. ESRD population. Increasing age, White race, and male gender are associated with higher mortality. Cause of ESRD is also an important predictor of mortality (Fig. 4). Patients with diabetes as the cause of ESRD have close to twice the mortality risk as patients with ESRD due to glomerulonephritis. Patients with ESRD due to hypertension have intermediate mortality rates.

Comorbidity

The prevalence of various comorbid conditions is high among patients treated for ESRD, and their presence has been shown to be associated with worse survival (Table 1). For example, by chart review, 45% of patients in a U.S. national random sample of HD patients had CAD (defined as a prior history of CAD, myocardial infarction, abnormal angiogram, angioplasty or coronary artery bypass graft) which is associated with a 44% higher risk of mortality compared to those without CAD, adjusted for demographics and other comorbid conditions.

An ankle–arm blood pressure index of less than 0.9, a sensitive and specific measure of peripheral vascular disease, was shown to be present among 35% of HD patients and was associated with more than a sevenfold increased risk of cardiovascular mortality. In another study, echocardiograms performed on a cohort of 433 patients starting dialysis found the presence of LVH in 74%, which was associated with a higher risk of mortality.

Among patients starting dialysis, low serum albumin has consistently been shown to be one of the strongest predic-

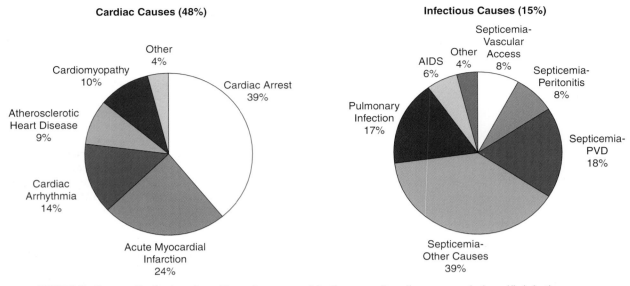

Cardiac Causes (48%)

Infectious Causes (15%)

FIGURE 3 Percent distribution of specific cardiac causes of death among all cardiac causes and of specific infectious causes of death for all infectious deaths for all ESRD patients. Data from the *U.S. Renal Data System 1999 Annual Data Report*. National Institutes of Health, National Institute of Diabetes and Digestive and Kidney Diseases, Bethesda, Maryland, 1999.

tors of mortality. Although it is too simplistic to equate albumin with nutritional status as it is affected by many other factors, other measures of nutrition have also been predictive of mortality among ESRD patients. In a U.S. national random sample of 3400 patients starting HD, patients who were undernourished (14%) had a 26% higher risk of mortality. In another large prospective cohort study of patients starting continuous ambulatory peritoneal dialysis (CAPD), worsened nutritional status (as measured by subjective global assessment and percent lean body mass) was associated with an increased relative risk of death. Low serum creatinine, also felt to be a measure of reduced muscle mass possibly due to malnutrition, has been shown to

be predictive of elevated mortality risk. Furthermore, a more recent study found increasing body weight for height to be associated with lower mortality. These data suggest that greater attention to nutritional therapy may be beneficial to patients with ESRD, although it may be that a patient's nutritional status is simply a measure of other comorbidity.

Socioeconomic Status

Socioeconomic factors have also been shown to predict mortality. Previous studies have found higher mortality to be associated with lower income, lack of family support, and living alone, although this is not always the case.

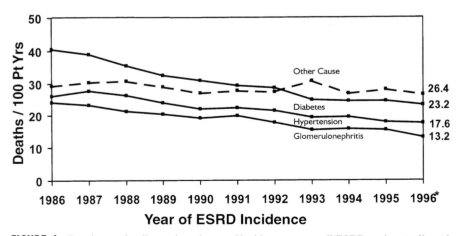

FIGURE 4 Death rates by diagnosis and year of incidence among all ESRD patients, adjusted for age, race and sex. *1996 follow-up is preliminary. Reproduced from the *U.S. Renal Data System 1999 Annual Data Report*. National Institutes of Health, National Institute of Diabetes and Digestive and Kidney Diseases, Bethesda, Maryland, 1999.

TABLE I

Prevalence and Relative Mortality Risk of Comorbid Conditions among U.S. Hemodialysis Patients, 1991

Comorbid conditions	Prevalence (%)	Relative mortality risk
Coronary artery disease	45	1.44
Congestive heart failure	42	1.62
Arrhythmia	31	1.51
Peripheral vascular disease	22	1.62
Cerebrovascular disease	16	1.31
Chronic obstructive lung disease	12	1.62
Neoplasm	9	1.32

Modality

A patient who develops end stage renal failure must choose between several end stage renal replacement therapy options. Broadly classified, these include two main types of dialysis (HD and PD) and transplantation. Several factors require consideration when choosing a treatment modality, including coexistent disease, the social or living circumstances of the patient, as well as preferences and beliefs regarding the treatment options. Relative outcomes associated with these modalities are also important in the decision process.

Survival rates for transplanted patients are better than those of dialysis patients, however patient selection obviously plays a role. A study comparing survival of transplanted patients to those who were receiving dialysis after being included on the transplant waiting list found substantially better survival among transplanted patients.

Recipients of cadaveric transplants have lower survival than those of living related transplants. In 1996, 1-year survival was 98% for living related transplants and 96% for cadaveric transplants. Among transplanted patients, there has been an overall trend to improved survival over the past decade.

In U.S. studies of long-term outcome data published in the mid 1990s, there were observations of higher mortality associated with PD than HD among selected subgroups of dialysis patients. Coinciding with these results were observations that a higher dose of PD, as determined by urea removal, was associated with improved patient survival. Since then there have been substantial changes in the prescription of PD dose with greater attention paid to dialysis adequacy and individualization of therapy. Owing to feasibility issues, there continues to be no randomized controlled trial and therefore no conclusive studies on comparative mortality outcomes by these two modalities. More recent epidemiologic studies comparing PD versus HD mortality have observed a general trend to better survival among PD treated patients initially after starting dialysis followed by a gradual move to equivalency with HD and then, an association with worse mortality in the longer term. It is unclear if the early advantage for PD is a true effect or if it is due to observed selection advantages among PD treated patients. Recent practice guidelines have suggested early initiation of dialysis with PD (in escalating doses as necessary) and eventual switch to HD if and when dialysis dose becomes inadequate with PD because of continuing decline in residual renal function. The two modalities will probably continue to evolve more as complementary than competitive treatments particularly if these guidelines become widely adopted.

Treatment Parameters

Several treatment parameters have been shown in epidemiologic studies to be associated with mortality. In several studies, lower dose of dialysis as determined by urea removal either as Kt/V or urea reduction ratio among HD treated patients and weekly Kt/V or creatinine clearance among PD treated patients was associated with higher mortality. The use of unmodified cellulosic membranes has also been associated with higher mortality than with potentially more biocompatible modified cellulosic or synthetic membranes. However, to date no clinical trials have been done to sort out if these treatment factors as opposed to other confounding factors (e.g., dialysis facility quality) are responsible for the worse outcomes. A large multicenter National Institutes of Health sponsored clinical trial comparing high-versus conventional-dose dialysis is currently in progress.

MORBIDITY

Relatively few U.S. studies which comprehensively quantitate and characterize the occurrence of morbid events among the ESRD population in a prospective fashion are available. Descriptions have more frequently been retrospective and have used number of hospital admissions, length of admission, or total number of hospitalized days/calendar year as measures of morbidity. To date, most published reports are not cause-specific and therefore also do not discriminate, for example, between a hospitalization for access surgery and one for a complication of ESRD. Limitations imposed by Medicare eligibility rules and health insurance and geographic location must also be considered.

USRDS data indicate that the morbidity of the dialysis population is also substantial. In 1997, on average, dialysis patients were admitted to hospital 1.41 times/year and were confined to hospital for 10.8 days/year. Among patients less than age 65, 43% of patients had no admissions. However 8% had 5 or more. Ten percent were admitted for over 30 days/year. Overall, however, there has been a trend for decreasing hospitalization days/patient over the past few years.

In one study of over 500 HD patients that did report cause-specific hospitalization, over 25% of admissions were dialysis access related (vascular access declotting, replacement, infection, or PD catheter placement). The second most frequent reason for admission was cardiovascular followed by gastrointestinal or metabolic disorders. The remainder was due to a variety of less frequent causes. In another study, the probability of requiring hospitalization for a myocardial infarction or angina was approximately 10%/year. There was a similar probability of developing pulmonary edema requiring hospitalization or ultrafiltration.

Hospitalization rates increase by patient age, as expected. Females have consistently been shown to have higher hospitalization rates than males. African-Americans are hospitalized more than Whites both early and late in life, with this pattern being more pronounced for males than females. In general, Asians have lower rates than the other racial subgroups. Rates for diabetics are higher than those for nondiabetics in all age groups. There are also substantial differences in hospitalization by geographic region, with the highest rates in the South Central, Middle Atlantic, and Northeast regions. The factors responsible for these observed differences are not clear.

As one would expect, the presence of comorbid conditions including angina, congestive heart failure, peripheral vascular disease, low serum albumin, and decreased activity level have been associated with increased hospital utilization. Hospitalization rates are slightly lower among PD treated compared to HD treated patients until age 20 and after age 70, but slightly higher in each age group in between. However, until a recent stabilization, hospitalization rates were gradually falling for PD patients, most likely owing to technical improvements in this modality, while those for HD patients have remained relatively stable. Patients with arteriovenous fistulas also have fewer hospitalizations than those with prostratic grafts.

TECHNIQUE SURVIVAL

The probability of failure of the chosen modality for renal replacement therapy may be an important factor in a patient's modality decision. Among dialytic techniques, there is a substantially higher failure rate among patients treated with PD compared to HD. Among patients treated with HD, less than 5% have switched to PD at 2 years whereas among patients initially treated with PD, approximately 15% have switched to HD. Failure on PD is most frequently due to peritonitis, exit site or tunnel infections, but can also be due to other CAPD related complications, inadequate dialysis due to loss of residual renal function or decreases in membrane clearance, or social reasons.

Among patients who receive a transplant, renal allograft survival is dependent on donor source, cadaveric or living down (Fig. 5). Five-year total adjusted graft survival was 75.8 and 61% for living related and cadaveric transplants, respectively. Graft survival has improved steadily over the past decade. Factors which have been identified as predictors of worse graft survival include donor age over 55 or less than 10 years, the amount of time between donor organ retrieval and transplantation, older recipient age, human leukocyte antigen (HLA) mismatch, and female donor. Post-transplantation factors which predict worse graft survival include absence of immediate graft function, a need for dialysis at 1 week after transplantation, rejection at hospital discharge, and elevated serum creatinine at hospital discharge. The use of cyclosporine and OKT3 monoclonal antibody have increased the rate of graft survival at 1 year. Newer immunosuppressives such as tacrolimus and mycophenolate mofetil are associated with a reduction in acute rejection episodes.

QUALITY OF LIFE

Quality of life, a more refined outcome measure than morbidity and mortality, is an important factor in the assessment of the various treatment choices among patients with ESRD. Interest in factors affecting and how best to improve quality of life has increased tremendously in the past several years. This is in part because the quality of life experienced by ESRD patients, as among patients with many other chronic illnesses is often significantly compromised. The renal failure itself, the disease that resulted in renal failure, and the high degree of associated comorbidity are likely contributing factors. Dialysis patients often complain of fatigue, lack of energy, anorexia, depression, decreased libido, musculoskeletal symptoms, and pruritus.

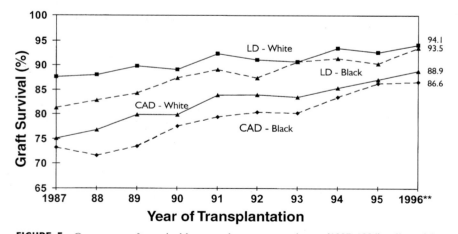

FIGURE 5 One-year graft survival by race, donor type, and year (1987–1996), adjusted for age, sex, cause of ESRD, among first transplants only. LRD = Living related renal transplant, CAD = Cadaveric renal transplant. ** 1996 follow-up is preliminary. Reproduced from the *U.S. Renal Data System 1999 Annual Data Report*. National Institutes of Health, National Institute of Diabetes and Digestive and Kidney Diseases, Bethesda, Maryland, 1999.

HD is usually required three times a week for 3 to 4 hr, and can be accompanied by various physical discomforts including nausea, dizziness, headaches, and lack of energy during or after dialysis. Dietary restrictions are strict and involvement in work, social, and recreational activities is frequently reduced. PD requires frequent dialysate exchanges and may be complicated by peritonitis or catheter tunnel infections. Renal transplant patients may experience side effects of immunosuppressive therapy including infection, acne, hirsuitism, and increased weight. Medical complications, financial pressures, marital discord, sexual dysfunction, emotional stress, and anxiety about loss or death are common, regardless of modality choice.

The measurement of quality of life—the self-assessed value of an individual's health experiences—is a complex multidimensional concept typically measured by a number of domains including physical functioning, social functioning, psychologic or emotional well-being, physical symptoms, cognitive function, vocational functioning, and overall satisfaction with health. It has been measured by both generic and ESRD specific quality of life instruments. Numerous studies have documented poor quality of life in patients with ESRD. For example, between 30 and 50% of patients on chronic dialysis are reported to have impaired physical performance capacity, and up to 70% have moderate to severe levels of emotional stress. Quality of life varies by demographic factors, comorbidity, underlying disease, and mode of treatment. It is inferior among patients with comorbid conditions and those with diabetes as a cause of renal failure. Among the ESRD modality choices, transplantation appears to offer substantially better quality of life than HD as shown by two prospective studies which compared quality of life of dialysis patients while on the transplant waiting list and the same patients after transplantation. There are less conclusive data on which dialysis modality type offers the best quality of life. Both longitudinal studies and a randomized clinical trial have found superior quality of life among dialysis patients treated with recombinant human erythropoietin (EPO).

REHABILITATION

When Medicare coverage for ESRD began in 1973, the expectation was that many of those whose lives were prolonged would contribute to society through work and taxes. However, since then the patient population has changed dramatically with the acceptance of older and sicker patients and now the majority are not gainfully employed. Consequently, rehabilitation no longer can be judged by employment alone, but must address the level of function of the patient before ESRD and their return to a comparable status.

Participation in an exercise program has been advocated to enhance rehabilitation outcome. To the extent possible, transplantation should be encouraged among suitable patients. In a prospective study, the proportion of ESRD patients employed increased from 30% before transplantation (on dialysis) to 45% 2 years after they were transplantation. This is probably because their more flexible schedule allowed them to engage in employment as well as because of improved physical and mental abilities. As health care costs rise the vocational and functional rehabilitation of patients undergoing dialysis or transplantation is receiving more attention by Congress and the public.

COST

Currently approximately 93% of U.S. ESRD patients have their treatment covered by Medicare. The estimated total monetary cost of treating ESRD in the United States in 1997, was $15.64 billion, of which the portion paid by Medicare was $11.76 billion. This includes the cost of dialysis and hospitalizations (each approximately 40% of total cost) as well as supplies, covered medications, physician fees, etc. (20% of total cost). Average Medicare spending/patient year was $43,000. On average, the total cost/patient (Medicare, other insurance, patient obligations, etc.) is approximately 20–25% higher. There is substantial variation by modality. Yearly Medicare costs (averaged for first and subsequent years) were $52,000 for HD, $45,000 for PD, and $18,000 for transplanted patients. Among transplanted patients, first year cost is substantially greater than subsequent years as it includes the cost of organ retrieval, transplantation, and initial hospitalization. In a prospective study comparing dialysis to transplantation, the cost of dialysis care pretransplant and the cost of the first year after transplant was similar. At 2 years, transplantation was clearly associated with better quality of life and was less costly than dialysis among all subgroups.

Annual costs for all ESRD patients rise steadily with age, primarily because of the decline in transplantation rate with increasing age. Diabetic patients are considerably more costly to treat than nondiabetics. Medicare payments are slightly higher for females than males in most age categories. Payments for African-Americans are higher than for whites among patients less than 65, again in part due to lower transplantation rates.

Bibliography

Bloembergen WE, Port FK, Mauger EA, Wolfe RA: A comparison of mortality between patients treated with hemodialysis and peritoneal dialysis. *J Am Soc Nephrol* 6:177–183, 1995.

Canadian Erythropoietin Study Group: Association between recombinant human erythropoietin and quality of life and exercise capacity of patients receiving haemodialysis. *Br Med J* 300:573–578, 1990.

Canada–USA (CANUSA) Peritoneal Dialysis Study Group: Adequacy of dialysis and nutrition in continuous peritoneal dialysis: Association with clinical outcomes. *J Am Soc Nephrol* 7:198–207, 1996.

Churchill DN, Taylor DW, Cook RJ, *et al.:* Canadian hemodialysis morbidity study. *Am J Kidney Dis* 19:214–234, 1992.

Evans RW, Manninen DL, Garrison LP, Jr, *et al.:* The quality of life of patients with end-stage renal disease. *N Engl J Med* 312:553–559, 1985.

Excerpts from U.S. Renal Data System 1999 Annual Data Report, Chapters on: Causes of Death; Patient Mortality and Survival; Hospitalization; Renal Transplantation: Access and Outcomes; The Economic Cost of ESRD and Medicare Spending for Alternative Modalities of Treatment. National Institutes of Health, National Institite of Diabetes and Digestive and Kidney Diseases, Bethesda, MD, 1996. *Am J Kidney Dis* 28:S1–S165, 1996.

Hakim RM, Held PJ, Stannard D, Wolfe RA, Port FK, Daugirdas JT, Agodoa L: The effect of the dialysis membrane on mortality of chronic hemodialysis patients (CHD) in the U.S. *Kidney Int* 50:566–570, 1996.

Held PJ, Port FK, Wolfe RA, Stannard DC, Daugirdas JT, Bloembergen WE, Greer JW, Hakim RM: The dose of hemodialysis and patient mortality. *Kidney Int* 50:550–556, 1996.

Jones KR: Factors associated with hospitalization in a sample of chronic hemodialysis patients. *Health Serv Res* 26:671–699, 1991.

Laupacis A, Keown PA, Pus N, Krueger H, Ferguson B, Wong C, Muirhead N: A study of the quality of life and cost utility of renal transplantation. *Kidney Int* 50:235–242, 1996.

Owen WF, Lew NL, Liu Y, Lowrie EG, Lazarus JM: The urea reduction ratio and serum albumin concentration as predictors of mortality in patients undergoing hemodialysis. *N Engl J Med* 329:1001–1006, 1993.

Port FK: Morbidity and mortality in dialysis patients. *Kidney Int* 46:1728–1737, 1994.

Rocco MV, Soucie JM, Reboussin DM, McClellan WM: Risk factors for hospital utilization in chronic dialysis patients. *J Am Soc Nephrol* 7:889–896, 1996.

Russell JD, Beecroft ML, Ludwin D, Churchill DW: The quality of life in renal transplantation—a prospective study. *Transplantation* 54:656–660, 1992.

Terasaki PI, Yuge J, Cecka JM, Gjertson DW, Takemoto S, Cho YW: Thirty-year tends in clinical transplantation. In: Terasaki PI, Cecka JM (eds) *Clinical Transplants 1993*. UCLA Tissue Typing Laboratory, Los Angeles, 1994.

Vonesh EF, Moran J: Mortality in end-stage renal disease: A reassessment of differences between patients treated with hemodialysis and peritoneal dialysis. *J Am Soc Nephrol* 10: 354–365, 1999.

Wolfe RA, Gaylin DS, Port FK, Held PJ, Wood CL: Using USRDS generated mortality tables to compare local ESRD mortality rates with national rates. *Kidney Int* 42:991–996, 1992.

Wolfe RA, Held PH, Hulbert-Shearon TE, Agodoa LYC, Port FK: A critical examination of trends in outcomes over the last decade. *Am J Kidney Dis* 32:S9–S15, 1998.

Wolfe RA, Ashby VB, Milford EL, Ojo AO, Ettenger RE, Agodoa LY, Held PJ, Port FK: Comparison of mortality in all patients on dialysis, patients on dialysis awaiting transplantation, and recipients of a first cadaveric transplant. *N Engl J Med* 341: 1725–1730, 1999.

NUTRITION AND RENAL DISEASE

T. ALP IKIZLER

During progression of chronic renal failure (CRF), the requirements and utilization of different nutrients change significantly. These changes ultimately phase renal failure patients at higher risk for protein–calorie malnutrition. In addition, the presence of protein–calorie malnutrition is an important predictor of poor outcome in these patients. Understanding the applicable nutritional principles and the available methods for improving nutritional status of these patients is essential.

NUTRIENT METABOLISM IN RENAL FAILURE

Protein Metabolism and Requirements

Chronic Renal Failure Patients

In general, the minimal daily protein requirement is one that maintains a neutral nitrogen balance and prevents malnutrition; this has been estimated to be a daily protein intake of approximately 0.6 g/kg in healthy individuals, with a safe level of protein intake equivalent to the minimal requirement plus 2 standard deviations, or approximately 0.75 g/kg/day. One of the most significant findings of advanced renal failure is a decrease in appetite. Several studies have indicated that CRF patients spontaneously restrict their dietary protein intake, with levels less than 0.6 g/kg/day when glomerular filtration rate is less than 10 mL/min. Other markers of malnutrition such as decreasing weight also correlate with decreasing renal function and dietary protein intake, suggesting that anorexia predisposes CRF patients to malnutrition. Accumulation of uremic toxins may not be the sole course of decreased dietary nutrient intake. Table 1 depicts some of the factors that can cause decreased nutrient intake as well as other potential mechanisms that can cause protein calorie malnutrition in renal failure patients. Patients with renal failure secondary to diabetes

TABLE I
Factors Associated with Decreased Nutritional Status of Chronic Renal Failure Patients

Increased protein and energy requirements
  Losses of nutrients (amino acids and/or proteins) during dialysis
  Increased resting energy expenditure
Decreased protein and calorie intake
  Anorexia
  Frequent hospitalizations
  Inadequate dialysis dose
  Comorbidities (diabetes mellitus, GI diseases, ongoing inflammatory response)
  Multiple medications
Increased catabolism/decreased anabolism
  Dialysis induced catabolism
    Bioincompatible hemodialysis membranes
  Amino acid abnormalities
  Metabolic acidosis
  Hormonal derangements
    Hyperparathyroidism
    Insulin and growth hormone resistance

mellitus are likely to be more prone to malnutrition because of dietary restrictions and gastrointestinal symptoms such as gastroparesis, nausea, and vomiting, as well as bacterial overgrowth in the gut and pancreatic insufficiency. Depression, which is commonly seen in CRF patients is also associated with anorexia. In addition, CRF patients are usually prescribed a large number of medications, particularly sedatives, phosphate binders, and iron supplements, which are also associated with gastrointestinal complications. Finally, the socioeconomic status of the patients, their lack of mobility, as well as their age, are other predisposing factors for decreased dietary protein intake.

Protein Restriction in Chronic Renal Failure Patients

Dietary protein restriction has been recommended as a therapeutic approach for retarding the progression of chronic renal failure. The results of several recent studies on this subject are conflicting. The results of the largest clinical trial, The Modification of Diet in Renal Disease (MDRD) did not demonstrate a benefit of dietary protein restriction on progression of renal disease. On the other hand, three recent meta-analyses indicate that such diets may be beneficial in slowing the progression, albeit to a small extent. If such diets are to be used, it is important to assure that patients are not out at risk for malnutrition. In the MDRD study, there were only minor changes in nutritional markers in the low-protein diet groups suggesting that under close observation, protein restricted diets provided with or without supplements of essential amino acids or their keto-analogs will maintain nutritional status. However, the dedicated dietitian involvement with heavy emphasis on maintenance of caloric intake, used in the MDRD study is not available to the majority of patients with chronic renal failure; thus, such dietary interventions should be tried only in highly motivated and closely supervised patients. Table 2 lists the recommended dietary prescriptions for protein intakes for patients at different stages of renal failure.

Chronic Dialysis Patients

Several dialysis related factors predispose chronic dialysis patients to negative nitrogen balance (Table 1). There are inevitable losses of amino acids during both hemodialysis (HD) and peritoneal dialysis (PD), ranging from 5 to 8 g of amino acids/HD session and 5–12 g/day of amino acids during PD. Losses may be higher with high flux HD or when peritonitis is present. The absorption of glucose during PD may also predispose patients to anorexia due to the development of satiety. In addition, a feeling of fullness may be related to the fluid in the peri-

TABLE 2
Recommended Intakes of Protein, Energy, and Minerals in Renal Failure

	Protein	Energy	Phosphorus	Sodium
Chronic renal failure				
Mild to moderate (GFR >25 mL/min)	No restriction	No Restriction	600–800 mg/day	<2 g/day[a]
Advanced (GFR <25 mL/min)	0.60–0.75 g/k/day[b]	35 kcal/kg/day[c]	600–800 mg/day[d]	<2 g/day
End stage renal disease				
Hemodialysis	>1.2 g/kg/day	35 kcal/kg/day[c]	600–800 mg/day[d]	<2 g/day
Peritoneal dialysis	>1.3 g/kg/day	35 kcal/kg/day[c]	600–800 mg/day[d]	<2 g/day
Acute renal failure				
Predialysis	1.0–1.2 g/kd/day	35 kcal/kg/day	600–800 mg/day[e]	<2 g/day
Dialysis	1.2–1.4 g/kg/day	35 kcal/kg/day	600–800 mg/day[e]	<2 g/day

[a]If hypertensive.
[b]With close supervision and frequent dietary counseling.
[c]30 kcal/kg/day for individuals 60 years and older.
[d]Along with phosphate binders, as needed.
[e]If phosphorus >5.5 mg/dL.

toneal cavity. One of the most important factors affecting the nutritional status of dialysis patients is the dose of dialysis. The results of a large multicenter study in PD patients showed a positive relationship between increasing amounts of dialysis and nutritional status. It was reported that decreasing serum albumin concentrations and worsening nutrition according to subjective global assessment were predictive of higher mortality and increasing hospitalizations.

Amino Acid Metabolism

Chronic renal failure patients have well-defined abnormalities in their plasma and to a lesser extent in their muscle amino acid profiles. Commonly, essential amino acid concentrations are low and nonessential amino acid concentrations high. The etiology of this abnormal profile is multifactorial. The progressive loss of renal tissue, where metabolism of several amino acids takes place, is an important factor. Specifically, glycine and phenylalanine concentrations are elevated, and serine, tyrosine, and histidine concentrations are decreased. Plasma and muscle concentrations of branched-chain amino acids (valine, leucine, and isoleucine) are reduced in chronic dialysis patients. Among these, valine displays the greatest reduction. In contrast, plasma citrulline, cystine, aspartate, methionine, and both 1- and 3-methylhistidine levels are increased. Although inadequate dietary intake is a possible factor in abnormal essential amino acid profiles, certain abnormalities occur even in the presence of adequate dietary nutrient intake indicating, that the uremic milieu has an additional effect. Indeed, it has been suggested that the metabolic acidosis which is commonly seen in uremic patients plays an important role in increased oxidation of branched-chain amino acids.

Energy Metabolism

The minimum energy requirement of renal failure patients is less well-defined (Table 2). This requirement is dependent on the resting energy expenditure, the activity level of the patient, and other ongoing illnesses. Resting energy expenditure is elevated in chronic dialysis patients compared to age, sex, and body mass index matched normal controls and is further increased during the HD procedure when catabolism is at maximum due to amino acid losses. The recommended energy intake is 35 kcal/kg/day for both chronic dialysis patients and CRF patients not yet on renal replacement therapy.

Lipid Metabolism

Dyslipidemia is quite common in CRF patients, and abnormalities in lipid profiles can be detected in patients once renal function begins to deteriorate suggesting that uremia is associated with lipid disorders. The presence of nephrotic syndrome or other comorbidities such as diabetes mellitus and liver disease as well as the use of medications altering lipid metabolism further contribute to the dyslipidemia seen in renal failure.

In hemodialysis patients, the most common abnormalities are elevated serum triglycerides, very-low-density lipoproteins, and decreased low-(LDL) and high-density (HDL) lipoproteins. The increased triglyceride component is thought to be related to increased levels of apoCIII, an inhibitor of lipoprotein lipase. A substantial number of chronic hemodialysis patients also have elevated lipoprotein (a) [Lp(a)] levels. Patients on PD exhibit higher concentrations of serum cholesterol, triglyceride, LDL cholesterol, and apoB even though the mechanisms that alter the lipid metabolism are similar to chronic hemodialysis patients. This is thought to be related to increased protein losses through the peritoneum and the glucose load supplied by dialysate. They also exhibit higher concentrations of Lp(a). Whether these differences in dyslipidemia are clinically significant remains to be clarified.

Dyslipidemia and Cardiovascular Risk in Dialysis Patients

Cardiovascular death is the leading cause of mortality in chronic dialysis patients. Hypercholesterolemia and other abnormalities in lipid profile have been associated with increased risk of atherosclerosis and cardiovascular events in the general population. However, whether this relationship applies to chronic dialysis patients has not been well established. Indeed, large cross-sectional studies have identified that low cholesterol concentrations, rather than high cholesterol concentrations are associated with increased risk of mortality in chronic dialysis patients. In contrast, a large multicenter study showed that in a cohort of diabetic patients on HD, those who died from a cardiovascular event had higher median cholesterol, LDL cholesterol, LDL/HDL ratio, and apoB concentrations at the time of initiation of dialysis. It is generally accepted that chronic dialysis patients with known risk factors for atherosclerosis and cardiovascular events should be treated with an appropriate regimen, including lipid lowering agents when indicated. A cholesterol concentration higher than 240 mg/dL and/or LDL concentration higher than 130 mg/dL in the presence of other risk factors should be treated in chronic dialysis patients. Whether this approach influences the overall outcome in these patients remains to be proved.

Mineral, Vitamin, and Trace Element Requirements

Sodium intake should be restricted to less than 2 g/day in CRF patients with hypertension. The restriction is similar in dialysis patients (to control interdialytic weight gain and reduce thirst). Potassium intake should be less than 2 g/day in patients with advanced CRF (creatinine clearance <10 mL/min) and in HD patients. In early renal failure, restricting phosphorus intake to 600 to 800 mg/day is recommended. Since further restriction of dietary phosphorus in clinical settings is impractical, once the creatinine clearance falls below 30 mL/min, phosphate binders should be prescribed along with the dietary restriction. Use of calcium-containing binders will also provide the supplemental calcium needed in advanced renal failure. Similar recommendations are appropriate for HD patients.

Vitamin A concentrations are usually elevated in chronic dialysis patients, and intake of even small amounts leads to excessive accumulation. There have been several reports on the vitamin A toxicity in chronic dialysis patients, and therefore it should not be supplemented. Vitamin E levels in chronic dialysis patients are not well-defined, and there have been reports of increased, decreased, or unchanged concentrations. Therefore, it is not clear whether Vitamin E supplementation is required in chronic dialysis patients. Vitamin K supplementation is usually not recommended in chronic dialysis patients unless they are at high risk for developing vitamin K deficiency, as with prolonged hospitalization, with poor dietary intake, or antibiotic therapy. Vitamin D (and calcium/phosphorus) metabolism is discussed in detail in Chapter 63. The serum concentrations of the water soluble vitamins are reported to be low in chronic dialysis patients mainly owing to decreased dietary intake and increased removal during hemodialysis. Multivitamin preparation specifically designed for renal failure patients are available and useful for correcting these low concentrations without inducing vitamin A toxicity. Nevertheless, it is important to recognize that the daily requirements of vitamin B_6, folic acid, and ascorbic acid are often increased in chronic dialysis patients. Monitoring levels may be appropriate for patients at risk of vitamin deficiency.

The concentrations of most of the trace elements are mainly dependent on the degree of renal failure. Although there is an extensive list of trace elements that may have altered concentrations in body fluids in chronic dialysis patients, only a few are thought to be important. Serum aluminum is the most important trace element in chronic dialysis patients since elevated levels have been shown to be associated with dialysis dementia as well as bone disease. Aluminum intoxication can be caused either by use of inadequate purified water for HD (mostly eliminated with the use of reverse osmosis for water purification) or by use of phosphate binders that contain aluminum hydroxide. Since the prolonged ingestion of such binders is a risk factor for aluminum intoxication, patients consuming aluminum on a long-term basis should have repeated aluminum measurements. A serum aluminum concentration well below 30 μg/L is the desired level in chronic dialysis patients.

METABOLIC AND HORMONAL DERANGEMENTS IN CHRONIC RENAL FAILURE PATIENTS

Metabolic acidosis, which commonly accompanies progressive renal failure, also promotes malnutrition, by increased protein catabolism. During metabolic acidosis, muscle proteolysis is stimulated by an ATP-dependent pathway involving ubiquitin and proteasomes. Several hormonal derangements including insulin resistance, increased glucagon concentrations, and secondary hyperparathyroidism are also implicated as factors in the development of malnutrition in CRF. Increased concentrations of para-

thyroid hormone have been shown to enhance amino acid release from muscle tissue. More recently, abnormalities in the growth hormone and insulin-like growth factor 1 axis have been suggested as an important factor in the development of malnutrition in CRF patients. Although plasma concentrations of growth hormone actually increase during the progression of renal failure, probably due to its reduced renal clearance, more recent evidence suggests that uremia per se is associated with the development of resistance to growth hormone action at cellular levels. This blunted response would be expected to attenuate the anabolic actions of these hormones, specifically protein synthesis.

INDICES OF NUTRITIONAL STATUS IN RENAL FAILURE PATIENTS

Although practical methods to assess nutritional status are imperative, the appropriate interpretation of nutritional markers in renal failure patients remains a challenge. Several markers utilized for nutritional purposes are influenced by many non-nutritional factors. In CRF patients, relatively simple biochemical measures reflecting the visceral protein stores, such as serum albumin, creatinine, and blood urea nitrogen (BUN), as well as more complex and not commonly used parameters such as transferrin, prealbumin, and insulin-like growth factor 1 have been proposed as nutritional markers. Serum albumin is probably the most extensively examined nutritional index in almost all patient populations, probably owing to its ready availability and strong association with outcome. However, serum albumin concentration may be affected by other coexisting problems in addition to malnutrition. Specifically, serum albumin is a negative acute-phase reactant; therefore its serum concentration decreases sharply in response to inflammation and thus may not necessarily reflect the changes in nutritional status in acutely or chronically ill patients. Serum albumin concentration in CRF patients may also be affected by other non-nutritional factors, such as external losses (i.e., proteinuria), extravascular fluid volume, and other illnesses, that is, liver disease.

Anthropometric studies can be used for body composition analysis in CRF patients. More reliable and accurate methods of body composition analysis, such as prompt neutron activation analysis which measures total body nitrogen content and dual-energy X-ray absorptiometry require expensive equipment and are only available in specialized centers. Subjective Global Assessment is a more recently proposed method to evaluate the nutritional status of chronic renal failure patients. Its advantage is that it includes objective data (disease state, weight changes), several manifestations of poor nutritional status, and the clinical judgement of the involved physician. The limitations are heavy reliance on the clinical judgement and inability to tailor a specific nutritional intervention. Its utilities as a standard nutritional tool in renal failure is yet to be determined.

Estimation of dietary protein intake can also be used as a marker of overall nutritional status in the CRF patient.

Although dietary recall is a direct and simple measure of dietary protein intake, several studies have shown that this method lacks accuracy in estimating the actual intake. Therefore, other means of measuring dietary protein intake, such as 24-hr urine urea nitrogen excretion in CRF patients or protein catabolic rate calculations in dialysis patients, have been suggested as useful methods to estimate protein intake. However, these indirect estimations of dietary protein intake are valid only in stable patients, and may easily overestimate the actual intake in catabolic patients where endogenous protein breakdown may lead to a high urea nitrogen appearance.

EXTENT OF MALNUTRITION IN CHRONIC RENAL FAILURE PATIENTS

Virtually every study which has evaluated the nutritional status of CRF patients has reported some degree of malnutrition in this population. The prevalence of malnutrition has been estimated to range from approximately 20 to 60% in different studies using various nutritional parameters. In chronic renal failure patients not yet on maintenance dialysis, mild to severe malnutrition by subjective global assessment is reported in 44% of patients. Using the same method, the prevalence of moderate to severe malnutrition is reported at 30% in chronic HD patients and 40% in PD patients.

ASSOCIATION OF NUTRITION AND OUTCOME IN RENAL FAILURE

A number of studies have documented the increased mortality and morbidity in renal failure patients suffering from malnutrition. In a comprehensive study of prevalent chronic dialysis patients, serum albumin concentration was identified as the most powerful indicator of mortality. Even serum albumin concentrations of 3.5–4.0 g/dL (considered a normal value by most laboratories) resulted in an increased relative risk of death as compared to 4.0 g/dL or higher. In addition, decreases in serum creatinine (an indicator of muscle mass) and percent ideal body weight were also associated with increased risk of death in this patient population. Similar observations can be made for incident dialysis patients. Specifically, low serum creatinine and albumin concentrations at the time of initiation of maintenance dialysis are associated with increased risk of mortality and morbidity over the subsequent years on hemodialysis.

STRATEGIES FOR TREATMENT OF MALNUTRITION IN RENAL FAILURE PATIENTS

A list of general measures to prevent and/or to treat malnutrition in different stages of CRF is presented in Table 3. Considering the catabolic state associated with chronic uremia, it is clear that attempts to encourage patients to maintain an adequate protein and calorie intake are essential. Most of these patients continue their predialysis diets while on chronic renal replacement therapy. It is im-

portant to ensure that the dietary protein and calorie intake of these patients fulfill the increased requirements after initiation of dialysis. Repetitive comprehensive dietary counseling by an experienced dietitian is an important step to improve dietary intake, as well as detection of early signs of malnutrition. Similar efforts should be spent not only in outpatient settings, but also during hospitalizations of these patients, since hospitalized patients have even lower dietary protein and calorie intake.

Where dietary counseling to improve nutritional status is unsuccessful, other forms of supplementation such as enteral (including oral protein, amino acid, and energy supplementation, nasogastric feeding tubes, percutaneous endoscopic gastrostom or jejunostomy tubes) and intradialytic parenteral nutrition (IDPN) may be considered. Only a limited number of studies evaluating the effects of enteral supplementation in malnourished chronic dialysis patients are available. Furthermore, most of these studies are uncontrolled and small in scope, and they demonstrate only a variable degree of success. Therefore, it is usually a challenge to determine whether an enteral form of supplementation is effective and when to try more expensive and invasive measures such as IDPN.

Several reports have emphasized the effective use of IDPN as a potential therapeutic intervention in malnourished chronic dialysis patients. In a retrospective analysis of more than 1500 chronic HD patients treated with IDPN, decreasing risk of death with the use of IDPN was reported, particularly in patients with serum albumin concentrations below 3.5 g/dL and serum creatinine concentrations below 8 mg/dL. Studies using amino acid dialysate (AAD) in PD patients have provided conflicting results. In studies which suggested benefit from AAD, serum transferrin and total protein concentrations increased and plasma amino acid profiles tended toward normal with one or two exchanges of AAD. On the other hand, increase in BUN concentra-

TABLE 3

Interventions to Prevent and/or Treat Malnutrition in Renal Failure

Chronic renal failure patients
  Close supervision and nutritional counseling (especially for patients on protein restricted diets)
  Initiation of dialysis or renal transplant in advanced chronic renal failure patients with apparent protein–calorie malnutrition despite vigorous attempts

Maintenance dialysis patients
  Appropriate amount of dietary protein (>1.2 g/kg/day) and calorie (>35 kcal/kg/day) intake
  Optimal dose of dialysis (urea reduction ratio >70%)
  Use of biocompatible hemodialysis membranes
  Nutritional support in chronic dialysis patients who are unable to meet their dietary needs
    Oral supplements
    Tube feeds (if medically appropriate)
    Intradialytic parenteral nutritional supplements for hemodialysis patients
    Amino acid dialysate for peritoneal dialysis patients

tions associated with exacerbations of uremic symptoms as well as metabolic acidosis are potential complications of AAD. Overall, the available evidence suggests that IDPN and AAD may offer alternative methods of nutritional intervention in a group of dialysis patients in whom oral or enteral intake cannot be maintained. Unfortunately, most studies evaluating IDPN and AAD are retrospective, uncontrolled or short-term and subject to other design flaws. Until a controlled study comparing various forms of nutritional supplementation in similar patient groups is completed, one should be cautious in prescribing highly costly nutritional interventions.

NUTRITION IN ACUTE RENAL FAILURE

The nutritional hallmark of acute renal failure is excessive catabolism. Numerous studies have shown that the protein catabolic rate in ARF patients requiring dialytic support is much higher than that seen in other patient popu- lations; it can be massive. Several factors have been postulated as the underlying mechanism for the high rate of protein catabolism observed in ARF patients. Concurrent illnesses may initiate a sequence of catabolic events through several different processes. Specific cytokines including interleukins and tumor necrosis factor are stimulated during catabolic conditions such as sepsis and induce increased whole body protein breakdown. In addition to increased catabolism, ARF patients may also encounter a diminished utilization and incorporation of available nutrients.

Nutritional indices can be employed to identify malnourished ARF patients, design appropriate nutritional support, and assess the response to nutritional supplementation. In ARF, the major process contributing to poor nutritional status is the metabolic response to ongoing morbidity or catabolism, whereas in other states, malnutrition is largely a response to chronic starvation. The nutritional markers that correlate best with efficacy of nutritional therapy and patient outcome may be considerably different in these two separate disease states, and have not been well delineated in the ARF patient population. The determination of urea nitrogen appearance, and levels of biochemical markers such as serum albumin, prealbumin, and transfer-rin are influenced by many factors. Similarly, utilization of traditional measures of body composition such as anthropometry have limited application in ARF patients owing to major shifts in body water.

The actual requirements for protein and energy supplementation in ARF patients are not well-defined (Table 2). In clinical practice, the actual nutritional needs of the patient are frequently not determined. Measurement of urea nitrogen appearance, which reflects protein catabolism may be cumbersome in clinical settings, as is the measurement of energy expenditure. The fluid distribution and the fat free mass may be considerably altered in ARF patients, especially during the oligoanuric phase. In the presence of diminished utilization and clearance due to diminished renal function, excessive protein supplementation will result in increased accumulation of end products of protein and amino acid metabolism, that is, higher BUN concentrations. Provision of large quantities of nutrients requires more fluid administration and may predispose patients to fluid overload. Aggressive nutrition may also cause hyper-glycemia, hyperlipidemia, hyper- or hyponatremia, and abnormalities in amino acid profiles. Although most of these abnormalities can be managed by complementary dialytic support, the initiation, intensity, as well as the dose of dialysis treatment in ARF is an area of controversy in itself. In highly catabolic patients who are administered excessive nutritional supplementation, even dialysis cannot fully prevent the undesirable accumulation of nitrogen waste products.

Bibliography

Chertow GM, Ling J, Lew NL, et al.: The association of intradialytic parenteral nutrition with survival in hemodialysis patients. *Am J Kidney Dis* 24:912–920, 1994.

Ikizler TA, Greene J, Wingard RL, et al.: Spontaneous dietary protein intake during progression of chronic renal failure. *J Am Soc Nephrol* 6:1386–1391, 1995.

Ikizler TA, Hakim RM: Nutrition in end-stage renal disease. *Kidney Int* 50:343–357, 1996.

Ikizler TA, Himmelfarb J: Nutrition in acute renal failure. *Adv Renal Replacement Ther* 4(Suppl 1):54–63, 1997.

Ikizler TA, Wingard RL, Hakim RM: Interventions to treat malnutrition in dialysis patients: The role of the dose of dialysis, intradialytic parenteral nutrition, and growth hormone. *Am J Kidney Dis* 26:256–265, 1995.

Klahr S, Levey AS, Beck GJ, et al.: The effects of dietary protein restriction and blood-pressure control on the progression of chronic renal disease. *N Engl J Med* 330:877–884, 1994.

Kopple JD: The nutrition management of the patient with acute renal failure. *JPEN* 20:3–12, 1996.

Lowrie EG, Huang WH, Lew NL, Liu Y: The relative contribution of measured variables to death risk among hemodialysis patients. In E.A. Friedman EA (ed) *Death on Hemodialysis,* p. 121. Kluwer Academic Publishers, Amsterdam, *1994.*

Mitch WE, Goldberg AL: Mechanism of muscle wasting: The role of ubiquitin–proteasome pathway. *N Engl J Med* 335:1897–1905, 1997.

Parker III TF, Wingard RL, Husni L, et al.: Effect of the membrane biocompatibility on nutritional parameters in chronic hemodialysis patients. *Kidney Int* 49:551–556, 1996.

Qureshi AR, Alvestrand A, Danielsson A, et al.: Factors predicting malnutrition in hemodialysis patients: A cross-sectional study. *Kidney Int* 53:773–782, 1998.

Stenvinkel P, Heimburger O, Paultre F, et al.: Strong association between malnutrition, inflammation, and atherosclerosis in chronic renal failure. *Kidney Int* 55:1899–1911, 1999.

RENAL OSTEODYSTROPHY AND OTHER MUSCULOSKELETAL COMPLICATIONS OF CHRONIC RENAL FAILURE

JAMES A. DELMEZ

The term, renal osteodystrophy, is used in a generic sense to include all skeletal disorders that primarily occur in patients with renal failure. These include osteitis fibrosa, osteomalacia, mixed and adynamic bone lesions, and dialysis-related amyloidosis. Because the kidney plays a major role in mineral homeostasis, by maintaining external balance for calcium, phosphorus, magnesium, and pH, the occurrence of metabolic bone disease in patients with renal failure is predictable. For example, the kidneys are responsible for the excretion of phosphorus. With renal failure, phosphorus accumulates causing a reciprocal fall in calcium levels and, therefore, stimulation of parathyroid hormone (PTH) secretion. Phosphorus retention also decreases the renal 1α hydroxylation of 25-hydroxyvitamin D to give $1,25(OH)_2D$ (calcitriol), the most potent metabolite of vitamin D. Calcitriol stimulates intestinal calcium absorption and mobilization of calcium from bone. It also directly suppresses PTH release, independent of its calcemic effect. Low levels of calcitriol may, therefore result in malabsorption of calcium, hypocalcemia, and further stimulation of PTH secretion. In addition, the kidney is the main organ responsible for the excretion of aluminum and β_2-microglobulin, substances implicated in the induction of dialysis-related osteomalacia and amyloidosis, respectively. The pathophysiology of renal osteodystrophy has recently been better defined, making possible a rational approach to its prevention and treatment.

The types of bone diseases seen in patients with renal failure are divided (with the exception of amyloidosis) into those with accelerated rates of bone turnover (i.e., osteitis fibrosa and mixed lesions) due to persistently high levels of PTH and low bone turnover states (i.e., osteomalacia and adynamic lesions) due to aluminum toxicity or relatively low levels of PTH. Recent studies show that high turnover bone disease is the predominant lesion in patients treated with hemodialysis (50–60% of total), whereas low turnover is present in 60–70% of patients undergoing peritoneal dialysis.

OSTEITIS FIBROSA AND SECONDARY HYPERPARATHYROIDISM

High levels of PTH lead to the development of osteitis fibrosa. The histological features include increased number and activity of osteoclasts, increased bone resorption, and marrow fibrosis. In addition, osteoblastic activity is increased with an abnormally large amount of the bone surface involved in bone formation. This state of high bone turnover is also characterized by an increased quantity of unmineralized bone matrix (osteoid). It differs from normal lamellar osteoid in that there is a haphazard arrangement of collagen fibers giving the appearance of a woven straw basket. Although woven osteoid can be mineralized, the calcium is deposited as amorphous calcium–phosphate instead of hydroxyapatite. These features are shown in Fig. 1 and contrast markedly with the normal bone histology shown in Fig. 2.

Pathogenesis of Secondary Hyperparathyroidism

Although recent studies have shown that hyperparathyroidism may develop without hypocalcemia, it is well accepted that low levels of this cation stimulate PTH secretion. The factors that contribute to hypocalcemia and secondary hyperparathyroidism include phosphate retention, impaired vitamin D metabolism, skeletal resistance to the calcemic action of PTH, altered calcium-regulated PTH secretion, and decreased rates of degradation of PTH. The pathophysiological events are summarized in Fig. 3.

Phosphate Retention and Calcitriol Deficiency

The original explanation for the development of secondary hyperparathyroidism in patients with renal failure was the "trade-off hypothesis." As glomerular filtration rate (GFR) fell, it was reasoned that there would be a rise in serum phosphorus levels with a transient reciprocal fall in calcium concentrations. The latter would stimulate PTH secretion leading to a phosphaturia and a normal-

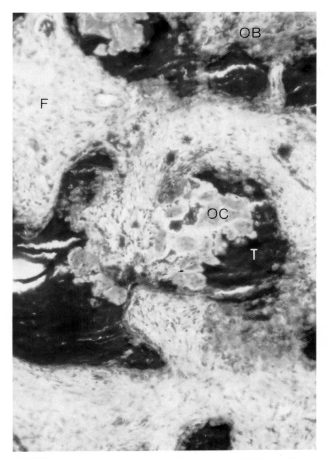

FIGURE I Histological features of severe osteitis fibrosa. Many multinucleated osteoclasts (OC) are actively resorbing trabecular bone (T) resulting in an irregular jagged surface. Osteoblasts (OB) are seen forming new bone surfaces. The marrow is replaced by fibrosis (F). (Courtesy of Steven L. Teitelbaum, M.D., original magnification ×40, modified Masson stain.)

ization of calcium and phosphorus levels. The trade-off was a normalization of phosphate levels at the cost of sustained PTH hypersecretion. Although hyperphosphatemia could not be consistently demonstrated in early renal failure, the hypothesis was supported by studies in animals and humans with mild renal failure showing that phosphate restriction in proportion to the decrease in GFR prevented or corrected the hyperparathyroid state.

More recent studies have shown that renal synthesis of calcitriol falls with worsening renal function, presumably because of declining renal mass. It is now appreciated that the principal effect of phosphorus restriction in early renal failure is to increase the renal production of calcitriol, resulting in near normal levels. However, as renal failure becomes advanced (GFR less than 20% of normal), hyperphosphatemia develops, leading to hypocalcemia and worsening hyperparathyroidism. Phosphate restriction no longer stimulates calcitriol synthesis, and calcitriol levels

remain low. Presumably, this is due to the limited am of residual renal mass available for synthesis. Howe PTH levels may still decline with phosphorus restricti independent of changes in calcium or calcitriol levels. This suggests that phosphorus may directly affect PTH secretion. This concept is supported by *in vitro* studies with parathyroid glands of normal rats where high phosphorus levels in the media stimulate PTH secretion. This process requires protein synthesis.

Calcium Malabsorption

In patients with a moderate degree of renal failure, calcitriol levels are either normal or slightly low. Calcium absorption is usually normal. In advanced renal failure, calcitriol deficiency may lead to impaired gastrointestinal absorption of calcium and negative calcium balance. Hypocalcemia is a potent stimulus for PTH secretion that, in turn, raises calcium levels toward normal by increasing bone resorption.

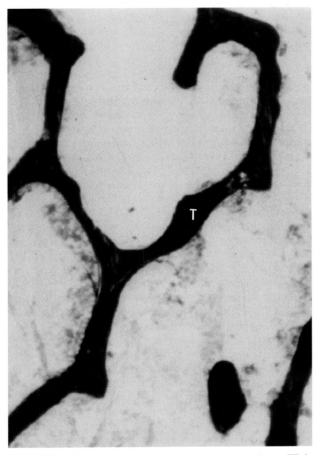

FIGURE 2 Normal bone histology. The trabecular bone (T) is fairly smooth without a prominence of osteoclasts or osteoblasts. No fibrosis or osteoid is seen. (Courtesy of Steven L. Teitelbaum, M.D., original magnification ×40, modified Masson stain.)

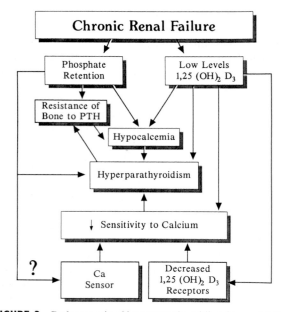

FIGURE 3 Pathogenesis of hyperparathyroidism in renal failure. From Slatopolsky E, Delmez J: Pathogenesis of secondary hyperparathyroidism. *Miner Electrolyte Metab* 21:91–96, 1995, with permission.

Skeletal Resistance to the Calcemic Action of PTH

The calcemic response to an infusion of PTH extract is less in hypocalcemic patients with renal insufficiency than in normal subjects or in patients with hypoparathyroidism. In experimental animals, prior parathyroidectomy corrects the defect. This suggests that some form of desensitization of the calcemic response to PTH occurs when the hormone is in excess. This would lead to a vicious cycle in renal failure where the impaired calcemic response leads to hypocalcemia, stimulating PTH secretion that would further impair the calcemic response of the bone. Phosphorus restriction improves the calcemic response to PTH via unclear mechanisms.

Altered Calcium-Regulated PTH Secretion

An insensitivity to the suppressive effects of calcium on PTH secretion has been shown *in vitro* in glands obtained from patients with chronic renal failure. The resistance to suppression by calcium may be overcome in a dose-dependent manner if the glands are incubated with calcitriol. Subsequent studies have shown that calcitriol reduces prepro-PTH messenger RNA levels by decreasing the rate of gene transcription. It has also been shown that there are a decreased number of calcitriol receptors in the uremic parathyroid gland that may promote a relative resistance to the steroid. Interestingly, the calcitriol receptor mRNA increases when the parathyroid gland is exposed to calcitriol. This suggests that calcitriol may upregulate its own receptor.

The low levels of calcitriol observed in patients with advanced renal failure could play a role in the abnormal secretion of PTH. Several studies have evaluated the PTH response to hypercalcemic suppression and hypocalcemic stimulation before and after intravenous calcitriol. Some, but not all investigators, have shown an increased sensitivity of the gland to ambient calcium levels following calcitriol.

A calcium receptor in parathyroid cell membranes has been cloned. By sensing extracellular calcium, the receptor regulates PTH secretion by changes in phosphoinositide turnover and cytosolic calcium levels. A decreased number of calcium receptors have been shown in glands of uremic patients. This may be another mechanism affecting the sensitivity of the parathyroid gland to calcium in renal failure. Uremic rats fed a high phosphorus diet have approximately half the number of calcium receptors compared to those on a low phosphorus diet.

Parathyroid Hyperplasia

Parathyroid hyperplasia is a prominent finding in uremic patients with severe secondary hyperparathyroidism. Little is known about the factors that lead to the cellular proliferation. Studies *in vivo* in uremic animals, however, suggest that calcitriol administration retards the development of parathyroid hyperplasia independent of changes in serum calcium levels. Hyperplasia, once established, is not reversed by short-term calcitriol treatment. Dietary phosphorus restriction also prevents parathyroid hyperplasia in uremic rats without affecting serum calcium or calcitriol concentrations. In uremic subjects with secondary hyperparathyroidism, monoclonal allelic losses on chromosome 11 have been demonstrated in the glands. This finding suggests that monoclonal transformation of previous hyperplasticly parathyroid tissue often occurs.

Diagnosis of Uremic Hyperparathyroidism

The diagnosis of severe hyperparathyroidism is made by the findings of high levels of PTH and radiographic changes of osteitis fibrosa. Typically, these features include subperiosteal erosions of the phalanges (see Fig. 4) and erosions at the proximal end of the tibia, the neck of the femur or humerus, and the inferior surface of the distal end of the clavicle. In the skull, there is a mottled and granular (salt and pepper) appearance with areas of resorption commonly associated with areas of osteosclerosis. Osteosclerosis is due to an increase in the thickness and number of trabeculae in spongy bone.

The correct interpretation of PTH levels in renal failure depends on an understanding of the metabolism of PTH and the specificity of the assay used to measure the hormone. PTH is primarily secreted as the intact hormone containing 84 amino acids. In the circulation, intact PTH undergoes degradation by the liver and kidneys, yielding biologically active amino- and biologically inactive middle region and carboxyl-terminal fragments. The removal of the latter two depends primarily, if not exclusively on glomerular filtration and subsequent reabsorption and degradation by the renal tubules. Therefore, in renal failure these fragments accumulate. This results in multiple forms of circulating PTH in which the concentration of bi-

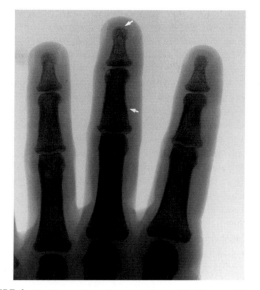

FIGURE 4 Radiographic changes of osteitis fibrosa. There are subperiosteal erosions of the phalanges and tuft (arrows).

ologically inactive fragments is about 100-fold greater than that of the biologically active amino-terminal fragments. To interpret PTH levels in renal failure, it is critical to know if the assay measures the intact, amino-terminal, middle, and/or carboxyl-terminal portions of the molecule. For example, if one uses an assay that measures the middle and carboxyl-terminal regions, the values associated with severe hyperparathyroidism may be 100-fold greater than the upper limits of normal determined in subjects with normal renal function. By contrast, results of an assay specific for the amino-terminal portion or intact PTH may suggest severe osteitis fibrosa when the results are 10 times the upper limits of normal. Most clinical centers have now adopted the intact PTH assay, and its use is encouraged. Without liver disease, the serum alkaline phosphatase levels often correlate with PTH and may confirm the presence of hyperparathyroidism. A bone biopsy may be necessary when the diagnosis is uncertain.

Prevention and Treatment of Uremic Hyperparathyroidism

Phosphorus Control

In early renal failure, phosphorus accumulation may be avoided by restriction of a dietary phosphorus intake to 600–800 mg/day. This generally involves limiting meats and dairy products. More strict dietary phosphorus restriction is usually impractical. When the GFR falls to less than 20–30 mL/min, hyperphosphatemia develops, and agents that bind phosphorus in the bowel are usually necessary. In the past, phosphorus binders containing aluminum were commonly used. It is now known that this metal may be absorbed and cause substantial toxicity (see later section Osteomalacia). Calcium-containing phosphorus binders

are now widely used. Agents such as calcium carbonate are most effective in binding phosphorus when given with meals in proportion to the usual phosphorus content of each meal. When calcium carbonate is ingested in the fasted state, less phosphorus is bound and more calcium is absorbed by the gastrointestinal tract. Since there is both patient to patient variability and variability from meal to meal in the same patient, a thorough dietary history and ongoing counseling are essential. Mismatching of the amount of calcium carbonate and phosphorus ingested may lead to inadequate phosphorus control or hypercalcemia. The usual starting dose is 500–1000 mg/day of elemental calcium (1250–2500 mg calcium carbonate), one to two pills/day, with further titration based on the resultant changes in calcium, phosphorus, and PTH levels. Recently, much interest has been focused on calcium acetate as a phosphorus binder. Acute studies have shown that this compound binds about twice as much phosphorus/calcium absorbed compared with calcium carbonate. Compared with calcium carbonate, one-half the amount of elemental calcium is usually effective. Unfortunately the decreased dose does not result in a lower incidence of hypercalcemia. In addition, because calcium acetate pills contain only 167 mg of elemental calcium, patients taking this preparation often require a greater number of pills/day. Thus, there may be no clinical advantage in using this preparation.

As patients begin dialysis therapy, the dietary protein requirements increase to more than 1 g/kg/day. This results in a requisite increase in dietary phosphorus to 800–1200 mg/day. Although hemodialysis removes approximately 1000 mg/treatment three times a week and continuous ambulatory peritoneal dialysis 300 mg/day, these effects are not sufficient to avoid the use of phosphorus binders in well-nourished patients. The physician may control the calcium fluxes during dialysis treatments by changing the concentration of calcium in the dialysate. A dialysate calcium concentration of 3.25–3.50 mEq/L (6.5–7.0 mg/dL, all ionized) causes a net influx of calcium to the patient. With the use of phosphorus binders containing calcium, there is a risk of developing hypercalcemia. If this occurs, the physician has the flexibility of decreasing the concentration of calcium in the dialysate to 2.5 mEq/L.

A phosphorus binder not containing calcium or aluminum, sevelamer hydrochloride, has been approved for use in patients undergoing dialysis. A lower incidence of hypercalcemia has been shown in hemodialysis patients treated with sevelamer hydrochloride compared to calcium acetate. Adequate control of phosphorus levels, however, may entail ingesting 5 or more g/day. The precise role for sevelamer hydrochloride in treating renal osteodystrophy remains to be determined. However, consideration for its use should be given in patients with uncontrolled hyperphosphatemia (phosphorus >7 mg/dL) or hypercalcemia, and to those treated with calcitriol.

Control of Calcium

As the GFR falls below 50 mL/min, there is impaired absorption of calcium by the gastrointestinal tract. This is due, in part, to the decreased renal synthesis of calcitriol. Administration of sufficient amounts of calcium to bind phosphorus may suffice in reversing the negative calcium balance. In patients with good control of phosphorus levels who nonetheless are hypocalcemic, calcium supplements may be added at night on an empty stomach. Alternatively, if the PTH levels are excessive, calcitriol may be started. Calcium and phosphorus levels must be monitored closely since there is a tendency for the development of hypercalcemia after several months. This is often heralded by a fall in alkaline phosphatase to the normal range. A similar approach is appropriate for patients treated with dialysis. Increasing the dialysate calcium to 3.5 mEq/L is an additional option to increase calcium levels.

Use of Vitamin D Sterols

Treatment with oral vitamin D, dihydrotachysterol, 25-hydroxyvitamin D, and calcitriol have all been shown to lessen symptoms of bone pain, improve bone histology, and lower PTH levels. All confer a risk of hypercalcemia. Vitamin D-induced hypercalcemia is particularly prolonged and may require weeks for resolution. The duration of hypercalcemia with calcitriol is usually 2 to 4 days. It is also the most potent metabolite of vitamin D in directly suppressing PTH secretion. Therefore, most consider it the vitamin D sterol of choice in suppressing hyperparathyroidism in renal failure. Calcitriol should not be used when hyperphosphatemia is present because a calcium–phosphorus product of greater than 75 (with each concentration expressed in mg/dL) may lead to the development of soft tissue calcifications. In addition, calcitriol increases the gastrointestinal absorption of phosphorus and may require an increase in the dose of phosphorus binders. Analogs of calcitriol that suppress PTH secretion, yet are possibly less active in raising calcium and phosphorus levels, have been developed. Two of such analogs, paricalcitol and doxercalciferol, are approved for use in the United States. The usual dose of intravenous paricalcitol is three to four times that of calcitriol. The initial recommended dose of doxercalciferol is 10 μg given orally three times a week. To date, there have been no published trials comparing the efficacy and safety of these analogs with calcitriol.

Many studies have demonstrated a marked suppression of PTH by administering 1.0–2.0 μg of calcitriol intravenously after each hemodialysis treatment three times a week. This suppression, which is greater than that observed with oral daily calcitriol, may be due to the very high serum levels achieved when the drug is given by this route. Pulse oral calcitriol (2–4 μg twice a week) also results in high levels and PTH suppression. This regimen is particular useful in patients treated with peritoneal dialysis in whom ready access to the circulation is not available. Whatever the route of administration and the dose, calcium and phosphorus levels should be carefully monitored during treatment with calcitriol.

The timing of the initiation of calcitriol and the dose of the drug depends, in part, on the intact PTH levels. Calcitriol should not be administered if the PTH levels are less than 250 pg/mL (or less than four times the upper limits of normal) for fear of inducing an adynamic bone lesion. In general, the more severe the hyperparathyroidism, the higher the dose. For values of 250 to 600 pg/mL, 1 to 2 μg of calcitriol (administered orally or intravenously) three times a week, should be considered. More severe hyperparathyroidism (600 to 1000 pg/mL) may require higher doses of 2 to 4 μg three times a week. In patients with extremely high PTH levels (>1000 pg/mL), doses as high as 4 to 6 μg may be necessary. To avoid oversuppression of the parathyroid glands, the dose should be decreased if the PTH levels decline to less than 250 pg/mL. If PTH levels do not fall into an acceptable range after 1 year of treatment, a surgical parathyroidectomy or parathyroid gland ablation by ethanol should be considered. The latter procedure involves the percutaneous injection of ethanol into the enlarged glands using ultrasound guidance. Although complications, such as recurrent laryngeal nerve palsy, are rare and transient, its use should be limited to centers with experience in the technique.

OSTEOMALACIA

Osteomalacia is characterized by histological findings of impaired mineralization activity and an increase in the osteoid seam width (see Fig. 5). Thus, in contrast to osteitis fibrosa, the rate of bone turnover is low. Patients often complain of bone and muscle pain, and spontaneous fractures occur in approximately 15% of those afflicted.

Pathogenesis of Osteomalacia

Although abnormalities of vitamin D metabolism (low calcitriol levels) and the presence of persistent metabolic acidosis may contribute to the development of osteomalacia, by far the most common cause in patients on dialysis is aluminum intoxication. Aluminum may accumulate due to contamination of the dialysate with this metal. With proper pretreatment of the tap water used to prepare dialysate, this route has diminished in relative importance. The main current source of aluminum accumulation is the ingestion of phosphorus binders containing aluminum. Because aluminum is normally excreted via urinary excretion, patients on dialysis are particularly prone to develop toxicity that, in its most severe state, encompasses dementia and premature death. Those with diabetes, prior parathyroidectomy, failed renal transplant, complete anuria, or a long history of consumption of large amounts of aluminum-containing phosphorus binders are at highest risk. Citrate increases absorption of aluminimum from the jiet. Uremic patients, consuming medications containing citrate (calcium citrate, Shohl's solution) along with those containing aluminum (Basaljel, Amphogel, Carafate) are particularly prone to aluminum accumulation.

Diagnosis of Osteomalacia

The diagnosis of osteomalacia is often difficult. The clinical setting of a large exposure to aluminum and bone pain suggests the diagnosis. Aluminum directly suppresses PTH secretion, and a low PTH level is characteristic but not uni-

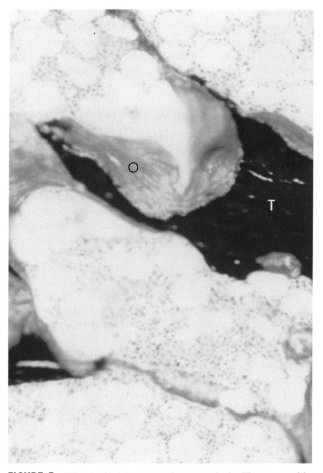

FIGURE 5 Histological features of osteomalacia. There are wide osteoid seams (O) surrounding trabecular bone (T). There is a paucity of osteoclasts and osteoblasts, thus reflecting a low rate of bone turnover. (Courtesy Steven L. Teitelbaum, M.D., original magnification ×40, modified Masson stain.)

versal. The radiographic findings of osteomalacia are not distinctive. Some data suggest that a basal serum aluminum level of >100 μg/L and an increment in aluminum level of >150 μg/L following chelation with deferoxamine (DFO) in combination with a low PTH level has a high predictive power for the presence of aluminum bone disease. For the test, 5–20 mg/kg is administered intravenously at the end of dialysis, and the serum aluminum is measured 24 to 48 hrs later. The "gold standard," however, remains the bone biopsy with appropriate staining for aluminum.

Prevention and Treatment of Osteomalacia Caused by Aluminum

Prevention of osteomalacia is critical with attention given to dialysate purity and avoidance of phosphorus binders containing aluminum, if possible. Chronic chelation therapy with DFO cures the osteomalacia, and follow-up biopsies usually show the development of osteitis fibrosa

of variable severity. The major mechanism for this is the removal of aluminum from the bone surface associated with marked increases in osteoblast number and rate of bone formation. A major problem with DFO treatment is the risk of fatal mucormycosis infections that occur in up to 5% of treated patients. DFO also binds iron, and the DFO–iron chelate can function as a siderophore to stimulate the growth of mucormycosis. An acute encephalopathy has also been described with DFO. Thus, the use of DFO should be restricted to those who have severe symptoms of aluminum intoxication and histological evidence of aluminum accumulation in the bone. Eliminating all aluminum-containing phosphorus binders and substituting one containing calcium may be effective in patients with mild symptoms. Over a period of 1 to 2 years, the aluminum burden will decrease as will the symptoms.

Adynamic Bone Lesions

Adynamic (also termed aplastic) bone lesions are characterized by decreased bone mineralization, with normal amounts of osteoid. In approximately 50% of cases, the cause is aluminum deposition. The treatment is the same as osteomalacia due to aluminum. Little is known about the etiology in the remaining half of patients. However, this lesion may be more common in patients treated with peritoneal dialysis, in the elderly, and in patients with diabetes. The PTH levels are generally <two to three times the upper limits of normal when measured with an intact PTH assay. It is likely that the lesion is the result of overzealous suppression of PTH. If so, some advocate allowing the PTH level to increase to four times the upper limits of normal. It should be noted, however, that patients with adynamic bone lesions not due to aluminum overload, report fewer symptoms of bone pain and myopathy and develop fewer fractures than those with either aluminum-related or osteitis fibrosa bone disease diagnosed by bone biopsy.

MIXED LESIONS

Some patients display histological evidence of both osteitis fibrosa and osteomalacia on a bone biopsy. Such patients frequently have high PTH levels and impaired bone formation and mineralization. Mixed renal osteodystrophy may be seen in patients with previously established osteodystrophy who are developing aluminum-related bone disease. The treatment is withdrawal of the aluminum exposure and aggressive treatment of the hyperparathyroidism.

Dialysis-Related Amyloidosis

It has long been known that there is an association between bone cysts, pathological fractures, arthritis, and carpal tunnel syndrome in patients treated with long-term dialysis. It is now clear that these are often due to the deposition of a form of amyloid unique to dialysis patients. This protein is composed of intact and modified β_2-microglobulin. This constant light chain of HLA class I antigens is excreted in the urine. Therefore, very high serum levels are uniformly seen in patients on dialysis. The amyloid is most frequently deposited in the flexor retinaculum of the wrist, entrapping the median nerve and causing carpal tunnel syndrome. The symptoms of hand pain can be relieved by a surgical release of the median nerve. The amyloid may also invade the synovium of joints causing pain, effusions, and erosive arthritis. Periarticular radiolucent bone cysts (Fig. 6), the result of the replacement of bone by amyloid, may result in pathological fracture. Once established, there is no proven treatment for the amyloid arthropathy. Use of high flux hemodialysis or hemodiafiltration removes some β_2-microglobulin and may delay the onset of the clinical expression of the disease. Early renal transplantation completely prevents the disease.

Renal Osteodystrophy Following Renal Transplantation

Following a successful renal transplant, the histological abnormalities of mild to moderately severe osteitis fibrosa usually resolve within a year. Severe hyperparathyroidism, however, may not completely resolve, and elevated PTH levels may persist for 5 to 10 years. Bone density of the lumbar vertebrae decreases due to the effect of steroids in impairing bone formation. A bisphosphonate, pamidronate [0.5 mg/kg intravenous], at the time of transplant and again 1 month later, may reduce the rate of bone loss. In those patients with osteomalacia, return of renal function allows

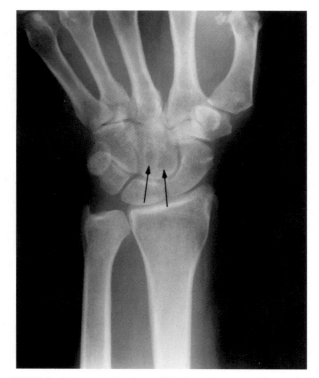

FIGURE 6 Bone cysts in a hemodialysis patient caused by amyloid infiltration of bone.

the removal of aluminum and, as a result, improvement in the bone histology. The symptoms of amyloid deposition often improve dramatically following transplantation, but the radiographic findings do not change. This suggests that the amyloid may be irreversibly bound to the tissue.

OVERALL APPROACH TO THE MANAGEMENT OF RENAL OSTEODYSTROPHY

Renal osteodystrophy is a dynamic process whose severity and even type of lesion may vary with time. In early renal failure, phosphorus restriction alone may suffice. With more severe renal failure, GFR less than 30 mL/min, calcium malabsorption should be countered by the administration of oral calcium with meals, if the phosphorus level is high, or at night if the phosphorus is normal. In the face of a calcium phosphorus product of greater than 75, the phosphorus should be initially lowered by the use of aluminum-containing phosphorus binders (maximum duration of 8 weeks) or sevelamer hydrochloride to prevent soft tissue calcifications. When the product has decreased below this value, calcium carbonate with meals should be substituted for the long-term binding of phosphorus. The target calcium and phosphorus levels are 9.5–10.5 and 4.5–5.5 mg/dL, respectively. Frequent monitoring of these values is necessary to avoid iatrogenic complications such as hypercalcemia. In hemodialysis patients, calcium and phosphorus levels should be determined monthly and PTH concentrations quarterly. The target intact PTH levels should be three to four times the upper limits of normal. Levels lower than the target range may cause a state of low bone turnover (adynamic bone lesion). Conversely, levels above this range may lead to osteitis fibrosa. The dose of calcium carbonate should be adjusted in relation to the calcium, phosphorus, and PTH levels. For example, if the calcium is 8.5 mg/dL, the phosphorus level acceptable, and the intact PTH concentration normal, one would consider doing nothing, lowering the dose of calcium carbonate, or decreasing the concentration of calcium in the dialysate. If, with the same levels of calcium and phosphorus, the PTH level is five times normal and progressively increasing, one would attempt a more aggressive approach. This may be achieved by increasing the dose of calcium given at night or by starting calcitriol therapy. When prescribing calcitriol, the calcium and phosphorus levels must be assessed more frequently. As with calcium carbonate, calcitriol should not be given in the presence of an elevated calcium phosphorus product. This presents a problem in the patient with severe hyperparathyroidism. In this situation, the patient's elevated serum calcium or phosphorus may be emanating from bone due to enhanced bone resorption. A surgical parathyroidectomy is often required. The other main indication for surgery is persistently high levels of PTH, corresponding to the presence of severe osteitis fibrosa, and bone pain. A bone biopsy is usually not required to make the diagnosis. If, however, the patient is at risk for the development of aluminum accumulation (see earlier), a bone biopsy may be warranted to confirm the diagnosis and exclude aluminum-related osteomalacia as a cause for the bone pain or hypercalcemia. At time of surgery, all four glands should be identified. Some surgeons will do a three and one-half gland parathyroidectomy; others will remove all glands and implant small pieces of one gland into the forearm to avoid future neck surgery if hyperparathyroidism recurs. The recurrence rates are probably the same for the two techniques (5–15%).

Bibliography

Andress DL, Keith MD, Norris C, *et al.:* Intravenous calcitriol in the treatment of refractory osteitis fibrosa of chronic renal failure. *N Engl J Med* 321:274–279, 1989.

Antonsen JE, Sherrard DJ, Andress DL: A cacimimetic agent acutely suppresses parathyroid hormone levels in patients with chronic renal failure. Rapid Communication. *Kidney Int* 53: 223–227, 1998.

Bleyer AJ, Burke SD, Dillon M, Garrett B, Kant KS, Lynch D, Rahman SN, Schoenfeld P, Teitelbaum I, Zeig S, Slatopolsky E: A comparison of the calcium-free phosphate binder sevelamer hydrochloride with calcium acetate in the treatment of hyperphosphatemia in hemodialysis patients. *Am J Kidney Dis* 33:694–701, 1999.

Block GA, Hulbert-Shearon TE, Levin NW, *et al.:* Association of serum phosphorus and calcium phosphate product with mortality risk in chronic hemodialysis patients: A national study. *Am J Kidney Dis* 31:607–617, 1998.

Boelaert JR, Fenves AZ, Coburn JW: Deferoxamine therapy and mucormycosis in dialysis patients; report of an international registry. *Am J Kidney Dis* 18:660–667, 1991.

Delmez JA, Slatopolsky E: Hyperphosphatemia: Its consequences and treatment in patients with chronic renal disease. *Am J Kidney Dis* 19:303–317, 1992.

Delmez JA, Tindira C, Grooms P, *et al.:* Parathyroid hormone suppression by intravenous 1,25-dihydroxyvitamin D: A role for increased sensitivity to calcium. *J Clin Invest* 83:1349–1355, 1989.

Fukuda N, Tanaka H, Tominaga Y, *et al.:* Decreased 1,25-dihydroxyvitamin D_3 receptor density is associated with a more severe form of parathyroid hyperplasia in chronic uremic patients. *J Clin Invest* 92:1436–1443, 1993.

Goodman WG, Belin T, Gales B, *et al.:* Calcium-regulated parathyroid hormone release in patients with mild or advanced secondary hyperparathyroidism. *Kidney Int* 48:1553–1558, 1995.

Hruska KA, Teitlebaum SL: Renal osteodystrophy. *N Engl J Med* 333:166–174, 1995.

Julian BA, Laskow DA, Dubovsky J, *et al.:* Rapid loss of vertebral mineral density after renal transplantation. *N Engl J Med* 325: 544–550, 1991.

Kakuta T, Fukagawa M, Fujisaki T, *et al.:* Prognosis of parathyroid function after successful percutaneous ethanol injection therapy guided by color Doppler flow mapping in chronic dialysis patients. *Am J Kidney Dis* 33:1091–1099, 1999.

Kifor O, Moore FD, Wang P, *et al.:* Reduced immunostaining for the extracellular Ca^{2+} sensing receptor in primary and uremic secondary hyperparathyroidism. *J Clin Endocrinol Metab* 81: 1598–1606, 1996.

Llach F, Keshav G, Goldblat MV, Lindberg JS, Sadler R, Delmez J, Arruda J, Lau A, Slatopolsky E: Suppression of parathyroid hormone secretion in hemodialysis patients by a novel vitamin D analogue: 19-nor-1,25-Dihydroxyvitamin D_2. *Am J Kidney Dis* 32:S48–S54, 1998.

Nebeker H, Andress D, Milliner D, *et al.:* Indirect methods for the diagnosis of aluminum bone disease: Plasma aluminum, the desferrioxamine infusion test, and serum iPTH. *Kidney Int* 18:S96–S99, 1986.

Sherrard DJ, Hercz G, Pei Y, *et al.:* The spectrum of bone disease in end-stage renal failure—An evolving disorder. *Kidney Int* 43:436–442, 1993.

Slatopolsky E, Weerts C, Lopez-Hilker S, *et al.:* Calcium carbonate as a phosphate binder in patients with chronic renal failure undergoing dialysis. *N Engl J Med* 315:157–161, 1986.

Slatopolsky E, Finch J, Denda M, *et al.:* Phosphorus restriction prevents parathyroid gland growth. *J Clin Invest* 97:2534–2540, 1996.

Szabo A, Merke J, Beier E, *et al.:* 1,25(OH)$_2$ vitamin D_3 inhibits parathyroid cell proliferation in experimental uremia. *Kidney Int* 35:1049–1056, 1989.

Tan AU, Levine BS, Mazess RB, Kyllo DM, Bishop CW, Knutson JC, Kleinman KS, Coburn JW: Effective suppression of parathyroid hormone by 1 alpha-hydroxy-vitamin D_2 in hemodialysis patients with moderate to severe secondary hyperparathyroidism. *Kidney Int* 51:317–327, 1997.

CARDIAC FUNCTION AND CARDIAC DISEASE IN RENAL FAILURE

ROBERT N. FOLEY, JULIAN R. WRIGHT, AND PATRICK S. PARFREY

Uremic pericarditis was a frequent cause of death before dialysis was available. Since the 1960s, cardiac disease has been shown repeatedly to be the major cause of death in end stage renal disease (ESRD). This is still the case today, with older and sicker patients being accepted for renal replacement therapy. The excessive cardiac mortality of ESRD crosses the divides of nationality, race, gender, and cause of ESRD. Cardiac disease also accounts for a substantial degree of comorbidity. Most studies in industrialized nations show that symptomatic ischemic heart disease and cardiac failure are present prior to initiation of ESRD therapy in over one-third of patients. About 10% of patients will develop one of these conditions every year after starting dialysis therapy.

EPIDEMIOLOGY

Prevalence

Echocardiographic left ventricular hypertrophy (LVH), coronary artery disease, and cardiac failure are conservatively estimated to be between two and five times more prevalent in ERSD patients compared to an age-matched general population.

Abnormalities of left ventricular structure and function are very common in patients starting renal replacement therapy. Studies show concentric LVH (where wall thickening occurs in response to pressure overload) was present in 39% of patients starting dialysis programs for ESRD. Twenty-seven percent of patients had left ventricular dilatation (increase in cavity size in response to volume overload), and 18% had systolic dysfunction (inadequate contractility, defined on echocardiography as a fractional shortening less than 25%). Several studies of patients with chronic renal failure (not yet dialysis-dependent) indicated that these abnormalities develop early in chronic renal failure and progress rapidly as renal function declines. In a patient population with progressive renal impairment, 27% of patients with creatinine clearance greater than 50 mL/min had LVH; this figure rose to 31% for clearances between 25 and 50 mL/min and 45% for clearances less than 25 mL/min.

Close to one-half of all hemodialysis patients in the United States have clinically evident ischemic heart disease. Silent coronary artery disease is also common in dialysis patients, especially in those with diabetes mellitus. The situation is confounded by the observation that over one-quarter of dialysis patients with typical angina have normal coronary arteriograms. Cardiac failure is also very common in dialysis patients; data from the U.S. Renal Data System registry suggest that almost one-half of all patients have a history of cardiac failure.

Risk Factors

Many of the traditional, Framingham-type parameters are also risk factors for cardiac disease in chronic uremia. Older age and diabetes mellitus have been consistently associated with mortality in ESRD patients. Paradoxically, *low* serum cholesterol and *low* blood pressure (BP) have been associated with mortality in large-scale epidemiological studies of dialysis patients. It is likely that low serum cholesterol levels reflect malnutrition, which has been shown to be a major predictor of mortality in most recent studies. In one study, even moderate degrees of hypertension were associated with progressive cardiac enlargement and subsequent cardiac failure. Two-thirds of all deaths were preceded by an admission for cardiac failure. After the development of cardiac failure low blood pressure was the single greatest predictor of subsequent mortality. Hypertension was also associated with the development of new symptomatic ischemic heart disease. These data suggest that the association between low blood pressure and mortality reflects the very high frequency of advanced cardiomyopathy in dialysis patients. They also suggest that aggressive management of hypertension (BP<140/90) is needed in patients without clinically apparent cardiac disease. Although a BP of <140/90 is an achievable target, the actual blood pressure target that minimizes cardiac risk in chronic uremia is not yet clear.

The data linking smoking to cardiac disease in ESRD are inconsistent. Some studies suggest that smoking is an independent mortality factor in ESRD. Smoking and diabetes appears to be a particularly adverse combination of risk factors.

Recent epidemiological data suggest that many factors related to the uremic state may be associated with cardiac disease. Several of these factors, especially anemia, hyperparathyroidism, and dose of dialysis are potentially amenable to correction. In addition, chronically uremic patients have an increased prevalence of mild–moderate hyperhomocysteinemia compared to patients with normal renal function.

Hyperhomocysteinemia appears to be a risk factor for cardiovascular mortality/morbidity in uremia. The mechanism by which hyperhomocysteinemia is atherogenic is yet to be elucidated, but endothelial cell injury is likely to be a factor. As yet, there is no evidence showing that treating hyperhomocysteinemia reduces cardiovascular disease in uremic patients. However, folic acid, vitamin B_6, and vitamin B_{12} combinations (as cofactors in the conversion of homocysteine to cystathionine) have been shown to lower levels of homocysteine in renal transplant patients. Elevated levels of serum lipoprotein (a) [Lp(a)] are also seen in patients with declining renal function. In high concentrations Lp(a), is associated with an increased incidence of cardiovascular disease. The kidney has a probable mechanism in catabolism of Lp(a), and therefore renal dysfunction may lead directly to a high serum Lp(a) concentration.

The effects of uremia on thrombogenesis and platelet function are complex. Elevated fibrinogen levels are associated with cardiovascular disease in patients with normal renal function. The epidemiological impact of fibrinogen levels in uremia, as well as altered antithrombin III, protein C, and protein S activity have yet to be determined. In addition, other effects such as platelet dysfunction occur in uremia, and therefore although uremia clearly affects thrombogenesis in many different ways, it cannot be thought of as simply a prothrombotic or antithrombotic state.

Prognosis

Systolic dysfunction, concentric LVH, and left ventricular (LV) dilatation are all strong and independent predictors of future cardiac failure, ischemic heart disease, and death in dialysis patients. The association between systolic dysfunction and mortality is immediate. In contrast, the impact of concentric LVH and LV dilatation on survival is only apparent after a lag phase of approximately 2 years, suggesting a possible time window to target interventions. It is very likely that these echocardiographic abnormalities lead to death via the intermediate step of cardiac failure.

Coronary artery disease predicts mortality independently of age and diabetes. It predisposes to systolic dysfunction and cardiac failure, which seem to be the major mediators of its adverse impact in ESRD patients. Clinically defined cardiac failure is a rapidly lethal condition in ESRD patients, much the same as it is in the general population. In one prospective cohort study, cardiac failure preceded two-thirds of all deaths of chronic dialysis patients with a median time interval between admission for cardiac failure and death of 13 months. It is often difficult to distinguish intrinsic cardiac dysfunction from salt and water excess in dialysis patients. It is thought that chronic salt and water excess can themselves lead to progressive cardiac failure, which adds to the diagnostic confusion. Many dialysis patients can tolerate vast amounts of extracellular fluid volume (ECFV) expansion without developing pulmonary edema. Although dialysis patients with normal hearts can develop pulmonary edema with the rapid accumulation of large amounts of salt and water, it is safer to assume cardiac dysfunction as opposed to simple ECFV expansion in patients who develop pulmonary edema. Patients with pulmonary edema should undergo further cardiac workup, initially by echocardiography. Noninvasive technology, such as inferior vena caval ultrasonography and bioimpedance monitoring, that can rapidly give an accurate assessment of ECFV status should be routinely available in the not-too-distant future. However, distinguishing cardiac failure from simple pulmonary edema, remains a difficult clinical problem.

Valvular dysfunction is common in dialysis patients. Some studies have noted mitral or aortic valvular abnormalities in one-half of all patients with chronic renal failure. Mild to moderate mitral regurgitation, usually secondary to LV dilatation, and calcification of the mitral valve are the most commonly reported abnormalities. The prevalence of hemodynamically important valvular dysfunction is not well described in the literature. In one study, approximately 10% of dialysis patients had hemodynamically important abnormalities of the mitral or aortic valves; the prognosis of these patients was determined by the degree of associated cardiomyopathy. Figure 1 shows survival of ESRD patients with the major clinical and structural manifestations of cardiac disease.

DIAGNOSIS

Cardiomyopathy

Chest X-rays and electrocardiographs are not sufficiently sensitive to detect cardiac enlargement. Echocardiography is noninvasive and relatively easy to perform. It gives information about cardiac dimensions, valve function, systolic function, and diastolic function. Cardiac magnetic resonance imaging shows great promise as a tool to measure cardiac dimensions, but it is not yet routinely available. Cardiomyopathy often progresses rapidly in chronic uremia, and many of the causes of this rapid progression are treatable. It is not clear how often echocardiography should be performed in chronic ESRD. Annual echocardiography is performed in many centers, partly as a tool to assess suitability for transplantation. There are, however, no comparative studies available to demonstrate the optimum use of echocardiography in chronic uremic patients, although it is clearly indicated when symptomatic cardiac dysfunction develops. It is important that echocardiography be carried out after ultrafiltration to as close to dry-weight as possible, preferably within 1 kg.

Ischemic Heart Disease

ESRD patients with symptoms of ischemic heart disease, diabetic patients, and older patients, undergoing pretransplant assessment should be formally evaluated for the

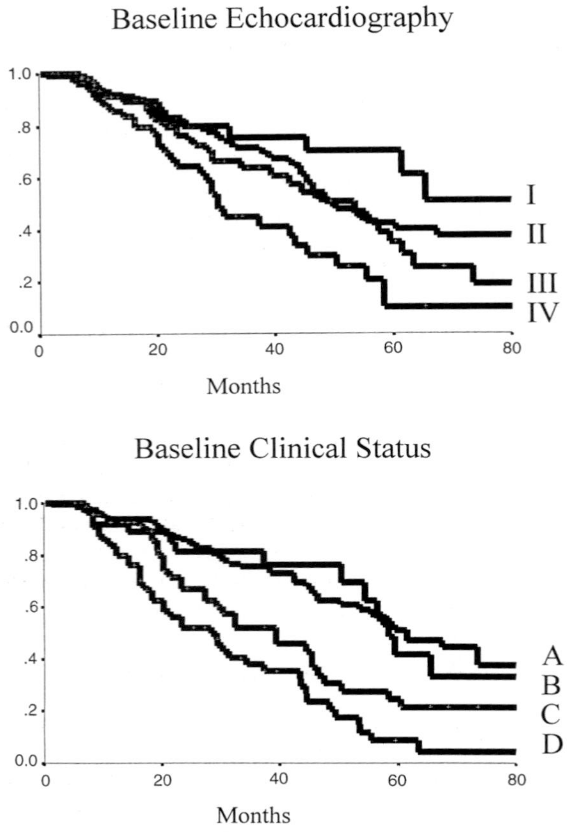

Baseline Echocardiography

Baseline Clinical Status

FIGURE 1 (Top) Survival according to baseline echocardiography in patients starting ESRD therapy. (I) Normal left ventricle. (II) Concentric LV hypertrophy. (III) LV dilatation. (IV) Systolic dysfunction. Data from Foley *et al.: J Am Soc Nephrol* 5:2024–2031, 1995; Parfrey *et al.: Nephrol Dial Transplant* 11:1277–1285, 1996. (Bottom) Survival according to presence or absence of ischemic heart disease and cardiac failure in patients starting ESRD therapy. (A) No ischemic heart disease, no cardiac failure. (B) Ischemic heart disease, no cardiac failure. (C) Cardiac failure, no ischemic heart disease. (D) Both ischemic heart disease and cardiac failure. Data from Harnett *et al.: Kidney Int* 47:884–890, 1995; Parfrey *et al.: Kidney Int* 49:1428–1434, 1996. With permission.

presence of coronary arterial narrowing. The role of noninvasive testing is still unclear. Exercise-based stress tests are often uninformative in ESRD patients, because most are unable to achieve an adequate level of exercise intensity. Of the other noninvasive screening tests available, adenosine thallium-201, dipyridamole thallium-201, and dobutamine stress echocardiography appear useful. Coronary arteriography, however, remains the gold standard. ESRD patients with symptomatic ischemic heart disease should be investigated with coronary arteriography if their physical state is such that revascularization would be seriously considered. The optimal approach to screening for coronary artery disease in asymptomatic renal transplant patients is a matter of dispute. One approach is to perform noninvasive screening on the following subgroups: patients

over 45 years, diabetics over 25 years, smokers, and those with ischemic changes on electrocardiography. Those who do not clearly have negative noninvasive screening tests should have arteriography.

TREATMENT

Risk Factor Management

The cardiac morbidity and mortality of uremic patients without coronary disease, or cardiomyopathy probably exceeds that of survivors of myocardial infarction in the general population. In the absence of high quality data from randomized controlled trials of modification of Framingham type risk factors, the following may be appropriate targets for all uremic patients, which should minimize the risk of new cardiac disease and the progression of existing cardiac disease: nonsmoking, euglycemia, blood pressure less than 120 systolic and 80 diastolic in patients who have not yet begun regular dialysis treatment, less than 140 mm Hg systolic and 90 mm Hg diastolic before each dialysis session, in hemodialysis patients, total serum cholesterol less than 200 mg/dL, LDL cholesterol less than 140 mg/dL, hemoglobin 11 to 12 g/dL, Kt/V >1.2 in hemodialysis patients, weekly Kt/V >2 in peritoneal dialysis patients, serum albumin >3.8 g/dL, serum calcium >2.2 mmol/L, PTH <200 ng/L.

At present there is no good evidence pointing to the superiority of any particular antihypertensive or lipid lowering strategy in this overall picture. However, in chronic renal failure patients, there is considerable evidence that angiotensin-converting enzyme (ACE) inhibitors may be the vasoactive agent of choice, because of their ability to retard the progression to end stage renal disease. Malnutrition is a major determinant of survival in dialysis patients; as most dialysis patients are already on restricted diets, the threshold for using pharmacological treatment for hyperlipidemia should be low. HMG-CoA-reductase inhibitors and fibrates are well tolerated and safe in patients with chronic renal failure. Erythropoietin (rHuEPO) is the agent of choice to treat renal anemia. Using rHuEPO in this manner will lead to an increase in blood pressure in up to one-third of patients; for most patients this increase in blood pressure is readily reversible with standard antihypertensive treatment. For most patients the benefits of partial correction of renal anemia outweigh the potential risks. The risks and benefits of normalizing hematocrit in hemodialysis patients with cardiac disease have recently been evaluated in a compensation trial. Epoetin was prescribed with the aim of maintaining a hematocrit of either 42 or 30%. Unexpectedly, there were more deaths and nonfatal myocardial infarctions in the group with normal hematocrit. In addition, patients with normalized hematocrit had a clear excess of arteriovenous access loss and an apparently small decrease in dialytic urea clearance. In uremic patients, anemia contributes to LVH, LV dilatation, higher cardiac morbidity and mortality, and lower quality of life. A recent trial randomly assigned hemodialysis patients with concentric LVH or LV dilatation to receive doses of epoetin required to achieve hemoglobin levels of 10 g/dL or 13.5 g/dL. A normal hemoglobin level did not lead to the regression of established LV dilatation in patients with concentric LVH. It did prevent the development of LV dilatation in those without this abnormality at study entry. In addition, the higher target hemoglobin was associated with clear quality of life benefits. Several ongoing trials should address the overlapping issues of target hemoglobin, patients groups likely to benefit from higher hemoglobin levels, and timing of these interventions. The efficacy and risks of routine antiplatelet and anticoagulants in this patient group have not been satisfactorily resolved.

Management of Coronary Artery Disease

As in the general population, antiplatelet therapy should be used unless otherwise contraindicated. Beta-blockers, calcium channel blockers, and nitrates are the cornerstones of symptomatic therapy. Risk factor management should be aggressive in this group. Patients should be encouraged to reach ideal body mass, stop smoking, and start a graded exercise program. Hypertension and hyperlipidemia should be aggressively managed. Beta-blockers should be prescribed unless contraindicated. Although full correction of anemia may ameliorate symptoms, such an approach has not been shown to increase longevity in this group, and has been associated with a clear excess of arteriovenous access loss; at present, the target hemoglobin for these patients should be in the range of 11–12 g/dL.

ESRD patients with symptoms of ischemic heart disease should have coronary arteriography. Dialysis patients fulfilling the anatomical and functional criteria used in the general population are likely to benefit from coronary revascularization. Generally accepted criteria include one, two, or three vessel disease with angina refractory to medical management, left main coronary artery disease, and triple-vessel disease associated with ventricular dysfunction or easily inducible ischemia. There is evidence that recurrence rates after coronary angioplasty are high in dialysis patients. The perioperative morbidity and mortality rates associated with coronary artery bypass surgery are higher in dialysis patients than in the general population. Most recent studies suggests that these rates are acceptable and justifiable on the basis of good subsequent survival rates. Evidence suggests that in the dialysis population, coronary artery bypass surgery is superior to angioplasty in terms of overall survival, cardiac death, and myocardial infarction, although prospective trials comparing revascularization procedures have not been undertaken.

Management of Cardiomyopathy

Eighty percent or more of dialysis patients have cardiomyopathy, which can progress rapidly. All patients who develop cardiac failure should have echocardiography to try to distinguish systolic from diastolic dysfunction. ACE-inhibitors, calcium channel blockers, and β-blockers form the cornerstone of treatment in concentric LVH. Based on data from the nonuremic population, we use ACE-inhibitors as the preferred initial therapy in patients with LV dilatation, systolic dysfunction, and symptomatic cardiac failure. It is not yet clear whether angiotensin II receptor antagonists are superior to ACE-inhibitors. Digoxin may benefit patients with cardiac failure in the presence of systolic dysfunction, but is best avoided in patients with diastolic dysfunction. Recent studies in the general population suggest that β-blockers and calcium channel antagonists may have a role as primary therapy for cardiac failure associated with both diastolic and systolic dysfunction. Such an approach should be done in consultation with a cardiologist. Nitrates are useful for symptomatic relief in frank cardiac failure, whether due to systolic or diastolic dysfunction. Although aldosterone inhibition is of value in patients with systolic dysfunction who have preserved renal function spironolactone has not been assessed in patients with chronic renal failure. The threat of hyperkalemia due to ACE-inhibitors or angiotensin II receptors in low renal clearance patients not yet on dialysis is considerable and likely to limit the use of spironolactone.

PERICARDITIS IN UREMIC PATIENTS

Clinically important pericarditis is now an infrequent occurrence, although small pericardial effusions are very common on echocardiography. Uremic pericarditis occurs in uremic individuals who have never received dialysis therapy. Pericarditis or pericardial tamponade may also occur in individuals already on dialysis. The uremic milieu is responsible for the former condition, although the specific culprits are unknown; the latter condition often has a viral etiology. About one-half of all patients who develop pericarditis while on dialysis therapy will clinically improve after intensified dialysis therapy with daily dialysis sessions of increased length, suggesting that uremia is causative in only a proportion of these cases.

Clinical Presentation

The major clinical findings are due to inflammation (precordial pain, dyspnea, fever, generalized systolic changes on electrocardiography) and fluid in the pericardial sac leading to a restriction to ventricular filling (fluid overload and intolerance of ultrafiltration). With large effusions, frank cardiac tamponade and cardiogenic shock may occur. It is more likely that a given volume of pericardial fluid will lead to cardiac tamponade when it accumulates quickly.

Echocardiography should be performed to estimate the volume of fluid within the pericardium. Intensification of dialysis therapy, with avoidance of heparin, and analgesia form the cornerstone of management. Some but not all authors recommend the use of nonsteroidal antiinflammatory agents. Surgical drainage is needed for large effusions (typically >250 mL) or where cardiac tamponade is imminent.

Bibliography

Besarab A, Bolton WK, Browne, Egrie JC, Nissenson AR, Akamoto DM, Schwab SJ, Goodkin DA: The effects of normal as compared with low hematocrit values in patients with cardiac disease who are receiving hemodialysis and epoetin. *N Engl J Med* 339:584–590, 1998.

Bloembergen WE, Stannard DC, Port FK, Wolfe RA, Pugh JA, Jones CA, Greer JW, Golper TA, Held PJ: Relationship of dose of hemodialysis and cause-specific mortality. *Kidney Int* 50:557–565, 1996.

Bostom AG, Lathrop L: Hyperhomocysteinemia in end-stage renal disease: Prevalence, etiology and potential relationship to arteriosclerotic outcomes. *Kidney Int* 52:10–20, 1997.

Churchill DN, Taylor DW, Cook RJ, La Plante P, Cartier P, Fay WP, Goldstein MB, Jindal K, Mandin H, McKenzie JK, Muirhead N, Parfrey PS, Posen GA, Slaughter D, Ulan RA, Werb R: Canadian hemodialysis morbidity study. *Am J Kidney Dis* 19:214–234, 1992.

Foley RN, Parfrey PS, Harnett JD, Kent GM, Murray DC, Barre PE: The progostic importance of left ventricular geometry in uremic cardiomyopathy. *J Am Soc Nephrol* 5:2024–2031, 1995.

Foley RN, Parfrey PS, Harnett JD, Kent GM, Martin CJ, Murray DC, Barre PE: Clinical and echocardiographic disease in end-stage renal disease: Prevalence, associations and prognosis. *Kidney Int* 47:186–192, 1995.

Foley RN, Parfrey PS, Morgan J, Barré PE, Campbell P, Cartier P, Coyle D, Fine A, Handa P, Kingma I, Lau CY, Levin A, Mendelssohn D, Muirhead N, Murphy B, Plante RK, Posen G, Wells, GA: The effect of complete vs partial correction of using epoetin on left ventricular structure in hemodialysis patients with asymptomatic cardiomyopathy. *J Am Soc Nephrol* 9:208A, 1998.

Harnett JD, Foley RN, Kent GM, Barre PE, Murray DC Parfrey PS: Congestive heart failure in dialysis patients: Prevalence, incidence, prognosis and risk factors. *Kidney Int* 47:884–890, 1995.

Herzog CA, Ma JZ, Collins AJ: Long-term outcome of dialysis patients in the United States with coronary revascularisation procedures. *Kidney Int* 56(1):324–332, 1999.

Levin A, Singer J, Thompson CR, Ross H, Lewis M: Prevalent left ventricular hypertrophy in the predialysis population: Identifying opportunities for intervention. *Am J Kidney Dis* 27:347–354, 1996.

Murphy SW, Parfrey PS: Screening for cardiovascular disease in dialysis patients. *Curr Opin Nephrol Hypertens* 5:532–540, 1996.

Oparil S: Treating multiple-risk hypertensive patients. *Am J Hypertens* 12(11):1215–1295, 1999.

Parfrey PS, Foley RN, Harnett JD, Kent GM, Murray DC, Barre PE: Outcome and risk factors of ischemic heart disease in chronic uremia. *Kidney Int* 49:1428–1434, 1996.

HEMATOLOGIC MANIFESTATIONS OF RENAL FAILURE

JONATHAN HIMMELFARB

ANEMIA

Pathogenesis

Normal erythropoiesis is primarily regulated by circulating erythropoietin. When erythropoietin binds to specific receptors on bone marrow erythroid progenitor cells, their proliferation, differentiation, and development into mature erythrocytes is enhanced. The kidney produces up to 90% of circulating erythropoietin, accounting for its pivotal role in erythropoiesis. Based on *in situ* hybridization techniques, the major site of erythropoietin production has been shown to be the renal peritubular interstitial fibroblast. Most ex-

tra renal erythropoietin is produced in the liver by centrilobular hepatocytes. However, extra renal erythropoietin production is rarely able to provide for significant erythropoiesis in an anephric state, suggesting that the liver is less sensitive than the kidney to hypoxic stimuli. The precise mechanisms by which hypoxia stimulates renal erythropoietin secretion remains incompletely understood.

The pathogenesis of anemia of chronic renal failure is multifactorial. Erythropoietin deficiency, shortened erythrocyte survival, the presence of uremic inhibitors of erythropoiesis, hemolysis, bleeding, and iron deficiency are all contributors. In normal subjects, circulating plasma erythropoietin levels are minute, but increase exponentially in response to anemia. In contrast, in anemic patients with progressive renal failure, the relationship between the degree of anemia and plasma erythropoietin is lost (Fig. 1). However, it is clear that the major cause of anemia in chronic renal failure is deficient erythropoietin production.

Support for the hypothesis that uremic toxins retained in the plasma inhibit bone marrow erythroid production rests on *in vitro* experiments demonstrating that uremic human serum blunts the growth of erythroid colony forming units (CFU-E). This *in vivo* erythroid inhibition has been thought to be due to polyamines such as spermine or putrescine as well as yet unidentified "middle molecules." More recent studies using human autologous cultured bone marrow cells have not demonstrated inhibition of erythroid progenitor cell growth by uremic serum. Furthermore, *in vivo* studies involving the infusion of recombinant erythropoietin into normal subjects and hemodialysis patients demonstrate that erythropoiesis, as quantitated by ferrokinetics and the reticulocyte response, are not blunted in subjects with chronic renal failure. Almost all patients with chronic renal failure, if iron replete and without inflammation or infection, will have an appropriate erythropoietic response to erythropoietin. Thus, current evidence suggests that uremic inhibitors of erythropoiesis play a minimal role if any in the pathogenesis of the anemia of chronic renal failure.

A decrease in erythrocyte survival has also been postulated to contribute to the anemia of chronic renal failure. Decreased erythrocyte survival in uremic patients may be related to reduced resistance to both complement-mediated erythrocyte lysis and oxidant stress. Erythrocyte survival is 60–90 days in uremic patients versus 120 days in normal individuals and generally does not improve with

dialysis therapy. The use of erythropoietin may also extend erythrocyte survival by preventing neocytolysis, a physiologic process by which the youngest erythrocytes in the circulation undergo hemolysis.

Laboratory and Clinical Manifestations of Anemia of Chronic Renal Disease

The anemia of chronic renal disease is morphologically a normocytic, normochromic anemia. Both the corrected reticulocyte count and serum erythropoietin levels are inappropriately low when compared to values seen in patients with similar degrees of anemia without renal failure. Iron parameters should be normal. The bone marrow examination is usually normal and is not usually necessary for the hematologic evaluation.

Patients with chronic renal failure who develop anemia should undergo screening for causes of anemia other than erythropoietin deficiency. This evaluation should include measurement of red blood cell (RBC) indices, reticulocyte count, iron parameters, and a test for stool occult blood. An abnormal platelet count or white blood cell count may reflect a more generalized disturbance of bone marrow function. Erythrocyte indices, reticulocyte counts, and iron parameters are helpful in detecting many anemias which are not due to erythropoietin deficiency. Microcytosis can reflect iron deficiency, aluminum intoxication, and certain hemogloblinopathies. Macrocytosis may be associated with vitamin B_{12} or folate deficiency.

As renal failure progresses there is an increased likelihood of developing anemia as diseased kidneys are unable to produce sufficient quantities of erythropoietin. Figure 2 depicts the relationship between the change in hematocrit and the serum creatinine in over 900 patients. While the mean hematocrit drops below 30 at a serum creatinine of approximately 6 mg/dL, there is considerable interpatient variation. There is even less correlation between the blood urea nitrogen (BUN) and hematocrit.

In patients whose renal failure is the result of polycystic kidney disease, the hemoglobin level and hematocrit may be higher than in patients with a comparable level of renal dysfunction due to other causes. On the other hand, patients who have undergone bilateral nephrectomies generally have more severe anemia than other patients on chronic dialysis therapy. Even when kidneys are devoid of excretory function, they usually retain some capability for erythropoietin biosynthesis.

Patients with severe anemia regardless of its etiology display signs and symptoms attributable to tissue hypoxia. However, many of the symptoms usually attributable to anemia may be clinically difficult to distinguish from symptoms related to uremia. For most patients, symptoms develop when the hematocrit decreases to 30 or less. Therapy is indicated at a higher level of hematocrit if angina pectoris or other significant symptoms develop. Younger patients often will adjust better to anemia. When anemia develops gradually, an intraerythrocytic increase in 2,3-diphosphoglycerate (2,3-DPG) occurs, which shifts the oxygen dissociation curve to the right and allows oxygen to be

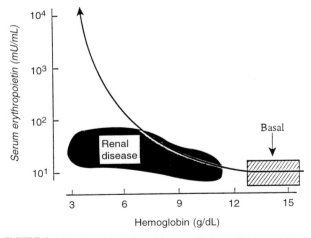

FIGURE 1 Erythropoietin levels in renal failure. The box entitled "basal" refers to serum erythropoietin levels in normal individuals. The upward arrow reflects the typical rise in serum erythropoietin levels in patients with anemia not due to chronic renal failure. Adapted from: Hillman RS, Ault KA: *Hematology in Clinical Practice.* McGraw-Hill, New York, 1995, with permission from the McGraw-Hill Companies.

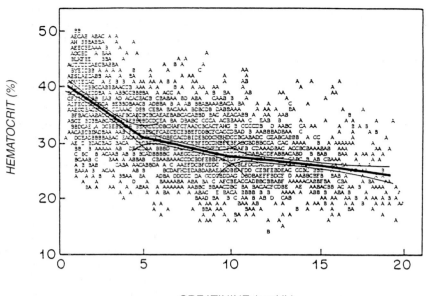

FIGURE 2 The change of hematocrit with creatinine in chronic renal failure. This figure represents approximately 4000 data points obtained from 911 patients followed without treatment with erythropoietin on dialysis. The 95% confidence limit of the slope is shown around each line. Each letter represents the number of data points at that value (e.g., A = 1 data point, B = 2 data points). Adapted from: Hakim RK Lazarus JM: Biochemical parameters in chronic renal failure. *Am J Kidney Dis* 11(3):238–247, 1988.

unloaded at the tissue level more readily. Thus, many patients may not be as severely symptomatic as might be expected from the degree of anemia. Additional cardiovascular compensatory mechanisms may also develop over time, thereby limiting symptoms directly attributed to anemia.

The symptoms of anemia include weakness, fatigue, and dyspnea, particularly with exertion. Decreased exercise tolerance is common, and many patients experience difficulty with concentration, attention span, and memory. Sexual dysfunction, cold intolerance, and anorexia may also be side effects related to anemia.

Treatment of Anemia

The therapeutic modalities available today for treatment of the anemia of renal disease include administration of recombinant erythropoietin, institution of renal replacement therapy including kidney transplantation, and packed red blood cell transfusions. The use of recombinant erythropoietin to treat the anemia of chronic renal failure has led to the recognition that the contribution of anemia to the morbidity of chronic renal failure is greater than formerly appreciated. The clinical benefits of improved tissue oxygenation have been quantitated to include improvements in exercise capacity, central nervous system function, endocrine and cardiac function, as well as a reduction in hospital admissions. The most important benefit in treating the

anemia of chronic renal disease may be in the reduction of cardiovascular morbidity and mortality.

Chronic anemia and consequent tissue hypoxia result in a compensatory increase in cardiac contractility which contributes to the development of left ventricular hypertrophy. The development of left ventricular hypertrophy with consequent diastolic dysfunction and myocardial ischemia is a risk factor for mortality in patients on dialysis therapy. Correction of the anemia of chronic renal failure generally results in improvement but not resolution of left ventricular hypertrophy. Anemia correction also lowers the rate of hospitalization for myocardial infarction and cardiac disease in general and markedly improves exercise capacity.

The use of erythropoietin to improve anemia in hemodialysis patients is also associated with improvement in cognitive function. This improvement has been quantitated both by documenting normalization of abnormal EEGs as well as improvement on neuropsychiatric testing.

Normalization of cerebral blood flow has also been demonstrated with improvement in anemia. These improvements in cognition have translated into a lessening of depression and improvements in quality of life indicators Endocrine changes also occur in response to erythropoietin therapy in chronic renal failure (see Chapter 66). Sexual function improves in some men after increase in hematocrit. Some (but not all) studies have demonstrated an increase in serum testosterone levels. Serum prolactin levels have decreased in some (but not all) male hemodialysis patients. Anemia may also play a role in growth retardation in pediatric patients.

Use of Recombinant Erythropoietin

The first clinical trials of recombinant human erythropoietin in hemodialysis patients began in 1985 and demonstrated a clear-cut relationship between the dose of erythropoietin and the rate of rise in hematocrit (Fig. 3). Erythropoietin responsiveness is dependent on dose, route, and frequency of parenteral administration. Absorption following subcutaneous administration of erythropoietin is incomplete. Subcutaneous erythropoietin administration results in a slower increase in serum erythropoietin levels with maintenance of a stable serum level for hours. Although intravenous erythropoietin administration has 100% bioavailability, most of the administered intravenous dose is probably biologically ineffective once the relatively small number of erythropoietin receptors are saturated on erythroid progenitor cells. As a result, subcutaneous dosing is more efficient. Several studies have demonstrated that 20–40% less erythropoietin is required to maintain a serum level of hematocrit with subcutaneous as opposed to intravenous dosing. Erythropoietin can also be administered intraperitoneally, which may be preferable for children treated with peritoneal dialysis.

It is currently recommended that the initial administration of erythropoietin for treatment of anemia in predialysis, peritoneal dialysis, and hemodialysis patients should be subcutaneous at a dose of 80–120 units/kg/week in two to three divided doses to achieve the target hematocrit (Fig. 3). Children less than 5 years of age frequently require higher doses than adults (300 units/kg/week). The site of erythropoietin injection should be rotated with each administration.

The appropriate target hemoglobin and hematocrit for patients with chronic renal failure on erythropoietin therapy remains incompletely defined. The original target hematocrit recommended by the U.S. Federal Drug Administration (FDA) in 1989 was 30–33%, which was subsequently widened to a target hematocrit range of 30–36% in June of 1994. Extensive evaluation by the National Kidney Foundation (NKF)- led to a recommended hematocrit of 33–36% with a corresponding hemoglobin target of 11–12 g/dL. This is the current generally accepted target. Several investigators have suggested that using erythropoietin to normalize hematocrit (target hematocrit 42), may have additional benefits in improving cardiac function, cognition, and quality of life. However, in a recent large prospective randomized trial, over 1200 long-term dialysis patients who had signs or symptoms of congestive heart failure or ischemic heart disease were randomized to receive erythropoietin to a target hematocrit of either $30 \pm 3\%$ or $42 \pm 3\%$ (Fig. 4). In an unexpected finding, the incidence of death and nonfatal myocardial infarction was higher in the normal as compared to low hematocrit group (relative risk 1.3, 95% confidence interval, 0.9 to 1.9). Results of a European and a Canadian trial addressing the same issue are not yet available. Given the results of the recently published trial, for the time being a target hematocrit of 33–36% or corresponding target hemoglobin of 11–12 g/dL appears prudent.

Use of Iron Therapy

A crucial aspect of erythropoietin therapy is the maintenance of adequate iron stores for the production of new erythrocytes. Normally, three-quarters of body iron is present in circulating erythrocytes, and one-quarter exists as storage iron primarily in the liver and bone marrow. Because the demands for iron by the erythroid marrow frequently exceed iron stores once erythropoietin therapy is initiated, iron supplementation is essential to assure adequate response. In the pre-erythropoietin era, advanced renal failure and its associated hypoproliferative anemia were frequently accompanied by excess storage iron. Since the widespread use of erythropoietin, iron overload is now uncommon, whereas iron deficiency has become quite common.

Iron status in patients receiving erythropoietin is monitored by measuring both the serum ferritin and the percent transferrin saturation. Serum ferritin and percent transferrin saturation are complimentary tests because they measure different pools of body iron. The serum ferritin is proportional to storage iron, and a low serum ferritin is highly specific for erythropoietin resistance. However, the serum ferritin is also an acute phase reactant that may be increase in the presence of acute or chronic inflammation. Thus, a low serum ferritin is a specific but not a sensitive marker for iron deficiency.

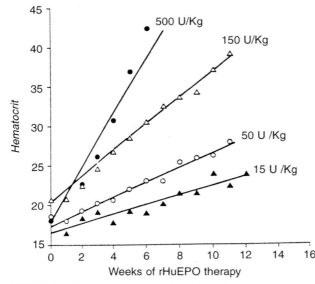

FIGURE 3 The response in hematocrit to erythropoietin therapy. Each line represents the response to the given dose of erythropoietin administered intravenously three times a week to hemodialysis patients. Adapted from: Eschbach JW, Egrie JC, Downing MR, Brown K Adamson JW: Correction of the anemia of end stage renal disease with recombinant human erythropoietin. *N Engl J Med* 316:73–78, 1987. Reprinted with permission. Copyright © 1987 Massachusetts Medical Society. All Rights reserved.

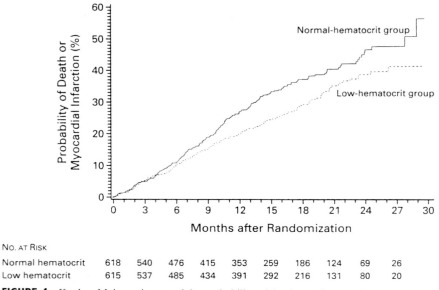

FIGURE 4 Kaplan–Meier estimates of the probability of death or a first nonfatal myocardial infarction in the normal-hematocrit and low-hematocrit groups. Adapted from: Besarab A, Bolton WY, Browne JK, Egrie JC, Nissenson AR, Okamoto DM, Schwab SJ, Goodkin DA: The effects of normal as compared with low hematocrit values in patients with cardiac disease who are receiving hemodialysis and epoietin. *N Engl J Med* 339:584–590, 1998. Copyright © 1998 Massachusetts Medical Society. All rights reserved.

In contrast, the percent transferrin saturation (measured as the serum iron divided by the total iron binding capacity multiplied by 100), reflects iron that is readily available for erythropoiesis. The transferrin molecule contains two receptors for molecular iron transported from storage iron sites to erythroid progenitor cells. The percent transferrin saturation is decreased with either absolute or functional iron deficiency. Functional iron deficiency exits when serum ferritin levels are >100 ng/mL, but patients have an augmented erythropoetic response to additional iron supplementation. Transferrin saturation appears to be a better predictor of iron responsiveness than the serum ferritin level. Other tests of iron status such as RBC ferritin or zinc protoporphyrin do not appear to increase diagnostic sensitivity or specificity and are less widely available. The gold standard test for iron status, bone marrow stainable iron, is invasive and expensive and need not be used on a routine basis. For optimal responsiveness to erythropoietin, current recommendations are that the serum ferritin should be maintained between 100 and 800 ng/mL, and the percent transferrin saturation should be maintained between 20 and 50%.

Iron can be administered either as oral iron salts or intravenously. When oral iron is used it should be given as 200 mg of elemental iron/day in two to three divided doses. For optimal absorption oral iron should be given more than 1 hr before meals or more than 2 hr after meals or ingestion of phosphate binders. In the majority of dialysis patients receiving erythropoietin, oral iron is insufficient to maintain adequate iron status, and intravenous iron is re-

quired. Iron dextran and ferric gluconate are the only forms of intravenous iron currently FDA approved in the United States. Anaphylactic reactions occur in 0.6% of intravenous iron dextran treated patients. Prior to initiating intravenous iron dextran therapy, a one time test dose of 25 mg must be given intravenously. However, anaphylactic reactions may occur in patients who have received any number of previous iron dextran injections. Iron dextran is frequently administered as a 100 mg doses with each hemodialysis treatment, with a total administered dose of 1000 mg. Some investigators now recommend that intravenous iron dextran be administered in 50–100 mg weekly doses continually in patients intolerant of oral iron salts or who cannot maintain adequate iron status with oral iron.

Recently, questions have been raised as to the safety of routine intravenous iron administration with the view that iron administration may result in increased risk of infection and cardiovascular complications. Iron is an important growth factor for bacteria, and organisms such as staphylococci have developed mechanisms to acquire iron during infection. Iron-overloaded hemodialysis patients may have defective phagocytic cell function and host defense. However, a recent large, multicenter, prospective study of risk factors for bacteremia in chronic hemodialysis patients did not identify iron overload (as measured by a high serum ferritin) as a risk factor for infection. It has also been suggested that the administration of high doses of intravenous iron would overwhelm plasma iron-binding capacity, leading to the presence of free ferrous iron in the plasma, which could increase oxidative stress. However, serum transferrin and other host defense mechanisms can handle a great deal of excess plasma iron without allowing free ferrous iron in the plasma. Thus, at the present time, the idea that intravenous iron administration contributes to septicemia or cardiovascular toxicity in chronic hemodialysis patients remains speculative. It may be prudent, however, to withhold intravenous iron therapy in dialysis patients with active infections.

Erythropoietin Resistance

True resistance to erythropoietin therapy for the treatment of chronic renal failure is rare (Table 1). In the largest clinical trial, over 96% of iron replete dialysis patients responded when erythropoietin was given at ~50 units/kg intravenously three times a week. The median dose of erythropoietin needed to maintain the target hematocrit was 75 units/kg intravenously three times a week. The most common cause of a poor response to erythropoietin is either an inadequate erythropoietin dose or the presence of iron deficiency. Other causes of erythropoietin resistance include the presence of inflammation or infection. Inflammation results in a deficient iron supply by blocking the release of iron from the reticuloendothelial system despite the presence of normal to increased iron stores and by decreasing oral iron absorption. Bone marrow fibrosis from osteitis fibrosa cystica as a consequence of hyperparathyroidism can cause true erythropoietin resistance. The definitive diagnosis of osteitis fibrosa cystica requires a bone biopsy, as hyperparathyroidism without osteitis fibrosa cystica does not blunt the effect of erythropoietin. Aluminum intoxication, now a rarity in maintenance dialysis patients, contributes to anemia by decreasing bone marrow hemoglobin synthesis. It can be suspected in the iron replete patient who has a low erythrocyte mean corpuscular volume and confirmed by measuring an increased serum aluminum level after deferoxamine administration or by positive staining for aluminum in a bone biopsy. Rarely, folate or vitamin B_{12} deficiency can be a cause of erythropoietin resistance. Resistance to erythropoietin therapy has also been documented due to anti-N_{form} hemolysis in patients with chronic formaldehyde exposure related to stenlization of reused dialyzers. Occult bleeding also needs to be considered in erythropoietin resistant patients.

TABLE I
Apparent Causes of EPO Resistance

Inadequate EPO dose

Inflammation

Osteitis fibrosa cystica

Aluminum intoxication

Folate deficiency

Severe malnutrition

Hemolysis or blood loss

Primary hematologic diseases

Side Effects of Erythropoietin Therapy

Early experiences suggested that accelerated hypertension, the development of seizures, and hyperkalemia frequently accompanied correction of anemia with erythropoietin therapy. However, extensive clinical experience has now demonstrated that the adverse effects of erythropoietin therapy are infrequent and generally manageable. The most frequent adverse effect is aggravation of hypertension in 20–30% of patients. An increase in blood pressure usually occurs in association with a rapid increase in hematocrit or at higher doses of erythropoietin. The development or worsening of hypertension is thought to be related to an increase in vascular wall reactivity as well as hemodynamic changes that occur as a consequence of increasing red cell mass. Endothelial cells have now been demonstrated to possess erythropoietin receptors, and infusion of erythropoietin *in vitro* can result in release of endothelin and an increase in vasoconstriction. Worsening hypertension associated with erythropoietin therapy can be treated by initiating or increasing antihypertensive therapy, by intensifying ultrafiltration in dialysis patients with evidence of volume expansion, or by reducing erythropoietin dose.

The initial multcenter study with erythropoietin in the United States noted a higher incidence of seizures during the first 3 months of the study compared to historical controls. These findings have not been confirmed subsequently. With the exception of patients with hypertensive encephalopathy, there does not appear to be evidence of increased seizures in patients in whom appropriate dose and titration recommendations are followed. A prior history of seizures is not considered a contraindication to the use of erythropoietin. While serious hyperkalemia was observed during the early clinical experiences, recent studies have not demonstrated a higher incidence of hyperkalemia in erythropoietin treated patients.

Whether increasing the hematocrit with erythropoietin increases the likelihood of developing vascular access thrombosis in hemodialysis patients remains controversial. Most studies have not demonstrated an increase in the rate of either native fistulae or prosthetic graft thrombosis when the hematocrit is kept at or below a target of 36%. An exception is the Canadian multicenter trial which suggested that erythropoietin increased the rate of thrombosis in synthetic grafts. Vascular access thrombosis clearly increases when hematocrits are normalized with erythropoietin therapy.

Erythrocytosis in Uremic Patients

Erythrocytosis is occasionally seen in previously anemic uremic patients who develop a renal cell carcinoma or large renal cyst and is occasionally seen in patients with polycystic kidney disease.

Erythrocytosis has also been reported to occur in up to 17% of renal transplant recipients. The pathogenesis of post-transplant erythrocytosis is poorly understood and is not usually related to higher circulating erythropoietin levels. Angiotensin converting enzyme inhibitors can often correct renal transplant erythrocytosis by an as yet undefined mechanism. Phosphodiesterase inhibitors such as theophylline can also correct post-transplant erythrocytosis. Because erythrocytosis of any etiology enhances the risks of thromboembolic disease, therapy for post-transplant erythrocytosis is recommended. Standard therapy includes discontinuation of cigarette smoking or diuretic use. Although serial phlebotomy has been the recognized standard of care, most transplant centers now use low-dose angiotensin converting enzyme (ACE) inhibitor therapy to successfully manage post-transplant erythrocytosis.

Platelet Dysfunction in Uremia

Clinical bleeding in patients with uremia is due to an acquired qualitative platelet defect and has best been correlated with a prolonged bleeding time. At present, however, there is no single unifying pathogenetic mechanism to explain the acquired platelet dysfunction seen in patients with uremia. The clinical bleeding tendency of patients with renal failure is generally improved by dialysis. Therefore, uremic toxins have been implicated as important mediators of the bleeding diathesis. However, the search for a specific uremic toxin that interferes with primary hemostasis has been elusive. Furthermore, the general experience has been that dialysis only incompletely corrects the prolonged bleeding time, and in some cases may actually transiently worsen the bleeding diathesis.

No single intrinsic defect in platelet function can be consistently linked to the bleeding tendency; uremic platelet dysfunction is thus considered a multifactorical disorder. Defects in *in vitro* platelet aggregability, diminished thromboxane A2 production, abnormal intracellular calcium mobilization, and increased intracellular cAMP have all been described in uremic platelets. Several studies have emphasized a defect in platelet adhesion to vascular subendothelium in uremic patients. Platelet adhesiveness to subendothelium depends on the cooperative interactions of platelet glycoproteins with von Willebrand's factor in the vascular wall. Platelet glycoprotein function is abnormal in hemodialysis patients. Fibrinogen fragments that interfere with platelet adhesion and aggregation may also accumulate in uremia. There are conflicting data as to whether patients with uremia have decreased von Willebrand's factor activity. Uremia may also be associated with increased release of endothelial prostacyclin and nitric oxide, both of which inhibit adhesion of platelets.

The mainstay of treatment of the bleeding diathesis of uremia has been dialysis, although it is not consistently effective. In addition to dialysis, a number of therapeutic approaches are available to correct the bleeding diathesis in patients who are experiencing serious bleeding complications. (Table 2). The synthetic vasopressin derivative desmopressin (or DDAVP) has been shown to shorten the bleeding time rapidly and improve clinical bleeding in uremia. The mechanism of action of DDAVP is thought to be related to release of large multimer von Willebrand's factor from endothelial cells and platelets, although this has not been conclusively demonstrated. A limitation to DDAVP therapy is the development of tachyphylaxis after two to three doses. Other therapeutic approaches have included the administration of cryoprecipitate or conjugated estrogens. Similar to DDAVP, the mechanism of action of these agents is thought to be related either to release of large von Willebrand's factor multimers or to endothelial functional changes. Unfortunately, all of these agents have variable clinical efficacy in uremia.

Increasing the hematocrit to above 30, either via packed red blood cell transfusions or the by use of erythropoietin, has been demonstrated to improve the bleeding time in most anemic patients. Although the primary pathogenetic mechanism of increasing the hematocrit in improving the bleeding time may be rheological, additional evidence suggests that increasing hemoglobin concentration may inactivate the platelet inhibiting effects of nitric oxide.

Leukocyte Dysfunction in Uremia

Infection remains a major cause of morbidity and mortality in the dialysis patient. Vascular access infections, particularly with *Staphylococcus* species, remains the leading source of serious infection in hemodialysis patients. Most infections in chronic hemodialysis patients are due to common catalase producing bacteria rather than to oppor-

TABLE 2
Treatment of Uremic Platelet Dysfunction

Therapy	Dose or goal	Onset	Duration	Comment
Increase hematocrit (EPO, RBC transfusion)	>30	Immediate	Prolonged	Highly effective
DDAVP	0.3 μg/kg intravenous	Immediate	4–8 hr	Rapid tachyphylaxis, use just before needed
Cryoprecipitate	10 units	1–4 hr	24 hr	Hepatitis, HIV risk
Conjugated estrogens	0.6 mg/kg/day × 5 days	6 hr	14 days	Hot flashes, HTN, abnormal LFTs

[a]HTN, hypertension; LFT, liver function test.

tunistic organisms. The pattern of infectious organisms in chronic dialysis patients is similar to patients with chronic granulomatous disease whose phagocytic cells lack the capability to produce reactive oxygen species.

The number and morphology of granulocytes in patients with uremia are normal except for a tendency toward hypersegmentation in some patients. Numerous studies have documented alterations in granulocyte function in patients with uremia or on chronic dialysis, including chemotaxis, granulocyte adherence, phagocytic capability, and reactive oxygen species production. Iron overload may contribute to phagocytic dysfunction.

In addition to changes in granulocyte function associated with uremia, it is now well documented that hemodialysis with cellulosic membranes results in complement mediated granulocyte activation and subsequent dysfunction. Changes in granulocyte function as a consequence of dialysis with cellulosic membranes include modulation of chemotactic receptors, changes in granulocyte reactive oxygen species production, alterations in granulocyte adherence, and alterations in granulocyte expression of cell adhesion molecules. A recent cohort study using the U.S. Renal Data System (USRDS) data base has demonstrated a correlation between the use of unmodified cellulosic dialysis membranes and the risk of mortality due to infection in chronic hemodialysis patients.

Changes in monocyte function as well as a reduction in number and function of lymphocytes in patients with uremia lead to altered immunity in this patient population. Evidence of altered immunity include alterations in T-cell-dependent humoral responses such as reduced responsiveness to vaccinations, diminished delayed hypersensitivity responses, and a dramatic attenuation of autoimmune disease activity with uremia. The chronic use of cellulosic dialysis membranes may also exacerbate the underlying defect in immunity in patients with uremia.

Bibliography

Besarab A, Kaiser JW, Frinak S: A study of parenteral iron regimens in hemodialysis patients. *Am J Kidney Dis* 34:21–28, 1999.

Besarab A, Bolton WK, Browne JK, Egrie JC, Nissenson AR, Okamoto DM, Schwab SJ, Goodkin DA: The effects of normal as compared with low hematocrit values in patients with cardiac disease who are receiving hemodialysis and erythropoietin. *N Engl J Med* 339:584–590, 1998.

Beusterein KM, Nissenson AR, Port FK, Kelly M, Steinwald B, Ware JF: The effects of recombinant human erythropoietin on functional health and well-being in chronic dialysis patients. *J Am Soc Nephrol* 7:763–773, 1996.

Churchill DN, Muirhead N, Goldstein M, *et al.*: Effect of recombinant human erythropoietin on hospitalization of hemodialysis patients. *Clin Nephrol* 43:184–188, 1995.

Eschbach JW, Haley NR, Egrie JC, Adamson JW: A comparison of the responses to recombinant human erythropoietin in normal and uremic subjects. *Kidney Int* 42:407–416, 1992.

Eschbach JW, Kelly MR, Haley NR, Abels RI, Adamson JW: Treatment of the anemia of progressive renal failure with recombinant human erythropoietin. *N Engl J Med* 321:158–163, 1989.

Eschbach JW, Egrie JC, Downing MR, Browne JK, Adamson JW: Correction of anemia of end stage renal disease with recombinant human erythropoietin: Results of a combined phase I and II clinical trial. *N Engl J Med* 316:73–78, 1987.

Fishbane S, Frei GL, Maesaka J: Reduction in recombinant human erythropoietin doses by the use of chronic intravenous iron supplementation. *Am J Kidney Dis* 26:41–46, 1995.

Foley RN, Parfrey PS, Harnett JD, Kent GM, Murray DC, Barre PE: The impact of anemia on cardiomyopathy, morbidity and mortality in end-stage renal disease. *Am J Kidney Dis* 28:53–61, 1996.

Goldblum SE, Reed WP: Host defenses and irnmunologic alterations associated with chronic hemodialysis. *Ann Intern Med* 93:597–613, 1980.

Hakim RM, Lazarus JM: Biochemical parameters in chronic renal failure. *Am J Kidney Dis* 11:238–247, 1988.

Kaufman JS, Reda DJ, Fye CL, Goldfarb DS, Henderson WG, Kleinman JG, Vaamonde CA: Subcutaneous compared with intravenous epoetin in patients receiving hemodialysis. *N Engl J Med* 339:578–583, 1998.

Lewis SL, Van Epps DE: Neutrophil and monocyte alterations in chronic dialysis patients. *Am J Kidney Dis* 9:381–395, 1987.

Owen WF: Optimizing the use of parenteral iron in end-stage renal disease patients: Focus on issues of infection and cardiovascular disease. *Am J Kidney Dis* 34:(4)S1–S52, 1999.

Powe NR, Griffiths RI, Watson AJ, *et al.*: Effect of recombinant ery-thropoietin on hospital admissions, readmissions, length of stay, and costs of dialysis patients. *J Am Soc Nephrol* 4:1455–1465, 1994.

Ratcliff PJ: Molecular biology of erythropoietin. *Kidney Int* 44:887–904, 1993.

Rice L, Alfrey CP, Driscoll T, Whitley CE, Hachey DL, Suki W: Neocytolysis contributes to the anemia of renal disease. *Am J Kidney Dis* 33:59–62, 1999.

Steiner RW, Coggins C, Carvalho ACA: Bleeding time in uremia: A useful test to assess clinical bleeding. *Am J Hematol* 7:107–117, 1979.

ENDOCRINE AND NEUROLOGICAL MANIFESTATIONS OF RENAL FAILURE

EUGENE C. KOVALIK

ENDOCRINE MANIFESTATIONS

Chronic renal failure (CRF), end stage renal disease (ESRD), and renal transplantation all affect the endocrine system. Problems include alterations in feedback mechanisms as well as production, transport, metabolism, elimination, and protein binding of hormones. Drug interactions may also be an issue (Tables 1 and 2). In addition, hormonal assays can give aberrant results in patients with renal disease, depending on whether the assay is specific for the hormone in question or cross-reacts with metabolites which normally are excreted by the kidney but accumulate with a falling glomerular filtration rate (GFR). Hormones that truly are elevated to some extent in chronic renal failure include growth hormone, prolactin, and catecholamines. Diagnosis of endocrine disease in renal patients must take into account all the aforementioned.

Hypothalamic–Hypophyseal Axes

Thyroid

Thyroid abnormalities have been well documented in CRF and ESRD patients. Up to 58% of uremic patients have evidence of a goiter by palpation, thought to be caused by an uncharacterized circulating goitrogen that accumulates as GFR falls. Total thyroxine (T_4) is either normal or decreased, and triiodothyronine (T_3) levels are depressed. Free T_4 levels may be low. The use of reverse T_3 (rT_3) to differentiate between hypothyroid states and the so-called euthyroid sick state is not helpful in patients with CRF since levels are often normal. Although binding globulin levels are normal, circulating inhibitors result in decreased globulin binding and interfere with the older resin uptake based tests of thyroid function. These abnormalities tend to worsen with the progression of renal disease. Thyroid stimulating hormone (TSH) tends to be normal despite the abnormalities in thyroid hormone levels and therefore is the best indicator of thyroid function, especially with the availability of ultrasensitive TSH assays. The basal metabolic rate is also normal.

Although TSH levels are normal in patients with CRF, subtle abnormalities exist in the hypothalamic–hypophyseal axis. Exogenous thyrotropin releasing hormone (TRH) stimulation results in a blunted TSH response. The usual nocturnal TSH surge is absent. TSH administration results in an increase in T_3 levels but not in the expected rise in T_4 levels. It has been postulated that two different problems occur in patients with CRF. First, there is an inappropriate response to decreased thyroid hormone levels due to a reset in the normal feedback loop to a lower level of TSH secretion for a given level of thyroid hormone. Second, thyroid gland resistance to TSH also occurs. For unknown reasons, the use of recombinant erythropoietin normalizes the TSH response to TRH but not the thyroid response to TSH. The mildly impaired thyroid axis may play a role in protecting the body by maintaining a positive nitrogen balance despite the uremic state. After renal transplantation, thyroid function tests normalize, although some patients may still have an abnormal TSH response to TRH because of glucocorticoid suppression of TSH secretion.

Growth Hormone

Although plasma growth hormone (GH) levels are elevated in patients with CRF and ESRD, due to both increased secretion and impaired clearance of the hormone, this change has no apparent clinical significance. Insulin-like growth factor (IGF) levels are normal. Dynamic testing of the GH axis demonstrates several abnormalities. Oral glucose loading does not suppress GH levels, whereas intravenous glucose, glucagon, or TRH paradoxically increase GH levels. Insulin induced hypoglycemia does not stimulate GH secretion. Growth hormone releasing hormone (GHRH) and L-dopa infusions also cause prolonged and exaggerated responses in GH secretion. Correction of anemia with erythropoietin corrects the paradoxical response to TRH and insulin induced hypoglycemia, although the prolonged GHRH response remains.

In children, uremia results in growth retardation despite normal or elevated GH and IGF levels. Contributing factors include protein malnutrition, chronic acidosis, recurrent infections, hyperparathyroidism, and decreased bioactive IGF. The assurance of adequate nutrition and dialysis as well as correction of acidosis and hyperparathyroidism improve growth. Renal transplantation does not by itself

TABLE I
Pathogenetic Mechanisms of Endocrine Dysfunction in Chronic Renal Failure[a]

Increased circulating hormone levels
  Impaired renal or extrarenal clearance (e.g., insulin, glucagon, PTH, calcitonin, prolactin)
  Increased secretion (e.g., PTH, aldosterone?)
  Accumulation of immunoassayable hormone fractions that may lack bioactivity (e.g., glucagon, PTH, calcitonin, prolactin)
Decreased circulating hormone levels
  Decreased secretion by diseased kidney (e.g., erythropoietin, renin, 1.25-dihydroxyvitamin D_3)
  Decreased secretion by other endocrine glands (e.g., testosterone, estrogen, progesterone)
Decreased sensitivity to hormones
  Altered target tissue response (e.g., insulin, glucagon, 1.25-dihydroxyvitamin D_3, erythropoietin, PTH)

[a] PTH, parathyroid hormone. From Mooradian AD: In: Becker KL (ed) *Principles and Practice of Endocrinology and Metabolism*, p. 1759. Lippincott, Philadelphia, 1995. With permission.

reverse the abnormal growth patterns observed in children, likely due to the effects of exogenous glucocorticoids used for immunosuppression. The availability and use of recombinant human growth hormone (rHGH) has greatly improved the well-being of children with CRF, restoring growth velocity and increasing muscle mass without adversely affecting epiphysial closure. rHGH does not affect glucose tolerance in children but does tend to aggravate preexisting hyperinsulinemia. The use of rHGH after renal transplantation in children also significantly improves growth.

TABLE 2
Directional Changes of Hormones in CRF[a]

Hypothalamopituitary axis
  GH $\uparrow$ prolactin $\uparrow$

Thyroid
  TT_4 N or $\downarrow$, FT_4 N or $\downarrow$
  TT_3 $\downarrow$, FT_3 $\downarrow$, rT_3 N, TSH N

Gonads
  Testosterone $\downarrow$, spermatogenesis $\downarrow$
  Estrogen N or $\downarrow$, progesterone $\downarrow$
  LH N or $\uparrow$, FSH N

Pancreas
  Insulin $\uparrow$, glucagon $\uparrow$

Adrenals
  Aldosterone N or $\downarrow$, cortisol N or $\uparrow$,
  ACTH N or $\uparrow$
  Catecholamine N or $\uparrow$

Kidney
  EPO $\downarrow$, renin $\downarrow$, 1.25 Vit D_3 $\downarrow$

[a] From Lim VS: In: Greenberg A (ed) *Primer on Kidney Diseases*, p. 315, Academic Press. San Diego, 1994. With permission.

Prolactin

Prolactin secretion is normally under inhibition via prolactin inhibitory factor (PIF) which, in turn, is controlled by dopaminergic neurons. Basal levels of prolactin are elevated up to six times normal in patients with CRF due to a decrease in dopaminergic activity. Many medications that have antidopaminergic effects also contribute to the increased prolactin levels by decreasing the tonic inhibitory effects of dopamine. The major effects of increased prolactin levels are reflected in the reproductive abnormalities observed in CRF and ESRD patients: gynecomastia, impotence, and amenorrhea. Bromocriptine can reduce prolactin levels, but its effectiveness in relieving symptoms has not been well established. Side effects lead to discontinuation of therapy in one-third of patients. Again, erythropoietin therapy can normalize prolactin levels and improve sexual dysfunction in men and menstrual regularity in women although the mechanism of the effect is not well established.

Any medications that can affect prolactin levels should be minimized or avoided if possible (i.e., α-methyldopa, phenothiazines, neuroleptics, metaclopramide, cisapride, and H_2 blockers, especially cimetidine) particularly if gynecomastia becomes painful or cosmetically displeasing for male patients. The pathogenesis of gynecomastia in men may also be related in part to an increased estrogen to androgen ratio as seen in male pubertal gynecomastia. Mammography should be performed since breast cancer does occur, although rarely, in men. Alternative therapies for gynecomastia in men include subcutaneous mastectomies or breast bud irradiation.

Glucocorticoids

Patients with CRF exhibit normal to elevated levels of adrenocorticotropin hormone (ACTH). The ACTH response to corticotropin releasing hormone (CRH) has been observed to be blunted or normal. Correction of anemia with erythropoietin can lead to an exaggerated ACTH response to CRH. The standard ACTH stimulation test for diagnosing hypocortisolism is not affected by the uremic state.

Basal cortisol levels in CRF patients are normal. Circadian rhythm of cortisol secretion remains intact. The usual oral low-dose 1 mg overnight or 2-day dexamethasone suppression tests used to evaluate hypercortisolism do not suppress cortisol levels in patients with CRF due, in part, to decreased oral absorption of the hormone and an altered set point of the axis. The 1 mg intravenous or 8 mg oral high-dose overnight dexamethasone test will suppress cortisol levels in CRF patients. Although insulin-induced hypoglycemia fails to raise serum cortisol levels, the response to major stress, such as surgery, remains preserved.

Gonadotropins

Males. Loss of libido, impotence, testicular atrophy, gynecomastia, and infertility may occur in males with CRF and ESRD. Testosterone is decreased and luteinizing hormone (LH) and follicle stimulating hormone (FSH) levels are elevated. Testosterone binding globulin levels are normal. Testicular biopsy reveals abnormal sperm maturation. Prolonged stimulation with human chorionic gonadotropin (HCG) can result in increased testosterone levels, suggesting some preservation of testicular reserve. The response to administration of luteinizing hormone releasing hormone (LHRH) is unpredictable; normal, blunted, and exaggerated, prolonged responses have all been observed. Thus it appears that both a central hypothalamic insensitivity and peripheral testicular failure exist in men with CRF and ESRD. Hyperprolactinemia and elevated parathyroid hormone (PTH) may contribute to the combined central and peripheral problem. Treatment with erythropoietin can improve symptomatology without actually affecting testosterone levels by increasing a patient's sense of well-being and by decreasing prolactin and PTH levels. Zinc deficiency has also been thought to contribute to the hypogonadism, although replacement therapy has yielded varying results. Renal transplantation reverses many of the symptoms. However, the hypogonadism may worsen as a consequence of immunosuppressive therapy.

Impotence problems may also be related to neuropathies or vasculopathies. Drugs that can contribute to impotence (such as β-blockers) should be discontinued or dose-reduced. Unfortunately, many patients fail to respond to these measures and require penile implants or vacuum erector devices. Due to their vasoconstrictor effects, cav-

ernous injections should be used with caution in severely hypertensive patients. Recently introduced sildenafil has significantly improved the ability to treat impotence. Figure 1 outlines an approach to sexual dysfunction in the male patient.

Females. Women with CRF and ESRD also develop problems with libido or inability to achieve orgasms. Approximately half of women on dialysis become amenorrheic, and those who still have menses find their periods progressively irregular and anovulatory as renal failure progresses. Less than 10% of women on dialysis have regular menses. FSH levels are normal with mildly elevated LH, resulting in an increased LH/FSH ratio, similar to prepubertal patterns, and a defect in the positive hypothalamic feedback mechanism in response to estrogen. This lack of positive feedback results in the failure of the mid-cycle LH and FSH surge to occur and hence, anovulation. Estradiol, estrone, progesterone, and testosterone levels are normal to low. Unlike premenopausal women, postmenopausal women have the expected increases in both LH and FSH. Hyperprolactinemia may also contribute to some of the abnormalities. Despite the above problems, women who have some remnant renal function and who are well dialyzed may rarely become pregnant and carry to term, although the fetus tends to be premature and small for gestational age (see Chapter 56). The use of estrogen replacement ther-

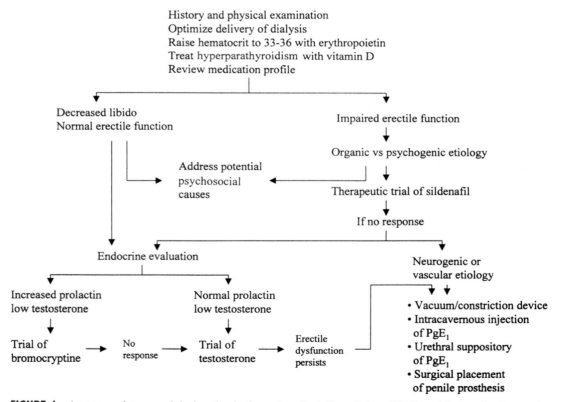

FIGURE 1 An approach to sexual dysfunction in the male patient. From Palmer BF: Sexual dysfunction in uremia. *J Am Soc Nephrol* 10:1384, 1999.

apy to decrease bone loss and cardiovascular risk in pre-menopausal CRF and ESRD women has not been investigated.

Transplantation rapidly restores fertility to premenopausal women. Ovulation can start within a month of transplantation. Appropriate counseling should be undertaken to stress the need for contraception. Current guidelines call for women who wish to become pregnant to wait 2 years with stable graft function (creatinine under 1.8 mg/dL), to be on minimal immunosupression, and to have easily controllable blood pressure. There are no good data on the use of oral contraceptives in the transplant patient group. Referral to a gynecologist should be made if this mode of contraception is considered due to the possible increased risk of thromboembolic disease. Figure 2 outlines an approach to sexual dysfunction in uremic women.

Carbohydrate Metabolism

Patients with CRF can develop what has been termed pseudodiabetes. The condition results from a combination of peripheral resistance to insulin, circulating inhibitors of insulin action, and abnormal islet cell insulin release. Dialysis corrects these defects. In contrast, diabetics with CRF and ESRD often find that their need for oral hypoglycemic agents or insulin decreases because of reduced insulin clearance by the kidney. In the case of type II, non-insulin dependent diabetics (NIDDM), where the problem is mostly due to peripheral insulin resistance, endogenous

insulin half-life is prolonged resulting in a decreased or eliminated need for medication. In addition, the decreased clearance of oral hypoglycemic agents (primarily first generation sulfonylureas) can lead to prolonged hypoglycemia. Agents which are primarily hepatically metabolized (second generation sulfonylureas), or insulin, should be used to treat type II patients. Metformin is contraindicated in patients with CRF because of the increased risk of lactic acidosis, but newer agents which decrease peripheral insulin resistance (i.e., thiazolidinediones) appear safe. Type I, insulin dependent diabetics (IDDM) may need their insulin dose reduced, but never discontinued since the underlying problem is a lack of endogenous insulin production. Glycemic control can worsen in peritoneal dialysis patients because of the glucose load absorbed from the peritoneal dialysis fluid. Intraperitoneal insulin administration, based on a sliding scale, may facilitate management.

Spontaneous hypoglycemia can occur in CRF and ESRD patients due to malnutrition, impaired glycogenolysis, and carnitine deficiency. Although many patients have glucose intolerance, fasting hyperglycemia with a glucose value over 140 mg/dL suggests that frank diabetes mellitus is present. Glycosylated hemoglobin values may underestimate the degree of hyperglycemia due to the shortened erythrocyte life span seen in uremia.

Transplantation often reveals an underlying abnormality of glucose metabolism in patients due to the high doses of steroids used for immunosupression. Patients not previously thought to be diabetic can develop diabetes mellitus

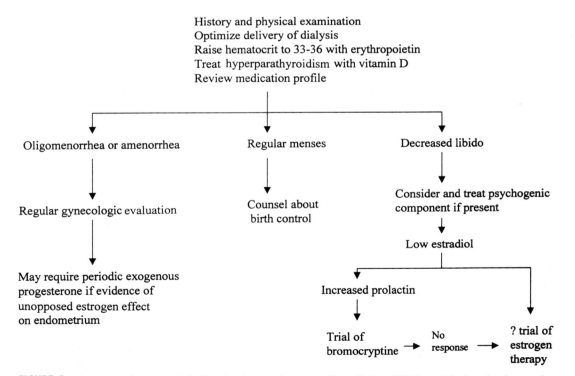

FIGURE 2 An approach to sexual dysfunction in uremic women. From Palmer BF: Sexual dysfunction in uremia. *J Am Soc Nephrol* 10:1386, 1999.

and require insulin therapy. Those already known to be diabetic may require conversion from an oral hypoglycemic agent to insulin or a significant increase in their insulin dosage due to steroid induced peripheral resistance to insulin action.

Mineralocorticoids

Due to the progressive loss of renal tissue with CRF, renin production is generally decreased with either normal to low aldosterone levels. The renin–angiotensin–aldosterone response to volume contraction or hypotension is blunted. Secondary to low renin levels, hyperkalemia becomes the most important stimulus for aldosterone secretion. Aldosterone in turn stimulates colonic loss of potassium, an often overlooked means of potassium removal in CRF patients. Measurements of renin levels are not particularly useful in CRF patients. Given the above findings, the finding of elevated aldosterone levels should raise the suspicion of primary hyperaldosteronism.

Adrenal Medulla

Basal levels of catecholamines in CRF and dialysis patients are elevated because of a number of factors: decreased degradation, decreased neuronal reuptake, and impaired renal clearance of metabolites. Hemodialysis treatments remove catecholamines, but not in sufficient amounts to cause intradialytic hypotension. The diagnosis of pheochromocytoma is difficult in patients with CRF. Suppression testing has not been validated in this setting. The combination of high levels of catecholamines and appropriate radiologic studies should be used together to make the diagnosis.

Lipid Abnormalities

Patients with CRF and ESRD infrequently have hypercholesterolemia or elevated levels of low density lipoprotein (LDL), but hypertriglyceridemia is observed in half of these patients. Conversely, levels of intermediate density lipoprotein (IDL) and small dense LDL are increased due to poor clearance. Low levels of high density lipoprotein (HDL) are also common. Nephrotic patients are an exception: they have elevated levels of all these lipid fractions. Heparin administration during hemodialysis causes release of both hepatic and endothelial lipoprotein lipase, resulting in a depletion of stores and worsening of triglyceride (TG) levels, particularly of highly atherogenic triglyceride rich remnant particles.

Elevated lipoprotein (a) [Lp(a)] and homocysteine levels are considered to be independent risk factors for atherosclerosis. Studies of Lp(a) levels demonstrate increased levels in CRF and ESRD patients, but the isoform distribution is similar to that of non-renal failure patients. Homocysteine levels are elevated in 75–90% of peritoneal and hemodialysis patients. Isotope studies suggest that in hemodialysis patients, hyperhomocysteinemia is due to a decrease in homocysteine remethylation to methionine rather than defects in the transsulfuration pathway. The hyperhomocysteinemia seen in hemodialysis patients has been estimated to lead to a 4% increase in access thrombosis risk for every 1 $\mu M/L$ increase in homocysteine levels.

Until further data are available, treatment of lipid disorders in CRF and dialysis patients should follow general guidelines used in patients with normal renal function. Patients with elevated LDL levels should be started on diet therapy and then advanced to pharmacological therapy. Bile acid resins binders such as cholestyramine and colestipol, should be avoided since they may worsen hypertriglyceridemia. Fibric acid derivatives such as gemfibrozil clinofibrate are relatively contraindicated in CRF and ESRD patients since they are cleared primarily by the kidney, and their accumulation increases the risk of rhabdomyolysis. The safest agents are the HMG-CoA reductase inhibitors. They are particularly useful in nephrotic patients to decrease LDL levels and reduce cardiovascular risk. High doses may increase the risk of myalgias and rhabdomyolysis and require close patient follow-up. Because of its many side effects such as insulin resistance and gastric irritation, nicotinic acid is not a good lipid lowering agent in the CRF population, and experience with its use is limited. Data on the use of probucol are lacking.

Studies have demonstrated the possible protective effects of vitamin E and folic acid in cardiac patients with normal renal function. Studies also suggest that elevated LDL levels, particularly oxidized LDL, can hasten the progression of CRF to ESRD. Because these agents act either

TABLE 3
Neurological Manifestations of Uremia

Predialysis	
Uremic encephalopathy	Acute CNS signs and symptoms of uremia
	Asterixis usually present
	Indication to initiate dialysis
Postdialysis	
Dialysis disequilibrium syndrome	Idiogenic osmoles result in brain-to-plasma osmolar gradient
	Caused by aggressive initial HD treatments
Dialysis dementia	Epidemic, endemic, and childhood forms
	Aluminum associated with epidemic form
	Frequently fatal
	Prevented by deionization of dialysis water and restriction of oral aluminum
	Avoid citrate and aluminum compounds
	Deferoxamine chelation therapy
Intellectual function	Generally impaired
Peripheral neuropathy	Motor and sensory impairment
Autonomic dysfunction	Postural hypotension, impaired sweating, gastrointestinal disturbances, impotence

as antioxidants (vitamin E) or by reducing homocysteine levels (folic acid), they should be safe to use in the CRF population as a means to reduce cardiac risk and theoretically slow the progression of cardiac disease. The dose of folic acid to reduce hyperhomocysteinemia is 4–5 mg/day. Vitamin C also acts as an antioxidant. Unfortunately, it is relatively contraindicated in CRF and ESRD patients because its metabolic by-product (oxalate) is renally excreted and can result in elevated serum oxalate levels or hyperoxaluria with renal calcification in CRF and ESRD patients.

As in dialysis patients, cardiovascular disease is the major cause of death in the transplant population, and every effort should be made to reduce risk factors. However, renal transplant patients should be considered separately from other CRF patients when it come to lipid abnormalities. Total cholesterol, TG, LDL, oxidized LDL, Lp(a), and homocysteine levels are elevated, whereas HDL levels are variable. In addition to the increased cardiac risk of post-transplant lipid abnormalities, some evidence suggests that hyperlipidemia may also contribute to chronic graft rejection.

Treatment of lipid abnormalities in transplant patients is similar to that of CRF patients. Bile resin binders should be avoided because they interfere with cyclosporine absorption. Gemfibrozil has an increased risk of causing rhabdomyolysis. HMG-CoA reductase inhibitors have been used in studies on transplant patients. But again, higher doses should be used with caution. Simvastatin and pravastatin have been employed in several studies without major side effects. At least one study has shown a reduction in acute rejection episodes using pravastatin. The use of vitamin E, vitamin C, and folic acid has not been investigated.

NEUROLOGICAL MANIFESTATIONS

Nervous system dysfunction commonly occurs in patients with renal disease. The spectrum of abnormalities includes mild to severe alterations in the sensorium, cognitive dysfunction, generalized weakness, and neuropathies. These problems can occur prior to the initiation of dialytic therapy and can progress despite adequate renal replacement therapy. Others respond well to dialysis and renal transplantation.

Uremic Encephalopathy

The term uremic encephalopathy refers to the central neurological signs and symptoms that result from a decline in renal function. The threshold for development of uremic encephalopathy is a fall in GFR to a level below 10% of normal. Symptoms are more severe and abrupt in onset when associated with acute rather than chronic renal failure. Psychomotor behavior, cognition, memory, speech, perception, and emotion can all be affected. In this respect, uremic encephalopathy resembles and can be difficult to distinguish from organic brain syndromes due to other etiologies.

Uremic encephalopathy should be suspected in patients with renal failure if there are clinical signs and symptoms consistent with central nervous system deterioration. However, overlap with symptoms resulting from other intercurrent illnesses or drug toxicities complicates diagnosis. In patients with both advanced liver and renal diseases, particularly those with hepatorenal syndrome, it is often difficult to determine whether the encephalopathy is due to hepatic or renal causes or both. In such patients the blood urea nitrogen (BUN) and serum creatinine do not always adequately reflect the degree of renal function impairment. Mildly elevated BUN and creatinine levels may underestimate the severity of renal failure due to malnutrition and/or a diminished capacity to generate urea and creatinine. The diagnosis may be made by exclusion if other causes such as hypercalcemia, hyper- or hyponatremia, hyper- or hypoglycemia, hypoxia, and hypercapnia are excluded, or in retrospect after improvement is observed in response to dialysis or other specific therapy.

The initial neurological presentation of patients with acute renal failure may include signs of psychosis, lassitude, and lethargy with disorientation and confusion occurring later. Physical findings may include cranial nerve signs, nystagmus, dysarthria, abnormal gait and motor signs manifested by weakness (both symmetric and asymmetric), fasciculations, and asymmetrical variation in deep tendon reflexes. These findings may progress to asterixis and hyperreflexia with unsustained clonus at the ankle. Spontaneous myoclonus may be present and has the same import as asterixis. If uremia is left untreated and allowed to progress, seizures and coma often supervene.

Electroencephalograms (EEG) in patients with acute renal failure are generally grossly abnormal when the diagnosis of acute renal failure is first made, and they are not usually improved by dialysis during the first few weeks of treatment. After approximately 6 months of dialysis treatments, the EEG tends to normalize. Completely normal tracings may not be reached until the patient receives a kidney transplant or recovers renal function. Despite the presence of these EEG abnormalities, it is not a tool used in diagnosing uremic encephalopathy since it cannot be rapidly obtained and because similar findings can be seen in other toxic and metabolic encephalopathies.

Pathogenesis

Although many factors may contribute to uremic encephalopathy, no precise correlation exists between the degree of encephalopathy and any of the commonly measured blood chemistries associated with renal dysfunction (BUN, creatinine, bicarbonate, or pH). There are numerous potential or putative uremic toxins, including parathyroid hormone (PTH) and nitrogenous wastes (see Chapter 58).

Peripheral Neuropathies

Neuropathy of some degree is probably present in about 65% of patients with CRF and ESRD. The findings may be subtle, and abnormal nerve conduction may be present in the absence of symptoms or physical findings. Specific questions about paresthesias, diminished sensation, sexual dysfunction, or presyncope may elicit a history of sensory neuropathy or postural hypotension that can be confirmed by careful physical examination. Uremic neuropathy is a distal, symmetrical, mixed polyneuropathy that belongs to a group known as dying-back polyneuropathies or central peripheral axonopathies. Uremic neuropathy is also associated with a secondary demyelinating process in the posterior columns of the spinal cord and the central nervous system. Motor and sensory modalities are both generally affected, and the lower extremities are more severely involved than are the upper extremities. Clinically, uremic neuropathy cannot easily be distinguished from the neuropathies associated with diabetes mellitus, chronic alcoholism, and other nutritional deficiency states. The occurrence of uremic neuropathy bears no relationship to the type of underlying kidney disease. However, some disorders including amyloidosis, multiple myeloma, systemic lupus erythematosus, polyarteritis nodosa, diabetes mellitus, and hepatic failure can cause both peripheral neuropathy and renal disease.

In severe symmetrical polyneuropathies, a generalized loss of peripheral nerve function may occur. Dysfunction is usually maximal distally and is characterized by a mixed motor and sensory polyneuropathy often resulting in weakness and wasting in the arms and legs. There may also be distal sensory changes in a "glove and stocking" distribution. Isolated or multiple isolated lesions of the peripheral nerves are designated as mononeuropathies. Motor nerve conduction velocity has very limited utility in detecting moderately impaired peripheral nerve function in CRF and ESRD patients due to a daily test variability of up to 20%. Sensory nerve conduction velocity testing is more sensitive, but too painful to be widely employed.

The etiology of uremic neuropathy has not been established. Although many have been implicated, no single uremic toxin can explain all the observed abnormalities of peripheral nerve function. Uremic neuropathy may, in part, also be related to anatomical nerve damage of unknown etiology and to the cumulative effects of multiple toxic agents over months to years.

Symptoms and Signs

The restless-leg syndrome is a common early manifestation of chronic renal failure. Clinically, patients experience sensations such as crawling, prickling, and pruritus in their lower extremities. The sensations are generally worse distally and are usually more prominent in the evening. Patients are awakened because they cannot find a comfortable leg position. The burning-foot syndrome, which is present in less than 10% of patients with chronic renal failure, actually represents swelling and tenderness of the distal lower extremities. The physical signs of peripheral nerve dysfunction often begin with loss of deep tendon reflexes, particularly in the ankle and knee. Sensory modalities which are lost include pain, light touch, vibration, and pressure.

Treatment

No one treatment appears to be effective, likely due to the multifactorial etiologies of the neuropathies. Analgesics (nonsteroidal agents, opiates, quinine, and muscle relaxants), anticonvulsants (such as gabapentin and carbamazepine), antidepressants (such as tricyclics), anxiolytics (such as benzodiazepams), and antiarrythmics have all been utilized. There is no reliable evidence to suggest that increasing the intensity of dialysis in ESRD patients ameliorates symptoms, although every effort should be made to ensure adequate dialysis therapy.

Autonomic and Cranial Nerve Dysfunction

Autonomic dysfunction is quite common in CRF and is usually associated with postural hypotension, impaired sweating, impotence, gastrointestinal motility disturbances, and an abnormal Valsalva maneuver. Hemodialysis associated hypotension is often associated with autonomic insufficiency especially in patients with diabetes or amyloidosis. Hand-grip dynamometer, heart rate response to Valsalva, beat to beat heart rate respiratory variability, and vascular response to norepinephrine infusion can all be used to evaluate autonomic dysfunction.

Cranial nerve involvement in uremia often manifests as transient nystagmus, miosis, heterophoria, and facial asymmetry. Eighth nerve involvement including both auditory and vestibular function is common and must be distinguished from deafness due to hereditary nephritis and drug ototoxicity such as that caused by aminoglycosides or high-dose furosemide.

Intellectual Dysfunction

Intellectual dysfunction is not well characterized and is without distinctive anatomical lesions. Based on psychological testing, progressive renal insufficiency is associated with organic-like loss of intellectual function. Because patients are often older, they are also susceptible to other conditions that can cause a decline in intellectual function such as Alzheimer's or multi-infarct dementia and chronic alcoholism. It is often quite difficult to establish a clear etiology for the declining function.

Complications of Dialysis Therapy
Dialysis Disequilibrium Syndrome

Several central nervous system disorders may occur as a consequence of dialytic therapy. One such disorder is dialysis disequilibrium syndrome (DDS), which can occur acutely in patients who have recently initiated hemodialysis, usually after the first several treatments. The symptom complex is quite variable and may include muscle cramps, anorexia, restlessness, dizziness, headache, nausea, emesis, blurred vision, muscular twitching, disorientation, hypertension, tremors, seizures, and obtundation. It occurs most often in the elderly and in children. The syndrome is generally associated with intense initiation of hemodialysis, but is rarely seen today due to a more gradual initiation of hemodialysis. Dialysis disequilibrium has not been described in peritoneal dialysis patients.

DDS is thought to be a result of overly rapid correction of plasma osmolality resulting in cerebral edema. As renal failure develops, the brain increases intracellular osmolality to protect itself from the associated hyperosmolality. If brain osmolality did not increase, the brain would lose water and shrink. Such a reduction in brain volume is undesirable as it can lead to intracranial hemorrhage. The brain increases intracellular osmolality by generating intracellular organic acids, amino acids, methylamines, and polyols, or so-called "idiogenic osmoles." A similar process occurs with hyperglycemia and hypernatremia. Thus, any treatment, such as hemodialysis, that acutely lowers plasma osmolality without allowing adequate time for the removal of neuronal intracellular idiogenic osmoles runs the risk of establishing a substantial brain-to-plasma osmolar gradient, which can result in brain water uptake and cerebral edema. To avoid DDS, nephrologists typically select an initial dialysis prescription that is deliberately inefficient in order to permit a gradual lowering of the plasma/central nervous system osmolar gradient and allow the brain to dissipate the idiogenic osmoles. With subsequent treatments, both the duration of dialysis and the blood flow rate through the dialyzer are increased. Other measures include ultrafiltration followed by dialysis, use of bicarbonate instead of acetate as the dialysate base, and the addition of mannitol, glycerol, or glucose osmoles to the dialysate solution or as intravenous bolus injections.

Dialysis Dementia

Dialysis dementia is a progressive, frequently fatal neurological disease which is seen almost exclusively in patients who are being treated with chronic hemodialysis. Dialysis dementia can occur in isolation or in association with osteomalacia, proximal myopathy, and anemia.

Dialysis dementia occurs in three settings: an epidemic form, a sporadic form, and with childhood renal disease. Initial symptoms of this disorder include dysarthria, apraxia, slurring of speech with stuttering, and hesitancy. Later in the course of the disease, symptoms progress to personality changes, psychosis, myoclonus, seizures, and eventually dementia and death within 6 months after the onset of symptoms. The diagnosis of dialysis dementia depends on the presence of the typical clinical picture, the characteristic EEG findings (multifocal bursts of high-amplitude delta activity with spikes and sharp waves) and, most importantly, exclusion of other causes of central nervous system dysfunction.

The epidemic form of dialysis dementia has now been linked to aluminum (*vide infra*). It occurred in dialysis units that did not use water purification techniques such as reverse osmosis or deionization that would remove aluminum from source water. Dialysate aluminum concentra-

tions were thus high, and patients were dosed with aluminum during hemodialysis. Numerous patients in these units developed dialysis dementia along with painful fracturing osteomalacia. This disorder disappeared once its relationship to aluminum exposure was established and water purification standards were upgraded. The sporadic form occurred in patients who had been on chronic hemodialysis for more than 2 years and was also thought to be due to long-term aluminum exposure.

Dialysis dementia has also been reported in children with renal failure. Many received high doses of aluminum containing phosphate binders, but some were neither on dialysis nor exposed to aluminum. Therefore, encephalopathy in such children cannot be ascribed to aluminum alone, and may represent developmental neurological defects resulting from exposure of the growing brain to the uremic milieu.

Role of Aluminum in Dialysis Dementia

Aluminum content in brain is more than threefold greater in patients with dialysis dementia than in those on chronic hemodialysis without dementia. Increased aluminum levels in CRF and ESRD are due both to an increase in gastrointestinal absorption and a decrease in renal elimination. Normally, only a minimal amount of orally administered aluminum is absorbed and later excreted by the kidneys. For unknown reasons, absorption appears to be increased in patients with renal failure which, when coupled with the decrease in excretion, leads to toxicity. Aluminum sources include drinking water and medications (such as aluminum containing antacids, citrate, and sucralfate containing preparations which increase aluminum absorption from the gastrointestinal tract). Prior to the routine deionization of the water used in hemodialysis, most of the aluminum in dialysis patients came from dialysate water. Aluminum is clearly responsible for the development of the epidemic form of dialysis dementia. However, whether aluminum plays an important role in the other types of dialysis dementia (sporadic, childhood) is still unresolved. Deionization of dialysate water not only removes aluminum but also cadmium, mercury, lead, manganese, copper, nickel, thallium, boron, and tin. Thus, not only aluminum, but several other trace elements and minerals may be involved in the pathogenesis of dialysis dementia. Fortunately, with improved water treatment and the elimination of routine use of aluminum containing antacids, the incidence of dialysis dementia has fallen markedly.

Treatment

Although diazepam or clonazepam appear to be useful in controlling initial seizure activity associated with the disease, the drugs usually become ineffective and do not appear to alter the usually fatal outcome. Improvement in symptoms has been reported in several patients treated with desferrioxamine which, when given intravenously, chelates aluminum and promotes its removal during hemodialysis.

Bibliography

Andreoti SP, Bergstein JM, Sherrard DJ: Aluminum intoxication from aluminum containing phosphate binders in children with azotemia not undergoing dialysis. *N Engl J Med* 310:1079–1084, 1984.

Arieff AL: Dialysis disequilibrium syndrome: Current concepts on pathogenesis and prevention. *Kidney Int* 45:629–635, 1994.

Arnaud CD: Hyperparathyroidism and renal failure. *Kidney Int* 4:89–95, 1973.

Bostom AG, Gohh RY, Tsai MY, *et al.:* Excess prevalence of fasting and postmethionine-loading hyperhomocysteinemia in stable renal transplant recipients. *Atheroscler Thromb Vasc Biol* 17(10):1894–1900, 1997.

Deck KA, Fischer B, Hillen H: Studies on cortisol metabolism during hemodialysis. *Eur J Clin Invest* 9:203–207, 1979.

Fraser CL, Arieff Al: Nervous system complications in uremia. *Ann Intern Med* 109:143–153, 1988.

Fraser CL, Arieff Al: Nervous system manifestations of renal failure. In: Schrier RW, Gottschalk CW (eds) *Diseases of the Kidney,* 5th Ed., pp. 2625–2646. Little, Brown, Boston, 1997.

Grundy SM: Management of hyperlipidemia of kidney disease. *Kidney Int* 37:847–853, 1990.

Haffner D, Nissel R, Wuhl E, *et al.:* Metabolic effects of long-term growth hormone treatment in pubertal children with chronic renal failure and after kidney transplantation. *Pediatr Res* 43(2): 209–215, 1998.

Holdsworth S, Atkins RC, Kretser DM: The pituitary–testicular axis in men with chronic renal failure. *N Engl J Med* 296(22): 1245–1249, 1977.

Katznelson S, Wilkinson AH, Kobashigawa, JA, *et al.:* The effect of pravastatin on acute rejection after kidney transplantation—A pilot study. *Transplantation* 61(10):1469–1474, 1996.

Kokot F, Wiecek A, Grzeszczak W, *et al.:* Influence of erythropoietin treatment on function of the pituitary–adrenal axis and somatotropin secretion in hemodialyzed patients. *Clin Nephrol* 33(5):241–246, 1990.

Lim VS: Reproductive function in patients with renal insufficiency. *Am J Kidney Dis* 9(4):363–367, 1987.

Lim VS, Flanigan MJ, Zavala DC, *et al.:* Protective adaptation of low serum triiodothyronine in patients with chronic renal failure. *Kidney Int* 28:541–549, 1985.

Massey ZA, Kasiske BL: Post-transplant hyperlipidemia: Mechanisms and management. *J Am Soc Nephrol* 7:971–977, 1996.

Mooradian AD: Endocrine dysfunction due to renal disease. In: Becker KL (ed) *Principles and Practice of Endocrinology and Metabolism,* pp. 1759–1762. Lippincott, Philadelphia, 1995.

Moustapha A, Gupta A, Robinson K, *et al.:* Prevalence and determinants of hyperhomocysteinemia in hemodialysis and peritoneal dialysis. *Kidney Int* 55:1470–1475, 1999.

Palmer BF: Sexual dysfunction in uremia. *J Am Soc Nephrol* 10:1381–1388, 1999.

Ramirez G, Butcher DE, Newton JL, *et al.:* Bromocriptine and the hypothalamic hypophyseal function in patients with chronic renal failure on chronic hemodialysis. *Am J Kidney Dis* 6(2): 111–118, 1985.

Ramirez G: Abnormalities in the hypothalamic–hypophyseal axes in patients with chronic renal failure. *Semin Dial* 7(2):138–146, 1994.

Schaefer RM, Kokot F, Geiger H, *et al.:* Improved sexual function in hemodialysis patients on recombinant erythropoietin: A possible role for prolactin. *Clin Nephrol* 31(1):1–5, 1989.

Sechi LA, Zingaro L, Catena C, *et al.:* Lipoprotein (a) and apolipoprotein (a) isoforms and proteinuria in patients with moderate real failure. *Kidney Int* 56:1049–1057, 1999.

Shemin D, Lapane KL, Bausserman L, *et al.:* Plasma homocysteine and hemodialysis access thrombosis: A prospective study. *J Am Soc Nephrol* 10:1095–1099, 1999.

Slatapolsky E, Martin K, Hruska K: Parathyroid hormone metabolism and Its potential as a uremic toxin. *Am J Physiol* 238: F1–F12, 1980.

van Guldener C, Kulik W, Berger R, *et al.:* Homocysteine and methionine metabolism in ESRD: A stable isotope study. *Kidney Int* 56:1064–1071, 1999.

67

THE EVALUATION OF PROSPECTIVE RENAL TRANSPLANT RECIPIENTS

BERTRAM L. KASISKE

INITIAL ASSESSMENT

Transplantation is the treatment of choice for end stage renal disease (ESRD). Once it is apparent that a patient will develop ESRD, transplantation should be considered, since it is sometimes possible to perform preemptive transplantation before initiating maintenance dialysis. Patients should be referred to a nephrologist as soon as it appears that treatment for ESRD may someday be necessary. Prior to acceptance for transplantation, a careful evaluation should determine if the patient is prepared not only for immunosuppression and its consequences, but also for surgery.

The evaluation should begin with a brief history and physical examination, so that obvious contraindications to transplantation can obviate the need for other, more expensive or invasive tests. There is no absolute age that precludes transplantation, but physiologic age and overall health status should be carefully considered in individuals who are over 60. Patients should also be screened for severe pulmonary disease that might greatly increase the risk of surgery. Obesity per se is rarely a contraindication to transplantation, but obesity increases morbidity and may increase the rate of graft failure. Therefore, weight reduction should be attempted prior to transplantation. Baseline laboratory evaluation should include a complete blood count with differential, routine serum chemistries, and a lipoprotein profile.

Patients with diabetes require special consideration. Cardiovascular complications are particularly common among diabetics, and may greatly increase the risk of transplant surgery. Diabetic patients should undergo a cardiac stress test as part of the transplant evaluation. In addition, some diabetic patients may be candidates for simultaneous pancreas–kidney (SPK) transplantation. In particular, patients with difficult to control diabetes may want to consider a SPK transplant. Although there are no controlled clinical trials showing that SPK reduces the long-term complications of diabetes compared to kidney transplantation alone, a successful SPK can improve the quality of life for some patients. Most agree that a diabetic with a potential living donor should generally undergo kidney transplantation alone, since living-donor graft survival is superior to cadaveric graft survival. However, a successful living-donor kidney transplant can be followed by a cadaveric pancreas transplant.

CANCER

Immunosuppression may favor the growth of malignant tumors, and an active malignancy is usually an absolute contraindication to transplantation. Exceptions may be locally invasive basal or squamous cell skin carcinomas and adequately treated cervical dysplasia. All patients should undergo routine screening with a physical examination, chest X ray, and stool hemoccult. Individuals over age 50 should also have flexible sigmoidoscopy. Women should have up-to-date mammography, pelvic examination, and Pap test following guidelines established in the general population.

Although immunosuppression may increase the risk of cancer recurrence, it is not necessary to deny transplantation to a patient who has had a tumor that was cured. Data from registries, although imperfect, provide some guidance on the chances of recurrence of different malignant tumors. A patient who has been free from all evidence of malignancy for 2 years has about a 47% chance of recurrence after renal transplantation. Although a 5-year waiting period would reduce this to 13%, it is probably unreasonable to demand that all patients wait 5 years. Individual tumors behave differently, and guidelines address how different tumors in potential transplant candidates should be approached.

INFECTIONS

Immunosuppression greatly increases the risk for life-threatening infections. Immunizations for influenza (yearly), pneumococcus, and hepatitis B are mandatory. Since the response to hepatitis B vaccine is reduced in patients with ESRD, many use a double dose or increase the number of inoculations beyond the recommended three. In addition, it may be prudent to first check for the presence of antibodies to hepatitis B core antigen or surface antigen, and to recheck after vaccination. If there is no response, vaccination can be repeated. In general, the effectiveness of these vaccinations is not well documented in ESRD, but their potential benefits outweigh their negligible risks. Patients should also be screened for infections that may become problematic with immunosuppression. Sites of occult infection include the lung, urinary tract, and dialysis catheters. Dialysis-related peritonitis within 3 to 4 weeks is a relative contraindication to transplantation. Patients should be screened for human immunodeficiency virus (HIV). A recent survey of transplant centers found that 88% would not offer a cadaveric, and 91% would not offer a living donor transplant to a patient who was HIV positive. There are theoretical reasons for and against transplanting an HIV-positive individual who has quiescent disease. Transplant rejection may stimulate viral replication in T cells. On the other hand, some immunosuppressive agents such as cyclosporine and mycophenolate mofetil may have antiviral activity. To date, no large series of patients has been reported.

Tuberculosis is common in the ESRD population, and may be asymptomatic. Screening should include a high index of suspicion, a chest X ray, and a purified protein derivative (PPD) skin test, unless there is already a history of a positive skin test. High-risk individuals are those: (1) with a past history of active disease, (2) from a high-risk population, and (3) with an abnormal chest X ray consistent with active or inactive tuberculosis. High-risk individuals should receive prophylactic therapy. Most authors recommend prophylaxis for 6–12 months, but it probably is not necessary to delay transplantation once therapy has begun.

Although cytomegalovirus (CMV) infection is common and is often transmitted with the transplanted organ, the presence of CMV antibodies in donors and recipients should not preclude transplantation. Some centers routinely use prophylactic therapy with hyperimmune globulin, ganciclovir, acyclovir, or valacyclovir for recipients of kidneys from CMV-seropositive donors. Potential recipients who are seronegative for the varicella-zoster virus are at risk for disseminated infection, and should be identified before transplantation. Patients from tropical regions should be screened for *Strongyloides stercolaris*. Viral hepatitis should also be considered in the pretransplant evaluation (see later).

LIVER DISEASE

Liver failure is a major cause of morbidity and mortality after renal transplantation, and transplant candidates should be carefully screened for liver disease. The A and E viruses do not cause chronic liver disease in transplant recipients, whereas hepatitis B virus (HBV) and hepatitis C virus (HCV) are common causes of chronic active hepatitis posttransplant. Transplant recipients who are hepatitis B surface antigen (HBsAg) positive are at increased risk of dying in the posttransplant period, however, HBsAg per se is not a contraindication to transplantation. Patients who are HBsAg positive and have serologic evidence of viral replication (by polymerase chain reaction assay or the presence of e-antigen) should probably forego transplantation. Likewise, HBsAg positive patients who also have hepatitis D (fortunately rare) develop severe liver disease and should not receive a transplant. Otherwise, HBsAg positive patients with elevated liver enzymes should undergo biopsy, and those with chronic active hepatitis may wish to stay on dialysis due to the increased risk of disease progression with immunosuppression. Fortunately, the incidence of HBV is declining in the ESRD population, largely due to effective vaccination and isolation procedures.

Although the natural history of HCV is less well defined, patients who are HCV antibody positive should undergo liver biopsy if enzymes are elevated, and possibly even if enzymes are not elevated, since disease may occur without enzyme elevation in patients with ESRD. Patients with HCV and evidence of viral replication (by polymerase chain reaction) and/or chronic active hepatitis on biopsy are probably at increased risk for progressive liver disease after transplantation. Antiviral therapy (interferon α) has been used in an attempt to induce a remission in ESRD patients with HBV or HCV viral hepatitis, and thereby allow renal transplantation. Although the long-term results of antiviral therapy in patients with ESRD are unclear, the number of patients who remain in remission after such therapy appears to be small.

CARDIOVASCULAR DISEASE

Ischemic heart disease (IHD) is a major cause of death after renal transplantation. All patients should be evaluated for possible IHD as part of the routine history and physical examination, chest X ray, and electrocardiogram. Patients with a history of IHD, or with signs and symptoms suggestive of IHD, should undergo a more thorough evaluation with noninvasive stress testing and/or angiography. Asymptomatic patients with multiple risk factors for IHD should also have noninvasive stress testing. The best noninvasive stress test remains to be defined. However, scintigraphy (with exercise or dipyridamole) and echocardiography (with exercise or dobutamine) may have reasonably high positive and negative predictive values in ESRD patients. Patients with critical coronary artery lesions should undergo revascularization prior to transplantation. All patients should be encouraged to reduce their risk of cardiovascular disease by managing known risk factors. In particular, patients should be encouraged to stop smoking.

CEREBROVASCULAR DISEASE

There is also an increased risk of atherosclerotic cerebrovascular disease complications after renal transplantation. Patients with a history of transient ischemic attacks or other cerebral vascular disease events should be evaluated for possible treatment and should be symptom-free for at least 6 months before surgery. Whether asymptomatic patients should undergo screening with a carotid ultrasound examination is unclear. In the general population, controlled clinical trials have shown that the success of prophylactic carotid endarterectomy is dependent on the center and on the selection of patients. Similarly, whether to treat patients who have asymptomatic carotid bruits with aspirin and risk factor intervention, or to use carotid ultrasound to select individuals for prophylactic endarterectomy is a decision that must be tailored to the patient and the center.

PSYCHOSOCIAL EVALUATION

Transplant candidates should be screened for cognitive or psychological impairments that may interfere with their ability to give informed consent. Failure to adhere to immunosuppressive therapy is a major cause of renal allograft failure, and the psychological assessment should also attempt to identify patients who are at risk. However, reliably identifying patients who will not adhere to therapy is difficult at best, and care should be exercised to avoid unjustifiably refusing transplantation. Most centers require patients with a history of chemical dependency to undergo treatment and demonstrate a period of abstinence prior to transplantation. Major psychiatric disorders are usually apparent during the routine pretransplant evaluation, and appropriate psychiatric care can be sought.

UROLOGIC EVALUATION

Evidence for possible chronic infection and/or incomplete bladder emptying should be sought on history and physical examination. In the absence of such evidence, a routine voiding cystourethrogram is not necessary. High-risk patients, for example, diabetics, can be screened by obtaining a postvoid residual urine volume. If the postvoid urine volume is greater than 100 mL, a voiding cystourethrogram and further urologic evaluation can be obtained. For patients with a ureteral diversion, every effort should be made to overcome the need for the diversion. Occasional patients may need to use intermittent self-catheterization for optimal bladder drainage. Indications for pretransplant nephrectomy include: reflux associated with chronic infection, polycystic kidneys that are too large to allow placement of the allograft or have infected cysts, severe nephrotic syndrome, nephrolithiasis associated with infection, renal carcinoma, and difficult-to-control hypertension.

RECURRENT RENAL DISEASE RISK

It is difficult to estimate the frequency with which diseases recur. Most recurrent disease is silent, and the incidence of recurrence depends on how often allograft biopsies are obtained. Although recurrence is common (Table 1), it does not often lead to graft failure, and the threat of recurrence is rarely a contraindication for transplantation. Idiopathic, focal, segmental glomerulosclerosis (FSGS) is the most common, clinically problematic disease to recur. Some centers may be reluctant to transplant individuals who have already lost one allograft to recurrent FSGS, since these patients have a 40–50% chance of losing another. However, it has recently been shown that approximately half of the FSGS recurrences will go into remission with plasmapheresis, giving new hope to these individuals.

Secondary amyloidosis (amyloid AA) can be expected to recur in the allograft in 20–30% of cases and is associated with a high incidence of cardiovascular complications. Five-year graft survival has been reported to be reduced to 66%, compared to 86% for controls. Nevertheless, patients and allografts may survive for years after trans-

TABLE I
Recurrent Renal Disease

Underlying disease	Rate of recurrence (%)
Focal segmental glomerulosclerosis	25–50
Membranoproliferative glomerulonephritis type I	20–30
Membranoproliferative glomerulonephritis type II (dense deposit disease)	90–100
Membranous nephropathy	5–10
IgA nephropathy	40–50
Henoch–Schönlein purpura	75–90
Antiglomerular basement membrane nephritis	10–25
Hemolytic–uremic syndrome/thrombotic thrombocytopenic purpura	10–25
Diabetes	100

plantation, and therefore secondary amyloidosis is not an absolute contraindication to transplantation. In general, the underlying plasma cell dyscrasia causing primary amyloidosis (amyloid AL) should be successfully treated before considering renal transplantation, however, preliminary reports suggest that simultaneous bone marrow and renal transplantation may someday be an option for such patients. Patients with primary oxalosis (once thought to be an absolute contraindication to transplantation) should be considered for preemptive transplantation with aggressive orthophosphate and pyridoxine therapy, with or without liver transplantation to provide a source of the deficient enzyme. Although diabetic nephropathy recurs in the allograft, the rate of progression is generally slow enough to make this an unusual cause of graft failure. One-year graft survival in patients with sickle cell nephropathy was recently reported to be 78%, that is, not different than that of controls. Finally, patients with Alport's syndrome have a small chance of developing antiglomerular basement membrane disease after transplantation, but this risk should not preclude transplantation.

GASTROINTESTINAL EVALUATION

Patients with symptomatic, recurrent cholecystitis should undergo cholecystectomy, because cholecystitis in an immunocompromised transplant recipient may be more severe and more difficult to diagnose and treat. However, most centers no longer routinely screen all patients with ultrasound, and most no longer perform cholecystectomy for asymptomatic cholelithiasis. Similarly, patients with symptomatic diverticulitis may be considered for partial colectomy, but most centers do not conduct screening and surgery for asymptomatic diverticular disease. Peptic ulcer disease is common in the posttransplant period. However, it can usually be managed medically, and most centers do not routinely perform endoscopy as part of the pretransplant evaluation.

BLOOD AND TISSUE TYPING

Three major immunologic barriers to transplantation need to be addressed: (1) Transplants should not generally cross ABO blood group barriers. (2) The degree of matching at the major histocompatibility (MHC) loci A, B, and DR correlate with long-term graft survival and is used in the United Network Network for Organ Sharing (UNOS) point system for cadaveric organ allocation (see later). (3) The presence of preformed antibodies and how broadly they react to a random panel of antigens from the general population is directly correlated to the likelihood of a positive cross-match when an organ becomes available, and is also used in the UNOS kidney allocation scheme (Table 2). Blood and MHC tissue type is determined when it is apparent that the patient will be a suitable transplant candidate. Serum is collected at the initial evaluation and at least quarterly to measure preformed antibodies. An estimate of the number of preformed antibodies is made by reacting the potential recipient's blood against a panel of lymphocytes from a random sample of the general population. The percentage of cells that react is called the percent panel reactive antibody (PRA). A high PRA indicates that it will be more difficult to find a donor with a negative cross-match for that recipient. A high PRA is also associated with decreased graft survival, even if the final cross-match is negative (see later). A recipient's PRA may fall over time, especially if blood transfusions are avoided.

As a final screen, the recipient's most recent serum is tested against donor tissue, since a positive cross-match indicates the presence of pre-formed antibodies that can cause hyperacute rejection. Not all reacting antibodies cause hyperacute rejection, so other laboratory tests are also performed to determine whether the recipient's reacting antibody should preclude transplantation. Usually, the serum with the highest previous PRA is also tested at

TABLE 2
Synopsis of the UNOS Point System for Kidney Allocation

Criteria	Points
ABO blood group O kidneys to O recipients	None[a]
Zero antigen mismatch (mandatory sharing)	None[a]
Time waiting since listing	
Relative (least to most)	0 to 1
Each year	1
Number of B or DR antigen mismatches	
Zero	7
One	5
Two	2
Panel reactive antibody level >80%	4
Medical urgency (local arrangement only)	None[a]
Pediatric age (years)	
<11	4
≥11 and <18	3
Patient has donated an organ or organ segment	4

[a]No points awarded, but affects allocation. For a details visit the UNOS web site at http://www.unos.org.

the time of final cross matching. Recipients with a negative cross-match, but a positive "historical" cross-match may be transplanted, but some studies indicate that the risk of graft failure is increased. Since it may be difficult to find a suitable donor for patients with a high PRA, some centers have experimented with plasmapheresis and other antibody removing techniques in an attempt to allow such patients to be transplanted.

ALLOCATION OF CADAVERIC ORGANS

Around the world, cadaveric organs are shared in both national and international programs. For example, in much of Europe (Austria, Belgium, Germany, Luxembourg, and the Netherlands), the Eurotransplant Kidney Allocation System allocates kidneys according to blood group and a point system based on MHC matching (double points for children), waiting time, distance from retrieval site to transplant center, and the national balance between previously imported and exported kidneys. In Scandinavia (Iceland, Norway, Sweden, Finland, and Denmark) Scandiatransplant requires members to exchange kidneys according to blood group and MHC matching. Other organ exchange organizations in Europe include Hellenic Transplant (Greece), Swiss Transplant (Switzerland), Etablissement Français des Greffes (France), United Kingdom Transplant Support Service Authority (United Kingdom), Lusotransplant (Portugal), and Organización Nacional de Trasplantes (Spain).

In the United States, once a patient is ready for transplant surgery, he or she can be placed on the UNOS waiting list to receive a cadaveric kidney. UNOS rules prohibit adult patients from receiving waiting time on the list until the creatinine clearance is 20 mL/min or less. Kidneys are usually allocated based on the UNOS point system (Table 2). Occasionally, UNOS may allow a center to transplant kidneys outside of the point system, usually for research purposes. The UNOS point system is designed to balance equity with efficiency. Equity demands that all patients be given the same access to transplantable organs, regardless of race, ethnicity, gender, or socioeconomic status. Efficiency dictates that kidneys are given to the patients who are likely to benefit the most, usually patients in whom the longest graft survival can be expected. Unfortunately, the goals of equity and efficiency often conflict. Although the UNOS point system is designed to allocate organs, the final decision to accept a particular organ once it is offered rests in the hands of the patient's physician.

Although the median waiting time for people listed in 1995 was 31.6 months (95% confidence interval 30.6–33.0 months), waiting time varies substantially according to a patient's ABO blood group. For patients listed in 1994 (most recent year for complete data) the median waiting time was 27.2 months (26.3–28.1), but for those with ABO blood group O, median waiting time was 33.3 (31.9–35.0) months, for A it was 17.9 (17.3–18.8) months, for B it was 43.4 (41.0–47.0) months, and for AB it was only 9.3 (8.0–11.0) months. It would be even more disadvantageous for patients who are blood group O if A, B, and AB blood group patients could also compete for O kidneys, so UNOS has established that all O kidneys must go to O recipients (Table 2). Points awarded for waiting time and points given for having preformed antibodies (preformed antibodies make it more difficult to find a cross-match negative kidney) are designed to make the system equitable. On the other hand, points are also assigned for how well matched a kidney is according to MHC antigens, since grafts that are better matched are, on average, more likely to survive longer.

Usually, a kidney is first offered locally, then if there is no suitable donor, it is offered regionally and then nationally. This scheme is designed to minimize the time it takes to ship kidneys; since prolonged cold ischemia time may delay graft function and possibly decrease graft survival. On the other hand, the long-term survival of kidneys with zero MHC antigen mismatches (there are two A, two B, and two DR MHC antigens) overrides concerns for increased cold ischemia time. Therefore, there is a mandatory policy that a kidney must be shipped anywhere in the United States if there is a cross-match negative recipient with zero MHC antigen mismatches. The only exception to the zero-antigen mismatch rule is a recipient of a simultaneous kidney and nonrenal organ transplant. Kidneys can voluntarily go to a recipient of a simultaneous kidney and nonrenal organ transplant with fewer points, although the receiving center must then pay the kidney back at a future date. Unfortunately, someone waiting only for a kidney may wait longer because a kidney that may have gone to them went instead to a simultaneous nonrenal organ recipient, and because another kidney that may have gone to them was shipped somewhere else as a payback.

LIVING DONORS

With the growing cadaveric donor shortage, a greater emphasis is being placed on living donations. Kidneys from living donors generally survive longer than cadaveric kidneys. The duration of graft survival based on the source of the donor kidney is, on average, identical twin > two-haplotype-matched sibling > one-haplotype-matched sibling or parent = zero-haplotype-matched sibling = distantly related or unrelated (emotionally related) living donor > cadaveric kidney. Living donor kidneys have the added advantages of allowing preemptive transplantation and sparing more kidneys for individuals who do not have suitable living donors.

Potential living (blood-related and emotionally related) donors should be counseled regarding both the short- and long-term risks of donation. In a survey of transplant centers, mortality from donation was estimated to be 0.03%, while major morbidity was 0.23%. The recent introduction of laproscopic nephrectomy at many centers has substantially reduced the morbidity of kidney donation, without compromising long-term outcomes for the recipient. With regard to long-term risk for the donor, a meta-analysis of 48 studies including 3124 patients and 1703 controls found little evidence of progressive renal dysfunction among normal individuals with only one kidney. Although there was

a small increase in blood pressure, this increase was not enough to raise the prevalence of hypertension in patients who had a single kidney. There was also a statistically significant increase in proteinuria, but the increase was probably too small to be of clinical relevance.

In general, proteinuria greater than 200 mg/24 hr should be considered a contraindication to donation. Microhematuria and pyuria should be investigated to rule out underlying renal disease that would preclude donation. Renal function should generally be normal, after adjusting for gender, age, and possible dietary influences on glomerular filtration rate.

Blood typing and cross matching are often the first steps in evaluating a living donor. If a potential donor and recipient are blood group compatible and cross-match negative, further evaluation can then be carried out. This should include a psychological evaluation to ensure that the donation is truly voluntary and that the patient can give an informed consent. A complete medical evaluation should also be carried out to uncover conditions that would increase the risk of surgery. Potential donors should be screened for conditions such as hypertension that may be made worse by having only one kidney. How diligently to test for possible incipient diabetes in donors with a positive family history or other risk factors for diabetes is controversial. This is because the effect of having one kidney on the rate of progression of diabetic nephropathy (if diabetes occurred) is uncertain. It is reasonable to screen with a fasting and 2-hr, postprandial blood glucose. Consideration should be given to the risk of inherited renal diseases such as autosomal dominant polycystic kidney disease and hereditary nephritis. Finally, the medical evaluation should ensure that the donor is free of diseases that could be transmitted with the kidney, including malignancies, HIV, viral hepatitis, and tuberculosis.

If there is more than one potential living donor, selection should be based on both medical and nonmedical factors, and good matching need not be the only determinant of donor choice. Although the best donor is usually a member of the recipient's immediate family, most centers would consider an emotionally related donor. Once a potential donor has been selected and evaluated, the final step is usually arteriography or an equivalent imaging technique to define the renal vasculature and to look for potential anatomic abnormalities.

THE TRANSPLANT PROCEDURE

The kidney is most often placed retroperitoneally in the iliac fossa. The renal artery is usually anastomosed (end-to-end) with the internal iliac artery. Different techniques are available for dealing with multiple renal arteries and atherosclerosis in the recipient's iliac artery. The renal vein is usually anastomosed (end-to-end) with the external iliac vein. The ureter is implanted via a long submucosal tunnel into the bladder. In general, this surgical approach has made the transplant procedure relatively routine, although immunosuppression delays wound healing and increases the risk of postoperative infection.

Bibliography

Bia MJ, Ramos EL, Danovitch GM, Gaston RS, Harmon WE, Leichtman AB, Lundin PA, Neylan J, Kasiske BL: Evaluation of living renal donors. The current practice of US transplant centers. *Transplantation* 60:322–327, 1995.

Cecka JM: The UNOS Scientific Registry. In: Cecka JM, Terasaki PI (eds), *Clinical Transplants 1998*, PP. 1–16. UCLA Tissue Typing Laboratory, Los Angeles, 1999.

De Meester J, Persijn GG, Wujciak T, Opelz G, Vanrenterghem Y: The new Eurotransplant Kidney Allocation System: Report one year after implementation. Eurotransplant International Foundation. *Transplantation* 66:1154–1159, 1998.

Heering P, Hetzel R, Grabensee B, Opelz G: Renal transplantation in secondary systemic amyloidosis. *Clin Transplant* 12:159–164, 1998.

Kasiske BL, Ma JZ, Louis TA, Swan SK: Long-term effects of reduced renal mass in humans. *Kidney Int* 48:814–819, 1995.

Kasiske BL, Ramos EL, Gaston RS, Bia MJ, Danovitch GM, Bowen PA, Lundin PA, Murphy K: The evaluation of renal transplant candidates: Clinical practice guidelines. *J Am Soc Nephrol* 6:1–34, 1995.

Kasiske BL, Ravenscraft M, Ramos EL, Gaston RS, Bia MJ, Danovitch GM. The evaluation of living renal transplant donors: Clinical practice guidelines. *J Am Soc Nephrol* 7:2288–2313, 1996.

Madsen M, Asmundsson P, Brekke IB, Hockerstedt K, Kirkegaard P, Persson NH, Tufveson G: Scandiatransplant: Organ transplantation in the Nordic countries 1996. *Transplant Proc* 29:3084–3090, 1997.

Ramos EL, Kasiske BL, Alexander SR, Danovitch GM, Harmon WE, Kahana L, Kiresuk TJ, Neylan JF: The evaluation of candidates for renal transplantation: The current practice of U.S. transplant centers. *Transplantation* 57:490–497, 1994.

Spital A: Should all human immunodeficiency virus-infected patients with end-stage renal disease be excluded from transplantation? The views of U.S. transplant centers. *Transplantation* 65:1187–1191, 1998.

United Network for Organ Sharing: *Scientific Registry and Organ Procurement and Transplantation Network Annual Report 1998.* United Network for Organ Sharing. Electronic citation: http//www.unos.org. 1999.

68

RENAL TRANSPLANTATION: IMMUNOSUPPRESSION AND POSTOPERATIVE MANAGEMENT

DOUGLAS J. NORMAN

Renal transplantation is the preferred treatment for end stage renal disease. Survival with a kidney transplant exceeds survival on dialysis while waiting for a transplant. In 1998, 12,166 kidney transplants were performed in the United States. Of these, 4153 came from living donors, and approximately 14% of the living donors were unrelated. Typical 1-year patient survivals are 98% and 95% for living-related donor and cadaveric donor recipients, respectively. One-year graft survivals are 95% for living-related donor transplants and 90% for cadaveric donor transplants. The half-lives are 16.7 years and 10.4 years for living donor and cadaveric donor kidneys, respectively. The success of kidney transplantation has led to a greatly lengthened national list of patients requesting a transplant. At the end of 1999, there were 43,995 patients on waiting lists at the 252 transplant centers in the United States.

RATIONALE FOR IMMUNOSUPPRESSION

To achieve long-term graft survival requires measures that counter the immune response. The key mediators of allograft damage are antibodies, produced by activated B lymphocytes, and cytolytic cells derived from T lymphocytes. Immunosuppression strategies are increasingly being directed against specific elements of the immune response. Potential targets for immunosuppression are: (1) B and T lymphocytes; (2) accessory cells including tissue macrophages, monocytes, and endothelial cells; (3) cytokines including a variety of growth and differentiation factors, and (4) adhesion molecules and receptors that promote cell-to-cell contacts and interactions. To date, the most successful immunosuppressive drugs are those directed to antigen recognition, cytokine production, cytokine-mediated cell activation, and DNA replication.

The most natural way to diminish the strength of the immune response is to match recipients and donors for the major histocompatibility (MHC) antigens. MHC antigens, known as HLA, are coded by the short arm of chromosome 6. Both class I (HLA A, B, C) and class II (HLA DP, DQ, DR) antigens are major targets of the immune response. If all the genes in the HLA regions are matched, which is only achievable among siblings who inherit the same paternal and maternal chromosomes 6 (a two haplotype match), the half-life of renal allografts is at least 25 years. If a living-related donor with a match for neither or one of the two haplotypes is used, the reported half-life is 14 years. The worst survival, with an 8-year half-life, is with cadaveric organs from donors who have two HLA A, two HLA B, and two HLA DR antigens mismatched (a six-antigen mismatch) with the recipients. Among cadaver recipients, however, there is a stepwise increase in graft survival with decreased antigen mismatching. The half-life for zero-antigen mismatched cadaver donor allografts is approximately 16 years.

The goal of clinical tissue typing is to ensure an adequate tissue match and a negative pretransplant cross match. Although practice guidelines require a negative cross match, there is no such requirement for a good antigen match and, unfortunately, only 10 to 20% of cadaver organs are transplanted into well-matched recipients.

CLASSIFICATION OF ALLOGRAFT REJECTION

Following transplantation, episodes of renal dysfunction may occur. Three distinct syndromes of rejection have unique pathology, immunopathogenesis, and clinical presentations. Hyperacute rejection is caused by preformed antidonor antibodies present in the serum of the recipient at the moment of transplantation. Excised allografts demonstrate fibrin thrombi in the glomerular capillaries and small vessels, vasculitis, and necrosis. Acute rejections often occur in the first 3 months after transplantation. They are caused by T cells via direct cytotoxicity, and by T cells and macrophages via local cytokine release (delayed-type hypersensitivity). The pathological appearance of acute rejection is a mononuclear interstitial cell infiltrate with tubulitis (lymphocytes invading renal tubules), and sometimes with endothelial damage suggestive of a vascular rejection. Glomeruli are spared. These rejections are usually reversible by using a pulse of corticosteroids or anti-T-cell antibody. Chronic rejection is generally progressive and refractory to immunosuppressive therapy. Its pathological appearance consists of vascular intimal thickening and occlusion, interstitial fibrosis, and glomerulosclerosis. Chronic rejection is likely triggered by endothelial cell damage leading to smooth muscle cell proliferation and fibrosis. Acute rejection episodes might begin this process; their oc-

currence correlates directly with long-term graft survival. A variant of chronic rejection, transplant glomerulopathy, is characterized by glomerular capillary loop thickening and proteinuria.

OTHER CAUSES OF ALLOGRAFT LOSS

Other factors may contribute to the pathological process that is best termed as chronic allograft failure. Hyperfiltration damage occurs when the glomerular filtration rate of a renal allograft falls below 20% of normal and may contribute to the further loss of kidney function. Factors that reduce the number of functioning nephrons and contribute to chronic allograft failure include the following: (1) advanced donor age, female donor sex, African-American donor ancestry, and small donor size; (2) preexisting renal damage in the donor from hypertension, lipids, drugs, or other illness; (3) complications occurring around the time of organ harvesting such as the cause of death of the donor, hypotensive episodes, cardiac arrest, and the use of nephrotoxic drugs prior to the declaration of brain death; and (4) nonrejection damage that can supervene in an allograft after transplantation due to hypertension, infections, nephrotoxic drugs, etc. In addition, some forms of glomerulonephritis may occur after transplantation and are a relative contraindication to retransplantation (see Chapter 67).

GENERAL POSTTRANSPLANT CARE

Posttransplant in-hospital surgical care of a transplant patient begins with management of the wound, drains, urinary catheter, central venous line, gastrointestinal function, diet, and ambulation. Routine medical care includes dialysis if the allograft does not function at once, fluid and electrolyte management, blood pressure control, infection surveillance, renal function monitoring, and immunosuppression. The pharmacist and transplant coordinator play important roles in teaching the patient about drug use, drug interactions, and side effects, providing pivotal education about the posttransplant routine, and preparing the patient for outpatient follow-up. This team approach to transplant patient management, combining input from the physician, surgeon, nurses, social worker, and pharmacist, is key to the success of transplantation.

Management of patients posttransplantation requires special attention to renal function. Renal dysfunction episodes result from a variety of causes, depending on timing after transplant. In general, the most common causes of renal dysfunction in the immediate postoperative period include anatomical problems related to the surgical procedure and renal preservation problems related to cadaveric donor management. With the use of sensitive cross-matching techniques and strong initial immunosuppression, rejection episodes are uncommon. The radionuclide renal scan is probably the most useful single diagnostic test for renal dysfunction in this setting, because it can demonstrate a urinary leak, ureteral obstruction, intrarenal infarct, vascular accident, acute tubular necrosis, and rejection. Acute rejection becomes a consideration 2 or 3 weeks after transplant, especially when induction immunosuppression with an antilymphocyte antibody is not used. The classic signs and symptoms of acute rejection including graft swelling, pain, and tenderness seldom develop now that stronger immunosuppressive drugs are being used. Rejection typically presents as only a rise in the serum creatinine level, without accompanying signs and symptoms.

Causes of renal dysfunction other than anatomical problems and rejection must always be considered, especially after the immediate postoperative period. These include cyclosporine or tacrolimus nephrotoxicity, urinary tract infection, hypersensitivity reaction to a penicillin or other drug, volume depletion from diuretic use or hyperglycemia, or other drug effect such as that of trimethoprim or cimetidine to decrease creatinine secretion. A careful history, physical, and laboratory examination will often disclose the cause of dysfunction. If cyclosporine or tacrolimus nephrotoxicity are suspected, it is often helpful to hold the evening dose of the drug and repeat the serum creatinine the next morning. Acute nephrotoxicity of these drugs is usually rapidly reversible. If such an evaluation does not provide a diagnosis, a renal allograft biopsy is the definitive diagnostic tool. As the biopsy is generally performed under ultrasound guidance, additional information about obstruction and presence of an extrarenal fluid collection, such as a lymphocele, is also provided. Also, Doppler studies obtained in ultrasound can reveal vascular problems with the renal artery.

The trend in transplant medicine has been to use the allograft biopsy more often to evaluate renal dysfunction episodes. As the serum creatinine is an insensitive measure of glomerular filtration rate and a poor predictor of interstitial disease, even small increases in the serum creatinine may have significance. Certainly, during the first 3 months after transplant, a 25% increase in the serum creatinine, in the absence of the aforementioned nonrejection causes of renal dysfunction, warrants a renal allograft biopsy. When a previous biopsy has shown advanced changes of chronic allograft nephropathy, in which case it is unlikely that a biopsy will demonstrate a treatable lesion, progressive renal insufficiency usually does not warrant another biopsy. Some centers use fine-needle aspiration of the allograft with cytologic examination in lieu of biopsies.

IMMUNOSUPPRESSIVE DRUGS

Immunosuppression is the cornerstone of a successful kidney transplantation. The evolution of immunosuppression during the past decade has been extraordinarily brisk and will likely continue at an accelerated pace. Immunosuppressive drugs can be divided into a few broad categories. The classic monoclonal (anti-CD3) and polyclonal antibodies are anti-target-recognition drugs that prevent antigen recognition by T cells. Newer antibodies prevent the binding of interleukin 2 (IL-2) to its receptor on activated lymphocytes. Currently available antibodies are basically of three types. The polyclonal antibodies are made in horses, (Atgam), or in rabbits, (Thymoglobulin), and are directed to

multiple different leukocyte surface molecules. They deplete peripheral lymphocytes, and in the case of Thymoglobulin, can cause long-term lymphocyte depletion. The monoclonal anti-CD3 antibody, muromonab CD3, is a fully murine monoclonal antibody, directed to T cells, that causes rapidly reversible T-cell depletion. It also removes the T-cell receptor and its associated molecules, known collectively as CD3, from the cell surface. The new monoclonal anti-IL-2 receptor (IL-2R) antibodies are part human and part mouse. These are daclizumab, a humanized (90% human) monoclonal antibody, and basiliximab, a chimeric (70% human) monoclonal antibody. Both of these antibodies are directed to the α chain of the high-affinity IL-2R. The α chain is increased 20-fold on activated T cells, making these antibodies more selective for activated T cells than for resting T cells. Compared with murine monoclonal antibodies, humanized or chimeric antibodies have two potential advantages, a longer serum half-life and an absence of human antibody production against them.

Cyclosporine and tacrolimus are calcineurin inhibitors. On entering a cell, these drugs combine in the cytoplasm with binding proteins (immunophilins) called cyclophilin and FK binding protein (FKBP), respectively, and inhibit calcineurin. Calcineurin is a phosphatase that, on cell activation, eliminates phosphates from serine or threonine residues on nuclear factor of activated T cells (NFAT). Dephosphorylation allows NFAT to cross the nuclear membrane and begin transcription of the IL-2 gene. Key steps leading to the immunosuppressive effects of these drugs are the binding of cyclosporine or tacrolimus to their specific immunophilin, blockade of calcineurin, and prevention of the transcription of cytokine genes, particularly IL-2. Sirolimus prevents IL-2-driven cell activation via a mechanism that is still not fully elucidated. Sirolimus binds FKBP and has the theoretical potential of antagonizing the effect of tacrolimus. However, because there is an abundance of FKBP there are no clinical consequences of using tacrolimus and sirolimus together.

Azathioprine, cyclophosphamide, mycophenolate mofetil, methotrexate, and brequinar sodium inhibit normal cell proliferation. They block enzymes vital to purine or pyrimidine production and therefore, to DNA replication. Finally, corticosteroids are both antiinflammatory and immunosuppressive.

As a rule, immunosuppressive drugs are given in combination. Typically, a calcineurin inhibitor (cyclosporine or tacrolimus), a purine synthesis inhibitor (azathioprine or mycophenolate mofetil), and an antiinflammatory drug (corticosteroids) will be employed together. The availability of a number of immunosuppressive drugs allows the transplant physician to select drugs based on patient characteristics. For example, tacrolimus is the calcineurin inhibitor of choice for women because it does not cause hirsutism. Mycophenolate mofetil should be used for high-immunological-risk patients because it is more potent than azathioprine; in low-immunological-risk patients, it might cause overimmunosuppression. The anti-IL-2R antibodies may be less potent than the polyclonal antibodies or OKT3, and may best be used in the low-immunological-risk group.

The side effects and toxicities of the immunosuppressive drugs are listed in Table 1.

PHASES OF IMMUNOSUPPRESSION

Three distinct phases of immunosuppression follow kidney transplantation: (1) induction, (2) maintenance, and (3) antirejection treatment. Immunosuppression induction requires drugs that are powerful yet specific for cells that initiate and effect the allograft-directed immune response. The induction phase begins with the transplant or, in the case of living donor transplantation, during the week before the transplant, and continues for 1 to 3 months after the transplant. The immune response is strongest when it encounters the allograft initially. Passenger leukocytes from the graft flow to regional lymph nodes and directly activate the immune response. Strong immunosuppression is required during this period, which is, unfortunately, also the time at which a patient is at greatest risk for bacterial wound, lung, and urinary tract infections. Therefore, drugs that promote delayed wound healing or broadly affect all leukocyte function are potentially dangerous. Moreover, during the first 5 to 7 days after transplant, exposure to high doses of potentially nephrotoxic drugs such as cyclosporine or tacrolimus, which can exacerbate preservation-induced organ damage, should be minimized if possible. Antibodies directed to lymphocytes, in combination with corticosteroids, a purine synthesis inhibitor, and the delayed use of calcineurin inhibitor, are widely used for induction. Several drugs are available, including muromonab CD3, Atgam, Thymoglobulin, daclizumab, and basiliximab. All have been proven effective for induction of immunosuppression. They prevent early rejection episodes that would otherwise require high doses of corticosteroids. A meta-analysis of the use of muromonab CD3 and polyclonal antilymphocyte antibodies demonstrated an improvement in long-term graft survival. Such meta-analyses are not yet available for the anti-IL-2R antibodies, and the individual studies have not demonstrated a significant benefit to graft survival. It appears that outcomes with the latter antibodies are improved if a calcineurin inhibitor is used concomitantly. Target levels and doses of the calcineurin inhibitors are usually 25 to 50% higher during the induction phase, and are reduced after approximately 3 months in patients who are rejection-free. Corticosteroid use is also higher during the induction phase than during the maintenance phase of immunosuppression. Because of the adverse effects of acute rejection episodes on long-term graft survival, a recent goal of induction immunosuppression has become the prevention of most rejection episodes.

Many different approaches to induction of immunosuppression are used among the approximately 250 kidney transplant programs in the United States. For those centers that employ antibody induction, some reserve the anti-IL-2R antibodies for low-immunologic-risk patients and give the more potent antibodies to the higher risk patients. Others use the anti-IL-2R antibodies in all patients. Still others favor the use of the more potent antibodies for most patients and avoid altogether the early use of a calcineurin inhibitor. Not all centers use antibodies for induction, and this is particularly true for low-immunological-risk patients. Induction of immunosuppression can also be accomplished with an intravenous calcineurin inhibitor, generally cyclosporine, a purine synthesis inhibitor, and corticosteroids. Benefits of this approach are a lower incidence of viral infections and posttransplant lymphoproliferative disease, and a lower cost. The risk is a higher incidence of early rejection.

TABLE I
Individual Immunosuppressive Drug Toxicities

Corticosteroids	Adrenal suppression; decreased intestinal absorption and increased renal excretion of calcium; weight gain and redistribution of fat to the abdomen, face ("moon face"), and neck ("buffalo hump"); osteoporosis; osteonecrosis; myopathy; delayed wound healing; hyperlipidemia; accelerated atherosclerosis; diabetes mellitus; cataracts; acne; hirsutism; growth retardation in children
Cyclosporine	Nephrotoxicity; hypertension; hirsutism; gingival hyperplasia; neurotoxicity including tremor, dysesthesia, and seizures; hepatotoxicity; hyperuricemia; diabetes
Tacrolimus	Nephrotoxicity; neurotoxicity including tremors, headaches, disorientation, and dysesthesias; gastrointestinal hypersensitivity, diabetes mellitus; alopecia
Mycophenolate mofetil	Myelosuppression; gastrointestinal toxicity
Azathioprine	Myelosuppression; pancreatitis; alopecia; hepatotoxicity; veno-occlusive liver disease
Muromonab CD3	Cytokine release syndrome (mediated by tumor necrosis factor, γ-interferon, IL-6 and other cytokines) including fever, chills, nausea, diarrhea, encephalopathy, pulmonary edema (capillary leak syndrome), and nephropathy; human antimouse antibody production in approximately 75% of patients (high titer in 10 to 20%)
Atgam	Thrombocytopenia; leukopenia; serum sickness; human antiequine antibody production in 75% of patients
Thymoglobulin	Leukopenia; prolonged lymphopenia; thrombocytopenia; serum sickness; human antirabbit antibody production in 75% of patients
Basiliximab and daclizumab	None reported

Immunosuppression maintenance generally requires lower doses of the same drugs, except for the antilymphocyte preparations, which are not used for maintenance therapy. The use of lower doses of the drugs is possible because the body adapts to the organ after the donor passenger leukocytes have been destroyed or dispersed. The goal of maintenance immunosuppression is to prevent chronic rejection while minimizing the adverse effects of long-term immunosuppression. The maintenance phase begins after 3 months and continues for life. Immunosuppressive drugs can never be discontinued because of a very high risk of rejection without them, even many years after transplant. During this phase most patients receive either cyclosporine or tacrolimus, and either mycophenolate mofetil or azathioprine. Cyclosporine and tacrolimus are generally considered to be of equal potency, although tacrolimus may be more potent for preventing acute rejection episodes. The side effects of these drugs differ, and some are more tolerable to men than women. For example, cyclosporine causes hirsutism. However, tacrolimus can cause diabetes, especially in African-Americans and patients of Hispanic ancestry. Mycophenolate mofetil has been shown to be more potent than azathioprine for preventing acute rejection episodes, although no difference on graft survival after 5 years resulted. Although most transplant centers are currently using mycophenolate mofetil exclusively, other centers prefer to use azathioprine in low-immunologic-risk patients because it is cheaper and causes fewer infections and side effects. Some centers substitute azathioprine for mycophenolate mofetil after a year. Prednisone is used in various amounts according to local tradition, and in some centers it is tapered off completely after the patient has proven to be stable, generally about a year after transplant.

The third phase of immunosuppression is antirejection treatment. Following the introduction of new immunosuppressive maintenance drugs, such as tacrolimus and mycophenolate mofetil, and especially when antilymphocyte antibodies such as Atgam, basiliximab, daclizumab, muromonab CD3, or Thymoglobulin have been employed, the incidence of acute rejection episodes has declined dramatically. Acute cell-mediated rejections occur most frequently during the first 3 months after transplantation and after major sensitizing events such as infections, trauma, surgery, or noncompliance with medications. First-line treatment of acute rejections is usually with an increased dose of corticosteroids given either intravenously or orally. Treatment of steroid-resistant or steroid-dependent rejections requires Atgam, muromonab CD3, or Thymoglobulin. These are generally effective for 75 to 80% of steroid-resistant rejections when administered for 7 to 14 days. Mild rejections can be treated by increasing the dose of calcineurin inhibitor and/or purine synthesis inhibitor. Moderate-severe rejections can be treated by switching from azathioprine to mycophenolate mofetil, or from cyclosporine to tacrolimus, in addition to using cortocosteroids or antibodies.

Standard maintenance doses of the most commonly used drugs are as follows: azathioprine (1 to 2 mg/kg once a day); mycophenolate mofetil (2 g in two or three divided daily doses); cyclosporine (4 to 8 mg/kg in one or two divided daily doses); tacrolimus (0.15 mg/kg in two divided daily doses); and prednisone (0.10 mg/kg once a day, or alternatively, 0.2 mg/kg every other day). Cyclosporine and tacrolimus therapies are monitored with drug levels. Desired drug levels vary according to assay used and frequency of dosing.

POSTTRANSPLANT INFECTION

Infection may result from overimmunosuppression. In the immediate postoperative period, the most common infections are bacterial urinary tract, pulmonary, wound, and intravenous line related infections. These can be avoided, or mitigated by careful anticipation and use of preventive measures. Opportunistic infections can occur at any time after transplantation, but generally they develop when immunosuppression is most intense, such as during the first few months after transplant and following treated episodes of rejection.

Herpes simplex is commonly activated by immunosuppression but can be prevented by acyclovir prophylaxis. Cytomegalovirus (CMV) is a particular problem when a CMV-seronegative recipient receives an organ from a seropositive donor. Approximately 80% of such patients will develop CMV disease ranging from fever alone to pneumonitis, hepatitis, and enteritis. Reactivation-CMV disease also occasionally occurs in seropositive recipients with prior CMV infection but is generally much less severe than the primary form. It may be difficult to distinguish CMV shedding in the urine, saliva, or bronchoalveolar lavage fluid from true infection. Rapid diagnostic tests for CMV include the Shell-Vial test, an overnight assay that detects viral antigen using a monoclonal antibody, and a CMV polymerase chain reaction (PCR) test that detects viral nucleic acid sequences in tissue or blood cells. The standard culture is the least useful because the result is available only after 2 or 3 weeks. CMV is most likely to occur between 1 and 6 months after transplant. Treatment with ganciclovir is usually very effective and patients rarely die of CMV disease, although significant morbidity and expense can result. Active CMV may present during a rejection; reduction of immunosuppression during active disease may promote rejection. Various preventive measures such as the use of valacyclovir, CMV immune globulin, and ganciclovir are available. Both valacyclovir and ganciclovir have been proven to prevent most CMV disease when given for 3 to 6 months after transplant. CMV immune globulin is an expensive adjunctive therapy that can further reduce the incidence of CMV. A typical protocol for the prophylactic use of antiviral agents is to use ganciclovir for 1 month after transplantation in recipients who are CMV-seropositive and for 3 months in recipients who are CMV-seronegative with a CMV seropositive donor. If both the recipient and donor are CMV seronegative, it is unnecessary to use antiviral prophylaxis.

Preemptive therapy with ganciclovir in patients identified to be infected with CMV, using frequent testing for CMV DNA or antigens in peripheral blood cells, is not considered to be cost-effective. The most effective, and least expensive way to prevent a primary CMV infection, which generally is more serious than reactivation disease, is by seromatching, that is, the avoidance of transplanting a seronegative recipient with a kidney from a seropositive donor. However, most transplant centers view this as impractical.

Hepatitis C (HCV) is not a contraindication to renal transplantation unless there is evidence of cirrhosis on a liver biopsy. HCV has occasionally progressed to cirrhosis after transplantation, and the use of immunosuppression may accelerate the course of disease. It is likely that antiviral drugs will be available in the future for eradicating or preventing the progression of HCV.

The transplant physician must also be vigilant regarding the development of other rarer diseases such as *Pneumocystis carinii, Listeria, Legionella, Toxoplasma gondii,* and *Cryptococcus* meningitis. The incidence of *Pneumocystis* and *Legionella* infection has been reduced by the routine use of postoperative trimethoprim–sulfamethoxazole prophylaxis. Community-acquired infections such as the common cold, influenza, *S. pneumoniae* pneumonia, *Chlamydia,* diarrheal syndromes, and sexually transmitted diseases can also affect transplant patients. All prospective transplant patients should be vaccinated against hepatitis A and B and varicella (if not already immune), tetanus, diphtheria, and pneumococcal disease. Like any other infectious diseases, these are potentially much more serious in immunosuppressed patients; the benefit of prevention is obvious.

POSTTRANSPLANT MALIGNANCIES

Neoplasia may also result from excessive immunosuppression. The incidence rates of most malignancies are probably increased among transplant patients, although lymphomas and skin cancers are increased severalfold. Approximately 1% of kidney transplant patients develop lymphoma and approximately 5% develop skin cancer. B-cell lymphomas are the most common, are often associated with Epstein-Barr virus and, if identified early, can sometimes be successfully treated by a drastic reduction in immunosuppression. If a reduction in immunosuppression is unsuccessful, local radiation and chemotherapy are also used. Prolonged or repeated courses of antilymphocyte antibodies, as well as high doses of immunosuppression are generally thought to place a transplant patient at greater risk for developing lymphoma. Both squamous cell and basal cell carcinomas should be anticipated in transplant patients, and appropriate referrals made to a dermatologist for evaluation of suspicious skin lesions. Many solid tumors that become manifest clinically after a transplant were actually present beforehand; age appropriate surveillance should be conducted prior to the transplant. Rarely, tumors are inadvertently transplanted with the allograft. Their discovery should prompt immediate discontinuation of immunosuppression.

POSTTRANSPLANT HYPERTENSION

Posttransplant hypertension is common and often requires multiple-drug therapy. Although essential hypertension and cyclosporine are the usual causes, allograft renal artery stenosis and excessive renin production by the na-

tive kidneys should always be considered. Calcium channel blockers are usually the first-line therapy for hypertension for several reasons, including a demonstrated reversal of the reduction in renal plasma flow and glomerular filtration rate (GFR) induced experimentally by cyclosporine and a possible direct immunosuppressive effect. Verapamil and diltiazem decrease the metabolism of cyclosporine and raise its blood levels. Nifedipine can independently cause gingival hypertrophy. Angiotensin converting enzyme inhibitors, α- and β-adrenergic blockers can also be used effectively in renal transplant patients.

POSTTRANSPLANT HYPERLIPIDEMIA

As a result of using prednisone and cyclosporine, many patients will develop hyperlipidemia following transplantation. Generally, transplant physicians delay the treatment of hyperlipidemia until the prednisone dose has been tapered to maintenance levels, because the problem may disappear or lessen. However, recent data from the heart transplant literature indicating that HMG-CoA reductase inhibitors improve outcome by reducing the incidence of both acute and chronic rejection, by an unknown mechanism, suggest that these drugs should be used earlier. After the prednisone dose has been tapered to low levels (e.g., 0.1 mg/kg/day), further reductions or discontinuation of prednisone altogether have generally not had any additional effect on lowering lipid levels. Because tacrolimus does not cause hyperlipidemia, one must consider conversion from cyclosporine to this drug if posttransplant hyperlipidemia is severe. Sirolimus can elevate both cholesterol and triglyceride levels, sometimes severely. Dietary maneuvers should always be a part of any attempt to lower a patient's lipid levels.

POSTTRANSPLANT HYPERCALCEMIA

In patients who have had long-standing renal failure, the parathyroid glands are often quite hyperplastic, and it may take months to years for them to regress to normal activity. The usual practice is to wait for this to happen, unless a patient is symptomatic from hyperparathyroidism. Occasionally, a posttransplant patient will develop significant and symptomatic hypercalcemia. In this case, early surgery should be considered.

OTHER POSTTRANSPLANT COMPLICATIONS

Some patients develop diabetes mellitus after transplantation because of steroid, tacrolimus, or cyclosporine use. Many of these patients require insulin. Urinary tract infection and *Pneumocystis* prophylaxis are generally prescribed for 3 to 4 months after transplant, and both goals can be accomplished with trimethoprim–sulfamethoxazole, one double-strength tablet every Monday, Wednesday, and Friday. Hypophosphatemia and hypomagnesemia are both very common following renal transplantation because of renal tubular abnormalities induced by cyclosporine, as well as hyperparathyroidism and other causes. These minerals should be replaced as needed. Calcium, alendronate, vitamin D, and calcium-sparing diuretics might reduce the severity of osteopenia. Erythrocytosis may result from excessive erythropoietin production by the allograft or native kidneys. Phlebotomy may be required; however, most patients respond to angiotensin converting enzyme inhibitors (see Chapter 65).

POSTTRANSPLANT DRUG PRESCRIPTIONS

Numerous drugs may have adverse effects in transplant patients. Nonsteroidal antiinflammatory drugs often cause precipitous and protracted declines in GFR, presumably because they block production of vasodilator prostaglandins that counter the renal vasoconstriction induced by cyclosporine. Allopurinol, a xanthine oxidase inhibitor, inhibits breakdown of 6-mercaptopurine, the active metabolite of azathioprine and increases its marrow-suppressive effect. Together, these effects complicate management of cyclosporine-induced gout. Intra-articular steroid injections, temporary increases in oral prednisone dosing, colchicine, and judicious coadministration of azathioprine and allopurinol may be necessary. Erythromycin, ketoconazole, fluconazole, itraconazole, diltiazem, nicardipine, verapamil, and methylprednisolone may interfere with cyclosporine degradation. Rifampin, phenytoin, phenobarbital, nafcillin, and carbamazepine accelerate cyclosporine metabolism. Cyclosporine levels should be closely monitored, and a need for dosage adjustment should be anticipated when these agents are prescribed. Because transplant patients are typically receiving numerous medications, and because of the propensity for adverse interactions among them, the physician should be especially vigilant when altering the medication regimen of transplant patients.

MANAGEMENT OF A FAILED RENAL ALLOGRAFT

When a renal allograft fails and a patient returns to dialysis, a decision must be made regarding discontinuation of immunosuppression and removal of the allograft. A retained allograft that is uncovered by immunosuppression can become inflamed causing local and even systemic symptoms. A more serious consequence of a retained allograft is the development of anti-HLA antibodies. If a patient desires retransplantation, these antibodies can be devastating. In general, most allografts that are lost acutely to rejection are removed, and immunosuppression is discontinued with a short taper of the prednisone. Allografts that are lost to chronic rejection can be retained if immunosuppressive drugs are continued (usually azathioprine and prednisone because they are inexpensive), if the patient is interested in being retransplanted, and if anti-HLA antibodies are absent so that it is likely that a kidney will be found within months. For sensitized patients in whom the wait for a subsequent transplant will be long, continuing the immunosuppression becomes too risky, and it is wiser to remove the kidney and discontinue the drugs. If the patient is not a candidate for retransplantation and the allograft was lost to a chronic process, it is reasonable to discontinue immunosuppression and observe the patient. A spike in anti-HLA antibodies occurs in about 25% of patients after the removal of an allograft if immunosuppression is discontinued immediately. Therefore, if there is no major risk of continuing immunosuppression, the drugs can be continued for 1 month before tapering. It has not been proved that this prevents antibody formation.

OUTCOME OF RETRANSPLANTATION

The survival of second transplants is clearly inferior to that of first transplants. If a previous graft was lost to rejection within 3 months of transplant, the outcome of a retransplant is especially poor. However, patients who keep their first grafts for more than 1 year do well with a second one and should not be denied that opportunity. The cause of a poorer survival with a retransplant is usually undetected sensitization. Patients receiving a second transplant are at high-risk for failure and are usually given more potent immunosuppression and certainly require the use of sensitive cross-matching techniques.

Bibliography

Andresdottir MB, Hoitsma AJ, Assmann KJ, et al.: The impact of recurrent glomerulonephritis on graft survival in recipients of human histocompatibility leukocyte antigen-identical living-related donor grafts. *Transplantation* 68:623–627, 1999.

Basar H, Soran A, Shapiro R, et al.: Renal transplantation in recipients over the age of 60: The impact of donor age. *Transplantation* 67:1191–1193, 1999.

Brennan DC, Flavin K, Lowell JA, et al.: A randomized, double-blinded comparison of Thymoglobulin versus Atgam for induction immunosuppressive therapy in adult renal transplant recipients. *Transplantation* 67:1011–1018, 1999.

Burlingham WJ, Grailer AP, Heisey DM, et al.: The effect of tolerance to noninherited maternal HLA antigens on the survival of renal transplants from sibling donors [see comments]. *N Engl J Med* 339:1657–1664, 1998.

Cho YW, Terasaki PI, Cecka JM, et al.: Transplantation of kidneys from donors whose hearts have stopped beating. *N Engl J Med* 338:221–225, 1998.

Dantal J, Hourmant M, Cantarovich D, et al.: Effect of long-term immunosuppression in kidney-graft recipients on cancer incidence: Randomised comparison of two cyclosporin regimens. *Lancet* 351:623–628, 1998.

Dean DE, Kamath S, Peddi VR, et al.: A blinded retrospective analysis of renal allograft pathology using the Banff schema: Implications for clinical management. *Transplantation* 68:642–645, 1999.

Fuller A, Profaizer T, Roberts L, et al.: Repeat donor HLA-DR mismatches in renal transplantation: Is the increased failure rate caused by noncytotoxic HLA-DR alloantibodies? *Transplantation* 68:589–591, 1999.

Hariharan S, Adams MB, Brennan DC, et al.: Recurrent and de novo glomerular disease after renal transplantation: A report from Renal Allograft Disease Registry (RADR). *Transplantation* 68:635–641, 1999.

Kuypers DR, Chapman JR, O'Connell PJ, et al.: Predictors of renal transplant histology at three months. *Transplantation* 67:1222–1230, 1999.

Lowance D, Neumayer HH, Legendre CM, et al.: Valacyclovir for the prevention of cytomegalovirus disease after renal transplantation. International Valacyclovir Cytomegalovirus Prophylaxis Transplantation Study Group. *N Engl J Med* 340:1462–1470, 1999.

Nashan B, Moore R, Amlot P, *et al.:* Randomised trial of basiliximab versus placebo for control of acute cellular rejection in renal allograft recipients. CHIB 201 International Study Group. *Lancet* 350:1193–1198, 1997.

Raiz LR, Kilty KM, Henry ML, *et al.:* Medication compliance following renal transplantation. *Transplantation* 68:51–55, 1999.

Ratcliffe PJ, Dudley CR, Higgins RM, *et al.:* Randomised controlled trial of steroid withdrawal in renal transplant recipients receiving triple immunosuppression. *Lancet* 348:643–648, 1996.

Schnuelle P, van der Woude FJ: Should A2 kidneys be transplanted into B or O recipients? *Lancet* 351:1675–1676, 1998.

Slakey DP, Wood JC, Hender D, *et al.:* Laparoscopic living donor nephrectomy: Advantages of the hand-assisted method. *Transplantation* 68:581–583, 1999.

Smets YF, Westendorp RG, van der Pijl JW, *et al.:* Effect of simultaneous pancreas–kidney transplantation on mortality of patients with type-1 diabetes mellitus and end-stage renal failure. *Lancet* 353:1915–1919, 1999.

Vincenti F, Kirkman R, Light S, *et al.:* Interleukin-2-receptor blockade with daclizumab to prevent acute rejection in renal transplantation. Daclizumab Triple Therapy Study Group. *N Engl J Med* 338:161–165, 1998.

SECTION 11

HYPERTENSION

69

PATHOGENESIS OF HYPERTENSION

CHRISTOPHER S. WILCOX

Hypertension implies either an increased cardiac output (CO) or total peripheral resistance (TPR). Often human essential hypertension developing in young adults is initiated by an increase in CO; the blood pressure (BP) is labile and the heart rate is increased. Later, the BP increases further owing to a rise in TPR with the restoration of a normal CO. Therefore, most patients encountered in clinical practice with sustained hypertension have an excessive TPR. This is due initially to increased vasoconstriction of resistance vessels but, over time and with aging, structural components of vascular resistance contribute.

Left ventricular systole creates a shock wave that is reflected back from the peripheral resistance vessels. During early diastole, this wave reaches the ascending aorta where it produces the dicrotic notch. With aging and loss of elasticity, the pressure wave is transmitted more rapidly out and back through the arterial tree. Eventually, the wave in the aorta coincides with the upstroke of the aortic systolic pressure wave, leading to an abrupt increase in the height of the systolic pressure. This accounts for the frequent finding of isolated, or predominant, systolic hypertension in the elderly. In contrast, systolic hypertension in the young usually reflects an enhanced cardiac contractility.

PATHOPHYSIOLOGY OF HYPERTENSION

When a normal subject arises, there is an abrupt fall in venous return and CO of 30–50% that elicits a baroreflex response. The ensuing contraction of resistance vessels buffers blood pressure acutely, whereas the contraction of capacitance vessels restores venous return. The outcome is only a small fall in systolic, and rise in diastolic, BP with a modest rise in heart rate. During prolonged standing, increased renal sympathetic nerve activity enhances the reabsorption of NaCl and fluid by the renal tubules, and the release of renin from the juxtaglomerular apparatus, with the subsequent generation of angiotensin II (Ang II) and aldosterone, which further maintain BP and the fullness of the circulation. In contrast, the BP of patients with autonomic insufficiency declines progressively on standing, often to the point of syncope. Since a stable blood pressure is so critical for efficient function of the brain, heart, and kidneys, it is not a surprise that evolution has provided multiple and coordinated BP regulatory processes. Therefore, the understanding of a sustained change in blood pressure, such as hypertension, requires knowledge of a number of interrelated pathophysiologic processes. The most important of these are discussed later.

Renal Mechanisms and Salt Balance

The kidney has a unique role in BP regulation. Renal salt and water retention sufficient to increase the extracellular fluid (ECF) and blood volumes (BV) enhances venous return, leading to a rise in CO and BP. In fact, the kidney is so effective in excreting excess NaCl and fluid during periods of surfeit, or retaining them during periods of deficit, that the ECV and BV vary less than 15% with changes in salt intake. Consequently, the role of body fluids in hypertension is subtle. For example, a 10-fold increase in daily NaCl intake in normal subjects leads to an increase in body fluids of less than 1 L and causes only a trivial increase in BP. Conversely, a diet with no salt content leads to the loss of approximately 1 L of body fluid over 3–5 days and only a trivial fall in BP. Quite different effects are seen in patients with renal insufficiency whose body fluid volumes and BP increase quite predictably with the level of salt intake. The degree of this "salt sensitive" component to BP increases progressively with loss of kidney function. It is most prominent in patients with primary vascular or glomerular diseases of the kidney. Among normotensive subjects, a modest salt sensitive component to BP is apparent in about 30% and appears to be genetically determined. About 50% of patients with hypertension and normal renal function manifest salt sensitivity. Salt sensitive hypertension is particularly common among African-Americans, the elderly, or those with impaired renal function. It is generally associated with a lower level of plasma renin activity (PRA).

What underlies salt sensitivity? Normally the kidneys are exquisitely sensitive even to small changes in BP. For example, a rise in mean arterial pressure (MAP) of 1–3 mm Hg leads to a subtle increase in renal NaCl and fluid elimination. This "pressure natriuresis" also conserves NaCl and fluid during decreases in BP. It is rapid, quantitative, fundamental for normal homeostasis, and is due primarily to changes in tubular NaCl reabsorption rather than renal blood flow or glomerular filtration rate (GFR). The latter are indeed accurately autoregulated in healthy kidneys across a wide range of BPs. Two primary mechanisms of pressure natriuresis have been identified. First, a rise in renal perfusion pressure causes hemodynamic changes within the kidney that result in parallel increases in renal interstitial hydraulic pressure that impair fluid uptake into the bloodstream. Therefore, NaCl and fluid reabsorption is diminished. Second, the degree of stretch of the afferent arteriole regulates the secretion of renin into the bloodstream, and hence the generation of Ang II. Therefore, an increase in BP increases the afferent arteriolar stretch, and reduces Ang II levels. Ang II coordinates the body's salt and fluid retention mechanisms. It stimulates thirst and enhances NaCl and fluid reabsorption in the proximal, loop, and distal nephron segments. By stimulating aldosterone and inhibiting atrial natriuretic peptic (ANP) secretion, Ang II further enhances reabsorption in the distal nephron. Thus, for normal homeostasis, an increase in BP should be matched by a decrease in PRA. It follows that a normal or elevated value for PRA in hypertension is effectively "inappropriate" for the level of BP and is thereby contributing to the maintenance of hypertension.

The relationship between BP and long-term changes in salt balance, and the role of the renin–angiotensin–aldosterone (RAA) system, are shown diagrammatically in Figure 1. Normal human subjects challenged with an increase in salt intake have only a modest and transient rise in MAP because the highly effective pressure natriuresis mechanism rapidly increases renal NaCl and fluid elimination sufficiently to restore a normal blood volume and BP. Expressed quantitatively in Fig. 1, the slope of the increase in NaCl excretion with BP is almost vertical. The steepness of this slope reflects the important effects of reciprocal changes in PRA with BP that dictate appropriate changes in salt handling by the kidney. Thus, when the RAA system is artificially fixed, the slope of the pressure natriuresis relationship flattens. For example, an infusion of Ang II into a normal subject raises the BP. Since Ang II is being infused, the kidney cannot reduce Ang II levels appropriately by reducing renin secretion. Therefore, the pressure natriuresis mechanism is prevented, and the BP elevation is sustained without a full renal compensation. In contrast, normal subjects treated with an angiotensin converting enzyme inhibitor (ACEI) to block Ang II generation have a fall in BP. Again, the kidney cannot dictate an appropriate rise in Ang II and aldosterone levels that would be required to retain sufficient NaCl and fluid to buffer the fall in BP. Thus, when the RAA system is fixed the BP becomes highly "salt sensitive" (Fig. 1). These studies demonstrate the unique role of the RAA system in long-term BP regulation and its importance in isolating the BP from the effects of changes in NaCl intake.

Three compelling lines of evidence implicate the kidney and RAA system in long-term BP regulation. First, transplantation studies between genetically hypertensive and normotensive rat strains show that normotensive animals receiving a kidney from a hypertensive animal become hypertensive and vice versa. Similarly, human renal transplant recipients become hypertensive if they receive a kidney from a hypertensive donor. Apparently, the kidney in hypertension is programmed to retain salt and water inappropriately for a normal level of BP, thereby resetting the pressure natriuresis to a higher level of BP and dictating the appearance of hypertension in the recipient. Second is the observation that blockade of Ang II generation with an ACEI or of AngII action on type 1 (AT_1) receptors with an angiotensin receptor blocker (ARB) or of aldosterone receptors with an aldosterone antagonist reduces BP by 5–20%. The fall in BP is greatest in those with elevated PRA values and is enhanced by dietary salt restriction (Fig. 1). Third, is the observation that nearly 90% of patients approaching end stage renal disease (ESRD) because of kidney failure have hypertension.

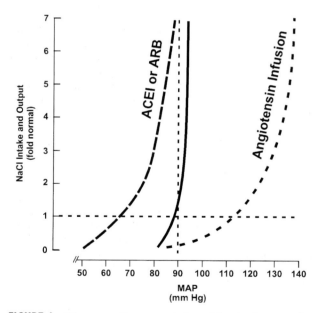

FIGURE 1 Diagrammatic representation of the steady-state relationship between sodium excretion, relative to intake, and mean arterial pressure (MAP) in normal subjects (solid line), and those given an angiotensin converting enzyme inhibitor (ACEI) or angiotensin receptor blocker (ARB) (long dashes) or an infusion of angiotensin II (short dashes) to prevent adaptive changes in angiotensin II levels. See text to explanation. Drawn from data from Guyton AC, Hall JE, Coleman TG, Manning RD: The dominant role of the kidneys in the long-term regulation of arterial pressure in normal and hypertensive states. In: Laragh JH, Brenner BM (eds) *Hypertension, Pathophysiology, Diagnosis and Management*, pp. 1029–1052. Raven, New York, 1990, with permission.

Total Body Autoregulation

An increase in CO necessarily increases peripheral blood flow. However, each organ has intrinsic mechanisms that adapt blood flow to its metabolic needs. Therefore, over time, an increase in CO is translated into an increase in TPR. Organ blood flow is maintained but hypertension becomes sustained. This "total body autoregulation" is demonstrated in human subjects given salt retaining mineralocorticosteroid hormones. An initial rise in CO is translated in most into sustained hypertension and a raised TPR over 5–15 days.

Structural Components to Hypertension

Hypertension causes hypertrophic or remodeling changes in distributing and resistance vessels and the heart and fibrotic and sclerotic changes in the kidney glomeruli and interstitium. Hypertrophy of resistance vessels limits the lumen:wall diameter and dictates a fixed component to TPR. This is evident as a higher TPR of hypertensive, compared to normotensive, subjects during maximal vasodilatation. Moreover, thickened and hypertrophied resistance vessels have greater reductions in vessel diameter during agonist stimulation. This is apparent as an increase in vascular reactivity to pressor agents. Sclerotic and fibrotic changes in renal glomeruli and interstitium, combined with hypertrophy of the afferent arterioles, limits the sensing of BP in the juxtaglomerular apparatus and interstitium of the kidney. This blunts renin release and pressure natriuresis and thereby contributes to salt sensitivity and sustained hypertension. Rats receiving intermittent weak electrical stimulation of the hypothalamus to raise their BP respond initially with an abrupt increase in BP, and an abrupt reduction after the cessation of the stimulus. However, after about 6 weeks, the baseline BP increases in parallel with the appearance of hypertrophy of their resistance vessels. These structural components may explain why it often takes some weeks or months to achieve maximal antihypertensive action from a drug or from correction of a renal artery stenosis. Vascular and left ventricular hypertrophy is largely, but not completely, reversible during treatment of hypertension whereas fibrotic and sclerotic changes unfortunately are not.

Sympathetic Nervous System, Brain, and Baroreflexes

A rise in BP elicits a baroreflex-induced reduction in tone of the sympathetic nervous system and an increase in tone of the parasympathetic nervous system. Paradoxically, human hypertension is often associated with an increase in heart rate, maintained or increased plasma catecholamine levels, and an increase in directly measured sympathetic nerve discharges despite the stimulus to the baroreceptors. What is the cause of this inappropriate activation of the sympathetic nervous systems in hypertension? First, studies in animals show that the baroreflex "resets" to the ambient level of BP after 2–5 days. It no longer continues to "fight" the elevated BP but defends it at the new elevated level. This adaptation occurs within the baroreceptors themselves. Second, central mechanisms in animal models of hypertension have been identified that alter the gain of the baroreflex process, and therefore the sympathetic tone, in hypertension. The importance of central mechanisms in human hypertension is apparent from the effectiveness of drugs, such as clonidine, that act within the brain to decrease the sympathetic tone. Third, with aging and atherosclerosis, the walls of the carotid sinus and other baroreflex sensing sites becomes less distensible. Therefore, the BP is less effective in stretching the afferent nerve endings, and the sensitivity of the baroreflex is

diminished. This may explain the enhanced sympathetic nerve activity and plasma catecholamines that are characteristic of elderly hypertensive subjects.

Endothelium and Oxidative Stress

Calcium metabolizing agonists such as bradykinin or acetylcholine, or sheer forces produced by the flow of blood, elicit the release of endothelium-dependent relaxing factors (EDRFs). These include nitric oxide (NO) and prostacyclin (PGI_2). NO has a half-life of only a few seconds due to inactivation by reactive oxygen species such as oxygen radicals (O_2^-). Animal models and humans with essential hypertension have defects in EDRF responses of peripheral vessels, and diminished NO generation. One underlying mechanism is oxidative stress; excessive O_2^- formation effectively inactivates NO, leading to a functional NO deficiency. In the kidney, NO inhibits renal NaCl reabsorption. Therefore, NO deficiency could not only induce vasoconstriction but also diminish the renal pressure natriuresis compensation. Functional NO deficiency in large blood vessels of hypertensive animals contributes to vascular damage and atherosclerosis.

Specific Genetic Theories

Studies in mice with targeted disruption of individual genes, or insertions of extra copies of genes, provide direct evidence for critical regulatory roles for certain gene products in hypertension. Deletions of the gene for endothelial NO synthase (NOS) or atrial natriuretic peptide (ANP) lead to salt-dependent hypertension in mice. These are compelling examples of circumstances where deletion of a single gene can sustain hypertension. However, studies with genetically altered mice sometimes produce results that are not in keeping with what might be predicted based on clinical experience. For instance, the addition of extra copies of the ACE gene has no effect on blood pressure. Presently, compelling evidence for individual gene defects in human essential hypertension is lacking. However, certain rare, specific forms of hereditary hypertension are due to single gene defects. For example, dexamethasone-suppressible hyperaldosteronism is due to a chimeric rearrangement of a gene encoding aldosterone synthase that renders aldosterone synthesis responsive to adrenocorticotrophic hormone. Liddle's syndrome is due to a mutation in the gene encoding one component of the endothelial sodium channel that is expressed in the distal convoluted tubule. The mutated form has lost its normal regulation, leading to a permanent "open state" of the sodium channel. This dictates inappropriate renal NaCl retention and salt-sensitive, low renin hypertension.

AGENTS IMPLICATED IN HYPERTENSION

Alterations in the synthesis, secretion, degradation, or action of numerous substances are implicated in certain categories of hypertension. The most important of these are described below.

Renin, Angiotensin II, and Aldosterone

The PRA is not appropriately suppressed in the majority of patients with essential hypertension. It is actually increased in approximately 15%. These subjects with normal and high renin hypertension have a greater antihypertensive response to single agent therapy with an ACEI or ARB than patients with low renin hypertension. The RAA system is particularly important in the maintenance of BP in patients with renovascular hypertension, although its importance wanes during the chronic phase when structural alterations in blood vessels or damage in the kidney, dictate an RAA-independent component to the hypertension.

Sympathetic Nervous Systems and Catecholamines

Pheochromocytoma is a catecholamine-secreting tumor, often in the adrenal medulla, that increases plasma catecholamines 10- to 1000-fold. However, even such extraordinary increases in pressor amines are rarely fatal because the renal pressure natriuresis mechanism is intact and reduces the blood volume, thereby limiting the rise in BP. Indeed, such patients can have orthostatic hypotension between episodes of catecholamine secretion.

An increased sympathetic nerve tone to resistance vessels in human essential hypertension causes α_1-mediated vasoconstriction to blood vessels and β-mediated increases in contractility and output of the heart. Increased sympathetic nerve discharge to the kidney leads to α_1-mediated enhancement of NaCl reabsorption and β-mediated renin release.

Dopamine

This hormone is synthesized in the brain and renal tubular epithelial cells independent of sympathetic nerves. In the kidney, dopamine synthesis is enhanced during volume expansion and contributes to decreased reabsorption of NaCl, especially in the proximal tubule. Defects in tubular dopamine responsiveness are apparent in genetic models of hypertension, but its role in human essential hypertension is unclear. Dopamine, acting on type I (DA1) receptors, lowers BP and increases renal blood flow and NaCl excretion in normal human subjects.

Arachidonate Metabolites

Arachidonic acid is a normal constituent of phospholipids in cell membranes. On release by phospholipases that are activated by agents such as Ang II, arachidonate is metabolized by three enzymes. Cyclooxygenase generates unstable intermediates whose subsequent metabolism by specific enzymes yields prostaglandins that are either vasodilator (e.g., PGI_2), vasoconstrictor (e.g., thromboxane), or of mixed effect [e.g. prostaglandin E_2 (PGE_2)]. Metabolism by cytochrome P450 monooxygenase yields 20-hydroxyeicosatetranoic acid (20-HETE) that is a vasoconstrictor of blood vessels but inhibits tubular NaCl reabsorption. Metabolism by epoxygenase leads to epoxyeicosatrienic acids (EETs) that are powerful vasodilators and may mediate an endothelium-dependent hyperpolarizing response in resistance vessels. Arachidonate metabolites act primarily as modulating agents in normal physiology. Their role in human essential hypertension remains elusive.

L-Arginine–Nitric Oxide Pathway

NO is generated by three isoforms of NOS that are widely expressed in the body. NO interacts with many iron-centered enzymes. Activation of guanylylcylase generates cyclic guanasine monophosphate (cGMP) that is a powerful vasorelaxant and inhibits NaCl reabsorption in the kidney. Defects in NO generation in the endothelium of human essential hypertension may contribute to increased peripheral resistance, whereas defects in renal NO generation may contribute to inappropriate renal NaCl retention and salt sensitivity. Recent studies have shown defects in conversion of [^{15}N]-labeled arginine to [^{15}N]-labeled NO in hypertensive human subjects and those with chronic renal failure.

Reactive Oxygen Species

The incomplete reduction of molecular oxygen, either by the respiratory chain during cellular respiration, or by oxidases such as NOS yields reactive oxygen species (ROS) including O_2^-. These are short lived, but highly reactive intermediates. Reaction of O_2^- with NO leads to its bioinactivation and generates peroxynitrite ($ONOO^-$) that can have long-lasting effects through nitrosylation reactions. Reaction of ROS with lipids leads to oxidized low density lipoprotein (LDL) that promotes atherosclerosis. ROS are hard to quantitate but indirect evidence suggests that hypertension is a state of oxidative stress. Drugs that reduce O_2^- level reduce BP in animal models of hypertension.

Endothelins

These are produced by vascular endothelial cells, renal tubular epithelial cells, and elsewhere. They act on discrete receptors that mediate either sustained increases in vascular resistance or the release of NO. Endothelin potentiates the vasoconstriction accompanying Ang II infusion or blockade of NOS. Endothelin is released by hypoxia, specific agonists such as Ang II, and cytokines. Nonspecific blockade of endothelin receptors lowers BP in models of volume-expanded hypertension. The role of endothelin in human essential hypertension is presently unclear.

Atrial Natriuretic Peptide

ANP is released from the heart during atrial stretch and acts on receptors that increase GFR, decrease NaCl reabsorption in the distal nephron, and inhibit renin secretion. ANP is released during volume expansion and contributes to the natriuretic response. Its role in essential hypertension is unclear. Endopeptidase inhibitors that block ANP degradation are natriuretic and antihypertensive.

PATHOGENESIS OF HYPERTENSION IN KIDNEY DISEASE

The prevalence of salt-sensitive hypertension increases in proportion to the fall in GFR during renal failure. Hypertension is almost universal in patients with renal insufficiency due to primary glomerular or vascular disease, whereas those with primary tubulointerstitial disease are often normotensive or, occasionally, salt losing.

With declining nephron number, chronic renal insufficiency limits the ability to adjust NaCl excretion rapidly and quantitatively. The role of ECF volume expansion is apparent from the facility of hemodialysis to lower BP, often to normotensive levels, in patients with ESRD.

Additional mechanisms besides primary renal fluid retention contribute to the increased TPR and hypertension in patients with renal disease. The RAA system is often inappropriately stimulated. Apparently, the ESRD kidney generates abnormal renal afferent nerve input that entrains an increased sympathetic nerve discharge that is reversed by bilateral nephrectomy. Plasma levels of endothelin increase with renal failure. Endothelin likely contributes to vasoconstriction. Renal failure induces oxidative stress which contributes to vascular disease and impaired EDRF responses. Additionally, a decreased generation of NO from L-arginine relates to the accumulation of asymmetric dimethylarginine (ADMA) that inhibits NOS. ADMA is removed by hemodialysis.

Hypertension in renal insufficiency is multifactorial. A degree of volume expansion and salt sensitivity is of predominant importance. Pressor mechanisms mediated by Ang II, catecholamines, or endothelin are more potent during volume expansion. This may underlie the importance of these systems in the ESRD patients. Finally, many of the pathways that contribute to hypertension in ESRD, such as impaired NO generation and excessive production of endothelins and ROS, also contribute to atherosclerosis, cardiac hypertrophy, and progressive renal fibrosis and sclerosis. Indeed, in poorly treated hypertension, renal damage leads to further hypertension that itself engenders further renal damage generating a vicious spiral culminating in accelerated hypertension, progressive renal disease, and the requirement for renal replacement therapy. Therefore, rational management of hypertension in renal insufficiency often first entails vigorous salt-depleting therapy with a salt-restricted diet and diuretic therapy. Patients frequently require additional therapy to combat the enhanced vasoconstriction and to attempt to slow the rate of progression of renal insufficiency.

Bibliography

Brady HR, Wilcox CS (eds): *Therapy in Nephrology and Hypertension.* Saunders, Philadelphia, 1998.

Folkow B: The "structural factor" in hypertension with special emphasis on the hypertrophic adaptations of the systemic resistance vessels. In: Laragh JH, Brenner BM (eds) *Hypertension, Pathophysiology, Diagnosis and Management,* pp. 565–582. Raven, New York, 1990.

Guyton AC, Hall JE, Coleman TG, Manning RD: The dominant role of the kidneys in the long-term regulation of arterial pressure in normal and hypertensive states. In: Laragh JH, Brenner BM (eds) *Hypertension, Pathophysiology, Diagnosis and Management,* pp. 1029–1052. Raven, New York, 1990.

JNC VI: The sixth report of the Joint National Committee on Detection, Evaluation and Treatment of High Blood Pressure. *Arch Intern Med* 153:154–183, 1993.

Wilcox CS: Management of hypertension in patients with renal disease. In: Smith TW (ed) *Cardiovascular Therapeutics,* pp. 538–545. Saunders, Philadelphia, 1996.

Wilcox CS, Schrier RW (eds): *Atlas of Diseases of the Kidney: Hypertension and the Kidney.* Current Medicine, Philadelphia, 1998.

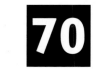

ESSENTIAL HYPERTENSION

JOSEPH V. NALLY, JR.

Hypertension is one of the most common problems in clinical medicine in the United States and is the leading indication for both physician office visits and prescription drugs. Essential or primary hypertension is the sustained elevation of systemic arterial pressure without a readily definable etiology. It is by far the most common form of hypertension, accounting for more than 90% of the nearly 50 million Americans with hypertension. This increase in

TABLE I

Classification of Blood Pressure and Recommendations for Follow-up for Adults Age 18 and Older[a]

Category	Systolic (mm Hg)		Diastolic (mm Hg)	Follow-up
Optimal	<120	and	<80	
Normal	<130	and	<85	Recheck in 2 years
High-normal	130–139	or	85–89	Recheck in 1 year
Hypertension				
Stage 1	140–159	or	90–99	Confirm in 2 months
Stage 2	160–179	or	100–109	Evaluate within 1 month
Stage 3	≥180	or	≥110	Immediate evaluation

[a]Adapted from JNC VI.

arterial pressure is a major risk factor for cardiovascular disease. Consequently, there has been a tremendous effort over the past two decades to identify and effectively treat patients with this "silent killer."

DEFINITION OF HYPERTENSION

There is no strict definition of hypertension, yet arbitrary limits have been proposed to identify increasing cardiovascular risk as a function of the elevation of systemic blood pressure. Initial efforts by the World Health Organization (WHO) suggested that blood pressure determinations greater than 160/95 mm Hg defined hypertension and increasing risk. In the United States, the 1984 report of the Joint National Committee on Detection, Evaluation, and Treatment of High Blood Pressure (JNC III) determined that cardiovascular risk increases at a lower threshold and established a limit of 140/90 mm Hg averaged over repeated measurements on three separate visits. The Sixth Report of the JNC (JNC VI) recognized the importance of systolic hypertension correlating with increased cardiovascular risk and proposed a definition of blood pressure (BP) determinations based on both the systolic and diastolic readings. The JNC VI report also redefined "normal" BP (i.e., <140/90 mm Hg) as optimal (<120/80 mm Hg), normal, or high normal, as cardiovascular risk correlates with BP determinations below 140/90 mm Hg. Table 1 summarizes these various levels of blood pressure determinations and the JNC VI recommendations for patient follow-up or referral.

PREVALENCE AND CARDIOVASCULAR RISK

The most exhaustive source of data for the prevalence of hypertension, hypertension awareness and control in the U.S. population emanates from the National Health and Nutrition Examination Survey (NHANES). Population surveys regarding hypertension were performed during several time periods from 1976 to 1994. For these studies, three blood pressure determinations were taken at a single visit, and individuals were questioned about their blood pressure and/or antihypertensive therapy. NHANES employed the JNC definition of hypertension, that is, systolic

blood pressure >140 mm Hg, diastolic blood pressure >90 mm Hg, or currently taking antihypertensive medications. Using these criteria, approximately 50 million Americans were deemed hypertensive. As seen in Table 2, there had been a gratifying increase in patient awareness, use of antihypertensive therapy, and control of BP, but this success has not been sustained more recently. Since the inception of the National High Blood Pressure Education Program (NHBPEP) in 1972, there has been a concomitant decrease in age-adjusted cardiovascular mortality rates, with a marked reduction in deaths from coronary heart disease (about 50%) and stroke (about 57%) over the past two decades. Nevertheless, the JNC VI report issued some notes of caution because BP control rates remain low, and the prevalence of congestive heart failure, renal failure, and stroke are increasing.

Special subsets within a population have an increased risk of hypertension. Both age and race are important variables. Blood pressure, especially systolic blood pressure, increases with age such that hypertension is quite common in the elderly. Over 50% of adults older than 65

TABLE 2

Trends in the Awareness, Treatment, and Control of High Blood Pressure in Adults: United States, 1976–1994[a]

	NHANES II (1976–1980) (%)	NHANES III (Phase 1) (1988–1991) (%)	NHANES III (Phase 2) (1991–1994) (%)
Awareness	51.0	73.0	68.4
Treated	31.0	55.0	53.6
Controlled[b]	10.0	29.0	27.4

[a]Adults age 18 to 74 years with systolic blood pressure (SBP) ≥140 mm Hg or diastolic blood pressure (DBP) ≥90 mm Hg or taking antihypertensive medication

[b]SBP <140 mm Hg and DBP <90 mm Hg. Source: Adapted from Burt V, Cutler JA, Higgins M, et al. Trends in the prevalence, awareness, treatment, and control of hypertension in the adult US population: Data from the health examination surveys, 1960 to 1991. *Hypertension* 25:305–313, 1995. Unpublished data from the National Center for Health Statistics, 1997 (NHANES III, Phase 2).

have a systolic blood pressure greater than 140 or diastolic blood pressure greater than 90. Isolated systolic hypertension, defined as systolic pressure >140 and diastolic pressure <90, is particularly problematic in the elderly population. Isolated systolic hypertension confers the same cardiovascular risk of stroke, congestive heart failure, and coronary heart disease as does combined systolic/diastolic hypertension. During the recent trials of isolated systolic hypertension in the elderly, active treatment with diuretic or long-acting dihydropyridine calcium antagonist significantly reduced stroke and coronary heart disease. Active treatment of systolic/diastolic hypertension in the elderly in the Swedish Trial in Old Patients with Hypertension (STOP-Hypertension) and the Medical Research Council (MRC) trial with a diuretic- and β-blocker-based regimen significantly reduced all cardiovascular mortality. Overall, the elderly have a greater prevalence of hypertension, yet they benefit from active antihypertensive therapy.

Race is also an important variable regarding the prevalence and target organ effects of elevated systemic pressure. Hypertension is nearly twice as common in African-Americans, and rates of more severe hypertension (diastolic blood pressure >105) are severalfold higher than in their White counterparts. Furthermore, for a given level of hypertension, African-Americans tend to have more target organ damage with left ventricular hypertrophy (LVH), strokes, and renal insufficiency.

Overall, cardiovascular risk in the entire population increases with elevation of systemic pressure above an "optimal" of 120/80. Simply stated, "the higher the pressure. . . the higher the risk." For example, a sustained elevation of diastolic pressure of 5–6 mm Hg increases the risk of stroke by 34% and the risk of coronary heart disease by 21%. Conversely, reduction of blood pressure by a similar degree during large-scale antihypertensive studies has lowered the rate of stroke by approximately 40%, although it only reduced coronary heart disease by about 14%. Additional cardiovascular risk factors such as hyperlipidemia, diabetes mellitus, smoking, and LVH may coexist with hypertension in any given patient. The goal of antihypertensive therapy in the twenty-first century is both the reduction of systemic blood pressure and the simultaneous modification of other cardiovascular risk factors. Increasingly, LVH has been identified as an independent risk factor for coronary heart disease and congestive heart failure. A recent meta-analysis suggests that different classes of antihypertensive agents may reduce blood pressure equally well, but have a variable effect on the regression of LVH. Whether regression of LVH in the short term translates into reduced patient morbidity and mortality remains to be determined.

To date, the incidence of end stage renal disease (ESRD) attributed to hypertension and nephrosclerosis has increased and remains a leading cause of renal failure in the African-American community. The question of which antihypertensive agents could have a renal protective effect remains unclear. The Afro-American Study of Kidney Disease (AASKD) has been initiated to address this important issue.

CLASSIFICATION OF HYPERTENSION

Over 90% of all patients with high blood pressure presenting to their primary care physician will have essential hypertension, as the cause of their hypertension is not readily definable. A classification of hypertension is outlined in Table 3, with the estimates of prevalence of the various forms of hypertension within the general population also listed. As seen in the table, approximately 5–10% of patients may have secondary forms of hypertension. Renal parenchymal disease is the most common medical condition associated with hypertension. Renovascular hypertension is the most common potentially remediable form of hypertension. Primary aldosteronism, pheochromocytoma, and Cushing's syndrome are seen less frequently. Note that use of oral contraceptives, excesses of alcohol, and cocaine abuse present potentially reversible causes of hypertension.

PATHOPHYSIOLOGY

Simply stated, blood pressure is the product of cardiac output and total peripheral resistance (TPR), that is,

$$BP = CO \times \overline{TPR}$$

TABLE 3
Classification of Hypertension

	Prevalence(%)
Essential (primary) hypertension	90–95
Secondary hypertension	5–10
Renal	2.5–6.0
Renal parenchymal disease	
Polycystic kidney disease	
Urinary tract obstruction	
Renin-producing tumor	
Liddle's syndrome	
Renovascular hypertension	0.2–4.0
or renal infarction	
Coarctation of the aorta	
Endocrine	1–2
Oral contraceptives	
Adrenal	
Primary aldosteronism	
Cushing's syndrome	
Pheochromocytoma	
Congenital adrenal hyperplasia	
Glucocorticoid remediable HBP	
(11 β-hydroxylase deficiency)	
Thyroid (hypo- and hyper-)	
Hypercalcemia	
Hyperparathyroidism	
Exogenous hormones—glucocorticoids,	
mineralocorticoids, sympathomimetics	
Pregnancy-induced hypertension	
Neurogenic	
Alcohol, cocaine, and medications	
(cyclosporine A, erythropoietin)	

Nearly all forms of sustained clinical hypertension are due to an elevation of TPR in the face of a normal or mildly depressed cardiac output. This simple concept is important to grasp in order to appreciate the intricacies of pathophysiology and implications for therapeutic intervention. In over 90% of cases, the precise cause of hypertension is not readily definable, and the patient is said to have idiopathic or essential hypertension. The etiology of essential hypertension is a heterogeneous mixture of complex interactions of heredity/environmental factors, sodium homeostasis, the renin–angiotensin system, sympathetic nervous system, and other factors which are incompletely understood. A detailed discussion of the pathophysiology of hypertension is found in Chapter 69.

CLINICAL PRESENTATION

Hypertension is often discovered in an asymptomatic individual as a result of a community screening program or during an evaluation for another clinical problem. As noted previously, the systemic pressure should be persistently elevated on at least three different occasions before labeling a patient as "hypertensive." The next important decision is the extent of the diagnostic evaluation required. Three key questions need to be addressed:

1. What is the cause of hypertension? Specifically, is there a potentially reversible form of secondary hypertension?
2. Is there evidence for target organ damage?
3. Are there coexistent cardiovascular risk factors?

All patients should undergo a thorough medical history and physical examination and have a selected laboratory evaluation to address these three important questions. The JNC VI report emphasizes that all hypertensive patients should be "staged" based on their systolic and diastolic BP determinations (Table 1). Furthermore, it is recommended that the physician note whether clinically evident target organ damage (or diabetes mellitus) is present or absent (see Table 4), because therapeutic recommendations will be based on this classification. The following evaluation is recommended by JNC VI.

Medical History

A detailed medical history should include the following:

- Known duration and level of blood pressure elevation
- Antihypertensive therapy, results and side effects
- History of cardiovascular, cerebrovascular, or renal disease and knowledge of diabetes, hyperlipidemia, or gout
- Symptoms suggesting secondary hypertension
- Family history of hypertension
- Family history of premature atherosclerotic heart disease, stroke, diabetes, or hyperlipidemia
- History of weight gain, smoking, physical activity, or mental stress
- Dietary assessment including salt, fat, and alcohol use
- Thorough medication history—especially oral

TABLE 4

Components of Cardiovascular Risk Stratification in Patients with Hypertension[a]

Major risk factors	Target organ damage/clinical cardiovascular disease
Smoking	Heart disease
Dyslipidemia	Left ventricular hypertrophy
Diabetes mellitus	Angina/prior myocardial infarction
Age older than 60 years	Prior coronary revascularization
Gender (men and postmenopausal women)	Heart failure
	Stroke or transient ischemic attack
Family history of cardiovascular disease: women under age 65 or men under age 55	Nephropathy
	Peripheral arterial disease
	Retinopathy

[a]Source: JNC VI.

contraceptives, steroids, nonsteroidal antiinflammatory drugs (NSAIDS), cold remedies, appetite suppressants, tricyclic antidepressants, MAO inhibitors, cyclosporine, erythropoietin, cocaine

Blood Pressure Measurements

The patient must refrain from smoking, caffeine, and exogenous adrenergic stimulants for 30–60 min. The patient should be resting comfortably (seated or supine) in a quiet room for at least 5 min. Using the appropriate equipment and cuff size (15 cm wide cuff with bladder size 80% of arm circumference), two or more BP measurements separated by 2 min should be obtained and then repeated after standing for at least 2 min. During the initial exam, verify blood pressure in the contralateral arm (if different, the higher value should be used).

Physical Exam

A thorough examination is required to search for evidence of target organ damage (see Table 4) or a cause of secondary hypertension. The initial exam should include the following:

- Height and weight
- Fundoscopic exam (with pupil dilatation if necessary) for arteriolar narrowing, arteriovenous nicking, hemorrhages, exudates, or papilledema (see Table 5)
- Examination of the neck for carotid bruits, jugular venous distension, thyroid gland enlargement
- Examination of the heart for rhythm, displaced point of maximal impulse, murmur, or congestive heart failure
- Examination of the abdomen for bruits, large kidneys, masses, or abnormal aortic pulsations
- Examination of the extremities for decreased or absent pulses, bruits, or edema
- Neurologic assessment

TABLE 5
Simplified Classification of Hypertensive Retinopathy

| Group | Retinal arterioles | | Hemorrhages | Exudates | Papilledema |
	Sclerosis	Narrowing grade			
1	<1	0–4	−	−	−
2	1 or more	0–4	±	−	−
3	0–4	0–4	±	+	−
4	0–4	0–4	±	±	+

Routine Laboratory Evaluation

The JNC VI has recommended that a few laboratory tests should be performed routinely prior to initiating therapy. These studies include: urinalysis, serum chemistry profile (fasting blood sugar, potassium, creatinine, calcium, uric acid), cholesterol/triglyceride profile, and electrocardiogram (EKG). The purpose of this testing is to screen for secondary causes of hypertension, cardiovascular risk factors, and existent cardiovascular disease. Although the echocardiogram is a more sensitive test than the EKG for detecting LVH, routine echocardiography is not recommended because of cost concerns. In the diabetic hypertensive population, the presence of microalbuminuria may be predictive of the increased risk of renal or cardiovascular disease. Additional laboratory testing for secondary forms of hypertension may be required if clinical suspicion exists.

Searching for Remediable Forms of Hypertension

In general, patients with essential hypertension present during midlife (35–55 years of age) with mild to moderate hypertension, mild or no target organ damage, and frequently have a family history of hypertension. However, a common exception is the young African-American male with essential hypertension who may present with severe hypertension and significant renal impairment or LVH. Table 6 summarizes the clinical features that are "atypical" for essential hypertension and should alert the physician to possible sec-

ondary forms of hypertension. Five to ten percent of all hypertensive patients may have definable forms of secondary hypertension, as outlined in Table 3. For example, patients with edema and proteinuria may have renal parenchymal disease requiring further evaluation. Patients with a family history of renal disease and hypertension who have a normal urinalysis should undergo renal ultrasonography to screen for polycystic kidney disease. Others with severe or resistant hypertension and/or an abdominal bruit may be candidates to screen for renovascular hypertension. (See Chapter 71). Coarctation of the aorta should be excluded by careful examination with blood pressures measured in the upper and lower extremities.

In selected cases, adrenal causes of hypertension should be considered as potentially remediable forms of hypertension. Patients with a symptom complex suggestive of pheochromocytoma (episodic hypertension, sweats, headaches, etc.) may be evaluated with plasma catecholamines, urinary vanillylmandelic acid/metanephrines, or a clonidine suppression test. Clinical clues suggesting Cushing's syndrome may be investigated with a dexamethesone suppression test and adrenocorticotrophic hormone (ACTH) measurement. Alternatively, patients with unprovoked hypokalemia and metabolic alkalosis may be screened biochemically for aldosterone overproduction. If a biochemical abnormality is suggestive of adrenal hyperfunction in these three states, the adrenal glands should be imaged with thin-cut computerized tomography.

TABLE 6
Features Suggesting Secondary Hypertension

Clinical features
Age of onset <30 or >55
Abrupt onset, severe hypertension (≥stage 3)
Hypertension resistant to effective medical therapy
Target organ damage (TOD)
Fundi with acute hemorrhages/exudates
Renal dysfunction
Left ventricular hypertrophy
Features indicative of secondary hypertension
Unprovoked hypokalemia
Abdominal bruit or diffuse atherosclerosis
ACE inhibitor-induced renal dysfunction
Labile hypertension, sweats, tremor, headache
Family history of renal disease
Palpable polycystic kidneys

THERAPY

The overall goal of antihypertensive therapy for patients with essential hypertension is to reduce cardiovascular morbidity and mortality. The goal of therapy may be best met by both lowering elevated systemic pressure and favorably modifying other cardiovascular risk factors. Specifics of nonpharmacologic and pharmacologic therapy in the management of the hypertensive patient are detailed in Chapter 72.

Bibliography
Bravo EL: Pheochromocytoma and mineralocorticoid hypertension. In: Glassock RJ (eds) *Current Therapy in Nephrology and Hypertension*, 4th Ed., pp. 330–334. Mosby-Year Book, St. Louis, 1998.
Bravo EL: Evolving concepts in the pathophysiology, diagnosis, and treatment of pheochromocytoma. *Endocr Rev* 15:356–368, 1998.

Breslin DJ, Gifford RW, Fairbairn JF, *et al.:* Prognostic importance of ophthalmoscopic findings in essential hypertension. *JAMA* 195: 335–338, 1996.

Burt VL, Whelton P, Roccella EJ, *et al.:* Prevalence of hypertension in the US adult population. Results from the Third National Health and Nutrition Examination Survey, 1988–1991. *Hypertension* 25:305–313, 1995.

Dahlöf B, Lindholm LH, Hansson L, *et al.:* Morbidity and mortality in the Swedish Trial in Old Patients with Hypertension (STOP-Hypertension). *Lancet* 338:1281–1284, 1991.

Kannel WB, Wilson WF: Cardiovascular risk factors and hypertension. In: Izzo JL, Jr, Black HR (eds) *Hypertension Primer,* 2nd Ed., pp. 199–202. American Heart Association, Dallas, Texas, 1999.

Kaplan NM: *Clinical Hypertension,* 7th Ed. Williams & Wilkins, New York, 1997.

MRC Working Party: Medical Research Council trial of treatment of hypertension in older adults: Principal results. *Br Med J* 304: 405–412, 1992.

Neaton JD, Kuller L, Stamler J, *et al.:* Impact of systolic and diastolic blood pressure on cardiovascular mortality. In: Laragh JH, Brenner BM (eds) *Hypertension: Pathophysiology, Diagnosis and Management,* 2nd Ed., pp. 127–144. Raven, New York, 1995.

Savage PJ, Pressel SL, Curb JD, *et al.:* Influence of long-term, low-dose, diuretic-based, antihypertensive therapy on glucose, lipid, uric acid, and potassium levels in older men and women with isolated systolic hypertension: The Systolic Hypertension in the Elderly Program. SHEP Cooperative Research Group. *Arch Intern Med* 158:741–751, 1998.

Schmieder RE, Martus P, Klingbeil A: Reversal of left ventricular hypertrophy in essential hypertension. A meta-analysis of randomized double-blind studies. *JAMA* 275:1507–1513, 1996.

HEP Cooperative Research Group: Prevention of stroke by antihypertensive drug treatment in older persons with isolated systolic hypertension. Final results of the Systolic Hypertension in the Elderly Program (SHEP). *JAMA* 265:3255–3264, 1991.

The Sixth Report of the Joint National Committee on Detection, Evaluation, and Treatment of High Blood Pressure. *Arch Intern Med* 157:2413–2446, 1997.

Tuomilehto J, Rastenyte D, Birkenhager WH, *et al.:* Effects of calcium-channel blockade in older patients with diabetes and systolic hypertension. Systolic Hypertension in Europe Trial Investigators. *N Engl J Med* 340:677–684, 1999.

71

RENOVASCULAR HYPERTENSION

LAURA P. SVETKEY AND PRESTON KLASSEN

Renovascular hypertension is a potentially curable form of high blood pressure. Its treatment, with angioplasty, stenting, or surgery, provides the opportunity to prevent cardiovascular morbidity and mortality due to hypertension and to avoid the expense and potential morbidity of life-long pharmacotherapy for hypertension. Therefore, hypertension due to renal artery stenosis should be identified and treated whenever possible.

DEFINITION

Renovascular hypertension (RVH) is defined as high blood pressure secondary to renal artery stenosis. In clinical practice the diagnosis is made retrospectively, that is, one can conclude that a patient has RVH if hypertension improves after correction of a renal artery stenosis. Improvement in blood pressure, as defined by the Cooperative Study of Renovascular Hypertension, means that previously elevated blood pressure becomes normal without antihypertensive medication, or that less medication is required to control blood pressure. Hypertension does not have to be cured to make the diagnosis of RVH.

Any process that narrows a main renal artery can cause RVH. In this discussion, renal artery stenosis (RAS) will generally refer to narrowing of a main renal artery, although stenosis of a branch or accessory artery may occasionally be responsible for RVH. In the United States, 70–80% of stenoses are due to atherosclerotic lesions, usually a manifestation of generalized atherosclerosis obliterans. The majority of atherosclerotic stenoses are ostial in location and involve extensions of bulky aortic plaques extending into the renal artery takeoff. Nonostial lesions also occur and involve the main trunk of the renal artery and occasionally its branches. Fibromuscular dysplasia (FMD) is the second most common cause of RAS, accounting for approximately 15–20% of all cases. Rarely, stenosis may be due to neurofibromatosis, radiation fibrosis, extrinsic compression, embolism, congenital anomaly, and Takayasu's disease.

Experimental studies indicate that the amount of cross-sectional obstruction required to produce significant hemodynamic change leading to hypertension and renal parenchymal injury is at least 75–80%, but the critical value in humans is unknown. Although it is often difficult to determine the true extent of an obstruction with two-dimensional angiography, most institutions use a cutoff of >50% or >70% stenosis to indicate a hemodynamically significant lesion.

PATHOPHYSIOLOGY

Knowledge of the pathophysiology of RVH comes primarily from experimental animal models; mechanisms of RVH in humans are presumed to be similar. The Goldblatt two-kidney, one-clip model best represents the condition of unilateral RAS and involves hypersecretion of renin by the ischemic kidney as a result of decreased perfusion pressure and delivery of sodium to the macula densa. Renin secretion increases circulating levels of the powerful vasoconstrictor angiotensin II as well as aldosterone. The sympathetic system is also activated by elevated angiotensin II and plays a role in maintaining hypertension. Euvolemia is maintained because the contralateral kidney exhibits normal perfusion and a pressure natriuresis. Human bilateral RAS shares some features of the two-kidney, one-clip model. However, patients with bilateral disease also tend to have intravascular volume excess, evidenced by higher cardiac output, flash pulmonary edema, and a diuretic phase after revascularization.

The relationship between the renin–angiotensin system and blood pressure in RVH evolves through three distinct phases (Fig. 1). In the first phase, seen in experimental models, acute stenosis results in rising renin levels and a parallel increase in blood pressure. After a period of time, renin levels fall and may approach the normal range but blood pressure remains elevated. This transitional phase exhibits a heightened vascular response to lower levels of angiotensin II. During both the acute and transition phases,

hypertension is responsive to removal of the stenosis, antiotensin II blockade, or removal of the affected kidney. Over months to years, there is a gradual progression to a chronic phase in which correction of the stenosis does not ameliorate hypertension. Elevated blood pressure is maintained as a result of long-standing hypertension-induced changes in the renal parenchyma. The clinical significance of this final phase is that RVH present for a prolonged period of time is less likely to benefit from attempts at revascularization.

EPIDEMIOLOGY

The prevalence of RVH among the hypertensive population is approximately 1%, with estimates ranging from 0.5 to 5.0%. Based on clinical criteria, however, a subset of the hypertensive population that has a higher prevalence, approximately 25–40%, can easily be selected. In particular, malignant hypertension or history of hypertensive emergency, abrupt onset of hypertension at age <20 or >50, hypertension refractory to aggressive medical therapy, an abdominal bruit, concurrent renal insufficiency, hypotension or an increase in serum creatinine with angiotensin converting enzyme (ACE) inhibition, and asymmetry of kidney size are all indicators that suggest the presence of RVH. RVH has been reported to be extremely rare in the African-American population. However, when appropriate clinically selected groups are examined by arteriography, African-Americans have a similar prevalence to White patients. Atherosclerotic renovascular disease has a high enough frequency in both sexes that gender should not be used to determine whether to proceed with invasive testing. Severe hypertension in a young female may raise the suspicion of RVH due to FMD. Tobacco use is a risk factor for general atherosclerosis as well as FMD, although smoking is too widely prevalent to be useful in distinguishing RVH from essential hypertension. Physicians should use the clinical history and exam to determine if a patient is at low, intermediate, or high risk for RVH (Table 1). Those at low risk do not need further workup. Patients with a high degree of suspicion for RVH should proceed directly to arteriography. It is the group of patients with intermediate risk that are selected for noninvasive testing to determine the need for further invasive tests.

NATURAL HISTORY

Retrospective angiographic studies and more recent reports suggest that atherosclerotic RAS is a progressive disorder. The rate of progression appears to be related to the degree of the initial stenosis; lesions with a greater degree of stenosis have a higher chance of progressing. RAS may play a role in morbidity and mortality independent of its effect on blood pressure. For example, within a population of patients undergoing cardiac catheterization, those with >50% RAS have a significantly lower 4-year survival compared to patients without RAS. These data suggest that RAS may be involved in morbidity and mortality, either

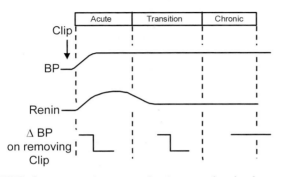

FIGURE 1 Phases of renovascular hypertension in the two-kidney, one-clip Goldblatt rat.

TABLE I
Clinical Index of Suspicion for RVH

Low (<5%)—no further testing indicated
  Borderline, mild, or moderate hypertension in the absence of
  other clinical clues

Moderate (5–15%)—obtain noninvasive testing to screen for
RVH/RAS
  Severe hypertension (diastolic BP greater than 120 mm Hg)
  Hypertension refractory to standard therapy
  Abrupt onset of sustained, moderate to severe hypertension
    at age <20 or >50 years
  Moderate hypertension (diastolic BP greater than 105 mm Hg)
    in a smoker, a patient with evidence of occlusive vascular
    disease (cerebrovascular, coronary, peripheral), or a patient
    with unexplained but stable elevation of serum creatinine
  Normalization of blood pressure by an angiotensin converting
    enzyme inhibitor in a patient with moderate or severe
    hypertension, particularly in a smoker or patient with recent
    onset of hypertension. (Absence of blood pressure response
    does not rule out RVH.)

High (>25%)—Proceed directly to arteriography
  Severe hypertension (diastolic BP greater than 120 mm Hg)
    with either progressive renal insufficiency or refractoriness
    to aggressive treatment (particularly in a patient who has
    been a smoker or has other evidence of occlusive arterial
    disease)
  Accelerated or malignant hypertension (grade III or IV
    retinopathy)
  Hypertension with a suggestive abdominal bruit (long,
    high-pitched, and localized to the region of the renal artery)
  Hypertension with recent elevation of serum creatinine, either
    unexplained or reversibly induced by an angiotensin
    converting enzyme inhibitor
  Moderate to severe hypertension with incidentally detected
    asymmetry of renal size

[a]Table adapted with permission from Mann SJ, Pickering TG:
Detection of renovascular hypertension. State of the art: 1992.
Ann Inter Med 117:845–853, 1992.

etiologically or as a marker for athersclerotic disease else-where. In addition, attention is now directed at the role RAS plays in ischemic parenchymal damage leading to renal insufficiency and end stage renal disease (ESRD). Without prospective data, it is difficult to determine the exact impact of RAS as an etiology of ESRD. However, retrospective investigations have suggested it accounts for 12–15%, raising the possibility of prevention of ESRD through revascularization. The importance of revascularization is highlighted by anecdotal reports of dialysis-dependent patients recovering renal function after correction of atherosclerotic RAS.

DIAGNOSTIC TESTS

The gold standard of diagnosis for RVH is blood pressure response to interventional therapy, an assessment that can only be made retrospectively. In clinical practice, however, diagnostic tests are used to detect RAS, which is a necessary precondition for the diagnosis of RVH. The gold standard for documenting renal artery stenosis is conventional contrast arteriography of the renal arteries. For patients with a moderate clinical suspicion of RVH, the risk and expense of invasive testing may not be warranted, and in these instances noninvasive testing is utilized. In addition, a few noninvasive procedures [captopril renography, duplex ultrasound, and magnetic resonance angiography (MRA)] have been advocated by some as having sensitivity and specificity high enough to justify directly proceeding to percutaneous revascularization. Many tests previously used to screen for RAS, such as plasma renin activity and the captopril provocation test, have been discarded due to low sensitivity and specificity compared to angiography. One of the most persistent dilemmas regarding RVH is determining which noninvasive test offers the best chance of resolving whether or not the condition is present. Because of differences in definitions, patient selection, and use of arteriography across studies, comparison of different techniques is difficult. Institutions report widely varying results for some tests, underscoring the fact that many techniques are operator-dependent. Until recently, the noninvasive diagnostic procedure of choice was captopril renography. Advances in ultrasound and magnetic resonance imaging are challenging this convention and require consideration.

ACE Inhibitor-Stimulated Renography

In the setting of RVH, both glomerular filtration rate and renal plasma flow depend on angiotensin II-mediated constriction of the glomerular efferent arteriole. Treatment with an ACE inhibitor antagonizes this vasoconstriction and decreases renal uptake and excretion of radiopharmaceuticals. A renogram is considered abnormal at baseline if there is evidence of asymmetric function, or if uptake or excretion of the marker is delayed. RAS is suspected if the abnormalities are exacerbated by ACE inhibition. Review of the literature suggests that sensitivity of captopril renography is approximately 88–92%, and specificity is slightly higher. A wide range exists, however, with some institutions reporting sensitivities near 70%. Moreover, the accuracy of this test is significantly reduced in the setting of renal insufficiency, a common finding in this population. Accuracy may also be reduced in bilateral disease. A positive renogram is strongly supportive of a diagnosis of RAS and is an indication for arteriography and intervention if an anatomic lesion is confirmed. In patients with normal renal function and a 10 to 20% likelihood of RAS based on clinical assessment, a negative renogram may be sufficient to rule out RAS.

Duplex Ultrasound

Clinicians occasionally use standard ultrasound to detect asymmetry in kidney size as a clue to renovascular disease. However, it is likely that by the time there has been sufficient loss of renal parenchyma distal to a unilateral stenosis to lead to renal asymmetry, revascularization has little to offer. In addition, there may be no asymmetry with bilateral stenosis. The use of color-flow Doppler in the diagnosis of RVH is an attempt to combine anatomic information from ultrasound with hemodynamic information from Doppler. This technique is seriously limited by its failure to visualize the proximal main renal artery in 25% of cases. In addition, small accessory and secondary renal arteries are often not detected. Duplex ultrasound is technically demanding, highly operator-dependent, and time-consuming. The high sensitivity and specificity reported from some research centers has not been duplicated in other centers. Recent advances in Doppler ultrasonography include the introduction of ultrasound contrast agents, such as microbubble echoenhancers, thereby improving the ability to visualize the renal arteries. These new developments may enhance the future utility of ultrasound as a screening tool in RVH.

Magnetic Resonance Angiography

MRA is a noninvasive modality that provides information about both anatomy and blood flow (Fig. 2). Compared to arteriography, MRA with three-dimensional gadolinium contrast scanning (3D-Gd) appears to have excellent sensitivity (>95%) and specificity (>90) for detecting stenosis of a main renal artery. The ability to accurately detect smaller accessory renal arteries is clearly lower, with aggregate sensitivity probably below 90% (although specificity is improved). In addition, prior studies have looked mainly at proximal renal artery stenosis, making this modality potentially less useful in the case of fibromuscular dysplasia where lesions are often at branch arteries. Along with providing anatomic information, MRA

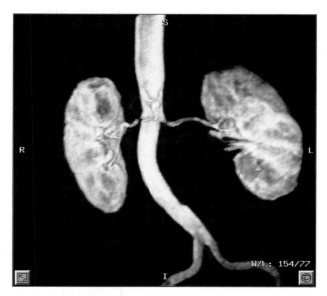

FIGURE 2 Magnetic resonance angiogram demonstrating high grade (>75%) ostial stenosis of the right renal artery and high grade near-ostial stenosis on the left. The left kidney measures 8 cm and the right 9.5 cm in length. Cortical thinning of the right upper, left lower, and left upper pole is also present.

techniques have been used to give information on the functional significance of stenotic lesions. The high cost of MRA is an important issue, but there has been no formal cost analysis of different diagnostic strategies. Although MRA has yet to be widely accepted as the noninvasive procedure of choice, it has supplanted renography in a number of institutions. In addition, MRA may offer a reasonable alternative to conventional arteriography in patients with high pretest probability of stenosis but who are also at high risk for contrast-related complications.

DIAGNOSTIC STRATEGY

The utility of any given test for screening and diagnosis of RVH will depend on the prevalence of RVH in the population being evaluated (the pretest probability) and on the sensitivity and specificity of the test. Even an excellent screening test, for example, one with 90% sensitivity and 90% specificity, will provide little help if the prior probability of RVH is low. If one assumes that unselected hypertensives have a 5% chance of having RVH, this hypothetical test will increase that likelihood to 32% if it is positive, leaving 68% of those with an abnormal test with a false positive result. A negative test will essentially rule out RVH (negative predictive value = 99%), but the likelihood that RVH was absent was 95% before the test.

Because of these limitations of diagnostic tests that perform well, Mann and Pickering have suggested a strategy, somewhat modified here, for selecting patients for further evaluation (Table 1). This strategy involves the definition of subgroups, based on the clinical suspicion (pretest probability) of RVH.

If a patient has a history of malignant hypertension, history of renal failure following ACE inhibitor, or the presence of an abdominal or flank bruit, the likelihood of finding RAS is greater than 30%, and one should proceed directly to angiography. In addition, if the motivation to find RAS is extremely high, for instance if a patient has severe hypertension (JNC-6 stage 3) that is difficult to control in the setting of progressive renal insufficiency, or if the patient has moderate hypertension (stage 2) and is unable to tolerate any antihypertensive regimen, then it is reasonable to proceed directly to angiography. In some circumstances with high pretest probability, such as coexistent renal disease or other relative contraindication to arteriography, it may be preferable to perform MRA first.

At the other end of the spectrum, if a patient has borderline or mild hypertension (stage 1) that is easily controlled, and none of the clinical clues previously discussed are present, then no further workup is indicated.

Diagnostic difficulties arise in patients with clinical clues that lead to an intermediate pretest probability of RVH. This group comprises, for example, those with severe hypertension without history of a malignant or accelerated phase, abrupt onset of hypertension very early or very late in life, sudden increase in the severity of chronic hypertension, and unexplained renal insufficiency, especially if there is evidence of vascular disease elsewhere. In this sub-group, a noninvasive test may be helpful and the physician must choose between MRA, ACE inhibitor renography, or Doppler ultrasonography. The choice of test may depend in part on the experience of the institution. For example, some centers have excellent results with Doppler ultrasonography, whereas many others do not. Overall, MRA offers high sensitivity, can be used in renal insufficiency, and provides anatomic evaluation along with information regarding blood flow and filtration rates. These characteristics make MRA a powerful test that should become the primary noninvasive diagnostic modality in the search for RAS in patients with intermediate probability of stenosis.

TREATMENT

Once RAS has been demonstrated, the options for management include renal artery angioplasty, arterial stenting, surgery, and medical therapy. In addition to the treatment of hypertension, preservation of renal function has become an important goal of revascularization. Even when hypertension is not cured (probably the majority of cases), revascularization with angioplasty, stenting, or surgery often results in decreased blood pressure or decreased antihypertensive medication.

Angioplasty

Advantages of percutaneous transluminal renal angioplasty (PTA) over surgery include the avoidance of general anesthesia, shorter hospitalization, and potential ability to repeat the procedure if needed. Complications, though rare, include contrast-induced renal failure, atheroemboli, rupture or dissection of the renal artery, thrombotic occlusion of the vessel, pseudoaneurysm, and hematoma. Cardiovascular events including myocardial infarction, stroke, and flash pulmonary edema have also been reported. The overall mortality in most studies is quite low, approximately 0–2%. Overall, the data suggest that the technical success of dilating an atherosclerotic lesion is quite good for nonstial plaques, on the order of 70–90%. Ostial lesions involve extensions of bulky aortic plaque and are prone to elastic recoil, causing a lower rate of technical success (approximately 30–60%) and higher rates of restenosis. When successful, angioplasty improves or cures renovascular hypertension due to atherosclerosis in 55–70% of cases. Complete cures, however, occur in less than 10% of patients. Stenosis due to FMD responds favorably in 60–100% of cases, with 20–60% cured. In patients with renal insufficiency, successful angioplasty improves or stabilizes kidney function in more than 50% of cases.

The main limitations of PTA are primary failure and subsequent restenosis. Primary failure occurs if the balloon catheter cannot be passed beyond the lesion. In addition, even when the procedure can be performed, angiography performed immediately after dilatation occasionally demonstrates persistent stenosis. These problems will be detected at the time of the procedure, and

should lead to alternative treatment (either repeat PTA, stenting, or surgical revascularization). After successful angioplasty, restenosis will occur over the following year in approximately 20%, with slightly higher rates in patients with atherosclerotic than FMD lesions. When restenosis occurs following PRA, a second angioplasty is often successful, but stenting or surgical revascularization may ultimately be necessary. Angioplasty is the procedure of choice in RAS due to FMD and may be useful in nonstial atherosclerotic lesions.

Renal Artery Stenting

The introduction of stents has markedly improved success rates in relieving ostial RAS. Stenting results in 95–100% initial patency in ostial lesions, with similar rates of success for more distal lesions that have failed renal artery angioplasty alone. Reported restenosis rates vary widely (from 6 to 65%) but are less than angioplasty alone. Hypertension is improved or cured in 40 to 70% of cases, with about 10% representing complete cure. Renal function improves or stabilizes in 66 to 95% of cases. Approximately 20 to 25% of patients experience worsening renal function. Because of the increased patency rates with good clinical response and similar complications to angioplasty, primary renal artery stenting is the revascularization procedure of choice in most patients with ostial atherosclerotic RAS.

Surgical Correction

Bypass procedures are the most common surgical treatment used for RAS. The technical success of vascular reconstruction is high, and restenosis rates are usually less than 10%. Operative mortality is higher than that of percutaneous procedures, ranging from 3 to 20%. Hypertension associated with atherosclerotic RAS shows improvement or cure in 60 to 90% of patients. Improvement or stabilization of renal function occurs in over 80% of patients. Surgery is preferable over percutaneous revascularization when revascularization is critical (e.g., uncontrollable hypertension) and few surgical risk factors are present. Surgery remains a primary therapy for distal disease and many cases of total renal artery occlusion with a viable kidney. It is also a secondary approach for patients who have failed initial attempts with angioplasty or stenting.

Medical Therapy

The development of powerful antihypertensive medications raises the possibility that medical management would be sufficient to control blood pressure in the setting of RAS. There have been three reports of randomized trials comparing angioplasty to medical therapy, but none involved the use of stents. The first two studies involved small numbers of patients with short follow-up times (6 months). No differences in blood pressure or renal function were seen between the angioplasty and medical therapy groups. The largest trial randomized 106 patients with

RAS to receive angioplasty or medical therapy. Although the angioplasty group took fewer antihypertensive medications, according to an intention-to-treat analysis there were no differences in blood pressure or renal function at 12 months. The analysis of this trial is hampered by the fact that 22 of 50 patients assigned to medical therapy eventually underwent angioplasty during the follow-up period because of persistent hypertension or deteriorating renal function. These studies suggest that angioplasty does not result in dramatic clinical improvement compared to medical therapy. However, the reality that many patients in the medical therapy group did undergo an interventional procedure underscores the belief that anatomic correction of RAS represents the best chance to restore normal hemodynamic and vasoactive relationships in the kidney. In summary, relief of renal artery stenosis by angioplasty with or without stenting is likely to improve blood pressure control and may preserve renal parenchyma, but the superiority of revascularization over medical therapy has not been definitively established.

Bibliography

Bonelli FS, McKusick MA, Textor SC, *et al.:* Renal artery angioplasty: Technical results and clinical outcome in 320 patients. *Mayo Clin Proc* 70:1041–1052, 1995.

Conlon PJ, O'Riordan E, Kalra PA: New insights into the epidemiologic and clinical manifestations of atherosclerotic renovascular disease. *Am J Kidney Dis* 35:573–587, 2000.

Dorros G, Jaff M, Mathiak L, *et al.:* Four-year follow-up of Palmaz–Schatz stent revascularization as treatment for atherosclerotic renal artery stenosis. *Circulation* 98:642–647, 1998.

Isles CG, Robertson S, Hill D: Management of renovascular disease: A review of renal artery stenting in ten studies. *Q J Med* 92:159–167, 1999.

Lencioni R, Pinto S, Napoli V, Bartolozzi C: Noninvasive assessment of renal artery stenosis: Current imaging protocols and futures, directions in ultrasonography. *J Computer Assisted Tomography* 23(Suppl 1):S95–S100, 1993.

Mailloux LU, Napolitano B, Bellucci AG, Vernace M, Wilkes BM, Mossey RT: Renal vascular disease causing end-stage renal disease, incidence, clinical correlates, and outcomes: A 20-year clinical experience. *Am J Kidney Dis* 24:622–629, 1994.

Mann SJ, Pickering TG: Detection of renovascular hypertension: State of the art, 1992. *Ann Intern Med* 117:845–853, 1992.

Martinez-Maldonado M: Pathophysiology of renovascular hypertension. *Hypertension* 17:707–719, 1991.

Nally JV, Jr, Olin JW, Lammert GK: Advances in noninvasive screening for renovascular disease. *Clev Clin J Med* 61:328–336, 1994.

Novick AC: Surgical revascularization for renovascular hypertension and preservation of renal function. In: Laragh JH, Brenner BM (eds) *Hypertension: Pathophysiology, Diagnosis, and Management,* pp. 2055–2068. Raven, New York, 1995.

Olin JW, Piedmonte MR, Young JR, DeAnna S, Grubb M, Childs MB: The utility of duplex ultrasound scanning of the renal arteries for diagnosing significant renal artery stenosis. *Ann Intern Med* 122:833–838, 1995.

Ramsay LE, Waller PC: Blood pressure response to percutaneous transluminal angioplasty for renovascular hypertension: An overview of published series. *Br Med J (Clin Res* Ed.) 300:569–572, 1990.

Rimmer JM, Gennari FJ: Atherosclerotic renovascular disease and progressive renal failure. *Ann Intern Med* 118:712–719, 1993.

Schoenberg SO, Prince MR, Knopp MV, Allenberg JR: Renal MR angiography. *Magnetic Resonance Imaging Clinics of North America* 6:351–370, 1998.

Svetkey LP, Kadir S, Dunnick NR, Smith SR, Duham CB, Lambert M, Klotman PE: Similar prevalence of renovascular hypertension in selected blacks and whites. *Hypertension* 17:678–683, 1991.

Tuttle KR, Chouinard RF, Webber JT, Dahlstrom LR, Short RA, Henneberry KJ, Dunham LA, Raabe RD: Treatment of atherosclerotic ostial renal artery stenosis with the intravascular stent. *Am J Kidney Dis* 32:611–622, 1998.

van Jaarsveld BC, Krijnen P, Pieterman H, Derkx FH, Deinum J, Postma CT, Dees A, Woittiez AJ, Bartelink AK, Man in 't Veld AJ, Schalekamp MA: The effect of balloon angioplasty on hypertension in atherosclerotic renal-artery stenosis. *N Engl J Med* 342:1007–1014, 2000.

72

THERAPY OF HYPERTENSION

JOHN M. FLACK

By definition, hypertension is present when there is a persistent elevation of either systolic blood pressure (SBP) ($\geq$140 mm Hg) or diastolic blood pressure (DPB) ($\geq$90 mm Hg), or when a patient is taking antihypertensive medication [regardless of the blood pressure (BP) level]. However, persons with diabetes, heart failure, and renal disease are now considered hypertensive at 130/85 mm Hg. The blood pressure level correlates directly with the magnitude of risk for clinical sequelae such as premature death, stroke, myocardial infarction, congestive heart failure, renal insufficiency, dementia, and peripheral vascular disease. Table 1 in Chapter 70 displays the blood pressure classification from the sixth report of the Joint National Committee on the Detection Treatment and Evaluation of High Blood Pressure expert panel. The scheme determines hypertension stage according to the highest pressure—either systolic or diastolic. The preponderance of epidemiological data suggests that systolic, not diastolic, blood pressure is the primary determinant of pressure-related risk.

RATIONALE FOR TREATMENT

A compelling case can be made for pharmacological treatment of elevated blood pressure. Pharmacological blood pressure lowering reduces the risk of premature cardiovascular morbid and fatal events as well as all-cause mortality. Antihypertensive drug therapy has also been shown to prevent the gradual progression of mild hypertension to more severe elevations of blood pressure. Early treatment of hypertension favorably impacts long-term clinical risk, in part, by preventing the development of pressure-related target organ damage. The risk of cardiovascular disease morbidity and mortality is severalfold higher when pressure-related target organ damage (i.e., elevated serum creatinine, left ventricular hypertrophy) is present than when it is not, even at identical levels of blood pressure. In addition, new evidence suggests that hypertension treatment reduces the risk of recurrent stroke among stroke survivors. Also, preinfarct hypertension treatment lessens the risk of recurrent myocardial infarctron (MI) in MI survivors. Though many antihypertensive drugs have dose-related side effects, it is not well appreciated that drug-treated hypertensive patients actually feel better subjectively (i.e., improved quality of life and fewer pressure-related symptoms) after successful blood pressure lowering. The evidence in support of this thesis is compelling.

GENERAL THERAPEUTIC PRINCIPLES

Several important therapeutic principles should be considered in treating hypertensive patients. In most hypertensives there is little to be gained from the pursuit of rapid blood pressure control. The most important therapeutic goal for the vast majority is to prescribe a combination of appropriate lifestyle modifications (weight loss, salt and alcohol restriction, and increased physical activity) plus the lowest doses of drug(s) that allow blood pressure normalization over the long term. In addition, the intensity of antihypertensive drug therapy required to reach goal blood pressure relates inversely to the success achieved with lifestyle interventions.

The erroneous clinical perception that diastolic blood pressure is the predominant pressure mediator of clinical risk contributes to physician hesitancy to intensify treatment to normalize systolic blood pressure once diastolic blood pressure has been lowered below 90 mm Hg. Drug acquisition costs also usually increase at higher dose levels. In certain instances, cost is a major barrier to patient compliance with prescribed drug therapies. The clinician and nursing staff should routinely ask patients whether they can afford the prescribed medications. Drug acquisition costs are but one consideration, albeit an important one, when formulating a hypertension disease management strategy. Table 1 lists several therapeutic strategies that have the potential to minimize hypertension treatment costs.

Establish a Goal Blood Pressure

Establishing a minimum goal blood pressure is an extremely important consideration prior to the initiation of antihypertensive drug therapy. In most uncomplicated hypertensive patients, the target blood pressure level minimally will be <140/90 mm Hg. Nevertheless, in selected high-risk subgroups (heart failure, renal insufficiency, diabetes), the minimum target blood pressure is lower (<130/85 mm Hg). The minimum blood pressure target is yet lower (<125/75 mm Hg) for hypertensives with $\geq$1 g of proteinuria/24 hr. The Treatment of Mild Hypertension Study (TOMHS) findings support more stringent goal blood pressure (<130/85 mm Hg) for uncomplicated stage

TABLE I
Strategies to Minimize Treatment Costs during Hypertension Treatment

Utilize diuretics, especially when taking >2 nondiuretic agents

Wait 4–6 weeks before uptitrating antihypertensive agents

Consider generic agents

Consider combination drugs in patients requiring polypharmacy

Consider reserpine

1 diastolic hypertensives. In TOMHS, drug-related hypertensives (also prescribed a multifactorial lifestyle intervention) had an average blood pressure of 140/91 mm Hg at baseline. After 4 years of treatment in this group, blood pressure averaged 127/79 mm Hg versus 133/82 mm Hg in TOMHS participants receiving only the multifactorial lifestyle intervention. The incidence of major and minor clinical events was 11.1% in the drug-treatment group versus 16.2% in those receiving only lifestyle modification.

Initiate Lifestyle Interventions

Lifestyle interventions such as weight loss, sodium and alcohol restriction, and increased physical activity all lower blood pressure when used alone or in combination. However, weight loss has the most significant impact on BP lowering of the aforementioned lifestyle interventions. The recently reported Dietary Approaches to Stop Hypertension (DASH) study documented that diets rich in fruits and vegetables lowered both cuff and ambulatory blood pressure. In addition, a diet enriched with fruits, vegetables, and low-fat dairy products that provided reduced saturated and total fat intake lowered BP even more. According to the most recent JNC VI report, lifestyle interventions are appropriately prescribed as initial therapy in many hypertensive patients. That is, those with BP <160/100 mm Hg in the absence of renal insufficiency, heart failure, and/or diabetes mellitus. However, in these high-risk patients, lifestyle modification(s) should be used as the initial therapeutic intervention, concurrently with antihypertensive drug therapy, when BP consistently exceeds 130/85 mm Hg.

Clinical Implications of Drug Pharmacokinetics

Drug pharmacokinetic profiles influence both the time to onset of maximal blood pressure lowering as well as the degree of protection against loss of blood pressure control during the interval between missed medication dose and the next dose taken. The terminal drug half-life in general, though not always, correlates directly with both the duration of blood pressure lowering and the time to reach steady-state drug levels. Drugs with a longer duration of action tend to have a delayed onset of maximal blood pressure lowering compared to drugs with a shorter duration of action. However, once steady-state drug levels have been achieved, long duration of action drugs

provide superior blood pressure control throughout the 24-hr dosing interval and also have a slow offset of action that minimizes the loss of blood pressure control when medication doses are missed. Pharmacokinetic considerations are important, as only 60% of hypertensives who take antihypertensive medications over the long term do so without missing scheduled doses. These considerations are particularly important factors in differentiating drugs within a therapeutic class.

Frequency of Monitoring/Drug Titration

A reasonable time frame for attainment of normal blood pressure levels should be measured in months, not days or weeks. In most patients, it matters little over the long term if blood pressure control is achieved in 4 months as opposed to 4 weeks. Long-acting antihypertensive drugs usually take up to 4 to 6 weeks to fully manifest their maximal blood pressure lowering effect. Thus, in most hypertensives, dose increases or medication changes should be undertaken no more frequently than every 6 weeks. This strategy will facilitate attainment of goal blood pressure with a minimum of office visits and also will minimize the likelihood of precipitating symptoms attributable to rapid blood pressure lowering. Nevertheless, if a patient manifests insignificant blood pressure lowering during the first few weeks of therapy, the likelihood of a meaningful blood pressure response over the ensuing weeks is low. A reasonable strategy at this point is to titrate the dose upward, add another medication, or stop the current medication and switch to another drug. Potential problems with rapid blood pressure lowering are listed in Table 2.

Side Effects

Both the patient and physician usually attribute subjective side effects experienced by drug-treated hypertensives to antihypertensive medication, because hypertension has long been considered an asymptomatic condition. How-

TABLE 2
The Potential Hazards of a Hypertension Disease Management Approach Utilizing Rapid Upward Titration of Antihypertensive Agents and Frequent Office Visits to Accomplish Rapid Blood Pressure Lowering

Subjective side effects
    Dose-related
        Correlate with rapidity of BP fall

Target organ ischemia
            Angina pectoris, MI, TIA, or stroke

Higher total cost of care
    Increased drug doses
    Unnecessary office visits
    Excessive medication changes
    Excessive patient monitoring

Note: MI, myocardial infarction; TIA, transient ischemic attack.

TABLE 3

Constellation of Symptoms Reported More Often in Hypertensives with Elevated Blood Pressures Compared to Drug-Treated Hypertensives with Lower Blood Pressure Levels

Headache

Fatigue/weakness

Lack of stamina, poor exercise tolerance

Cardiac awareness

Dizziness

Nervousness

Sleep disturbance

Chest pain

Shortness of breath

Tinnitus

ever, there is considerable evidence that hypertensive patients do indeed experience a constellation of symptoms (Table 3) that correlate with the blood pressure level. Even though antihypertensive drugs can cause symptoms, they appear to alleviate more symptoms than they cause, as drug-treated hypertensives report fewer subjective side effects than placebo-treated individuals with higher blood pressure levels. Pressure-related symptoms such as weakness and fatigue not only relate to the blood pressure level, but may also occur in a time-limited manner after rapid blood pressure lowering. The symptomatic drug-treated hypertensive is relatively common in clinical practice as fewer than 50% of drug-treated hypertensives attain blood pressure levels <140/90 mm Hg.

ANTIHYPERTENSIVE DRUG SELECTION

Monotherapy

The clinician must have reasonable expectations about the likelihood of blood pressure normalization with monotherapy. If expectations are unrealistic, then subsequent therapeutic decisions will be misguided and therefore unlikely to result in blood pressure normalization. Furthermore, the lack of therapeutic success will frus-

trate both the patient and physician. The probability of achieving blood pressure normalization with monotherapy in the overall hypertensive population ranges between 50 and 60%. Two or fewer drugs will control about 85 to 90% of all hypertensives, whereas three or more drugs will be required for blood pressure normalization in the remainder. The probability of blood pressure normalization with monotherapy is significantly influenced by the magnitude of the pretreatment blood pressure elevation. The Sixth Joint National Committee blood pressure classification scheme can thus be quite useful in guiding therapeutic decisions (Table 4). A common clinical mistake is to expect monotherapy to normalize blood pressure levels in hypertensives with "high" stage 2 or stage 3 hypertension. If, however, an adequately dosed therapeutic trial of monotherapy of sufficient duration is undertaken and unsuccessful at these high blood pressure levels, then a more effective strategy will be to add a second drug when monotherapy fails. However, if a second drug from an additional drug class is substituted, it is also likely that this agent will fail to normalize blood pressure. In this situation, drug substitution leads to extra office visits, excessive patient monitoring, and unnecessary changes in their therapeutic regimen, all of which contribute to a higher total cost of care. Conversely, in "high" stage 2 or higher hypertension, *initial* monotherapy still remains a viable *initial* treatment strategy even though the probability of ultimately achieving blood pressure control with a single drug is low. Initiation of treatment with low-dose combination therapy is also a reasonable option. Table 5 displays the advantages and disadvantages of the major antihypertensive drug classes.

Diuretics

Thiazide diuretics are the most commonly prescribed diuretics for hypertension treatment. Monotherapy with thiazide diuretics effectively lowers blood pressure with a similar degree of efficacy in both African-American and White hypertensives. Thiazides are, however, ineffective when the glomerular filtration rate is <40 mL/min; a clinical rule of thumb is that thiazides should be avoided when serum creatinine levels are ≥2–3 mg/dL. Current recommendations are to prescribe 25 mg/day or less.

TABLE 4

An Adaptation of the JNC V Blood Pressure Classification Scheme That Describes Therapeutic Options When Monotherapy Fails to Lower Blood Pressure to <140/90 mm Hg According to Patients Initial Blood Pressure Level

	SBP (mm Hg)	DBP (mm Hg)	When monotherapy is unsuccessful
Stage 1	140–159	90–99	Switch drugs
Stage 2			
"low"	160–169	100–104	Switch drugs; however, consider adding a second drug
"high"	170–179	105–109	Add a second drug
Stage 3–4	≥180	≥110	Add a second drug; however, consider two-drug treatment initially

Doses as low as 6.25 mg/day have been shown to effectively lower blood pressure. These agents are cheap, as drug acquisition costs can be as low as pennies per day. The absence of a diuretic is perhaps the most common cause of resistant hypertension in patients treated with complex (>2) antihypertensive drug regimens. The relatively long drug half-lives of thiazides (chlorthalidone > hydrochlorothiazide) is a favorable pharmacokinetic characteristic for long-term hypertension management. Thiazides have dose-related side effects such as hypokalemia (<3.5 mEq/L), hypomagnesemia, and hyperuricemia. Hypokalemia is the most common metabolic side effect, occurring in 30 to 35% of diuretic-treated hypertensives consuming an ad libitum sodium diet. The likelihood of hypokalemia can be reduced by these non-mutually exclusive strategies: (1) reduce the diuretic dose; (2) lower intake of dietary sodium; or (3) add a potassium sparing diuretic or potassium supplement. Thiazides can impair free water clearance and thus can occasionally cause hyponatremia in older hypertensives. These agents also cause modest lipid disturbances, as they raise cholesterol levels ~6% and triglyceride levels approximately 15%, while leaving high-density lipoprotein levels unaffected. Thiazides also can adversely affect glycemic control; however, this can usually be avoided by preventing potassium depletion. These agents are the worst offending drug class for causing sexual dysfunction in men. Loop diuretics, metolazone, and indapamide maintain their blood pressure lowering efficacy in patients with compromised renal function. Though loop diuretics are more potent diuretics than the thiazides, these agents lower blood pressure less effectively than thiazides in individuals with normal renal function. Diuretics are especially useful in hypertensives with congestive heart failure. Potassium sparing diuretics (triamterene, amiloride) are often used in combination with thiazide diuretics for minimizing hypokalemia and added blood pressure control. Aldosterone antagonists are currently enjoying a resurgence in their use. These agents (spironolactone, eplerenone) may be used effectively as monotherapy or as components of complex drug regimens.

β-Blockers

β-blockers are a heterogeneous group of drugs, which can be subclassified according to their relative affinity for β-receptor subtypes, the presence or absence of intrinsic sympathomimetic activity, and their lipophilicity. β-blockers can be categorized as: (1) nonselective (β_1 and β_2) (i.e., nadolol, propranolol, timolol), (2) cardioselective (β_1) (i.e., atenolol, metoprolol), (3) cardioselective with intrinsic sympathomimetic activity (acebutolol), (4) nonselective with intrinsic sympathomimetic activity (i.e., pindolol), or (5) α–β blocker (labetalol, carvedilol). β_1 receptors are the predominant β receptor subtype in the heart, whereas β_2 receptors predominate in the lung and peripheral blood vessels. Nevertheless, both receptor subtypes are found in target organs. Cardioselective β_1 β-blockers have theoretical advantages in patients with bronchospastic lung disease as

nonselective β-blockers (β_1 and β_2) are more prone to incite bronchospasm. However, because target tissues are not populated by distinct β-receptor subtypes, even cardioselective β-blockers can cause bronchospasm and should be avoided in patients with lung disease. β-blockers (without intrinsic sympathomimetic activity) should be a favored antihypertensive therapy in the postmyocardial infarction patients because of their proven cardioprotection and their ability to lower mortality. Likewise these nonintrinsic sympathomimetic activity β-blockers are particularly useful in the hypertensive patient with either angina pectoris or migraine headaches. Lipophilicity, particularly at higher β-blocker doses, may predispose to central nervous system side effects. The lipophilicity of commonly used β-blockers in rank order is propranolol > metoprolol > timolol > acebutolol > atenolol. These agents are highly effective blood pressure lowering agents when used alone or in combination with diuretics. In the calcium antagonist group, only the dihydropyridines are suitable for combination therapy with β-blockers. β-blockers reduce cardiac output by approximately 20 to 25%; thus, these agents have been associated with low cardiac output symptoms such as weakness, fatigue, and poor exercise tolerance. β-blockers can also worsen symptomatic peripheral vascular disease, have been linked to depression, and can lower high-density lipoproteins while raising triglycerides. The adverse lipid effects are less pronounced with intrinsic sympathomimetic activity β-blockers. Less lipophilic β-blockers may cause less depression because they poorly traverse the blood–brain barrier into the central nervous system. β-blockers should be used with caution in hypoglycemia-prone diabetics because they: (1) blunt the tachycardia accompanying hypoglycemia, and (2) delay the metabolic recovery from hypoglycemia. There are new and promising data suggesting the incremental benefit of low-dose β-blockade [on top of diuretics, digitalis, and angiotensin converting enzyme (ACE) inhibitors] in patients with congestive heart failure. However, β-blocker therapy should only be initiated in persons with stable heart failure. Abrupt discontinuation of these agents can lead to rebound hypertension and a heightened risk for myocardial infarction.

Angiotensin Converting Enzyme Inhibitors

Angiotensin converting enzyme inhibitors are particularly useful in diabetic hypertensives with proteinuria as well as in hypertensives with congestive heart failure and in those who have survived myocardial infarction. ACE inhibitors have also been shown to forestall the occurrence of microalbuminuria in persons with type 2 diabetes without pretreatment albuminuria. These agents are metabolically neutral [lipids, glucose, and electrolytes remain unchanged in most patients], do not cause male erectile dysfunction, and have no effect on fasting glucose even though they modestly improve insulin sensitivity. The major side effect of this drug class is cough, which occurs in ~9% of hypertensives taking these agents. Angioedema is a potentially life-threatening side effect occurring in approximately 3/1000 ACE inhibitor-treated patients. An-

TABLE 5
Advantage and Disadvantage of Seven Commonly Used Antihypertensive Drug Classes[a]

Advantages	Disadvantages
Angiotensin converting enzyme (ACE) inhibitors	
Renoprotective in type 1 diabetes	Cough (~9%)
Profoundly antiproteinuric	Rare angioedema (~3/1000)
↓ Morbidity and mortality and symptomatic improvement in CHF patient	Rare hyperkalemia
	Higher dose requirements in some African-Americans
↓ Ventricular remodeling and mortality post-MI	BP lowering effect very sensitive to level of dietary sodium intake
Leftward shift of pressure–natriuresis curve	Teratogenicity after first trimester of pregnancy
Safely combined with antihypertensives, especially diuretics or calcium antagonists.	
α_1 Antagonists	
Positive effect on all lipoprotein fractions	Orthostatic hypotension (particularly in elderly, in combination with other vasodilators, in the setting of autonomic dysfunction and in volume depleted patients)
Improved insulin sensitivity (fasting glucose unchanged)	
Unchanged to improved sexual function in men	Slightly higher doses needed in African-Americans
Blunts thiazide-induced rise in cholesterol	Modest plasma volume expansion
Improves maximal urine flow in men with BPH	
Angiotensin II (AT$_1$) receptor antagonists	
Lesser peak BP lowering compared to ACEs	Relatively flat BP dose–response curve
Nearly complete blockage of A-II effect	Limited data available in African-Americans
No known effect on enkephalins and substance P	Rare hyperkalemia (less than with ACE inhibitors)
Augments tissue bradykinin	Potentially teratogenic
Uricosuric (losartan)	
Profoundly antiproteinuric	
Metabolically neutral	
Rare angioedema (less than with ACE inhibitors)	
No cough	
β-Blockers	
Differential cardiac and hemodynamic effects	Can worsen CHF; however, at low doses may improve CHF
Proven to lower morbidity and mortality post-MI	Low cardiac output symptoms
Selected agents useful in patients with migraine or angina	Can worsen or precipitate depression
	Bronchospasm
	Can aggravate PVD symptoms
	Lowers HDL and raises TGs
	Delays recovery from and masks symptoms of hypoglycemia
	Abrupt discontinuation can lead to rebound hypertension
	Male erectile dysfunction (mostly older β-blockers)
Calcium antagonists	
Unqualified efficacy profile (African-Americans, diabetics, elderly)	Immediately post-MI or during unstable angina (short-acting dihydropyridines) may increase CHD risk
Heterogeneous electrophysiologic, inotropic, hemodynamic, chronotropic, and SNS effects	Rate-limiting CBs can worsen CHF and ↑ mortality in patients with systolic heart failure
Useful in diastolic dysfunction	Side effect profile varies (constipation—verapamil, pedal edema, and vasodilatory symptoms—dihydropyridines)
Metabolically neutral	
Minimal erectile dysfunction in men	Combined use of rate-limiting calcium antagonist with β-blockers can result in profound bradycardia and depression of myocardial contractility
BP lowering effect is robust in setting of high dietary sodium intake	
BP lowering effect not attenuated by NSAIDs	
Central adrenergic inhibitors	
Relatively cheap	Sedation
Useful in hypertensive urgencies (clonidine)	Depression (high-dose reserpine)
Methyldopa is drug of choice for pregnant women	Orthostatic hypotension
	Decreased heart rate (clonidine)
	Frequent skin irritation (clonidine patch), dry mouth
	Abrupt discontinuation can lead to rebound hypertension
	Positive Coombs test in ~15% (methyldopa)

(continues)

TABLE 5 *(continued)*

Advantages	Disadvantages
Direct vasodilators	
Relatively cheap	Best suited for adjunctive therapy
Effective in severe hypertension (minoxidil > hydralazine)	Salt and water retention necessitate use of loop diuretics
	Reflex tachycardia necessitates use of rate-limiting CCB or β-blocker
	Do not regress LVH
	Lupus-like syndrome (>200 mg/day of hydralazine)
	Hirsutism (minoxidil)
	Edema (minoxidil)
Diuretics	
Cheap acquisition cost	Thiazides are ineffective when GFR <40 mL/min
Highly effective and lowers BP similarly in all demographic groups	Dose-related hypokalemia
	Hypomagnesemia
Proven to lower BP-related morbidity and mortality	Raises cholesterol and triglycerides
Enhances the BP lowering effect of all other BP drugs	Glucose intolerance especially in setting of K^+ depletion
Chlorthalidone and metolazone have relatively long half-lives	Increased uric acid
	Male erectile dysfunction in men
	"Hidden" costs of metabolic monitoring

*BP, blood pressure; BPH, benign prostatic hyperplasia; ACE, angiotensin converting enzyme inhibitors; A-II, angiotensin II; CCBs, calcium channel blockers; CHD, coronary heart disease; CHF, congestive heart failure; HDL, high-density lipoprotein; PVD, peripheral vascular disease; TG, triglycerides, SNS, sympathetic nervous system; NSAIDs, nonsteroidal antiinflammatory drugs; MI, myocardial infarction; LVH, left ventricular hypertrophy; GFR, glomerular filtration rate; CB, channel blockers.

gioedema can occur months after the initiation of ACE inhibitor therapy. The incidence of hyperkalemia in all ACE inhibitor-treated hypertensives is less than 1%. However, those with renal insufficiency and/or diabetes mellitus as well as those treated with nonsteroidal antiinflammatory drugs, potassium-sparing diuretics, potassium supplements, and/or heparin have a higher risk. ACE inhibitors should be avoided in patients with bilateral renal artery stenosis and should be used cautiously in patients with unilateral renal artery stenosis because of the risk of iatrogenic renal failure. African-Americans, particularly those with high intake of dietary sodium, may require higher doses of these agents to achieve blood pressure control. The combined use of ACE inhibitors with either a diuretic or a calcium antagonist appears to be highly efficacious and well tolerated. ACE inhibitors also blunt thiazide-induced hypokalemia. These agents are potentially teratogenic (after first trimester) and should therefore be avoided during pregnancy or when pregnancy is either planned or likely. Women of childbearing potential should be counseled to use contraceptives while taking ACE inhibitors and should be changed to another agent if they are attempting to become pregnant or if pregnancy is likely.

α_1 Antagonists

α_1 antagonists improve insulin sensitivity and cause modest favorable changes in all blood lipoproteins, making them desirable in hypertensives with either diabetes mellitus or dyslipidemia. These are preferred agents in older men with benign prostatic hyperplasia as they improve maximum urine flow rates in a dose-dependent manner.

This drug class either does not affect or modestly improves erectile function in men. Doses required to achieve blood pressure control are slightly higher in African-American hypertensives than in White hypertensives. These agents can precipitate or worsen orthostatic hypotension. Thus the clinician should routinely take orthostatic blood pressure measurements in at-risk groups including older persons, diabetics, sedentary individuals, and hypertensives concurrently treated with diuretics, central adrenergic inhibitors, or combined $\alpha-\beta$ blockers. These agents are particularly useful in combination drug regimens required in high-risk hypertensive subgroups such as in persons with type 2 diabetes.

Calcium Antagonists

Calcium antagonists are a heterogenous class of vasoactive compounds, which effectively lower blood pressure in all racial, ethnic, and demographic groups. These agents have variable hemodynamic, inotropic, chronotropic, and neurohumoral effects. There is essentially no role for short-acting calcium antagonists in the long-term therapy of hypertension. Short-acting nifedipine, occasionally, can be useful for acute blood pressure lowering during legitimate hypertensive urgencies, although recent evidence suggests caution when using this agent for this indication. Calcium antagonists also can be subclassified as either rate limiting (verapamil, diltiazem) or dihydropyridine (i.e., nifedipine, amlodipine, felodipine). Rate-limiting calcium antagonists, in contrast to the dihydropyridines, have atrioventricular nodal blocking properties and generally should not be used in combination with β-blockers, nor should they be used in patients with impaired systolic heart function. Dihydropyridine calcium antagonists are more potent peripheral vasodilators and therefore do not depress myocardial contractility. Lower extremity edema can occur with any calcium antagonist, though it most typically occurs with the dihydropyridines. Neither rate limiting nor dihydropyridine calcium antagonists should be prescribed to patients with sick sinus syndrome unless a functioning ventricular pacemaker is in place.

Angiotensin Receptor Antagonists

Angiotensin receptor antagonists are well tolerated as monotherapy and have been most extensively studied in combination with diuretics. These agents are metabolically neutral and do not cause erectile dysfunction in men. Like the ACE inhibitors, angiotensin receptor antagonists antagonize the renin–angiotensin–aldosterone system (though at a different site). Unlike the ACE inhibitors, angiotensin receptor antagonists do not cause cough. Anecdotal reports of angioedema with angiotensin receptor antagonists have, however, now surfaced, though the incidence is probably lower than with the ACE inhibitors. Similar to the ACE inhibitors, these agents should be avoided in individuals with bilateral renal artery stenosis and used cautiously in patients with unilateral renal artery stenosis. These agents should also be used with caution in hyperkalemia-prone individuals, though they are less likely to cause hyperkalemia than the ACE inhibitors. These agents are the logical alternative therapy for ACE-intolerant patients, most notably, in heart failure and diabetes mellitus. Similar to the ACE inhibitors, angiotensin receptor antagonists should be avoided during pregnancy or when pregnancy is planned, because of potential teratogenicity.

Central Adrenergic Inhibitors

Central adrenergic inhibitors (i.e., clonidine, methyldopa) are most useful for adjunctive antihypertensive therapy. These agents effectively lower blood pressure and also cause regression of left ventricular hypertrophy. However, sedation, dry mouth, and orthostatic hypotension limit patient acceptance of these agents. Abrupt discontinuation of these drugs can lead to rebound hypertension making these agents less than ideal therapeutic selections for patients with known noncompliance. The use of these agents in combination with β-blockers should be discouraged because of the risk of bradycardia. Methyldopa is the antihypertensive agent of choice in hypertensive pregnant women. These agents are typically used as adjunctive therapy in complex drug regimens.

Direct Vasodilators

Direct vasodilators (i.e., minoxidil, hydralazine) are uncommonly used as monotherapy, mostly because they evoke marked arterial vasodilatation and thus cause reflexive activation of the sympathetic nervous system. This leads to both salt and water retention as well as tachycar-

dia. The latter raises myocardial oxygen consumption and therefore can precipitate new or worsen preexisting coronary ischemia in patients with coronary heart disease. These agents are most effectively used in combination with diuretics and β-blockers or a rate-limiting calcium antagonist. Lower extremity edema may complicate minoxidil therapy even when potent diuretics are simultaneously prescribed.

Vasopeptidase Inhibitors

Fastidotril and omapatrilat are representative agents of this new class of antihypertensive compounds. These agents potently lower blood pressure via simultaneous inhibition of ACE and neutral endopeptidase. Omapatrilat is the vasopeptidase inhibitor that will first be released for general use.

Combination Therapy

Almost 50% of all hypertensives and most stage 2 or higher hypertensives will require more than a single antihypertensive agent to achieve blood pressure normalization. Thus, physicians should become familiar with the clinical scenarios when combination therapy will likely be needed. In "high" stage 2 or higher hypertensives, it is reasonable for physicians to consider initiating antihypertensive therapy with two drugs. Dual drug therapy can be initiated either by prescription of two separate pills or by prescribing a single combination pill. The combined blood pressure lowering effect of two drugs at low-to-moderate doses usually exceeds the magnitude of blood pressure lowering obtainable by upward titration of either drug alone to its maximum dose and with fewer side effects. Figure 1 shows useful therapeutic combinations of antihyper-

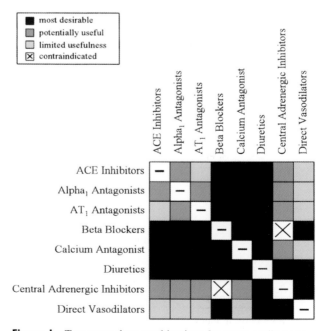

Figure I   Two-agent drug combinations for seven antihypertensive drug classes according to their relative clinical utility.

tensive drugs. Certain drug classes may, however, be "preferred" in complex drug regimens. Preferred drugs are (1) those that are initially prescribed and pushed to their maximally tolerated (or minimally effective dose) and (2) agents that are continued even when it does not control BP as monotherapy. Drug classes are usually conferred "preferred" status based on the ability to treat concomitant conditions in addition to hypertension as well as because of evidence of human target-organ protection. A few select examples of the concept of preferred therapeutic choices are displayed in Table 6.

THERAPEUTIC CONSIDERATIONS FOR SPECIAL POPULATIONS

African-Americans

African-Americans have a premature onset of hypertension that is associated with a greater burden of pressure-related target organ damage (i.e., microalbuminuria, left ventricular hypertrophy, elevated serum creatinine) compared to Whites. The clinician will frequently encounter severe hypertension (stages 2 to 3) with concomitant diabetes mellitus and other cardiovascular conditions (i.e., stroke) in the hypertensive African-American. Obesity, particularly among African-American women, contributes to the high frequency of salt sensitivity and intermediate blood pressure phenotype that correlates with higher antihypertensive drug requirements. Persuasive data indicate that even modest reductions in dietary sodium intake (<135 mmol/day) will augment the hypotensive effect of virtually all antihypertensive drugs in all hypertensives, though more so in African-Americans.

Diuretics will often be required to achieve blood pressure normalization given the higher prevalence of renal insufficiency and reduced natriuretic capacity in African-Americans. Nevertheless, African-Americans should be viewed as individuals for whom the most appropriate antihypertensive drug therapy is chosen based on considerations (i.e., concomitant diseases, drug synergy/interactions, renal function) unique to that individual. It is an outdated concept that race should be the primary consideration when selecting antihypertensive drug therapy for any individual. Nevertheless, monotherapy with diuretics and cal-

cium antagonists has been shown to result in greater blood pressure lowering in African-Americans compared to other commonly used nondiuretic drug classes (i.e., ACE inhibitors, α-antagonists, and β-blockers). However, the clinician should not generalize these data to an individual and therefore presume a lack of blood pressure lowering efficacy solely, or even mostly, because of their race or ethnicity. When an adequately dosed therapeutic trial of sufficient duration is undertaken, most African-Americans will have a meaningful blood pressure response to antihypertensive agents from any of the commonly used drug classes. A lower therapeutic blood pressure goal [<130/85 mm Hg] will be appropriate for many hypertensive African-Americans because of concurrent diabetes, renal insufficiency, and heart failure.

The Elderly

Although some clinicians have been hesitant to initiate antihypertensive therapy in older individuals (≥60 years), the totality of evidence from epidemiological studies and clinical trials documents that older patients have a higher risk for pressure-related clinical events than younger hypertensives at any given blood pressure level. Moreover, drug-treated older hypertensives take their antihypertensive medication and comply with lifestyle modifications (i.e., weight loss, salt and alcohol restrictions) as well or better than their younger counterparts. Elderly hypertensives actually manifest more impressive reductions in pressure-related complications within a shorter time frame compared to younger hypertensives. Concomitant cardiovascular conditions (i.e., diabetes mellitus, vascular disease, renal insufficiency), noncardiovascular chronic conditions, and poverty are more common in older compared to younger hypertensives. In part because of impaired baroreceptor reflexes, older hypertensives are prone to develop orthostatic hypotension and should therefore be checked for postural hypotension. If present, then the standing blood pressure should be used to guide therapeutic decisions. The clinician should have a heightened suspicion for the presence of orthostatic hypertension in older hypertensives treated with α_1 antagonists, diuretics, and/or central adrenergic inhibitors.

Renal Insufficiency

Hypertension is a risk factor for renal insufficiency, and in turn, renal insufficiency irrespective of etiology causes hypertension. Approximately 85% of individuals with renal insufficiency also have hypertension. Diabetes mellitus and hypertension account for over one-half of all cases of end stage renal disease. The major therapeutic goal for individuals with hypertension associated with renal impairment is to set and subsequently achieve an aggressive therapeutic blood pressure goal (<130/85 mm Hg) over many weeks to months. The average number of drugs needed to achieve blood pressure control in this hypertensive subgroup is 4.3; thus, therapeutic debates that focus on choices of a single agent are mostly superfluous given that complex drug regimens are the rule. Limited renal natriuretic

TABLE 6
Examples of Preferred Antihypertensive Drugs

Condition	Drug(s)
Diabetes mellitus with proteinuria	ACE inhibitors, AT$_1$ receptor antagonists[a]
Heart failure	ACE inhibitors, AT$_1$ receptor antagonists[a], β-blockers, diuretics[b]
Angina pectoris	β-blockers (without ISA[c]), calcium antagonists
Benign prostatic hyperplasia	α_1 antagonists

[a]ACE inhibitor intolerant patients.
[b]Preferred as adjunctive therapy.
[c]ISA, intrinsic sympathomimetic activity.

TABLE 7

Drugs Commonly Used in Hypertensive Urgencies and Emergencies

Drug	Dose schedule	Duration	Comment
Oral			
Clonidine	0.1 mg initially then 0.1 mg every 2 hr until a maximum dose of 0.7 mg reached	3–12 hr	Onset of action is within 30 to 45 min; peak BP lowering 3 to 4 hr post dose; side effects include sedation, dry mouth, and orthostatic hypotension; can dramatically lower BP in volume-depleted and older patients; CBF, CO, pulse rate, and PVR all reduced; favor use when SNS tone is high (i.e., abrupt cessation of β-blockers, alcohol/drug withdrawal); avoid use in CHF or in setting of greater than first degree heart block.
Nifedipine	10 mg po or sublingual, repeat after 1 hr, maximum total dose = 20 mg	4–6 hr	Onset of action is 10–15 min; peak BP lowering occurs 1.0–1.5 hr post dose; abrupt onset of action evokes SNS activation which can lead to reflex tachycardia thus increasing myocardial oxygen demand with precipitation or worsening of coronary ischemia; should be avoided in patients with unstable angina pectoris, MI, or aortic stenosis; only short-acting formulation is useful in HTN urgencies.
Captopril	6.25–25.00 mg po or chewed; maximum total dose = 25 mg		Onset of BP lowering within 15 to 30 min after po dosing; peak BP lowering occurs 1–2 hr post dose; BP lowering effect will likely be blunted in setting of volume overload; however, rapid and excessive BP reductions can occur in volume-depleted patients; preload and afterload are decreased and CBF preserved; avoid use in bilateral renal artery stenosis and in patients with a history of ACE inhibitor-induced angioedema.
Intravenous Sodium nitroprusside	0.25 to 8 μg/kg/min^{-1} with titration every 5 min	<5 min	Rapid onset (seconds) and offset of action allow precise titration of BP response; very potent; balanced preload and afterload reduction; increases CO thus desirable in CHF; may, however, cause a "coronary steal" syndrome and precipitate or worsen coronary ischemia; hypoxemia may result from intrapulmonary shunting; activates SNS, thus avoid in aortic dissection; raises ICP; thiocyanate and cyanide toxicity can occur.
Nitroglycerine	5–200 mg/min	<5 min	Onset and offset of action is within minutes; reduces preload and, at higher doses, afterload; shunts blood flow into the subendocardium, an ischemia-prone area, intravenous agent of choice for treating severe hypertension in setting of MI, unstable angina, or in individuals with known CHD; also desirable in setting of pulmonary edema and CHF; occasionally causes bradycardia; raises ICP; also, may result in excessive BP lowering in setting of volume-depletion; causes methemoglobinemia rarely.
Labetalol	Bolus: 20–40 mg every 20–30 min continuous infusion: 0.5–2.0 mg/min; maximum dose = 200–300 mg/24 hr.	2–6 hr	BP response is variable thus precise titration not possible; onset of action is rapid, however, offset of action takes hours; CBF is preserved; avoid use in setting of bronchospastic lung disease or CHF; excessive BP lowering can occur in setting of volume depletion; monitor for orthostatic hypotension; useful in hypertensive emergencies attributable to cocaine ingestion, though cocaine-induced coronary vasoconstriction is not reversed.
Nicardipine	2–4 mg/hr with titration every 15 min; when goal BP attained lower infusion to 4 mg/hr	>4 hr	Onset of action is within 15 min; offset of action takes hours; avoid in setting of ongoing coronary ischemia (MI, unstable angina pectoris) and in aortic dissection, unless combined with β-blockade; maintains or increases CO in CHF; potent dilatory effect on coronary arteries; reduces cerebral vasospasm and may improve neurological outcomes, therefore, this agent is specifically indicated in subarachnoid hemorrhage.
Enalapril	0.625–1.250 mg every 6 hr; reduce initial dose by 50% in patients on diuretics or if renally impaired.	~6 hr	Onset of action is within 15 min; offset of action takes hours; reduces both preload and afterload and dilates coronary vessels; thus is a desirable agent in CHF and CHD patients with severe hypertension; CBF maintained; avoid in bilateral renal artery stenosis and in patients with a history of ACE inhibitor-induced angioedema; can result in excessive BP lowering in volume-depleted patients.

(continues)

TABLE 7 (*continued*)

Drug	Dose schedule	Duration	Comment
Furosemide	May initiate treatment with doses as low as 5–10 mg if renal function is normal; 20–40 mg in CHF; if renal function abnormal may need to dose much higher	~4.5 hr	Onset of action is within 15 min; initiates peripheral venous pooling, resulting in preload reduction followed by a diuresis, the latter being maximal at 1.5 hr; favor when severe HTN is complicated by CHF, pulmonary edema, and/or renal insufficiency; avoid in setting of dehydration; use cautiously in conjunction with aminoglycosides because of ototoxicity; need to monitor glucose and electrolytes, especially potassium and magnesium. Can lower BP when used alone but mostly used to potentiate other agents.
Fenoldopam	Initial intravenous infusion of 0.03–0.10 mg/ kg/min with titration increments of 0.05–0.10 mg/ kg/min no sooner than every 15 min. Do not bolus intravenously.	Peak effect ~15 min postinitiation of infusion	Onset of action is within the first 5 min while the offset of action is over 15–30 min. Fenoldopam causes a natriuresis and diuresis. Kaliuresis also occurs, most notably in persons with renal insufficiency. Renal function improves as renal blood flow, glomerular filtration rate, and urine flow increases. This agent does not cross the blood–brain barrier. Must observe for volume depletion and hypokalemia. Allergic reactions can occur in sulfite sensitive persons. Fenoldopam causes transient increases in intraocular pressure. Partial tolerance may occur with prolonged high doses. Avoid concurrent use of β-blockers.

ACE, angiotensin converting enzyme; BP, blood pressure; CBF, cerebral blood, low; CHD, coronary heart disease; CHF, congestive heart failure; CO, cardiac output; HTN, hypertensive; ICP, intracranial pressure; MI, myocardial infraction; PVR, peripheral vascular resistance; SNS, sympathetic nervous system.

A breif description of the pharmacokinetic, hemodynamic, and clinical indications and contraindications is provided for each drug.

capacity, routine utilization of complex drug regimens, and the frequent use of drugs (i.e., ACE inhibitors), which can cause hyperkalemia are important reasons to use diuretics (loop diuretics or metolazone) in hypertensive patients with compromised renal function. Potassium sparing diuretics and potassium supplements should be used with considerable caution, if at all, in these patients, particularly when ACE inhibitors, angiotensin receptor antagonists, or nonsteroidal antiinflammatory drugs are concurrently prescribed. ACE inhibitors, and perhaps angiotensin receptor antagonists, are particularly useful, because in addition to being antiproteinuric, they antagonize the renal renin–angiotensin system which appears to be pathophysiologically linked to the characteristic structural and functional renal abnormalities found in experimental models of renal injury (see Chapter 58). Nonsteroidal antiinflammatory drugs also further augment the risk for hyperkalemia. In hypertensives with renal impairment, simply lowering blood pressure can lead to a rise in creatinine which, in most instances is followed by a subsequent fall in creatinine to pretreatment or lower levels. ACE inhibitors and perhaps angiotensin receptor antagonists can incite a precipitous decline in renal function as evidenced by a rise in creatinine in patients with critical bilateral renal stenosis or unilateral stenosis in a solitary kidney.

Diabetes Mellitus

Over 50% of diabetics are hypertensive. Diabetic hypertensives usually manifest disproportionate elevations in systolic compared to diastolic blood pressure and more often than not will require complex multidrug regimens to achieve blood pressure normalization. The long-term target blood pressure should minimally be <130/85 mm Hg

in this high-risk group. Roughly one-third of diabetics have hyporeninemic hypoaldosteronism (type IV renal tubular acidosis), a condition which attenuates renal potassium secretion. Thus, diabetic hypertensives should be regularly checked for hyperkalemia, particularly when potassium-sparing diuretics, potassium supplements, nonsteroidal antiinflammatory drugs, ACE inhibitors, or angiotensin receptor antagonists are prescribed. If blood pressure normalization is to be achieved, diuretics will often be required in complex drug regimens (>2 drugs). Diuretics augment renal potassium secretion because the reduction in plasma volume causes secondary hyperaldosteronism. Several major hypertension drug treatment trials (Hypertension Detection and Follow-up Program and the Systolic Hypertension in the Elderly Program) have documented a similar percent reduction in risk for pressure-related clinical events in diabetics and nondiabetics when treated with diuretic-based regimens. ACE inhibitors have proved to be renoprotective in type I diabetics with proteinuria and thus should be utilized in such patients even in the absence of established hypertension. Though the risk of end stage renal disease is much lower in type II diabetics, (lifetime risk ~8%) compared to type I diabetic, the former accounts for the overwhelming majority of diabetes-related end stage renal disease cases. A reasonable clinical extrapolation is that ACE inhibitors should also be preferred antihypertensive agents in type II diabetics with and, perhaps, in those without proteinuria. Angiotensin receptor antagonists, such as the ACE inhibitors, are antiproteinuric, although long-term clinical outcome studies are lacking with the former. α_1 antagonists, like the ACE inhibitors, improve insulin sensitivity and additionally have a favorable impact on all blood lipoprotein fractions. (See Chapter 28 for an in-depth discussion of treatment of the diabetic hypertensive). It is well established that hypertension treatment reduces the risk of both micro- and macrovascular complications in this high-risk population. ACE inhibitors, diuretics, and calcium antagonist-based treatment regimens all have been shown to lower risk for cardiovascular renal disease in hypertensive persons with diabetes mellitus.

HYPERTENSIVE URGENCIES AND EMERGENCIES

Hypertensive Urgencies

A hypertensive urgency can be defined as a blood pressure elevation in the absence of ongoing major pressure-related symptoms that is high enough to engender concerns regarding the new onset or worsening of pressure-related target organ damage (i.e., congestive heart failure, new or progressive renal insufficiency, neurological symptoms) unless blood pressure is lowered over the ensuing hours to days. Hypertensive urgencies represent the most common indication for which acute blood pressure lowering therapy is undertaken. In true hypertensive emergencies, blood pressure levels usually exceed 210 mm Hg systolic or 130 mm Hg diastolic. A sizable proportion of hypertensives treated acutely to lower blood pressure have only uncontrolled hypertension, not a legitimate hypertensive urgency. In minimally symptomatic hypertensives with less severe blood pressure elevations, the short-term risks of treatment (Table 2) clearly exceed the potential benefits of immediate blood pressure lowering. However, blood pressure levels higher than the aforementioned cut-points do not automatically warrant acute therapeutic intervention. Treatment when indicated is usually via the oral route (Table 7). Oral therapy can be conveniently administered in a wide range of clinical settings. However, the blood pressure response to oral therapy is unpredictable. In special clinical situations (i.e., postoperative period, intractable epistaxis), hypertensive urgencies are most appropriately treated with intravenous medications.

Malignant/Accelerated Hypertension

The incidence of both malignant and accelerated hypertension has steadily declined, mainly because of increasingly effective treatment of chronic hypertension. The clinical presentation of both entities can be quite dramatic, leading to devastating clinical consequences including death and serious long-term disability unless recognized and treated appropriately. Although these two hypertensive emergencies can be distinguished on clinical grounds, they portend a similar ominous prognosis. The 1-year survival rate in untreated accelerated malignant hypertension is only 20%; however, 5-year survival rates are over 90% after successful treatment. Blood pressure is usually higher than 200/130 mm Hg. Patients typically present with one or more of the following: severe headaches, blurred vision, focal neurological symptoms, nystagmus, extensor plantar reflexes, congestive heart failure, and/or renal failure. The funduscopic examination routinely confirms severe retinopathy (bilateral hemor-

rhages and exudates). Papilledema is, however, required to make the diagnosis of malignant hypertension. Abrupt cessation of either β-blockers or central adrenergic inhibitors can also lead to a rebound in blood pressure to much higher than pretreatment levels and thus may present as a hypertensive emergency. Patients with malignant or accelerated hypertension should always be treated with intravenous medications (Table 7) in a setting where close patient monitoring is feasible (i.e., intensive care unit). Intravenous sodium nitroprusside and nitroglycerin are the most commonly used effective therapies for hypertensive emergencies. The major advantage of these agents is that their onset and offset of action occurs within seconds to minutes, allowing for precise titration of the infusion according to the blood pressure response. The therapeutic goal for these patients is not blood pressure normalization but rather a gradual reduction of mean arterial pressure [(2 × diastolic blood pressure) + systolic blood pressure)/3] of no more than 15 to 20% over the first hour or so of treatment. Systolic and diastolic blood pressure should not be lowered below 170 and 110 mm Hg, respectively. Gradual and cautious blood pressure lowering will minimize the probability of iatrogenic target organ ischemia as a consequence of vital organ hypoperfusion. In special situations such as unstable angina pectoris, congestive heart failure, pulmonary edema, or aortic dissection a lower target blood pressure may be justified. Secondary causes of hypertension such as critical renal artery stenosis, glomerulonephritis, Cushing's syndrome, and pheochromocytoma should be sought in patients presenting with malignant or accelerated hypertension.

Chronic Hypertension in the Hospital Setting

The clinician should have a relatively high threshold for prescribing acute blood pressure lowering therapy, even via the oral route, in asymptomatic to minimally symptomatic hospitalized hypertensives with poorly controlled blood pressure. Potentially reversible causes for elevated blood pressure such as pain, hypoxia, hypercarbia, hypoglycemia, pulmonary edema, and status epilepticus should be considered. Withdrawal from alcohol or drugs or even rebound hypertension attributable to prior abrupt discontinuation of either β-blockers or central adrenergic inhibitors may underlie blood pressure elevation in hospitalized patients. Infusion of saline containing intravenous fluids should be minimized and dietary sodium restricted to 2g (88 mmol)/day or less. If no reversible cause of elevated blood pressure is identified, and the blood pressure level is high enough, then the approach to treatment is virtually identical to that utilized in hypertensive urgencies. Hospitalized patients are prone to orthostatic hypertension because of prolonged bed rest. Thus, if feasible, blood pressure should be periodically measured in both the seated or supine and upright positions. Automated blood pressure measurement devices should be regularly calibrated against a mercury manometer to ensure their accuracy. Most hospitalized patients will be optimally treated simply with intensification of their ambulatory blood pressure medication regimen. The tendency to titrate drugs every day or so on hospital rounds can result in excessive blood pressure lowering, leading to side effects and/or target organ ischemia. The ultimate therapeutic goal in hospitalized patients with poor blood pressure control is to keep blood pressure under levels that are likely to incite target organ damage over the short term. Thus, blood pressure normalization (<140/90 mm Hg), per se, is not the usual therapeutic goal. In minimally symptomatic patients with elevated blood pressure, the pressure levels triggering physician notification should be stated in the admission orders. The blood pressure level should be high enough (210/120 mm Hg) to minimize the likelihood of unnecessary and potentially harmful therapy being prescribed for acute blood pressure lowering.

Bibliography

Abdelwahab W, Frishman W, Landau A: Management of hypertensive urgencies and emergencies. *Ther Rev* 35:747–762, 1995.

Appel LJ, Moore TJ, Obarzanek E, *et al.*: A clinical trial of the effects of dietary patterns on blood pressure. DASH Collaborative Research Group. *N Engl J Med* 336(16):1117–1124, 1997.

Bertowitz DR, Ash AS, Hickey EC, *et al.*: Inadequate management of blood pressure in a hypertensive population. *N Engl J Med* 339:1957–1963, 1998.

Calhoun DA, Oparil S: Treatment of hypertensive crisis. *N Engl J Med* 323(17):1177–1183, 1990.

Epstein M, Bakris G: Newer approaches to antihypertensive therapy. *Arch Intern Med* 156:1969–1978, 1996.

Feigin VL, Rinkel GJ, Algra A, Vermeulen M, van Gijn J: Calcium antagonists in patients with aneurysmal subarachnoid hemorrhage: A systematic review. *Neurology* 50(4):876–883, 1998.

Flack JM: Optical blood pressure on medication. *Curr Hypertens Rep* 1:381–386, 1999.

Flack JM, Cushman W: Evidence of the efficacy of low-dose diuretic monotherapy. *Am J Med* 101(Suppl 3A):53S–60S, 1996.

Flack JM, McVeigh GE, Grimm RH, Jr: Hypertension therapy in the elderly. *Curr Opin Nephrol* 2:386–394, 1993.

Flack JM, Neaton JD, Daniels B, *et al.*: Ethnicity and renal disease: Lesson from multiple risk factor intervention trial and the treatment of mild hypertension study. *Am J Kidney Dis* 21(4):31–40, 1993.

Flack JM, Mensah, McVeigh GE, *et al.*: Diagnosis, evaluation and management of hypertension in an ambulatory clinic setting. *J Clin Outcome Manage* 2(5):1–21, 1995.

Flack JM, Neaton J, Grimm RH, Jr, *et al.*: Blood pressure and mortality among men with prior myocardial infarction. *Circulation* 92:2437–2445, 1995.

Flack JM, Novikov SV, Ferrario CM: Benefits of adherence to antihypertensive drug therapy. *Eur Heart J* 17(a):16–20, 1996.

Flack JM, Yunis C, Preisser J, Holmes CB, *et al.*: The rapidity of drug dose escalation influences blood pressure response and side effect burden in hypertensives: The quinapril titration interval management evaluation [ATIME] study. *Arch Intern Med* 160(12):1842–1847, 2000.

Grimm RH, Jr, Flack JM, Grandits GA, *et al.*: Long-term effects on plasma lipids of diet and drugs to treat hypertension. *JAMA* 275:1549–1556, 1996.

Hansson L, Zanchetti A, Carruthers SG, *et al.*: Effects of intensive blood pressure lowering and low-dose aspirin in patients with hypertension: Principal results of hypertension optimal treatment [HOT] randomised trial. *Lancet* 351:1755–1762, 1998.

Joint National Committee: The sixth report of the Joint National Committee on Detection, Evaluation and Treatment of High Blood Pressure (JNC VI). *Arch Intern Med* 157(21):2413–2446, 1997.

Lewis CE, Grandits GA, Flack JM, *et al.*: Efficacy and tolerance of antihypertensive treatment in men and women with stage 1 diastolic hypertension. *Arch Intern Med* 156:377–385, 1996.

Meredith PA: Therapeutic implications of drug holidays. *Eur Heart J* 17(Suppl A):21–24, 1996.

Moore TJ, Vollmer WM, Appel LJ, *et al.*: Effect of dietary patterns on ambulatory blood pressure: Results from the dietary Approaches to Stop Hypertension (DASH) trial. DASH collaborative Research Group. *Hypertension* 34(3):472–477, 1999.

National High Blood Pressure Education Program: 1995 Update of the Working Group Reports on Chronic Renal Failure and Renovascular Hypertension. *Arch Intern Med* 156:1928–1947, 1996.

Neaton JD, Grimm RH, Jr, Prines RJ, *et al.*: Treatment of mild Hypertension Study (TOMHS) final results. *JAMA* 270:713–724, 1993.

Staessen JA, Fagar DR, Thijs L, *et al.*: Randomised double-blind comparison of placebo and active treatment for older patients with isolated systolic hypertension: The systolic hypertension in Europe [Syst-Eur] Trial Investigators. *Lancet* 350:757–764, 1997.

UK Prospective Diabetes Study Group: Tight blood pressure control and risk of macrovascular and microvascular complications in type 2 diabetes UKPDS 38. *Br Med J* 317:703–713, 1998.

INDEX

Proximal tubule
  function, 9
  genetic disorders of transport, 20–22
Pseudohypoparathyroidism,
    hypocalcemia association, 109
Pyramid, anatomy, 4

R

Radiocontrast agents, nephrotoxicity
    induction, 255
Radionuclide imaging, overview of renal
    imaging, 49–50
Relapsing polychondritis, renal
    involvement, 211
Renal artery, anatomy, 5
Renal artery stenosis, *see also*
    Renovascular hypertension
  renal alkalosis, 85
  treatment
    angioplasty, 484
    bypass, 484
    pharmacotherapy, 484–485
    stenting, 484
Renal biopsy
  adequacy of sample, 142–143
  complications, 142
  contraindications, 141
  frequency of diagnoses, 141–142
  indications, 141
  lupus glomerulonephritis, 205–207
  microscopy, 142
  systemic sclerosis, 209–210
  technique, 142
Renal failure, *see also* Acute renal
    failure; Chronic renal failure
  drug prescription principles
    dialysis and drug dosage adjustment
      continuous ambulatory peritoneal
        dialysis, 295
      continuous renal replacement
        therapy, 295
      hemodialysis, 294–295, 404
    dosimetry, 293–294
    drug–drug interactions, 294
    drug level monitoring, 294
    intraperitoneal drug
      pharmacokinetics, 295
    parent drugs and active metabolites,
      291–292
    pharmacokinetic changes, 290–292
    plasma protein binding of drugs, 291
  hypercalcemia association, 111
  hyperphosphatemia association, 114
  metabolic acidosis, 77
  nutrient metabolism
    amino acids, 422
    energy metabolism, 422
    lipids, 422
    minerals, 422–423
    protein
      chronic renal failure patient
        requirements and protein
        restriction, 420–421
      dialysis patients, 421–422

trace elements, 423
    vitamins, 423
  potassium adaptation, 99
  urinary tract infection in patients, 359
Renal osteodystrophy
  amyloidosis from dialysis, 431–432
  management guidelines, 432–433
  osteitis fibrosa
    diagnosis, 428–429
    histology, 426
    pathogenesis of secondary
      hyperparathyroidism
      calcitriol deficiency, 427
      calcium malabsorption, 427
      hormone secretion alterations,
        428
      overview, 426
      parathyroid hyperplasia, 428
      phosphate retention, 426–427
      skeletal resistance to hormonal
        calcemic action, 428
    prevention and treatment
      calcium control, 429–430
      phosphorous control, 429
      vitamin D therapy, 430
  osteomalacia
    adynamic bone lesions, 431
    diagnosis, 430–431
    histology, 430
    pathogenesis, 430
    prevention and treatment, 431
  overview of disorders, 426
  renal posttransplantation period, 432
Renal transplantation
  allocation
    cadaveric organs, 458–459
    United Network for Organ Sharing
      scheme, 458
  allograft failure
    causes, 461
    management, 466
  donor evaluation, 459
  drug prescription, 466
  evaluation of prospective patients
    cancer screening, 455
    cardiovascular disease, 456
    cerebrovascular disease, 456
    diabetics, 455
    gastrointestinal evaluation, 457
    infections, 455–456
    initial assessment, 455
    liver disease, 456
    psychosocial evaluation, 457
    recurrent renal disease risk, 457
    typing of blood and tissue, 458
    urologic evaluation, 457
  failure rates, 418
  hypercalcemia association, 111
  hypophosphatemia association, 113
  immunosuppression
    drugs, 462–463
    phases, 463–464
    rationale, 460–461
  posttransplant care, 461–462

posttransplant problems
    hypercalcemia, 465
    hyperlipidemia, 465
    hypertension, 465
    infection, 464–465
    malignancy, 465
    mineral deficiency, 465–466
  pregnancy, 373
  quality of life factors, 418–419
  rehabilitation, 419
  rejection classification, 461
  renal imaging, 53
  renal osteodystrophy, 432
  retransplantation outcomes, 466
  survival rates, 417, 460
  technique, 459
Renal tubular acidosis (RTA), *see*
    Metabolic acidosis
Renal vein lesions, renal imaging, 53
Renin
  aging effects, 380
  blood pressure regulation, 471–472,
    474
  cirrhosis, renal function abnormalities,
    186–187
  congestive heart failure, 180
  control of release, 13
  renal synthesis, 3
  sodium excretion regulation, 13
Renovascular hypertension (RVH)
  course, 481–482
  definition, 480–481
  diagnosis
    angiotensin-converting enzyme
      inhibitor-stimulated
      renography, 482
    duplex ultrasound, 482–483
    magnetic resonance angiography,
      483
    overview, 482
    strategy, 483–484
  epidemiology, 481
  pathophysiology, 481
  treatment of renal artery stenosis
    angioplasty, 484
    bypass, 484
    pharmacotherapy, 484–485
    stenting, 484
Respiratory acidosis
  clinical manifestations, 88–89
  definition, 87
  diagnosis, 89
  etiology
    acute disease, 88
    chronic disease, 88–89
  pathophysiology, 87
  secondary physiological response,
    87–88
  treatment, 89–90
Respiratory alkalosis
  clinical manifestations, 92
  definition, 90
  diagnosis, 92
  etiology, 91–92
  pathophysiology, 90–91